Davidson's Principles and Practice of Medicine

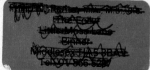

The Editor

JOHN MACLEOD

M.B., Ch.B., F.R.C.P.Edin.

Head of University Department of Medicine, Western General Hospital, Edinburgh
Consultant Physician, Western General Hospital, Edinburgh
Consultant Physician, Royal Edinburgh Hospital
Consultant Physician, Clinic for Rheumatic Diseases, Royal Infirmary, Edinburgh

The Contributors

Primarily from the Departments of Medicine and
Therapeutics, University of Edinburgh, but also
from other University Departments in Britain,
Africa, Australia and Canada.

Davidson's Principles and Practice of Medicine

A TEXTBOOK FOR STUDENTS AND DOCTORS

EDITED BY

John Macleod

TWELFTH EDITION

CHURCHILL LIVINGSTONE
EDINBURGH LONDON AND NEW YORK 1977

CHURCHILL LIVINGSTONE
Medical Division of Longman Group Limited

Distributed in the United States of America by Longman Inc., 19 West
44th Street, New York, N.Y. 10036 and by associated companies,
branches and representatives throughout the world.

First Edition	1952
Reprinted	1953
Second Edition	1954
Reprinted	1955
Third Edition	1956
Reprinted	1957
Fourth Edition	1958
Reprinted	1959
Fifth Edition	1960
Reprinted	1961
Sixth Edition	1962
Reprinted	1963
Seventh Edition	1964
Reprinted	1965
First ELBS Edition published	1965
Eighth Edition	1966
Reprinted	1968
ELBS Edition of Eighth Edition	1967
ELBS Edition reprinted	1968
Ninth Edition	1968
Reprinted	1969
Reprinted	1970
ELBS Edition of Ninth Edition	1968
ELBS Edition reprinted	1970
Tenth Edition	1971
Reprinted	1972
ELBS Edition of Tenth Edition	1971
ELBS Edition reprinted	1971
ELBS Edition reprinted	1972
ELBS Edition reprinted	1973
Eleventh Edition	1974
Reprinted	1976
ELBS Edition of Eleventh Edition	1974
ELBS Edition reprinted	1975
ELBS Edition reprinted	1976
Twelfth Edition (including Tropical Diseases)	1977
ELBS Edition of Twelfth Edition	1977

ISBN 0 443 01622 4 (cased)
ISBN 0 443 01566 X (limp)

British Library Cataloguing in Publication Data
Davidson, *Sir* Stanley
  Davidson's principles and practice of medicine.
  12th ed.
  1. Pathology 2. Medicine
  I. Macleod, John, b. 1915 II. Principles and
  practice of medicine
  616 RB111 77–30073

Printed in Great Britain by Pitman Press, Bath

Preface to the Twelfth Edition

With this new production, *Davidson's Principles and Practice of Medicine* will have appeared in 12 editions and over 20 reprints since it was first published a quarter of a century ago. The book has established an international reputation, and not only is it used extensively throughout the English speaking world but it has also been translated into Spanish, Italian, Greek and Croato-serbian. This continuing success is a remarkable tribute to the genius and vision of Sir Stanley Davidson and the editorial policy he instituted, but we are acutely aware that if the book is to retain its unique place in the field of medical education, it must be kept completely up to date in terms of both content and approach. This objective has, we hope, been achieved by consensus support for a progressive editorial policy and by the regular recruitment of younger authors.

There are major changes in the 12th edition. The chapters on genetics, diseases of the cardiovascular system, diseases of the liver and biliary tract, psychiatry and tropical diseases have been entirely or largely rewritten. Extensive changes have also been made throughout the remainder of the text to keep pace with new developments in rapidly advancing disciplines.

Tropical diseases have always figured prominently in 'Davidson'. At first, only those conditions were included which might be encountered in temperate climates or were of particular educational value. The demand for the textbook in Africa and Asia led to the publication in 1964 of a *Tropical Diseases Supplement* which is now in its 5th edition. In 1965 the parent textbook and the supplement were published together in Africa and Asia in a large paperback, at a greatly reduced price, under the auspices of the English Language Book Society. This joint publication has appeared in seven editions. Now the *Tropical Diseases Supplement* has been incorporated with the parent book, thus ensuring that all readers will have at least some knowledge of human needs and medical problems in countries other than their own. A more prosaic reason for this change in policy is that economies effected by publishing one textbook instead of three will enable the price to be kept at a modest level despite increasing costs at every stage of production.

Although much new material has been included, it has nevertheless proved possible to shorten the book by some 60 pages mainly by discarding what has been superseded. A close interrelationship has also been established with the 4th edition of *Clinical Examination*, in which several of the contributors and the editor participate.

The opening chapters of the 12th edition deal with fundamental general factors in disease such as genetics, immunology, infection, nutrition and electrolyte balance. These are followed by accounts of diseases of the various systems and by outlines of psychiatry and acute poisoning. The final chapter, on tropical disease and helminthic infections, ends with a short section on the promotion of health and prevention of disease, re-emphasising the prominence given to prophylaxis in every chapter. In recognition of the fact that education must be a continuing process, many of the chapters conclude with brief comments on prospects for the immediate future.

The task of preparing the 12th edition has been made easier for the editor and contributors by the pleasure and satisfaction derived from working as a team, by the stimulus provided by new authors and by the challenge of constructive criticism from students and doctors all over the world. Our primary objective, as before, has been to ensure that the book provides a rational and easily comprehensible basis for the practice of medicine, and we hope that it will continue to make as substantial a contribution to the education of medical students, both undergraduate and postgraduate, in the future as it has done in the past.

Edinburgh, 1977   *John Macleod*

Acknowledgments

We have had generous help from many colleagues and we would like to express our thanks especially to Professor B. E. C. Nordin, Dr Roger Whitehead and Miss Erica Wheeler (nutrition), Mr C. V. Ruckley (thromboembolism), Dr D. H. Cummack (radiographs of alimentary tract), Dr A. J. Keay (cystic fibrosis of the pancreas), Dr J. F. Cullen (diabetic retinopathy), Dr H. A. Reid (snake bite), Dr D. A. Warrell (climate and altitude), Mr. J. E. Pizer (line drawings), Drs Donald Bain and Alison McCallum (proof reading) and Greta Proven and Pat Hollis (preparation of manuscript). Other acknowledgments are made in the text.

To Ellen Green we are particularly indebted for maintaining efficient and harmonious relationships between publishers, printers and editor.

List of Contributors

ALLAN, N. C., M.B., Ch.B., F.R.C.P.Edin., F.R.C.P.Path.
Senior Lecturer, University Department of Medicine, Western General Hospital, Edinburgh and formerly of University of Ibadan, Nigeria. Consultant Haematologist, Western General Hospital, Edinburgh.
Blood Disorders in the Tropics.

BAIRD, JOYCE D., M.A., M.B., Ch.B.Aberd., M.R.C.P.Edin.
Senior Lecturer, University Department of Medicine, Western General Hospital, Edinburgh and Hon. Consultant Physician, Western General Hospital, Edinburgh.
Diabetes Mellitus and other Metabolic Disorders.

BRYCESON, A. D. M., M.D., F.R.C.P.Edin., D.T.M. and H.
Senior Lecturer, London School of Hygiene and Tropical Medicine. Consulting Physician, Hospital for Tropical Diseases. Consultant in Tropical Dermatology, St John's Hospital for Diseases of the Skin, London.
Tropical Diseases and Helminthic Infections.

CREAN, GERARD P., Ph.D., F.R.C.P.Edin.
Hon. Lecturer in Medicine, University of Glasgow (Western Infirmary). Consultant Physician, Southern General Hospital, Glasgow. Physician-in-charge, The Gastrointestinal Centre, Southern General Hospital, Glasgow.
Diseases of the Alimentary Tract and Pancreas.

DUTHIE, J. J. R., M.B., Ch.B., F.R.C.P.Edin.
Lately Professor of Medicine (Rheumatology), University of Edinburgh. Hon. Consultant Physician, Northern General Hospital. Physician-in-charge, Rheumatic Diseases Unit, Northern General Hospital, Edinburgh.
Diseases of Connective Tissues, Joints and Bones.

EMERY, A. E. H., M.D., Ph.D., D.Sc., F.R.C.P.Edin., M.F.C.M., F.R.S.Edin.
Professor of Human Genetics (Western General Hospital), University of Edinburgh. Consultant in Medical Genetics, Lothian Health Board, Scotland.
Genetic Factors in Disease.

FINLAYSON, N. D. C., Ph.D., M.B., Ch.B., M.R.C.P.Edin., M.R.C.P.Lond.
Physician, Gastrointestinal and Liver Service, The Royal Infirmary, Edinburgh.
Diseases of the Liver and Biliary Tract.

FRENCH, E. B., B.A., M.B., B.Chir.Cantab., F.R.C.P.Edin., F.R.C.P.Lond.
Lately Reader, University Department of Medicine and Hon. Consultant Physician, Western General Hospital, Edinburgh.
Infection and Disease.

GEDDES, A. M., M.B., Ch.B., F.R.C.P.Edin., M.R.C.P.Lond.
Senior Clinical Lecturer and Tutor in Infectious Diseases, University of

Birmingham. Consultant Physician, Department of Communicable and Tropical Diseases, East Birmingham Hospital, Birmingham.
Infection and Disease.

GIRDWOOD, R. H., M.D., Ph.D., F.R.C.P.Edin., F.R.C.P.Lond., F.R.C.Path.
Dean of the Faculty of Medicine and Professor of Therapeutics, University of Edinburgh. Hon. Consultant Physician, Royal Infirmary, Edinburgh.
Diseases of the Blood and Blood-forming Organs.

GOULD, J. C., B.Sc., M.D., F.R.C.P.Edin., F.Inst.Biol., F.R.C.Path., F.F.C.M., F.R.S.Edin.
Director of the Central Microbiological Laboratories, Edinburgh.
Infection and Disease.

GRANT, I. W. B., M.B., Ch.B., F.R.C.P.Edin.
Senior Lecturer, University Department of Medicine, Western General Hospital, Edinburgh. Consultant Physician, Respiratory Unit, Northern General Hospital, Edinburgh.
Diseases of the Respiratory System.

HORNE, N. W., M.B., Ch.B., F.R.C.P.Edin.
Hon. Senior Lecturer, Department of Respiratory Diseases and Tuberculosis, University of Edinburgh. Consultant Physician, Chest Unit, City Hospital, Edinburgh.
Diseases of the Respiratory System.

INNES, JAMES, M.D., F.R.C.P.Edin.
Senior Lecturer in Medicine, University of Edinburgh. Consultant Physician, Royal Infirmary, Edinburgh.
Diseases of the Blood and Blood-forming Organs.

IRVINE, W. J., D.Sc., M.B., Ch.B., F.R.C.P.E., M.R.C.Path.
Reader, Department of Therapeutics, University of Edinburgh. Consultant Physician, Royal Infirmary, Edinburgh.
Immunological Factors in Disease; Diseases of the Endocrine System.

JULIAN, D. G., M.A., M.D., F.R.C.P.Edin., F.R.C.P.Lond., F.R.A.C.P.
British Heart Foundation Professor of Cardiology, University of Newcastle-upon-Tyne. Consultant Cardiologist, Freeman Hospital, Newcastle-upon-Tyne.
Diseases of the Cardiovascular System.

LAWSON, A. A. H., M.D., F.R.C.P.Edin.
Consultant Physician, Milesmark Hospital, Dunfermline and to associated hospitals in West Fife District, Fife. Postgraduate Tutor for West Fife, Postgraduate Board for Medicine, University of Edinburgh; member of the Clinical Teaching Staff, Department of Medicine, Royal Infirmary, Edinburgh.
Acute Poisoning.

McCORMICK, J. N., M.B., Ch.B., M.R.C.P.Edin.
Hon. Senior Lecturer, Departments of Medicine and Bacteriology, University of Edinburgh. Consultant Physician, Rheumatic Diseases Unit, Northern General

Hospital, Edinburgh.
Diseases of Connective Tissues, Joints and Bones.

McHardy, G. J. R., M.A., B.Sc., B.M., F.R.C.P.Edin., F.R.C.P.Lond.
Senior Lecturer, Department of Respiratory Diseases and Tuberculosis, University of Edinburgh. Consultant Physician, Chest Unit, City Hospital, Edinburgh. Consultant Clinical Respiratory Physiologist, City Hospital and Western General Hospital, Edinburgh.
Diseases of the Respiratory System.

McManus, J. P. A., M.B., Ch.B., F.R.C.P.Edin.
Professor of Medicine and Director of Gastroenterology, University of Laval, Quebec, Canada. Formerly Senior Lecturer, Department of Medicine, and Consultant Physician, Gastrointestinal Unit, Western General Hospital, Edinburgh.
Diseases of the Liver and Biliary Tract.

Matthew, Henry, M.D., F.R.C.P.Edin.
Lately Senior Lecturer, Department of Therapeutics, University of Edinburgh. Consultant Physician, Royal Infirmary, Edinburgh. Physician-in-charge, Area Poisoning Treatment Centre, Royal Infirmary, Edinburgh. Director, Scottish Poisons Information Bureau.
Acute Poisoning.

Matthews, M. B., M.A., M.D.Cantab., F.R.C.P.Edin., F.R.C.P.Lond.
Senior Lecturer, University Department of Medicine, Western General Hospital, Edinburgh. Consultant Cardiologist, Western General Hospital, Edinburgh.
Diseases of the Cardiovascular System.

Mawdsley, C., M.D., F.R.C.P.Edin., F.R.C.P.Lond.
Senior Lecturer in Medical Neurology, University of Edinburgh. Hon. Consultant Neurologist, Royal Infirmary and Northern General Hospital, Edinburgh.
Diseases of the Nervous System.

Richmond, John, M.D., F.R.C.P.Edin., F.R.C.P.Lond.
Professor of Medicine, University of Sheffield. Hon. Consultant Physician, Sheffield Area Health Authority (Teaching).
Diseases of the Liver and Biliary Tract.

Robson, J. S., M.D., F.R.C.P.Edin.
Professor of Medicine (Royal Infirmary), University of Edinburgh. Hon. Consultant Physician, Royal Infirmary, Edinburgh.
Disturbances in Water and Electrolyte Balance and in Hydrogen Ion Concentration.
Diseases of the Kidney and Urinary System.

Shearman, D. J. C., Ph.D., M.B., Ch.B., F.R.C.P.Edin.
Mortlock Professor of Medicine, University of Adelaide and Head of the Professorial Medical Unit, Royal Adelaide Hospital, Australia.
Diseases of the Alimentary Tract and Pancreas.

SIMPSON, J. A., M.D.Glasg., F.R.C.P.Edin., F.R.C.P.Lond., F.R.C.P.Glasg., F.R.S.Edin.
Professor of Neurology, University of Glasgow. Senior Neurologist, Institute of Neurological Sciences, Southern General Hospital and Consultant Neurologist, Western Infirmary, Glasgow.
Diseases of the Nervous System.

SMALL, W. P., V.R.D., M.B., Ch.B., Ch.M., F.R.C.S.Edin., F.R.C.P.Edin.
Consultant Surgeon, Gastrointestinal Unit, Western General Hospital, Edinburgh.
Diseases of the Alimentary Tract and Pancreas.

STRONG, J. A., M.B.E., M.A., M.D.Dubl., F.R.C.P.Edin., F.R.C.P. Lond., F.R.S.Edin.
Professor of Medicine (Western General Hospital), University of Edinburgh. Hon. Consultant Physician, Western General Hospital, Edinburgh. Hon. Consultant Physician, Medical Research Council Clinical and Population Cytogenetics Research Unit.
Diseases of the Endocrine System, including Diabetes Mellitus; Obesity.

TRUSWELL, A. S., M.D., F.R.C.P.Lond., M.F.C.M.
Professor of Nutrition and Dietetics, Queen Elizabeth College, University of London. Hon. Consultant Physician in Nutrition, Charing Cross Hospital Medical School, London.
Nutritional Factors in Disease.

WALTON, H. J., Ph.D., M.D., F.R.C.P.Edin., D.P.M.
Professor of Psychiatry, University of Edinburgh. Director, University Department of Psychiatry, Western General Hospital. Hon. Consultant Psychiatrist, Royal Edinburgh Hospital.
Psychiatry.

WRIGHT, F. J., M.A., M.D.Cantab., F.R.C.P.Edin., F.R.C.P.Lond., D.T.M. & H. Eng.
Lately Head of Medical Department, Kilimanjaro Christian Medical Centre, Moshi, Tanzania. Hon. Senior Lecturer in Medicine, University of Dar es Salaam, Tanzania. Formerly Senior Lecturer in Diseases of Tropical Climates, University of Edinburgh and Government Medical Specialist, Kenya.
Tropical Diseases and Helminthic Infections.

Contents

1. Genetic Factors in Disease

In recent years there has been an increasing awareness of the importance of genetic factors in the aetiology and pathogenesis of many disorders affecting man. Perhaps of more importance is that this knowledge has also led to possible means of prevention of such disorders through genetic counselling and antenatal diagnosis.

At the turn of the century morbidity and mortality in infancy and childhood could largely be attributed to environmental factors such as infections and nutritional deficiencies. With advances in medicine these problems are decreasing, at least in the developed countries, while others, in which genetic factors are largely or even entirely responsible, are becoming more obvious. In a survey carried out in Newcastle in 1970, no less than 42 per cent of childhood deaths could be attributed to diseases which are genetic in causation. The contribution of genetic factors to mortality and morbidity in adults is more difficult to assess but is also increasing.

It is useful to consider human disease as forming a spectrum at one end of which we have those diseases which are entirely genetic in origin and in which environmental factors play little if any part. This group of disorders includes *chromosomal abnormalities* and so-called *unifactorial disorders*. The latter are due to single gene defects (Mendelian factors); though individually rare there are over a thousand of them. They are usually serious disorders; they often present at birth or in childhood, though notable exceptions are Huntington's chorea, myotonic dystrophy and polyposis coli. The mode of inheritance is straightforward and follows Mendelian principles, and the risks of occurrence in relatives are high. For the vast majority of these unifactorial disorders there is as yet no effective treatment and prevention is the main approach to the problem.

At the other end of the spectrum are those diseases such as infections and nutritional deficiencies which are entirely environmental in aetiology. In the middle of the spectrum are many common conditions which are partly genetic and partly environmental in causation, so-called *multifactorial disorders*. These include many congenital malformations (such as congenital dislocation of the hip, club foot, congenital pyloric stenosis, congenital heart disease, anencephaly and spina bifida), 'diseases of modern society' (diabetes mellitus, essential hypertension, coronary artery disease) and possibly certain psychiatric disorders (such as schizophrenia and manic-depressive psychosis). In multifactorial disorders the genetic component is complex, probably involving in each case many genes. The risks to relatives are usually low.

Chemical Basis of Inheritance

Within the nucleus of every cell are the chromosomes which bear the genes which carry genetic information. Deoxyribonucleic acid (DNA) is the essential component of hereditary material and it is within the DNA of the gene that genetic information is stored.

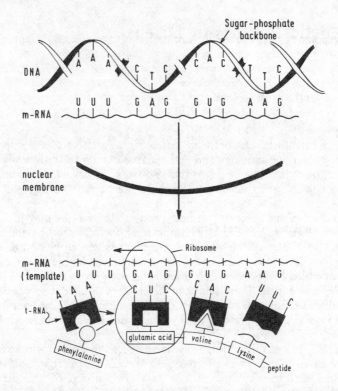

Fig. 1.1 Translation of genetic information into protein synthesis. Guanine (G) pairs with cytosine (C) and adenine (A) with thymine (T) or uracil (U).

DNA is composed of two polynucleotide chains, twisted together to form a double helix (Fig. 1.1). Each nucleotide is composed of a nitrogenous base, a sugar molecule (deoxyribose) and a phosphate molecule. The nitrogenous bases in DNA are adenine and guanine (purines) and cytosine and thymine (pyrimidines). The arrangement of the bases is not random: a purine in one chain always pairs with a pyrimidine on the other chain. There is also specific base pairing: guanine in one chain always pairs with cytosine in the other chain and adenine always pairs with thymine. This is the Watson-Crick model of DNA. It is postulated that at nuclear division the two strands of the DNA molecule separate and as a result of specific base pairing each chain then builds its complement. In this way, when a cell divides, genetic information is conserved and transmitted to each daughter cell.

The primary action of the gene is to synthesise protein by various combinations of 20 different amino acids. Genetic information is stored within the DNA molecule in the form of a triplet code such that a sequence of three bases determines the structure of one amino acid.

Whereas DNA is found mainly in the chromosomes, ribonucleic acid (RNA) is found mainly in the nucleolus and the cytoplasm. RNA has a structure similar to DNA (Fig. 1.1): both nucleic acids contain adenine, guanine and cytosine but thymine is replaced by uracil in RNA and the latter contains the sugar ribose. The information stored in the DNA code of the gene is transmitted to a particular type of RNA, so-called messenger-RNA (m-RNA). Each m-RNA is formed by a particular gene, such that every base in the m-RNA molecule is complementary to a corresponding base in the DNA of the gene: cytosine with guanine, thymine with adenine but adenine with uracil since the latter replaces thymine in RNA. The m-RNA then migrates out of the nucleus into the cytoplasm where it becomes associated with the ribosomes which are the site of protein synthesis. In the ribosomes the m-RNA forms the template or mould for arranging particular amino acids in sequence. In the cytoplasm there is yet another form of RNA referred to as transfer -RNA (t-RNA). Each amino acid in the cytoplasm becomes attached to a particular t-RNA. The other end of the t-RNA molecule consists of three bases which combine with complementary bases on the m-RNA. Thus a particular triplet in the m-RNA is related through t-RNA to specific amino acid. The ribosome moves along the m-RNA in a zipper-like fashion, the assembled amino acids linking up to form a polypeptide chain.

Structural and Control Genes. There are essentially two types of gene: structural genes which are responsible for the synthesis of specific proteins such as haemoglobin, collagen and enzymes, and control genes which are thought to modify the action of structural genes.

A change (mutation) of a base pair of the DNA molecule may result in any one of a number of possible effects. If the altered triplet codes for the same amino acid then of course the change will go undetected. Possibly 20 to 25 per cent of all possible single base changes are of this type. Alternatively a single base mutation may result in a triplet which codes for a different amino acid resulting in an altered protein. The latter may retain its biological activity (e.g. enzyme activity) but have altered physico-chemical properties such as electrophoretic mobility or stability so that it is more rapidly broken down. This is the case in many of the abnormal haemoglobinopathies in which the aberrant haemoglobin can be detected by its altered electrophoretic mobility. However the substitution of a different amino acid may result in reduced or even absent biological activity. In inborn errors of metabolism therefore the level of a particular enzyme may be reduced because it is not synthesised, or it is synthesised but has reduced activity or because of its instability it is more rapidly broken down.

Chromosomes and Chromosomal Disorders

Chromosome Structure and Number. Among higher animals each species bears within the nucleus of its cells a set of chromosomes which is characteristic both in number and in morphology for that species. Each nucleus in the somatic cells of man contains a set of 46 chromosomes. Two of these chromosomes determine the sex of the individual and are therefore known as *sex chromosomes*; the remaining 44 chromosomes are known as *autosomes*.

The DNA of higher organisms is coated with histone and non-histone proteins. This produces a deoxyribonucleoprotein fibre (chromatin) which forms the basic unit of chromosome structure. Although much information on the structure of chromosomes has been acquired by the use of a variety of techniques which include chemical analysis, X-ray diffraction, electronmicroscopy and autoradiography, the detailed nature of their structure still remains a subject of dispute. Several models have been put forward to explain the way in which the DNA and other chromosomal constituents are arranged but none are entirely satisfactory.

Chromosomes are in a suitable state for detailed study only during specific intervals within the period of cell division, for it is during these periods that the chromosomes become contracted, thicker and more readily stained. Chromosomes in the resting nucleus do not take up most stains in a satisfactory way.

Each chromosome has a point along its length, a constriction, known as the *centromere* which divides the chromosome into two arms which are usually unequal in length. The chromosomes also differ in their overall length. Further by using certain stains each chromosome can be shown to have a specific banding pattern. By these criteria it is now possible to identify individual chromosomes.

The chromosomal complement of any nucleus is composed of two sets of chromosomes which are arranged in pairs. Because the two members of any given pair (with the exception of the sex chromosomes) resemble one another they are said to be *homologous*. One homologue of any pair is derived from one parent and its partner from the other parent. Thus man has 22 pairs of homologous chromosomes (autosomes) and one pair of sex chromosomes.

During gametogenesis the number of chromosomes is halved in order that the number of chromosomes remains constant and is not doubled at each conception. Thus somatic cell nuclei contain twice as many chromosomes as gametes and with respect to their chromosome complement are said to be *diploid*, whereas gametes are said to be *haploid*.

The two sex chromosomes of the female are identical and are referred to as *X chromosomes*. The sex chromosomes of the male, however, are not identical. One of the pair resembles the X chromosome seen in females while the other is much smaller, differs considerably in morphology and is referred to as a *Y chromosome*. Thus the sex chromosome constitution is XX in a female and XY in a male. In the female each ovum bears one or other of the X chromosomes, whereas in the male the sperms bear either an X or a Y chromosome. At fertilisation an ovum therefore has an equal chance of being fertilised by either an X or a Y bearing sperm. It is for this reason that the sex ratio is approximately (not exactly) unity at birth.

Mitosis. Unlike highly differentiated cells such as neurones, the cells of many tissues in the body repeatedly undergo division. In fact some cells, such as those of the intestinal tract and bone marrow, continue to divide throughout the life of an individual. For the error rate in cell division to remain as low as it is, nuclear division must be extremely well regulated. The process by which nuclei divide to produce two identical daughter nuclei is known as *mitosis*. During mitosis each chromosome divides into two so that the number of chromosomes in each daughter nucleus is the same as in the parent cell. Though mitosis is a continuous process, one step merging imperceptibly into the next, it can be divided into stages for ease of description. These stages are known as interphase, prophase, metaphase, anaphase and telophase (Fig. 1.2).

Interphase is the resting stage between nuclear divisions when the chromosomes are loosely coiled and difficult to visualise. By the end of interphase each chromosome has divided longitudinally into two daughter chromosomes, or *chromatids*, which remain attached to each other at the centromere.

During *prophase*, the chromosomes take up stains more readily and therefore become easier to visualise. By the end of prophase the nucleoli are no longer visible and each chromatid is a tightly coiled structure which is closely aligned to its partner.

Metaphase begins with the disappearance of the nuclear membrane and the for-

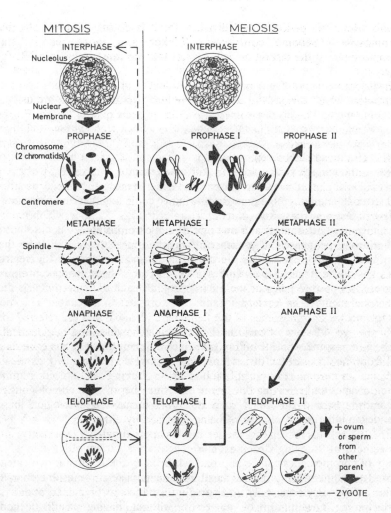

Fig. 1.2 Stages of mitosis and meiosis.

mation of the spindle apparatus, which consists of a number of minute 'threads' which run from one pole of the nucleus to the other. The chromosomes become orientated around the centre of the nucleus in the equatorial plane. Each chromosome is attached to the spindle by means of its centromere. The spindle is responsible for the movement of the chromosomes during mitosis.

During *anaphase* the centromere of each chromosome divides into two, each half 'repels' the other and the chromatids move apart towards opposite poles of the spindle. When the chromatids reach the poles they form two separate but identical groups.

Telophase begins as the daughter chromosomes arrive at the poles of the spindle. The two groups of chromosomes become surrounded by a new nuclear membrane and gradually become less visible.

Cell division is completed by cleavage of the cytoplasm. New cell membranes develop and the nuclei of the two daughter cells re-enter the interphase stage. Thus at the end of mitosis a cell has divided into two daughter cells each with an identical genetic constitution.

Meiosis. The process by which the chromosome number is halved during gametogenesis is known as meiosis. Although meiosis involves two division stages, the chromosomes divide only once, each gamete normally receiving either of a pair of homologous chromosomes.

Each of the two steps in meiosis has a prophase, metaphase, anaphase and telophase stage as in mitosis (Fig. 1.2). The prophase of the first stage is very long. It is thought that DNA replication has already taken place by the onset of this stage, although each chromosome still appears morphologically to be a single thread. During prophase the chromosomes become more contracted, as a result of tighter coiling, and homologous chromosomes come together and pair along their length. Then a process known as *crossing-over* may occur in which there is an exchange of genetic material between chromatids of homologous chromosomes.

Following prophase the sequence of events is essentially similar to that occurring in mitosis, except that during this first meiotic division the centromere does not divide. Instead the members of each pair of homologous chromosomes migrate to opposite poles of the nucleus so that each daughter nucleus receives only one member of each pair and therefore bears a haploid chromosome complement.

In the second stage of meiosis the centromere divides and the chromatids of each chromosome separate and migrate into different nuclei. Thus each daughter cell from the first meiotic division has in turn divided to form two identical cells. Meiosis therefore results in each gamete having a haploid number of chromosomes and receiving one or the other member of each homologous pair of chromosomes and the genes it bears. This forms the cytological basis for Mendelian inheritance.

Methods of Studying Chromosomes. There are a variety of ways in which the study of chromosomes can be approached. Broadly these fall into two categories: those techniques which are used to study the complete chromosome complement of an individual, or those which enable information to be gained about the sex chromosome constitution of a person without having to do a complete chromosome analysis.

Since it is only during critical stages of the mitotic or meiotic cycle that the chromosomes are in a suitable state to study, chromosome analysis requires the provision of a large number of cells which are actively dividing. Meiotic studies can of course be done only on specimens of tissue obtained from the gonads. Mitotic studies, on the other hand, can be made on a variety of different and more easily available tissues, e.g. directly from cells which are rapidly dividing *in vivo*, as in bone marrow. More commonly, however, specimens are obtained from tissues which are not rapidly dividing *in vivo* but are much more accessible to study, such as skin and blood leucocytes, and the cells are stimulated to divide *in vitro* by the addition of phytohaemagglutinin. The addition of colchicine arrests cell division at the metaphase stage when the chromosomes are most suitable for study. The use of hypotonic solutions causes the cells to swell, disperses the chromosomes and makes them easier to study and count (Fig. 1.3). Finally the material is stained (e.g. with Giemsa) to demonstrate the banding patterns of the chromosomes. A suitable metaphase spread is then photographed through a high power microscope and the individual chromosomes are cut out from the

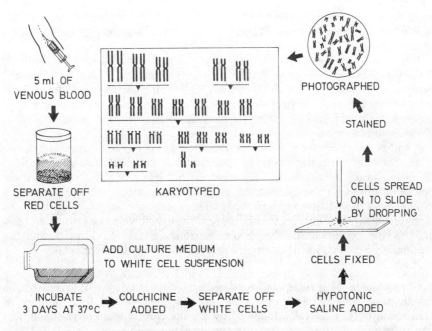

Fig. 1.3 Preparation of a karyotype.

photograph. The chromosomes are then arranged in an orderly fashion, in homologous pairs, to produce a standard arrangement known as a *karyotype*.

Methods are available for studying the sex chromosome constitution of an individual without having to resort to the costly and time-consuming process of preparing and analysing the complete karyotype. These are the study of sex-chromatin and 'drumsticks' in polymorphonuclear leucocytes in females and fluorescent bodies in males.

Female nuclei contain a distinctive mass of nuclear chromatin characteristically situated close to the nuclear membrane, the *sex chromatin* or 'Barr-body', which represents a genetically inactive X chromosome. In the female inactivation of one X chromosome in normal cells is a random process so that either the paternal or maternal X chromosome can be inactivated in any particular cell of the same animal. The cell nuclei of all the tissues in a human female contain a sex-chromatin body, but for convenience the most suitable cells for study are those of the buccal mucosa. The inside of the cheek is gently scraped with a spatula and the cells obtained spread onto a glass slide (*buccal smear*). These cells are then fixed and stained and can be examined for the presence of sex-chromatin bodies. Sex-chromatin bodies are seen in 30 to 60 per cent of nuclei of a normal female. Since only one X chromosome is active per cell, then the number of sex-chromatin bodies (inactivated X chromosomes) is one less than the total number of X chromosomes. Thus a normal female has one sex chromatin body, a patient with XO Turner's syndrome (p. 12) has no sex-chromatin bodies (chromatin negative) and a patient who has Klinefelter's syndrome (p. 10) with three X chromosomes (XXXY) has two sex chromatin bodies.

In suitably stained smears of peripheral blood about 3 per cent of the polymorphonuclear leucocytes of females show a small accessory nuclear lobule, which resembles a drumstick and projects from the main mass of the nuclear lobes. This is not seen in polymorphs from normal males, or females with an XO sex-chromosome constitution. The number of drumsticks is not, however, related to the number of X chromosomes.

Interphase nuclei of cells from males exhibit a fluorescent spot called the F body (or Y-chromatin) when stained with quinacrine; the number of F bodies represents the number of Y chromosomes. The technique can be adapted for use with buccal smears and so provides a method of assessing the number of Y chromosomes comparable with the sex-chromatin method of studying X chromosomes.

It can be seen, therefore, that these techniques are complementary and by combining them the sex chromosome constitution of an individual can be determined with ease, speed and accuracy. This is extremely useful clinically in the investigation of patients with abnormalities of sexual development or infertility, or for use in large-scale population surveys. Apart from these more common applications these techniques are also being used in new fields involving the separation of X and Y bearing sperm (half of human sperms contain an F body and are presumably Y bearing) and the determination of the sex of an unborn child.

Chromosome Nomenclature. A shorthand notation is used to describe a karyotype in the simplest way. This consists first of the total number of chromosomes (in numerals), followed by the sex chromosome constitution, and finally by any abnormalities that are present. Thus a normal male is 46, XY; a normal female is 46, XX. A girl with Turner's syndrome may be 45, XO and a boy with Klinefelter's syndrome, 47, XXY. The short and long arms of any chromosome are designated 'p' and 'q' respectively. A (+) or (−) sign is placed before an appropriate symbol where it means an additional or missing whole chromosome, but after a symbol when it refers only to part of a chromosome. Thus a boy with Down's syndrome is 47, XY, + 21 and a boy with part of the short arm of chromosome 5 missing is 46, XY, 5 p −.

Chromosomal Disorders

Specific chromosomal abnormalities are associated with recognised diseases or clinical syndromes in man. These include Down's syndrome (mongolism), abnormalities of sexual development (Turner's and Klinefelter's syndromes), syndromes of multiple congenital malformations (13- and 18-trisomies), spontaneous abortions, personality disorders (XYY and XXX etc.), chronic myeloid leukaemia and ataxia telangiectasia.

It has been found that 1 in every 200 live-born babies has a gross abnormality of chromosome number or structure. High as this figure is, it does not indicate fully the frequency with which chromosomal anomalies occur at fertilisation, for in a study of spontaneous abortions chromosomal aberrations occurred in over 30 per cent. Many of these chromosomal anomalies are rarely found in live-born babies and are therefore presumably lethal and the cause of a significant number of early abortions.

Chromosomal abnormalities can be divided into those which involve the autosomes and those which involve the sex chromosomes. These can be further divided into abnormalities of number and of structure. Numerical abnormalities arise when one or more chromosomes are either lost or gained, a phenomenon referred to as *aneuploidy*. When a whole set of chromosomes is gained the phenomenon is known as *polyploidy* and is not compatible with survival in man. The loss of a whole autosome, *monosomy*, also appears to be lethal in man. The addition of an extra chromosome, so resulting in three chromosomes instead of two (*trisomy*), seems, however, to result in less severe effects.

Autosomal abnormalities. Trisomy of a number of different autosomes have now been reported in man; the most common is trisomy-21 which results in Down's syndrome. The two other well-recognised syndromes (trisomy-13 and trisomy-18) occur far less frequently than Down's syndrome. They are both more severe in effect and usually result in death within the infant period.

Down's syndrome occurs in about 1 in 700 live-births. Individuals with this syndrome have a flat face with widely spaced and upward slanting eyes, epicanthic folds, brachycephaly, malformed ears, broad and/or short neck, and a single, transverse palmar crease. They are invariably mentally retarded, but have a pleasant, quiet personality and show a great fondness for music. This condition is also associated with an increased frequency of both congenital visceral anomalies, particularly congenital heart disease, and acute leukaemia. Although the mortality rate of these patients is high within the first year of life, many now survive into adulthood and there are several reports of women with Down's syndrome having children; on average half their offspring are normal and half have Down's syndrome.

About 95 per cent of cases of Down's syndrome are due to regular trisomy-21 which arises as a result of non-disjunction during meiosis. Normally during meiosis the two homologous chromosomes of any pair separate and pass into different gametes. Occasionally an accident occurs and the chromosomes fail to separate, both members of the pair passing into the same gamete. If such a gamete is then fertilised by a normal gamete the resulting zygote will possess an additional chromosome. All the trisomy syndromes are found to have a significant relationship to maternal age, the frequency of trisomic births increasing with increasing maternal age. It is thought that perhaps some effect of ageing in the ova of older mothers makes them more prone to non-disjunction. There have been reports, however, of trisomy-21 recurring in some families, which suggests that the phenomenon of non-disjunction may be under genetic control at least in these rare families.

About one per cent of cases of Down's syndrome are *mosaics*, that is, they possess two different cell lines, one of which has a normal chromosome constitution, the other an extra chromosome 21. This arises as a result of non-disjunction occurring at or after the first zygotic division and is very rarely inherited. The clinical picture may often be considerably modified in some of these cases.

About four per cent of cases of Down's syndrome result from a phenomenon known as *translocation*, in which there is an exchange of segments between different chromosomes. The mechanism is thought to be that two chromosomes lying close to one another suffer simultaneous breaks followed by an exchange of chromosomal material. For example, in Down's syndrome a large part of chromosome 21 may be united with part of chromosome 15. A carrier of such a translocation (who has only 45 chromosomes) produces four types of gametes. A gamete may contain a normal chromosome 15 and a normal chromosome 21, in which case the resulting offspring will be normal. Or a gamete may contain a translocation (15/21), in which case the resulting offspring will have only 45 chromosomes and will be a carrier like the parent. Or a gamete may contain the translocation and a normal chromosome 21, in which case the offspring will have 46 chromosomes but in effect will be trisomic for chromosome 21 and will therefore have Down's syndrome. Finally a gamete may contain a chromosome 15 but no chromosome 21; this would produce a zygote monosomic for chromosome 21 which is lethal and would presumably result in an abortion. Theoretically, therefore, a carrier of such a translocation has a 1 in 3 chance of having a child with Down's syndrome, but for reasons which are not clear the actual risk is much less. In Down's syndrome the translocation usually involves an exchange of material between chromosomes 13, 14 or 15 and chromosome 21. Rarely there may be an exchange between chromosomes 21 and 22 or even between two 21s.

OTHER AUTOSOMAL ABNORMALITIES. *Deletions* arise when a segment of a chromosome has been lost. New techniques have led to the demonstration of deletions involving a number of autosomes and an increasing number of these are being associated with clinically recognisable syndromes, examples of which are summarised in Table 1.1. Other rarer forms of chromosomal abnormalities are *ring chromosomes* and *isochromosomes*. Ring chromosomes involving both autosomes and sex chromosomes have been described; they are thought to be formed when two ends of a chromosome have been deleted and the broken (more 'sticky') ends fuse to form a ring. In effect ring chromosomes are manifest as deletions and in shorthand they are represented as an 'r'. An isochromosome is formed when the centromere divides horizontally instead of longitudinally resulting in a chromosome consisting of either two long arms or of two short arms.

The *Philadelphia chromosome* (Ph¹) is an *acquired* chromosomal abnormality associated with chronic myeloid leukaemia. It is a translocation involving chromosome 22 and another autosome, usually chromosome 9.

Sex Chromosome Abnormalities. Numerical abnormalities of the sex chromosomes are more common than with the autosomes, and in general they produce less severe effects. They are brought about by the same phenomenon of non-disjunction. As with the autosomes, abnormalities of structure also occur although they are far less common than the numerical anomalies.

Klinefelter's syndrome was the first sex chromosome aneuploidy to be demonstrated in man. Affected males have an extra X chromosome resulting in an XXY sex chromosome constitution or as many as four X chromosomes may be present; an extra Y chromosome may also be present on occasions resulting in an XXYY sex chromosome constitution. The main clinical features are eunuchoid body proportions, sterility (due to azoospermia), hypogonadism, gynaecomastia and often mental retardation. There appears to be a relationship between mental retardation and the number of X chromosomes in both males and females. In Klinefelter's syndrome all individuals with an XXXY sex chromosome constitution are mentally retarded, whereas this is so in only about one-quarter of those with XXY sex chromosome constitution. Like the autosomal trisomies, Klinefelter's syndrome is found to occur more frequently in the sons of older mothers.

The XYY sex chromosome constitution is another sex chromosome aneuploidy in the male. Such men are reported to occur with increased frequency amongst inmates of institutions for the mentally retarded with criminal tendencies. It has been shown by various surveys that between two and five per cent of such populations may be XYY. However, the exact relationship of this chromosomal anomaly with either mental retardation or criminal tendencies is uncertain es-

Table 1.1 Autosomal abnormalities associated with recognised clinical syndromes

Chromosome abnormality	Syndrome	Clinical features
trisomy-21 translocation 13–15/21 translocation 22/21 translocation 21/21	Down's	characteristic facies mental retardation hypotonia congenital heart disease Simian palmar crease
trisomy-8	——	moderate mental retardation concomitant strabismus clinodactyly other skeletal defects
trisomy-9	——	abnormal facies skeletal abnormalities hypoplastic genitalia congenital heart disease
trisomy-13	Patau's	motor and mental retardation microcephaly microphthalmia cleft palate/hare lip polydactyly congenital heart disease
trisomy-18	Edwards'	motor and mental retardation flexion deformities of fingers micrognathia 'rocker-bottom' feet congenital heart disease
trisomy-22	——	mental and motor retardation microcephaly abnormal facies and ears
trisomy-4p	——	abnormal facies digital anomalies foot deformities
trisomy-9p	——	abnormal facies large, low-set ears mental retardation incurved and short V digit
4p—	——	mental retardation abnormal facies cleft palate coloboma epilepsy hypospadias scalp defects
5p—	Cri du chat	mental retardation microcephaly hypertelorism characteristic cry
13q— 13r	——	mental and motor retardation abnormal facies microcephaly abnormal thumbs abnormal ears
18q—	De Grouchy's	mental retardation 'carp-mouth' abnormal ears tapering fingers
18p—	De Grouchy's	mental retardation ocular abnormalities *(Continued)*

Table 1.1 (*continued*)

Chromosome abnormality	Syndrome	Clinical features
	De Grouchy's (*continued*)	abnormal ears dental decay CNS abnormalities
18r	——	combination of 18p — and 18q — features
21 q— (G deletion syndrome I)	'anti- mongolism'	antimongoloid slant of eyes hypertonia micrognathia growth retardation skeletal malformations
22q — (G deletion syndrome II)	——	epicanthic folds hypotonia syndactyly retarded development

pecially as XYY individuals have been found amongst the normal general population.

Turner's syndrome was the first aneuploidy to be described in females. An XO sex chromosome constitution is the commonest abnormality in this disorder, but clinical features of Turner's syndrome may also result from iso-chromosomes, deletions, and rings involving the X chromosome. This abnormality must arise by non-disjunction, but unlike Klinefelter's syndrome, Turner's syndrome does not show a relationship with maternal age. The main clinical features are shortness of stature, primary amenorrhoea, lack of secondary sex characteristics and a variety of congenital abnormalities such as webbing of the neck, increased carrying-angle of the forearm (cubitus valgus) and coarctation of the aorta. Although, overall, patients with Turner's syndrome have a significantly lower I.Q. than normal, marked retardation is uncommon and the discrepancy is mainly in the performance aspect of their I.Q.

Females have also been described with three or even four X-chromosomes (XXX, XXXX); they may occasionally be mentally subnormal or have psychiatric disorders, but in all other respects appear to be healthy. All children born to XXX females have so far been reported to be normal.

Unifactorial Inheritance

These disorders are due to defects of a single gene, i.e. to a primary error in the DNA code. They are inherited in a simple fashion, following Mendelian laws. The risk of their recurring in a family may therefore be accurately predicted on theoretical grounds making genetic counselling more straightforward.

These disorders may be subdivided according to the chromosome on which the abnormal (or mutant) gene is situated and also by the nature of the trait itself. Thus a trait which is determined by a gene situated on an autosome is said to be inherited as an *autosomal* trait, and this may be either *dominant* or *recessive*. A trait determined by a gene situated on one of the sex chromosomes is said to be *sex-linked* and may also be either dominant or recessive.

Autosomal Dominant Inheritance. A dominant trait is one which is manifested in the *heterozygote*. In other words a person exhibiting an autosomal dominant trait possesses both the mutant gene and the normal gene, the presence of only one mutant gene being necessary for the trait to be manifested in the carrier. If the disorder is common, then some affected individuals could be *homozygotes* (i.e. the case), then affected individuals are almost always heterozygotes. It should be noted that the normal and abnormal genes are known as *alleles*, i.e. they are alternative forms of the same gene.

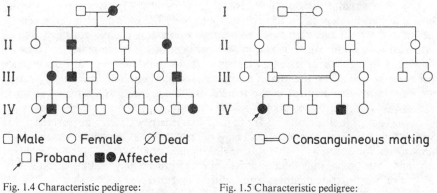

□ Male ○ Female ∅ Dead □━○ Consanguineous mating
◢□ Proband ■●Affected

Fig. 1.4 Characteristic pedigree: autosomal dominant trait.

Fig. 1.5 Characteristic pedigree: autosomal recessive trait.

Usually persons affected with an autosomal dominant trait are found to have an affected parent, the trait being transmitted from one generation to the next in a family, as illustrated in Figure 1.4. This is not always the case, however; sometimes the disorder may appear suddenly in a family when no members of previous generations have been affected. This may be due to illegitimacy, to one parent being so minimally affected that they passed unnoticed, or more commonly to the occurrence of a new mutation. This may complicate genetic counselling and is a problem which arises particularly in conditions inherited in a dominant fashion. In diseases which are severe, affected individuals seldom have children because they are either infertile or do not survive to reach reproductive age. In such conditions the disease will eventually become extinct in affected families and is maintained in the population only by fresh mutations. Achondroplasia is one of the forms of short-limbed dwarfism and is inherited as an autosomal dominant trait. In one large study it was shown that affected individuals exhibited a marked reduction in reproductive fitness. It is not surprising, therefore, that a high proportion of cases are the result of new mutations.

In conditions which do not have a marked effect on survival it is often possible to trace the conditions through many generations of a family. Such a condition is the adult form of polycystic disease of the kidneys. Although affected individuals may eventually die from chronic renal failure, they often show no symptoms or signs of the disease until early middle life when they have already had their family and run the risk of transmitting the trait to their children.

In autosomal dominant conditions, if an affected individual marries a normal person, then on average half their children will be similarly affected. This arises because the affected individual produces gametes, half of which contain the normal gene and the other half contain the mutant gene. The normal partner produces gametes all of which contain the normal gene. Thus at fertilisation the normal partner's gametes have an equal chance of uniting with a gamete carrying either a normal or an abnormal gene with the result that at conception there is a 1 in 2 chance of producing an affected individual. Because of the smaller size of modern families, by chance all the children of an affected individual may be normal, or similarly by chance again all his children may be affected. It is on average that half the offspring of an affected individual will be affected.

Autosomal dominant conditions affect both males and females. Sometimes, however, the sexes are not affected with equal frequency: the gene shows sex influence. For example, idiopathic haemochromatosis (p. 456) is a chronic disease characterised by deposition of excess iron in body tissues as a result of a genetic defect in the mechanism governing iron absorption. It is usually considered to be inherited as a dominant trait and yet 80 per cent of cases are male. This sex influence is thought to be due (at least in part) to the differences in iron balance between the two sexes, the loss of iron during menstruation and pregnancy acting as a protective mechanism in the female. In its extreme form, when one sex is exclusively affected, this is known as *sex limitation*.

Some autosomal dominant traits are extremely variable in severity, this variability in clinical manifestation being referred to as *expressivity*. Osteogenesis imperfecta, for example, is an autosomal dominant condition in which affected individuals may have only blue sclerae, whereas others may exhibit the full syndrome of blue sclerae, deafness and multiple fractures.

Occasionally an individual may carry a mutant gene and yet not exhibit any of its effects; the gene is then said to be *non-penetrant*. This phenomenon explains situations where dominant mutant traits appear to have 'skipped' generations in certain families. This variation in expression of a mutant gene results both from the modifying influence of other genes and from environmental factors. The degree of penetrance of a gene is that proportion of heterozygotes who express the gene in any degree, however mild. For a gene to be *fully penetrant* its effects must be manifest to some degree in all individuals who carry the gene. The phenomenon of varying penetrance can give rise to problems when estimating recurrence risks in order to give genetic advice. For example, tuberous sclerosis (epiloia) is inherited as a dominant trait but is not always penetrant. This condition is characterised by adenoma sebaceum (small papules over the cheeks and nose), epilepsy and mental retardation of varying severity. Some individuals carrying the gene may be so mildly affected as to pass as normal and so produce an apparently 'skipped' generation. However, it is unusual to find a proven carrier (e.g. with an affected child and an affected parent) who does not show at least some evidence of the disease, such as a few typical papules on the face.

Autosomal Recessive Inheritance. Autosomal recessive traits also affect both males and females. Unlike dominant traits, recessive traits are manifest only in the homozygous state, that is, in those individuals who possess a double dose of the mutant gene. Heterozygotes who possess only one mutant gene are usually perfectly healthy. Similarly the offspring of an affected person are usually normal, because most recessive conditions are so rare that it would be most unlikely that an affected person would marry a person heterozygous for the same mutant gene. In the even more unlikely event of two persons homozygous for the same recessive trait marrying, all their children would be affected. In general, however, both parents and offspring of a person homozygous for a rare recessive gene will be healthy. Characteristically in recessive traits affected individuals cannot be traced from one generation to the next and if more than one member of a family is affected they are usually sibs, i.e. brothers and sisters. The pedigree of an autosomal recessive trait (Fig. 1.5), therefore, differs from that of a dominant trait.

At conception there is a 1 in 4 chance that any child of two heterozygous parents will be affected. Each parent produces gametes of two types, one bearing the normal gene and the other bearing the mutant gene. At conception, therefore, one-quarter of the offspring will be normal, one-half will be healthy heterozygotes and one-quarter will be affected. These are average figures; by chance all the offspring of such a couple might be affected, or similarly all their offspring might be normal. It has been calculated theoretically that in marriages between two heterozygotes, in 75 per cent of families with only one child that child will be unaffected, in 56 per cent of families with two children both children will be unaffected, but in only 32 per cent of families with four children will all four children be unaffected.

When dealing with rare recessive diseases the parents of affected individuals are often found to be related, because such individuals are more likely to have inherited the same mutant gene from an ancestor they have in common. The chance that first cousins will carry the same recessive gene is 1 in 8, but the chance that two unrelated individuals will carry the same recessive gene is very much lower and depends on the frequency of the particular gene in the population. In general the rarer the gene the greater the frequency of consanguinity amongst the parents of affected individuals.

At present roughly 1 in 200 marriages in Britain is between first cousins, so that giving advice on the genetic consequences of cousin marriages is a problem with which geneticists are frequently faced. Several extensive studies have shown that among the offspring of consanguineous matings there is an increased perinatal mortality rate together with an increased frequency of both congenital abnormalities and mental retardation, but the actual risks are small and in fact only slightly greater than in the general population. The situation is quite different, however, if there is a family history of a recessive disorder, when the risks will be greatly increased.

Many conditions show an autosomal recessive mode of inheritance and include, for example, many inborn errors of metabolism, some types of deaf-mutism and some types of congenital blindness. The commonest autosomal recessive trait known in Western Europe is fibrocystic disease of the pancreas (p. 388) which affects one in every 2,000 births.

Sex-linked Inheritance. Conditions determined by genes situated on either of the sex chromosomes are said to be inherited as sex-linked traits. Genes carried on the X chromosome are said to be X-linked, those on the Y chromosome being Y-linked.

Y-linkage of a gene implies that only males would be affected and that all the sons of an affected male would inherit the gene. With the possible exception of hairy ears, there are no proven examples of Y-linked single gene disorders in man. Thus all known sex-linked conditions are due to genes on the X chromosome. As with autosomal traits these conditions may be either dominant or recessive.

X-linked dominant conditions are manifest both in females who are heterozygous for the mutant gene and in males who carry the mutant gene on their single X chromosome. The pedigree of an X-linked dominant trait (Fig. 1.6) can superficially resemble that of an autosomal dominant trait, but there is a fundamental difference. Although an affected female will transmit the trait to half her offspring of either sex, an affected male will transmit the trait to all of his daughters but to none of his sons. There will therefore be an excess of females in families exhibiting such conditions. There are few X-linked dominant disorders but a

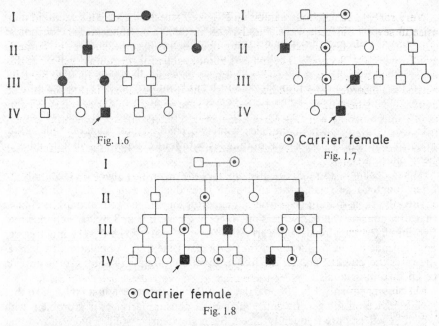

Fig. 1.6

⊙ Carrier female
Fig. 1.7

⊙ Carrier female
Fig. 1.8

Fig. 1.6 Characteristic pedigree: X-linked dominant trait.
Fig. 1.7 Characteristic pedigree: X-linked recessive trait when affected males do not reproduce (e.g. Duchenne muscular dystrophy).
Fig. 1.8 Characteristic pedigree: X-linked recessive trait when affected males do reproduce (e.g. haemophilia).

notable example is one form of vitamin D resistant rickets (p. 121).

An X-linked recessive condition is caused by a gene carried on the X chromosome and is manifest in females only when the gene is in the homozygous state. In males, a mutant gene present on the single X chromosome is always manifest because it is unopposed by the modifying effect of a normal gene on the second X chromosome, as happens in females. As with autosomal recessive conditions, the heterozygous carrier is usually healthy. Conditions inherited in this way therefore predominantly affect males and are transmitted by healthy female carriers (Fig. 1.7). In those conditions where affected males may survive to have children, the condition will also be transmitted by affected males (Fig. 1.8).

Haemophilia is the best known example of an X-linked recessive trait. Whereas in the past most boys with this disease died at an early age, with improvements in treatment most now survive. If an affected man marries a normal woman, then all his daughters will be carriers but none of his sons will be affected. An X-linked trait is never transmitted from father to son. This is because a man transmits his only X chromosome (which if he is affected bears the mutant gene) to each of his daughters but his Y chromosome to each of his sons.

If a woman carrying an X-linked recessive trait marries a normal man, then half of her sons will be affected and half of her daughters will be carriers because each of her children has an equal chance of inheriting from her either the normal X chromosome or the one bearing the mutant gene.

Duchenne muscular dystrophy (p. 754) is inherited as an X-linked recessive trait and because affected boys die young, it is transmitted solely by healthy female carriers.

Very rarely a female may exhibit an X-linked recessive trait. This situation may arise in several different ways. Firstly, she may have an abnormal chromosomal constitution resulting in her only having one X chromosome, such as in Turner's syndrome (XO). Secondly, she may be homozygous for the mutant gene, but this is very unlikely with rare recessive disorders because she would have to have inherited the disorder from both her parents. The third possibility is that she may be a 'manifesting heterozygote'. If, by chance, in the majority of her cells it is the normal X chromosome which is inactivated, then a female heterozygote may exhibit the trait. Careful examination of carriers of Duchenne muscular dystrophy sometimes reveals varying degrees of weakness in the same groups of muscles that are weak in affected boys.

The modes of inheritance for some unifactorial disorders are given in Table 1.2.

Table 1.2 Mode of inheritance of some unifactorial disorders

Autosomal dominant	Autosomal recessive	X-linked recessive
Achondroplasia	Albinism	Christmas disease
Dubin–Johnson syndrome	Ataxia telangiectasia	Glucose-6-phosphate
Facioscapulohumeral	Congenital adrenal	dehydrogenase deficiency
muscular dystrophy	hyperplasia	Haemophilia
Gilbert's disease	Congenital goitrous	Hunter's syndrome
Haemochromatosis—	cretinism	Nephrogenic diabetes
adult type	Crigler–Najjar syndrome	insipidus
Haemoglobinopathies	Cystic fibrosis of	Pseudohypertrophic
Hereditary spherocytosis	pancreas	muscular dystrophy (Duchenne)
Huntington's	Fanconi's syndrome	
chorea	Friedreich's ataxia	
Hyperlipoproteinaemia	Galactosaemia	
Type II	Gaucher's disease	
Marfan's syndrome	Glycogen storage diseases	
Myotonia congenita	Hurler's syndrome	
Myotonic dystrophy	Limb girdle muscular	
Neurofibromatosis	dystrophy (Erb)	
Osteogenesis imperfecta	Niemann–Pick disease	
Polycystic disease	Phenylketonuria	
of kidneys (adult	Pendred's syndrome	
form)	Tay–Sachs disease	
Polyposis of colon		
Porphyria, acute		
intermittent		
Rotor syndrome		
Tuberous sclerosis		

Multifactorial Inheritance

Many human characteristics can be measured and if the values are plotted against the number of individuals in the population with each particular value then a bell-shaped or normal frequency distribution curve is found (Fig. 1.9). This applies to such characteristics as intelligence, stature, weight, skin colour and blood pressure. Some of these traits may be largely environmentally determined, such as weight, whereas others are largely genetically determined, such as stature and intelligence. In each case many genes are probably involved. Characteristics which are due to many genes plus the effects of environment are said to be inherited on a *multifactorial* basis.

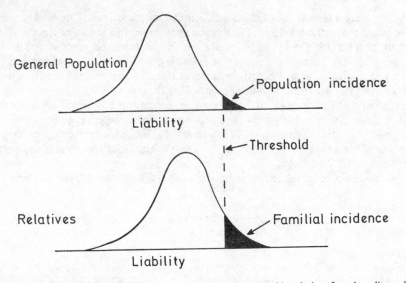

Fig. 1.9 Hypothetical curve of liability in the general population and in relatives for a hereditary disorder in which the genetic predisposition is multifactorial.

It is now believed that many common disorders are inherited in this way. In such conditions it is assumed that there is some underlying graded attribute which is related to causation. This is referred to as the individual's *liability*, which includes not only his genetic predisposition but also the environmental factors which render him more or less likely to develop the disease. It is assumed that the curve of liability has a normal distribution in the general population. In one simple model (Fig. 1.9), it is believed that there is a *threshold* value such that all affected individuals have a liability above this value and all unaffected individuals have a liability below this value. Relatives of affected individuals have a higher average liability than the population average so the curve of liability for relatives is shifted to the right. In the general population the proportion above the threshold is the population incidence and among relatives the proportion above the threshold is the familial incidence. Such a model can be used to explain the familial incidence of such disorders as essential hypertension, coronary artery disease, peptic ulceration and many of the commoner congenital malformations.

There are several consequences of such a model. Familial incidence will be greater among the relatives of more severely affected individuals because presumably they are more extreme deviants along the curve of liability and the number of abnormal genes segregating in such families is greater than in families in which individuals are less severely affected. Thus in hare lip with or without cleft palate the proportion of affected sibs and children is roughly 6 per cent when the index patient has double hare lip and cleft palate, but only 2·5 per cent if the index patient has a single hare lip. By similar reasoning it would be expected that the incidence among sibs born subsequent to the index patient would be greater the more affected relatives there were in the family. In spina bifida, for example, the incidence of this condition, or the related disorder anencephaly, in sibs born after one affected child is roughly 5 per cent, but the incidence rises to 10 per cent after the birth of two affected children. This is quite different from the situation in unifactorial disorders where the risk to subsequent sibs remains constant irrespective of the number of affected individuals in the family (e.g. 1 in 4 for an autosomal recessive trait). Finally as a consequence of this model it might be expected that when there is a sex difference in the population incidence, the relatives of the less frequently affected sex would be more often affected. The reason for this is that in the less frequently affected sex, when individuals are affected they are presumably more extreme deviants along the curve of liability and possess more abnormal genes. Thus in congenital pyloric stenosis, which is 5 times commoner in boys than girls, the proportions of affected relatives of male index patients are roughly 5·5 per cent for sons and 2·4 per cent for daughters, but 19·4 per cent for sons and 7·3 per cent for daughters when the index patient is a female.

Though it is not possible to measure liability to a particular disease it is possible to estimate how much of the aetiology can be ascribed to genetic factors as opposed to environmental factors. This is referred to as the *heritability*, which may be defined as that proportion of the total variation which is due to genetic factors and is therefore expressed as a percentage. The greater the value for the heritability the greater the contribution of genetic factors to aetiology. The heritability for a particular disorder is calculated from the known incidences of the disorder in the general population and in relatives, usually first-degree relatives (sibs, parents and children), or from knowing the incidences in identical (monozygotic) and non-identical (dizygotic) twins. It should be appreciated that heritability is estimated from the degree of resemblance between relatives and this may in part be due to sharing of a common environment. Thus it is important to derive estimates from different kinds of relatives, and not sibs alone, and to measure the frequency of the condition in relatives reared or living apart and in unrelated individuals living together, such as spouses, in order to assess the possible effects of common environmental factors.

Some estimates of heritability are given in Table 1.3. The values, though approximate, do indicate that genetic factors are of more importance in aetiology in asthma, schizophrenia and early onset diabetes than in, for example, peptic ulcer.

Assessment of the incidence of disease in relatives not only provides an estimate of heritability, and therefore of the contribution of genetic factors to aetiology, but is essential for genetic counselling. It is on such knowledge that empiric risks are based (p. 21).

Table 1.3 Estimates of heritability for various multifactorial disorders

Disorder	Incidence (%)	Heritability (%)
Schizophrenia	1	85
Asthma	4	80
Cleft lip ± cleft palate	0·1	76
Pyloric stenosis (congenital)	0·3	75
Diabetes mellitus: early onset	0·2	75
late onset	2–3	35
Ankylosing spondylitis	0·2	70
Club foot (congenital)	0·1	68
Coronary artery disease	3	65
Hypertension (essential)	5	62
Dislocation of hip (congenital)	0·1	60
Anencephaly and spina bifida	0·5	60
Peptic ulcer	4	37
Congenital heart disease (all types)	0·5	35

Prevention of Genetic Disease

Since there is at present no effective treatment for most genetic disorders the role of the medical practitioner lies mainly in the prevention of such conditions through genetic counselling. This involves providing advice on the chances of recurrence of a genetic disorder in the children of either healthy parents who already have an affected child, or when one of the parents or a near relative is affected with a disease which is known to be inherited.

In chromosomal disorders if the parents have normal karyotypes, i.e. do not carry a translocation which in the unbalanced state would cause abnormality, then the chances of recurrence are usually low. The most important chromosomal disorder from this point of view is Down's syndrome. The risk of having a child with Down's syndrome is about 1 in 100 in women who have previously had an affected child, and at least 1 in 50 in women over the age of 40. However, the risks are higher if one of the parents carries a chromosome translocation (Table 1.4).

Table 1.4 Recurrence risks of Down's syndrome due to various chromosome aberations.
C = Carrier, N = Normal

| Patient | Karyotypes | | Recurrence risk (%) |
	Father	Mother	
Translocation:			
21/13–15	N	C	10–15
	C	N	5
21/22	N	C	10–15
	C	N	5
21/21	N	C	100
	C	N	100
Trisomy 21	N	N	1
Translocation or mosaic	N	N	1

In unifactorial disorders the chances of recurrence are based on Mendelian principles. As we have seen, for example, for a fully penetrant autosomal dominant disorder there is a 1 in 2 chance of recurrence in any child of an affected parent. However, if both parents are healthy an affected child must be the result of a new mutation and the chances of recurrence in subsequent children are negligible. If parents have had a child with an autosomal recessive disorder the chance of recurrence in subsequent children is 1 in 4. Should such a child survive there is very little chance of its having affected children. Finally, with X-linked recessive disorders there is a 1 in 2 chance that any son of a known carrier will be affected and a 1 in 2 chance that any daughter will be a carrier. All the daughters of an affected male will be carriers.

In recent years the most important advance in the prevention of X-linked disorders has been the development of tests for detecting healthy female carriers of such disorders as Duchenne muscular dystrophy and haemophilia. An urgent problem at present is the need for reliable methods for detecting symptomless, preclinical cases of autosomal dominant disorders such as Huntington's chorea, polyposis coli, polycystic kidney disease and myotonic dystrophy in which symptoms often do not develop until the third or fourth decade of life. If such tests should become available it would be possible for individuals likely to become affected, and therefore transmit the disease to their children, to receive advice before they had a family.

In multifactorial disorders risks of recurrence cannot be predicted from Mendelian principles but have to be determined by studying the frequency of the condition among the relatives of affected individuals. Examples of risk figures, derived in this way (so-called *empiric* risks), for some relatively common conditions are given in Table 1.5.

Table 1.5 Empiric risks (in %) for some common disorders

Disorder	Incidence	Sex ratio M:F	Normal parents having a second affected child	Affected parent having an affected child	Affected parent having a second affected child
Anencephaly	0·20	1:2	5*	—	—
Cleft palate only	0·04	2:3	2	7	15
Cleft lip ± cleft palate	0·10	3:2	4	4	10
Club foot	0·10	2:1	3	3	10
Cong. heart disease (all types)	0·50	—	1–4	1–4	—
Diabetes mellitus (early onset)	0·20	1:1	8	8	10
Dislocation of hip	0·07	1:6	4	4	10
Epilepsy ('idiopathic')	0·50	1:1	5	5	10
Hirschsprung's disease	0·02	4:1			
male index			2	—	—
female index			8	—	—
Manic-depressive psychosis	0·40	2:3	—	10–15	—
Mental retardation ('idiopathic')	0·30	1:1	3–5	—	—
Profound childhood deafness	0·10	1:1	10	6	—
Pyloric stenosis	0·30	5:1			
male index			2	4	13
female index			10	17	38
Schizophrenia	1–2	1:1	—	16	—
Scoliosis (idiopathic, adolescent)	0·22	1:6	7	5	—
Spina bifida	0·30	2:3	5*	3*	—

* Anencephaly or spina bifida

Genetic Advice

The first step in giving genetic advice is to establish a precise diagnosis, secondly to be certain that the disorder in question is genetic and thirdly to verify the presence or absence of the disease in relatives. Without a precise diagnosis it is not possible to give reliable genetic counselling since certain disorders though superficially similar may be inherited differently. For example Hunter's syndrome and Hurler's syndrome both present similar clinical features of 'gargoylism' but whereas clouding of the cornea does not occur in the former condition it is present in the latter. Further, Hunter's syndrome is an X-linked recessive trait and therefore the unaffected sister of an affected boy may be at risk of having affected children. Hurler's syndrome on the other hand is an autosomal recessive disorder and only affects sibs. In this condition there is therefore no chance of an unaffected sister having affected children, provided she does not marry a near relative who might also carry the mutant gene.

It is always advisable to check that the disease in question is in fact genetic and not due to some environmental factor (i.e. a *phenocopy*). For example congenital deafness is often due to a rare recessive gene but it may also result from intrauterine infection with rubella during the first three months of pregnancy which may also cause other abnormalities in the fetus such as congenital heart disease and eye defects. If it can be shown in a particular case that congenital deafness was due to maternal rubella then there would be no chance of recurrence in subsequent children. It is therefore important before giving genetic advice to ask about the possibility of maternal exposure to radiation, drugs or infections during pregnancy and details of any birth trauma which might possibly account for the disorder in question.

Factors which influence the parents' decision whether or not they will accept a risk of having an affected child include the severity of the abnormality, whether or not there is an effective treatment, the actual risk, their religious attitude and possibly their socioeconomic status. In general, however, parents usually accept the risk of having an affected child if this is less than one in 20 but do not accept a risk of greater than one in 10 if the disease is serious.

Antenatal Diagnosis. Family limitation is not the only course of action open to parents who are found to be at high risk of having a child with a serious genetic disorder. Other possibilities include artificial insemination by donor (if the father is affected with a dominant disorder, or if both parents are heterozygous for a rare recessive gene) and antenatal diagnosis with selective abortion of affected fetuses. This is possible by studying cells present in amniotic fluid or the amniotic fluid itself. About 5 to 10 ml of fluid is removed by transabdominal amniocentesis around the 15th week of gestation. The specimen is centrifuged and the uncultured cells (which are derived largely from the fetal skin) may be studied to determine the sex of the fetus by fluorescent (F-body) and sex-chromatin studies, though it is advisable to confirm the sex of the fetus by also culturing the cells for full karyotype analysis. This is valuable in X-linked disorders which cannot yet be diagnosed *in utero* (e.g. Duchenne muscular dystrophy). In this way a known carrier mother can be guaranteed a daughter who will not be affected (though she might be a carrier), for if the fetus is a male the parents may decide on termination since there is a one in two chance the fetus could be affected. Amniotic fluid cells can also be cultured and from the study of this material it is possible not only to sex the fetus but also to diagnose cytogenetic abnormalities and certain inborn errors of metabolism in the fetus. At present the main application of such studies is in the antenatal diagnosis of Down's syndrome and many centres now offer amniocentesis to all pregnant women over the age of 40 because of their increased risk of having a child with this disorder. Finally anencephaly and open spina bifida are associated with raised levels of alphafetoprotein in amniotic fluid and these disorders may therefore also be diagnosed *in utero*.

Conclusion. The main contribution which genetics can make to medicine is in understanding more about the aetiology of certain disorders and in preventing such disorders through genetic counselling.

In genetic counselling it is not sufficient merely to quote risk figures. As far as possible the nature and cause of the disease should be explained to parents and any feelings of guilt should be removed. Since genetic counselling may have profound long-term effects on a family such advice must never be given without careful appraisal of all the factors involved if the needs of the individual are to be met. Genetic counselling, like many other aspects of medicine, is as much an art as a science.

A. E. H. Emery

Further reading:

Emery, A. E. H. (1973). *Antenatal Diagnosis of Genetic Disease*. Edinburgh: Churchill Livingstone.
Emery, A. E. H. (1975). *Elements of Medical Genetics*. 4th edition. Edinburgh: Churchill Livingstone.
Emery, A. E. H. (1976). *Methodology in Medical Genetics*. Edinburgh: Churchill Livingstone.

2. Immunological Factors in Disease

THE science of immunology arose from the study of man's resistance to infection. The most striking feature of this resistance is the specific nature of its enhancement in individuals following infection. Thus, antigenic stimulation and antibody production began to be elucidated in the context of infectious disease and immunity to it. Terms such as 'immunology', 'immunisation' and 'specific immune response' are derived from these origins.

It soon appeared that such specific 'immune' responses might also confer unpleasant and sometimes dangerous hypersensitivity to subsequent exposure to the provoking antigen. Resistance to infection is not an essential feature of the immune response; for example, bacteria may induce antibodies which have no obvious protective value and immune responses are often evoked by injection of intrinsically harmless non-living organic substances, such as serum protein from another individual or species. After exposure to antigen the individual develops a changed reactivity. The ability to develop specific immunity to infection is only one consequence of a wider capacity in the individual to recognise and to respond specifically to the foreignness of a wide range of biological substances that are not normally present in his own tissues. Immunology is the study of what this 'changed reactivity' or allergy is in terms of cellular biochemistry, how it is brought about, and how it is regulated both quantitatively and qualitatively. In the present chapter an account of current concepts of the physiology of the immune system is given in order that the clinical application of immunology may be understood in such diverse conditions as infection, asthma, drug reactions and certain endocrine, gastrointestinal, haematological and connective tissue disorders.

The Immune System

The antigenicity of a substance (i.e. its ability to induce an immune response) is determined by one or more specific molecular groups on its structure known as antigenic determinants. When immunocompetent lymphocytes recognise a foreign substance (antigen) they respond by undergoing transformation into lymphoblasts and then into antibody-producing plasma cells or lymphocytes as indicated in Figure 2.2. It is considered that the population of antibody-producing cells arises by random mutation and that a single cell will then react to produce a family of cells (clone) with a specific function. Essential to this concept is that random mutation of lymphocytes allows the production of cells that are capable of responding to all antigens, although a single cell can react to only one antigen. Antibody-production is a special example of protein synthesis, i.e. the putting together of amino acids to form protein molecules, in this instance, immunoglobulins, and the replication of this process according to a pattern. Its special feature is that it involves a synthesis that can be varied on demand to produce different antibodies capable of reacting to any of the many different antigenic determinants.

If antigenic material (either part of self or a foreign substance) comes into contact with the cells of the antibody-forming system at the stage before the cells have reached maturity, e.g. in fetal life, the result is a failure of response rather than stimulation of antibody formation or other form of immune response against the antigen concerned. This is referred to as immunological tolerance to the antigen. Probably for this reason an individual does not normally show an immune response against components of his own tissues. In the abnormal situation where an immune reaction does occur to a component of the body's own tissues, the reaction is referred to as autoimmune.

The importance of transplantation in modern surgery gave a great impetus to the study of tolerance. The antigens that give rise to the immune response that results in rejection of a tissue allograft are known as histocompatibility or transplantation antigens. They are genetically determined and in each species can be grouped with a number of complex genetic systems. The major histocompatibility system in man is known as HLA. Histocompatibility antigens are found on most tissues, but differ quantitatively in their distribution on these tissues. HLA is the most polymorphic genetic system yet defined in man and is situated on chromosome 6. The antigens of the system are present on leucocytes and platelets in peripheral blood but not on erythrocytes, and can be detected either by serological techniques or in lymphocyte culture.

The antigens which are detected serologically can be divided into three series and within each series the antigens behave as if they were determined by mutually exclusive alleles. Under the new nomenclature the first series of antigens are called HLA-A, the second series HLA-B, and the third series HLA-C (Fig. 2.1). In addition a fourth series of antigens can be determined only by their ability to stimulate lymphocytes in culture (although their serological definition should be possible eventually) and this series is known as HLA-D. Well-defined antigens in each series are given a number e.g. HLA-A1, HLA-A2, etc., while less well-defined antigens are given the prefix W, e.g. HLA-AW19, HLA-AW30, etc. There are 20 defined specifications of the A series, 20 of the B series, 5 of the C series and 6 of the D series. Thus the possible combinations of alleles on a chromosome (this being known as a haplotype) is enormous, although certain alleles tend to occur together on the

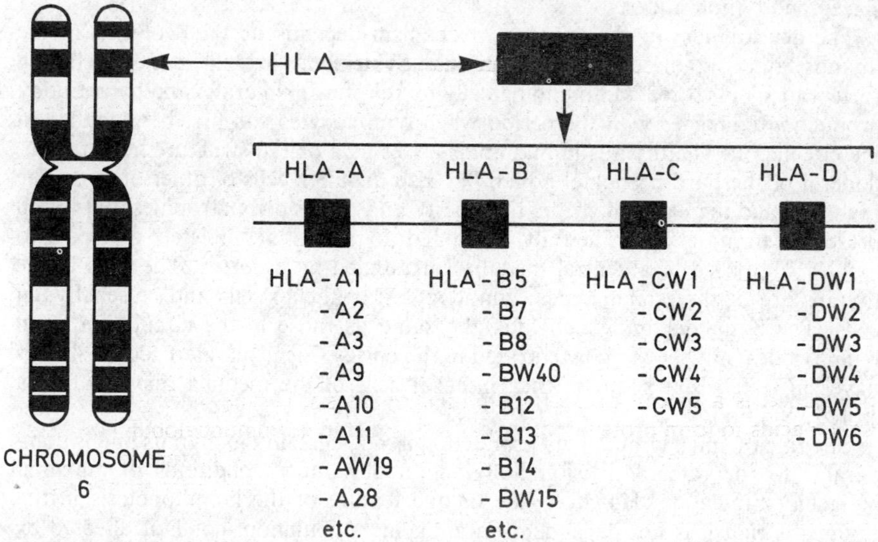

HLA-A	HLA-B	HLA-C	HLA-D
HLA-A1	HLA-B5	HLA-CW1	HLA-DW1
-A2	-B7	-CW2	-DW2
-A3	-B8	-CW3	-DW3
-A9	-BW40	-CW4	-DW4
-A10	-B12	-CW5	-DW5
-A11	-B13		-DW6
-AW19	-B14		
-A28	-BW15		
etc.	etc.		

CHROMOSOME 6

Fig. 2.1 The HLA system in man

chromosome, e.g. HLA-A1 and HLA-B8. Nevertheless, the chance of two unrelated people being identical for HLA is very low.

Skin grafts between HLA identical siblings show a marked prolongation of survival, while renal allografts between HLA identical siblings have very few rejection episodes and a 95 per cent survival at 3 years. However, in unrelated cadaver renal transplantion, true HLA identity is rare, and partial matching for HLA can offer only a modest improvement in survival figures.

A skin graft from a genetically different individual of the same species (allograft) applied for the first time becomes vascularised and appears healthy for 13 to 14 days, depending on the degree of genetic difference between the donor and the recipient. The circulation then begins to fail, the graft becomes infiltrated with inflammatory mononuclear cells, and later necrotises and sloughs. If a second similar graft is now applied to the same recipient there is an accelerated and greatly increased inflammatory reaction with rapid necrosis. Sloughing of the graft occurs within three to four days, indicative of the development at the first exposure of an active immunity to the antigens of the donor tissue. Even when there is a lapse of time after the first acquaintance with the antigen, the cells of the immune system retain a memory of the antigen and are stimulated rapidly by further contact with the antigen. This augmented and accelerated secondary response not only involves cell mediated immunity but is also well recognised in the classical immunology of bacterial infection in relation to the levels of circulating antibody.

COMPONENTS OF THE IMMUNE SYSTEM

The main cells involved in immune reactions are lymphocytes, plasma cells and macrophages. Anatomically, the immune system can be subdivided into the 'central' and 'peripheral' lymphoid tissues. The central lymphoid tissue consists of the thymus and the cloacal lymphoid organ in birds known as the bursa of Fabricius. In mammals the tonsils and the lymphoid tissue of the gut may well represent the analogue of the bursa of birds. The major peripheral lymphoid tissues are the spleen and lymph nodes.

The development of the immune mechanism depends on the evolution of the thymus and organised lymphoid tissues. The time at which a developing vertebrate can first react immunologically by rejecting skin grafts and by antibody production coincides with the period when lymphocytes can first be identified in the circulation. The thymus in mammals arises as a paired structure from the endoderm of the third branchial pouch but also acquires cells of other origins. The thymus gland increases in size until puberty and then slowly atrophies, but is still present even in old age. The fully developed thymus is incompletely divided into lobules composed of a central medulla surrounded by a cortex. The cells in the thymus are of three main types: lymphocytes, epithelial cells and mesenchymal cells. The lymphocytes, which look the same as those in the circulation or in lymph nodes, are heavily concentrated in the cortex. Electron microscopic studies have suggested that some of the epithelial cells of the medulla may contain a stored secretion.

The rate of small lymphocyte production is very high in the thymus and is comparable to the rate of division in lymph nodes under conditions of maximal antigenic stimulation. However, the unique feature of the lymphopoiesis in the thymus is that it is not dependent on antigenic stimulation, nor is it affected by resection of other lymphoid organs, partial thymectomy or by the presence of one or numerous thymus implants. This suggests that the primary stimulus for the proliferation of thymic lymphoid cells must arise from within the thymus itself.

Immune reactions are mediated by humoral or cellular mechanisms or by both. The humoral factor consists of antibody (immunoglobulin) secreted by plasma cells. The cellular component is made up of lymphocytes sensitised to specific antigens and reactive with those antigens without the presence of free antibody. In addition, certain lymphoid cells and monocytes, although not themselves specifically sensitised, can gain specificity in the presence of antibody or antigen-antibody complexes on the surface of the target cells or on their own surface. This is known as cell-mediated (K) antibody-dependent cytoxicity (CADC, type VI) reaction (p. 44). The lymphoid cells involved are referred to as killer or K cells.

Immunological responses mediated by humoral antibody and by cells both depend initially upon the activity of small lymphocytes which stem from precursors in the bone marrow. The main effect of neonatal thymectomy is to prevent the development of cell-mediated immunological reactions such as allograft rejection. In birds antibody production, but not cell-mediated reactions, is dependent on the bursa of Fabricius. These and other findings suggest that stem-cells originating in the bone marrow differentiate to form two main lymphocyte populations. One is dependent on the presence of the thymus (T lymphocytes) and is responsible for cell-mediated hypersensitivity. The other is independent of the thymus but dependent on the bursa of Fabricius or its equivalent in man (B lymphocytes, Fig. 2.2)

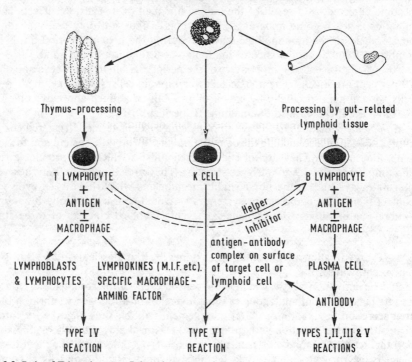

Fig. 2.2 Role of T lymphocytes, B lymphocytes and K cells in immunological responses. Many of these events involve active cell proliferation, but for simplicity this has not been shown. (From Irvine, *Proceedings of the Royal Society of Medicine*, 1974.)

and is responsible for humoral antibody synthesis. They also differ in their distribution and probably in their life span. T lymphocytes constitute a greater part of the pool of small lymphocytes that circulate in the blood, interstitial spaces and lymph and most of them have a relatively long life (months or years in man) while the B lymphocytes are more restricted to lymphoid tissue and most of them appear to be short-lived (several weeks). There is evidence for the existence of subclasses, presumably with differing functions, within these main classes; e.g. short-lived T lymphocytes and long-lived B lymphocytes. Thus immunological memory is achieved by the existence of long-lived T and B cells.

The thymus plays an essential role in inducing the differentiation of immunologically competent thymus-dependent lymphocytes (T cells) from non-competent precursors. This function is dependent upon the integrity of the epithelial cells in the thymic medulla which secrete a factor or hormone that effects this change.

Unlike thymectomy in the newborn, thymectomy in adult life leads to no immediate significant impairment of immuno-capacity although there may be some reduction in the population of lymphocytes in the peripheral blood, thoracic duct lymph, lymph nodes and spleen. If, however, the lymphoid system in the adult mouse is damaged or destroyed by ionising radiation, then the thymus is important for the anatomical and functional regeneration of this system. Furthermore, when animals thymectomised in adult life are challenged with a new antigen six or more months later, there is clear evidence of immunological deficiency. Presumably the adult thymus influences the development of an adequate population of long-lived immunologically competent cells. Only when this pool has become depleted, as a result of the limited life span of its cells, do defects in immune capacity become apparent. The thymus is thus not only essential for the development of the immunological system during the neonatal period but is also important for the maintenance of immunological function in the adult.

About 70 per cent of lymphocytes in the peripheral blood are T cells and about 20 per cent are B cells. The non-sensitised lymphoid cells that are neither T nor B cells but can gain specificity by means of antibody or antigen-antibody complexes (K cells) are included in the remaining 10 per cent.

Complement belongs to the group of plasma systems termed 'triggered enzyme cascades', which also include the coagulation and fibrinolytic system and the kinin generating system. They are all effector mechanisms which can produce a rapid and amplified response to a trigger stimulus. They are complex both in their reaction pathways and in the homeostatic mechanisms which have been evolved to control them. The complement system is activated characteristically by antigen-antibody interactions; the sequence of events involved consists of three stages (Fig. 2.3):

1. The generation of C3 splitting enzymes by the classical and by the alternative pathways.
2. The activation of C3, which is the central event of the complement sequence and its bulk reaction, analogous to the conversion of fibrinogen to fibrin in blood coagulation. The fixation of C3 at complement fixation sites (e.g. the Fc component of IgG after reaction with antigen, p. 31) is probably the system's most important activity. Bound C3 reacts with various receptors on phagocytic cells, platelets, erythrocytes and certain lymphocytes and retention of cells at complement fixation sites contributes largely to the activity of the complement system in inflammation. The generation of C3b leads to the activation of a self-amplifying

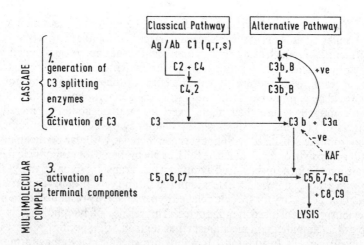

Fig. 2.3 The complement system. The bar over a component represents an activated state, usually enzymatic, generated during the complement sequence. B represents a factor of unknown nature which activates the alternative pathway. (*From Irvine, 1977*)

positive feedback cycle. This is damped by the action of the C3b inactivator (KAF Fig. 2.3).

3. The activation of the terminal components. This step is initiated by the activation of C5 which seems to be the last enzymic reaction in the complement sequence. Thereafter the remaining components (C6–C9) combine to form a multimolecular complex which mediates the most characteristic *in vitro* event of the complement system: the generation of membrane lesions leading to cell lysis.

MECHANISM OF THE IMMUNE RESPONSE

The recognition of antigen by B lymphocytes is believed to be mediated by antibody synthesised in the cell and bound into the surface membrane, the specificity of the antibody being determined by the genetic characteristics (programming) of the individual lymphocyte. T lymphocytes, on the other hand, do not have detectable antibody on their surface but have antibody-like receptors for antigens, the exact nature of which is not clear. In both instances combination with the appropriate antigen then triggers off the immunological response.

The induction of mitosis in T lymphocytes and their transformation to larger 'blast' cells (Fig. 2.2) may be effected both by specific antigens and by non-specific mitogens which include agents such as phytohaemagglutinin (PHA). It is likely that stimulation of mitosis in some T lymphocytes involves processing of the antigen by macrophages, possibly leading to presentation of antigen determinants at the surface of the macrophage. For example, lymphocyte preparations largely freed of phagocytic cells are unresponsive to certain antigens but activity can be restored by addition of macrophages. Lymphocytes in tissue-culture can be seen to wander incessantly and presumably identify the antigens of the cells over which they move in terms of their degree of 'fit' with the antibody on the lymphocyte surface. Likewise, in the body the T lymphocytes migrate through the tissues (immunological surveillance) permitting their sensitisation or transformation to blast cells by contact with antigen in the periphery, with or without the help of macrophages.

The T lymphocyte sensitised to a specific antigen undergoes blast transformation and proliferation on contact with the antigen. In addition, the interaction of antigen with T lymphocytes leads to the release of non specific soluble factors (lymphokines, Figs. 2.2 and 2.11) which bring about a number of tissue changes associated with cell-mediated hypersensitivity reactions. One of these factors inhibits the migration of macrophages in tissue culture. *In vivo* the effect of the migration inhibitory factor (MIF) would be to immobilise randomly wandering macrophages at the site of reaction with antigen, where they might exert a cytotoxic action or merely act as scavengers of cells already damaged by lymphocytes. Other non-specific factors released from the sensitised lymphocytes can increase vascular permeability, cause inhibition of growth or death of tissue cells, be chemotactic for mononuclear cells and stimulate mitosis in 'non-sensitised' lymphocytes. Transfer factor is a dialysable substance with a molecular weight of less than 10,000 and yet can apparently transfer the 'information' necessary for specific delayed hypersensitivity responses to be mounted by previously unsensitised lymphocytes. The release of lymphokines is another example of an amplification mechanism that augments the specific response initiated by relatively few cells. In addition to lymphokines, specific macrophage arming factor is released which renders macrophages cytostatic to cells bearing that particular antigen.

How B lymphocytes are stimulated to become the antibody-forming cells of the plasma cell line is not yet fully understood. A possible sequence of events is shown diagrammatically in Figure 2.4. Certain antigens are apparently capable of reacting directly with the corresponding antibody on the surface of a B lymphocyte to induce it to transform and proliferate into active antibody-producing cells (plasma cells). Such antigens generally have many antigenic determinants of the same specificity so that they can simultaneously trigger a number of receptors on the surface of the same B lymphocyte. Other antigens, or small doses of antigen, may have to be taken on to the surface of a macrophage, as mentioned above in relation to T lymphocytes, thus being more readily available for stimulating a B lymphocyte either directly or through the co-operation of a helper T lymphocyte.

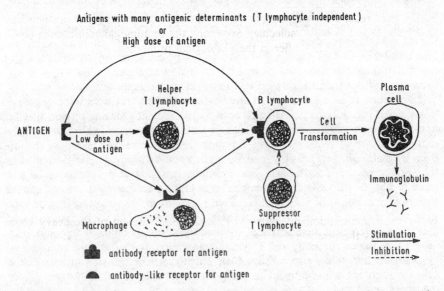

Fig. 2.4 Possible sequence of events in humoral antibody formation, illustrating co-operation between T lymphocytes, B lymphocytes and macrophages and role of suppressor T lymphocytes.

In this way a high local concentration of antigen is achieved during cell to cell contact with the B lymphocyte, thereby stimulating a greater number of receptor sites in a given cell than if the antigen were uniformly dispersed throughout the body fluids. Once stimulated, the cell undergoes division and produces the antibody that it is genetically programmed to do.

There is evidence for negative in addition to positive control of immunological mechanisms as indicated in Figure 2.4. A subpopulation of T lymphocytes (suppressor T cells) exists which can exert a suppressive effect on the synthesis of antibody by B cells. Relaxation of this control may play an important role in the development of autoimmunity (p. 45).

Another possible result of the interaction of certain types of antigens with the surface of a lymphocyte is that the cell is prevented from transforming for antibody formation and is functionally eliminated. The individual has immune tolerance to that particular antigen.

Observations *in vitro* and *in vivo* have shown that continued division of lymphoblasts ultimately gives rise to progeny with the morphological characteristics of small lymphocytes, and this expanded population of lymphocytes with the same antibody specificity as the original parent cells may provide a basis for the immunological memory referred to above and which is a feature of both cellular and humoral responses. The lymphocyte population is therefore a heterogeneous group of morphologically similar cells.

IMMUNOGLOBULINS

From the early days of immunology, antibodies have been described in terms of their various reactions with antigens as precipitins, lysins, antitoxins, agglutinins, etc. and it was believed that these effects were due to the same kind of antibody acting in different circumstances. It is now clear on two scores that not all antibodies reacting with the same antigen are of the same kind. Firstly, different antibodies may react with antigenic determinants of varying specificity on the same substance (e.g. a protein molecule). Secondly, the immunoglobulin classes (IgG, IgM, IgA, IgD and IgE) differ in their biological properties.

Structure of Immunoglobulins. Immunoglobulins are made up of distinct subunits held together in the whole molecule by disulphide (S-S) bonds (Fig. 2.5). The bonds can be broken by reducing agents, so that the molecule falls apart into pairs of polypeptide chains called light and heavy chains as determined by their molecular weights. Two types of light chain exist, K and L, of which individual immunoglobulins have only one type. The enzyme papain splits the immunoglobulin molecule into two antigen binding (Fab) fractions and one crystallisable fraction (Fc). The Fc fragment of the heavy chain is responsible for the antigenic differences between the classes of immunoglobulin which enables their ready quantitation by antisera. It is the Fc fragment of the heavy chain which carries the predominant part of the molecule responsible for complement activation or fixation. This depends upon changes in the configuration of the immunoglobulin molecule when reacting with antigen. The Fc fragment also contains sites for macrophage fixation and for fixation to the killer (K) lymphoid cells of Type VI reactions (Fig. 2.8).

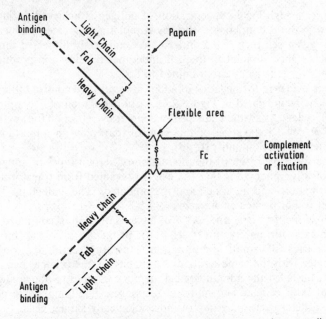

Fig. 2.5 Immunoglobulin structure. Note (1) Disulphide bond cleavage produces two light chains and two heavy chains. (2) The dotted line shows the site of papain cleavage producing two Fab portions and one Fc portion. (3) The amino acids that vary in sequence for different antibodies are shown as interrupted ends of the light and heavy chains and may represent the combining sites that determine the specificity of individual antibody molecules for their particular antigen.

CLASSIFICATION AND FUNCTIONS OF IMMUNOGLOBULINS

IgG. In healthy adults, the total IgG (about 80 g) accounts for 73 per cent of the immunoglobulins in normal serum and is distributed equally between the blood and interstitial tissues, about a quarter passing across the capillary walls each day and the same amount returning via the thoracic duct. In man, IgG is the only immunoglobulin that is transported across the placenta to reach the fetal circulation and provide the baby with passive immunisation during its early life. IgG antibody is particularly suited to neutralising soluble toxin such as that of *C. diphtheriae*.

IgM. The macro-molecular IgM is predominantly intravascular. It constitutes only seven per cent of the serum immunoglobulins and is made up of five immunoglobulin units linked with disulphide bonds to provide ten identical combining-sites instead of the two of IgG. IgM is especially effective in activating complement to produce immune lysis of foreign cells by digesting holes in the cell membranes at the sites where antibody has reacted. Fifty micrograms/100 ml of IgM antibody could destroy half the red cells in the circulation. IgM antibodies are much more efficient than IgG antibodies in linking particulate antigens together for agglutination and phagocytosis and would seem to be specially adapted for dealing with cell debris or bacteria in the bloodstream.

IgA, which accounts for 19 per cent of the total serum immunoglobulins, is preferentially secreted into colostrum, saliva, intestinal juice and respiratory

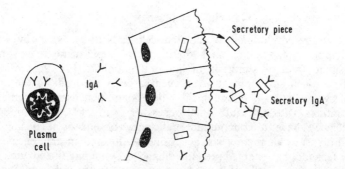

Fig. 2.6 The conversion of IgA produced by plasma cells (e.g. in the lamina propriae of the gut) to the more stable secretory IgA which bathes the mucous surfaces of the body.

secretions. The major sites of IgA synthesis are the laminae propriae underlying the mucous membranes throughout the respiratory tract and the gut. The monomer produced locally by plasma cells is largely taken up by the epithelial cells, when two of them link together and a secretory piece (Fig. 2.6) is added which protects the molecule from digestive enzymes. Secretory IgA is available right through to the colon and these antibodies are vital in the defence of the gut against enteroviruses, e.g. poliomyelitis. In general, IgA plays a major role as part of an antiseptic secretion over the mucous surfaces of the body.

IgD. These have some of the properties of the IgG globulins, although little is known of their exact role.

IgE. These have a very low serum level (250 pg/ml) and the distinctive property of possessing an affinity for cell surfaces. They are an integral part of immediate hypersensitivity reactions such as occur in hay fever and in some cases of asthma (p. 38). The Fc portions of the IgE antibodies combine with sites on the surface of mast cells especially in the nasopharynx and bronchi and also in the gut, leaving the antigen-combining sites freely available. The combination of antigen (in the circumstances sometimes referred to as reagin) with IgE antibody on the surface of the mast cell triggers the release of vasoactive substances which mediate anaphylactic (immediate hypersensitivity) reactions (Figs. 2.8 and 2.9). The physiological function of IgE antibodies is obscure but they may possibly have a role in the defence against helminths.

The mechanisms for the production and deployment of immunoglobulins are therefore well adapted to bring antibody into almost every milieu in the body where its presence may serve a useful function.

Immunodeficiency Disorders

So important are the immunological mechanisms for survival that it is not surprising that patients are rarely seen suffering from major defects. Deficiencies of the humoral and cellular components of the immunological system may occur separately or together. Figure 2.7 shows the probable sites of the primary defects in the immune system for a number of clinical patterns that have been recognised.

Combined Deficiency States

A block in the development of the stem-cell leads to deficiency in both the T and B lymphocyte systems and therefore to impairment of cell-mediated hypersensitivity and of synthesis of humoral antibody (Fig. 2.7, lesion 1). A failure of stem-cell development at an even earlier stage leads to the additional feature of agranulocytosis although the red cells and platelets are normal. About half the infants with the autosomal recessive form of severe combined immunodeficiency have a concomitant deficiency of adenosine deaminase, the aminohydrolyase which converts adenosine to inosine in the purine salvage pathway. This fact has enabled prenatal diagnosis by finding the enzyme deficiency in cultured amnion cells. It is not known at present precisely how the enzyme defect causes the deficiency but it appears to be causally related. Infants with either the autosomal or the X-linked types are incapable of limiting the most benign viral infections. Death has resulted from generalised chickenpox, measles with giant cell pneumonia, and in a few instances, from cytomegaloviral and adenoviral infection. Vaccination results in progressive, ultimately fatal vaccinia infection. BCG inoculation has also resulted in progressive BCG infection.

In the rare condition of ataxia telangiectasia (Fig. 2.7, lesion 6) there is a defect in the development of mesenchyme and the thymus fails to develop. There is also a partial failure of immunoglobulin production, particularly affecting IgA, but the reason for this is obscure.

Deficiency of Humoral Immunity

Selective primary deficiency of the B lymphocyte system occurs in X linked recessive hypo- or a-gammaglobulinaemia (Fig. 2.7, lesion 2). The lack of immunoglobulins is not absolute but the patient fails to respond to antigenic stimuli. However, cell mediated hypersensitivity and the capacity to react to a homograft are normal. It is not incompatible with survival for many years, though the patient is very susceptible to bacterial infections, particularly to pyogenic cocci.

There is also what is known as '*common, variable, unclassifiable immunodeficiency*'. Most patients with immunodeficiency have 'acquired' or 'late-onset' agammaglobulinaemia. Deterioration of T cell function may also be observed in some of these cases. B lymphocytes are usually, but not always, present in the circulation as detected by labelling with fluorescein conjugated immunoglobulin. Such B cells are absent in the X-linked form of agammaglobulinaemia. Quantification of immunoglobulins in the sera of patients with acquired agammaglobulinaemia usually reveals levels of IgG under 500 mg per 100 ml higher than those encountered in the sera of children with X-linked disease. Both IgA and IgM may also be detected in significant quantity in the sera of these patients. Lymph nodes lack plasma cells, but in lieu of the absence of follicles noted in X-linked agammaglobulinaemia, follicular hyperplasia may be evident.

Primary acquired agammaglobulinaemia has been found equally in males and females. They have an unusually high incidence of autoimmune disease, such as pernicious anaemia, haemolytic anaemia, etc. A prominent and frequent complication is a sprue-like syndrome and *Giardia lamblia* infection (p. 845) is common. Another distinguishing feature of the variable form is the frequent occurrence of non-caseating granulomas, especially in lungs, liver, spleen and skin.

As the different immunoglobulins have different functions, deficiencies might be

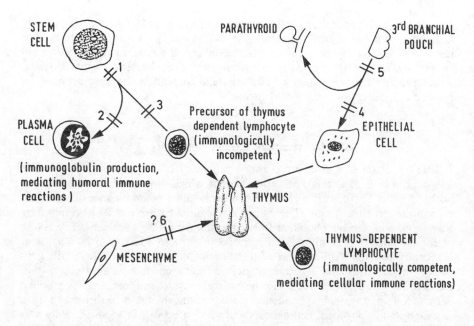

Fig. 2.7 The sites of developmental defects which lead to some of the immunodeficiency syndromes observed clinically.

Site of Defect	Clinical Syndrome
1	Severe combined immunodeficiency; thymic hypoplasia, lymphopenia and agammaglobulinaemia. Autosomal recessive or X-linked inheritance. Do not survive infancy, but variable therapeutic success has been achieved with fetal liver cell or fetal thymus transplants.
2	X-linked recessive agammaglobulinaemia; normal thymus, no lymphopenia and normal cell-mediated hypersensitivity. Recurrent infection with extracellular pyogenic pathogens. Treated effectively with gammaglobulin to maintain a serum level of 200 mg per 100 ml.
3, 4 & 5	Thymic hypoplasia and lymphopenia; normal immunoglobulins. Frequent fungal or viral infections. Usually die in infancy. In 5, Di George syndrome, absence of parathyroids presenting as tetany in the newborn can be dramatically reversed by transplants of fetal thymic tissue.
	Wiskott–Aldrich syndrome difficult to classify; X-linked; eczema, thrombocytopenia and recurrent infections; survival rare beyond first decade. There appears to be a progressive deterioration of thymus-dependent cellular immunity with concomitant changes in the lymph nodes. Serum IgM usually low; IgG and IgA normal or elevated. No unifying hypothesis explains the disparate elements of this syndrome yet most aspects have been ameliorated by the administration of transfer factor obtained from dialysis of normal donor lymphocytes (p. 30).
?6	Thymic hypoplasia–ataxia telangiectasia. May be part of a more widespread mesenchyne deficiency. Autosomal recessive inheritance. Difficult to classify.

expected to produce different clinical pictures. Thus IgM deficiency is possibly associated with meningococcal meningitis and lack of IgA with gastrointestinal or respiratory tract infections. In the absence of IgA the lowered resistance would permit invasion of the normally sterile upper gut by bacteria, some of which would produce decomposition of bile salts and thus affect the absorption of fat causing malabsorption with steatorrhoea.

Deficiency of Cellular Immunity

This condition is a selective primary deficiency of T lymphocytes (Fig. 2.7, lesions 3, 4 and 5) and is analogous to that which develops in thymectomised neonatal mice. There is severe lymphocytopenia and a predominance of reticulum cells in the lymphoid tissue. The patient's lymphocytes are unable to respond by transformation into lymphoblasts following stimulation with antigens. The failure of the patient's T lymphocytes to respond *in vitro* to PHA (p. 29) is a useful laboratory test for the detection of this type of defect. On account of the deficiency in cell mediated hypersensitivity, affected children cannot reject skin homografts and do not respond in the normal way to antigens such as monilia. Although immunoglobulin production is normal the child fails to thrive and there is wasting and diarrhoea. Candidiasis and viral infections arise and usually survival is brief.

Little is known about the role of cell-mediated immunity in acute and chronic viral infections. Its importance is emphasised by the fact that infants with thymic aplasia in whom the cell-mediated aspect is completely lacking are highly susceptible to viral infections, which usually prove fatal. It has frequently been noted that patients with agammaglobulinaemia but with normal thymic function do not suffer from severe disease in response to a number of viral infections.

The fact that there are deficient humoral antibody responses to some antigens in conditions associated with lesions at sites 3, 4 and 5 of Figure 2.7 exemplifies the existence of co-operation between T and B lymphocytes in relation to certain antigens as indicated in Figures 2.2 and 2.4.

Secondary Immunodeficiency

Maternal IgG is transferred across the placenta by active secretion to the fetus during the third trimester of pregnancy. Premature babies may thus have some degree of hypogammaglobulinaemia and prophylactic IgG treatment may reduce the incidence of infections. The production of immunoglobulins in the early years of life is well below that of adults and this may well explain the greatly increased susceptibility of the young to infection, particularly gastrointestinal and respiratory tract infection in relation to IgA deficiency. IgA is present in colostrum and there is evidence that breast feeding provides the infant with intestinal immunity and that IgA molecules largely survive passage through the gastrointestinal tract.

Immunoglobulin deficiency may arise also in adults as a result of abnormal metabolism of serum proteins as occurs in uraemic patients in whom susceptibility to infection is increased. Diseases such as sarcoidosis and Hodgkin's disease are associated with a depression mainly of cell-mediated hypersensitivity. Drugs depressing the immune system are discussed later.

Complement Deficiencies

Study of complement deficiency indicates that the principal activities of the complement system are related to protection against infectious disease. In the case of failure of C3 activation, syndromes are produced that are basically very similar to those of the antibody deficiency syndrome. Absence of the components of the classical pathway C3 convertase seem to cause a more subtle immunity deficiency where infection with essentially non-virulent organisms may give rise to immune complex disease. Deficiency of the late-acting complement components may be associated with an increased susceptibility to certain forms of bacterial infection, particularly *Neisseria*.

Treatment of Immunodeficiency. Immunoglobulin injections (0·250 g/kg body weight per week, consisting mainly of IgG) can provide effective protection against severe, recurrent pyogenic infections in patients with various types of hypo- or a-gammaglobulinaemia. Recently the transplantation of fragments of human fetal thymus has been effective in replacing the cellular immune deficiency in type 5 lesions as shown in Figure 2.7. Transfer factor has been effective in the Wiskott-Aldrich syndrome (Fig. 2.7).

Lymphoproliferative Disorders

Abnormal Immunoglobulin Synthesis

In various proliferative and neoplastic disorders, mainly of the reticuloendo-thelial system, discrete components of immunoglobulins, known as myeloma or M-proteins, may appear in the plasma. In an individual patient they belong to only one of the five immunoglobulin classes IgG, IgA, IgM, IgD, or IgE and contain light chains of either K or L type. Multiple myeloma represents the malignant proliferation of a clone of plasma cells synthesising a single species of immunoglobulin, but the counterpart in the T lymphocyte population has not been so well defined. Myeloma and Waldenstrom's macroglobulinaemia (p. 625) are the most important of these conditions and when associated with diseases the proteins may be designated G-, A-, or D-myeloma or M-macroglobulins. Abnormal proteins may also occur in the urine in these disorders. Bence Jones proteinuria is found in about 50 per cent of patients with myeloma and 15 per cent of those with macroglobulinaemia. It consists of light chains only, usually dimerised (two molecules attached together as a unit).

Heavy chain disease is a very rare disorder occurring in association with rapidly progressive lymphomas. A dimer of the IgG heavy chain resembling the Fc fragment is present in the plasma and urine.

Patients with abnormal immunoglobulin synthesis have an increased susceptibility to bacterial infections and particularly to pneumonia.

Types of Immune Reaction and their Relation to Human Disease

There are six types of immune reaction which may be harmful to the tissues (Fig. 2.8).

Type I— anaphylactic (immediate hypersensitivity, reagin-dependent, IgE)
Type II— cytotoxic antibody (humoral antibody, IgG, IgM)

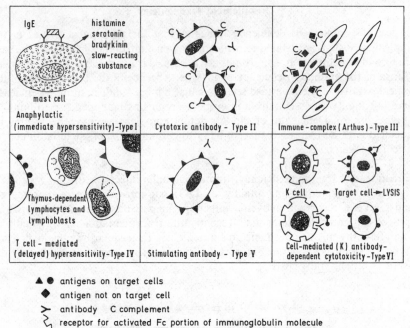

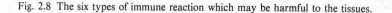

▲ ● antigens on target cells
◆ antigen not on target cell
⅄ antibody   C complement
⌇ receptor for activated Fc portion of immunoglobulin molecule
Ⅴ⋰ receptors on the surface of T lymphocytes directed against two antigens

Fig. 2.8 The six types of immune reaction which may be harmful to the tissues.

Type III—immune complex (Arthus)
Type IV—T cell-mediated (delayed) hypersensitivity
Type V— stimulating antibody
Type VI—cell-mediated (K) antibody-dependent cytotoxicity (CADC).

Anaphylactic (Immediate Hypersensitivity)—Type I Reactions

In man, only IgE (reaginic) antibodies are able to produce anaphylactic Type I reactions. As these antibodies adhere strongly to tissues (and particularly to mast-cells in the tissues) they are often called tissue-sensitising antibodies. Anaphylactic phenomena are caused by antigen–antibody reaction on the surface of the mast-cell activating a series of enzymes leading to the release of histamine and other agents from the mast-cells (Figs. 2.8 and 2.9). Individuals who have a hereditary predisposition to anaphylactic reactions are said to be atopic, as in some forms of asthma and in hay fever.

Previous usage of the term anaphylaxis emphasised the clinically severe form, anaphylactic shock, but current usage refers to the underlying mechanism and not to clinical severity. In man, anaphylactic reactions are of two types depending on the portal of entry of the antigen, local or systemic. Relatively mild symptoms occur when antigen–antibody reactions occur at an exposed mucosal surface. These reactions occur most commonly to pollens or animal dander and the symptoms may be limited to rhinorrhoea and conjunctivitis (Fig. 2.9). However, intense bronchospasm may be produced as a result of inhalation of the antigen. Patients with asthma induced by contact with antigens in this manner have levels of IgE immunoglobulin up to six times higher than that found in patients with asthma that is not induced in this way.

A second group of more severe reactions, referred to as *systemic anaphylaxis*, may occur rapidly if the antigen is injected parenterally, as in the case of a drug such as penicillin, foreign sera, or the sting of an insect. This is manifested in man by bronchospasm, laryngeal oedema resulting in extreme dyspnoea and cyanosis and a marked fall in blood pressure. There may also be nausea, vomiting and diarrhoea. Systemic anaphylaxis is a potentially fatal condition if not treated promptly with adrenaline, hydrocortisone and an antihistamine.

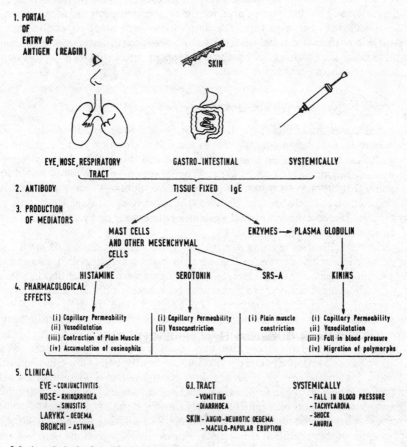

Fig. 2.9 Anaphylaxis. (Modified from Turk, 1972)

Urticaria, the formation of weal and flare lesions in the skin, is an anaphylactic phenomenon which can develop as a result of absorption of antigen through the intestinal tract. Common allergens are present in strawberries, nuts, egg and shell-fish. Cutaneous urticaria often occurs alone, but may be associated with other signs of generalised anaphylaxis. Not all uticaria is caused by an immune reaction. It is known that the pharmacological agents which cause urticaria can be released by other means, especially physical agents such as trauma or cold.

Most of the reactions found in anaphylaxis can be attributed to the release or activation of histamine, slow reacting substance-A, serotonin (5H-T) and the plasma kinins, bradykinin and kallidin. The kinins are simple peptides formed from plasma globulins by the enzymes, kallikrein, plasmin or trypsin. They cause increased capillary permeability, vasodilation and a fall in blood pressure. Bradykinin produces pain when injected into man. Another effect is to cause polymorphonuclear leucocytes to migrate from blood vessels and accumulate in the tissues (chemotaxis). Once they are formed the kinins are rapidly broken down by kininases present in the blood. Thus their accumulation at any site is controlled.

Intradermal testing in sensitised individuals is the most convenient *in vivo* method for the detection of specific IgE antibodies. A radioallergosorbent test (Phadebas RAST) has been introduced for the *in vitro* detection and quantitation of antigen specific IgE. The test is rapid and simple to perform. Small paper discs coated with specific antigen are supplied. Test serum is added, followed—after washing —with radiolabelled anti-IgE. The presence of specific IgE antibody in the test serum is associated with an uptake of isotope.

Cytotoxic (Humoral Antibody)—Type II Reactions

The clearest example of a Type II reaction (Fig. 2.8) as a cause of disease oc-curs in autoimmune haemolytic anaemia; red cell destruction is the result of ab-sorption of autoantibodies on to the cell surface and this can be demonstrated *in vitro* by the antiglobulin (Coombs') test. When antihuman globulin is added to a suspension of the patient's red cells that have antibody on their surfaces, agglutination of the cells occurs. *In vivo*, the altered or damaged red cells are destroyed by the reticuloendothelial system in the spleen or liver. Both IgG and IgM antibodies have been implicated.

Circulating antibodies reacting *in vitro* with other tissue components are a com-mon occurrence in a wide range of diseases in man, but their role in causing the corresponding disease is less clear. Another example of IgG antibodies being directly pathogenic is antibody to glomerular basement membrane in certain types of experimental glomerulonephritis in animals and in a rare type of glomerulonephritis in man associated with haemoptysis (Goodpasture's syn-drome, p. 478). Infusion of such antibodies into experimental animals rapidly induces glomerulonephritis and this mechanism may result in damage to a kidney transplant in a patient whose own kidneys had previously been destroyed by glomerulonephritis.

In other instances, current evidence would suggest that IgG antibodies may have only a weakly pathogenic effect. Thus, the occurrence of intrinsic factor anti-bodies in the circulation of a patient shows a strong correlation with Addisonian pernicious anaemia, but the role of the antibody in causing the gastric atrophy characteristic of this condition is not clear. For example, pernicious anaemia may occur in patients with marked hypogammaglobulinaemia. However, antibody reactive with the vitamin B_{12} binding site of intrinsic factor has been shown to be present in the gastric juice of some patients with pernicious anaemia: it may block the action of any remaining secretion of intrinsic factor with consequent malab-sorption of vitamin B_{12}.

There are circumstances in which IgG antibodies may be pathogenic only when combined with cell-mediated hypersensitivity or other forms of tissue damage. Thus in experimental orchitis in guinea-pigs neither circulating antibody nor cell-mediated hypersensitivity alone is sufficient to produce lesions and both types of immune reaction are necessary. Again complement-fixing IgG antibodies to thyroid secretory epithelium are a frequent occurrence in autoimmune thyroid disease but they seem to have little or no pathogenic role by themselves. These antibodies can be transmitted across the placenta with no evidence of damage to the fetal thyroid. Although at least one of these antibodies can bring about rapid destruction of trypsinised human thyroid cells *in vitro* in the presence of complement, *in vivo* it seems to have difficulty in reaching the intracellular antigens in the absence of some other damaging agent.

Finally, in other situations, antibodies detectable in the serum and often useful diagnostically, seem to have no discernible pathogenic role when acting on their own. For example, antibody to thyroglobulin is harmless to thyroid cells in tissue culture and infusion into animals produces at most a weak granulomatous reaction in the thyroid. A second example is the mitochondrial antibodies with no tissue specificity which occur most commonly in patients with primary biliary cirrhosis. However, antibody to thyroglobulin may play an important role in pathogenesis when part of a type VI reaction (p. 44).

In summary, antibodies detectable in the circulation or produced locally in certain tissues by infiltrating plasma cells may be directly responsible for certain diseases, while in other diseases such antibodies, although abundantly present and useful in diagnosis, do not seem to have a direct role on their own account.

Diagnostic methods. Those most widely used for the detection of antibodies in the serum are:

The Indirect Immunofluorescence Technique. This method is used to detect autoantibodies to nuclei (antinuclear factors), to the cytoplasm of thyroid cells, gastric parietal cells, adrenal cortical cells, steroid-producing cells in the ovary, pancreatic islet cells and to glomerular basement membrane. Cryostat sections of the appropriate tissue are incubated with serum and, after thorough washing, with fluorescein labelled antihuman Ig serum. They are then examined by fluorescence microscopy.

Complement Fixation Tests. Certain antigen–antibody reactions fix complement and the occurrence of such a reaction *in vitro* can be detected by determining whether complement, which had been added in a critical amount, is still present in the free form. An indicator system is used consisting of sheep red cells coated with horse or rabbit antibodies against the red cells. If complement has been fixed before the addition of the indicator system, it is no longer available to permit lysis of the sheep red cells. This technique forms the basis of the Wassermann reaction for syphilis, and the gonococcal complement fixation test; it is also used in the demonstration of antibodies against certain viruses and also for thyroid and gastric autoantibodies in serum.

Precipitation Test. This is used, for example, in the detection of antibodies to thyroglobulin in the differential diagnosis of thyroid disorders.

Tanned Red Cell or Latex Particle Agglutination. Sheep red cells are treated with tannic acid so that they can be coated with antigens (e.g. thyroglobulin). In the presence of the corresponding antibody the cells undergo agglutination. This provides a very sensitive and semi-quantitative method for the detection of certain serum antibodies, e.g. to thyroglobulin. Latex particles coated with human γ-globulin are used to detect the presence of the rheumatoid factor in patients' serum (p. 638).

Immune Complex (Arthus)—Type III Reactions

Immune complex reactions are induced by deposition of antigen–antibody complexes in the tissues, causing an inflammatory reaction via mediators such as complement which consists of a variety of proteins some of which are proteolytic enzymes. These are activated in turn and bring about an amplification of the immune process as shown in Figure 2.10. Thus the deposition of immune complexes causes the activation of complement which results in a polymorphonuclear inflammatory response and also damage to the cell membranes of adjacent tissues. Hydrolytic enzymes released from the granules of the leucocytes also contribute to the irreversible vascular damage which is the hallmark of this type of immune reaction.

The immune complex reaction can be induced in man by the intradermal injection of antigens if there is a high level of circulating IgG antibodies, for example by the intradermal injection of fungal antigens in pulmonary aspergillosis (p. 306) and of thermophilic actinomycetes in patients with the disease 'farmer's lung' (p. 307). Immune complex reactions in man are red and oedematous reaching maximum intensity between 4 and 12 hours after intradermal injection.

The systemic syndrome known as chronic serum sickness is based on an immune complex reaction and can be produced by a wide range of different antigens, such as antitetanus serum and especially drugs such as penicillin, streptomycin, sulphonamides and the thiouracils. It consists of skin rashes, fever, joint pains and often swelling of the regional lymph nodes. The duration of symptoms varies greatly. The illness is seldom serious, though it may give rise to much discomfort.

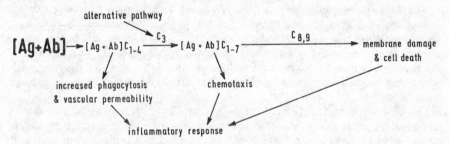

Fig. 2.10 The role of complement in immune-complex reactions. (Ag + Ab) = antigen + antibody immune complex deposited in tissue in the presence of moderate antigen excess. C = complement.

Glomerulonephritis can also be caused by an immune complex reaction. Thus, in the clinical entity of glomerulonephritis, there are at least two immune pathogenic mechanisms and, in all probability, numerous aetiological factors capable of initiating each. As described on page 40, in the rare glomerulonephritis produced by a Type II immune reaction antibodies react with glomerular basement membrane. In glomerulonephritis produced by an immune complex reaction the specificity of the antibodies is irrelevant; what is important is that antigen–antibody complexes of appropriate size are present in the circulation and are deposited in the glomerular capillary walls.

The only property of antigen–antibody complexes presently known to affect the localisation in vessels is size. Small complexes in great antigen excess tend to remain in the circulation whereas frank precipitates formed at equivalence or at antibody excess are rapidly taken up and disposed of by phagocytes. The intermediate-sized complexes formed in moderate antigen excess are still soluble but large enough to react with complement and are the most likely to be deposited in vessel walls and so induce inflammation. The vessel walls of the renal glomeruli are particularly vulnerable. Morphologically the trapped antigen–antibody complexes appear under the electron microscope as heaped-up lesions on the glomerular basement membrane (p. 477).

Immune complex reactions may or may not be related to autoimmunity. The antigen involved may be foreign to the body or it may be autogenous. Thus, poststreptococcal proliferative glomerulonephritis, at least as seen in children, is caused by the deposition of circulating non-glomerular antigen-antibody complexes. The best example of an autogenous immune complex reaction causing glomerulonephritis in man is that occurring in systemic lupus erythematosus. It is associated with the formation of antinuclear antibodies (particularly to DNA) and the deposition of these antibodies, nuclear antigens and complement in the renal glomerulus.

In addition to the above, lesions due to immune complexes occur in polyarteritis, viral hepatitis, the renal manifestations of infective endocarditis, the nephrotic syndrome in children with *P. malariae* infections, lepromatous leprosy, etc. Immune complex reactions thus occur in response to diverse antigens related particularly to micro-organisms, drugs and autogenous sources.

Cell-mediated (Delayed) Hypersensitivity—Type IV Reactions

Type IV reactions are those mediated by T lymphocytes and in which free antibody plays no part (Fig. 2.8). They are characteristically induced by infectious agents which are predominantly intracellular in the infected host, e.g. many viral infections such as measles, smallpox, herpes and some bacterial infections (tuberculosis, brucellosis, pertussis, and syphilis). The classical example of this reaction is the tuberculin response, in which the sensitised individual produces an inflammatory, indurated area consisting mainly of mononuclear cells and which gradually appears over 18 to 48 hours. The homograft reaction is believed to be predominantly produced by cell-mediated hypersensitivity in which the thymus-dependent lymphoblasts and lymphocytes are the main effector cells.

Type IV reactions can also occur by skin contact with a variety of substances ranging from nickel in brassière straps to drugs including penicillin. These substances are not themselves antigenic but become antigenic by co-valent binding to proteins in the skin. The hypersensitivity of the skin is generalised and may be detected by the application of a small patch test containing the substance anywhere on the body. Transfer of contact dermatitis has been achieved in animals and in man with lymphocytes from the thoracic duct and spleen. The clinical features of contact dermatitis include redness, swelling, vesiculation, scaling and exudation of fluid.

Autoimmune Disease. Evidence suggesting the importance of cell-mediated hypersensitivity as a cause of autoimmune disease can be summarised as follows:

1. The histology of the affected organs shows lymphocytic infiltration and atrophy, e.g. in Hashimoto thyroiditis, atrophic gastritis of Addisonian pernicious anaemia and idiopathic (autoimmune) adrenal failure.

2. Similar histological changes can be produced in animals by sterile methods that cause cell-mediated hypersensitivity in relation to the tissue antigens used for immunisation, e.g. injection into the foot pads of tissue antigen emulsified in Freund's adjuvant (p. 46).

3. When such diseases have been induced immunologically in experimental animals they can be transferred to normal animals by means of lymphocytes alone.

4. Positive *in vitro* tests supposedly for cell-mediated hypersensitivity have

been obtained with the lymphocytes from the peripheral blood of patients or of experimental animals with certain autoimmune diseases. These tests include the leucocyte migration inhibition test, transformation and cytotoxicity tests. As shown in Figure 2.2, when T lymphocytes that have been sensitised to a specific antigen come into contact with that antigen, the lymphocytes undergo blast transformation (which can be quantitated by measuring the uptake of tritiated thymidine) and among the lymphokines released is one that inhibits the migration of macrophages in tissue culture and supposedly *in vivo*. Cytotoxicity by lymphocytes is quantitated by measuring the release of isotopes from labelled chicken or sheep red cells coated with the appropriate antigen.

It must be emphasised, however, that the lymphocytes or lymphoid cells infiltrating affected tissues may be T, B or K cells and that until cell marker studies have been done on the affected tissues no statement can be made concerning the predominant cell type.

Stimulating Antibody—Type V Reaction

Certain IgG antibodies—and certain human specific TSH receptor antibodies are the best example—have the ability to stimulate their target cells rather than to inhibit or kill them (Fig. 2.8). Human specific thyroid-stimulating antibodies are the likely cause of thyrotoxicosis and their transfer across the placenta is the most probable explanation for neonatal hyperthyroidism.

Cell-Mediated (K) Antibody-Dependent Cytotoxicity (CADC)—Type VI Reaction

K cells may be defined as belonging to a subpopulation of lymphoid cells or monocytes which *in vitro* are able to lyse target cells coated with antibody. The cytotoxic reaction is complement-independent and is initiated through contact of the K cell with the Fc portion of the antibody molecule complexed with antigen on the surface of the target cells (Fig. 2.8). K cells may also be 'armed' through the Fc receptor with antigen–antibody complex which, if present in antibody excess, will be cytotoxic to target cells coated with that specific antigen. Should immune complexes be produced in the presence of excess antigen, there would be no free combining sites left on the antibody moiety to react with antigen on target surfaces so that this type of K cell would be ineffective (blocked). K cell mediated cytotoxic mechanisms may be important in the pathogenesis of autoimmune disease and in tumour rejection (p. 50). K cells are also involved in the defence against parasitic infections (e.g. schistosomiasis p. 894) where the size of the organism may be too large for effective phagocytosis.

Autoimmune Disease

Immune mechanisms may simply be part of a chain of events that leads to the final end product, the clinical manifestation of disease (Fig. 2.11). Thus a virus infection may initiate tissue damage or combine with a cell constituent to act as a hapten and thereby engender an autoimmune response in a susceptible individual. This may occur for example in insulin-dependent diabetes.

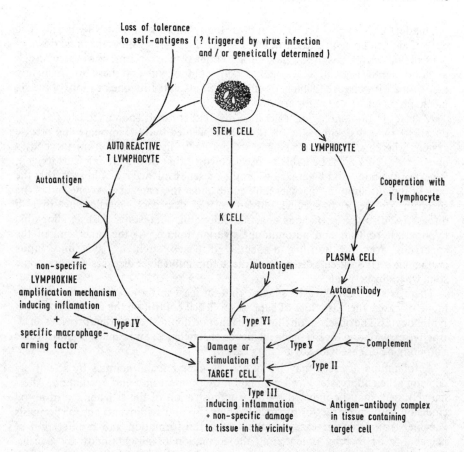

Fig. 2.11 Diagram representing the interactions of immune mechanisms types II–VI in the production of autoimmune disease. The different mechanisms may have greater importance in some diseases than in others. Thus type II reactions are predominant in autoimmune haemolytic anaemia, while types II, IV and VI are predominant in Hashimoto's thyroiditis, and probably type V in thyrotoxicosis.

The lymphokine and complement systems may be regarded as non-specific amplification mechanisms in order to boost the effect of a small number of specifically sensitised cells or a small amount of antibody interacting with the antigen at the target site. Specific macrophage arming factor may be regarded as a specific amplification mechanism.

WHY SHOULD AUTOIMMUNE REACTIONS OCCUR?

Defect in immunological tolerance. Normally a person or animal does not mount a significant immune response against its own body constituents because intricate controlling and suppressor mechanisms exist to prevent this happening. For example, it has been suggested that clones of immunocompetent cells capable of reacting with self-antigens are either eliminated or rendered unresponsive by early and continued exposure to antigen (p. 25). Unresponsiveness may exist either at the level of the helper T lymphocyte or at the level of the antibody-producing B lymphocyte or at both. If unresponsiveness exists only at the level of the helper T cell, autoantibody synthesis will occur when the requirement for T cell help is bypassed. As discussed on page 31 it has also been suggested that a subpopulation of T lymphocytes can suppress the synthesis of antibody by B cells. The dose of antigen presented to the immune system is also relevant to the breakdown of control (tolerance). In spite of these intricate control mechanisms, however, man can and does synthesise antibodies against body components and these are frequently associated with disease (clinical or subclinical) mediated by one or more of the six mechanisms illustrated in Figure 2.8.

A defect in immunological tolerance may either occur spontaneously or be induced by some exogenous factor. It could be argued that the intricate and precise system whereby foreign substances are normally distinguished from the body's own constituents must be liable to breakdown so that errors are made as to what is part of the body and what is not. On the present evidence it would seem that the bulk of the autoimmune diseases may come under this category. At one end of the spectrum are the organ-specific, but interrelated, disorders—autoimmune thyroid disease, Addisonian pernicious anaemia, idiopathic Addison's disease, idiopathic hypoparathyroidism and autoimmune ovarian failure. At the other end of the spectrum are the non-organ-specific diseases such as systemic lupus erythematosus. Sjögren's disease and the autoimmune liver diseases perhaps come somewhere in between.

There is some evidence to suggest that, at least in the organ-specific autoimmune diseases, there is a loss of suppressor T cell control on the function of the B lymphocytes. The observation that T cell function diminishes with age provides an attractive explanation for the rising incidence of subclinical and clinical organ-specific autoimmune disease with advancing years.

Autoimmune diseases may be induced in experimental animals by selectively depleting the suppressor T cell population by thymectomy and irradiation. Alternatively they may be induced by the administration of the self antigen in an oil emulsion with an extract of tubercle bacillus (Freund's adjuvent) and/or pertussis vaccine. Adjuvants increase lymphoblastic transformation and proliferation of helper T cells thereby potentiating the formation of autoantibody by B cells. Freund's adjuvant may in addition exert a carrier effect if it forms complexes with the host antigens (hapten effect).

Sequestrated Antigen. There are some antigens, such as those of the lens of the eye, that do not normally come into contact with the immunological system so that there has been no opportunity for immunological tolerance or self-recognition to develop. Injury to an eye may result in the escape of antigen with antibody formation as a physiological consequence and lead to immunological damage to the other eye (sympathetic ophthalmia). A further example of this is sperm, which if extravasated following unilateral blockage of the vas deferens may induce antibody formation and contribute to sterility. Sperm antibodies may also be produced following vasectomy in normal men.

Infection. In the hypersensitive host, invading micro-organisms may share antigen with certain of the host's tissues and induce the formation of antibodies which cross-react with these tissues. Possibly this may be an effect of antigen dosage. Thus the sharing of antigen between some Group A β-haemolytic streptococci and the heart may be relevant to rheumatic carditis. Likewise, the sharing of antigen between *Esch. coli* O14 and colon epithelium may be relevant to the pathogenesis of ulcerative colitis.

Drugs. Some drugs such as methyldopa seem to alter the immunological system so that antibodies develop that are reactive with red cells producing a positive Coombs' test and a haemolytic anaemia which is reversible on withdrawal of the drug. Alternatively it is possible that methyldopa in some way unmasks antigens present on the erythrocyte surface which do not under normal conditions stimulate antibody production. Other drugs such as procainamide are associated with the development of antinuclear antibodies.

Genetic Factors. When the breakdown of immunological tolerance seems to be spontaneous one asks whether it is genetically determined, whether it occurs by spontaneous mutation or whether it might be induced by some agent such as a virus that has so far escaped recognition at least in the human situation. It is known that there is a genetic factor operating in the autoimmune diseases of disordered immunological tolerance, but the exact mode of inheritance escapes clear definition. A characteristic feature of the autoimmune diseases is that the auto-antibodies are formed continually, at least over a period of years. By contrast, if a tissue is damaged by some other means—such as occurs in myocardial infarction, burns, etc.—in general the corresponding antibodies appear only temporarily.

The genetic factor could operate as a built-in defect in the immune system so that, usually later rather than sooner, tolerance breaks down according to a certain pattern. Alternatively, what may be genetically determined is susceptibility to an exogenous agent such as a virus, for which there is some evidence in a special strain of mice. However, there is as yet no convincing evidence that genetic susceptibility to a virus infection is the basis of autoimmune diseases in man except possibly in insulin-dependent diabetes. Whether or not there is an exogenous factor operating in man is a question that remains unanswered. Also unanswered is why immunological tolerance should break down according to certain patterns that clinicians recognise as interrelated diseases in which immune mechanisms seem to play an important part.

HLA AND DISEASE. During the past 10 years the immune response to many antigens has been shown to be genetically controlled in several species including man and this genetic control has been shown to be linked to the major histocompatibility system of these species. Some very strong associations between HLA and susceptibility to certain diseases have been described, especially the autoimmune diseases and certain other conditions with a probable allergic basis (Table 2.1). While most of the associations that have been described so far are in relation

Table 2.1 HLA associated disease

Disease	Antigen showing significant increase in frequency (p < 0·001)	% of patients with antigen	% of control population with antigen
Ankylosing spondylitis	HLA-B27	95	8
Active chronic hepatitis	HLA-B8	70	24
Idiopathic Addison's disease	HLA-B8	69	24
Insulin-dependent diabetes	HLA-B8	56	27
	HLA-BW15	33	18
Thyrotoxicosis	HLA-B8	50	24
Coeliac disease	HLA-B8	70	24
Myasthenia gravis	HLA-B8	60	24
Psoriasis	HLA-B13	18	4
	HLA-BW17	29	8

to the B series, it is now possible to determine, albeit crudely, antigens of the D series which stimulate allogeneic lymphocytes in mixed lymphocyte culture. As the analogous genetic locus in the mouse is in the same area as the genes controlling immune responsiveness, it is of interest that there appears to be a closer association with the linked HLA-D antigen than with the HLA-B antigen itself. Thus a closer association has been shown between insulin-dependent diabetes (characterised by autoimmunity to pancreatic islet cells) and HLA-DW3 than with HLA-B8. Very recently another system of antigens has been recognised which is analogous to the Ia (immune associated) antigens in the mouse. These antigens are detected serologically and are present on B lymphocytes. It may be that future research will show an even closer association between the occurrence of certain Ia genes and susceptibility to immunopathology.

Suppression of Immune Reactions or of their Effects

Antihistamines. When anaphylaxis presents as an acute clinical problem the immediate aim is to give drugs which antagonise the effects of the mediators. These antagonists are the antihistamines and various drugs which have opposite actions to the mediators.

The antihistamines occupy the same tissue receptors as histamine without providing any stimulus to the effector cells. In man, the intravenous injection of an antihistamine quickly produces adequate tissue concentrations. The weal, the erythema and the itch of acute urticaria are reduced but there is no consistent improvement in lung function in acute bronchial asthma. The failure of the antihistamines to relieve airways obstruction caused by an anaphylactic reaction has been attributed to high concentrations of histamine close to the smooth muscle cells. It may also be due to the presence of other mediators of the anaphylactic response. Bradykinin is rapidly inactivated in plasma by a kininase but its effects are not inhibited by antihistamines. No specific antagonists of bradykinin or SRS-A are known, although salicylates have been shown to suppress experimental anaphylaxis in guinea-pigs.

Disodium Cromoglycate. This compound (p. 305) is believed to inhibit the release of the mediators following the interaction of antigens (reagins) with IgE antibodies. It is partially effective in preventing the induction of asthma by specific antigens. If inhaled by an asthmatic subject before exposure to the antigen, protection may last for several hours, but if given after exposure to the antigen it has little effect.

Adrenaline and Related Drugs. In clinical emergencies drugs which act by producing effects which oppose the mediators are more effective than the antihistamines. Adrenaline, isoprenaline and aminophylline are efficient bronchodilators in acute bronchial asthma. Adrenaline also produces constriction of the arterioles in the skin and splanchnic area. Vascular permeability and oedema are reduced. Urticaria is relieved and where oedema threatens the airway, the risk of asphyxia is lessened. Despite their effectiveness these non-specific antagonists have serious disadvantages. They are antagonists in their own right, acting on receptors which differ from those occupied by the mediators, and their effects never precisely counteract those of the mediators. The dose of a sympathomimetic amine which relieves airways obstruction may produce tachycardia and palpitations even when the amine is administered as an inhaled aerosol.

Salbutamol does not have these disadvantages as it is more specific in its actions on β-adrenergic receptors in the bronchi.

Corticosteroids. Hydrocortisone or prednisolone produce improvement in status asthmaticus in a few hours. The mechanism is not known but is probably related to their anti-inflammatory actions and not to selective interference with any particular stage in the development of the anaphylactic response. Their use in Types II, III and IV immune reactions is discussed below.

Hyposensitisation. Anaphylactic individuals can be made less sensitive by multiple subcutaneous injections of antigen. Pollen antigens can be used to prevent the development of hay fever and asthma in some patients. Up to 50 subcutaneous injections may be given, gradually increasing the dose of antigen. Another technique is to suspend the antigen in an oily base. As a result of slower absorption the patient develops IgG antibodies against the antigen over a longer period. These antibodies have a higher avidity for the antigen than do IgE antibodies and are able to compete successfully for the antigen sites on the pollen, fragment of insect or whatever has induced the anaphylactic response. As reactions with the IgG antibodies do not take place at cell surfaces, anaphylactic phenomena are not produced. The reactions with the IgG antibodies do not have any harmful effect as the amount of IgG antibodies produced is not sufficient to cause an immune-complex (Type III) reaction. In this context the IgG antibodies are referred to as blocking antibodies.

Cytotoxic Drugs. The production of immunoglobulins and the cellular immune response are dependent upon the division of lymphoid cells. Drugs which interfere with dividing cells are therefore all potentially *immunosuppressive*. Such drugs were originally developed as antitumour agents and are generally referred to as cytotoxic drugs. Of these azathioprine, cyclophosphamide and methotrexate have been used as immunosuppressive drugs. Their side-effects of bone-marrow suppression and depletion of the intestinal epithelium are to be expected. In organ transplantation the use of azathioprine has become almost universal and it is under trial in the treatment of other diseases such as systemic lupus erythematosus, the autoimmune liver diseases and ulcerative colitis. When used in daily maintenance doses of 3 mg/kg body weight, azathioprine does not produce serious side-effects if renal function is satisfactory.

Antilymphocyte Serum. This substance, or a semipurified globulin containing the active fraction, is a potent agent for the suppression of cell-mediated immunity. It is prepared by immunising another species, usually the horse, with human lymphocytes. The precise mode of action is debatable but it interferes with the function of T lymphocytes while not affecting antibody formation to previously encountered antigens. Its main application has been in relation to organ transplantation. The major side-effects are the development of anaphylactic reactions to the injection of serum of another species and the development of antibodies to the antilymphocyte serum with deposition of immune complexes in the kidney and consequent renal damage. A further possible hazard, shared by other immunosuppressive agents, is an increased incidence of malignant tumours, such as lymphomas, possibly on account of the suppression of immunological surveillance of the body tissues which is part of the normal mechanism for the control of spontaneous tumours (see below).

Anti-D Immunoglobulin. The clearest example of interference with a specific immune response is the use of human anti-D immunoglobulin to prevent haemolytic disease of the newborn (p. 609).

'Anti-inflammatory Agents'. Drugs which interfere with the unwanted consequences of Types II, III and IV immune reactions include the corticosteroids and, to a lesser extent, salicylates. The corticosteroids may also partially suppress the development of immune responses, but when used in high dosage they have serious side-effects. Use is therefore being made of other 'anti-inflammatory' drugs such as indomethacin or phenylbutazone, sometimes in combination with a cytotoxic drug.

Thymectomy. The only human autoimmune disease for which thymectomy is regularly performed is myasthenia gravis (p. 753). Thymectomy has also been successful in infants with autoimmune haemolytic anaemia when other methods have failed. Apart from myasthenia gravis, thymectomy has not been helpful in relation to autoimmunity in adults, where it has been tried for example in systemic lupus erythematosus. Thymectomy as a treatment for autoimmune diseases other than myasthenia gravis may be effective only in childhood when the influence of the thymus on the immunological system is particularly important.

Cancer Immunology. Cancer cells lose some of the normal tissue-specific antigens and appear to gain some tumour-associated antigens which were not previously present in the cells from which they were derived. It used to be thought that the process of immunological surveillance destroys many early cancers by virtue of the recognition by the normal immune system of the 'foreignness' of tumour-associated antigens. However, immunodeficiency, either primary or iatrogenic, is mainly associated with tumours of the lymphoreticular tissues and not with cancer generally. It is now thought that it is more likely that the immune system is important in relation to the control of oncogenic viruses, rather than immune surveillance per se. Attempts have been made to augment the normal immune response so as to help ablate malignant growth after the bulk of the tumour has been removed or killed by conventional means. Immunisation with BCG and allogeneic irradiated malignant cells may be beneficial in acute myeloid leukaemia.

There is evidence which suggests that, in the presence of continued antigenic stimulation, macrophages, previously coated with specific macrophage arming factor, may become activated so that they are cytolytic to rapidly dividing (e.g. malignant) as opposed to normal cells. There is also increasing evidence which suggests that antigens from malignant tumours are released into the circulation in excess of the amount of antibody produced against the tumour; this situation of antigen excess would block Type VI cytotoxic reactions and thereby overcome one of the body's defences (p. 44). It is also likely that nonimmunological toxic factors may induce a state of relative immunodeficiency in cancer patients.

Although positive claims have been made, as yet there is no convincing evidence for an immunological test in relation to a common cancer antigen. Certain tumour associated macromolecules are, however, potentially useful as indicators of the presence or, in certain defined situations, the amount of tumour in a patient, e.g. cancer embryonic antigen (CEA) in colorectal cancer.

W. J. Irvine

Further reading:

Irvine, W. J. (1977) In *Companion to Medical Studies*. Vol. 2, ch. 23. Oxford, Blackwell.
Roitt, I. M. (1974) *Essential Immunology*. 2nd edition. Oxford: Blackwell.
Weir, D. M. (1973) *Immunology for Undergraduates*. 3rd edition. Edinburgh: Churchill Livingstone.

More detailed texts:

Gell, P. G. H., Coombs, R. R. A. & Lachman, P. J. (Eds.) (1975) *Clinical Aspects of Immunology*. 3rd edition. Oxford: Blackwell.
Hobart, M. J. & McConnell, I. (1975) *The Immune System*. Oxford: Blackwell.
Irvine, W. J. (Ed.) (1977) *Immunology in Clinical Medicine*. Oxford: Blackwell.

3. Infection and Disease

THE life and health of human beings, animals and plants are constantly threatened by parasites, particularly by micro-organisms—protozoa, fungi, bacteria and viruses, which after invasion of the tissues may produce infectious disease. In numerical terms this is the most important group of maladies affecting the human race. In areas where the full effect of modern medicine is felt, many of the more serious infectious diseases have almost vanished, e.g. typhoid, tuberculosis and poliomyelitis. While the mortality from infectious diseases is now low in Britain the morbidity remains high, and is responsible for much ill-health and absenteeism.

The control of infection cannot be fully effective without a knowledge of the nature of the infecting organism, the epidemiological factors involved in the source and spread of infection and the nature of the host's defences. A brief discussion of these follows, and thereafter the general features of infection and its prevention are considered.

Nature of the Micro-organism

Micro-organisms may be *saprophytic*, living an independent existence in soil and water, or in waste and dead material, and generally such organisms do not produce disease in man. There are exceptions, for example the toxins of *Clostridium botulinum* which may contaminate prepared foodstuffs and lead to toxaemia and even death. Bacteria normally saprophytic such as *Pseudomonas*, may be *opportunist pathogens* when they invade the tissues under exceptional conditions; such circumstances occur more frequently in hospital when the organism may survive even in antiseptics and be introduced into wounds or body cavities. Disturbance of the commensal flora of the body by antimicrobial agents may also allow the establishment of opportunist pathogens, such as *Candida* which can lead to thrush infection.

In contrast other micro-organisms are parasites living in close association with a host; some are highly adapted to local conditions on the surfaces of the body and are best described as *commensals* which under certain conditions may invade the tissues; other parasites play a more definite part in disease and are described as *pathogens*. There is of course no hard and fast dividing line and many pathogens exist in an apparently quiescent role as commensals.

Variation in Micro-organisms. As with other living creatures, micro-organisms adapt to their environment by changes in their genetic structure. Such adaptation can become apparent in a short time because of the high rate of growth and reproduction of micro-organisms. When the characters affected by these genetic changes are related to pathogenicity, virulence and resistance to antimicrobial agents, they are of importance in medicine and particularly in the management of individual patients. Amongst bacteria the mechanisms altering genetic structure may be extremely effective in bringing about rapid changes in resistance to one or more antibiotics. This especially applies to the Gram-negative coliform bacilli such as *Escherichia* and *Shigella*. Resistant bacteria have tended to increase in proportion to the amount of antibacterial agent used, particularly in closed environments such as hospitals.

Source of Infection. This is the site where the pathogen is growing and multiplying. Infection in man may be *autogenous* where the source is the patient himself, or *exogenous* and commonly derived from another person. Autogenous infection may result from recent colonisation of the host following contamination from an exogenous source. This frequently occurs in hospital where pathogenic staphylococci from the environment may colonise staff and patients and then cause infection in some of these persons.

Pathogenic micro-organisms are usually species specific and the human sources are patients who are in the incubation period, course or convalescent stage of infection, and carriers who are healthy but harbour pathogens which can be transmitted to others. Carriers may never have suffered from clinical infection or may be in the convalescent stage following an illness and, as after typhoid fever, may continue to excrete the causative organism for many years.

Animals may be the natural hosts of infections which can be spread to man (zoonoses), e.g. brucellosis from milk of cows or goats, leptospirosis from rodents, ornithosis from birds and frequently salmonellosis from birds or wild rodents.

A few infections arise from non-living sources. The soil is the apparent source of some bacteria, e.g. *Cl. botulinum* and *Cl. tetani* which cause human disease although ultimately many of these species are derived from animals. Fungi such as *Coccidioides* and *Blastomyces*, normally saprophytes in the soil, may produce systemic infection. An increasing number of organisms from inanimate sources, particularly fungi, are now recognised as playing a part in human disease.

Spread of Infection

(1) **Autogenous Sources.** An organism like *Staph. aureus*, may spread directly from the site on the skin at which it is growing as a commensal or it may involve different sites on the body surfaces. Similarly *Strept. pyogenes* from the nasopharynx may cause erysipelas of the face, or *Esch. coli* from the large bowel may pass from the anus to the urethra and invade the urinary tract. Alternatively the transmission may be by the bloodstream, as in infective endocarditis.

(2) **Exogenous Sources.** Micro-organisms may take a direct or indirect route from source to host. Examples of the former are venereal infections and skin diseases such as impetigo or scabies. Indirect routes of spread are:

(i) *Airborne Infection.* This includes transmission by airborne droplets and dust particles. During breathing and talking organisms present in the nasopharynx, throat and mouth are expelled in droplets of secretion which may be inhaled directly into the respiratory passages of new hosts. It is thus important to teach persons not to spit and to cover the mouth and nose with a clean handkerchief during coughing and sneezing. Medical attendants should wear suitable masks during operations, the dressing of wounds and on other occasions when the patient is at particular risk.

Organisms survive in a layer of protein derived from dried droplets; the smaller particles remain airborne while the larger settle on exposed surfaces and, along with other material derived from mineral sources, clothing, handkerchiefs, bedclothes, carpets and screens, and from human and animal surfaces, contribute to the dust and its microbial flora which may be inhaled or contaminate body surfaces or wounds. This mode of spread is especially important in streptococcal and staphylococcal infection in hospital and in the transmission of respiratory diseases.

The spread of diseases of the respiratory tract, meningococcal infection and many of the common infectious diseases of childhood is mainly airborne and is reduced by fresh air, sunlight and good ventilation. In hospitals and institutions there should be an adequate distance between beds, dust should be reduced by damp dusting and vacuum cleaning, and contaminated sources of particles such as bedclothes should be frequently cleaned or sterilised.

(ii) *Water-, Milk- and Food-borne Infection.* Pathogens transmitted by these vehicles are usually ingested and, as distribution may be wide and often simultaneous, epidemic outbreaks frequently occur, e.g. the enteric fevers and other salmonelloses, bacillary dysentery, cholera, hepatitis and enteroviral infections such as poliomyelitis. These infections are further disseminated by the faecal–oral route with the human hand as an important vehicle.

Water supplies may be contaminated from human or animal excreta; there may be faulty disposal of sewage and seepage from cracked drains may contaminate water in wells or pipes. Organisms such as leptospires from animals may contaminate water and invade the mucosa of man when he is immersed, e.g. in Weil's disease due to *Leptospira icterohaemorrhagiae.*

Infection from milk and food may be derived from the animals which provide them and transmit diseases such as brucellosis and salmonellosis. Possibly more common is the contamination of milk and food during collection, preparation and distribution by infective handlers, or by vermin or flies. Subsequent multiplication may take place so that large numbers of organisms are ingested. Milk- and food-borne disease can be prevented by strict public health control of the source and supply of these products. Hand washing, especially by food sorters, is a vital factor in the prevention of infection transmitted by the faecal–oral route.

(iii) *Transmission by Fomites.* Fomites is the term used to describe inanimate articles in the environment such as clothing, blankets, table ware, drinking glasses, instruments and furniture which frequently act as reservoirs for infection. Disinfection by physical and chemical measures is important in the prevention of spread of infection by fomites.

(iv) *Animal or Insect-borne Infection.* Many animals may aid the spread of disease in a purely mechanical way by coming into contact with sources and reservoirs of infection, e.g. flies becoming contaminated by faeces.

Blood-sucking insects may play a more specific part in the life cycle of a parasite, e.g. in plague where the rodent flea derives *P. pestis* from the blood of the infected animal and subsequently transmits it to other rodents and occasionally to man. The plague bacillus however goes through a growth cycle in the flea in which it also produces disease. Many widespread epidemic infections due to viruses, rickettsiae, bacteria and protozoa are spread by blood-sucking insects.

(v) *Instrument-borne Infection.* The medical and nursing professions may introduce infection through imperfect sterilisation of instruments, by the transfusion of blood, plasma or serum, or by the inoculation of contaminated material e.g. virus B hepatitis. Introduction of organisms into the bladder by catheterisation is invariable and infection may follow particularly if the instrument is indwelling. Accidental inoculation of organisms into the spinal canal carries a high chance of infection because of the poor defences of the cerebrospinal fluid; without due care an abscess in the buttock following intramuscular injection is all too common.

Incubation Period

The period of time which elapses between the invasion of the tissues by pathogens and the appearance of clinical symptoms and signs of infection is called the incubation period of the disease. Its duration varies: in diphtheria it is about three days, in measles about 10 days, in viral hepatitis type A two to six weeks, in type B two to six months, and in leprosy one to several years. The incubation period tends to be shorter when the inoculum is large.

Defence of the Human Host

Susceptibility to Infection. Both man and animals show group or individual differences in their liability to infection. Thus negroes with the sickle-cell trait whose red cells contain haemoglobin S are relatively immune to malaria (p. 823). Man and the guinea-pig may be infected by human and bovine strains of *Myco. tuberculosis* but are resistant to the avian strain. Many persons develop *Herpes simplex* infection in association with coryza or any other febrile illness or even following exposure to ultraviolet light.

Resistance to infection is also affected by age, environment and illness and its treatment. Thus infants during the first six months of life are relatively insusceptible to infection owing to transplacental-derived immunity (p. 32) and this may be augmented by breast feeding. An unfavourable environment may lower resistance to infection and pathogenic or saphrophytic organisms harboured by the individual may precipitate disease. Medical or surgical treatment may interfere with resistance to infection by reducing immunity, e.g. by the use of cytotoxic drugs or irradiation, or by destroying the physical barriers to invasion, e.g. by surgical operation or instrumentation.

First Line of Defence. The surface barrier presented by the intact skin, the lining of the respiratory and alimentary tracts and of the conjunctival sac is augmented by chemical defences in the secretions. Mucus acts mechanically but along with other secretions contains low concentrations of antibody and enzymes which inactivate and kill microbes which are not adapted to a commensal existence. Organisms on the surfaces are diluted by the flow of secretion, and anything which interferes with these secretions may increase the likelihood of invasion and infection.

The ciliated epithelium of the respiratory tract collects micro-organisms trapped in the mucus and carries them upwards eventually to be swallowed and killed by acid in the stomach. The alimentary tract is also protected from contaminating pathogens by the defence barrier of the commensal microflora. Removal of these commensals by chemotherapy can allow minority populations such as *Candida albicans* to flourish and cause thrush, or it may allow contaminating pathogens to establish themselves and produce infection, e.g. Staphylococcal enteritis.

Second Line of Defence. The first stage of infection is invasion of the tissues. Factors related to the pathogenicity of the micro-organism or accidental or surgical wounding allow penetration of the surfaces into the underlying tissues. Contamination of deeper tissues may occur directly after wounding and this bypasses the surface defences so that the deep or tissue defences are immediately called on. These defences are cellular, humoral and mechanical.

Cellular Defence. Immediately after invasion of the tissues, micro-organisms are phagocytosed by reticulo-endothelial cells, both wandering and tissue macrophages and polymorphonuclear leucocytes; these deal successfully with the great majority of incidents, but if the organism is virulent and multiplies faster than the rate of phagocytosis, it will dominate.

Humoral Defence. The role of antibodies has been described in the preceding chapter.

Mechanical Defence. In many infections a mechanical barrier forms against the spread of infection, e.g. the fibrin from the acute inflammatory reaction of a pyogenic infection, or the fibrous tissue around a tuberculous focus or a hydatid cyst. It should be remembered however that some organisms elaborate substances which weaken this defensive barrier, e.g. β-haemolytic streptococci may produce a fibrinolysin which dissolves fibrin, and hyaluronidase, a substance which enables the organisms or their products to spread more rapidly through the tissues.

Reactions of the Host to Specific Infections. The nature of the responses of the body and their intensity depend upon the type of infecting agent, its quantity and its virulence. Viral infections tend to excite a local lymphocytic reaction and a polymorph leucopenia with relative lymphocytosis in the blood. Rarely there is an initial polymorph leucocytosis. Some worm infections are associated with an eosinophilia. When the infection is bacterial, the character of the ensuing reaction varies. Pyogenic organisms (staphylococci, streptococci, pneumococci, meningococci, gonococci and *Esch. coli*) give rise to an acute local inflammation with the outpouring of neutrophil polymorphonuclear leucocytes, serum and fibrin and a general reaction of abrupt onset with pyrexia and polymorph leucocytosis. Typhoid and paratyphoid infections cause a local monocyte response, a polymorph leucopenia and a gradual increase of fever over several days. Whooping-cough induces a lymphocytosis. Tuberculosis and leprosy are more chronic infections, with a local reaction of lymphocytes and reticuloendothelial cells; fever is less marked or may be absent and there is seldom any change in the total or differential leucocyte count.

General Reaction of the Host. The course of an infection depends upon the patient's psychological, physical and nutritional state. An absence of fever and leucocytosis in pneumococcal pneumonia, for instance, indicates a poor response and a bad prognosis. This is especially liable to occur in elderly or alcoholic subjects. It has long been recognised that the mental attitude of the patient towards his affliction can affect his power of recovery. The doctor's ability to give confidence to the patient and the relatives is a very important part of treatment. That the endocrine glands may play an important role in the defence mechanism is suggested by the increased susceptibility to and mortality from infection in diabetes mellitus and in patients taking adrenocorticosteroid treatment.

Diagnosis of Infectious Disease

A knowledge of infections prevailing in the locality may be a valuable guide to diagnosis, e.g. when mumps is prevalent, the occurrence, without apparent cause, of acute epididymo-orchitis in an adult may be attributed to mumps with some confidence, a diagnosis which could not be made on clinical evidence alone. Mild or atypical infections may be correctly diagnosed on similar grounds, e.g. infectious hepatitis without jaundice occurring in a person who has been in contact with that disease. It is wise to enquire about contacts among the family, friends and workmates. Persons following certain occupations may be unduly exposed to infection, e.g. leptospirosis occurs in coal miners, pig farmers, sewer-workers and fish cleaners; anthrax occurs in tanners and in handlers of imported bone meal.

A recent history of laparotomy or of obscure abdominal pain should suggest subphrenic or intrahepatic abscess.

Residence or travel abroad within the previous year or two raises the possibility of malaria, amoebic abscess of the liver or other exotic disease.

In many infections a diagnosis beyond all reasonable doubt may be made on clinical grounds, e.g. measles, chickenpox, mumps and rheumatic fever. In others there may be doubt about the identity of the causal organism and demonstration of its presence is essential for diagnosis. Other considerations such as the tracing of a carrier may make it desirable to ascertain the precise strain of organism present.

The Laboratory Diagnosis of Infection. The causal organism may be identified in some instances microscopically in tissue, exudate or excreta, e.g. *N. gonorrhoeae* in urethral exudates, or *Myco. tuberculosis* in sputum. In the majority, however, it is necessary to isolate the organism in artificial culture, or more rarely in laboratory animals. In cases where these methods are inapplicable or unavailing, e.g. in many viral diseases or in the convalescent stages of infection, indirect means must be used to demonstrate specific antibody in the patient's serum.

Antibody is present in significant amounts from about 7 days after the onset of infection. The demonstration of specific antibody is of value in the diagnosis of toxoplasmosis, brucellosis, leptospirosis, syphilis, infectious mononucleosis and certain types of streptococcal and staphylococcal disease. The clinical value of serological tests is limited in most viral infections by the fact that recovery has often occurred before the result has been obtained, but such tests are of especial value in the exclusion of mumps and smallpox.

The significance of the isolation of certain micro-organisms may require further support by the demonstration of specific antibody, e.g. the mere isolation of an enterovirus from the faeces may be equivocal without an accompanying significant rise in corresponding antibody titre. As the normal range of antibody values is wide, at least two specimens should be examined at an interval of not less than 5 days so that a change in titre may be measured. In all cases the results of serological tests must be interpreted with a knowledge of the patient's occupation, history and clinical findings, previous immunisation and residence in endemic areas.

Differential Diagnosis of Infection. Most febrile illnesses are due to infection and often the diagnosis can be made by clinical examination alone. In other instances a diagnosis may require confirmation by haematological examination, radiography, isotope scanning, bacteriological investigation of blood or other body fluids, discharges or excreta. Often detection of specific antibodies in the serum may have to be undertaken before the diagnostic problems may be solved. Occasionally the cause of a febrile illness remains uncertain in spite of investigation and such a case is categorised PUO (pyrexia of unknown origin). In order to establish the diagnosis the following measures should be undertaken:

1. Retake the history; a symptom may have been overlooked or misinterpreted; enquire whether the patient has lived or travelled overseas.
2. Repeat the examination of the patient; new signs may have appeared while others could have been missed or their significance not appreciated. The throat and ears of children in particular should be inspected again.

3. Examine the urine repeatedly for protein, white and red blood cells and micro-organisms.
4. Inspect the temperature charts for evidence of some characteristic appearance such as the undulations seen in some cases of reticulosis (Pel-Ebstein fever) or the periodicity of malaria.
5. Review the results of laboratory investigations, thoroughly rescrutinise any radiographs and repeat such examinations as may seem necessary.

If the diagnosis is still uncertain, further tests will be required. These will be indicated by any new information obtained as a result of the clinical reassessment. It should be borne in mind that most problematic fevers are due to a common disorder with an unusual presentation. In the absence of clues, investigations should be planned in accordance with the most probable causes of PUO taking into account age, sex of the patient and the country in which the patient has been living. In Britain the more common causes of PUO are tumours (such as carcinoma with or without metastases, or Hodgkin's disease), infections (among which tuberculosis is important), connective tissue disorders and drug hypersensitivity. In the tropics and elsewhere a wide variety of infections must be considered; as a glance at the map on page 935 will demonstrate.

Mysterious fevers, particularly in patients who have some knowledge of medicine or nursing, may be due to deceit (factitious fever). Doubts should be raised if the skin of a supposedly febrile patient does not feel hot or if the general health does not deteriorate in spite of persistent fever. The occurrence of some bizarre symptom or sign may arouse suspicion that the temperature is being falsified. There are both subtle and simple techniques for doing this. The latter include holding the thermometer close to a hot water bottle or other source of heat, dipping it into a hot drink, applying friction to the bulb, or shaking it in a retrograde manner.

If the diagnosis remains obscure another opinion should be obtained, as reconsideration of the evidence by an unbiased observer may throw new light on the problem.

When a diagnosis still cannot be established and the patient's condition is deteriorating, various remedies, e.g. antibiotics, may be tried empirically in the hope of influencing the course of the disease. A therapeutic trial should not be regarded as a satisfactory diagnostic test and it can further obscure the diagnosis by suppressing but not curing the infection. It is most useful in suspected tuberculosis, for the combination of PAS and isoniazid (p. 292) is unlikely to influence fever of other origins.

The Prevention of Infection

The control of infection is largely based on three concepts:

1. *The host is separated from the parasite.* The oldest known public health measures employed isolation of the infected patient (source isolation) which remains an extremely important method of preventing the spread of infection, including that occurring in hospital. Isolation is carried to its most sophisticated development in pathogen free units (protective isolation) for the care of patients who are particularly prone to infection, e.g. those suffering from leukaemia under treatment with cytotoxic and corticosteroid drugs. The elimination of a disease from the community by finding, treating and isolating the sources of infection is an ideal which should always be vigorously pursued and it has met with considerable success in health campaigns against tuberculosis. It is soon expected to

lead to the extinction of smallpox. In highly developed countries many water- and food-borne diseases have been largely eliminated by good sanitation and other public health measures. Individuals who have been in contact with a serious and highly infectious disease like smallpox are placed in quarantine. The term is derived from the original period of 40 days of compulsory isolation of ships after leaving a port where diseases such as plague or cholera were raging. The duration of quarantine has come to be two days more than the maximum known incubation period of the disease in question. For the common infectious diseases of childhood, a period of observation has replaced quarantine. The probability of patients and known carriers acting as a source of infection can be reduced by isolation. Dependent upon the nature of the infection it may be necessary to disinfect or destroy surgical dressings, sputum, or excreta, to sterilise the clothing and utensils of patients and carriers, and to take precautions against spread by those attendant upon the patient, and by those concerned with the handling of food.

2. *The micro-organism is attacked.* Most bacterial infections and many other microbial diseases may be cured with antimicrobial agents. Microbes in the environment can be destroyed by physical and chemical agents.

Autogenous infection may be reduced by good personal hygiene and by the use of topical antibacterial preparations such as chlorhexophane and chlorhexidine, incorporated in soaps, creams or sprays. Endocarditis following dental extractions in patients with valvular disease of the heart can be prevented by prophylactic antibiotic therapy. Infection arising from operations on the alimentary tract may be reduced by preoperative chemotherapy.

In tropical diseases especially, complex biological cycles may be broken at many points and this eliminates the chance of spread. For example, malaria may be prevented by treating the whole population of an affected area, by prophylactic measures applied to all the persons at risk, by killing mosquitoes by insecticides or by attacking the larvae in their breeding grounds, and finally by eliminating the breeding grounds themselves.

3. *The resistance of the host is increased.* Apart from encouraging the maintenance of general health by adequate food, fresh air and exercise, sleep and good housing conditions, certain specific steps may be taken to increase resistance to infection. Active immunisation has been the most successful of these.

Active immunisation. In Britain parents should be advised to have their children immunised against whooping-cough, diphtheria, tetanus, measles and poliomyelitis (Table 3.1). Because of the risk of damage to the developing embryo or fetus if rubella should occur during pregnancy, it is recommended that rubella vaccine be given to all girls between 11 and 14 years and to non-pregnant women of child-bearing age who are found to be serologically negative for this antigen. Similarly, immunisation against tuberculosis should be given to all non-reactors to tuberculin during adolescence.

The indications for vaccination against influenza, enteric fevers, cholera, plague, typhus, yellow fever and rabies depend upon the likelihood of exposure or international health regulations (pp. 933, 934).

Passive Immunisation. An injection of specific antiserum will produce immunity for about six weeks only and should be followed by active immunisation with the appropriate antigen. The most common example of the use of antiserum is in protection against tetanus. Antitetanic serum is prepared from the horse, and its injec-

Table 3.1. Immunisation schedule generally followed in Britain

Age	Visits	Vaccine	Intervals
4–12 months	3	Three administrations of DTP + OPV	6–8 weeks and 4–6 months
12–24 months	1	Measles vaccination	
First year at school	1	Booster DT + OPV	
10–13 years	1	BCG for the Tuberculin negative	
Girls: 11–13 years	1	Rubella vaccination	
15–19 years or on leaving school	1	TT + OPV	

DTP = Diphtheria, tetanus, pertussis ('triple') vaccine.
OPV = Oral poliomyelitis vaccine.
DT = Diphtheria, tetanus vaccine.
TT = Tetanus toxoid.

tion induces the production of antibodies against horse serum. Subsequent injections of serum are therefore not only likely to be ineffective, but are also prone to cause sensitivity reactions, hence the need for following passive with active immunisation. These risks can be avoided by the use of hyperimmune human globulin.

DISEASES DUE TO INFECTION

Diseases due to infection are the commonest cause of ill health throughout the world. Organisms involved include bacteria, mycoplasmas, rickettsiae, viruses, protozoa, metazoa and fungi. The term infestation is now limited to ectoparasites, usually arthropods such as lice and fleas, which remain on the surface of the body but which may transmit a systemic infection. Protozoal infections such as malaria, amoebic dysentery, sleeping sickness and leishmaniasis and helminthiasis (worms) are of great importance in the tropics. Fungi causing ringworm and thrush occur all over the world but systemic infections with other fungi, such as coccidioidosis, histoplasmosis and the blastomycoses, are rare except in certain geographical locations.

The range of diseases caused by bacteria is large; streptococci and staphylococci are widespread and produce similar diseases throughout the world. Others such as the cholera vibrio and plague bacillus are locally endemic but may produce epidemics from time to time. Some bacterial infections may be acute such as diphtheria and tetanus, others chronic such as tuberculosis, syphilis and leprosy.

Organisms smaller than true bacteria, the rickettsiae which cause typhus fevers, the mycoplasmas of atypical pneumonia and the chlamydiae (bedsoniae) of psittacosis, lymphogranuloma and trachoma are now recognised to be widespread and are susceptible to chemotherapy. Thus most bacterial, protozoal and fungal infections can be successfully treated with antibiotics and chemotherapeutic agents provided that the appropriate drug is prescribed early in the disease. This emphasises the need for rapid and accurate diagnosis supplemented where necessary by specific tests to indicate the most effective therapeutic agent.

As yet few specific therapeutic measures are available for viral diseases, among which are the exanthemata—chickenpox, smallpox, measles and rubella; mumps and glandular fever; respiratory illnesses such as the common cold, pharyngitis and influenza; diseases of the nervous system such as rabies and other forms of encephalitis, poliomyelitis and choriomeningitis, and liver disorders such as infective hepatitis and yellow fever. The problem of chemotherapy is to control the growth and propagation of the virus without damage to the host cell on which it is so dependent. The number of viral infections for which prophylaxis is available is increasing in parallel with modern advances in virology and now there is preventative treatment for smallpox, rabies, yellow fever, poliomyelitis, measles and rubella. Several viral infections may be prevented temporarily by passive immunisation with human gammaglobulin.

Diseases due to infection which involve one system predominantly are described in the appropriate chapter in this book. Those infectious diseases which are limited to the tropics or are commoner there than in temperate regions are described in the section 'Tropical Diseases and Helminthic Infections'. The infectious diseases described here are:

BACTERIAL		VIRAL
Streptococcal infections	Tetanus	Measles
Staphylococcal infections	Brucellosis	Rubella
Whooping-cough	Meningococcal	Mumps
Diphtheria	infections	Chickenpox
Typhoid and paratyphoid fevers	Gonorrhoea	Smallpox
Bacterial food poisoning	Syphilis	
Bacillary dysentery	Leptospirosis	

Streptococcal Infections

Haemolytic streptococcal infection results in features which vary with the invasiveness of the organism, its capacity to produce toxins, the site involved and the reaction of the host. If the resistance is low and the invasive properties of the haemolytic streptococcus are high, a rapidly spreading erysipelas, or cellulitis, lymphangitis or bacteraemia, may result. The haemolytic streptococcus may produce a specific exotoxin causing a widespread punctate erythema. When the infection is associated with such a rash the syndrome is known as scarlet fever. The same type of streptococcus may produce in one person acute tonsillitis, in another scarlet fever and in a third erysipelas.

Scarlet Fever

Although scarlet fever is at present a mild disease, it may not necessarily remain so, as fluctuations in its severity have been recorded for the past two or three hundred years. The primary site of infection in scarlet fever is usually the pharynx or the tonsils but the disease may follow haemolytic streptococcal infection in other situations, e.g. in the genital tract after childbirth resulting in 'puerperal' scarlet fever or in wounds resulting in 'surgical' scarlet fever. It is transmitted by airborne infection, or more rarely by milk or ice-cream contaminated by streptococci. The disease is notifiable. The incubation period is about two to four days. Quarantine is not necessary.

Clinical Features. Scarlet fever occurs most commonly in children from 3 to 10 years of age. It has a sudden onset and the more severe cases present with a sore throat, shivering, pyrexia, headache, and vomiting. There is inflammation of the fauces; the tonsils are enlarged and may be covered with a follicular exudate which occasionally becomes confluent. The exudate may be distinguished from the membrane seen in diphtheria by its yellow appearance and the ease with which it is wiped off. There is tender enlargement of the tonsillar lymph nodes. The rash, which usually appears first behind the ears on the second day, rapidly becomes a generalised punctate erythema. It is most intense in the flexures of the arms and legs. The face is not affected by the rash, though it is usually flushed due to fever, and the region round the mouth is pale. The tongue is initially furred but shows prominent red papillae, an appearance known as the 'white strawberry' tongue. In two or three days the fur peels leaving the 'red strawberry' tongue. The rash fades in about one week and is succeeded by desquamation of the skin.

Complications. The complications are less common than formerly as a result of the mild form of the disease and the introduction of effective chemotherapy. Extension of infection along the Eustachian tubes may lead to acute suppurative otitis media. Suppurative cervical adenitis and sinusitis also occur. Rheumatic fever and acute nephritis are rare sequelae which develop two or three weeks after the onset of the illness and are due to hypersensitivity.

Diagnosis. *Infectious mononucleosis* (p. 615), *measles* (p. 81), and *rubella* (p. 82) may sometimes be mistaken for scarlet fever. Rashes resulting from *sensitivity to a drug* are more commonly encountered in adults than in children and may differ from scarlet fever in their persistence and distribution. In scarlet fever a profuse growth of haemolytic streptococci can usually be obtained from a throat swab. A high antistroptolysin O titre (ASO) may be demonstrated in the serum. Staphylococcal septicaemia can occasionally be associated with a scarlatiniform skin rash.

Treatment and Prevention. The treatment of scarlet fever is the same as for streptococcal sore throat. Most cases respond rapidly to phenoxymethylpenicillin (250 mg for children to 500 mg for adults every 6 hours for 7 days). An institutional epidemic calls for chemoprophylaxis with penicillin. Erythromycin is indicated for persons sensitive to penicillin.

Erysipelas

Erysipelas is an acute local haemolytic streptococcal infection of the skin. It occurs in both sexes and is much commoner in the elderly than in the young. The disease is notifiable. A quarantine period is not necessary.

Clinical Features. The onset is abrupt with local heat and pain in the infected region of the skin together with a general systemic upset. There is a rapidly spreading red patch of inflamed skin with much underlying oedema of the subcutaneous tissues. The edge of the patch is palpably raised and clearly defined and the lymph nodes draining the area become enlarged and tender. As the oedema subsides vesicles and bullae appear in the central part of the affected area. The face is involved in at least 80 per cent of all cases of erysipelas as a result of the spread of streptococci from the nose or throat.

Treatment. Erysipelas is usually brought under complete control within 48 hours of treatment with penicillin; hence the prognosis is now excellent for a disease which used to be very serious.

Staphylococcal Infections

Staph. aureus is responsible for a wide variety of suppurative conditions such as infected lacerations, styes, boils, carbuncles, abscesses, osteomyelitis, pneumonia, endocarditis, umbilical cord sepsis, necrotising enterocolitis and bacteraemia with pyaemic abscesses. Infection is derived from human or sometimes animal sources and the organisms can be grown from the nasopharynx and skin of up to 30 per cent of healthy persons. The staphylococcus is readily spread from these sites and from clothing to contaminate the dust in which it survives in the dry state for weeks or months. In hospital this organism is an important cause of wound infection, pneumonia and neonatal sepsis. Under suitable conditions it multiplies freely in food and milk and so is an important cause of food poisoning. However, many infections, particularly boils, carbuncles and abscesses, are due to autogenous infection.

Strains of *Staph. aureus* resistant to antibiotics have increased in number since these drugs were introduced. Such strains are more commonly acquired in hospital and may give rise to small epidemics of infection. Elsewhere the majority of strains are sensitive to antibiotics usually effective although the production of penicillinase by many precludes treatment with benzylpenicillin. *Necrotising enterocolitis* is usually the result of the unrestricted growth of drug-resistant staphylococci in the gut following the suppression of other organisms by chemotherapy. The diarrhoea, dehydration and peripheral circulatory failure may be so severe as to resemble cholera.

Boils are satisfactorily treated with an occlusive dressing or the local application of antiseptic agents. When the severity of the disease warrants antibiotic therapy, the choice depends on whether the infection has been acquired inside or outside hospital. In the latter case the organism may be sensitive to penicillin. If the illness is severe treatment should be commenced with the cloxacillins (p. 90), unless the patient is known to be allergic to the penicillins when clindamycin (p. 93). should be given.

All possible care must be taken to prevent the spread of staphylococcal infection and infective patients should be isolated and barrier-nursed.

Whooping-cough

Whooping-cough (pertussis) is a highly infectious disease caused by *Bordetella pertussis*. It is spread by droplet infection. Clinical diagnosis in the early and most infectious stage is virtually impossible so that epidemics are common. However, the incidence and severity of the disease have been decreasing over the last few years since the institution of more effective prophylactic measures. The disease is notifiable. The incubation period is 7 to 14 days to the catarrhal stage. A quarantine period is not necessary. Whooping-cough occurs at all ages but approximately 90 per cent of cases are children under 5 years of age.

Clinical Features. The first stage of whooping-cough consists of a highly infectious upper respiratory catarrh lasting about one week during which conjunctivitis, rhinitis and an unproductive cough are present. The distinctive paroxysmal stage follows and is characterised by severe bouts of coughing. The number of such paroxysms in 24 hours varies from an occasional attack to 40 or 50 and they are always more severe at night. Each paroxysm consists of a succession of short sharp coughs, gathering in speed and duration and ending in a deep inspiration during which the characteristic whoop may be heard. It may be absent in older children and in adults because the air passages are so much wider. During these paroxysms, the face becomes congested and cyanosed, the eyes bulge and the tongue is protruded to such an extent that ulceration of the frenum may occur from trauma by the lower teeth. The last paroxysm of a series frequently ends with expectoration of tenacious mucus and vomiting. The physical signs in the chest are those of bronchitis. The paroxysmal stage lasts from one to several weeks and is followed by the stage of convalescence during which the cough becomes less frequent and the sputum less tenacious. After the illness there is usually a lasting immunity. Second atypical attacks are sometimes seen in adults who, although not seriously ill, may be greatly distressed by the spasmodic coughing.

Complications. The most important complications of whooping-cough are pneumonia and segmental or lobar collapse which may be followed by bronchiectasis. Convulsions are of grave significance especially if they are frequent. Subconjunctival or periorbital haemorrhage, ulceration of the frenum of the tongue, and prolapse of the rectum are relatively unimportant results of the stress of coughing. Maternal antibody may be detected in cord blood, yet neonates are highly susceptible and the mortality is greatest in the first year of life.

Diagnosis. The diagnosis of whooping-cough is very difficult in the catarrhal stage when the disease is most infectious. It can be confirmed in the laboratory by the isolation of *Bord. pertussis* from per-nasal swabs (taken from the posterior wall of the nasopharynx on small swabs passed along the floor of the nose) or less frequently from cough-plates containing selective medium. Examination of the blood shows a lymphocytosis which, however, may not develop until the disease is well established. The diagnosis is easy in the paroxysmal stage when the whoop has developed, but by this time the danger of transmission of infection has largely disappeared.

Treatment. Ampicillin may reduce the severity of the infection if taken during the catarrhal stage. Antibiotics are of no value if the spasmodic stage has been reached and they should not be used unless secondary infection occurs. The milder case need not be kept in bed, and is better out of doors. A cough suppressant such as linctus methadone may be helpful in controlling the severity of paroxysms. When the illness is of long duration and vomiting is frequent, skilled nursing will be required to maintain nutrition, especially in infants and young children. Feeds are usually accepted and retained if they are given immediately after the vomiting which frequently follows a paroxysm of coughing.

Prevention. Active immunisation (p. 59) can occasionally cause convulsions or neurological damage and adverse publicity regarding this has led to a marked decrease in the number of children who are immunised against the disease. However, the adverse effects of the vaccine have to be balanced against the risk of contracting a potentially serious disease, especially in young children. It is important that the patient should be segregated as early as possible. Many of the deaths from whooping-cough occur in the first three months of life and hence very special care must be taken to avoid exposure of infants to the risk of contracting the disease. Contacts should be isolated on the first sign of catarrhal symptoms and per-nasal swabs taken.

Diphtheria

By 1946 diphtheria, which was formerly a common and lethal disease in Britain, became so rare as a result of prophylactic inoculation that many doctors have never seen it. Yet in many parts of the world diphtheria is still an important cause of illness.

Infection with *Corynebacterium diphtheriae* occurs most commonly in the upper respiratory tract and sore throat is frequently the presenting feature. The disease is usually spread by droplet infection from cases or carriers. The organisms remain localised at the site of infection and the serious consequences result from the absorption of a soluble exotoxin which damages the heart muscle and the nervous system.

The infection may occur rarely on the conjunctiva or the genital tract, or it may complicate wounds, abrasions or diseases of the skin.

The disease is notifiable. The average incubation period is two to four days. Quarantine is not necessary. Cases are isolated until cultures from six daily nose and throat swabs are negative.

Clinical Features. The diagnostic feature is the 'wash-leather' elevated membrane of variable extent on the tonsils with a well-defined edge and surrounded by a zone of inflammation. The membrane is firm and adherent. There may be swelling of the neck and tender enlargement of the lymph nodes. In the mildest infections, especially in the presence of a high degree of immunity, a membrane may never appear and the throat is merely slightly injected. In these circumstances, diagnosis cannot be made clinically but depends upon obtaining a positive culture from a throat swab.

The disease begins insidiously. The temperature is seldom much raised although tachycardia is usually marked. The infection may remain mild if the membrane is confined to the anterior nares or the larynx or the tonsils. With anterior nasal infection there is also nasal discharge often tinged with blood. In laryngeal diphtheria there is a husky voice, a high-pitched cough, and a danger of respiratory obstruction which can be fatal if tracheostomy is not carried out. Tonsillar diphtheria usually causes a sore throat. When the infection spreads towards the uvula, to the fauces and then to the nasopharynx, the patient is often gravely ill and apathetic. The complexion is pale, the pulse rapid and of poor volume and the blood pressure low. Death from peripheral circulatory failure may occur within the first 10 days. If there is haemorrhage from the throat and nose or into the skin, the disease is almost always fatal. Those who survive the earlier toxaemia may later develop arrhythmias or cardiac failure. Electrocardiographic changes are common and are due to myocarditis. These are reversible and there is no permanent damage to the heart in those who survive.

Involvement of the nervous system sometimes occurs, and after tonsillar or pharyngeal diphtheria it usually commences with palatal palsy on about the tenth day of the illness. The voice assumes a nasal quality, while regurgitation of fluids through the nose and sluggishness of palatal movements may be observed. Paralysis of accommodation soon follows and may be inferred from the patient's complaint of difficulty in reading small print. Such paralysis may occur irrespective of the site of infection. In myopes it may pass unnoticed.

A week or two later, though somewhat rarely, weakness and parasthaesia in the limbs due to polyneuritis may develop. In exceptional cases paralysis of the respiratory muscles may necessitate the use of a mechanical respirator. Recovery from such neuritis is always ultimately complete.

Differential Diagnosis. It must be emphasised that the diagnosis of diphtheria is primarily clinical, and laboratory confirmation may take several days. The differential diagnosis includes:

(1) *Streptococcal tonsillitis*, in which the onset is abrupt with high fever and the initial constitutional disturbance often severe. There is widespread inflammation of the throat, whereas the exudate, usually follicular but occasionally confluent, is always limited to the tonsils. It is yellowish-white in colour and is easily wiped off with a swab. *Strept. pyogenes* may be isolated on culture.

(2) *Infectious mononucleosis* which is frequently associated with an inflamed throat accompanied by exudate. There is often a petechial rash on the palate. The lymph nodes and spleen may enlarge. Sooner or later the characteristic atypical leucocytes appear. A positive Monospot test confirms the diagnosis.

(3) *Vincent's infection*, in which a foul smelling ulceromembranous lesion, often spreading from the gums, is present. Constitutional disturbance is absent or slight, and the presence of spirochaetes and fusiform bacilli may be demonstrated in a stained smear (p. 355).

(4) *Agranulocytosis, pancytopenia* or *acute leukaemia*, in any of which ulceration may occur in the throat, can be diagnosed by the characteristic blood changes.

(5) *Thrush* (p. 355) when extensive, may be distinguished from diphtheria by the white colour, by the presence of multiple outlying patches which resemble milk curds, and by the absence of cervical lymphadenitis or constitutional disturbance. Microscopic examination shows the presence of the fungus, *Candida albicans*.

Treatment. Upon making a clinical diagnosis of diphtheria, the case should be notified to the community medical authorities and sent urgently to a hospital for infectious diseases. Refined antitoxic serum (p. 32) should be injected intramuscularly without awaiting the report on a throat swab. Every moment of delay increases the danger to the patient, because toxin, once fixed to the tissues, can no longer be neutralised by antitoxin. However, horse serum, in which antitoxin is contained, being a foreign protein, is liable to cause undesirable reactions. Firstly, there may be an immediate anaphylactic reaction with dyspnoea, pallor and collapse or even death. Secondly, within 7 to 12 days serum sickness, with fever, urticaria and joint pains may occur. If there is a previous history of inoculation of horse serum, the symptoms commonly appear in three or four days. As anaphylaxis is potentially lethal, every patient must be asked whether they have ever had antiserum before and whether they suffer from any allergic disorder. In either case a small test injection of serum should be given half an hour before the full dose.

When a reaction does occur after the test dose in an allergic subject, rapid desensitisation must be undertaken with extreme caution. In all cases an ampoule of $\frac{1}{1000}$ adrenaline solution must be close at hand to deal with any immediate type of reaction ($0 \cdot 5$–$1 \cdot 0$ ml i.m.). An antihistamine is also given.

In a very severe case the risk of anaphylactic shock is outweighed by the mortal danger of diphtheritic toxaemia and up to 100,000 units of antitoxin should be injected intravenously if the test dose has not given rise to symptoms. For cases of moderate severity 16,000–32,000 units i.m. will suffice, and for mild cases 4,000–8,000 units.

Penicillin should be administered for one week to eliminate *C. diphtheriae*. Patients allergic to penicillin can be given erythromycin.

Complete rest is essential for at least three weeks owing to the danger of cardiac and circulatory failure. This period must be lengthened if there is evidence of myocardial involvement. After a moderate attack, judged by the clinical state, the patient may be fit for discharge in six or seven weeks. After severe attacks, patients may not be fit for three months, while those who develop polyneuritis may take six to nine months to recover.

Prevention. The mortality in diphtheria, combined with the fact that the risks and cost of treatment are considerable, emphasise the necessity for active immunisation. This should be given in accordance with the instructions on page 60.

If diphtheria occurs in a closed community, a daily examination of the throat of all contacts should be made during the incubation period and swabs taken for the detection of carriers and potential cases. Those with positive throat swabs or with the slightest suspicion of clinical diphtheria should be isolated and given erythromycin which is more effective than penicillin in eradicating the organism in carriers. All contacts should also be advised to have active immunisation or a booster dose of toxoid.

Cases, convalescents and healthy carriers are isolated until six daily throat swabs are negative on culture.

Typhoid and Paratyphoid Fevers
(*The Enteric Fevers*)

In many countries where sanitation is primitive, enteric fevers, which are transmitted by the faecal–oral route, are an important cause of illness. Elsewhere they are relatively rare. Nevertheless, outbreaks occur from time to time and the infection may be contracted by persons travelling abroad.

Aetiology. The enteric fevers are caused by infection with *Salmonella typhi* and *paratyphi* which are specific human pathogens. Other members of the Salmonella group, many of which cause infection in animals, produce disease in man ranging from mild food poisoning to more serious infection which may simulate many of the features of paratyphoid fever including bacteraemia. Typhoid and paratyphoid infections have a world-wide distribution and occur endemically wherever sanitation is poor and the water supply is liable to be contaminated by human excreta. In such regions flies may also transmit the disease. In Britain spread is usually by carriers, often food handlers, through the contamination of food, milk or water; infected shell fish are occasionally responsible for an outbreak. The bacilli may live in the gallbladder for months or years after clinical recovery and pass intermittently in the stools.

Pathogenesis. After a few days of bacteraemia, the bacilli localise mainly in the lymphoid tissue of the small intestine. The typical lesion is in the Peyer's patches and follicles. These swell at first, then ulcerate and ultimately heal, but during this sequence they may perforate or bleed. The mesenteric lymph nodes and spleen are enlarged.

The incubation period of typhoid fever is about 10 to 14 days; that of paratyphoid is somewhat shorter. The diseases are notifiable. Quarantine is not necessary, but contacts are kept under surveillance for three weeks.

Clinical Features. *Typhoid Fever.* The onset is insidious and it may be 3 or 4 days before the patient is forced to stay in bed. The temperature rises in a step-ladder fashion for 4 or 5 days, being higher at night than in the morning. There is malaise, with increasing headache, drowsiness and aching in the limbs. Cough and epistaxis are not uncommon; constipation is usually present although in children diarrhoea and vomiting may be prominent early in the illness. The pulse is often slower than would be expected from the height of the temperature. At the end of the first week the typical rash may appear on the upper abdomen and on the back as sparse slightly raised, rose-red spots which fade on pressure. After 2 or 3 days they disappear, to be succeeded sometimes by fresh crops of spots. About the seventh to tenth day of illness the spleen becomes palpable. It is soft and seldom extends more than one or two finger breadths below the costal margin. Often about this time constipation is succeeded by diarrhoea and generalised abdominal distension with tenderness in the right iliac fossa. Bronchitis may develop and there may be delirium. By the end of the second week the patient may be profoundly ill unless the disease is modified by antibiotic treatment. In the third week toxaemia increases and the patient may pass into coma and die. The prognosis may worsen at this stage due to haemorrhage from or perforation of the ulcerated Peyer's patches. In those who recover the temperature falls by lysis, the appetite returns, distension disappears, and strength improves. After an initial recovery recrudescence of the disease may occur.

Paratyphoid Fever. The most common variety in Britain is due to *S. paratyphi B*. The course tends to be shorter and milder than that of typhoid fever but the onset is often more abrupt with acute enteritis. The rash may be more abundant and the intestinal complications less frequent.

Complications of the Enteric Fevers. The dangerous complications of enteric fevers are those of haemorrhage and perforation which occur at the end of the second week or during the third week of the illness. The bleeding may be sudden and very severe. The features of shock suggesting that a haemorrhage has occurred are described on page 372. Perforation usually occurs from ulcers near the ileo-caecal valve. Additional complications may involve almost any viscus or system as a result of the septicaemia which is present during the first week. Pneumonia, thrombophlebitis, myocarditis, myositis, arthritis, periostitis, osteomyelitis, meningitis and cholecystitis are all recognised complications.

Diagnosis. In the first week of the disease the diagnosis may be very difficult as in this invasive stage with bacteraemia the symptoms are those of a generalised infection without localising features. In a suspected case, blood culture is the most important diagnostic method, particularly during the first week of the disease. During this period the organism may not grow from the stool and urine using selective media. The faeces will contain the organism more frequently during the second and third weeks. A white blood count may be helpful as there is typically a leucopenia.

Agglutinating antibodies to the causative organisms form after the second week of the disease (*Widal reaction*), but their detection is of limited value. Titres greater than 240 or significantly rising titres in unvaccinated persons can be more helpful in countries where the disease is rare; where it is common antibodies may result from previous infection. Antibodies to the 'Vi' antigens of *S. typhi* and *S. paratyphi* may be measured and are sometimes of use in detecting carriers of these organisms.

Treatment. The patient should be treated in bed and preferably in isolation. A high standard of nursing is required with special attention to the maintenance of nutrition and fluid intake, to the care of the mouth and to the prevention of pressure sores. Scrupulous precautions must be taken against the spread of infection by the provision of special gowns and adequate washing facilities by the bedside, and sterilisation of excreta and of articles used by the patient.

Chloramphenicol should be given for 14 days initially in a dose of 3 g daily, reducing to 2 g daily as the patient responds. Co-trimoxazole (p. 88) is an alternative to chloramphenicol in typhoid fever and is the drug of choice for paratyphoid fever. Even with effective chemotherapy there is still a danger of complications, of recrudescence of the disease and of the development of a carrier state. For at least three weeks the patient must be kept under careful supervision while healing of the bowel takes place. For the first few days a semifluid diet should be given, followed by a low roughage diet. A second course of chemotherapy must be given in the event of a relapse and this usually produces good results. The chronic carrier should be treated for several weeks with co-trimoxazole, as chloramphenicol has proved ineffective. In some cases cholecystectomy may be necessary.

The treatment of haemorrhage is described on page 372. Prior to the introduction of chloramphenicol the treatment of perforation was by immediate recourse to surgery, which carried a high mortality in the seriously ill. Such patients can be treated conservatively while chloramphenicol is continued, but advice from a surgeon should be sought as laparotomy may be indicated.

The patient should be considered as infective until six consecutive stools and urines are found to be negative on culture.

Prevention. Those who propose to travel or live in countries where enteric infections are endemic should be inoculated with vaccine containing killed *S. typhi* and *S. paratyphi* A and B (TAB) (p. 934).

Bacterial Food Poisoning

Food poisoning includes a number of disorders presenting with diarrhoea and vomiting due to acute gastroenteritis developing up to 48 hours after the consumption of food or drink. It is customary not to include under this term the enteric fevers (p. 67), dysenteries (p. 71) and cholera (p. 862) which are also spread by infected food and drink. In contrast to enteric fever which is relatively uncommon and cholera which has been almost unknown in Britain for the past 100 years, there is an increase in the reported incidence of bacterial food poisoning.

Food poisoning may also be due to intestinal allergy, e.g. to shellfish, or to children eating unripe fruit or other unsuitable foods. Rarely a poisonous substance may be eaten, e.g. *Amanita phalloides*, in mistake for a mushroom or a chemical poison in food may be unwittingly consumed. Examples of the latter range from barium carbonate used in baking in mistake for flour, to arsenic or powdered glass administered murderously in the tradition of the Borgias.

Food which has been placed in a container previously used for holding a chemical poison may be contaminated. Placing acid fruit juices in cheap enamel or zinc vessels may result in the liberation of antimony or zinc. Home-made wine kept in glazed earthenware containers may be the source of chronic lead poisoning.

Aetiology. Bacterial food poisoning is usually divided into the infection and toxin types.

INFECTION TYPE. The organisms mainly responsible belong to the Salmonella group whose source is certain birds, rodents, cattle and less frequently reptiles, such as pet tortoises. The domestic fowl is one of the commonest sources and modern methods of poultry husbandry involving battery-rearing and deep-freezing of carcasses encourage the spread and transmission of infection. *Salmonella typhimurium* causes at least three-quarters of the cases of food poisoning of the 'infection' type in Britain. Food may be contaminated with infected excreta of mice or rats, or infection may be transferred by flies or by human carriers employed in the handling of food. The size of the infecting dose of bacteria bears a close relationship to the speed of onset of symptoms and to the severity of the illness. This indicates the dangers of bacterial multiplication which may take place when food is contaminated and thereafter remains warm for many hours or days. The types of food which are particularly likely to be affected are twice-cooked meat dishes, stews, gravies, soups, custards, milk and synthetic cream. The danger of food poisoning is greatly reduced if such foods are kept in a refrigerator. Ducks tend to be carriers of salmonella organisms in the oviduct and alimentary tract, and duck's eggs are not suitable for the preparation of lightly cooked foods. Hen's eggs are rarely affected.

TOXIN TYPE. Such poisoning is most commonly caused by the enterotoxin of *Staph. aureus*. This frequently originates from a food handler suffering from a septic lesion. Incubation at a suitable temperature leads to growth of the organism and production of toxin which is relatively heat resistant and may not be destroyed by cooking. Strains of *Clostridium welchii*, many of them relatively resistant to heat, may contaminate certain foods, particularly meat. Pre-cooking of stews and pies may not destroy all the spores and the keeping of such food will lead to the formation of heat-stable toxins which can give rise to gastroenteritis, sometimes severe. Other bacteria may contaminate food without obvious spoilage and cause mild gastroenteritis.

Outbreaks of food poisoning affecting large numbers of persons occur in canteens, restaurants, hospitals and other institutions.

Clinical Features. The simultaneous occurrence of symptoms in more than one member of a household or institution often simplifies diagnosis. The incubation period is a useful pointer to the aetiology. If vomiting starts within 30 minutes of the ingestion of suspected food, it is likely to be due to a chemical poison; if it arises 12 to 48 hours later, it is probably due to a Salmonella infection. The incubation periods of staphylococcal and clostridial food poisoning are usually intermediate between these extremes being from 1 to 12 hours.

The severity of symptoms depends on the type and amount of the poisonous substance ingested. The principal symptoms are nausea, vomiting, diarrhoea and central abdominal colic. Staphylococcal food poisoning may be associated only with vomiting while diarrhoea and abdominal pain are more prominent with *Cl. welchii* toxins. In severe cases there may be prostration, collapse and signs of dehydration. In the chemical and toxin types of food poisoning the onset tends to be sudden and severe and the patient may rapidly become shocked. Recovery however usually occurs within 24 hours. In the infection type, symptoms develop more slowly and there is usually pyrexia and toxicity. The patient may be ill for several days. The stools are watery and offensive, and may contain blood and some mucus, in contrast to bacillary dysentery where there is also pus.

A rare cause of bacterial food poisoning is the ingestion of one of the most potent poisons known to man, namely the toxin produced by *Cl. botulinum*. Imperfectly treated tinned food or soup or preserved fish may be contaminated with the organism and be the source of the toxin. The clinical features differ from all other types of bacterial food poisoning and consist chiefly of vomiting, constipation, thirst and the secretion of viscid saliva and of ocular and pharyngeal pareses and aphonia. The mortality can be high.

Diagnosis. A specimen of the patient's stool or vomit together with the suspected food, if available, should be sent for culture. Organisms of the Salmonella group can usually be readily isolated. In more severe cases blood should be sent for culture. Notification of Salmonella infection and other types of food poisoning is compulsory in Britain.

Treatment. Most cases are mild and can be treated at home. Solid food should be withheld and the patient instructed to take fluids only. A teaspoonful of salt added to one pint of water flavoured with a small quantity of fruit juice provides a satisfactory oral replacement solution. Patients who are severely ill, collapsed or dehydrated require intravenous fluid therapy.

Symptoms normally pass off spontaneously in a day or two. When acute symptoms cease, semi-fluid low-roughage diet may be taken containing bread, butter, eggs, fish, soft puddings and jellies. To control diarrhoea, kaolin mixture may be given in 10 ml doses every 2 to 4 hours. Codeine phosphate 30 mg six-hourly is also useful.

Antibiotics should not be given for acute diarrhoea and vomiting as they are ineffective and frequently exacerbate symptoms. If salmonella bacteraemia is suspected or confirmed, ampicillin, 1 g every six hours should be given by intramuscular injection. Co-trimoxazole is a satisfactory alternative.

If the poisoning is thought to be due to a chemical or a poisonous food, the patient's stomach should be washed out with tepid water, using the technique described on page 803.

Prevention. In Salmonella food poisoning the carrier state persists on the average for about 14 days after infection but may be much longer, and the patient must not be allowed to handle food until he has stopped excreting the organism. A reduction in the high incidence of food poisoning can best be achieved by improving the standards of personal hygiene, especially in those handling food, and by stressing the importance of hand-washing after using the lavatory. Increasing facilities for low temperature storage of food which has to be kept for some hours or days before being consumed is of the greatest importance. It is essential to keep frozen poultry at room temperature for at least eight hours before cooking or pathogens at the centre may survive unharmed.

Dysentery

Dysentery is an acute inflammation of the large intestine characterised by diarrhoea with blood and mucus in stools. Its causes are bacillary, protozoal or helminthic infection. Amoebic dysentery is described on page 842 and schistosomiasis (Bilharziasis) on page 894.

Bacillary Dysentery

The bacilli belong to the genus *Shigella* of which there are three main pathogenic groups, *Shiga*, *Flexner* and *Sonne*, the last two having numerous strains. In Britain the majority of cases of bacillary dysentery in recent years have been caused by *Shigella sonnei*.

Epidemiology. Bacillary dysentery in endemic form is found all over the world. It occurs in epidemic form wherever there is a crowded population with poor sanitation, and thus has been a constant accompaniment of wars and natural catastrophies. Spread may occur by contaminated food or flies but contact through unwashed hands after defaecation is by far the most important factor. Lavatory chains and door handles may be contaminated even before hand washing is possible. Hence the modern provision of plenty of handbasins, disposable towels and hot air driers goes a long way towards the prevention of the faecal–oral spread of disease. Outbreaks are not uncommon in mental hospitals, residential schools and other closed institutions. The disease is notifiable.

Pathology. There is generalised inflammation of the large bowel which may extend to involve the lower part of the small intestine. Endoscopy shows that the mucosa is red and swollen, the submucous veins are obscured and mucopus is seen on the surface. Bleeding points appear readily at the touch of the endoscope. Ulcers may form and the adjacent lymph nodes are enlarged.

Clinical Features. There is great variation in severity. Sonne infections may be so mild as to escape detection and the patient remains ambulant with a few loose stools and perhaps a little colic. Flexner infections are usually more severe while Shiga dysentery may be fulminating and cause death within 48 hours.

In a moderately severe illness, the patient complains of diarrhoea, colicky hypogastric pain and tenesmus. The stools are usually small, and after the first few evacuations, contain blood and purulent exudate with little faecal material. There is frequently fever, with dehydration and weakness if the diarrhoea persists. On physical examination there will be tenderness over the colon more easily elicited in the left iliac fossa. In Sonne infection the patient may develop a febrile illness and diarrhoea may be mild or even absent; there is usually some headache and muscular aching.

In a very small minority of cases of dysentery the diarrhoea becomes chronic and the illness then becomes indistinguishable from chronic ulcerative colitis. Arthritis or iritis may occasionally complicate bacillary dysentery.

Diagnosis. Diagnosis depends on culture of faeces. Microscopic examination of the stool shows the presence of numerous pus cells. Bacillary dysentery must be differentiated from other causes of bloody diarrhoea especially ulcerative colitis. Amoebic and schistosomal infections usually have a less acute onset than bacillary dysentery.

Treatment and Prevention. The patient frequently retires to bed with bacillary dysentery of any severity. Mild cases, however, who may remain ambulant, should preferably be confined to the home to prevent spread of infection. Diarrhoea may be controlled by codeine or kaolin. A fluid or semifluid low-roughage diet should be given depending on the severity of the diarrhoea but if this is severe, it will be necessary to replace the water and electrolyte loss by intravenous therapy.

Bacillary dysentery is usually a self-limiting disease and antibiotics or sulphonamides are not indicated in most cases. In severe infections, especially those caused by Shiga or Flexner strains, ampicillin 500 mg 6 hourly or co-trimoxazole two tablets twice daily should be given. In Britain the majority of shigellae are now sulphonamide-resistant although in tropical countries sulphonamides are still of value in severe bacillary dysentery. When they are used, an ample intake of fluids must be ensured in order to guard against anuria due to the precipitation of crystals in the kidneys.

The prevention of faecal contamination of food and milk, the isolation of cases, and the identification of carriers, are methods which are theoretically important but may be difficult to apply except in limited outbreaks. Hand-washing is very important.

Tetanus

This disease results from infection with *Clostridium tetani*, which exists as a commensal in the gut of man and domestic animals and is found in cultivated soils. Infection enters the body through wounds, often trivial, such as those caused by a splinter, a nail in the boot or a garden fork or following septic infection such as a dirty abrasion or a whitlow. The disease is thus most commonly found in agricultural workers and gardeners. If childbirth takes place in an unhygienic environment *tetanus neonatorum* may result from infection of the umbilical stump or the mother may develop the disease. Tetanus is still one of the major killers of adults, children and neonates in the tropics.

In circumstances unfavourable to the growth of the organism, spores are formed and these may remain dormant for years. Spores germinate and bacilli multiply only in the anaerobic conditions which occur in areas of tissue necrosis or if the oxygen tension is low as a result of the presence of other organisms, particularly aerobic ones. The bacilli remain localised but produce an exotoxin with an affinity for motor nerve endings and motor nerve cells. Involvement of the former by direct spread causes local tetanus. The anterior horn cells are affected after the exotoxin has passed into the blood stream and their involvement results in rigidity and convulsions. Symptoms first appear from two days to several weeks after injury—the shorter the incubation period, the more severe the attacks and the outcome may well be fatal with an incubation period of only a few days.

Clinical Features. Much the most important early symptom is trismus—a painless spasm of the masseter muscles which causes difficulty in opening the mouth and in masticating, hence the name, 'lockjaw'. This tonic rigidity spreads to involve in turn the muscles of the face, neck and trunk. Contraction of the frontalis and the muscles at the angles of the mouth gives rise to the 'risus sardonicus'. There is rigidity of the muscles of the neck and trunk of varying degree. The back is usually slightly arched and the board-like abdominal wall resembles that seen a few hours after the perforation of a peptic ulcer, but there is little or no tenderness. In the more severe cases sudden violent spasms lasting for a few seconds to 3 or 4 minutes occur spontaneously or may be induced by diverse stimuli such as moving the patient, knocking the bed or making a noise. These convulsions are painful, exhausting and of very serious significance, especially if they appear soon after the onset of symptoms. They gradually increase in frequency and severity for about one week and the patient may die from exhaustion, from asphyxia or from aspiration pneumonia. In less severe cases convulsions may not commence for about a week after the first sign of rigidity and in very mild infections they may never appear.

Rarely the only manifestation of the disease may be *local tetanus*—stiffness or spasm of the muscles near the infected wound—and the prognosis is good if treatment is commenced at this stage. If local tetanus follows wounds of the head and neck, the resulting irritation or paralysis of cranial nerves may resemble tuberculous meningitis or polioencephalitis and in cases of doubt the cerebrospinal fluid should be examined; in tetanus it is normal. Lumbar punctures should be avoided except in cases of real doubt.

The diagnosis is made on clinical grounds. It is rarely possible to isolate the infecting organism from the original locus of entry. Spasm of the masseters due to dental abscess, septic throat or other causes is painful, in contradistinction to tetanus.

Prognosis. The mortality in countries where tetanus is common is nearly 100 per cent in the newborn and around 40 per cent for others, being worse for young children and the elderly. Even with all modern aids, as described below, the mortality is still considerable.

Treatment. Treatment should be begun as soon as possible and because of the technical difficulties and the seriousness of the complications, this should be undertaken in hospital. The essentials are as follows:

1. PREVENTION OF FURTHER ABSORPTION OF TOXIN FROM THE WOUND. A single intravenous injection of immune serum containing 20,000 i.u. of antitoxin should be given immediately the diagnosis is suspected. Whenever possible *human* antitetanus globulin should be used. The wound requires to be thoroughly cleaned and drained if there is evidence of necrotic tissue, foreign body or sepsis. Surgery should not be undertaken until 1 hour after the injection of antitoxin. Benzylpenicillin should be administered in doses of 300 mg 6 hourly as it is effective against *Cl. tetani*.

2. CONTROL OF SPASMS

(*a*) *General Measures.* The patient should lie in a quiet darkened room on a flat comfortable bed, with the bedclothes supported by a cradle. A notice should be put outside the door requesting silence. All necessary manipulation of the patient should be done gently and with due warning, for unexpected stimuli are particularly liable to provoke spasms. Expert nursing is of supreme importance.

(*b*) *Sedatives and Antispasmodics.* In most cases spasms may be prevented by diazepam. In more serious cases curare should be given intravenously, but only when facilities for assisted respiration are available. The aim of such measures is to control spasms which are terrifying, exhausting and occasionally fatal from asphyxia.

3. GENERAL MEASURES. Sufficient food and fluids are of vital importance to enable the patient to survive an ordeal which may be prolonged and violent. In milder cases it may be possible for the patient to swallow fluids or to tolerate a stomach tube left *in situ*. If oral treatment is impossible, intravenous feeding should be commenced without delay. Aspiration of bronchial secretions and antibiotic treatment of pneumonia may be necessary.

Prevention. Active immunisation should be given in accordance with the in-structions on page 60.

Contaminated injuries must be treated by debridement. The immediate danger of tetanus can be greatly reduced by the injection of a large dose of a long-acting preparation of penicillin followed by a 10-day course of oral penicillin. If wound sepsis is present cloxacillin should be given as penicillin may be inactivated by penicillinase produced by staphylococci. When the risk of tetanus is judged to be present, further protection may be given by a subcutaneous injection of 250 units of human tetanus antitoxin, and an intramuscular injection of toxoid which should be repeated one month and six months later. For those already protected a booster dose of toxoid should be given.

Brucellosis
(Undulant Fever; Malta Fever; Abortus Fever)

Undulant fever is caused in Britain by infection with *Brucella abortus* which is usually spread to man by the ingestion of raw milk from infected cattle. It is also an occupational hazard of veterinary surgeons, laboratory personnel, slaughter-house workers and others. In Malta, the disease is due to *Br. melitensis* and is transmitted by infected goat's milk. In the USA and the Far East *Br. suis* acquired from pigs may be the causative organism. The disease is not notifiable. The incubation period is about 3 weeks.

Clinical Features. The disease commences as a blood stream infection and the clinical manifestations are gradual in onset and variable. The symptoms in order of frequency are sweating, weakness, headache, anorexia, pain in limbs and back, constipation, rigors, cough, sore throat, and joint pains. The spleen may be palpable. The temperature characteristically shows undulations, during which febrile and afebrile periods alternate over periods of a week or so. In other cases the pyrexia may be continuous and sweating profuse. Untreated, the disease may last for a few days or continue for many months, and in the latter case the patient often becomes extremely depressed or irritable. Neutropenia and lymphocytosis usually occur in the more severe cases. Subacute arthritis of one or more joints may develop and occasionally radiological changes due to osteomyelitis of a vertebra can be demonstrated.

The diagnosis of undulant fever is most readily confirmed by agglutination and complement-fixation tests. Blood culture in special media should be attempted but it is rarely positive in *Br. abortus* infections in man. Other conditions causing prolonged fever must be considered in differential diagnosis (p. 57).

Treatment. Tetracycline 500 mg 6 hourly for 21 days is usually effective in the acute uncomplicated case, but for the chronic or relapsing disease a daily dose should be given of tetracycline (1 g), streptomycin (1 g) and sulphadimidine (4 g) for 2 or 3 weeks. Co-trimoxazole is also effective.

Prophylaxis. Undulant fever is prevented by the boiling or pasteurisation of all milk used for human consumption, as *Br. abortus* is readily destroyed by heat. The disease in animals is being eradicated in Britain by methods which have already succeeded in parts of Europe.

Meningococcal Infections

Infections caused by the Gram-negative diplococcus, *Neisseria meningitidis*, are serious and not infrequently fatal. In the Sudan savanna belt of Africa special climatic conditions predispose to annual outbreaks of 10,000 to 100,000 cases. Spread is by the airborne route and epidemics occur, particularly in cramped living conditions or when the climate is hot and dry. The organism invades through the nasopharynx producing bacteraemia and usually also pyogenic meningitis. The meningococcus is the commonest cause of bacterial meningitis in Britain where an increasing proportion of meningococci have become sulphonamide-resistant; fortunately, all strains remain sensitive to penicillin.

Clinical Features. The disease may present in a fulminating form with abrupt onset and prostration associated with shock and a widespread purpuric rash. The progression of the infection may be relentless even with chemotherapy and the patient can die within hours of the first symptom as a result of haemorrhage into the adrenal glands (p. 541). Disseminated intravascular coagulation (p. 634) can also occur in the course of meningococcal infections.

Meningitis (p. 713) is a much commoner presentation. Upper respiratory symptoms for 1 to 2 days are followed by fever, vomiting, headache and usually a petechial rash. This frequently starts with a few lesions on the buttocks spreading to involve limbs and trunk. The spots can remain petechial but occasionally large purpuric areas may form. The patient, often a child, is febrile and toxic, and signs of meningeal irritation are common. Convulsions may occur, especially in babies.

Chronic meningococcaemia is a rare condition in which the patient can be unwell for weeks or even months with recurrent fever, sweating, joint pains and transient rash.

Diagnosis. There is a polymorph leucocytosis. The CSF is turbid due to the presence of many polymorphs, the protein content is raised and the glucose reduced. The diagnosis is confirmed bacteriologically by culture of *N. meningitidis* from blood or CSF. The CSF should be stained by Gram's method when intracellular bean-shaped diplococci may be seen. However, in a proportion of cases, particularly if the patient has been treated with an antibiotic prior to admission to hospital, Gram stain and culture of CSF may be unhelpful and an early clinical diagnosis is therefore of the utmost importance in a disease which can be so rapidly fatal.

Treatment and Prevention. Benzylpenicillin, given initially by intravenous injection, is the antibiotic of choice for meningococcal infection. Because of superior penetration of the 'blood–brain barrier' sulphadimidine is frequently given as well as penicillin, but this is not necessary. An intravenous infusion should be set up and shock treated (p. 193). Intravascular coagulation may be an indication for heparin therapy (p. 634).

Close contacts of patients with meningococcal infections, especially children, should be given a 5-day course of sulphadimidine (p. 88).

Venereal Disease

Venereal diseases are almost invariably contracted during coitus. Gonorrhoea and other forms of urethritis are common in Britain, but syphilis is relatively rare.

Chancroid (p. 869) and granuloma venereum (p. 854) are frequent in the tropics. About half of the male cases of venereal disease result from homosexual contacts.

Gonorrhoea

Gonorrhoea is due to infection of the mucous membrane of the genitourinary tract with *Neisseria gonorrhoeae*. The eyes, anal canal, rectum and throat may also be infected. The incubation period is about 3 to 10 days.

Clinical Features. In the male the infection starts in the anterior part of the urethra and tends to spread to the prostate and occasionally to the bladder or the epididymes. There is dysuria and a white or yellow discharge from the urethra. If untreated or inadequately treated the discharge becomes less copious or intermittent, or may be observed only on waking from sleep—a condition known as gleet.

In females the infection is mainly in the urethra, the cervix uteri and the Bartholinian glands. At the onset there is dysuria, vaginal discharge and some swelling of the vulva. The symptoms may be trivial and pass unnoticed. Extension up the genital tract leads to cervicitis and acute salpingitis. Infection of the conjunctiva of infants born of infected mothers causes a profuse purulent discharge and often damage to sight. This condition, known as *ophthalmia neonatorum*, is now rare in this country, but was formerly a frequent cause of blindness. Systemic spread of gonorrhoea may cause acute or chronic arthritis (p. 639) and iritis. Gonococcal septicaemia may occur and can be associated with skin lesions. These vary from discrete violaceous papules or vesicles to haemorrhagic papules and pustules, often surrounded by a zone of erythema.

Diagnosis. The clinical diagnosis is confirmed by the demonstration of intracellular Gram-negative kidney-shaped diplococci in pus from the infected areas. Culture of the exudate on the appropriate medium gives a much higher percentage of positive diagnoses than reliance on microscopic examinations alone and is essential for medicolegal purposes.

Treatment. A single injection of 2·4 g (2·4 million units) of procaine penicillin is usually sufficient to cure most infections. For refractory infections or those in which the gonococci have been shown to be relatively resistant to penicillin, twice this dose plus 1 g probenecid is indicated. Tetracycline, spectinomycin or kanamycin are effective alternatives for patients allergic to penicillin or infected with penicillin-resistant gonococci. Gonococcal conjunctivitis responds to penicillin solution instilled into the conjunctival sac. It should also be given intramuscularly. In women, infection with *Trichomonas vaginalis* is also commonly present and requires treatment with metronidazole (Flagyl) 200 mg thrice daily by mouth for 7 days. It is essential to establish that cure of gonorrhoea and any accompanying infection is complete by culturing secretions from the infected area. The presence of syphilis acquired at the same time as gonorrhoea may be obscured by chemotherapy; it is obligatory that serological tests for syphilis should be carried out 3 months after treatment.

Non-specific Urethritis

In Britain urethritis in males is more commonly due to organisms other than the gonococcus. Many cases are due to infection with mycoplasmas or chlamydiae but in a considerable number of patients no organism can be detected. Treatment is with tetracycline. Non-specific urethritis also occurs in Reiter's disease (p. 639).

Syphilis

This is a chronic infection due to *Treponema pallidum*. It is convenient to describe untreated syphilis in three stages—primary, secondary and tertiary. It must be realised, however, that the disease is generalised and continuous from the time of infection, and that it may be almost completely latent during its long course which may last for over 30 years.

Clinical Manifestations. PRIMARY STAGE. The primary lesion (chancre) develops at the site of infection. It occurs usually on the genitals, but it may be found on the lips, in the mouth, at the anus, or on a finger. The incubation period is 10 days to 10 weeks. A small painless indurated swelling forms and usually ulcerates. The regional lymph nodes are enlarged, firm, painless, and seldom suppurate.

SECONDARY STAGE. The primary lesions tend to heal, and from about the third to sixth month evidence of generalised infection becomes apparent. The patient may have malaise, headaches, sore throat and low irregular fever.

Four cardinal signs must be remembered, though any of them may be absent.

(1) *Cutaneous Rashes*. The most common early rash is a faint macular erythema which may be perceptible only in a good light. Later the rashes are characteristically polymorphic, symmetrical, of a dull red colour, do not itch and may become scaly.

(2) *Condylomata*. In moist areas, such as in the perineum, the lesions become heaped up and are known as condylomata; they contain spirochaetes and are highly infective.

(3) *Mucous Patches*. The mucous membranes of the mouth are commonly affected by shallow ulcers with a narrow red edge and a surface covered by a thin whitish membrane. Their appearance has given rise to the descriptive term of snail track ulcers. They are highly infective.

(4) *Lymphadenopathy*. There may be generalised painless enlargement of the lymph nodes.

In over 30 per cent of cases changes occur in the cerebrospinal fluid, indicating that there has been some involvement of the central nervous system; the clinical features of meningitis may be present, accompanied sometimes by cranial nerve palsies. Rarely there may be clinical evidence of involvement of any other part of the body. After several months the secondary changes gradually disappear to be followed by a latent period lasting from 2 to 30 years.

TERTIARY STAGE. In this stage lesions appear almost anywhere, but particularly in the skin and subcutaneous tissues, bone, tongue, testes, liver, aorta (p. 242) and central nervous system (p. 716). The affected structure is infiltrated with granulation tissue containing plasma cells and lymphocytes. There is endarteritis obliterans which causes necrosis. The formation of a localised necrotic swelling, which is characteristically painless, is known as a gumma.

Congenital Syphilis. The fetus may contract syphilis from an infected mother. There is then no primary stage. The damage done may be such that the child is born dead or skin eruptions may be present at birth. The child may appear to be normal at birth but fails to thrive, and within a few months presents with rashes, and signs of syphilitic disease of bone, liver, kidneys and other organs. In yet a third group of cases the overt manifestations may be delayed until late childhood, when such findings appear as deformities of bone and teeth, iritis, keratitis, juvenile tabes or general paralysis.

Congenital syphilis is now rare, as treatment of a syphilitic woman during pregnancy will ensure the birth of a normal baby.

Diagnosis. In the primary and early secondary stages, the spirochaete may be demonstrated in serum from the chancre, condylomata or mucous patches. The serological tests for syphilis become positive from about the fourth week of the disease onwards and are invariably strongly positive by the end of the third month in untreated cases. It should be realised that non-specific antigen is used in the usual serological screening tests—Wassermann (WR), Kahn and Venereal Disease Research Laboratory (VDRL) tests. Hence the specificity and sensitivity of such tests is variable. False positive tests may be found temporarily in glandular fever, systemic lupus erythematosus and other generalised diseases, while negative tests may be observed in many patients with late syphilis. For conclusive results additional tests which use specific treponemal antigen, e.g. fluorescent treponemal antibody (FTA) and treponemal immobilisation tests (TPI), may be required.

Treatment. *T. pallidum*, though very sensitive to benzylpenicillin, has to be exposed to it for longer periods than most micro-organisms if a spirochaeticidal effect is to be obtained. Hence the longer-acting forms of penicillin such as procaine penicillin are used. A patient suffering from early primary (sero-negative) syphilis requires 600 mg procaine penicillin daily for 10 consecutive days. For sero-positive primary cases and for secondary syphilis double this dosage should be given for 20 days. Several such courses may be required for patients with tertiary syphilis. If the patient is allergic to penicillin, tetracycline should be used.

Leptospirosis

Although over 100 serotypes of leptospires have been identified only *Leptospira icterohaemorrhagiae* and *L. canicola* have been shown to cause human disease in Britain.

The natural host of *Weil's disease*, caused by *L. icterohaemorrhagiae*, is the rat. An infected rat's urine contains the organisms which can penetrate the skin or mucosa of a man. Fish cleaners, farm workers, veterinarians, and vagrants are those most at risk. Immersion in canals or stagnant water may also result in sporadic infection.

Infection by *L. canicola*, which is contracted from dogs and pigs, usually presents as aseptic meningitis or pyrexia of unknown origin. It is not often associated with jaundice and is a less severe disease in contrast to Weil's disease.

Pathology. In patients dying from Weil's disease, there is a combination of hepatic, renal and cardiac failure. The changes in the liver are non-specific; in severe cases, there may be centrilobular and even massive necrosis. Oedema and inflammatory exudate lead to intralobular biliary stasis. In the kidneys, the glomeruli are usually spared, but the tubules are affected and contain haemoglobin and myoglobin casts. The main findings in the myocardium are focal haemorrhages, interstitial oedema and cellular infiltration. A similar picture is seen in skeletal muscle.

Clinical Features. The average incubation period is 10 days, the range being 4 to 21 days. A high proportion of infections are subclinical or cause a mild undiagnosed fever. In the more severe infections the illness begins abruptly with headache, severe myalgia, pyrexia, conjunctival suffusion, anorexia and vomiting. Infrequently, there are skin rashes or petechiae and enlargement of the liver and spleen.

After about a week leptospiral antibodies appear in the blood. The temperature falls by lysis and is usually normal for 2 or 3 days. In the majority of patients, there is further pyrexia for a few days and transient meningism (p. 714) followed by prompt recovery. In other cases, especially those caused by *L. icterohaemorrhagiae*, during this phase, hepatitis, tubular necrosis, myocarditis and meningitis may occur. The cause of these serious complications is uncertain but cell damage from immune complexes is a possible explanation.

Hepatitis is indicated by epigastric pain, tenderness in the right upper quadrant of the abdomen and jaundice. In severe cases, jaundice deepens, there is marked anorexia, vomiting and a haemorrhagic tendency. The condition may progress to acute liver necrosis (p. 443). *Renal tubular necrosis* may lead to acute renal failure (p. 495). *Myocarditis* is suggested by tachycardia, fall in blood pressure and cardiac enlargement. The development of profound hypotension, arrhythmias and cardiac failure are ominous signs. *Meningitis* causes severe headache, neck stiffness and a positive Kernig's sign (p. 714) and is the usual clinical picture in *L. canicola* infections.

By the third and fourth week of the illness, the majority of patients enter the convalescent phase. When there has been serious involvement of the liver, kidneys and heart, mortality in Weil's disease is in the region of 15 to 20 per cent. Those who recover do so completely.

Laboratory Data. Most patients with leptospirosis show a polymorphonuclear leucocytosis. When there is liver involvement, liver function tests indicate a mild hepatocellular jaundice with an intrahepatic obstructive element; bilirubin and urobilinogen are present in the urine. In patients with renal failure the urine contains protein, red blood cells and cellular and granular casts; in severe cases the rise in blood urea is progressive. In myocarditis there is electrocardiographic evidence of conduction disturbances and arrhythmias. Meningitis is characterised by an increase of lymphocytes in the cerebrospinal fluid with little or no rise in protein; xanthochromia may be observed in the jaundiced patient. Apart from the few patients developing severe haemorrhagic pneumonia, scattered opacities probably due to haemorrhage are seen on radiography of the chest in 10 to 20 per cent of cases.

The diagnosis is made by culturing the organism from the blood in the first week or from the urine in the second and third weeks. Alternatively, blood or urine specimens may be inoculated into a guinea-pig. From the second week onwards, a rising titre of specific leptospiral antibodies is found. The titre may not reach diagnostic levels in those cases treated promptly.

Treatment. Leptospires are sensitive to penicillin *in vitro*. Benzylpenicillin, 600 mg (1 million units) 6 hourly for 7 days is effective provided it is given early enough and in adequate doses; it shortens the average illness and reduces the incidence of complications. Penicillin is of doubtful value if treatment is initiated late in the infection. Appropriate fluid replacement is important during the period of acute illness. In severely affected patients supportive treatment for acute liver necrosis, acute renal failure, arrhythmias and cardiac failure may be required.

Measles

Measles (morbilli) is a viral disease which spreads by droplet infection. One attack confers a high degree of immunity. Most people suffer from measles in childhood, and a mother who has had the disease confers passive immunity on her infant for the first six months of life. Measles is very severe in many tropical countries with a high mortality. The disease is notifiable in England but not in Scotland. The incubation period is about 10 days to the commencement of the catarrhal stage. A quarantine period is not necessary.

Clinical Features. *Catarrhal Stage.* Measles commences in much the same way as a common cold. There is an acute febrile onset, with nasal catarrh, sneezing, redness of the conjunctivae, some swelling of the eyelids and watering of the eyes. In addition a short cough, hoarseness of the voice due to laryngitis, and photophobia usually appear by the second day. At this stage, a diagnosis of measles may be made from the presence of Koplik's spots on the mucous membrane of the mouth. These are small white spots surrounded by a narrow zone of inflammation. Though often numerous on the inside of the cheeks, they may be sparse and confined to the region around the opening of the parotid duct. The disease is highly infectious during the catarrhal stage and the child is miserable and irritable.

Exanthematous Stage. After 3 or 4 days of the catarrhal stage, the diagnostic Koplik's spots disappear while the dark red macular or maculopapular skin rash develops. The rash is first seen at the back of the ears and at the junction of the forehead and the hair. Within a few hours there is invasion of the whole skin area, and there is usually some accentuation of fever. As the spots rapidly become more numerous they fuse to form the characteristic blotchy appearance of measles. The face is ordinarily the most densely covered area. When the rash is fully erupted in 2 or 3 days, it tends to deepen in colour and then fade into a faint brown staining followed by a fine desquamation of the skin. The malaise and the fever subside as the rash fades.

Complications. Convulsions occur in young children and are commonest as the rash is appearing. Secondary infection by haemolytic streptococci, pneumococci or staphylococci is sometimes responsible for the development of otitis media and pneumonia which are particularly dangerous in the first 18 months of life. Persistent conjunctivitis may be followed by corneal ulceration which, if neglected, may result in impairment of vision. Stomatitis, gastroenteritis, appendicitis and encephalitis (pp. 721 and 728) may also occur.

Diagnosis. Considerable difficulty may arise in those cases in which a prodromal rash indistinguishable from *scarlet fever* develops in the catarrhal stage. However, in measles Koplik's spots are present and the eyes have the appearance of those of a child that has recently been crying. The differential diagnosis from *rubella* is discussed on page 82. It is important to remember that *drug rashes* are common and may simulate closely the eruption of measles, rubella or scarlet fever.

Treatment. The patient should be isolated if possible and excluded from school for 14 days from the appearance of the rash. Most cases of measles, in spite of the high temperature, remain uncomplicated, and antibiotics should be prescribed only for unequivocal bacterial complications. Contacts should be examined daily for the first sign of infection.

Prevention. ACTIVE IMMUNISATION. One injection of live attenuated measles virus should be given subcutaneously in children over one year old who have not had the disease. This may be followed by a mild febrile disturbance.

PASSIVE IMMUNISATION. Human immunoglobulin, given intramuscularly, is recommended for the prevention or attenuation of measles, particularly for contacts under 18 months of age and for debilitated children. The dose is 250 mg for children under one year old and 500 mg for those over this age.

German Measles

German measles (rubella) is a viral disease which spreads by droplet infection. One attack confers a high degree of immunity. It tends to affect older children, adolescents and young adults and spreads less readily than measles. The disease in children is trivial. In adults the illness may be more severe, but of short duration and of little importance except when it develops in a woman during the first four months of pregnancy. In such cases the child may be born with a congenital malformation such as a cardiac or mental defect, cataract or deafness. The risk of damage to the fetus by the rubella virus varies from over 50 per cent during the first 4 weeks of pregnancy to virtually zero after the end of the fourth month. The disease is not notifiable. The incubation period is usually about 18 days. A quarantine period is not necessary.

Clinical Features. In children the constitutional symptoms are so slight that the illness is rarely suspected until the rash is seen. The spots are pink macules which appear first behind the ears and on the forehead. The rash spreads rapidly, first to the trunk and then to the limbs. A minor degree of conjunctival suffusion is common. Slightly tender enlargement of the suboccipital lymph nodes is usual and these appear before the rash or even in its absence. Sometimes many groups of lymph nodes are affected and the tip of the spleen may be palpable. In adolescents and adults the onset may be acute with fever and generalised aches, but even then the illness lasts for only 2 or 3 days.

Complications. Polyarthritis, affecting especially the smaller joints, is undoubtedly the commonest complication and it is seen mostly in adult women. Encephalomyelitis and thrombocytopenic purpura are very rare. Complete recovery from all of them is the rule.

Diagnosis. The disease may be distinguished from *measles* by its trivial nature, its brief duration, the pink colour of the rash, the absence of Koplik's spots and the presence of enlargement of cervical lymph nodes. The morphology of the rash of rubella may vary from one epidemic to another. Sometimes there is a close resemblance to the punctate erythema of *scarlet fever*, but in rubella the circumoral region is not spared. *Infectious mononucleosis* is another disease which should be considered in the differential diagnosis (p. 615). *Rashes due to drugs* may have a similar appearance and since they commonly occur, enquiry should always be made in regard to the taking of medicines.

The diagnosis can be confirmed by isolation of the virus from the throat or by demonstration of a rising titre of antibodies in the blood.

Treatment. No treatment is available. Indeed none is required except for non-immune women who are exposed to infection during the first four months of pregnancy. Then human immunoglobulin should be given at once, though its efficacy in protecting the fetus is in doubt. It is advisable to vaccinate all girls between their 11th and 13th birthdays who have not had the disease. Women of child-bearing age who are found to be serologically negative should also be offered vaccine provided that they are not pregnant and are willing to avoid pregnancy for eight weeks after vaccination.

If infection is known to have occurred during the first 16 weeks of pregnancy there is such a high chance of fetal abnormality that termination should be recommended.

Mumps

Mumps is caused by a virus which spreads by droplet infection and affects mainly children of school age and young adults. The infectivity rate is not high and there is serological evidence that 30–40 per cent of infections are clinically inapparent. The incubation period is about 18 days. A quarantine period is not necessary.

Clinical Features. Malaise, fever, trismus and pain near the angle of the jaw is soon followed by tender swelling of one or both parotid glands. Indeed, parotid swelling alone is often the first feature. The submandibular salivary glands may also be involved. The swollen glands subside in a few days, and may be succeeded by swelling of a previously unaffected gland. Orchitis occurs in about one in four males who develop mumps after puberty; it is usually on one side only, but if it is bilateral, sterility may be a sequel. Obscure abdominal pain may be due to pancreatitis or oöphoritis. Acute lymphocytic meningitis is another mode of presentation. Encephalomyelitis is rare.

Diagnosis. Most cases of mumps can be diagnosed on clinical grounds alone, but the diagnosis can be confirmed in doubtful cases by the demonstration of specific antibodies, or the virus may be cultured from the saliva, or from the cerebrospinal fluid in meningitis. Suppurative parotitis is distinguished by the circumstances of onset in an old, frail, ill, febrile or dehydrated patient in whom oral hygiene is poor, and confirmed by obtaining pus from the parotid duct. Calculous obstruction of the parotid duct is rare; it is relatively common in the submandibular duct where the stone can often be felt. Sarcoidosis may cause enlargement of the parotid glands and is usually painless and accompanied by other signs especially uveitis.

Treatment. Oral hygiene is important when the mouth is very dry due to lack of saliva. Difficulty in opening the mouth may necessitate feeding through a straw. Apart from the relief of symptoms as they appear, no other treatment is necessary. Orchitis can be relieved by the administration of prednisolone for a few days without apparent danger of dissemination of infection. Cases of mumps should be isolated until the gland last affected has subsided.

Chickenpox

Chickenpox (varicella) is a viral infection which spreads by droplets from the upper respiratory tract or by contamination from the discharge from ruptured lesions of the skin or through contact with herpes zoster (p. 723). Herpes zoster is due to reactivation of infection with chickenpox virus. It may be accompanied by a varicelliform rash. Chickenpox is highly infectious and chiefly affects children under 10 years of age. Most children are little incommoded by this disease but, as often happens with viral infections, adults may develop a more severe illness including a prodromal rash. A suspicion of smallpox may easily be aroused. Second attacks are very rare. In patients on long-term steroid therapy the disease may be severe or even fatal. Most recorded fatalities have been suffering from leukaemia and it is probable that the blood disorder has been the major factor in reducing resistance to the virus. The disease is not notifiable. The incubation period is about a fortnight. A quarantine period is not necessary.

Clinical Features. Constitutional symptoms are usually brief and mild, and the first sign of the disease is often the appearance of the rash. Lesions are sometimes present on the palate before the characteristic rash appears on the trunk on the second day of the illness. Then the face and finally the limbs are involved. The spots

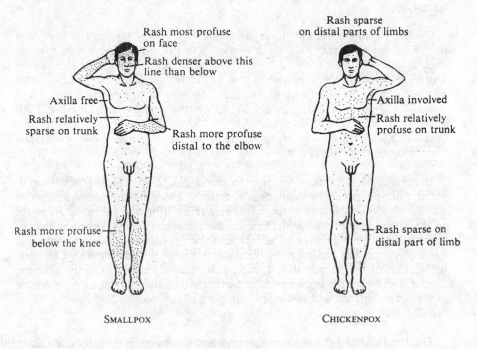

SMALLPOX

Rash most profuse on face
Rash denser above this line than below
Axilla free
Rash relatively sparse on trunk
Rash more profuse distal to the elbow
Rash more profuse below the knee

CHICKENPOX

Rash sparse on distal parts of limbs
Axilla involved
Rash relatively profuse on trunk
Rash sparse on distal part of limb

Fig. 3.1 Smallpox: Note *peripheral* distribution of the rash. Chickenpox: Note *central* distribution of the rash.

reach their maximum density upon the trunk, and are more sparse on the periphery of the limbs. The axillae should be inspected as this region is almost invariably affected, while in smallpox the reverse is true (Fig. 3.1). Macules appear first and within a few hours the lesions become papular and then vesicular. The vesicles are unilocular, very superficial and thin-walled. The shape is elliptical rather than spherical. Within 24 hours the lesions become pustular. The vesicles and pustules are so fragile that they may be ruptured by the chafing of garments. Damage from scratching is also frequent, since itching may be troublesome. Whether or not the pustules rupture, they dry up in a few days to form scabs. The spots appear in crops, so that lesions at all stages of development are seen in any area at the same time. The course of the disease is usually uneventful.

Complications. The only common complication is secondary infection of the lesions by staphylococci and streptococci. Acute demyelinating encephalomyelitis may occur (p. 728). Chickenpox pneumonia (p. 276) or myocarditis may also rarely cause a very serious illness.

Diagnosis. Although the typical case of chickenpox presents no diagnostic problem it is important to remember that great difficulty may be encountered in cases of modified smallpox and variola minor. When the rash has fully developed, however, the peripheral distribution of the lesions in smallpox is preserved. Serious consideration of the possibility of smallpox must be given to apparent cases of chickenpox occurring in patients who have just returned from an endemic area or during an outbreak of smallpox. Typical variola major may be distinguished by certain features which contrast with those of chickenpox. In smallpox

(a) there is a prodromal illness of 2 to 4 days;
(b) the density of the lesions is greatest at the periphery, the rash is relatively profuse on convex and exposed surfaces, and the axillae are not affected (Fig. 3.1);
(c) the spots are deep-set, multilocular, circular lesions and are present predominantly at a single stage of development.

Treatment. No treatment is required in the majority of cases. At the first sign of secondary infection a local antiseptic should be applied to the skin, e.g. chlorhexidine (Hibitane). If bacterial infection progresses, an appropriate antibiotic should be prescribed. Children who lack natural immunity owing to leukaemia, immunological deficiency, or treatment with corticosteroid or cytotoxic drugs, and who have been in contact with chickenpox should be given an injection of human anti-chickenpox gammaglobulin.

Spread of infection can be prevented by isolation of the patient and the sterilisation of all soiled articles, but the disease is usually so mild that in domiciliary practice these precautions are not normally required.

Smallpox

The virus of variola major (severe or 'classical' smallpox) causes a highly infectious and frequently fatal disease which spreads by droplet infection from the respiratory tract or by contamination with material from the skin lesions. There are also two variants of this virus: (1) variola minor virus causes a much milder disease, which is similar in its clinical features and mode of spread, but is seldom fatal; (2) vaccinia virus (cowpox) is seldom the cause of systemic disease, and cannot be spread readily from one person to another. Immune antibodies to all these viruses are developed in response to infection by any one of them, though vaccinia gives rise to a less permanent immunity than an attack of variola. Smallpox has been eliminated from Britain, where it was at one time a terrible scourge, but it may be re-introduced from abroad. Smallpox still exists in Ethiopia; the World Health Organisation has eradicated the disease elsewhere. The incubation period of smallpox is usually 12 days (extremes 7 to 16 days). The quarantine period is 18 days.

Clinical Features. In Britain there may be a history of contact or knowledge that the disease has recently been introduced into the country or that the patient has just come from abroad. In a known suspect, the disease must be considered at the onset of any febrile illness within the quarantine period, and it can be excluded only by the certain knowledge of a recent successful vaccination. Variola major begins abruptly with severe systemic disturbances which antedate the appearance of the characteristic rash. The principal symptoms of the *prodromal illness* are malaise, shivering, frontal headache, pain in the back, sore throat, cough and hoarseness of the voice. A fleeting erythematous or morbilliform rash is sometimes seen, but petechial or purpuric rashes at this stage indicate that the disease will probably be fatal. Vesicles may form on the buccal, faucial, pharyngeal, laryngeal and nasal mucosa and are soon transformed into shallow grey ulcers. On the second or third day of the illness the characteristic *skin eruption* of smallpox appears. The order of the development and the distribution of the lesions are of the utmost importance in diagnosis. Macules appear first on the forehead and the wrists, then the arms, the trunk—especially the back—then the legs. The lesions are more dense on the extremities and on the extensor surfaces than on the concavities and the flexor surfaces, and the axillae in particular are spared. The hands and forearms, the feet and legs, and the upper part of the face are covered more densely than the upper arms, the thighs and the lower part of the face (Fig. 3.1). The density of the rash is always greater upon the limbs and forehead than upon the trunk, though the back and, to a lesser extent, the abdomen may be extensively affected in a severe case. The rash develops in a regular sequence. Macules turn to deep-set, dark-pink papules in a matter of hours. The final appearance of papules may take 2 or 3 days. The conversion of papules to vesicles then commences with those lesions which were first to appear, and the whole process may take a further 24 hours. The vesicles feel hard and are not easily ruptured, for they are deep-set and multilocular. The outline of the lesions is circular. After about 2 days the vesicular stage merges into the pustular stage. The pustules are surrounded by a zone of erythema at first, but this gradually disappears. During the ensuing 8 or 9 days the pustules gradually dry up to form dark-brown or almost black scabs. These separate after several days leaving pitted scars or 'pocks'.

After the initial fever and the outbreak of the rash, the patient improves and the temperature may fall to normal for a short period. During the pustular stage, however, the temperature rises again and the patient becomes extremely toxic. The severity of this recrudescence is proportional to the extent of the rash. The patient is in a miserable state, for in addition to feeling exceedingly ill, there is oedema of the skin and ulceration of the conjunctivae, mouth, throat, larynx and trachea; a concomitant pneumonia is common.

Complications. Heart and circulatory failure may result from toxaemia. Secondary bacterial invasion of the ulcerated respiratory tract gives rise to bronchitis and pneumonia. There may be delirium or convulsions, and encephalomyelitis may occur. Lesions of the conjunctiva may lead to corneal ulcer and impairment or loss of vision. Mortality in major smallpox approaches 40 per cent.

Differential Diagnosis. A typical case of smallpox presents little diagnostic difficulty. It is essential, however, to emphasise that the diagnosis of variola major developing in a patient who is partially immune owing to previous vaccination (modified smallpox) may present the greatest difficulties. In variola minor or in modified smallpox the prodromal illness is less severe and the secondary fever is slight or absent. The rash may be sparse and considerably modified in many of its features, but the distribution of the lesions is nearly always typical.

The chief differential diagnosis is from chickenpox, and the points of distinction have already been mentioned on page 85.

Treatment. General nursing care by attendants who have been recently vaccinated is the essence of treatment. The prevention of secondary infection by special care in the hygiene of the mouth and of the skin is of importance; when infection occurs appropriate antibacterial therapy must be employed. When the last scab has been shed the patient is no longer infectious.

Prevention. Effective vaccination programmes, the isolation of cases and the quarantine of contacts are measures which are expected soon to eliminate smallpox for ever. International regulations for vaccination are given on page 933. Vaccination is contraindicated in the presence of active skin diseases, especially infantile eczema, owing to the probable development of generalised vaccinia, which may be fatal. Should generalised vaccinia occur, the outlook can be improved by the injection of human antivaccinial immunoglobulin. Other contraindications to smallpox vaccination include pregnancy, coricosteroid or immuno-suppressive therapy and leukaemia.

CHEMOTHERAPY OF INFECTIONS

The concept of chemotherapy is almost as old as the science of bacteriology. Attempts were made in the late nineteenth century to treat infections such as tuberculosis by the injection of other organisms or their products. The ability of one micro-organism to interfere with the growth of another is called antibiosis and is due to specific diffusible metabolic products termed *antibiotics*.

Early in the twentieth century Ehrlich synthesised drugs such as trypan red and organic arsenical compounds which were antiprotozoal and antispirochaetal. However, it was not until Domagk and Trefouel in 1935 demonstrated the therapeutic effect of sulphanilamide that systemic antibacterial chemotherapy became available. Penicillin, the first antibiotic suitable for systemic use, was introduced in 1940. Since then methodical research has produced a wide range of antibiotics and a variety of chemotherapeutic agents such as metronidazole, trimethoprim, dapsone and isoniazid. A general term for all of these substances is *antimicrobial agent*. Effective chemotherapy is now available against all known bacteria, rickettsiae, mycoplasmas and chlamydiae. Many specific antiprotozoal compounds are used in the treatment of diseases such as sleeping sickness, kala azar, malaria and amoebic dysentery. Topical antifungal agents are widely prescribed, but fully effective, non-toxic, antifungal drugs have not yet been found for use in systemic infection. Antimicrobial agents active against viruses have also been discovered but few have been successful therapeutically.

The Sulphonamides

Although the sulphonamides have been superseded in many countries by antibiotics, their usefulness has been greatly extended by the introduction of co-trimoxazole, a combination of a sulphonamide and trimethoprim. This compound is, however, relatively expensive compared with other sulphonamides. The preparations most suitable for clinical use are the *short-acting sulphonamides*, e.g. sulphadimidine. It is rapidly absorbed and quickly excreted in the urine in a soluble form. Administration is every 4 to 8 hours, by mouth; a preparation is also available for intravenous or intramuscular administration.

The most common indication for the use of sulphonamides is acute cystitis. A dose of 1 g, 8 hourly is adequate since the drugs give high concentrations in the urine. If this fails, treatment with other antibacterial agents, selected on the basis of laboratory culture, should be undertaken. Sulphonamides have long been used in the treatment of meningococcal infection, particularly meningitis; unfortunately the incidence of resistant strains is increasing and therefore penicillin is now used in treating this condition.

Non-absorbable sulphonamides such as succinylsulphathiazole are used, frequently combined with neomycin, to control the growth of organisms in the lower bowel, e.g. in preoperative preparation of the colon.

Adverse Effects. Sulphonamides have a wide range of potential hazards, but with the short-acting group these are probably no greater than with many other groups of antimicrobial agents. Rashes, fever, agranulocytosis, haematuria and anuria are sometimes encountered. The risks of haematuria and anuria can be decreased by ensuring an adequate output of alkaline urine. Serious but rare complications are haemolytic anaemia, purpura and pancytopenia. Glucose-6-phosphate dehydrogenase deficiency (p. 821) is a contraindication to the use of sulphonamides, as haemolysis may be induced. The Stevens–Johnson syndrome (erythema multiforme and ulceration of mucous membranes) may be induced by sulphonamide and can be fatal. When any of the above complications develop the drug must be stopped immediately. Cyanosis due to methaemoglobinaemia, and nausea and vomiting, which were commonly encountered with earlier preparations, rarely occur with the newer, short-acting forms.

Sulphonamides can detach protein-bound drugs such as warfarin and sulphonylurea antidiabetic agents and thereby cause overdosage.

Sulphonamide preparations applied to the skin are liable to cause light sensitivity which may persist for a number of years; they should not be used topically.

Co-trimoxazole. The two components of this compound, trimethoprim and sulphamethoxazole, act by inhibiting enzymes at two successive stages in the synthesis of para-aminobenzoic acid to folic acid and DNA. Co-trimoxazole is thus bactericidal whereas sulphonamide is bacteriostatic and it is particularly useful in exacerbations of chronic bronchitis and infections of the urinary tract. It is also effective in the treatment of invasive Salmonella infections and typhoid carriers. The adult dose is 2 tablets twice daily and there is a preparation for intravenous infusion.

The adverse effects are those of the sulphonamides but the clinician must also be on the alert for possible haematological reactions to trimethoprim including megaloblastic anaemia due to folate deficiency and also thrombocytopenia. The compound should not be given to pregnant women and care should be taken in the elderly, the chronic sick and others who may be folate-deficient; its prolonged use should be accompanied by monthly blood counts.

The Penicillins

All penicillins are bactericidal and the range of activity of the group is wide as both Gram-positive and certain Gram-negative organisms are sensitive to individual penicillins. The outstanding adverse effect is the risk of inducing a hypersensitivity reaction. Even so the penicillins are the most useful antibiotics at present available.

The principal penicillins are:

1. *Benzylpenicillin*, which is the original and most active penicillin; it must be given by injection. Its action can be prolonged by combining it with procaine—*procaine penicillin* and an even longer-acting form is *benzathine penicillin*.

2. *Phenoxymethylpenicillin*, which is absorbed when administered by mouth.

3. *Cloxacillin*, which is not inactivated by staphylococcal penicillinase and is reserved for the treatment of severe staphylococcal infections resistant to benzylpenicillin. *Flucloxacillin* is better absorbed than cloxacillin when given by mouth.

4. *Ampicillin* and its analogue *amoxycillin*, which are effective against Gram-negative bacilli, in contrast to the other penicillins whose activity is largely limited to Gram-positive organisms and Gram-negative cocci.

5. *Carbenicillin* is a broad spectrum penicillin which is effective against *Ps. aeruginosa*.

Benzylpenicillin. Benzylpenicillin is rapidly absorbed following intramuscular injection and is excreted by the kidneys within a few hours. A dose of 300 mg (half a million units) 6- or 8-hourly will suffice for most infections due to sensitive organisms. Large intramuscular or intravenous (up to 12 million units daily) doses may be required to achieve therapeutic concentrations within deep-seated or walled-off foci of infection, as occurs in infective endocarditis or lung abscess. The intramuscular injection of large doses is painful. Probenecid, 2 g daily by mouth will raise the blood level of penicillin by delaying its excretion by the kidney and allow smaller doses to be used.

Benzylpenicillin remains the antibiotic of choice for the treatment of pneumococcal, meningococcal and streptococcal infections, gonorrhoea and syphilis, yaws, diphtheria, tetanus, gas gangrene, anthrax and actinomycosis. It is also indicated for infections caused by penicillin-sensitive strains of *Staph. aureus*.

Penicillin is also used prophylactically. Benzylpenicillin is given to patients with valvular heart disease before a dental extraction to reduce the risk of infective endocarditis (p. 209). It is also given to prevent gas gangrene and tetanus after high amputations of ischaemic legs and for wounds containing dirt and devitalised tissue.

Benzylpenicillin passes in very small quantities into cerebrospinal fluid or pleural, pericardial or joint spaces. In the presence of inflammation its diffusion to these sites is greater. Benzylpenicillin may be given by local injection when treating severe infections of the meninges, joints, pleura or pericardium.

Procaine Penicillin and Benzathine Penicillin. These are long-acting penicillins given by injection and used in the treatment of gonorrhoea and the treponemal diseases, syphilis and yaws. *Procaine penicillin* in aqueous suspension, in a dose of 600 mg (1 million units) intramuscularly once daily, is relatively painless and will maintain an adequate blood level for 24 hours. *Benzathine penicillin* has a duration of action of 3 to 4 days. A single injection of 600,000 units has proved to be an effective cure for yaws, but the blood levels are inadequate for acute infections such as pneumonia. It can be used for the prophylaxis of rheumatic fever in patients who cannot be relied upon to take oral penicillin.

Phenoxymethylpenicillin is relatively unaffected by the acidity of the stomach and frequent oral administration will produce reasonable blood levels. The usual dose of phenoxymethylpenicillin is 500 mg every 4 to 6 hours, taken half an hour before meals to ensure maximum absorption. In patients who are seriously ill or vomiting, intramuscular benzylpenicillin is essential because of uncertainties in absorption. During recovery oral therapy may be substituted in such patients.

Phenoxymethylpenicillin is indicated for minor streptococcal infections and for pneumococcal pneumonia after initial therapy with benzylpenicillin. It is used prophylactically on a long-term basis following an attack of rheumatic fever to prevent recurrences. In addition to the obvious advantages of oral administration, severe anaphylactic reactions are rare when the antibiotic is given by mouth.

Cloxacillin. Unlike benzylpenicillin, this semisynthetic penicillin is unaffected by staphylococcal penicillinase. Cloxacillin should be kept in reserve for the treatment of severe infection caused by staphylococci resistant to benzylpenicillin. It can be given orally in a dose of 500 mg 6-hourly, but for seriously ill patients treatment should be initiated by the intramuscular injection of 1 g every 4 hours. Cloxacillin cannot be prescribed if the patient is allergic to benzylpenicillin. In these circumstances erythromycin or lincomycin should be used.

Flucloxacillin has an identical antibacterial range to cloxacillin. It is preferable for oral therapy as its absorption is more reliable.

Ampicillin. This is a semisynthetic penicillin which is effective by mouth and which has a bactericidal action against Gram-positive organisms and also a variety of Gram-negative organisms, including salmonellae, shigellae, *H. influenzae* and certain strains of *Esch. coli* and *Proteus*. It is inactivated by staphylococcal penicillinase. Ampicillin is of value in urinary tract infections due to *Esch. coli* and *Proteus* and in exacerbations of chronic bronchitis. It is a less effective alternative to chloramphenicol in enteric fever but is preferable in the treatment of Salmonella carriers. The dose is 250 mg to 1 g, 4- to 8-hourly by mouth. Preparations for injection are also available. Maculopapular rashes occur in approximately 5 per cent of all patients given ampicillin and in over 90 per cent of patients with infectious mononucleosis; this antibiotic should not therefore be prescribed for sore throats which may be due to glandular fever.

Amoxycillin is an analogue of ampicillin which has a similar antibacterial range but is better absorbed from the gastrointestinal tract. Amoxycillin is much more costly than ampicillin.

Carbenicillin. This has a wider range of activity than ampicillin against Gram-negative organisms and, in particular, is active against most, but not all strains of *Ps. aeruginosa*. Unfortunately, carbenicillin can be given only by injection and its administration by the intramuscular route is painful as large quantities are necessary. The standard dose for urinary tract infections is 1 g every 6 hours but up to 30 g per day by intravenous injection may be required for systemic *Ps. aeruginosa* infections, the incidence of which has increased in recent years, especially in debilitated patients and in urological wards. This antibiotic is very expensive.

Carfecillin is the phenol ester of carbenicillin and when given by mouth, it is absorbed and split into carbenicillin and the ester moiety. It may be used for lower urinary tract infections particularly those due to *Ps. aeruginosa*.

Adverse Effects of the Penicillins

An increasing number of patients have acquired hypersensitivity to the systemic administration of the penicillins. This takes the form of urticaria and pyrexia or of an acute anaphylactic reaction which has occasionally proved fatal. The factors responsible for sensitisation can be either a degradation product of the penicillin 'nucleus' or protein residues from the manufacturing process. In the former case the patient will be allergic to all the penicillins and none should be used again. In the latter case, cross-allergenicity between all penicillins does not necessarily occur. Ampicillin, for example, commonly produces a maculopapular rash which differs from penicillin-induced urticaria and is specific for ampicillin alone. It is almost certainly unrelated to true penicillin allergy and is therefore not a contraindication to future treatment with other penicillins. The patient should always be asked about previous allergy to any form of penicillin before treatment is commenced as a severe reaction may be provoked by the administration of only a few milligrams. Patients who suffer from bronchial asthma or are hypersensitive to other drugs are particularly liable to become allergic to penicillin.

Skin sensitisation may result from topical applications of any antibiotic, but is so frequent with penicillin that it should never be applied locally.

Although penicillin is otherwise a safe antibiotic, its accumulation in patients with renal failure may lead to encephalopathy, so that dosage in these circumstances must be guided by the blood levels. The injectable preparations of all penicillins are formulated as sodium or potassium salts and hypernatraemia or hyperkalaemia can also result if large doses are given to patients with renal failure. Great care should be taken with the intrathecal administration of penicillin as fatal encephalopathy can occur if the dose is excessive.

It is important to avoid accidental intravenous administration when injecting procaine penicillin intramuscularly as this may result in a very severe reaction consisting of a sensation of impending death, paraesthesiae and confusion lasting up to an hour and followed by exhaustion and anxiety.

Erythromycin

Erythromycin has a fairly wide range of antibacterial activity but its main indication is in the treatment of streptococcal and pneumococcal infections in patients hypersensitive to penicillin. Its use in hospital is limited by the development of resistant organisms. Erythromycin is prescribed in a dosage of 250–500 mg by mouth every 6 hours. A parenteral preparation is also available. Jaundice occasionally occurs with erythromycin estolate but clears on withdrawal of the antibiotic. Allergic reactions to erythromycin are rare. Being well tolerated and easily administered it is useful for the treatment of respiratory infections in children in domiciliary practice. It is the best antibiotic for diphtheria carriers.

The Cephalosporins

The cephalosporins are structurally similar to penicillin but have a wide range of activity against both Gram-positive and Gram-negative bacteria. Hypersensitivity reactions occasionally occur and a small number of people are allergic to both the cephalosporins and the penicillins. Because resistant staphylococci may emerge if they are used freely, the cephalosporins are best reserved for situations where the use of other antibiotics is limited. *Cephaloridine* is given by injection in doses of 250–500 mg 6-hourly. In severe infections doses of up to 6 g daily, limited to 4 g for patients over 50 years, can be used if renal function is normal. Cephaloridine is well tolerated; however, it is excreted unchanged in the urine and renal tubular damage may occur if large doses are given or if there is pre-existing renal disease. Frusemide should not be given simultaneously as there is evidence that it enhances the nephrotoxicity of cephaloridine. Other cephalosporins include *cephalexin*, which is given by mouth in doses of 250–500 mg 6 hourly.

The Tetracyclines

Tetracycline, oxytetracycline and *chlortetracycline* are very closely related bacteriostatic agents which for practical purposes have an identical range of activity. The adult dose is 250–500 mg 6 hourly before meals. *Demethylchlortetracycline* and *methacycline* attain higher and more prolonged blood levels and hence may be given less frequently. These advantages, however, are balanced by their higher degree of binding to plasma proteins and their cost.

The tetracyclines inhibit the growth of a wide range of Gram-positive and Gram-negative bacteria and are particularly useful in the treatment of acute exacerbations of chronic bronchitis, but their value may be limited by an increase in tetracycline-resistant pneumococci and *H. influenzae*. The tetracyclines are also active against the rickettsia (typhus fevers), *Coxiella burneti* (Q-fever), *Mycoplasma pneumoniae* (atypical pneumonia) and chlamydia (lymphgranuloma venereum, psittacosis).

The tetracyclines are also employed systemically in the treatment of acne vulgaris and rosacea where their beneficial effect is almost certainly not due solely to their antibacterial action. Chlortetracycline is used for the local treatment of skin infections as it does not cause cutaneous sensitisation.

Adverse Effects. Many of the normal commensals of the alimentary tract are sensitive to the tetracyclines and are inhibited when these antibiotics are administered. Insensitive organisms then multiply and cause 'superinfection'. This occurs particularly with fungi such as *Candida albicans* which cause oral, alimentary or vaginal thrush (p. 355). In hospital, superinfection with resistant staphylococci may occur and the ensuing enteritis, septicaemia or pneumonia can be fatal. Fortunately this is a rare complication of tetracycline therapy. Superinfection following the use of the tetracyclines emphasises that an antibiotic with a wide range of activity should not be prescribed if an appropriate 'narrow-spectrum' antibiotic is available. The tetracyclines quite commonly cause mild diarrhoea. Tetracyclines chelate with calcium; they interfere with the development of bone and stain growing teeth. Accordingly the use of tetracyclines is contraindicated in childhood and in pregnancy.

The tetracyclines can also exacerbate renal failure and should not be given to patients with disease of the kidneys.

Chloramphenicol

Chloramphenicol has a range of activity similar to that of the tetracyclines with the important difference that it is effective in enteric fever. It is more active than the tetracyclines against *H. influenzae* and is the antibiotic of choice in meningitis and epiglottitis due to this organism. The daily dose for an adult is 1–3 g. Preparations for parenteral administration are also available. Chloramphenicol eye drops and ointment are indicated for purulent conjunctivitis.

Adverse Effects. As with the tetracyclines, chloramphenicol may cause diarrhoea. Much more serious, although fortunately rare, are blood dyscrasias. This antibiotic has in its chemical structure a benzene ring of the type known to cause bone marrow aplasia. Although pancytopenia due to chloramphenicol is very uncommon, it is almost invariably fatal; this antibiotic should be used systemically only for the treatment of typhoid fever and *H. influenzae* infections and in other conditions if there is no alternative therapy.

Chloramphenicol should never be given to premature infants and very rarely to the newborn because of the risk of the development of the frequently fatal '*grey syndrome*'. This is a state of peripheral circulatory failure caused by the very high blood levels of chloramphenicol due to its inadequate conjugation in the liver at this age.

The Lincomycins

Lincomycin and *Clindamycin* (7-chlorolincomycin) resemble erythromycin in activity and are effective against penicillinase-producing *Staph. aureus*. They penetrate well into bone and are therefore particularly useful in osteomyelitis and infective arthritis. The lincomycins are also the antibiotics of choice for the treatment of *Bacteroides* infections which cause local suppuration often related to the intestinal tract, e.g. pelvic abscess. The dose of lincomycin is 500 mg 6 hourly and clindamycin 300 mg 6-hourly, orally or by injection.

Clindamycin is at least five times more active than lincomycin against staphylococci; it is better absorbed from the gut and seldom causes diarrhoea. The lincomycins can rarely produce a pseudomembranous ulcerating colitis which may be severe and occasionally fatal.

Sodium Fusidate

This sodium salt of fusidic acid is highly bactericidal against staphylococci and is useful in infections caused by penicillin-resistant organisms. Like the lincomycins it is well concentrated in bone. Sodium fusidate is given orally in doses of 250–500 mg thrice daily, is rapidly absorbed, attains high tissue levels and is reasonably well tolerated, although nausea and vomiting are not uncommon during therapy. An intravenous preparation is available. This antibiotic is expensive and is principally indicated for bone infections due to staphylococci.

The Aminoglycoside Antibiotics

Streptomycin, Kanamycin, Gentamicin, Tobramycin, Amikacin and Neomycin

These have similar chemical structures, pharmacological actions and adverse effects. They are not absorbed and for systemic treatment must be given by injection.

The outstanding property of *streptomycin* is its bactericidal effect on the tubercle bacillus. It is given in conjunction with two other antituberculous drugs and this triple therapy prevents the emergence of resistant strains (p. 292). For long-term therapy the daily dose of streptomycin should not exceed 1 g. Streptomycin is the antibiotic of choice in plague and other tropical infections. Its use in infections due to Gram-negative bacilli is restricted by the rapid development of bacterial resistance. When infective endocarditis is due to an organism relatively resistant to penicillin, such as *Strept. faecalis*, good results may be obtained by combining streptomycin with large doses of benzylpenicillin or ampicillin.

Kanamycin is active against many Gram-negative bacilli and resistance develops much more slowly than with streptomycin. It should be reserved for the treatment of serious infection such as peritonitis or bacteraemia due to Gram-negative bacteria, e.g. *Esch. coli* or *Proteus* species. It is also used in the treatment of gonorrhoea due to organisms of reduced penicillin sensitivity. The dose should not normally exceed 250 mg 6 hourly by intramuscular injection.

Gentamicin has a range of activity similar to kanamycin but has the very important additional advantage of being effective against *Ps. aeruginosa*. It is also active against penicillin-resistant staphylococci but inactive against streptococci and most anaerobic organisms. The dose depends on renal function and the age and weight of the patient. Up to 7·5 mg per kilogram body weight per 24 hours in divided doses is required for serious infections but 2 mg per kg is sufficient for uncomplicated urinary tract infections. *Tobramycin* is more active than gentamicin against *Ps. aeruginosa*.

Amikacin is a recently introduced antibiotic active against certain Gram-negative bacilli resistant to gentamycin.

Neomycin is too toxic to be given parenterally but local applications containing neomycin are used in infections of the skin and eye. Neomycin is used for the preoperative preparation of the large bowel and also in hepatic encephalopathy to reduce the numbers of colonic bacteria.

Adverse Effects. The outstanding toxic effect of all the aminoglycosides is on the eighth cranial nerve. With streptomycin and gentamicin the vestibular division is initially affected with resultant vertigo and incoordination. Later, deafness may also occur. Kanamycin tends to cause deafness first. Aminoglycosides, especially gentamicin, should not be administered together with the diuretic ethacrynic acid, as both can cause eighth nerve damage and additive ototoxicity may result from the combination. The ototoxicity of the aminoglycosides is related to the age of the patient, the serum level of the antibiotic and the duration of administration. The aminoglycosides are principally excreted from the body by the kidneys and the risk of toxicity is increased when there is impairment of renal function. In such cases serum levels of the antibiotic must be monitored and the frequency of dosage adjusted accordingly. Sensitivity rashes and fever occur in about 5 per cent of patients treated with streptomycin. Desensitisation is indicated if it is essential to continue with the antibiotic. Application of neomycin to the skin may cause hypersensitivity.

The Polymyxins

Colistin (Polymyxin E) is the most important member of this group. Its principal use is in *Ps. aeruginosa* infections of the urinary tract in which treatment with carbenicillin has failed. It is given by intramuscular injection in a dose of 1–3 million units 8 hourly depending on the weight of the patient and renal function.

Colistin is sometimes prescribed orally in *Esch. coli* gastroenteritis of infants. All polymyxins are nephrotoxic and may also cause paraesthesiae and ataxia although these side-effects are rare with colistin.

Nitrofurantoin and Nalidixic Acid

The use of these two unrelated chemotherapeutic agents is limited to the treatment of infections of the urinary tract. They are active against the common Gram-negative bacilli such as *Esch. coli* and Proteus and are administered by mouth. The dose of nitrofurantoin is 100 mg 3 or 4 times a day and that of nalidixic acid 1 g 3 times a day. Nausea and vomiting are common during nitrofurantoin therapy while photosensitivity skin reactions occasionally occur with nalidixic acid. Both drugs are potentially neurotoxic. Nitrofurantoin can cause peripheral neuropathy especially if there is renal failure and nalidixic acid may produce increase in intracranial pressure in babies.

Antimicrobial Agents Effective against Fungi

Nystatin. This antibiotic is effective against *Candida albicans*. Nystatin is not absorbed when given by mouth and cannot be administered parenterally because of its low solubility. A suspension, tablets and pessaries are available for the treatment of oral, intestinal and vaginal thrush respectively.

Amphotericin B. This antibiotic is indicated only for the treatment of severe systemic fungal infections. It is given in gradually increasing doses by intravenous injection (p. 299). Its adverse effects include fever, vomiting, thrombophlebitis and a rise in blood urea.

There are many polyene antibiotics, but apart from nystatin and amphotericin only *candicidin* and *natamycin* have any clinical application, the former in vaginal thrush and the latter by inhalation for the treatment of aspergillosis (p. 299).

Griseofulvin. This antibiotic is effective in dermatophyte infection such as ringworm of the skin, hair and nails where it appears to be taken up by newly formed keratin. Superficial skin lesions respond quickly but many months of treatment may be required to eradicate infection from the nails. The antibiotic is given in a dosage of 250 mg (child) to 500 mg (adult) daily and is well tolerated.

Antiviral Chemotherapy

The success of antibacterial chemotherapy has not been matched in viral diseases where only a very few infections are at the present time susceptible to drug therapy. During the relatively long incubation period of many viral infections, replication of the virus is almost complete before clinical features appear, maximal cell damage has occurred and the disease is well advanced. The intracellular position of the micro-organism further complicates chemotherapy. There are, however, three compounds which, although expensive, are of some therapeutic value.

Idoxuridine. This interferes by competitive inhibition with viral DNA metabolism and is effective in the treatment of infections caused by viruses of the herpes group. It is used topically in *Herpes simplex* infections of the cornea, skin and genitalia. Idoxuridine is also used in the treatment of herpes zoster where frequent local applications to the rash appear to reduce the duration of the skin lesions and decrease the incidence of postherpetic neuralgia. It is an expensive drug.

Cytarabine (*Cytosine arabinoside*). This also acts on viral DNA and has been used for the treatment of disseminated *H. simplex* infections and severe attacks of shingles such as generalised zoster and zoster encephalitis. It is also used in acute leukaemia. Adenine arabinoside is a promising new antiviral agent.

Selection of Antimicrobial Agent

In addition to knowledge about the properties of the available antimicrobial agents important considerations in the choice of effective chemotherapy are the nature and site of the infection, adverse effects and cost.

The Nature and Site of the Infection. In instances where the nature of the infection can be reliably predicted from the clinical features of the illness, treatment can proceed without isolation of the causative organism. For example, acute follicular tonsillitis and lobar pneumonia are sufficiently characteristic on clinical examination to allow the causative organism and its antibiotic sensitivity to be assumed with a high degree of probability and the appropriate antibiotic (penicillin) given. In acute exacerbations of chronic bronchitis the causative organisms are almost always pneumococci and *Haemophilus influenzae* and the use of ampicillin or co-trimoxazole is indicated without specific laboratory diagnosis.

Where there is uncertainty about the nature of the infection a bacteriological diagnosis should be made so that the appropriate antibiotic can be given. If the organism is one such as *Strept. pyogenes*, which has a predictable susceptibility to the generally used antimicrobial agents, no further laboratory sensitivity tests are necessary.

Sensitivity tests will be required for a minority of bacteria known to vary in their susceptibility to antimicrobial agents. The acquisition of resistance occurs particularly with staphylococci, Gram-negative bacilli and tubercle bacilli. Once the sensitivity of the organism has been determined, it is relatively rare for this to change in the course of treatment. However, there is not a complete correlation between the results of sensitivity tests and the response to chemotherapy and sometimes clinical judgement may indicate a different drug from that recommended by the bacteriologist.

When sensitivity tests indicate that several antimicrobial agents are effective it is advisable in the first instance to select one that is bactericidal in order that the organisms are killed rapidly; bacteriostatic drugs suppress the growth of the organism while the natural defence mechanisms of the body dispose of it. The choice is probably of no great significance in the majority of infections but may be important in the treatment of bacteraemia and in patients with deficient defence mechanisms.

The use of two or more antibacterial drugs is only occasionally of proven value. Thus ideally in tuberculosis three agents are prescribed so as to reduce the emergence of resistant strains. Combinations of antibiotics with differing ranges of activity may also be used to treat infections due to more than one species of micro-organism or where it is believed that the effect of the combination of drugs is more potent than an equivalent amount of any one of the compounds acting alone. This has been described as 'synergy'; an example of this is co-trimoxazole which is the combination of trimethoprim with sulphamethoxazole. Unfortunately there have been relatively few clinical trials which have compared the efficacy of combinations of antibiotics with single drugs so that the use of combinations remains somewhat empirical. Whenever possible their choice should be specifically directed by bacteriological diagnosis and accompanying sensitivity tests.

The selection of an antimicrobial agent is also determined by the site of the infection. The principles involved are discussed when the treatment of individual systems is described.

THE CHEMOTHERAPY OF BACTERAEMIA. In many patients in whom bacteraemia is suspected, treatment must be started without any knowledge of the causative organism or its susceptibility to antibacterial drugs as delay in instituting treatment while awaiting a bacteriological diagnosis may lead to the death of the patient. Initially therefore antimicrobial therapy must cover both Gram-positive and Gram-negative organisms and either a wide range antibiotic or a suitable combination of agents may be employed. The cephalosporins (p. 92) and gentamicin (p. 94) have a wide range of activity and can be given singly. Alternatively ampicillin (500 mg 6 hourly) plus cloxacillin (1 g 6 hourly) can be used. Gentamicin combined with penicillin or lincomycin is valuable for the treatment of fulminating undiagnosed infections such as suspected septicaemia in patients with a poor resistance, e.g. those suffering from leukaemia.

Where Gram-positive cocci are the cause of the infection, benzylpenicillin should be given if the organism is known to be sensitive to penicillin. Flucloxacillin is indicated if penicillinase-producing staphylococci are responsible for the infection. If the patient is allergic to penicillin or the organism is resistant to cloxacillin, the next choice is clindamycin.

Following the identification of the infecting organism and its antibiotic sensitivity, the drug or combination of drugs specifically indicated should be given along with other measures for the treatment of circulatory failure, dehydration and intravascular coagulation (p. 634).

Selection of Antimicrobial Agents in Relation to Adverse Effects. Before prescribing an antimicrobial agent enquiry should be made about any previous allergic reactions. Pregnant women and children should not be given tetracyclines. Co-trimoxazole is also best avoided in pregnancy and this compound, together with other sulphonamides, must not be given to patients with glucose-6-phosphate dehydrogenase deficiency as haemolysis may be precipitated. Chloramphenicol should be prescribed only in the circumstances described on page 93 and is contraindicated in the neonate. Ampicillin must not be given to patients suffering from glandular fever and the aminoglycoside antibiotics should be used with caution in patients with renal disease and in the elderly.

Cost. The chemotherapy of infections can be very expensive, especially when newly introduced preparations are used. Unusual antibiotics should not be prescribed without due reason as the difference in cost can be over a hundred-fold.

Conclusion

General Principles in the Use of Antimicrobial Agents

1. Antibiotics must not be prescribed unless absolutely necessary. They should not be given for trivial infections such as minor skin sepsis or gastroenteritis and, with very few exceptions (p. 95), they are ineffective in viral disease.

2. Serious infections should be treated whenever possible with bactericidal as opposed to bacteriostatic preparations and initially with parenteral agents. Although the average recommended dose of an antibiotic is sufficient for the treatment of the majority of infections, higher dosage may be necessary when the condition is serious.

3. Many acute infections such as streptococcal tonsillitis and pneumococcal pneumonia which are caused by organisms of predictable sensitivity can be treated without assistance from the laboratory. Laboratory aid is however required for bacteraemia, recurrent infections and those caused by less common pathogens.

4. Well established and usually cheaper antibiotics are preferable to new and generally more expensive preparations unless there is some commanding reason to choose otherwise.

5. Antibiotics with a relatively limited range of activity such as benzylpenicillin are preferable to broad-spectrum compounds like tetracycline, so as to reduce the danger of superinfection.

6. There are very few indications for combinations of antibiotics (p. 96) or prophylactic antibiotics.

7. Many adverse effects and even death may result from the use of antibiotics, and their careless prescription is to be deplored.

E. B. FRENCH
A. M. GEDDES
J. C. GOULD

Further reading:

Christie, A. B. (1974) *Infectious Diseases: Epidemiology and Clinical Practice.* 2nd edition. Edinburgh: Churchill Livingstone.

Cruickshank, R. (1973) *Medical Microbiology.* 12th edition. Edinburgh: Churchill Livingstone.

Garrod, L. P., O'Grady, F. & Lambert, H. P. (1973) *Antibiotic and Chemotherapy.* 4th edition. Edinburgh: Churchill Livingstone.

4. Nutritional Factors in Disease

Although man has used foods for ritual purposes and attributed magical properties to some of them since the beginning of history, the science of nutrition has nearly all originated in the twentieth century. The concept of vitamins was introduced around 1912; the cure of human rickets with vitamin D was established in 1922; nicotinamide was first used to treat pellagra in 1938. Kwashiorkor was originally reported in 1932 from an obscure African hospital, but medical science did not become aware of its importance until 1952. Human zinc deficiency was not established until 1972.

The world's population is estimated to have reached 4,000,000,000 by 1976 and presents the greatest threat to mankind. This explosive growth in population is due not to increased fertility but to the remarkable reduction in the death rate that has been achieved in recent decades. The most obvious effects of overpopulation are actual shortage of food for many poor people in underdeveloped communities and ever rising food costs in industrial countries. Some 400 million people are undernourished, many of them children. Famines are occurring most of the time in one part of the world or another. Agricultural production is hampered by bad climates, soil erosion, lack of fertilisers, antiquated farming methods, political upheavals and war. The situation will continue to deteriorate unless national programmes of population control and family planning based on modern contraceptive techniques are effectively put into operation. Food production can be further increased by the application of science to peasant agriculture but nothing will be gained if machines displace people from the land and increase the numbers of unemployed in the developing countries. A knowledge of nutrition has three uses in clinical medicine:

1. Elsewhere in this book diseases are described the multiple causes of which may include what or how people eat over long periods; among these are dental caries, coronary heart disease, diabetes mellitus, and even some of the carcinomas, e.g. of the liver and of the colon. These diseases take a long time to develop and the precise importance of one factor such as diet involves discussion and sometimes controversy. Details are not appropriate to a clinical primer and may be sought in a textbook of nutrition (p. 151).

2. For some diseases, modification of the diet (therapeutic dietetics) is valuable treatment. In gluten enteropathy and phenylketonuria the correct diet is of vital importance. For other diseases like chronic renal failure and diabetes mellitus appropriate adjustment of the diet forms a major aspect of the management. Principles of the therapeutic diets are described in the respective places in this book. Space does not allow inclusion of a full set of diet sheets; those for obesity and diabetes appear on pages 939–946. For other diet sheets the reader is referred to a textbook of nutrition (p. 151).

3. There are diseases which result primarily from disturbed nutrition; these are described in this chapter. It should be stressed that these primary nutritional diseases seldom present in pure form. Where food is short in quantity or defective in

quality all the members of a community are not equally affected. People with physical (or mental) diseases are likely to succumb first. Nutritional diseases thus often have a predisposing illness and when this is prominent the resulting malnutrition is spoken of as conditioned or secondary. Furthermore someone who has one type of malnutrition is likely to have another; sometimes it is possible to find clinical or biochemical signs of six or more nutrient deficiencies in the same patient. For this reason treatment should never be confined to large intakes of the nutrient whose deficiency is the most prominent clinical feature. Lastly malnourished patients are liable to complications, particularly certain infections. These may be the presenting illness or they may occur in modified form because the malnutrition has suppressed some of their characteristic features. They should be sought out and treated.

Much of the skill in diagnosing patients with malnutrition consists in being aware of and disentangling predisposing illnesses, other types of malnutrition and complicating illnesses. Only when this is done can treatment be fully effective.

Aetiology of Nutritional Disorders

There are five essential types of nutritional disorders:

1. *Quantitative Dietary Deficiency.* Not enough food results in undernutrition or when more severe, frank starvation.

2. *Qualitative Dietary Deficiency.* Wrong food results in malnutrition. The term 'malnutrition' should be restricted to those nutritional disorders, e.g. rickets and scurvy, which are due to lack of specific chemical components (nutrients) of a proper diet.

3. *Quantitative Overnutrition.* Too much food results in obesity.

4. *Qualitative Overnutrition.* This is due to too much of one food component, e.g. hypervitaminosis D (p. 122) and siderosis (p. 113).

5. *Effects of Natural Toxins in Foods.* Some foods contain small amounts of toxic substances which can lead to disease if a person or community has to rely too heavily on a single foodstuff, e.g. lathyrism (p. 141).

Social and Economic Causes of Nutritional Disorders. Even in countries where food can be purchased, ample in quantity and quality, nutritional disorders arise because of poverty, prejudice, ignorance or bad housekeeping often caused by bad housing. The old, the solitary and children are most often affected.

Pathological Causes of Nutritional Disorders. CONDITIONED MALNUTRITION. Even with an ample income, an adequate home and a knowledge of dietetics, a patient may develop a nutritioned disorder through some other disease which 'conditions' (facilitates) it in one or more of the following ways.

DEFECTIVE INTAKE OF FOOD. (*a*) *Loss of appetite* may be an important symptom of organic disease, e.g. cancer of the stomach, and also of psychogenic disease, e.g. anorexia nervosa. (*b*) *Persistent vomiting* from any cause. (*c*) *Food fads*, e.g. in very strict vegetarians (vegans). (*d*) *Alcohol* provides calories but no essential nutrients. Chronic alcoholics suffer from malnutrition more often than undernutrition. (*e*) *Unbalanced therapeutic diets*, e.g. diets for digestive diseases may lack ascorbic acid unless care is taken to provide it. (*f*) *Prolonged parenteral feeding* with intravenous glucose after surgical operations may precipitate acute deficiencies of the vitamin B complex.

DEFECTIVE DIGESTION AND ABSORPTION. (a) *Achlorhydria* is a contributory factor in the causation of iron deficiency anaemia. (b) *Steatorrhoea* leads to malabsorption. (c) *Intestinal hurry* due to surgical short circuits, etc. may impair digestion. In starving people the ingestion of unsuitable foods often causes intestinal hurry and intensifies their plight. (d) *Antibiotics*, if their administration is prolonged, may interfere with the synthesis of vitamins by intestinal bacteria.

DEFECTIVE UTILISATION. (a) *Cirrhosis* of the liver may interfere with the proper utilisation of ingested nutrients, e.g. of protein and vitamin K. (b) *Malignancy*, in some unknown way, may produce a state of undernutrition despite an adequate diet. The same may be true of tuberculosis and other prolonged infections. (c) In *renal failure* vitamin D is not converted to the active metabolite (p. 118). (d) Some *drugs*, e.g. anticonvulsants, are antagonists of folate and of vitamin D (e) Inborn errors of metabolism may interfere with nutrients, e.g. Hartnup disease leads to pellagrous signs on ordinary diets (p. 134).

LOSS OF NUTRIENTS FROM THE BODY. (a) In the *nephrotic syndrome* there is loss of protein in the urine. (b) In *diabetes mellitus* uncontrolled glycosuria causes undernutrition. (c) In *excessive menstrual bleeding* (menorrhagia) secondary iron deficiency anaemia is common. (d) In severe or chronic *diarrhoea* potassium is lost.

INCREASED NUTRITIONAL NEEDS. (a) In pregnancy, lactation and adolescence (especially after an illness in the last named), and for those engaged in hard physical work, particularly in cold climates, the usual diet may be insufficient. (b) In fevers and hyperthyroidism the increased metabolism calls for more calories. (c) After burns, fractures and major surgery, there is an increased catabolism of protein and ascorbic acid.

ENERGY-YIELDING NUTRIENTS

Carbohydrates. These usually provide the greater part of the energy in a normal diet, but no individual carbohydrate is an absolute dietary necessity in the sense that the body needs it but cannot make it for itself from other nutrients. If the carbohydrate intake is less than 100 g per day ketosis is likely to occur.

Fats. With their high caloric value, fats are useful to people with a large energy expenditure; moreover they are helpful in cooking and making food appetising. Though rats need linoleic or arachidonic acids in their diet, *essential fatty acid deficiency* is rare in man. It has been demonstrated in patients who have been fed intravenously for long periods without fat emulsions. There is a scaly dermatitis and eicosatrienoic acid accumulates in plasma lipids. Essential fatty acids are precursors for the synthesis of prostaglandins.

Proteins. Proteins provide amino acids, of which eight are essential for normal protein synthesis and for maintaining nitrogen balance in adults. These are termed *essential amino acids* because the body cannot make them for itself and so must obtain them from the diet. They are methionine, lysine, tryptophan, phenylalanine, leucine, isoleucine, threonine, and valine. There is evidence that histidine and perhaps arginine are needed for growth in infants.

The 'biological value' of different proteins depends on the relative proportions of essential amino acids they contain. Proteins of animal origin, particularly from milk, eggs and meat, are generally of higher biological value than the proteins of vegetable origin. Most vegetable proteins are deficient in one or more of the essential amino acids; but it is possible to have a diet of mixed vegetable proteins with high biological value if the principle of *supplementation* is used. For example cereals, e.g. wheat, contain about 10 per cent protein and are relatively deficient in lysine. Legumes contain around 20 per cent of protein which is relatively deficient in methionine. If two parts of wheat are mixed (or eaten) with one part of legume, a food results which contains 13 per cent of a protein of high biological value. This happens because cereals contain enough methionine and legumes enough lysine to supplement the other component of the mixture.

The usual recommended allowance for an adequate protein intake is 10 per cent of the total calories. The minimum requirement is less, around 40 g per day of good biological value protein for an adult.

Energy Requirements

Requirements for energy (calories) vary widely, even among apparently similar individuals. 'Recommended Allowances' provide only an approximation for an individual. The UK Department of Health and Social Security recommended in 1969 that 3,000 kcal is adequate for a moderately active man and 2,200 kcal for a moderately active woman. Slightly lower figures are recommended by the Food and Nutrition Board of the USA.

The population of Britain, including infants, children and adults, probably needs an overall average *intake* of 2,500 kcal/head/day. In order that the population may actually consume this amount, the food retailed in the shops must provide more to allow for household wastage. The food supplies of Britain ordinarily provide around 3,000 *retail* kcal/head/day. It is this shop-value of our food supplies that is sometimes discussed in Press and Parliament and often confused with average physiological requirements.

Undernutrition and Starvation

Starvation may conveniently be defined as undernutrition of sufficient severity to warrant in-patient treatment in hospital; the body weight may be reduced to 75 per cent of normal or less.

Undernutrition and starvation arise (1) when there is not enough food to eat, for instance in times of famine, (2) when there is severe disease of the digestive tract, preventing the absorption of nutrients, as in the malabsorption syndrome and cancer of the oesophagus or (3) when there is a toxaemia which prevents normal metabolism of nutrients by the tissues often with anorexia also, e.g. in renal or hepatic failure or in severe and long-continued infections. In all these circumstances there is wasting of the body with much loss of both muscle and fat. This gives rise to a clinical picture with an underlying morbid anatomy and chemical pathology which is essentially similar whatever the primary cause.

Clinical Features. When the caloric value of the diet is inadequate, adults lose weight, and children cease to grow or even lose weight. The loss may be rapid at first, but tends to slow down and become stabilised at a lower level because the body is able to adapt itself, at least partly, to an insufficient intake of food. This adaptation is possible because (*a*) the bulk of the muscles and glands is reduced in size, requiring less energy for their maintenance, (b) the basal metabolism of the tissues is reduced, (c) the body, being lighter, requires less mechanical work to move it about, and (d) unnecessary voluntary movements are curtailed.

The patient becomes thin and the skin lax, most noticeably over the upper arm and abdomen. The skin is thin, dry, inelastic and often cynanosed at the extremities. The hair becomes dull, dry and inflexible ('staring' hair). The eyes are dull and sunken, yet the wasting of orbital tissues may give them an unusual prominence. The heart is reduced in size and there is often bradycardia and a reduced systolic blood pressure. Atrophy of the small intestine is present and may be severe, in which case the inability to digest and absorb nutrients requires great care during refeeding. In severe cases, once diarrhoea has begun, the loss of fluid in the stools causes grave disturbances in water and salt balance.

Loss of 2–4 kg of body water in the urine is a characteristic immediate response to severe calorie or carbohydrate restriction. It is probably related to depletion of glycogen which has water-holding properties. This phenomenon probably explains why reducing diets for obesity are so successful for the first few days. Eventually, dependent 'famine' oedema begins to appear. This results from prolonged intake of insufficient food. It is often preceded by a period of nocturnal polyuria. Famine oedema is not necessarily associated with any fall in the level of plasma proteins, but is due rather to wasting of tissues without a corresponding loss of body water. A mild normocytic, normochromic anaemia is common, due to a reduction in the red cell population without corresponding alteration in the plasma volume.

Seriously underfed patients are weak and sometimes suffer from attacks of syncope. Hypothermia should be looked for with a low-reading thermometer. Psychological symptoms frequently occur in starving people. Mental restlessness, irritability and indifference to the troubles of others may be combined with physical apathy. Undernourished individuals are susceptible to infections like bronchopneumonia as well as to diarrhoea and starving groups in famines have often had high mortalities from epidemics, e.g. of typhus or cholera.

Diagnosis. In times of famine the signs of starvation may be all too obvious, and other causes of emaciation can be overlooked. However, a similar clinical picture may be produced by the cachexia of advanced cancer, tuberculosis, other severe chronic infections, malabsorption and late chronic cardiac or respiratory failure. It is also seen in young children with protein calorie malnutrition (PCM).

Famine oedema must be distinguished from other primary causes of oedema, eg. cardiac, renal or hepatic and from the oedema of PCM and beriberi. The diagnosis of undernutrition depends on (a) careful enquiry into the social, economic and dietary history and a knowledge of local food conditions, and (b) evidence of recent weight loss and the other clinical features mentioned above.

The severity of the starvation can be assessed by working out the patient's weight for height as a percentage of the estimated normal for the population (Table 18.2, p. 948). Starvation is severe and dangerous when weight is less than 70 per cent of normal.

Treatment. In mild undernutrition, all that is needed is suitable food. Its management is more an administrative than a medical problem. When the patient suffering from starvation is seriously ill the nature of the treatment depends essentially on the facilities available.

Most famine victims, because of alimentary dysfunction, cannot deal with large quantities of food. The patient's desire for food may be immense and no guide to his digestive capacities. Limitation of the food intake is essential if there is nutritional diarrhoea or a severe degree of nutritional cachexia.

The choice of food needs care. In advanced cases only bland food can be tolerated by the thin-walled intestines lacking essential digestive enzymes. Skimmed milk may not be well tolerated if the patient has deficient intestinal lactase activity. It is also advisable to give foods with which the patient is familiar.

The ideal diet to start with is one based on the patient's staple cereal and some sucrose or glucose together with moderate amounts of bland, protein-rich food, e.g. milk powder and some fat or oil. Small feeds should be given at frequent intervals and new foods added one at a time to see that they do not increase diarrhoea. It is advisable to give a multivitamin preparation. With refeeding there may be some increase in oedema, unless the supply of salt is restricted.

There may come a time when a patient with severe starvation refuses all food, although fully rational. The outlook is then very grave. Feeding of milk and other fluids through a stomach tube then provides the only hope.

Prognosis. Physical and psychological recovery is usually complete if sufficient calories are provided for cases of primary undernutrition. When irreversible changes have developed in the heart and small intestine, as occurs in severe starvation, the prognosis is poor.

Prevention. This rests with the social, economic and agricultural legislators and executives. Famines from crop failure can be greatly alleviated by advanced contingency planning. Those caused by a natural disaster like an earthquake are unexpected: the outcome depends on how well the country's administration stands up to the strain. Famines resulting from war are the most difficult. The problems of prevention and relief of famine are discussed in a book published by the Swedish Nutrition Foundation (p. 151).

Protein-Calorie Malnutrition
(PROTEIN-ENERGY MALNUTRITION)

Aetiology and Classification. Protein-calorie malnutrition (PCM) in early childhood is now regarded as a spectrum of disease. At one end there is *kwashiorkor* in which the essential feature is deficiency of protein with relatively adequate calorie intake. At the other end is *nutritional marasmus* which is total inanition of the infant, usually under 1 year of age, and is due to a severe and prolonged restriction of all food, i.e. calories and protein as well as other nutrients. In the middle of the spectrum is *marasmic kwashiorkor* in which children have some clinical features of both disorders.

Some children adapt to prolonged calorie and/or protein shortage by *nutritional dwarfism*. The most prevalent of all the varieties of PCM is *mild to moderate PCM* or the underweight child (see Table 4.1, p. 110). Children with one form of PCM often shift to another form. Thus a child with mild to moderate PCM may develop kwashiorkor after an infection. When such a child is treated and loses oedema he may look marasmic.

The incidence of PCM in its various forms is high in India and Southeast Asia, in most parts of Africa and the Middle East, in the Caribbean Islands and in South and Central America. PCM is the most important dietary deficiency disease in the world, affecting tens of millions of children; hence it will be described in detail.

Table 4.1 Classification of PCM

	Body weight as percentage of international standard for age	Oedema	Deficit in weight for height
Kwashiorkor	80–60	+	+
Marasmic kwashiorkor	<60	+	+ +
Marasmus	<60	0	+ +
Nutritional dwarfing	<60	0	minimal
Underweight child	80–60	0	+

Based on Joint FAO/WHO Committee on Nutrition. 8th Report, 1971 (with modifications in weight/height column).

Kwashiorkor

Cicely Williams in 1933 was the first to record that 'some amino acid or protein deficiency' might be an aetiological factor in kwashiorkor, the name given to this disease by the Ga tribe living in and around Accra, the capital of Ghana.

Aetiology. Kwashiorkor typically arises when, after prolonged breast feeding, the child is weaned on to a traditional family diet, which is low in protein, such as cassava, plantain or yam or a cereal diet which is refined and diluted (Fig. 4.1, p. 110). There is little or no milk and custom, sometimes reinforced by taboos, determines that the limited supply of foods of animal origin is given to the men of the family, or the small amount of high protein food is in a sauce, which is made with hot peppers or spices and unsuitable for young children. In many rural areas, where kwashiorkor is endemic, the food supply becomes scarce each year before the harvest; at this 'hungry season' the incidence of kwashiorkor and other nutritional diseases increases.

If the customary diet of a population is limited in protein and in calories to around the levels of minimum requirements, a child may be in moderate health until his protein requirements are raised by an infection. Gastroenteritis, measles and malaria are all notorious precipitating causes of kwashiorkor.

Pathology. The insufficient supply of amino acids leads to inadequate protein synthesis, which impairs tissue replacement and development of organs and reduces synthesis of enzymes and plasma proteins. Some enzymes and tissues are more severely affected than others, particularly those with a rapid turnover.

The total protein content of the body may be as low as 60 per cent of normal for height, while the water content is increased. The failure to synthesise plasma albumin reduces the concentration to around 15 g/l. By contrast the plasma gammaglobulin is usually well maintained. A failure to synthesise digestive enzymes is frequently present, including those secreted by the pancreas and the mucosa of the small intestine (especially lactase). This may be partially responsible for the gastrointestinal upsets and diarrhoea which are so commonly present and which cause marked electrolyte disturbances due to loss of potassium and magnesium in the stools. The protein content of the liver is greatly reduced, while the lipid content is much increased.

Clinical Features. *Failure of Growth.* The child's weight is usually well below standard for his age (Table 18.1, p. 947) but the deficit may be masked by *oedema* from hypoalbuminaemia. This usually affects the feet but may also be found in the hands and face. Ascites and pleural effusions are usually slight and, if detected clinically, suggest the presence of an infection such as tuberculosis.

Muscles and Fat. The muscles are wasted. This is particularly noticeable around the chest and the upper arm; the wasting of the legs and around the hips is frequently concealed by oedema. Subcutaneous fat is often plentiful in children whose diets have provided ample energy but little protein. If the disease has resulted from a restriction of both calories and protein, muscle wasting and an almost complete lack of subcutaneous fat is the most striking feature, but the feet are oedematous ('marasmic kwashiorkor').

Mental Changes. The child is apathetic and miserable.

Hair. This is nearly always affected in African children; in Asiatics the changes are less frequent. The hair becomes fine, straight and is often sparse. The hair of African children may show a variety of pigmentary changes from brown and reddish to grey, blond or even white. The extent of these changes in the hair is not an indication of the severity of the disease. They are sometimes pronounced in children who have been unwell for a long time but never seriously ill. Children with long straight black hair may show a pale band across the hair, corresponding to an earlier episode of kwashiorkor. This is the 'flag sign'.

Skin. Alterations in the skin are usually present, especially in severe cases. These include pigmentation, desquamation and ulceration. In moderate cases the dermatosis resembles crazy paving. A severe case may look like an extensive burn. The legs, buttocks and perineum are most frequently involved, but any region may be affected. This is in contrast to pellagra (p. 134) in which the dermatosis occurs mainly on the exposed surfaces. The skin lesions are determined in part by associated vitamin deficiencies and in part by infections and trauma. Healing is accompanied by desquamation.

Mucous Membranes. Angular stomatitis, cheilosis and a smooth tongue are commonly seen, as is ulceration around the anus.

Liver. This may be enlarged and extend down to the umbilicus but the liver can be fatty without being clinically remarkable. Hepatosplenomegaly from malaria and other causes is common in the tropics.

Gastrointestinal System. Anorexia is usually present and sometimes vomiting; there is usually diarrhoea, with the passage of stools containing undigested food. This feature may be secondary to failure of the pancreas to secrete digestive enzymes, to intestinal mucosal atrophy or to an associated gastroenteritis.

Anaemia. Some degree of anaemia is frequently present. It often becomes worse during treatment. The degree of anaemia and its nature are largely determined by associated infections and other dietary deficiencies.

Differential Diagnosis. A variety of diseases may be confused with kwashiorkor. Chronic dysentery, abdominal tuberculosis, coeliac disease, infantile pellagra and beriberi, fibrocystic disease of the pancreas and nephritis are diseases which have clinical features in common with kwashiorkor. Hookworm infection with anaemia and oedema may resemble kwashiorkor in many respects. The age of onset, the dietary and social history, characteristic skin and hair lesions, normal urine and the response to protein therapy should help to distinguish kwashiorkor.

Treatment. GENERAL MEASURES. An easily digested diet which provides adequate amounts of protein, minerals and vitamins with extra calories for 'catch-up growth' is essential. Milk is a good base, and the most convenient locally available form may be used. If skimmed milk is given, however, it is necessary to include additional fat. Plant protein mixtures, such as Incaparina or CSM (corn-soya-dried milk), may also be used.

Severely ill children may be unable to maintain their body temperature even in the tropics, especially where there is a large fall of atmospheric temperature at night. Heated rooms or electric blankets are essential for such cases. Vitamins A and D, B complex and C and therapeutic doses of iron should be given. If dermatosis is severe the skin should be cleaned and carefully protected. The child's weight tends to fall during the first days of treatment due to loss of oedema fluid. Initiation of cure is indicated by increasing appetite, improvement in general condition, loss of oedema and rise of plasma albumin.

DIETS FOR SEVERE CASES. All the major units with research experience of kwashiorkor have evolved somewhat different therapeutic diets, depending on local availability of and preferences for weaning foods. The principle of all the regimes is to work up to protein intakes of 3 to 4 g/kg/day and energy intakes of 150 kcal/kg/day or more. For the first day or two, if the child is unable to feed from a spoon, a polythene tube passed through the nose into the stomach will be necessary. A recipe successfully used in Jamaica is:

Either		*or*	
dried whole milk	115 g	dried skimmed milk	90 g
sugar	66 g	sugar	90 g
vegetable oil	53 g	vegetable oil	80 g
water to make to	1 *l*	water to make to	1 *l*

This is offered *ad lib* in 5 to 6 feeds per day up to a maximum of 240 kcal/kg/day. The mixture contains 135 kcal and 3·1 g protein per 100 ml. A child recovering from kwashiorkor, unless his progress is retarded by infection, will accept very high calorie intakes until his weight approaches the normal value for his height.

Anorexia may be serious, but often can be overcome by feeding the child very slowly in the mother's lap and by giving frequent feeds. Food may be taken better cold than hot. If the diarrhoea appears to be made worse on feeds containing skimmed milk, lactose intolerance may be present (p. 396). Such a child should respond to a mixture such as Casilan, cream, glucose and cereal.

As the clinical condition improves and the child attains normal weight for height, he may be given the local diet in frequent feeds, care being taken to introduce a variety of plant and animal protein foods and maintain the fat content of the diet.

Infants may lose 1–4 g of potassium chloride in the stools in one day if there is severe diarrhoea. The effect of the resulting potassium depletion on the myocardium may cause sudden death. Potassium should be given by mouth as a routine to all infants admitted with kwashiorkor. Depending on the age and weight of the child and the severity of the diarrhoea, the dose should be from 0·5 to 1 g of potassium chloride dissolved in water and added to three or four feeds each day. There is little or no danger of potassium intoxication when the mixture is given by mouth in these doses. Some centres also give magnesium.

PARENTERAL THERAPY. For very ill patients in a well-equipped and well-staffed hospital, who are suffering from marked dehydration, hypoglycaemia, acid-base disturbance or electrolyte imbalance, parenteral therapy with solutions such as half isotonic Darrow's solution with 2·5 per cent dextrose may be a life-saving measure which should be started prior to the beginning of dietetic treatment. Likewise, for severe anaemia from any cause, small slow transfusions of packed erythrocytes are of great value. In developing countries facilities for these measures are not available for the majority of severe cases of PCM.

VITAMINS. Vitamin A deficiency with xerophthalmia and keratomalacia (p. 117) occurs in from 1 to 70 per cent of severe cases of PCM. This is a major cause of preventable blindness in developing countries. All kwashiorkor patients should receive moderate amounts of vitamin A routinely, e.g. in a fish liver oil concentrate or multivitamin syrup, and if xerophthalmia is suspected 30 mg should be given for 3 days.

Biochemical signs of thiamin and niacin deficiencies are commonly associated with kwashiorkor in countries where rice or maize respectively are the staple weaning foods. Folate deficiency is also fairly frequent. It would therefore be wise to give B vitamins routinely. Children with PCM have often been indoors out of the sun for weeks and a minority of cases have associated rickets (p. 119). Vitamin K_1 in a single intramuscular dose of 10 mg should be given if there is any purpura or bleeding or if a surgical procedure is required. Therapeutic diets for kwashiorkor tend to be low in vitamin C.

INFECTIONS AND COMPLICATIONS. The usual signs of infection like pyrexia may not appear. Because infections are so common some authorities give e.g. penicillin and a sulphonamide routinely to all patients. Many of these children harbour worms. However, all anthelmintics are potentially toxic and must be used with due care in patients who are seriously ill. If anaemia from hookworm is so severe as to endanger life, small transfusions with packed cells should be given and will probably restore the child's condition sufficiently to permit appropriate treatment later. Iron-deficiency anaemia, which is frequently present due to dietary deficiency of protein and iron and as a consequence of infections, requires appropriate treatment. Less commonly a megaloblastic anaemia is present which responds excellently to folic acid. Antimalarial drugs in both prophylactic and therapeutic doses are well tolerated. The possibility of tuberculosis should always be considered, particularly if the child does not make the expected progress to recovery.

CONVALESCENCE. When a child who has had severe kwashiorkor comes to be discharged from hospital he is still usually well below normal weight and height for his age. At this stage 'catch-up' (supernormal) growth is possible and obviously desirable, but it will not occur unless the child is in a favourable environment and getting all the food he will eat. If home conditions are difficult some simple convalescent home or nutritional rehabilitation centre (p. 151) would be ideal where available. In any case follow up should be arranged to ascertain that the child does not deteriorate.

MILD KWASHIORKOR AND FOLLOW-UP CASES. Most cases have to be treated outside hospital. Dried skimmed milk sprinkled over the food is recommended if available or a local protein food mixture. Mothers should be given instruction in regard to hygiene and methods of feeding. The doctor should try to arrange help for socioeconomic problems where possible. A well-run nutrition rehabilitation centre can be very effective in treating these children at modest cost.

Prognosis. Severe kwashiorkor has a mortality of around 20 per cent even in a well equipped hospital. Most deaths occur in the first week or 10 days. Jaundice, petechiae and stupor are bad prognostic signs. The usual causes of death are intercurrent infections and severe malnutrition, including potassium deficiency. The availability of medical care is another factor influencing prognosis.

In the long term, follow-up studies have shown that the fatty liver of acute kwashiorkor does not progress to cirrhosis. Physical growth of the brain is retarded in children who suffer from severe PCM in the first year or two of life. There is circumstantial evidence that intelligence may be impaired, particularly if the child goes home to an environment in which catch-up growth cannot occur. Hence the great importance of trying to arrange the best possible conditions for a child's nutrition and mental development after leaving hospital.

Prevention. Ignorance and poverty are two main factors responsible for kwashiorkor. Every effort should be made to alleviate these causes. Education in nutrition, the introduction of improved farming methods and measures to reduce infections in young children, are all important. In each country careful thought must be given to the provision of protein-rich foods made from local crops which are suitable both for infant feeding and for supplementing diets low in protein. Cameron and Hofvander (p. 151) give over a hundred recommended weaning recipes from many developing countries.

Even small amounts of food of animal origin, such as dried milk, egg, a little meat or concentrates of fish protein, are of great value when mixed with high protein vegetable foods. Although milk powder is a convenient source of protein it is only essential for treating severe kwashiorkor. The disease can, and often has to be prevented by appropriate combinations of local foods, e.g. cereals and legumes or groundnuts.

Education of parents, particularly mothers, in regard to the value of foods and best methods of preparing them, especially at the time of weaning, is invaluable. Much is being done to alleviate this disorder by the establishment or extension of Child Welfare Clinics and Health Centres where free or subsidised skimmed milk powder or a protein food mixture is supplied, advice on diet given, and where diseases liable to lead to kwashiorkor are prevented or treated. At the same time and place the advantages to mother and child of wider spacing of births should be carefully explained and contraceptive measures provided.

Nutritional Marasmus

The importance of nutritional marasmus as a cause of mortality and morbidity in infants is still not fully appreciated. In some developing countries marasmus is of greater clinical importance than kwashiorkor. It affects principally infants under 1 year of age in contrast to kwashiorkor which is chiefly encountered between 1 and 4 years of age. Marasmus is more likely to occur in poor people in underdeveloped countries who live in cities, while kwashiorkor occurs more frequently in those living in rural areas. The factors which predispose to marasmus are a rapid succession of pregnancies, and early and often abrupt weaning, followed by dirty artificial feeding of the infants with very dilute milk or milk products given in inadequate amounts to avoid expense. Thus the diet is low in both calories and protein. In addition unsatisfactory home conditions make the preparation of uncontaminated feeds almost impossible. Repeated infections therefore develop, especially of the gastrointestinal tract, which the mother often

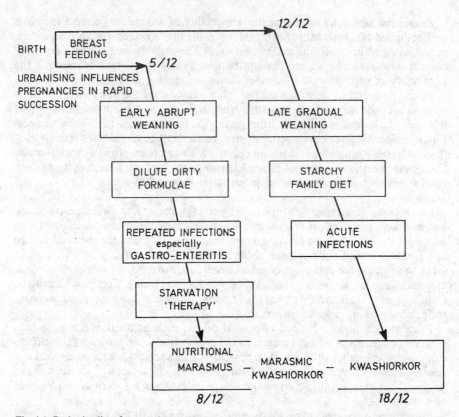

Fig. 4.1 Paths leading from early weaning to nutritional marasmus and from protracted breast feeding to kwashiorkor. (By courtesy of Dr D. S. McLaren and the editor of the *Lancet*.)

treats with water, rice water or some other non-nutritious fluid (Fig. 4.1).

The most important cause of marasmus, early weaning, is in contrast to the late weaning, often extending over two years, which is characteristic of kwashiorkor. The mother may be induced to stop breast feeding for various reasons, including the presence of infection in herself or in the infant. She may have been influenced by advertisements which advocate the advantages of artificial food products. One reason for stopping breast feeding is economic pressure on the mother to go out and work. Another reason is pregnancy; there is widespread belief among un-educated women in developing countries that the milk of a pregnant woman is bad for her child.

Clinical Features. The two constant features of marasmus are: (1) retardation of growth and reduction of weight which is much more marked than that of length, and (2) wasting of muscles and subcutaneous fat which gives the infant a wizened, old appearance. There is usually watery diarrhoea or semi-solid, bulky, acid stools. In contrast to kwashiorkor, oedema is absent and the characteristic changes in the hair and skin, apathy and anorexia are seldom encountered. The abdomen may be distended with gas but the liver is not fatty. A careful search must be made for chronic infection like tuberculosis which predisposes to marasmus. The features of associated vitamin disorders such as angular stomatitis or keratomalacia, may develop, as may a deficiency of minerals, especially potassium and magnesium. Dehydration frequently occurs as a consequence of gastrointestinal infection.

Treatment and Prevention. In the acute stage of marasmus survival depends primarily on the efficiency with which measures can be applied to combat dehydration and restore electrolyte balance. In addition the child must be given a satisfactory diet along similar lines to those described for kwashiorkor. A longer refeeding period is usually required because the marasmic child is more severely wasted. The mortality rate during treatment is similar to that of kwashiorkor.

Prevention is a complex and difficult problem. Education of mothers so that they will continue breast feeding for as long as possible is of the greatest importance. Further research is urgently needed into improved methods of feeding both healthy and ill infants in developing countries. The epidemiology of the failure of lactation and the control of infection in infants are other important matters requiring further investigation. It is probable that in the future marasmus will become of increasing clinical importance in developing countries as a consequence of a continuing decline in breast feeding and the urbanisation of uneducated families, socially insecure and living in poor, insanitary houses and with insufficient money to buy adequate supplements of milk or milk substitutes.

Nutritional Dwarfing

Some children adapt to very prolonged mild to moderate calorie and/or protein deficiency by a proportional failure of growth. They are light in weight and short in stature but have superficially normal body proportions and subcutaneous fat. Such children are more prone to infections than normal. Unless the weight for age of such a child is checked against normal standards (Table 18.1, p. 947) it is easy for the doctor in a busy clinic to miss this form of PCM.

Mild to Moderate PCM (The Underweight Child)

For every florid case of kwashiorkor or marasmus there are several children in the community with mild to moderate PCM. The situation is like an iceberg. There is more malnutrition below the surface than is recognisable on clinical inspection. The children with subclinical PCM can however be detected by their weight for age, which is less than 80 per cent of the international standard (Table 18.1). In areas where kwashiorkor is the predominant florid form of PCM, subclinical cases have reduced plasma albumin and sometimes other biochemical signs of protein deficiency ('prekwashiorkor'). In parts of many developing countries surveys may show up to 5 per cent of children under 5 years with signs and symptoms of kwashiorkor or marasmus while up to 50 per cent are underweight.

The great importance of mild to moderate PCM is that these children are growing up smaller than their potential and they are very susceptible to gastroenteritis and respiratory infections, which in turn can precipitate frank malnutrition. Mild to moderate PCM is probably the major underlying reason why the one to four year mortality in a developing country can be 30 to 40 times higher than in Europe or North America. Official statistics record most of these deaths as due simply to infections.

WATER, ELECTROLYTES AND MINERALS

The normal distribution of water and electrolytes in the body and the disturbances which result when their intake or output is diminished or increased are discussed in detail on pages 152 to 164.

Twelve elements are clearly essential for man, as they are for other animals; deficiency disease is known for each but may not always result from an inadequate diet. The elements are sodium (p. 153), potassium (p. 156), magnesium (p. 159), calcium, phosphorus, iron, sulphur, iodine, zinc, copper and chromium. Fluoride appears to be essential for rats and optimal intakes reduce dental caries. Cobalt is physiologically active only in the form of vitamin B_{12}.

In addition manganese, tin, vanadium, molybdenum, selenium, nickel and silicon have been shown, by highly artificial isolator systems, to be essential for animals. Human deficiency disease is not known for any of these minor trace elements.

Elements of Importance in Human Nutrition

Calcium. The body of an adult normally contains about 1,200 g of calcium. At least 99 per cent of this is present in the skeleton, where calcium salts (chiefly hydroxyapatite $Ca_{10}(PO_4)_6(OH)_2$) held in a cellular matrix provide the hard structure of the bones and teeth. Obviously all of this calcium comes from the diet. Among common foods, the calcium-containing protein of milk (caseinogen) is much the richest source, which is one reason why milk and cheese are especially valuable for growing children. Half a litre of cow's milk contains about 0·6 g of calcium. Most other foods contribute much smaller amounts. However, peas, beans, other vegetables and particularly cereal grains are frequently the chief contributors because of the large amounts eaten.

Drinking water can provide significant amounts of calcium. In Britain the average intake from this source is about 75 mg Ca/day; but the variations are large: from none in water from peaty, acidic hill lochs in Scotland to 200 mg or even more in water obtained from wells sunk in chalk or limestone.

Absorption. The problem of calcium absorption is extremely complicated. It is not known why 70 to 80 per cent of the calcium in the food is normally excreted in the faeces. Calcium absorption may be impaired either by lack of vitamin D, by any conditions causing small intestinal hurry, by the combination of calcium with excess fatty acids to form insoluble soaps in steatorrhoea, or by certain substances in the diet which can form insoluble salts with calcium. These include foods rich in oxalic acid (e.g. spinach) and phytic acid which is present in the outer layers of cereal grains. Hence 'wholemeal' bread contains more phytic acid than white. To overcome the influence of phytic acid, calcium carbonate has been added to flour in Britain.

Daily Recommended Intakes of Calcium. The Department of Health and Social Security (UK) recommended in 1969 a daily intake of 500 mg for adult men and women, rising to 1,200 mg during pregnancy and lactation. For adolescent boys and girls the recommended intake was from 600 to 700 mg daily.

In many parts of Africa and Asia children develop healthy bones and adults remain in calcium balance despite calcium intakes which may be no more than half the above recommendations. Abundant sunshine possibly produces this effect. However a daily intake of 1,000 mg should be taken during pregnancy and lactation.

Deficiency of calcium and vitamin D go hand in hand and are best considered together (p. 118).

Phosphorus. Eighty-five per cent of the phosphorus is normally present in the bones in combination with calcium. The remainder is chiefly in the cells. Phosphorus is essential for most metabolic processes.

Phosphorus is present in all natural foods, though in refined and processed foods the phosphorus content may be greatly reduced. The best sources are those foods that also contain good amounts of calcium and protein. Phosphorus normally presents no problem for the dietitian. A useful working rule is 'take care of the calcium and the phosphorus will look after itself. Phosphorus depletion can occur in man from prolonged and excessive intake of aluminium hydroxide antacids. The features are weakness, anorexia, malaise and bone pains.

Iron. A good mixed diet with average amounts of meat and vegetables contains about 12–15 mg of iron. Cheap monotonous high carbohydrate diets based on refined wheat flour contain much less. Foods which are particularly rich in iron are meat, liver, eggs, wholemeal cereals, oatmeal, peas, beans and lentils. The availability of the iron varies in different foods. Tests in man with ^{59}Fe incorporated into foods have shown that iron is absorbed well from meat, haemoglobin and wine, moderately from pulses and poorly from eggs. Absorption is enhanced in iron deficient individuals. An account of the measures for the prevention and treatment of iron deficiency anaemia is given on page 599. Next to obesity this is probably the most important nutritional cause of ill-health in Britain and other prosperous countries.

Siderosis. Dietary iron overload is seen in South African Bantu men who cook and brew beer in iron pots. They may ingest as much as 100 mg of iron per day. Iron accumulates in the liver and when severe can lead to cirrhosis. A similar condition has been described in other countries following excessive indulgence in cheap wines which can contain 30 mg of iron per litre.

Iodine. Simple enlargement of the thyroid gland attributed to lack of iodine in the food occurs particularly in mountainous regions far from the sea. Other factors may also contribute to the causation of simple goitre (p. 529).

Sources. Iodine in small amounts is widely distributed in living matter. Seafoods are the only rich source in the diet. Vegetables and milk may contain useful amounts.

Prophylactic Uses. The prophylactis requirement is around 150 μg/day. The Medical Research Council recommends the addition of potassium iodide to all table salt in Britain as this has been proved to be highly successful in reducing the incidence of simple goitre in Switzerland, the USA and other parts of the world. Regrettably the legislation required to enforce this recommendation in Britain has not yet been enacted.

Fluoride. Fluoride has recently been shown to be an indispensable nutrient for rats. Its regular presence in minute amounts in human bones and teeth and its influence on the prevention of dental caries justifies its inclusion as an element of importance in human nutrition.

Sources. Most adults ingest between 1 and 3 mg of fluoride daily. The chief source is usually drinking water, which, if it contains 1 part per million (p.p.m.) of fluoride, will supply 1–2 mg/day. Soft waters usually contain no fluoride, whilst very hard waters may contain over 10 p.p.m. Compared with this source, the fluoride in foodstuffs is of little importance. Very few contain more than 1 p.p.m.; the exceptions are sea-fish which may contain 5–10 p.p.m. and tea. In Britain and Australia, where people drink tea frequently, the adult intake from this source may be as much as 3 mg daily.

Use of Fluoride in the Prevention of Dental Caries. Epidemiological studies in many parts of the world have established that where the natural water supply contains fluoride in amounts of 1 p.p.m. or more, the incidence of dental caries is lower than in comparable areas where the water contains only traces of the element.

Floride becomes deposited in the enamel surface of the developing teeth of children. Such teeth are unusually resistant to caries for reasons not yet fully understood; it may be that traces of fluoride in the enamel discourage the growth of acid-forming bacteria. Alternatively, the calcium hydroxyapatite of the enamel may be rendered more resistant to organic acids by combination with traces of the element. It should be noted that fluoride is not deposited in fully developed adult teeth, so that little benefit to adults can be expected when they begin for the first time to drink water containing traces of fluoride.

The deliberate addition of traces of fluoride to those public water supplies which are deficient is now a widespread practice throughout North America where at least 75 million people are now drinking fluoridated water. In at least 30 other countries similar projects have been started.

In view of the widespread incidence of caries throughout Britain, the case for the addition of fluoride up to 1 p.p.m. to the water supplies of those areas where it is lacking has been strongly supported by carefully controlled trials. Many expert committees have examined the evidence and conclude that fluoridation of water at 1 p.p.m. is safe (Report of the Royal College of Physicians, 1976). Regrettably some local authorities are not yet adding fluoride to their water supplies.

Fluorosis in Man. In parts of the world where the water fluoride is high (over 3 to 5 p.p.m.) mottling of the teeth is common. The enamel loses its lustre and becomes rough. Bands of brown pigmentation separate patches as white as chalk. Small pits may be present on the surface. Mottling is usually best seen on the incisors of the upper jaw. The effect is purely cosmetic; fluorotic teeth are resistant to caries and not usually associated with any evidence of skeletal fluorosis, or with any impairment of health.

Chronic Fluoride Poisoning. This occurs in several localities in India, China, Argentina, East and South Africa, where the water supply contains over 10 p.p.m. fluoride. Fluorine poisoning has also occurred as an industrial hazard among workers handling fluorine-containing minerals such as cryolite, used in smelting aluminium. The main clinical features are referable to the skeleton which shows sclerosis of bone, especially of the spine, pelvis and limbs, and calcification of ligaments and tendinous insertions of muscles.

Sulphur. This is mainly supplied by the S-containing amino acids in the diet—methionine and cysteine; effects of its deficiency are therefore inseparable from those of protein.

Zinc. A syndrome has recently been described in Egypt and Iran of dwarfism and hypogonadism in late teenage boys. Serum zinc was low and prolonged treatment with zinc sulphate (27 mg Zn per day) was accompanied by accelerated growth and sexual maturation. The cause is thought to be interference with zinc absorption by phytate in unleavened bread, which is the staple diet.

Other Minerals. *Copper* deficiency occasionally occurs in young children; the main features are anaemia, neutropenia, retarded growth and skeletal rarefaction. *Chromium* facilitates the action of insulin. Deficiency has been reported in some children with protein calorie malnutrition. For further information see sodium (p. 153), potassium (p. 156), and magnesium (p. 159).

THE VITAMINS

Although vitamin deficiency disorders are now uncommon in Britain they deserve consideration in detail because they are still widespread in many parts of the world. Even in industrial countries certain types of people are known to have chances of developing some vitamin deficiency. Doctors should be ready to diagnose these treatable conditions in their early stages.

Vitamins are organic substances in food which are required in small amounts but which cannot be synthesised in adequate quantities. A large number of substances conforming to this definition have been recognised by feeding tests on animals, but deficiencies of only 12 vitamins have, so far, been demonstrated to have clinical effects in man. These are:

Fat-soluble	Water-soluble	
Vitamin A	Vitamin C—Ascorbic acid	
Vitamin D		Thiamin
Vitamin E		Niacin
Vitamin K	Vitamin B	Riboflavin
	complex	Pyridoxine
		Biotin
		Cobalamins (B_{12})
		Folate

Pantothenic acid, which is a major component of coenzyme A, also appears to be essential, but human deficiency disease has not been reported, perhaps because the vitamin is widely distributed in foods.

Factors influencing the Utilisation of Vitamins

Availability. Not all of a vitamin may be in absorbable form. For instance niacin in maize is bound in such a way that it is not absorbed from the gut. Fat-soluble vitamins may be deficient if dietary fat is not eaten or absorbed.

Antivitamins. These are known to be present in some natural foods, e.g. thiaminase in raw fish. Some synthetic antagonists of the vitamins are used as drugs in the therapy of neoplasms (e.g. methotrexate, p. 619) or of infections (e.g. pyrimethamine, p. 840). Neoplastic cells and micro-organisms are much more sensitive than normal cells but with high doses of the antivitamin a conditioned vitamin deficiency can occur.

Provitamins. Substances occur in foods which are not themselves vitamins but are capable of conversion into vitamins in the course of digestion. Thus some of the carotenes are provitamins of vitamin A and, to some extent at least, the amino acid tryptophan can be converted to niacin.

Biosynthesis in the Gut. The normal bacterial flora of the gut is capable of synthesising significant amounts of vitamin K. Bacteria are also capable of extracting vitamins from the ingested food and retaining them until excreted in the faeces. Except for vitamin K and probably biotin, bacteria are more likely to reduce than to increase the amounts of vitamins available for absorption, as is demonstrated in bacterial colonisation of the small intestine (p. 396).

Biosynthesis in the Skin. Vitamin D need not be provided in the diet if the skin is regularly exposed to adequate sunshine (p. 118).

These considerations indicate how difficult it may be in practice to define the nutritive value of a diet simply from chemical analysis of its vitamin content.

Vitamin A—Retinol

Retinol is found only in foods of animal origin. Animals obtain the vitamin from its precursors or provitamins—some of the carotenoid pigments. The conversion of even the best of these, β carotene, into retinol in the human small intestinal wall is only 30 per cent efficient. The absorption of both retinol and carotene is facilitated by fats and bile salts. It seems likely that retinol has a place in the metabolism of all human cells, but the precise way that it behaves is not yet explained in biochemical terms except in the retina.

Dietary Sources. Retinol is chiefly found in milk, butter, cheese, egg yolk, liver and some of the fatty fish. The liver oils of fish are the richest natural sources but these are used as nutritional supplements rather than foods.

Carotene is widely distributed among plant foods. It is found chiefly in green vegetables in association with chlorophyll, so that the green outer leaves of vegetables like cabbage and lettuce are good sources. Other useful sources are yellow and red fruits and vegetables. Vegetable oils are devoid of vitamin A activity except red palm oil which is extensively produced in West Africa, Malaysia and Brazil. This oil is a rich source of carotene. In Britain and some other countries retinol is added artificially to margarine to provide the same concentration as that of good quality summer butter. Both retinol and carotene are stable to ordinary cooking methods, though some loss may occur at temperatures above 100°C as when butter or palm oil is used for frying.

Recommended daily intakes of retinol are $300\,\mu g$ for infants and young children, $500-600\,\mu g$ for children of 9 to 15 years, $750\,\mu g$ for adolescents and adults, and $1,200\,\mu g$ for lactating women (1 μg retinol = 3 of the old i.u.) In many parts of the world most or all of the requirements are obtained from carotenoids in vegetable foods. Because only approximately $\frac{1}{3}$ of β carotene is absorbed into the intestinal wall and then only $\frac{1}{2}$ of this is converted into retinol, 1 μg retinol equivalent (=1 μg retinol) is now taken as = 6 $\mu g\,\beta$ carotene. Healthy adults in Britain have large stores of 90 to 150 mg retinol in their livers.

Pathology. Deficiency of the vitamin results in morphological changes in the epithelial surfaces of all parts of the body. The cells undergo squamous metaplasia whereby they become flattened and heaped one upon another. The sebaceous glands and hair follicles of the skin and the tear glands of the eye become blocked with horny plugs of keratin so that their secretions diminish. The lack of tears and the heaping up of epithelium on the scleral conjunctiva and cornea produce xerophthalmia. When softening, ulceration and necrosis of the cornea develop, the condition is referred to as keratomalacia.

Night Blindness

Retinol is an essential component of the pigment rhodopsin (visual purple) on which vision in dim light depends. Hence lack of retinol may result in impairment of 'dark adaptation' which can be measured by means of an adaptometer. Night blindness is common, as also is vitamin A deficiency, in poor people living in underdeveloped countries; it can occur in the malabsorption syndrome in affluent countries. In such cases it responds excellently to retinol. Fatigue and anxiety states may cause persons to complain of night blindness. It may also result from organic disease of the eye such as retinitis pigmentosa. The diagnosis of vitamin A deficiency is supported by low plasma vitamin A concentration and is confirmed by marked improvement in dark adaptation following therapeutic doses of the vitamin.

Xerosis Conjunctivae, Bitôt's Spots and Xerophthalmia

The earliest sign of xerosis conjunctivae is a dry, thickened and pigmented bulbar conjunctiva. The pigmentation gives the conjunctiva a peculiar smoky appearance. Bitôt's spots are glistening white plaques formed of desquamated thickened conjunctival epithelium, usually triangular in shape and firmly adherent to the underlying conjunctiva. Xerosis conjunctivae and Bitôt's spots are certainly common in children whose diet is deficient in vitamin A but they also occur in children whose intake of the vitamin is satisfactory. When dryness spreads to the cornea it takes on a dull, hazy, lacklustre appearance due to keratinisation, and xerophthalmia is said to be present.

In young children, xerophthalmia is almost always attributable to recent vitamin A deficiency and is usually associated with PCM. In older children and in adults its interpretation is less simple. Exposure to dust and glare may produce similar changes. They should, however, always call attention to the diet. Xerophthalmia is very important in young children because once the cornea is involved the process can rapidly progress to keratomalacia.

Keratomalacia

This disease causes blindness among Indians, Indonesians and other rice-eating people of Asia; it also occurs in parts of Africa, the Middle East and Latin America. In Europe and North America it is very rare. Children between the ages of 1 and 5 years are most commonly affected. It only occurs in persons who have been living for long periods on diets almost entirely devoid of vitamin A. The disease is frequently associated with PCM.

The earliest manifestations are night blindness and xerophthalmia. Later the cornea undergoes necrosis and ulceration. Unless early and adequate treatment is given, there is a grave risk of blindness or death from associated diseases.

Treatment. A good all round diet and attention to any associated infection is essential for the treatment of the above disorders. In xerophthalmia or severe adult cases of night blindness the administration of vitamin A in a dose of 30 mg retinol (100,000 i.u.) daily for three days should be started immediately. It is recommended that half the dose should be given orally in the form of halibut or similar rich fish oil and half intramuscularly as retinol acetate or palmitate, in order to ensure that the patient is actually getting the vitamin. The practice of instilling cod-liver oil directly into the eye is not recommended. During convalescence 9 mg of retinol daily in the form of fish-liver oil orally is adequate.

For the prevention and treatment of secondary bacterial infection, antibiotics are of value. Local treatment of the eye will be required only if disorganisation is already present, in which case the services of an ophthalmic surgeon should be obtained.

Prevention. Doctors and nurses working in the tropics, who may have been trained in Europe or North America, should make sure they are familiar with the appearances of xerophthalmia. If in doubt it is better to give a short course of vitamin A treatment. Pregnant women should be advised to eat dark green leafy vegetables. This helps to build up stores of retinol in the fetal liver. They should also be taught to give such vegetables or locally available yellow or orange fruits to their babies. In some countries where keratomalacia is a major cause of blindness, e.g. in India, single prophylactic oral doses of 60 mg retinol are being tried in young children. On the world scale vitamin A deficiency is one of the seven most common causes of blindness, the others being trachoma, onchocerciasis, gonococcal ophthalmia, accidents, cataract and glaucoma.

Follicular Keratosis

In this condition the hair follicles are blocked with horny plugs of keratin, rendering the skin surface rough and dry like the skin of a toad. The typical distribution is over the backs of the upper arms and the fronts of the thighs. Therapeutic trials in Africa have repeatedly shown a striking clinical improvement in follicular keratosis when patients are given halibut liver oil or red palm oil. Nevertheless, it is not a specific sign of vitamin A deficiency, since it occurs not uncommonly in people who, by every other criterion, are adequately nourished in respect of vitamin A.

Vitamin D

Vitamin D_2 (ergocalciferol) is manufactured by the action of ultraviolet light on ergosterol, a sterol found in fungi and yeasts. When the term 'calciferol' is used in clinical practice it refers to ergocalciferol. Although widely used in therapeutics, it occurs very rarely in nature. *Vitamin D_3 (cholecalciferol)* is the natural form of the vitamin which occurs in man and other animals. It is formed in the skin by the action of ultraviolet light on 7-dehydrocholesterol. The vitamin is present in very high concentrations in fish-liver oils. The material originally described as vitamin D_1 was subsequently found to be an impure mixture of sterols.

Metabolism and Mode of Action. Ingested vitamin D requires bile and probably fatty acids for its absorption. In most people it is probable that a larger portion of the vitamin D supply is normally formed by ultraviolet irradiation of 7-dehydrocholesterol in the skin. Exposure of the face of a European infant to sunshine for a few hours a week produces sufficient vitamin D to prevent rickets. It has been suggested that the pigment in the skin of coloured people living in the tropics protects them from the liability to vitamin D intoxication. On the other hand their skin pigment may make them more susceptible to rickets and osteomalacia when they emigrate to higher latitudes where the intensity of sunlight and people's exposure to it are relatively small. Unlike vitamin A, stores of vitamin D in the body are not large: only a little is stored in the liver and moderate amounts in adipose tissue.

Cholecalciferol is not the active form of the vitamin. It is converted in the liver to 25-hydroxycholecalciferol. In the kidney, it is further hydroxylated to 1,25-dihydroxycholecalciferol, which is several times more potent than cholecalciferol. It stimulates the synthesis in the small intestinal epithelial cells of a specific calcium transport protein, which facilitates calcium absorption and hence ensures an adequate concentration of mineral at the growing and active sites of the bones. Here calcium comes in contact with inorganic phosphates, liberated from organic phosphates under the influence of phosphatase produced by the osteoblasts. The calcium phosphate thus formed is then used to calcify new bone. It is possible that vitamin D has an additional direct stimulating action on bone but the mechanism underlying this is uncertain. In states of vitamin D deficiency the characteristic change in the bones is a reduced calcium phosphate content, and in developing bone this is particularly prominent at the growing points.

Dietary Sources. The sources of the natural vitamin are all fat-containing animal products. The richest sources are fatty fish and their liver oils, some of which contain thousands of micrograms of vitamin D per 100 g. Vitamin D is also present in much smaller quantities in dairy products such as butter and eggs. In Britain vitaminised margarine is the most reliable food source of the vitamin for adults: 1 ounce (28 g) contains nearly the daily requirement. Milk has a very small content of vitamin D, meat and white fish have insignificant amounts and cereals, vegetables and fruit have none.

The recommended daily dietary intake for infants and children up to 5 years of age and for pregnant or lactating women is 10 μg. For older children and adults about 2·5 μg is adequate (1 μg = 40 i.u.).

Rickets

Rickets is a disease of calcium and phosphorus metabolism which occurs when infants or children obtain insufficient vitamin D. It is still an important clinical problem in some developing countries, especially in large towns and cities. Infants in their first year are mainly affected due to an inadequate intake of vitamin D because of the low content of this vitamin in both human and animal milk and the failure to provide them with a supplement of vitamin D in any form. In addition, for various social and cultural reasons, their mothers wrap them up in clothes which prevents their exposure to sunlight. By the second year the infant is able to crawl about in the sunshine and spontaneous healing usually occurs. In contrast the age-group mainly affected in Britain and other affluent countries is from 1 to 3 years and sometimes older, and the disease is now uncommon. This is the result of a variety of measures which have led to greatly improved standards of nutrition and housing. Of particular importance are the satisfactory supply of milk, the distribution of cod-liver oil and other sources of vitamin D and the fortification with vitamin D of preparations of dried milk, margarine and some proprietary cereal foods. That it would be rash to suggest that any of these measures is now redundant is clearly indicated by reports of limited outbreaks of clinical rickets in Asian immigrant children in the large cities and occasionally in underprivileged and neglected white children. Rickets in British Asian children seems to arise from a combination of little exposure of the skin to sunlight and very low dietary intakes of vitamin D. High phytate intakes in chapatti flour may contribute by inhibiting calcium absorption. The disease is also liable to occur in premature babies.

Chemical Pathology. Serum calcium tends to fall from its normal level of 2·12–2·62 mmol/l (8·5–10·5 mg/100 ml) of which approximately 50 per cent is available in the ionised form. More commonly the serum phosphate falls from the normal value. This is thought to be due to the activity of the parathyroid glands which respond to a slight reduction in serum calcium by increasing the excretion of phosphorus in the urine.

Clinical rickets may occur when the levels of calcium and phosphorus in the serum are still within normal limits. A diagnostic change is an increase in serum alkaline phosphatase. This enzyme is formed by the osteoblasts which accumulate in the osteoid tissue at the growing points of the bones. These cells, unable to make bone without a sufficient supply of calcium, probably liberate into the circulation the excess of this enzyme which they cannot use. Some specialised laboratories can now measure plasma 25-hydroxycholecalciferol. Its concentration is very low or zero in rickets.

Clinical Features. The infant with rickets has often received sufficient calories and may appear well nourished, but is restless, fretful and pale, with flabby and toneless muscles. Excessive sweating of the head is common. The abdomen is distended. The infant is prone to respiratory infections and gastrointestinal upsets. Development is delayed so that the teeth often erupt late and there is failure to sit up, stand, crawl and walk at the normal ages.

The bony changes are the most characteristic signs of rickets. In general there is extension and widening of the epiphyses at the growing points, where cartilage meets bone. The earliest bony lesion, however, is often craniotabes—small round unossified areas in the membranous bones of the skull, yielding to the pressure of the finger, with a crackling feeling, like a ping-pong ball. This sign is of particular value in the diagnosis of rickets in developing countries where the disease is common in infants under 1 year of age. It usually disappears within 12 months of birth. Two other early signs are enlargement of the epiphyses at the lower end of the radius and at the costochondral junctions of the ribs, the latter known as the 'rickety rosary'. Later there may be 'bossing' of the frontal and parietal bones and delayed closure of the anterior fontanelle. Later still, there may be deformities of the chest such as pigeon chest and Harrison's sulcus.

If rickets continues into the second or third year of life deformities such as kyphosis develop as a result of the new gravitational and muscular strains, caused by sitting up and crawling. At the same time there may be enlargement of the lower ends of the femur, tibia and fibula. When the rachitic child begins to walk, deformities of the shafts of the leg bones develop, so that 'knock knees' or 'bow legs' are added to the clinical picture. Pelvic deformities may follow and lead later to serious difficulties at childbirth.

When there is a reduction in the level of ionised serum calcium, infantile tetany may result, with spasm of the hands and feet and of the vocal cords. The latter causes a high-piched distressing cry and great difficulty in breathing. Epileptic fits may also occur.

Radiological examination of the wrist will show characteristic changes at the epiphyses; the outline of the joint is blurred and hazy, and the epiphyseal line becomes broadened. In older children, the classical concave 'saucer' deformity is shown. A raised level of serum alkaline phosphatase should give further support to the diagnosis. However, the alkaline phosphatase may be unchanged when rickets and PCM occur together and, on the other hand, occasional normal children with no dietary or clinical evidence of rickets may have enzyme levels above the expected range.

Treatment. The two essentials of treatment are the provision of a supplement of vitamin D and an ample intake of calcium.

A therapeutic dose of vitamin D varies from 25 to 125 μg (1,000–5,000 i.u.) daily, depending on the severity of the disease and age of the child. In contrast, the prophylactic dose is 10 μg or less daily depending on the sunlight. The B.P. preparation of cod-liver oil contains approximately 10 μg per 5 ml plastic spoonful. Children can be given halibut-liver oil in a very small dose (1 ml) since it contains 30 times the vitamin D concentrations of cod-liver oil. Many proprietary preparations are available which contain standard amounts of vitamins A and D, dispensed as capsules or palatable syrups.

For severe cases needing 125 μg or more daily, synthetic calciferol is useful. The B.P. calciferol solution contains 75 μg of vitamin D per ml.

In times of social upheaval, such as may be occasioned by war, floods or pestilence, when a young child may be seen once by an emergency medical service and perhaps not again for months, a single massive dose of vitamin D, e.g. 3·75 mg, can be given by mouth with reasonable safety and curative effects. The daily administration of small doses is the method recommended for normal practice, because of the danger of overdosage (p. 122).

In addition to vitamin D, rachitic infants and children require an ample supply of calcium, the best source of which is milk. At least half a litre should be taken daily by a young child with rickets. For a severe case a supplement of calcium tablets should also be given such as calcium gluconate or calcium gluconate effervescent (B.P.C.), one or two tablets dissolved in a glass of water three times a day. Each tablet contains 1 g calcium gluconate.

For treatment of tetany see page 534.

Vitamin D and diet are not the whole solution to the treatment of rickets. An attempt must be made to improve the hygienic environment of the child. Unnecessary clothing should not be worn and the child should be allowed as much as possible into the sunshine, particularly in countries where supplements of vitamin D are not provided.

PROGRESS. The earliest evidence of healing in rickets is provided by radiological examination of the growing ends of the bones. The levels of calcium and phosphorus in the serum provide an inconstant and unreliable guide. A more constant change is a decrease in the raised serum alkaline phosphatase level but this does not usually occur for several weeks after treatment is initiated; the therapeutic dose of vitamin D should be continued so long as the phosphatase level remains elevated; thereafter it may gradually be reduced to the prophylactic dose of 10 μg daily.

VITAMIN D RESISTANT RICKETS. Occasionally cases of rickets are encountered which are resistant to ordinary therapeutic doses of vitamin D. The disease persists into late childhood ('late rickets') or even adult life, producing the clinical appearance of osteomalacia, unless adequately treated. One cause of this syndrome is defective reabsorption of phosphate as occurs in uncommon congenital disorders of the renal tubules e.g. the Fanconi syndrome (p. 471). A similar state may sometimes arise as a conditioned deficiency resulting from malabsorption of vitamin D or from chronic renal failure in which renal formation of the active metabolite from cholecalciferol is impaired. Whatever the cause, treatment consists in giving large doses of vitamin D by mouth together with calcium salts. The initial dose of calciferol may be 1·25–3·75 mg daily (1–3 B.P. strong calciferol tablets) but it should be reduced at the first suspicion of toxic symptoms.

HYPERVITAMINOSIS D. In the case of vitamin D it is possible to have too much of a good thing. Large doses are toxic and cause hypercalcaemia. The symptoms include nausea, vomiting, constipation, drowsiness and signs of renal failure; metastatic calcification in the arteries, kidneys and other tissues may occur. Since renal damage may develop before clinical signs of toxicity appear, it is recommended that all patients on large doses of vitamin D should have their serum calcium level checked regularly at three-monthly intervals and if this is found to be above $2 \cdot 62$ mmol/l ($10 \cdot 5$ mg/100 ml) it is an early indication of overdosage.

Prognosis. Rickets is not a fatal disease *per se*, but the untreated rachitic child is always at risk of infections, notably bronchopneumonia. The skeletal changes, if mild in degree, usually tend to heal spontaneously as the child gets older, but in severe cases pigeon chest, spinal curvature, knock knees, bow legs or pelvic deformities persist. With early and sufficient treatment these changes are entirely avoided.

Prevention. The provision of adequate milk for children, the clearing of slums, the building of new housing estates and smoke abatement schemes are basic prophylactic measures which must be continued. In addition mothers must be educated in the need to keep their infants and children in the sunshine as much as possible. Nevertheless, for reasons already stated and particularly in northern countries, the supply of the vitamin from this source is uncertain and attention must be paid to the dietary supply. It must be remembered that none of the common foods in a child's diet is a good source of vitamin D. Practical experience shows that the majority of children benefit by receiving a daily supplement of about 10 μg, preferably in the form of some natural source such as cod-liver oil, which also provides useful amounts of vitamin A. In temperate climates at least, this should be continued summer and winter for the first 5 years of life.

It is necessary to consider how much vitamin D the infant is getting from other sources. Some proprietary cereal foods for infants are 'fortified' with vitamin D by the manufacturers, as in British margarine (p. 119). Not only is there no advantage in giving infants and young children more than 10 μg of vitamin D daily *from all sources* for prophylactic purposes, but there is a distinct possibility that higher doses given over a long period could predispose to infantile hypercalcaemia, a form of hypervitaminosis D. It should be noted, however, that the prophylactic dose of vitamin D for premature infants should be twice that for full-term infants and it should be started within 2 weeks of birth.

Osteomalacia and Osteoporosis

Osteomalacia, which means softening of bone, is primarily due to a deficiency of vitamin D, and to a lesser extent of calcium, or both. This results in a failure to lay down calcium and phosphorus in the organic matrix of bone. Hence the ratio of calcium phosphate to matrix is reduced. The progressive decalcification of the bones leads to the replacement of bony substance with soft osteoid tissue.

Osteoporosis, which is an atrophy of bone, is believed to be due to defective formation of bone matrix which leads to a reduction in the total mass of bone. In other words osteoporosis may be defined as a disorder of too little bone of normal composition. In contrast to osteomalacia the ratio of calcium phosphate to matrix is normal.

New bone has to be formed in adults because, like other tissues, bone is continually and slowly turning over by resorption and replacement. Both osteoporosis and osteomalacia occur in old people in all countries.

Osteomalacia

Aetiology. Osteomalacia is the adult counterpart of rickets. In its fully developed form as it occurs in women in purdah in oriental countries, it causes great deformity and suffering. Such women are of the child-bearing age, live on poor cereal diets devoid of milk, are kept indoors and seldom see the sun, and become depleted of calcium by repeated pregnancies. In oriental countries the onset often coincides with the first pregnancy, a remission occurring after delivery, but symptoms return with each succeeding pregnancy. In Scotland and in other countries where osteomalacia is a relatively common disease in old people, especially women, the disease may be due to malabsorption from any cause, including previous gastrointestinal operations especially partial gastrectomy, or to direct dietary deficiency of vitamin D. Chronic renal disorders are a less important cause.

Epileptics who have to take anticonvulsants for years are likely to develop osteomalacia; these drugs increase the catabolism of cholecalciferol by liver microsomes.

Clinical Features. Skeletal pain is usually present and persistent and ranges from a dull ache to severe pain. Sites frequently affected are the ribs, sacrum, lower lumbar vertebrae, pelvis and legs. Bone tenderness on pressure is common. Muscular weakness is often present and the patient may find difficulty in climbing stairs or getting out of a chair. A waddling gait is not unusual. Tetany may be manifested by carpopedal spasm and facial twitching. Spontaneous fractures may occur, independent of the pseudo-fractures described below. The biochemical changes in the blood are the same as those in rickets.

Radiological examination shows rarefaction of bone and commonly translucent bands (pseudo-fractures, Looser's zones), often symmetrical, at points submitted to stress. Common sites are the ribs, the axillary border of the scapula, the pubic rami and the medial cortex of the upper femur. Looser's zones are diagnostic of osteomalacia.

Histological examination of stained undecalcified sections of bone obtained by biopsy may be required as this shows unequivocally the presence of excess osteoid tissue.

Treatment. This is essentially the same as for rickets when osteomalacia is primarily due to defective intake, namely 25 to 125 μg vitamin D daily; the response is usually dramatic. If there is evidence of malabsorption the dose should be 1·25 mg daily and it may have to be given intramuscularly at weekly intervals. If the disease is secondary to renal disorders double or treble this dose may be necessary. Maintenance treatment with vitamin D will be required for all cases of osteomalacia in which the cause cannot be removed. In addition a good diet should be given which includes milk. A supplement of calcium should be given orally, namely one to two tablets of calcium gluconate (B.P.) thrice daily or preferably one Sandocal tablet three times a day in a glass of water. Within 4 to 8 weeks of starting treatment the pain and weakness have usually disappeared. The decision to reduce or discontinue the dose of vitamin D and calcium is based on the improvement in the clinical features and the disappearance of biochemical and radiological abnormalities. The dangers of vitamin D intoxication should be kept in mind.

Prevention. With improved education and better standards of living the disease is now much rarer in many Asian towns where previously it was common. Free access to sunshine and an adequate intake of dairy produce, supplemented when necessary with fish-liver oil, will prevent nutritional osteomalacia. Particular attention to these prophylactic measures should be given to inmates of geriatric and mental hospitals and to old people living alone whose exposure to sunshine is limited and also to those who have had gastric surgery. Epileptic patients on long-term anticonvulsant therapy should be given prophylactic doses of vitamin D.

Osteoporosis

Osteoporosis is the commonest metabolic disease of bone and is found most frequently in elderly women when it is known as postmenopausal osteoporosis. It may occur in elderly men (senile osteoporosis) and rarely in younger people (idiopathic osteoporosis). There is a wide variation in the geographical and racial incidence of generalised osteoporosis. For example, in the United States it is more prevalent in Caucasians than in Negroes.

Aetiology. A physiological decrease in skeletal mass occurs in all persons from the age of 40 to 50 onwards; the process is more marked in women, and in some individuals it would appear to be accelerated by factors which are largely unknown. In postmenopausal women there is a failure of oestrogen secretion and in men diminished androgen formation may contribute. It would appear unlikely that simple dietary deficiency has a primary role in the aetiology.

Inadequate physical activity promotes generalised osteoporosis and may, in part at least, account for the high incidence of this condition in affluent societies. Immobilisation by splinting, inflammation or pain is the main cause of local osteoporosis.

Generalised osteoporosis may be secondary to prolonged treatment with adrenal corticosteroids; it occurs in various endocrine disorders, notably Cushing's syndrome and hypogonadism, and also in severe malnutrition and chronic renal disease. Osteoporosis, like anaemia, may therefore be the end result of a number of diverse processes.

Pathology. The histological appearances are in keeping with Albright's original conception of a primary osteoblastic hypoplasia. The bone is deficient in quantity but there is no abnormality of its quality or architecture, in contrast to osteomalacia where there are abnormally large amounts of osteoid tissue.

Clinical Features. The patient is usually an elderly woman who is otherwise healthy. There may be no disability despite obvious radiological abnormality. In others there are episodes of severe pain usually due to fractures of the brittle bones often occurring after minimal trauma. The lumbar and thoracic vertebrae, the neck of the femur, the upper end of the humerus and the lower end of the radius are the commonest sites of fracture. Healing is not impaired and as it occurs pain usually subsides. More persistent backache is a later feature of osteoporosis due to progressive compression or collapse of several vertebrae. This may result in loss of stature and in kyphosis. Persistent pain elsewhere is not a feature of osteoporosis but is more characteristic of osteomalacia, Paget's disease or skeletal metastases. In contrast to these conditions there is also a tendency for spontaneous improvement to occur in osteoporosis. Idiopathic osteoporosis is occasionally found in younger persons in whom it also tends to be self-limiting.

The radiological changes are more marked in the bones of the axial skeleton than in the limbs; they consist of loss of bone density, reduction in the number and size of trabeculae and thinning of the cortex. The upper and lower surfaces of the lumbar and thoracic vertebral bodies become biconcave, and later compression or collapse causes anterior wedging.

The calcium, phosphorus and alkaline phosphatase levels in the blood are normal in contrast to osteomalacia.

Treatment. The physiological decline in skeletal mass, the obscure aetiology of idiopathic osteoporosis and its tendency to remission, together with the need for long-term assessment, make therapeutic measures very difficult to evaluate. None has as yet been proved to be clearly effective.

The patient should know that the natural history of the disease is characterised by spontaneous improvement and that suitable regular exercise is beneficial. Immobilisation following a fracture should be limited to the part involved and accompanied by graduated remedial exercises. The patient should remain ambulant if symptoms permit. The use of spinal supports is undesirable.

Cyclical oestrogen therapy (p. 554) may be prescribed for otherwise healthy postmenopausal women. The use of testosterone in males for senile osteoporosis is extremely dubious. Some authorities believe that the best all-purpose treatment for generalised osteoporosis is vitamin D, 250 μg daily. On general principles, at least an adequate intake of vitamin D and calcium should be ensured. Cows' milk is the best source of the latter, half a litre providing about 20 g of protein and 600 mg of calcium, but obesity must be avoided and, if present, corrected. It should be borne in mind that osteomalacia can coexist with osteoporosis especially in patients with a fracture of the neck of the femur. Any primary factor such as excessive corticosteroid therapy or endocrine disease should be corrected if possible.

Vitamin E

Alpha-tocopherol is the most potent of eight related substances with vitamin E activity. It is found in vegetable oils, eggs, butter, wholemeal cereals and broccoli and peas.

Vitamin E prevents oxidation of polyunsaturated fatty acids in cell membranes. The main feature of human deficiency is a mild haemolytic anaemia. This has been described only in premature infants and a few cases of the malabsorption syndrome.

There is no scientific justification for self-medication with vitamin E in the belief that this will increase energy, and virility.

Vitamin K

Vitamin K is required for the formation in the liver of prothrombin and factors VII, IX and X, which are necessary for the normal clotting of blood (p. 626). It exists in nature in two forms, vitamin K_1 and vitamin K_2. Vitamin K_1 (phytomenadione) is soluble in fat solvents but only slightly in water. It is found in leafy vegetables and is available in pure form as a pharmaceutical preparation.

Foods of animal origin, including fish-liver oils, are poor sources unless they have undergone extensive bacterial putrefaction, with formation of one of the vitamin K_2 series. Adequate amounts are normally supplied in the average diet and bacterial synthesis occurs within the colon, but it is not clear how the vitamin K_2 so formed is absorbed.

The therapeutic uses of vitamin K_1 are discussed on page 633.

Vitamin C—Ascorbic Acid

Chemistry and Physiological Action. Ascorbic acid is a simple sugar. It is the most active reducing agent found in living tissues and is easily and reversibly oxidised to dehydro-ascorbic acid. Its highest concentration in the body is in the adrenal cortex. Stress and corticotrophin lead to a loss of ascorbic acid from the cortex. The presumption, therefore, is that ascorbic acid is intimately concerned in bodily reactions to stress, though in a manner as yet obscure. Man is one of the few animals that cannot synthesise his own ascorbic acid from glucose.

Dietary Sources. Blackcurrants, citrus fruits, berries and green vegetables are the richest sources. Foods of animal origin contain very little except for liver and glandular tissue. Dried cereals and pulses contain no ascorbic acid.

Ascorbic acid is very easily destroyed by heat, alkalis such as sodium bicarbonate, traces of copper or by an oxidase liberated by damage to plant tissues. Ascorbic acid is very soluble in water. For these reasons many traditional methods of cooking reduce or eliminate it from the diet. A satisfactory daily intake is 30 mg.

Scurvy

Aetiology. In 1497 Vasco da Gama sailed round the Cape of Good Hope and established a trading centre on the Malabar coast. Scurvy occurred among his crew on the voyage and 100 out of his 160 men died. For the next 300 years scurvy was a major factor determining the success or failure of all sea ventures until it was recognised that it results from the prolonged consumption of a diet devoid of fresh fruit and vegetables. Such diets are principally deficient in ascorbic acid, the cause of scurvy, but can also be deficient in iron, vitamin A and folic acid and sometimes protein. Thus, although ascorbic acid will relieve the predominant signs of the disease, it does not always cure the patient.

Sporadic cases of scurvy continue to arise in Britain in infants as a result of ignorance, poverty and maternal neglect and also amongst old people, especially men living alone with neither the opportunity nor the aptitude to feed themselves properly. Scurvy appears to be a rare disease in infants and children in most subtropical countries but it may be seen in infants who are weaned prematurely. It is more likely to occur in arid regions of the world in times of drought, as in Arabia and parts of India after a failure of the monsoon rains.

Pathology. Ascorbic acid deficiency results in defective formation of collagen in connective tissue because of failure of hydroxylation of proline to hydroxyproline, the characteristic amino acid of collagen. There is in consequence delayed healing of wounds and there may be defective osteoid tissue in children. There are also capillary haemorrhages and sub-normal platelet stickiness.

Clinical Features. ADULT SCURVY. The pathognomic sign is the swollen and spongy gums particularly in the region of the papillae between the teeth, sometimes producing the appearance of 'scurvy buds'. These are livid in colour and bleed on the slightest touch. The teeth may become loose and even fall out in severe cases. There is always some infection; indeed this seems necessary for the production of the scorbutic gingival appearances since volunteers suffering from experimental deficiency did not develop it if their gums were previously healthy. Associated with the infection there is an offensive foetor. In patients without teeth the gums appear normal.

The first sign of cutaneous bleeding is often found on the lower thighs, just above the knees. These haemorrhages are perifollicular—tiny points of bleeding around the orifice of a hair follicle. There is a heaping-up of keratin-like material on the surface around the mouth of the follicle, through which a deformed 'corkscrew' hair characteristically projects. Perifollicular haemorrhages are often followed by petechial haemorrhages, developing independently of the hair follicles, which are usually first seen on the feet and ankles. Thereafter large spontaneous bruises (ecchymoses) may arise almost anywhere in the body, but usually first in the lower extremities, producing the characteristic 'woody leg'. Haemorrhage may occur into joints, into a nerve sheath, under the nails or conjunctiva, into the gastrointestinal tract or there may be epistaxis. Scurvy can present with any of these features. By the time the disease is fully developed the patient is usually anaemic.

Another characteristic of scurvy is that fresh wounds fail to heal—a feature that the surgeon has to bear in mind. Osteoporosis of the spine has been reported in prolonged cases in adults.

Before the changes in the gums and skin appear, the patient has usually felt feeble and listless for some weeks or months. If hard work is expected of him, he may have been suspected of malingering, through absence of clinical signs suggesting disease and hence the gravity of his condition may not have been appreciated. Yet he may die suddenly and without warning apparently from cardiac failure.

The dietary and social history is helpful in doubtful cases. Old, solitary people may insist that they fend very well for themselves, but careful questioning, or an inspection of the larder, will reveal that they do not bother to purchase fresh fruit or vegetables. In other instances the proper foods may be purchased but they are so badly cooked that in fact the diet is made scorbutic.

INFANTILE SCURVY. The main clinical features are lassitude, anaemia, painful limbs and enlargement of the costochondral junctions. Until the teeth have erupted, scorbutic infants do not develop gingivitis. When this occurs the gums have the classical appearance of 'scurvy buds'. The first sign of bleeding is usually a large subperiosteal haemorrhage immediately overlying one of the long bones—frequently the femur—producing the characteristic 'frog-legs' position. This gives rise to intense pain, especially on movement. The infant may cry continuously and agonisingly, and scream even louder when lifted.

Special Investigations. Ascorbic acid can be estimated with relative ease in plasma. This is useful only in excluding the diagnosis since the plasma level of the vitamin falls to very low levels long before the disease develops. A better index of the tissue reserves of the vitamin is its concentration in the white blood cells or the platelets. If this is very low, the diagnosis of scurvy is practically certain.

Differential Diagnosis. The distinctive appearance of the gums must be distinguished from other causes of gingivitis (p. 354). The diagnosis of scurvy is most difficult in people who are edentulous, for then the clinician does not have the changes in the gums to guide him.

The perifollicular haemorrhages of scurvy are distinctive in appearance but if only petechiae are visible, other causes of purpura must be excluded (p. 627).

Scurvy in infants and children may sometimes be mistaken for rheumatic fever or osteomyelitis, because of the pain caused by a subperiosteal haemorrhage in immediate relation to one of the long bones. The refusal of the child to use one leg may cause the disease to be mistaken for poliomyelitis.

Treatment. Because of the danger of sudden death, synthetic ascorbic acid should be given at once in adequate amounts. Parenteral treatment has no advantage over oral administration. The aim should be to saturate the body with ascorbic acid with as little delay as possible. The normal body contains about 1·5 g of the vitamin, so that a dose of 250 mg by mouth four times daily should achieve this within a few days, despite a considerable loss in the urine which quickly follows each dose.

Once the danger of sudden death is averted, attention should be paid to correcting the general deficiencies of the patient's former diet. A liberal diet, including fresh fruit and as much properly cooked vegetables as are available and the patient will accept, should be given. If the patient is anaemic iron and sometimes folic acid are indicated.

With adequate treatment no patient dies of scurvy and recovery is usually rapid and complete.

Prevention. Fruit juice should be given for the first 2 years of life, especially to bottle-fed infants.

No simple administrative means has been found of preventing scurvy among the old and solitary, who are largely unresponsive to education. Should the physician be unable to stimulate such a person to take fruit and vegetables, he should at least insist on one 25 mg tablet of synthetic ascorbic acid being taken daily. Alternatively a mass dose can be given at longer intervals—say, 500 mg on the first day of every month.

Special provision against scurvy is desirable for any group of people living on packed, preserved rations for any length of time such as explorers or armed forces operating in a barren territory. They should take synthetic ascorbic acid tablets with them. In default of such supplies antiscorbutic remedies can often be prepared from green herbs on the spot such as scurvy grass which grows on seashores, infusions of pine needles or sprouting peas and beans whose germination is produced by spreading the dried pulses under wet cloths.

ASCORBIC ACID AND THE COMMON COLD. It has been claimed that ascorbic acid in doses of 1–2 g daily will prevent the common cold. If it does, this is a pharmacological and not a vitamin effect as coryza is not a manifestation of scurvy. It is inadvisable for people to dose themselves with large quantities of ascorbic acid as this favours the formation of oxalate stones in the urinary tract and could have other adverse effects.

Thiamin—Vitamin B₁

Thiamin salts are readily soluble in water but not in fat. Thiamin pyrophosphate (TPP) is an essential coenzyme for the decarboxylation of pyruvate to acetyl coenzyme A. This is the bridge between anaerobic glycolysis and the tricarboxylic acid (Krebs) cycle. TPP is also the coenzyme for transketolase in the hexose monophosphate shunt pathway and for decarboxylation of α-ketoglutarate to succinate in the Krebs cycle. Consequently when thiamine is deficient (a) the cells cannot utilise glucose aerobically; this is likely to affect the nervous system first, since it depends entirely on glucose for its energy requirements; (b) there is accumulation of pyruvic acid and of lactic acid derived from it, which produce vasodilatation and increase cardiac output. High carbohydrate diets predispose to and aggravate thiamin deficiency.

In man thiamin deficiency can produce cardiomyopathy and/or peripheral neuropathy and/or encephalopathy. These occur in various combinations in wet and dry beriberi, infantile beriberi and Wernicke's encephalopathy.

Dietary Sources. Pulses, pork, liver, nuts, the germ of cereals and yeast, are the only rich sources. Dried brewer's yeast, yeast extract (Marmite) and the bran of rice and wheat have all been used in the treatment of beriberi. Green vegetables, roots, fruits, flesh foods and dairy produce (except butter) contain small amounts of the vitamin. It is not found in butter or in vegetable or animal oils. In the refining of sugar and many cereal products (wheat, rice) nearly all the naturally occurring vitamin may be removed; there is also none in spirits.

As thiamin is readily soluble in water, considerable amounts may be lost when vegetables are cooked in an excess of water which is afterwards discarded. It is relatively stable below 100°C provided that the medium is slightly acid, as in baking with yeast. But if baking powder is used, or if soda is added in the cooking of vegetables, almost all the vitamin may be destroyed. The loss of thiamin in the cooking of an ordinary mixed diet is usually around 25 per cent. Modern processes for freezing, canning and dehydrating food result in only small losses. Unlike vitamin A, thiamin is not stored in the body to any appreciable extent; hence symptoms due to deficiency may develop within a few weeks.

The recommended daily intake is 0·4 mg/1,000 kcal or about 1·2 mg in an adult male.

Beriberi

Beriberi is a nutritional disorder formerly widespread in South and East Asia. The word comes from the Singhalese language and means 'I cannot', signifying that the patient is too ill to do anything. It has almost disappeared from prosperous Asian countries such as Japan, Taiwan and Malaysia and from big cities such as Hong Kong, Manila and Singapore. Oriental beriberi is usually caused by eating diets in which most of the calories are derived from polished, i.e. highly milled, rice. The disorder is often precipitated by infections, hard physical labour or pregnancy and lactation. In Britain and North America occasional cases of beriberi heart disease are seen, usually in alcoholics who have been consuming little but alcohol for some weeks.

Chemical and Pathological Findings. Owing to a lack of thiamin, carbohydrates are incompletely metabolised and there is an accumulation of lactic and pyruvic acids in the tissues and body fluids. The local accumulation of these metabolites causes dilatation of peripheral blood vessels, as in normal exercise. In beriberi this vasodilatation may be extreme, so that fluid leaks out through the capillaries, producing oedema. At the same time the blood flows rapidly through the dilated peripheral circulation. There is a high cardiac output and as the disease progresses the heart dilates because the myocardium is both overworked and unable to use glucose efficiently as an energy substrate. Cardiac failure accentuates the oedema. Sudden death may result. Microscopic examination usually shows loss of striation of myocardial fibres, which are also finely vacuolated and often fragmented and separated by oedema.

In dry beriberi there is severe wasting of muscles. In long-standing cases there is degeneration and demyelination of both sensory and motor nerves. The vagus and other autonomic nerves may be affected. In dry beriberi the level of blood pyruvate is usually within normal limits.

In Wernicke's encephalopathy there are foci of congestion and petechial haemorrhage in the upper part of the mid-brain, the hypothalamus, and the walls of the third ventricle. The corpora mammillaria are always involved and this is believed to account for defects of memory.

Clinical Features. The *early* symptoms and signs are common to wet and dry beriberi. The onset is usually insidious, though sometimes precipitated by unaccustomed exertion or a febrile illness. There is anorexia and malaise, associated with heaviness and weakness of the legs. There may be a little oedema of the legs or face and the patient may complain of precordial pain and palpitations. The pulse is usually full and moderately increased in rate. There may be complaints of 'pins and needles' and numbness in the legs. The tendon jerks are usually sluggish, and the calf muscles may be tender on pressure. Hypoaesthesia or anaesthesia of the skin, especially over the tibiae, is common. In areas where beriberi is endemic such a condition may persist for months or even years with only minor alterations in the symptoms. The patients are only mildly incapacitated and many continue to earn their living even as manual labourers, but at a very low level of efficiency. At any time this chronic malady may develop into either of the severe forms.

WET BERIBERI. Oedema is the most notable feature and may develop rapidly to involve not only the legs but also the face, trunk and serous cavities. Palpitations and breathlessness are marked. There may be pain in the legs after walking. This is probably due to the accumulation of lactic acid. The neck veins become distended and pulsate freely. The heart is enlarged. There is usually tachycardia and an increase in pulse pressure. While the circulation is well maintained, the skin is warm owing to the vasodilatation; as heart failure advances, the skin becomes cold and cyanotic. The mind is usually clear. Electrocardiograms often show no changes except sinus tachycardia but in some cases there are inverted T waves or evidence of disturbed conduction.

DRY BERIBERI. The essential feature is a polyneuropathy (p. 139). The muscles become progressively weak and wasted, and walking becomes increasingly difficult. The thin, even emaciated patient needs at first one stick, then two, and may finally become bedridden. The disease is essentially a chronic one, which may be arrested at any stage by improving the diet. Bedridden patients and those with severe cachexia are very susceptible to infections. Patients with dry beriberi are always liable to a sudden onset of oedema which may be due to a variety of dietary causes, e.g. lack of thiamin, protein or calories.

INFANTILE BERIBERI. This is seen in areas where adult beriberi is endemic. It occurs in breast-fed infants, usually between the second and fifth months. Although the mothers of such infants must have been eating a diet and secreting milk with a low thiamin content, classical signs of beriberi are stated to be absent in 50 per cent of them. The illness usually starts acutely and is rapidly fatal, if not promptly treated. The mother may have noticed that the infant is restless, often cries, is passing less urine than normal and shows signs of puffiness. The infant then may suddenly become cyanosed with dyspnoea and tachycardia and die within 24 to 48 hours. Other serious signs are convulsions and coma. In severe cases partial or complete aphonia is characteristic and is usually preceded by the infant's cry becoming thin with a plaintive whine. Infantile beriberi was formerly the chief cause of death between 2 to 6 months of age in rice-eating rural areas in Southeast Asia, and it may still be important in isolated areas.

WERNICKE'S ENCEPHALOPATHY. This syndrome may be associated with other forms of beriberi but in Europe and the USA most commonly occurs in alcoholics. It usually presents as an acute psychiatric problem with disorientation, faulty memory, confabulation, delusions and abnormal behaviour; a group of mental symptoms called *Korsakoff's psychosis*. Confusion may progress to stupor or coma. The predominant signs are the loss of pupillary reflexes and of extra-ocular movements. Nystagmus is an early feature.

Laboratory Diagnosis. Pyruvic or lactic acids can be measured in the blood but they are not elevated in the more chronic forms of beriberi and if they are increased are not specific. The best laboratory test is measurement of transketolase activity in red cells with and without added thiamin pyrophosphate *in vitro*. The test requires fresh red cells and blood must be taken before thiamin treatment is started. A grossly abnormal result appears to be specific for beriberi or Wernicke's encephalopathy.

Differential Diagnosis. In endemic areas the diagnosis of beriberi is usually not difficult. Outside these areas the diagnosis should be considered if there is a history of a poor diet associated with alcoholism or based on polished rice or other refined cereal.

In mild and chronic cases there may be few or no physical signs and the diagnosis may have to depend on the interpretation of symptoms and the dietary history, often inaccurately described. In prisons and labour forces, such patients may be accused of malingering. The symptoms also closely resemble those of anxiety states.

The oedema of wet beriberi must be distinguished from that associated with hepatic and renal disease, cardiac failure and PCM. The warm extremities in cardiac beriberi and the absence of protein in the urine are useful diagnostic points. Famine oedema should seldom be a diagnostic difficulty if a proper dietary history is taken. Wet beriberi and famine oedema seldom occur together in adults.

Heart failure due to beriberi must be distinguished from that due to other causes, notably the high output failure of hyperthyroidism and severe anaemia. A history of alcoholism or a poor diet, often a surprisingly normal ECG and sometimes an associated peripheral neuropathy are valuable pointers to beriberi. If in doubt the patient should be given 50 to 100 mg of thiamin parenterally, preferably before other therapy has been started. Beriberi responds dramatically.

The features of dry beriberi are sometimes indistinguishable on clinical examination from other forms of nutritional, infective and toxic polyneuropathy (p. 750). The differential diagnosis is accordingly based on the presence or absence of a history of nutritional deficiency and of such aetiological factors as alcoholism, the ingestion of toxic substances or an infective illness. The disease may be confused with neural leprosy in areas where this is endemic (p. 856).

The diagnosis of infantile beriberi may be difficult. Neither oedema nor paralysis is an early sign and sudden death may occur before either is present. In cases of doubt the presence of minimal signs or symptoms of beriberi in the mother may decide the issue.

The possibility of Wernicke's encephalopathy should always be borne in mind in the presence of any acute psychosis, especially when this develops in a patient who is an alcoholic.

Treatment. *Wet Beriberi.* Treatment must be started as soon as the diagnosis is made, because fatal heart failure may occur suddenly. Complete rest is essential and thiamin should be given in amounts of 50 mg intramuscularly and continued for three days. Thereafter oral treatment in a dose of 10 mg three times a day should be continued until convalescence is established.

The prompt response of a patient with beriberi to thiamin is one of the most dramatic events of medicine. Within a few hours the breathing is easier, the pulse-rate slower, the extremities cooler and a rapid diuresis begins to dispose of the oedema. In a few days the size of the heart is restored to normal. Muscular pain and tenderness are also dramatically improved. The ECG may show characteristic paradoxical changes while the patient improves. In a typical case the tracing is normal while heart failure is severe, then as recovery starts T wave inversions appear over the right ventricle for a few days.

Dry Beriberi. The treatment is that of a nutritional polyneuropathy as described on page 139.

Wernicke's Encephalopathy. The ophthalmoplegia and nystagmus respond within hours to thiamin. The confusional state takes longer to clear, usually passing through the stage of Korsakoff's psychosis with confabulation for several days. Some impairment of memory may persist.

Infantile Beriberi. The simplest way to treat infantile beriberi is via the mother's milk. The mother should receive 10 mg thiamin hydrochloride twice daily—in severe cases by injection. In addition the infant must be given thiamin starting with 20 mg intramuscularly.

Associated Deficiencies. Other deficiencies in the patient's diet may include protein, vitamin A, nicotinic acid and riboflavin. In the early stages the other B vitamins should be supplied, e.g. as tablets, and a good protein intake given. Thereafter a mixed diet with less emphasis on rice is needed.

In all forms of beriberi, preoccupation with dietary treatment should not divert attention from the necessity of good nursing, management of associated infections, physiotherapy and subsequent rehabilitation.

Prevention. In principle all that is necessary in endemic areas is to prevent the production of over-milled rice or wheat. In practice, however, there are many difficulties in the control of milling processes and in persuading people to change their customary diet. Nevertheless improvement in milling practices has probably played an important part in reducing the incidence of beriberi.

Wherever possible, it is desirable to reduce the proportion of rice in the diet and encourage the growing of alternative crops and the consumption of other foods. Much can sometimes be done with small gardens properly cultivated. The substitution of parboiled rice for highly milled rice also greatly reduces the incidence of beriberi. Parboiling is the term used to indicate that unhusked rice has been steamed or boiled after preliminary soaking. If this is done before the rice is milled the greater portion of the vitamin B complex is conserved. Ignorance of the relative nutritional values of different foods is a contributory factor and can only be overcome by better education, improvement in social and economic conditions and establishing many more maternal and child health services.

In Western countries the prevention of beriberi and Wernicke's encephalopathy is related to the control of alcoholism.

Niacin

(Nicotinic Acid and Nicotinamide)

Nicotinamide is an essential part of the two important pyridine nucleotides, NAD and NADP which are hydrogen-accepting coenzymes for dehydrogenases at many steps in the pathways of glucose oxidation. NAD is also the coenzyme for alcohol dehydrogenase. Nicotinic acid (niacin) is readily converted in the body into the amide. For nutritional purposes the two have equal biological activity and are considered together in foods under the generic term 'niacin'. Both are water-soluble and resistant to heat.

Dietary Sources. Niacin is widely distributed in plant and animal foods, but only in relatively small amounts, except in meat (especially the organs), fish, wholemeal cereals and pulses. Removal of the bran in milling cereals reduces their niacin to low levels. Coffee is also a useful source. A cup of good coffee provides about 1 mg of niacin. In a normal Western European diet about half the nicotinic acid content is provided by meat and fish.

Cooking causes little destruction of niacin but considerable amounts may be lost in the cooking water and 'drippings' from cooked meat if these are discarded. In a mixed diet, from 15 to 25 per cent of the niacin of the cooked foodstuffs may be lost in this way. Commercial processing and storage of foodstuffs cause little loss.

A special feature of this vitamin is that it is normally synthesised in the body in limited amounts from the amino acid tryptophan; 60 mg of tryptophan yields 1 mg of nicotinamide. For this reason niacin equivalents in a diet are calculated by adding together the niacin plus $\frac{1}{60}$ of the tryptophan intake (in mg). The recommended daily intake is 18 mg of niacin equivalents in adult males.

Pellagra

Pellagra is a nutritional disease endemic among poor peasants who subsist chiefly on maize (American corn). The greater part of the niacin in maize is in a bound form, niacytin, which is unavailable to the consumer. Moreover the principal protein of maize, zein, is deficient in the essential amino acid tryptophan.

Pellagra is a relatively new disease, unknown to classical and mediaeval physicians. It has occurred all over the world, wherever maize is the staple cereal, e.g. the southern states of the USA, Africa and Southern Europe and also in certain regions in India, Asia and Latin America. In recent years pellagra has disappeared from many countries where it was once endemic; in areas where it remains the incidence is much less than formerly. An exception is southern Africa where big outbreaks occur in the spring and summer in certain Bantu areas.

Isolated cases of pellagra occur among people who are not dependent on maize. It is found as a complication of chronic alcoholism and has been reported in patients with renal failure on very low protein diets which had not been supplemented with B complex vitamins. Any chronic disease of the gastro-intestinal tract, leading to malabsorption, may result in the development of pellagra. In the rare inborn error of metabolism, *Hartnup disease*, tryptophan absorption is impaired and there is a pellagrous dermatitis with neurological abnormalities which respond to nicotinamide.

Pathology. In addition to dermatitis, the mucous membranes of the alimentary tract and vagina usually show abnormal epithelium with underlying inflammation. Small mucous cysts are seen in the colon and sometimes ulcers. In the nervous system there may be chromatolysis of ganglion cells and patchy demyelination in the spinal cord.

Clinical Features. *General.* Pellagra can develop in only 6 to 8 weeks on diets very deficient in niacin and tryptophan. The patient is often underweight, and presents the general features of poor nutrition. Pellagra has been called the disease of the three D's: dermatitis, diarrhoea and dementia.

Skin. The diagnosis is generally first suggested by the appearance of the skin. Characteristically, there is an erythema resembling severe sunburn, appearing symmetrically over the parts of the body exposed to sunlight. Local trauma or irritation of the skin may also determine the site of the lesion. The affected areas are well demarcated from normal skin. They are at first red and slightly swollen; they may itch and burn. In acute cases the skin lesions may progress to vesiculation, cracking, exudation and crusting with ulceration and sometimes secondary infection; but in chronic cases the dermatitis occurs as a roughening and thickening of the skin with dryness, scaling and a brown pigmentation. Dermatitis of the vulva, perineum and perianal area are usually present. Nasolabial dyssebacea is sometimes seen (p. 136).

Pellagra may sometimes occur without any apparent involvement of the skin if the patient has been confined indoors. This variety is sometimes called 'pellagra sine pellagra' and should be remembered if unexplained delirium or dementia is found in a person who has been taking a poor diet for a prolonged period.

Alimentary Tract. Diarrhoea is common but not always present. There may be anorexia, nausea, dysphagia and dyspepsia. The tongue characteristically has a 'raw beef' appearance—red, swollen and painful. Glossitis is an early symptom and may precede the skin lesions. The mouth is sore and often shows angular stomatitis and cheilosis (p. 136). It is probable that a non-infective inflammation extends throughout the gastrointestinal tract and accounts for the diarrhoea which is characteristically profuse and watery, sometimes with blood and mucus in the stools.

Nervous System. In the milder cases the symptoms consist chiefly of weakness, anxiety, depression, irritability and failure of concentration; in severe cases delirium is the most common mental disturbance in the acute form of the disease and dementia in the chronic form. Because of these changes, chronic pellagrins may be admitted to mental hospitals.

Treatment. Nicotinamide is given in a dose of 100 mg every 4 to 6 hours by mouth, although a smaller dose is likely to be effective. The vitamin is rapidly absorbed from the stomach, despite severe digestive disorders. There is therefore no indication for giving it parenterally. The response to nicotinamide is usually dramatic; within 24 hours the erythema of the skin diminishes, the tongue becomes paler and less painful and the diarrhoea ceases. Often there is also striking improvement in the patient's behaviour and mental attitude.

Nicotinamide alone is usually insufficient to restore health. Some of the features found in pellagra are clearly the result of associated nutritional deficiencies. First, a relatively low intake of protein and the amino acid tryptophan is an essential condition for development of the disease, and hypoalbuminaemia is common. Secondly, anaemia may coexist, either of iron or folate deficiency type. Thirdly, deficiencies of other B complex vitamins are to be expected. Peripheral neuropathy may be caused by thiamin or pyridoxine deficiency, nasolabial dyssebacea and angular stomatitis by riboflavin deficiency and spinal cord lesions, when present, by vitamin B_{12} deficiency. Lastly the patient has usually lost weight. Nicotinamide treatment should therefore be supplemented with a nutritious diet, high in protein. Vitamin B complex tablets should be given and iron, folic acid and vitamin B_{12} may be necessary in addition for some cases. Alcohol should be forbidden.

Rest in bed and sedation are necessary for severely ill pellagrins, especially those with marked mental symptoms; they are often troublesome patients, so their behaviour must be tolerated with objective understanding of its cause. If the dermatitis is associated with much crusting or secondary infection, gentle washing with a bland solution is indicated. If the diarrhoea is severe enough to cause electrolyte disturbances parenteral fluids may be needed. Infection may well be present and require appropriate treatment.

Prognosis. In the endemic areas the majority of cases are mild, improving in the winter and relapsing with the increased sunshine in the spring. In long-standing cases there may be persistent mental, spinal cord and digestive disorders.

Occasionally a fulminating form develops, with fever and severe prostration which may be fatal. In the past, most of the deaths arose from secondary infections, notably tuberculosis and dysentery, or from emaciation due to general dietary failure, intensified by the diarrhoea.

Prevention. The fact that pellagra has vanished from the southern states of America, whereas before the Second World War it afflicted tens of thousands of poor country folk, demonstrates that the disease is preventable. Its disappearance has sometimes been attributed to the fortification of bread and maize meal with nicotinic acid, but this is only one of several factors which have produced this satisfactory result. The most likely reason is the general improvement in the economic state, education and nutrition of the population.

In Central America the peasants eat a staple diet of maize but pellagra is unusual. The reason is because of the traditional method of boiling the maize in lime water (dilute calcium hydroxide) before they make tortillas. It has been found that the indigestible niacytin is hydrolysed to free niacin in dilute alkali.

From the standpoint of agricultural policy, it is clearly wise to avoid too much dependence on a single cereal crop, such as maize, or to devote too great an acreage of fertile land to the cultivation of cash-crops, such as cotton or tobacco. Animal husbandry and cultivation of legumes should be encouraged in all areas where pellagra is endemic.

For the medical practitioner in such an area, without direct influence on agricultural policy, the best advice that he can give to people is to take as much animal products and legumes as they can afford. He will also do well to prescribe tablets of vitamin B complex for patients with a poor dietary history or skin signs suggesting early pellagra.

Riboflavin

Riboflavin is a constituent of the flavoproteins which are concerned with tissue oxidation. It is a yellow-green fluorescent compound soluble in water but not in fats. Though stable to boiling in acid solution, in alkaline solution it is decomposed by heat. It is also destroyed by exposure to light.

Dietary Sources. The best sources of riboflavin are liver, kidney, meat, cheese and eggs. Milk and green vegetables contain moderate amounts. It differs from other components of the vitamin B complex in that it occurs in good amounts in dairy produce, but is relatively lacking in cereal grains, especially when highly milled. It is also present in beer. Ordinary methods of cooking do not destroy the vitamin apart from losses that occur when the water in which vegetables have been boiled is discarded. If foods, especially milk, are left exposed to sunshine, large losses may occur. Marmite and Bovril are particularly rich sources of the natural vitamin. The recommended daily intake is 1·7 mg in adult males.

Disorders due to Riboflavin Deficiency

When human volunteers have been given diets very low in riboflavin, the most consistent clinical manifestations have been angular stomatitis, cheilosis and nasolabial seborrhoea; these responded to the addition of pure riboflavin to the deficient diet.

Angular Stomatitis. This is not specific for riboflavin deficiency. Deficiencies of niacin, pyridoxine and iron can all produce it. It can follow herpes febrilis at the angle of the mouth. In Britain the commonest cause is ill-fitting dentures, associated with candidiasis.

Cheilosis. Cheilosis is the name given to a zone of red, denuded epithelium at the line of closure of the lips. It has occurred in experimental pure niacin deficiency. It is often associated with angular stomatitis and frequently seen in pellagrins.

Nasolabial Seborrhoea or Dyssebacea. This is the term given to the appearance of enlarged follicles around the sides of the nose which are plugged with dry sebaceous material. This skin change is seen in some patients with pellagra.

Other Abnormalities. Vascularisation of the cornea, scrotal dermatitis, a magenta-coloured tongue and anaemia have been attributed to riboflavin deficiency but its place in their causation in man is controversial.

Riboflavin clearly plays a vital role in cellular oxidation and there are communities and individuals who have both minimal dietary intakes and very low concentrations in urine or blood. Yet it is surprising that the clinical effects of riboflavin deficiency are trivial and mostly non-specific. Features of riboflavin deficiency are most likely to be found in pellagrins and in malnourished rice-eaters in Southeast Asia. In the first situation they are overshadowed by niacin deficiency and in the second by thiamin or protein deficiency.

Treatment. The therapeutic dose of riboflavin is 5 mg three times a day by mouth. It gives the patient's urine a green fluorescence. For reasons discussed above, other B complex vitamins should also be given.

Pyridoxine—Vitamin B$_6$

Pyridoxine is not a single substance but consists of three closely related chemical compounds with similar physiological actions. The biologically active form of the vitamin is pyridoxal phosphate, the coenzyme for over 60 different enzyme systems, including aminotransferases which are involved in the metabolism of amino acids. Vitamin B$_6$ is widely distributed both in plants and animal tissues, reflecting its importance in the metabolism of many kinds of cell. Meat, liver, pulses, egg yolk, vegetables and the outer 'coats' (bran) of cereal grains are all good sources. The normal adult requirement is 2 mg per day.

Disorders due to Pyridoxine Deficiency

Although pyridoxine participates in several different steps in the metabolism of amino acids, and although a series of pathological changes in the skin, liver, blood vessels, nervous tissue and bone marrow have been produced experimentally in various animals, disorders due to deficiency of pyridoxine rarely occur in man, and then very seldom as a result of dietary deficiency.

Convulsions, which respond to pyridoxine, have been reported to occur in infants on artificial feeds of powdered milk deficient in pyridoxine. In adults dermatitis, cheilosis, glossitis and angular stomatitis have been produced by means of the pyridoxine inhibitor, 4-desoxy-pyridoxine. The peripheral neuropathy associated with isoniazid therapy is due to a conditioned pyridoxine deficiency. Some cases of sideroblastic anaemia (p. 601) respond to treatment with pyridoxine.

Biochemical features of pyridoxine deficiency can occur in women taking oral contraceptives, and it has been reported that the mild depression which affects a small proportion of such women may be relieved by pyridoxine.

Biotin

Biotin functions as coenzyme for several carboxylases. It is present in a number of different foods; the requirement is small (about 100 μg/day) and it can be synthesised by intestinal bacteria. Human deficiency is rare; it has occurred in adults who have taken for long periods large amounts of raw egg. Egg white contains an antagonist avidin. The clinical features include dermatitis. It is reported that the seborrhoeic dermatitis of infants responds to biotin.

Vitamin B$_{12}$—The Cobalamins

Vitamin B$_{12}$ is the name given to a group of cobalamins present only in foodstuffs of animal origin and in micro-organisms—bacteria and moulds—which alone seem capable of synthesising them and are probably the original source. Vitamin B$_{12}$ is the largest molecule essential for human nutrition (molecular weight about 1,350). Its absorption, which occurs in the ileum, is very poor unless gastric intrinsic factor is available. Healthy adults have body stores of about 3,000 μg. The normal requirement is about 2 μg per day. Consequently it takes several years before deficiency becomes manifest when ingestion or absorption of the vitamin ceases.

Deficiency of vitamin B$_{12}$ affects DNA synthesis so it is most severely felt in tissues where the cells are normally dividing rapidly, e.g. in the blood-forming tissues of the bone marrow and in the gastrointestinal tract. The nervous system is affected by a different biochemical mechanism. Methylmalonyl coenzyme A is normally metabolised by a vitamin B_{12}-dependent mutase. Consequently in deficiency odd numbered and branched-chain fatty acids accumulate in the myelin.

Disorders due to Vitamin B_{12} Deficiency

These disorders may rarely result from a strict vegetarian diet, but more commonly from lack of gastric intrinsic factor, either in Addisonian pernicious anaemia (p. 602) or after gastrectomy. They may also occur from bacterial colonisation of the small intestine (p. 396) or from disease of the ileum causing malabsorption of vitamin B_{12} (p. 392). The two principal effects of deficiency are megaloblastic anaemia and subacute combined degeneration of the spinal cord (p. 740). A subnormal serum vitamin B_{12} is valuable in making the diagnosis.

Folate

Dietary Sources. Fresh, leafy vegetables, liver and kidney are the best sources, with other green vegetables, pulses, nuts and some seafoods the next best. Beef, fresh fruits, root vegetables and wheaten flour contain a little, whilst milk, eggs and other meats are poor in folate. Considerable losses occur when vegetables are boiled for a long time.

Folate occurs in a variety of forms in foods with from one up to seven glutamate residues in the molecule. The polyglutamates may not be so well absorbed. The recommended daily intake is 0·4 mg of total folate in adults and double this during pregnancy.

Disorders due to Folate Deficiency

Deficiency of folate leads to megaloblastic anaemia and atrophic changes in parts of the gastrointestinal tract, e.g. the tongue, because folate derivatives are coenzymes for DNA synthesis.

Compared to the rarity of megaloblastic anaemias due to dietary deficiency of vitamin B_{12} in Britain, those due to an inadequate intake of folate are quite common and can develop in four to five months. They are especially likely to occur in pregnancy and in infancy, when requirements are increased. Conditioned deficiencies can occur in haemolytic diseases, are frequent in the malabsorption syndrome and are a complication of long-term anticonvulsant therapy for epilepsy.

In treatment a daily dose of 5–10 mg of folic acid by mouth is sufficient (p. 604). It must never be given in Addisonian or other B_{12} deficiency anaemias because it can aggravate or precipitate the neurological features of vitamin B_{12} deficiency.

Nutritional Neurological Syndromes

The nervous system is susceptible to damage from dietary causes. It is dependent on finely adjusted mechanisms requiring a source of energy derived only from carbohydrate of which it has no immediate store, and a variety of highly complicated enzyme systems which govern and control the use of this energy.

The various nutritional neuropathies are mostly chronic conditions in contrast to other nutritional disorders, such as the heart failure of beriberi and the haemorrhagic manifestations of scurvy, which respond dramatically to treatment with the appropriate vitamin. Nerve cells have limited powers of recovery compared with other cells; hence no sudden or striking diminution of symptoms or signs in any chronic disease of the nervous system with structural changes can be expected to follow nutritional therapy. Toxins in the diet play a part in the aetiology, which in some syndromes is more important than nutritional deficiency.

Classification

1. The lesion is predominantly in the peripheral nerves in:

   (a) The polyneuropathies of beriberi, alcoholism, and pregnancy.
   (b) The burning feet syndrome.

2. The lesion is predominantly in the central nervous system in:

   (a) The cord syndromes:

      (i) vitamin B_{12} neuropathy (subacute degeneration of the cord);
      (ii) tropical ataxic neuropathy;
      (iii) lathyrism and other causes of spastic paraplegia.

   (b) Nutritional amblyopia.
   (c) Wernicke's encephalopathy (p. 131).

Nutritional and Alcoholic Polyneuropathies

The polyneuropathy of dry Oriental beriberi is the classic example. It arises from the consumption of a poor diet composed chiefly of polished rice, but is not due to lack of any one single dietary nutrient. Nutritional neuropathies occur most frequently in thin, underfed people. In countries outside the tropics an essentially similar disease occurs not infrequently in chronic alcoholics and rarely during pregnancy when vomiting is a prominent feature, and in the malabsorption syndrome.

Thiamin deficiency is clearly important in the pathogenesis of both Oriental and alcoholic polyneuropathy. However, polyneuropathy can be produced in man by deficiency of pyridoxine, vitamin B_{12}, probably niacin and possibly pantothenic acid. In different clinical situations one or more of these may have been associated. Biochemical tests on the blood when the patient is seen do not necessarily reflect the nutritional status of the peripheral nerves when the process started. It should be borne in mind too that endogenous and exogenous toxins (p. 750) can produce a similar picture and isoniazid is more likely to cause neuropathy in malnourished people because it antagonises the action of pyridoxine.

The pathology and clinical features are similar to those of the polyneuropathy of dry beriberi (p. 130).

Treatment. This demands, first, attention to the patient's diet both in quantity and quality. The neurological lesions will not improve until the patient regains his strength, so every effort should be made to restore him to his original body weight. Plenty of protein—milk, eggs, meat, fish—is desirable, supplemented by generous doses of the vitamin B complex. If these are given as tablets care must be taken that all the vitamins are included. Some authorities prefer natural sources such as yeast or yeast extract (e.g. Marmite), rice bran or wheat germ. If the patient has anorexia, vomiting or malabsorption the vitamin B complex should be given by injection. Physiotherapy is very important and may need to be prolonged.

Burning Feet Syndrome

Outbreaks of this clinical syndrome have occurred in Europe, Central America, Africa and India among people living on very poor diets. It became very troublesome among European prisoners in the Far East during the Second World War.

The syndrome has usually been associated with a diet deficient in the B group of vitamins. Patients who suffer from it may also develop mucocutaneous signs suggesting riboflavin deficiency or nutritional amblyopia (p. 141), but rarely frank beriberi.

The earliest symptom is aching, burning or throbbing in the feet, followed by sharp, stabbing pains, which may spread up as far as the knee like an electric shock. They come on in paroxysms and are usually worse at night. Objective signs of neuropathy are seldom found unless the polyneuropathy of beriberi coexists.

The therapeutic response to pure vitamin preparations has been variable. Some patients have responded to pantothenic acid preparations, some to riboflavin or other B complex vitamins, some not to any combination of vitamins.

Vitamin B_{12} Neuropathy

Subacute Combined Degeneration of the Cord. Dysfunction or degeneration of the posterior and lateral columns of the spinal cord together with peripheral neuropathy usually occurs in association with Addisonian pernicious anaemia (p. 602). Less commonly it occurs after gastrectomy or in other causes of vitamin B_{12} malabsorption (p. 392). Rarely it arises from a lack of vitamin B_{12} in the diet, e.g. in some castes of strict Hindu and in vegans (vegetarians who eat no animal products of any kind). There may be little anaemia presumably because a vegetable diet supplies sufficient folic acid, which can correct the megaloblastic anaemia but not the neuropathy. Serum vitamin B_{12} is subnormal. The clinical features and treatment are discussed on pages 740–742.

Tropical Ataxic Neuropathy

Patients have been reported from Jamaica, Nigeria and East Africa with signs indicating a lesion in the posterior columns of the spinal cord. There is sensory ataxia and vibration sense in the legs is often lost. There may be associated amblyopia or deafness.

Although these patients have been eating a poor diet, and are often thin and may have muco-cutaneous signs of vitamin deficiency, recent investigations suggest that the probable cause is chronic cyanide ingestion from prolonged large intakes of certain foods, particularly cassava. Patients have been found to have high thiocyanate concentrations in their blood. Traditional methods of cooking, if properly followed, wash or boil off most of the cyanide in cassava. Patients may be expected to improve if changed to a balanced diet and vitamin B_{12} may help in detoxifying the cyanide in the body.

Spastic Paraplegia

Lathyrism. *Lathyrus sativus* is a drought-resistant pulse, widely grown in parts of India. If eaten in excessive amounts, it gives rise to lathyrism, a nutritional spastic paraplegia.

Epidemic lathyrism is associated with undernutrition since the pulse is eaten in large quantities only when the main crops have failed. If, because of drought, there is a poor crop of wheat, a useful harvest of lathyrus may be reaped. Eaten in small quantities, lathyrus seeds are a valuable food. But if they are the main source of energy, disease of the spinal cord may result. A neurotoxin has recently been isolated from lathyrus seeds, β-N-oxalyl-amino-L-alanine (BOAA).

The onset of paralysis is usually sudden and is often preceded by exertion or exposure to cold. The condition is a spastic paralysis of the lower limbs, due to a localised lesion of the lower parts of the pyramidal tracts. The motor nerves to the muscles of the trunk, upper limbs and sphincters are spared. The sensory nervous system is not involved. In severe cases the disease progresses to paraplegia, but in mild cases there is only stiffness and weakness of the legs and exaggerated knee and ankle jerks.

There is no specific treatment. All patients need a good diet. Minor cases may make a complete recovery following satisfactory dietary and physical rehabilitation. In most cases the pathological changes are irreversible and the patients drift into beggary and become a social problem.

Other Forms of Spastic Paraplegia. Spastic paraplegia of uncertain origin occurring in adults is not infrequently seen in various parts of Asia and Africa and in Jamaica. Toxins in plant foods or 'bush teas' have been suspected.

On the Pacific island of Guam there is an exceptionally high incidence of amyotrophic lateral sclerosis (p. 736). It has been suggested that this results from the indigenous population's regular consumption of cycad seeds.

Nutritional Amblyopia

A progressive failure of vision attributable to a retrobulbar neuropathy occurred amongst prisoners-of-war in the Far East in the Second World War. Similar amblyopias occasionally occur in beriberi, pellagra and subacute combined degeneration of the spinal cord. Cases have been reported in Nigeria and Jamaica. The patients appear to have had one feature in common, a period of months on diets grossly deficient in respect of many essential nutrients. A similar condition occurs in affluent communities in some heavy tobacco smokers (p. 675).

A typical history is that in over a period of three weeks or so there is a growing inability to see the colours of small objects. A mist obscures the central field of vision and gradually becomes so intense that it becomes impossible to recognise acquaintances. There is usually no pain. On examination of the visual fields a central or paracentral scotoma is present. The visual acuity varies greatly. On ophthalmoscopy there is temporal pallor of the optic discs in severe cases.

Oriental cases responded to a good diet supplemented with yeast or Marmite. Tobacco amblyopia is often effectively treated with hydroxocobalamin (p. 675). In Nigeria retrobulbar neuropathy and spinal ataxia occur together in people who subsist largely on cassava.

Nutritional Disorders of the Skin, Hair, Nails, Mouth and Eyes

Follicular keratosis (p. 118), xeroderma (dryness of the skin, cracked skin, crazy paving skin), pachyderma (elephant skin), atrophy of the skin, pigmentary changes of the skin and tropical ulcers are disorders of the skin and mucous membranes which are frequently seen in persons subsisting for long periods on unsatisfactory diets. In such individuals there may also be changes in the texture and colour of the hair (p. 106), and the finger nails may be thin, brittle or spoon-shaped (p. 598). Disorders of the eye may also be present (p. 116), and deficiency of nicotinic acid, riboflavin, vitamins B_6 and B_{12}, folate or iron may give rise to a nutritional glossitis and stomatitis. Until more is known about the chemical pathology of the skin, hair, nails and eyes it will continue to be difficult to assess the significance of certain clinical changes in these structures which are not infrequently seen in examination of underfed or malnourished people. Hence it would be unwise always to attribute these disorders solely to dietary deficiency. Undoubtedly exposure to dirt, heat, moisture, trauma and infection can contribute to their causation. The practical importance of these stigmata is that their presence in either an individual or a community should at once draw attention to the diet.

Biochemical Diagnosis and Subclinical Vitamin Deficiencies

Biochemical methods are an integral part of modern medical diagnosis. For example, plasma sodium and potassium concentrations are essential for the diagnosis and treatment of difficult electrolyte problems and serum or red cell folate and serum vitamin B_{12} concentrations are desirable before treating a patient with megaloblastic anaemia. Likewise with the other vitamins, biochemical tests have been developed which are more or less valuable. (a) for confirming the diagnosis of a deficiency disease in places where it is uncommonly seen or if the clinical picture is complicated or (b) in community surveys, for identifying individuals with subclinical vitamin deficiencies.

The tests which can be used for the major vitamins are listed in Table 4.2. As with other tests in chemical pathology there can be false positives and false negatives. Each result needs to be evaluated with critical understanding; for example, serum vitamin B_{12} is increased in acute hepatitis and alkaline phosphatase may not be elevated if rickets is accompanied by PCM.

In general when the dietary intake of a nutrient is inadequate the individual goes through three stages. The first stage is that of adaptation to the low intake. For example, urine excretion falls but there is no evidence of abnormal function or of depletion of the cells.

In the second stage there are in addition biochemical changes indicating either impaired function, e.g. reduced red cell transketolase activity in thiamin deficiency, or cellular depletion, e.g. reduced white cell ascorbic acid. But clinical manifestations of deficiency are absent or non-specific.

The third stage is that of clinical deficiency disease.

Most clinical biochemistry laboratories provide only some of the methods as a routine but others might be provided in special circumstances or, alternatively, specimens could be sent to a laboratory specialising in nutrition research.

Table 4.2 Biochemical methods for diagnosing nutritional status (protein and vitamins)

| Nutrient | Principal Methods | | Supplementary Methods |
	Indicating Reduced Intake	Indicating Impaired Function (IF) or Cell Depletion (CD)	
Protein	Urinary nitrogen	PLASMA ALBUMIN (IF)	Fasting plasma amino acid pattern
Vitamin A	PLASMA VITAMIN A (retinol) and PLASMA CAROTENE		
Thiamin	Urinary thiamin	RBC TRANSKETOLASE and TPP EFFECT* (IF)	Plasma pyruvate and lactate*
Riboflavin	Urinary riboflavin	RBC glutathione reductase and FAD effect (IF)*	RBC riboflavin
Niacin	URINE N′METHYL NICOTINAMIDE and 2-pyridone		Fasting plasma tryptophan
Pyridoxine	Urinary 4-pyridoxic acid	RBC glutamic oxalacetic transaminase and PP effect (IF)*	Urinary xanthurenic acid after tryptophan load*
Folic Acid	Plasma folate (Lactobacillus casei)	RED CELL FOLATE (CD) Haemoglobin, PCV and smear (IF)	Urinary FIGLU after histidine load* Bone marrow morphology
Vitamin B_{12}	PLASMA VITAMIN B_{12} (Euglena gracilis)	Haemoglobin, PCV and smear (IF)	Schilling test Bone marrow morphology
Ascorbic Acid	Plasma ascorbic acid	LEUCOCYTE ASCORBIC ACID (CD)	Urinary ascorbic acid
Vitamin D	Plasma 25-hydroxy-cholecalciferol	PLASMA ALKALINE PHOSPHATASE (IF)*	Serum calcium and inorganic phosphorus

Note: 1. The tests in capital letters are those most commonly used at present.
   2. Asterisk⁽*⁾ indicates value *increased* in deficiency.

PREVENTION OF NUTRITIONAL DEFICIENCIES

There are broadly three ways of approaching prevention:

1. *Increasing food consumption per head.* This requires increased production of food in the country or increased export earnings with which to import food. However, an overall increase of food in a country will be of little value unless the majority of people have jobs which provide sufficient money to buy the food they need. In addition effective national programmes of population control must be implemented in many countries. Doctors are likely to have more of a role to play in helping with birth control than with agricultural or economic planning.

2. *Nutrition education and food enrichment.* Education in nutrition consists of

teaching and motivating people to make a healthy choice of foods. It ranges from advising agricultural planners on which crops should be encouraged to teaching mothers how to feed their children and distribute food sensibly in the family, using what is available to them.

Where vitamin or mineral deficiencies occur, or could occur, food enrichment is one possible solution. This is used mostly in industrial countries; it is difficult to organise in developing countries where there are many small farmers who grow their own food. To be effective the enriched food should reach the potentially deficient segment of the population, so the choice of which staple food to enrich needs careful consideration. Addition of vitamins A and D to margarine and iodization of salt are good examples of useful food enrichment. The use of nutrients which are toxic in large amounts must be limited. Food enrichment should be supervised and monitored by the appropriate government ministry. It is not the answer to every nutritional deficiency even in industrial countries. We do not believe, for example, that further enrichment of bread with iron will solve the problem of iron deficiency anaemia. It is better dealt with by the third strategy.

3. *Health and medical action for vulnerable groups.* Many countries provide nutritious lunches for school children. Pregnant mothers should be given prophylactic doses of iron and folate; young children should be given small prophylactic doses of vitamin D or their mothers should expose them to sunlight regularly; women with menorrhagia and patients who have had gastric surgery should be given iron tablets from time to time, and so on. Doctors should be trained to anticipate the possibility of certain types of malnutrition in association with particular diseases.

In developing countries where most people do not have direct access to a doctor, maternal and child health clinics provide a centre for therapeutic, preventive and educational services at moderate cost, aimed at the most vulnerable sections of the community. In this setting nutrition and infection must be treated in an integrated way and can often be combined with family planning.

A. S. TRUSWELL

OBESITY

Obesity is the most common nutritional disorder in infants, children and adults in affluent societies, where it is responsible for more ill-health than all the vitamin deficiencies. The importance of obesity requires constant emphasis, not only because of the excess mortality it carries, but also because of numerous complications and the predisposition it creates to common and potentially serious conditions such as diabetes mellitus. It reduces the efficiency of those affected, it detracts from their ability to participate in many normal activities, and it is frequently associated with emotional and other psychological disturbances, all of which may interfere in a major way with the welfare of an individual, a family, or a community.

Obesity can be defined as an abnormal accumulation of fat in the stores of adipose tissue throughout the body. The size of the fat depot depends on two variables: the number of fat cells (adipocytes) and the amount of fat in these, but the methods of measuring each factor are at present unsuitable for general clinical application. A guide for therapeutic advice is based on the notion of a desirable weight, for any given height, to be maintained from early adult life onwards. A suitable working rule for the treatment of obesity is that patients should remain within 10 per cent of the desirable weight, a table for which is given on page 948.

Aetiology. *Genetic and Environmental Factors.* A genetic component can be identified in many cases but its mode of transmission and operation is still not clear. Environmental considerations such as the dietetic habits of the family and economic factors are also important.

Sex. The normal fat content of young adult women, approximately 15 per cent of body weight, is about twice that of young men. With advancing years, women are more prone to obesity than men. The gain in weight which usually occurs in pregnancy may not be corrected in the months after delivery. In addition, gain in weight at and after the menopause frequently aggravates a disability established in earlier years.

Appetite and Feeding Patterns. People who consume more calories than they require to match their energy output will gain weight. Excellent evidence exists in animal models to show that damage to hypothalamic centres can lead to obesity, and from this it is sometimes deduced that an imbalance between appetite and satiety centres in the hypothalamus leads to overeating. Rats made fat in this way and obese humans are less responsive than normal to satiety, that is, in knowing when to stop eating, and surprisingly, after deprivation from food, both eat less than normal controls. In this sense they are said to be under-responsive to 'internal cues'. By contrast, with free access to food both over-respond by eating an excess of foods they find particularly palatable, but eat less than normal controls when the food offered is unpalatable. Thus they are said to be hyper-responsive to 'external cues', in this case the attractiveness of the food offered.

Many people develop the habit, sometimes deliberately, of taking one large meal a day, rather than three or more smaller meals. There are grounds for suggesting that such a habit is more likely to be associated with obesity than a more evenly spaced intake of the same amount of food at intervals throughout the day.

Physical Activity. It is well recognised that physical activity is less in the obese than in the lean, though the amount of energy expended by an obese person on most tasks is likely to be more because of the extra weight to be moved. There is also evidence to suggest that below a certain level of exercise the relationship between appetite and energy requirement is more difficult to maintain.

Energy expenditure on walking is quite considerable: at $3\frac{1}{2}$ miles per hour a normal man would use about 300 calories per hour. Walking for one hour daily, this amounts to the equivalent of more than 1 kg of adipose tissue per month, by no means a negligible consideration in relation to energy balance.

Social and industrial trends have steadily diminished the need in the developed societies for energy expenditure, and while some maintain their interests and participation in physical recreation, the majority become spectators exclusively at an early age.

Energy Balance. It has sometimes been suggested that differences between the fat and the lean could be due to inordinately efficient absorption in the obese as compared with those of normal weight, or that the lean have a special mechanism denied to the obese for 'burning off' excess calories. Various factors, for example a fat mobilising substance, and an anorexigenic substance produced during exercise have also been postulated with the support of experimental work, to account for the difficulties of the obsese in maintaining a normal weight.

Endocrine Factors. These may contribute in a minor way to a patient's difficulties in maintaining a normal weight. For example, in Cushing's syndrome, adrenocortical hyperfunction is often associated with a gain in weight and an increase in body fat, mainly confined to the head, neck and trunk, but sparing the limbs. In pregnancy, endocrine factors contribute to the increase in weight. In hypothyroidism, diminished energy expenditure may be associated with gain in weight. In obesity, hyperinsulinism may aggravate the disability by promoting lipogenesis and inhibiting lipolysis. These endocrine variables, however, are certainly not primary considerations in most obese patients.

Psychological Factors. Obese patients are often psychologically disturbed, though it may be difficult to distinguish between cause and effect. Depressed or anxious patients or the emotionally deprived may seek relief in food. Many patients, especially younger adult females, are often greatly ashamed of their appearance and may be easier to treat than the older patient who has lost any ambition to recover a more youthful appearance.

Comment. No single factor can be held to be responsible for obesity. The simple general conclusion emerges that obesity represents an accumulation of energy in excess of requirements, and that weight reduction can be achieved only by reducing energy intake, by increasing output, or by a combination of the two.

Clinical Features. The diagnosis will be apparent from the patient's appearance and is confirmed by measurement of weight and height. The amount of surplus tissue can be estimated by reference to Table 18.2 (p. 948). The distribution of adipose tissue is variable, but measurement of the skin-fold thickness over the triceps muscle has been found to be useful. Special springloaded 'Harpenden' calipers are available for this purpose. Obesity is indicated by readings above 20 mm in a man and above 28 mm in a woman.

Complications. In addition to aesthetic considerations and psychological repercussions, obesity leads to mechanical disabilities, predisposes to metabolic and cardiovascular disorders and so reduces the expectancy of life.

Mechanical Disability. Flat feet and osteoarthrosis of the knees, hips and lumbar spine are more common in obese people, who are also less mobile and more accident prone. The abdominal muscles that support the viscera and those in the legs whose contractions promote venous return, are less efficient with consequent abdominal and diaphragmatic hernias and varicose veins. Adipose tissue around the trunk interferes with the mechanics of respiration and predisposes to bronchitis. Chronic infection of the skin occurs between folds of fat under the breasts and in the axillae (intertrigo).

Metabolic Disorders. Obesity may be associated with an elevated level of cholesterol and triglyceride in the blood. The obese are more prone to develop gall-stones than those of normal weight.

The association of obesity and diabetes mellitus is well recognised and is particularly important because of the increased morbidity and mortality that these two conditions carry. It applies mainly in the older group of diabetic patients, with adult or maturity-onset diabetes. Obesity is associated with increased insulin secretion and with increased resistance to the action of insulin; both of these are reversible with weight reduction. When diabetes has become manifest in an obese patient, it is sometimes possible to reverse the diabetic biochemical abnormalities by weight reduction alone.

Gout afflicts the obese more commonly than others.

Cardiovascular Disorders. Obese persons suffer from hypertension more commonly than those of normal weight. The work of the heart is increased by the added bulk of body tissue. This, coupled with the tendency to coronary atherosclerosis, accounts for the liability to angina pectoris and cardiac failure among obese people in middle life.

Life Expectancy. Obesity constitutes a poor risk from the standpoint of life insurance. The statistics of the Metropolitan Life Insurance Co. (U.S.A.) have shown that men aged 45 years who are of medium height and frame and weigh 90 kg, which is 16 kg above the average, can expect to live 4 years less than men of comparable build who weigh 68 kg, which is within the range of desirable weights. The risks with obesity in women are somewhat less.

Diagnosis. This very common disorder is frequently overlooked because the doctor is preoccupied by one of its many complications or simply ignores it because it is so familiar. Recording the patient's weight and height must be just as much a routine part of clinical examination as taking the blood pressure or testing the urine. People with small frames may appear to be of normal weight as judged by accepted standards, and yet may be obese; their obesity, often concentrated in the abdomen, is easily overlooked. Athletes in training are sometimes considerably overweight as judged by normal standards; their extra weight is due to muscular hypertrophy.

Obesity must be distinguished from a gain in weight due to occult oedema in cardiac failure or renal or hepatic disease. Oedema does not generally become manifest clinically until the extracellular fluid is increased by 10 per cent or more. In hypothyroidism there may be a sufficient accumulation of myxoedematous tissue to cause excessive weight.

Treatment. GENERAL CONSIDERATIONS. The most important single requirement in the management of obesity is education of the patient. The more they can be taught about the nature and behaviour of the disorder, the more likely are they to succeed. This makes heavy demands on the time, energy, skill and enthusiasm of the doctors, dietitians, and nurses who are called upon to supervise these patients. Most patients have already made attempts to reduce their weight either on their own responsibility, or on their doctors' advice, or as frequently happens now, with the support of lay groups run for the express purpose of helping patients to diet, for example 'Weight Watchers'. The number of patients requiring supervision is so great, the need for this support is so prolonged, and the success of some of these lay organisations compares so favourably with conventional medical methods, that until medical treatment has something considerably more effective to offer, it is justifiable to take advantage of the facilities provided by these groups. Most of these organisations refer members to their own doctors at the first suggestion of any untoward development.

However this supervision is arranged, it is most important for success that these patients should be given precise instructions as to how they should reorganise their dietary and other habits. It is essential also that they should remain under formal care, attending at frequent intervals, certainly no longer than 2 weeks at first.

Among the important lessons to be learned by obese patients is the need to manage the disorder themselves. Unlike most conditions for which they seek help, success does not depend upon operations, drugs, injections or other manipulations undertaken by the therapist, but rather on the ability of the patient to accept advice, to act upon it, and to persist indefinitely with some restrictions on dietary freedom.

The task will seem less formidable if rewards for achievement in weight reduction and maintenance are kept in front of the patient. In addition to improvement in health there are such advantages as the recovery of a more attractive figure, the ability to wear standard size garments and to take part in swimming and other activities without appearing conspicuous or even ridiculous. The physician's role is to provide advice and continuing support.

The basic requirement for the treatment of obesity is the regulation of the daily intake of energy sources. In the first instance an unweighted diet is used, but if this is not effective, the stricter discipline of a weighed diet, as might be prescribed for a diabetic, may need to be imposed occasionally. In some resistant cases anorectic drugs may provide temporary help. Obese patients who fail to respond to any of these measures require further investigation from both physical and psychological aspects and, exceptionally, intensive treatment under strict supervision in hospital.

THE CONSTRUCTION OF A WEIGHT-REDUCING DIET. Energy requirements have been given on page 102. An obese middle-aged housewife will usually lose weight satisfactorily on a diet providing 800–1,000 kcal/day, such as Diet No. 1 (p. 939). An obese man engaged in active physical work cannot tolerate a diet as low as 1,000 kcal/day. A satisfactory weight loss can be expected from a diet containing about 1,500 kcal/day. Diet No. 1 can be used for this purpose by the addition of 3 carbohydrate exchanges, 2 protein exchanges and $\frac{1}{2}$ a fat exchange (p. 941) and by increasing the milk allowance to 500 ml daily.

Protein. Dietary protein of 50 g/day is sufficient to maintain nitrogen balance. High protein diets may satisfy appetite more effectively than high carbohydrate diets, but they are expensive, they may not be particularly palatable after a time, they may have a high incidental content of fat, and are therefore seldom practicable.

Carbohydrate. The intake of foods rich in carbohydrate must be reduced since over-indulgence in such foods is common. Obese people seldom develop more than a trace of ketosis and never sufficient to cause symptoms as long as they consume small amounts of carbohydrate. In a diet of 1,000 kcal/day, 100 g of carbohydrate is a suitable allowance.

Fat. A diet containing 100 g of carbohydrate and 50 g of protein, cannot include more than 40–45 g of fat. This allowance of fat, though small, is sufficient to make the diet palatable.

Vitamins. A properly designed reducing diet should contain plenty of green vegetables and fruits, since they contain few calories, while their bulk helps to fill the stomach and relieve hunger; they also help to minimise the constipation common on a low food intake. Their vitamin A and vitamin C activity will be sufficient to meet the body's needs. With meat, fish and eggs in the diet and little or no refined cereals and sugar, it is improbable that deficiency of any component of the vitamin B complex will arise.

Minerals. The only minerals that need serious consideration are calcium and iron. Provided the diet includes 300 ml of skimmed milk, there is little likelihood of a negative calcium balance developing in an adult. The supply of iron is less sure and may call for the prescription of iron supplements.

Fluids and Salt. At one time patients were often advised to restrict their intake of water, but there is no logical reason for keeping fat patients thirsty. Sweetened 'juices' must be avoided, except those sold for diabetic patients, which have a low caloric content. *Alcoholic drinks* are also a source of calories and hence are best avoided, but if taken, a corresponding reduction in the diet is necessary.

In addition to liability to the usual causes of oedema, the obese are also particularly susceptible to water and salt retention. Diuretics should be used with discrimination in these patients, because potassium depletion is particularly liable to occur while they are on a reducing regimen. Salt restriction alone may be sufficient to alleviate oedema, but strict adherence to a reducing regimen will often relieve the oedema of obesity in any case. When diuretics are considered essential, potassium supplements should also be given.

MORE INTENSIVE DIETETIC TREATMENT. With an intelligent, co-operative patient who is determined to lose weight and who is only moderately obese all that may be necessary is to discuss the essentials of treatment described above and the kind of foods which must be avoided because of their high calorie content (p. 946). If this is not successful then more detailed instructions are necessary and the patient should be treated with an unweighed but measured diet such as Diet No. 1 (p. 939). This diet is, in general, suitable for the treatment of an overweight middle-aged housewife in Britain but it may be unsuitable in other circumstances and in other climates. Dietitians with knowledge of local eating habits can achieve a great deal of good by devising diets suitable to the established customs which provide about 1,000 kcal made up from about 100 g carbohydrate, 50–60 g protein and 40–45 g fat.

Failure to respond to the unweighed diet indicates that the patient requires the stricter regime provided by a weighed diet.

The dietetic regimes described above aim at achieving a rate of weight loss of just over 1 kg per week. Very fat patients will have to persist with such a regime for predictable periods before achieving their declared target weight. Slow progress may be disheartening and lead to treatment being abandoned. Provided there are no orthopaedic or cardiovascular complications, it is possible to increase the physical activities gradually and reduce the diet still further. Patients have been kept on diets providing only 400 kcal/day for periods of several weeks, whilst they walked 10 miles daily. This regime involved negative balances of the order of 3,000 kcal/day. The patients lost weight at rates of up to 3 kg per week yet remained healthy.

A period of several weeks of starvation in hospital, only water and non-caloric drinks with vitamin and mineral supplements being allowed, has been recommended for very obese patients who have failed to respond to orthodox treatment. Although the initial loss of weight may be marked the long-term results are no more satisfactory than other systems since many patients regain most of the weight lost when this strict regime is discontinued. However, it may be of value for selected patients, particularly as a demonstration of what can be achieved with sufficient discipline. Such a regime is contraindicated for older patients, especially if they have cardiovascular complications, and deaths have occasionally occurred. Ketosis may be troublesome in the early stages, and hyperuricaemia, sometimes accompanied by gout, may occur.

EXERCISE. Most obese patients lead sedentary lives and benefit from physical activity such as walking, swimming, gardening, provided it does not exceed their cardiovascular capacity. Regular daily exercise is much more valuable than episodic activity.

ANORECTIC DRUGS. These are no substitute for a dietary regime and should not be used at the beginning of treatment. If an obese person has failed to respond, one of the anorectic drugs may be prescribed for not longer than 6 weeks as they tend to lose their effect after regular use.

Unfortunately some of the more effective drugs used in the past, particularly amphetamines, are addictive and have been so widely abused that they are no longer recommended for the treatment of obesity. Fenfluramine does not have the disadvantages of amphetamines, but it is quite expensive. The dose is 20–40 mg twice daily before meals. Occasionally unpleasant side-effects are produced such as dry mouth, diarrhoea, dizziness and tiredness. Much more rarely confusion may become so marked that the drug has to be withdrawn.

Fenfluramine is a suitable anorectic drug for use in anxious patients who have become disheartened with the poor results achieved by diet alone. For patients of the lethargic type phentermine, 30 mg daily before breakfast, would be more suitable as it has a stimulating effect which may help the patient to persevere with the diet.

THYROXINE. The administration of thyroxine to euthyroid obese patients is not only useless but is potentially dangerous, especially if degenerative heart disease is present. It should be prescribed only if hypothyroidism coexists with obesity.

METHYL CELLULOSE. This is an indigestible substance which adds bulk to the diet. It distends the stomach and so may help to allay hunger. In clinical trials it has been shown to have little if any effect in promoting weight loss, and it is very doubtful if this product is of any value as an adjunct to dietary therapy.

SURGICAL TREATMENT. Operations such as small intestine bypass, aimed at inducing malabsorption, have been undertaken in some centres for the treatment of intractable cases of severe obesity. The side-effects, particularly diarrhoea, have sometimes been distressing. Wiring the jaws together to prevent eating has also been undertaken exceptionally. It seems unlikely that these experimental techniques will contribute substantially to the management of obesity in more than a very small minority of the most resistant cases.

Prognosis. It is easy for an obese person to lose up to 5 kg in weight. This accounts for the temporary successes of numerous popular 'slimming cures'. How difficult it is to achieve further losses is not generally realised. The published records of seven obesity clinics in the U.S.A. showed that satisfactory results ranged only from 12 to 28 per cent if the index of success was the loss of 12 kg or more.

Experience in many clinics has shown also that it is difficult for patients to maintain their reduced weight. The reasons for these poor results are not clear, but must be related to failure of motivation in the patient, and to the inadequacies of the methods at present available for the control of obesity.

Prevention of obesity. This must depend in part on the doctor who discerns when his patients (be they infants, children or adults) are gaining too much weight. For this purpose alone, one of the most useful records that a doctor can keep about his patients is a record of their weight, measured at regular intervals. The doctor's responsibility with an overweight patient, at any time, is advisory and educational: he must draw the attention of his patients to the dangers of obesity and to the appropriate methods of correcting it.

All the health agencies available should be mustered to support a steady campaign of education and persuasion of patients and potential patients on the need to avoid obesity. The antenatal services, infant welfare clinics, school health authorities, health visitors and many others to whom the public look for advice when they are in difficulties should serve as the medium for this educational programme.

J. A. STRONG
A. S. TRUSWELL

Further reading:

Cameron, M. & Hofvander, Y. (1971). *Manual on Feeding Infants and Young Children (for application in the developing areas of the world with special reference to home-made weaning foods).* New York: Protein-Calorie Advisory Group of the United Nations System.—Obtainable free of charge; write to 866 United Nations Plaza, New York, N.Y. 10017, U.S.A. Valuable recipes for nutritious home-made combinations of foods suitable for young children, which come from and can be applied in many different countries.

Davidson, Sir Stanley, Passmore, R., Brock, J. F. & Truswell, A. S. (1975). *Human Nutrition and Dietetics*, 6th edition. Edinburgh: Churchill Livingstone.—The standard textbook. Covers the whole field of nutrition in 60 chapters.

Department of Health and Social Security (1969). *Recommended Intakes of Nutrients for the United Kingdom.* Reports on Public Health and Medical Subjects No. 120. London: HMSO.—A revised version should be published in 1978.

British Medical Journal (1975). Editorial: Nutrition rehabilitation units. *British Medical Journal*, **4,** 246.—Introduces the reasons for and types of these units.

Garrow, J. S. (1974). *Energy Balance and Obesity in Man.* Amsterdam: North-Holland; New York: American Elsevier.—An admirably balanced book on the physiology of obesity. Thoughtful but readable.

Jelliffe, D. B. (1966). *The Assessment of the Nutritional Status of the Community (with special reference to field surveys in developing regions of the world).* WHO Monograph Series No. 53. Geneva: World Health Organization.—The best manual on the subject, with some good photographs.

McCance, R. A. & Widdowson, E. M. (1960) *The Composition of Foods.* Medical Research Council Special Report Series No. 297. London: HMSO.—British food tables: now being revised. Most large countries have prepared their own food composition tables.

Olson, R. E. (Ed.) (1975) *Protein-Calorie Malnutrition.* New York: The Nutrition Foundation and Academic Press.—The latest monograph: 30 chapters by different international experts mostly on scientific aspects.

Passmore, R., Nicol, B. M., Rao, M. N., Beaton, G. H. & De Maeyer, E. M. (1974) *Handbook on Human Nutritional Requirements.* Published as either FAO Nutritional Studies No. 28, Rome or WHO Monograph Series No. 61, Geneva.—An International handbook on requirements of the major nutrients.

Reichsman, F. (Ed.) (1972) *Hunger and Satiety in Health and Disease.* Basel: Karger.—Further reading in a difficult field.

Report of the Royal College of Physicians (1976) *Fluoride, Teeth and Health.* London: Pitman Medical.—A working party of the College reviews fluoridation of water and concludes that it is safe in a temperate climate.

Swedish Nutrition Foundation (1971) *Famine.* Uppsala: Almqvist and Wiksells.—Report of a symposium with international speakers. Scientific research papers on this topic are rare.

5. Disturbances in Water and Electrolyte Balance and in Hydrogen Ion Concentration

THE chemical events collectively called metabolism require the concentration of hydrogen ions and electrolytes to remain within narrow limits in the tissue cells and in the fluid which bathes them. Derangement of water and electrolyte balance and disturbances in hydrogen ion concentration occur in a wide variety of clinical conditions which are separately described in the appropriate chapters of this book. It is convenient, however, to summarise here the relevant physiological facts and to describe briefly the more common abnormalities. The kidney plays an important part in maintaining water, electrolyte and acid base balance; the details of the movements of ions that occur in the nephron are given on page 469.

Normal Distribution of Water and Electrolytes

Water. The body of a normal man of 65 kg contains approximately 40 litres of water. About 28 litres of this is intracellular, and 12 litres extracellular. The latter is composed of 9–10 litres of interstitial fluid and 2–3 litres of plasma. Using tritiated water, it has been shown in human subjects that water readily passes through almost all membranes of the body and permeates easily into all fluid compartments. Its final distribution between the compartments is determined by osmotic and hydrostatic pressures and under normal conditions the total amount of water in the body is kept remarkably constant.

Electrolytes. The inorganic ions dissolved in the body water include sodium, potassium, calcium, magnesium, chloride, phosphate, bicarbonate and sulphate. These are not dispersed in the same concentrations throughout the various body fluid compartments. Sodium and chloride are confined mainly to the extracellular fluids where they are present in average concentrations of 142 mmol/l and 100 m-mol/l respectively. These ions contribute the major part of the total osmolal concentration of the plasma and extracellular fluids. Potassium, magnesium, phosphate, and sulphate are present in highest concentration inside the cells where they maintain the osmolal concentration analogous to that of sodium and chloride in the extracellular fluids. In extracellular fluid potassium is present in a mean concentration of only 4·5 mmol/l and magnesium in a concentration of about 1 m-mol/l. Bicarbonate is found in the fluid outside the cells and in the tissue cells themselves in concentrations of 25 mmol/l and 10 mmol/l respectively. Hydrogen ions are present in a concentration of only 40 nanomol/l. They are present within cells at a higher concentration than in the extracellular fluids.

Because of the permeability of the capillaries, the concentration of electrolytes in the plasma and in the extracellular fluids in the tissue spaces is very similar. Interchange between these extracellular compartments is limited, however, in respect of protein molecules, the concentration of which is many times greater in the plasma than in the interstitial fluid. The volume of the plasma is largely the result of hydrostatic pressure which tends to force water outwards, and the osmotic pressure of the plasma proteins which draws water back into the vascular bed. In spite of the differences in the ionic pattern inside the cells as compared with that of the fluid which bathes them, under normal conditions the osmotic pressure is believed to be identical in extracellular and intracellular fluids. The differences in composition are established and maintained by the activity of ionic pumps within or near the cell membrane and are essential to life.

Disturbances in Water and Electrolyte Balance

The complexity of the composition of body fluids is reflected in the variety of disturbances that may occur in them either as a result of disease or as a consequence of therapeutic endeavour and drug administration. Such disturbances not only contribute to the clinical picture of many diseases, but are themselves a hindrance to recovery. For this reason it is important to maintain the chemical composition of the body fluids and correct as far as possible any derangements that may arise. It is also important that specific disturbances are recognised and appropriately treated. The labelling of such abnormalities in fluid and electrolyte balance simply as 'dehydration' and the indiscriminate use of intravenous isotonic, NaCl solution, i.e. 'normal' saline in an attempt to correct them is to be deprecated. The more common disturbances in water and electrolyte balance are as follows:

1. Sodium depletion
2. Primary water depletion
3. Potassium depletion
4. Potassium excess and intoxication
5. Magnesium deficiency and intoxication
6. Water intoxication
7. Sodium and water accumulation.

Sodium Depletion

Normal sodium (salt) balance depends upon an equality between the amounts of sodium excreted and ingested. In health and in temperate climates negligible amounts of sodium are lost in the stools and from the skin. In the absence of renal disease the kidneys possess considerable power to conserve sodium in the face of reduced intake and normal salt balance may be maintained with a very small daily intake. For these reasons sodium depletion generally occurs because of excessive loss of salt from the body rather than because of inadequate intake.

Because of the intimate relation of salt to water balance, loss of sodium is usually accompanied by a corresponding reduction in the water content of the body. *Pure* sodium depletion unattended by significant water loss is rare and probably occurs only as a result of abnormal loss of salt and water when an unrestricted intake of water has been permitted or encouraged. This may arise, for example, from excessive sweating in unfavourable environments when fluid loss is replenished by salt-free liquids. In these circumstances the change in total body water may be negligible in spite of a considerable deficit of body salt. More commonly, however, conditions giving rise to sodium depletion are attended by some degree of water loss and unless large amounts of salt-free fluids have been given, the depletion is really a *mixed* one, though the salt loss usually predominates over the water loss.

Causes of Depletion. In temperate regions predominant sodium depletion arises as a result of excessive loss of salt in the urine or because of increased loss of sodium-containing fluids from the gastrointestinal tract.

Failure of the kidney to conserve salt may develop because of intrinsic renal disease or inadequate hormonal control. Examples are found in some patients with pyelonephritis (i.e. 'salt-losing nephritis'), medullary cystic disease, the diuretic phase of acute renal failure of ischaemic origin, after the relief of urinary tract obstruction, Addison's disease and to a lesser extent in hypopituitarism. Excessive loss of salt in the urine together with water loss occurs in the osmotic diuresis of uncontrolled diabetes mellitus and chronic uraemia. If diabetic ketoacidosis develops, urinary sodium loss is further increased as the mechanism for hydrogen ion secretion is unable to cope with the severe degree of acidosis. Sodium depletion may also be induced by the excessive or prolonged use of diuretics.

Gastrointestinal causes of sodium depletion include all conditions involving external loss of salt-containing fluids, i.e. acute or chronic diarrhoea, intestinal fistulae, aspiration of gastrointestinal contents and vomiting. Considerable degrees of sodium loss also occur if sodium containing fluid is sequestered in dilated loops of intestine, i.e. ileus or in the peritoneal cavity as in ascites.

Sweating is a well-known cause of sodium depletion in tropical countries and often aggravates the degree of sodium depletion caused by disease (p. 832). Loss of sodium from the skin is also important in generalised dermatitis and in children suffering from cystic disease of the pancreas.

Consequences of Predominant Sodium Depletion. As sodium is predominantly extracellular, salt depletion quickly reduces the volume of the extracellular fluids. Any disproportionate loss of salt to that of water tends to render the extracellular fluids hypotonic. This tendency however is mitigated by two events, (1) the volume of water excreted in the urine is initially increased in order to restore the normal total osmolal concentration, and (2) some extracellular water migrates into the cells so that the threatened extracellular dilution is minimised. As a result, there is a further diminution in the volume of extracellular fluid, including plasma, while the water content of the cells may even increase. The fact that predominant salt depletion chiefly affects the volume of the extracellular fluid is responsible for many of the clinical features such as loss of elasticity of the skin, diminution of intra-ocular pressure and dryness of the tongue. Thirst is not a prominent complaint, and its absence may be due to the hypotonicity of the body fluids. The decrease in blood volume leads to a fall in blood pressure and in the rate of glomerular filtration; oliguria then occurs. The capacity of the body to rid itself of urea diminishes and uraemia develops. The pulse rate rises. Selective vasoconstriction diminishes the circulation through the skin so that the skin and the limbs become pale and cold. Although the plasma sodium concentration may be within normal limits, it may be reduced to 120 mmol/l or less in severe cases.

Treatment. The administration of water or of glucose in water in conditions associated with salt depletion is fraught with danger because the hypotonicity may be further aggravated. As more salt-free fluid is given, the kidneys respond by the excretion of large volumes of dilute urine in an attempt to restore the normal osmolal concentrations. The ill-effects of such treatment, moreover, are all too easily obscured by the conventional fluid balance chart which records only fluid intake and urine output, without reference to sodium balance. Adequate treatment consists of giving salt and water by mouth or an isotonic NaCl solution intravenously. The latter is required in all but very mild cases with normal blood pressure. Two to three litres of isotonic NaCl solution intravenously in 2 hours represents the usual adult requirements. In the more severe cases with marked circulatory impairment, deficits equivalent to 4–8 litres of isotonic NaCl solution occur. Such deficits should be repaired largely by isotonic sodium chloride. The first 2–3 litres should be given rapidly within the first 2–3 hours, the remainder being given within 24 to 48 hours. The best guides to the amount required are the disappearance of the signs of salt depletion and the restoration of normal blood pressure and pulse rate. Plasma sodium determinations are useful in controlling the treatment of severe cases, especially when the causative disease is likely to lead to continued salt loss, e.g. severe and persisting diarrhoea. Excessive administration of salt is to be avoided; the bases of the lungs should be frequently examined in order to detect crepitations, and the neck veins should be inspected to detect any increase in venous pressure. In severe cases it is often helpful to monitor the right atrial (central) venous pressure (p. 193).

Severe salt depletion is almost invariably associated with water depletion and disturbance in acid-base balance. Frequently potassium balance and occasionally magnesium metabolism are also disturbed. When accompanied by these disturbances the treatment of salt depletion requires to be modified accordingly.

Primary Water Depletion

Pure or predominant water depletion is one of the simplest of chemical disorders. The water content of the body is reduced both absolutely and relatively to the salt content, and the osmolal concentration of the extracellular fluids tends to rise. Between $\frac{1}{2}$–1 litre of water is lost daily from the body in the expired air and by evaporation from the skin. This daily loss continues irrespective of the water intake. The urine is the other main channel of excretion of water but its volume can be reduced if necessary by increasing its concentration up to a limit determined by renal concentrating ability and the amount of solute to be excreted.

Causes of Water Depletion. Primary water depletion occurs less commonly in clinical practice than sodium depletion and usually arises because water intake is reduced below an amount necessary to maintain balance. This is liable to occur in patients who suffer from dysphagia or have obstructive lesions of the oesophagus or more simply in those who are comatose, depressed or apathetic, as is common, for example, in the aged. Water deficit then occurs because the intake falls below the amount being lost from the lungs and the skin. This obligatory daily loss of water from the lungs and skin is increased by hyperpnoea, hyperthyroidism and in conditions associated with pyrexia. Excessive loss of water in the urine is a less common cause of water depletion but occurs in patients in whom the renal power of concentration is restricted, as for example in diabetes insipidus, hyperparathyroidism and in water-losing nephritis.

Relative water deficits may be induced by giving patients excessive protein or salt-containing artificial foods mixed with insufficient water. Newborn infants are especially susceptible to this danger as their power to concentrate the urine is not fully developed.

Consequences of Water Depletion. As water is lost from the body the extracellular fluid becomes hypertonic. Water then migrates from the cells in accordance with this increase in osmotic pressure and intracellular dehydration occurs. The overall body water loss is thus shared by the extracellular and intracellular fluids. For this reason the circulatory signs of dehydration are not so obvious as those of salt depletion. Thirst is usual unless the patient is senile or confused. The migration of water from the cells to the extracellular fluids helps to maintain the volume of the extracellular fluid nearly within normal limits for a time, so that the blood pressure, packed cell volume, and plasma and blood concentrations remain unaltered until considerable depletion has occurred. The patient, however, may exhibit mental confusion or complain of vertigo and difficulty in swallowing. In severe cases the skin and tissues acquire a curious 'doughy' consistency. Ultimately renal blood flow is reduced and the blood urea concentration rises. The plasma sodium concentration and the packed cell volume then become elevated.

Treatment. Water depletion should be treated by giving salt-free fluids. The use of isotonic sodium chloride solution is contraindicated. If the patient is conscious and is not vomiting, water should be given by mouth until thirst is quenched and thereafter amounts of between 1·2 to 2·5 litres per day are usually sufficient. If the patient is unable to swallow fluids in sufficient amounts, 5 per cent glucose in water should be given by intravenous infusion. The amount required varies with the degree of depletion. In moderately severe cases 2–4 litres of 5 per cent glucose in the course of 24 hours is usually sufficient. In severe water depletion 5–10 litres may be needed. The best guides to the amount of fluid required are the clinical improvement of the patient and the increase in the volume of urine, which should rise to about 1·5 litres per 24 hours. If water depletion is due to water-losing renal diseases, it may be necessary to continue to give large daily amounts of water.

It must be remembered that when water depletion is associated with salt loss, isotonic NaCl solution and water are both required and should be given together in amounts determined by clinical assessment of the relative degrees of the two deficiencies.

Potassium Depletion

Potassium depletion is responsible for various clinical features in a wide variety of disorders. Depending upon the daily intake, the healthy individual in potassium balance excretes about one-third of his daily potassium intake in the stools and two-thirds in the urine. The bulk of urinary potassium is excreted by the cells lining the distal renal tubules in response to the electrical potential gradient created by active sodium reabsorption and the presence of negatively charged anions within the tubular lumen that are not reabsorbed. Diffusion of potassium at this site is also affected by the acid-base state (Fig. 10.1, p. 469).

Causes of Potassium Depletion. Potassium depletion usually occurs as a result of excessive loss of potassium from the gastrointestinal tract or in the urine. Alimentary losses occur as a result of acute, severe or chronic diarrhoea, vomiting, fistulous drainage or gastric aspiration. The chronic use of laxatives is sometimes an underlying cause and is easily missed. Renal wastage of potassium is complex in its origin and occurs:

1. In circumstances which lower the efficiency of the cellular ionic pump throughout body cells.

2. In circumstances which favour the diffusion of potassium into the lumen of the distal tubule.

Almost all the potassium in the body lies within the cells, and circumstances which encourage its transfer to the extracellular fluid lead to increased urinary losses and ultimately to potassium depletion. Such circumstances include hypoxia, impaired oxidation of carbohydrate, water depletion and acidosis of metabolic or respiratory origin in which the buffering of H^+ within cells leads to the loss of K^+ from them.

The conditions which favour the diffusion of potassium into the distal tubule and so into the urine fall into two main categories:

1. Circumstances in which the transtubular PD becomes more negative facilitate diffusion. This mechanism is probably responsible in primary and secondary aldosteronism, Cushing's syndrome, renal artery stenosis, heart failure and disorders associated with hypoproteinaemia, in all of which there is increased Na^+ reabsorption. It may also be responsible when Na^+ reabsorption is increased as a result of drugs such as corticosteroids and carbenoxolone. Diuretics which increase the delivery of Na^+ to the most distal tubules also encourage K^+ loss in this way.

2. In many circumstances the rate of secretion of potassium is related inversely to the rate of H^+ excretion. Since both are secreted by the distal tubular cells it seems likely that their relative intracellular concentration determines this relationship. Thus carbonic anhydrase inhibitors such as acetazolamide, which reduce H^+ formation, increase urinary potassium loss. In renal tubular acidosis and metabolic alkalosis, in which tubular secretion of H^+ is also reduced, the urine is alkaline and potassium loss is increased.

Many elderly people who take a diet inadequate in potassium become mildly potassium-depleted. The precise mechanism is unknown but it is most likely due to continued urinary loss.

Consequences and Clinical Features of Potassium Depletion. Significant depletion of potassium may occur without alteration in the plasma potassium concentration and the diagnosis of intracellular potassium deficit is made difficult by the inaccessibility of the intracellular fluid to analysis. Biochemical evidence of potassium lack may be suggested by an elevation in plasma bicarbonate concentration or a diminution in plasma sodium concentration. These effects are believed to be due to the migration of hydrogen and sodium ions from the extracellular into the intracellular fluids.

Symptoms attributable to potassium deficiency include apathy, muscular weakness, mental confusion and abdominal distension. It is clear that such features arise in the course of many diseases. Nevertheless, their occurrence in circumstances which are known to lead to potassium deficiency, and their relief after potassium administration justify the diagnosis. Potassium depletion reduces the ability of the kidney to concentrate; hence polyuria and thirst commonly occur. Potassium depletion also gives rise to increased susceptibility to intoxication with digitalis. Severe potassium depletion lowers the cardiac output and this may give rise to oedema.

Potassium deficiency sufficiently severe to be associated with reduction of the plasma concentration is more easily recognised, but is less common than simple intracellular depletion. It may occur in any of the conditions mentioned above if the deficiency is severe enough and is particularly liable to develop in cases of diabetic ketoacidosis which have been vigorously treated with sodium containing solutions or glucose and insulin; this therapy causes a migration of potassium from the extracellular to the intracellular space with resulting hypokalaemia. The clinical picture of extracellular potassium deficit is characterised by generalised muscular weakness with paresis or flaccid paralysis and ileus. Paraesthaesiae are also frequently present. The electrocardiogram commonly shows a small T wave and ST depression. Death may occur if treatment is inadequate.

Treatment. Potassium depletion should be treated by giving a potassium salt orally or intravenously. The former route is more commonly used and is less dangerous than parenteral administration. The normal daily intake of potassium is about 2–3 g.

1. Established deficiencies of moderate severity (about 400 mmol) can be remedied by giving 10–15 g of potassium chloride per day orally, in divided doses for some days in addition to a diet rich in potassium, i.e. containing fruit and fruit juices.

Potassium chloride tablets, even when enteric coated, are sometimes irritating to the gastrointestinal tract. 'Slow release' tablets of potassium chloride are less troublesome in this respect, each tablet containing 600 mg of KCl. Some patients tolerate effervescent potassium tablets more readily and these appear to be less nauseating. Each tablet contains 250 mg of potassium. Some effervescent tablets contain chloride which is useful in correcting the metabolic alkalosis which is associated with potassium depletion and which is frequently due to concurrent chloride depletion (p. 168).

2. Intravenous infusions of potassium chloride are needed for patients who are unable to take potassium by mouth, but should be given only when the existence of hypokalaemia is established by chemical analysis. Such infusions should rarely be given in the presence of anuria or oliguria and only when facilities for repeated chemical analysis are available.

If oliguria is due to associated water and salt depletion these should be treated first. For intravenous administration, potassium chloride (1·5 g in sterile ampoules) can be conveniently added to 500 ml of isotonic NaCl or 5 per cent glucose solution. The solution then contains 40 mmol/l and should be given slowly over 2 to 3 hours. Repeated determinations of the plasma potassium are necessary to determine whether further infusions are required. Administration of potassium by mouth should be started as soon as possible, as the major portion of the deficit can be corrected only by this means. When the depletion of potassium has arisen because of persistent vomiting and is associated with alkalosis due to loss of gastric hydrochloric acid, potassium is conveniently given with sodium and ammonium chloride as described on page 169.

Prophylactic administration of potassium chloride (3–4 g daily) or effervescent potassium tablets should be given to patients who are being treated by drugs known to increase urinary loss of potassium. These include corticosteroids and many diuretics (p. 163).

Potassium Excess and Intoxication

Causes. Abnormal accumulation of potassium in the blood and extracellular fluid usually occurs in association with severe oliguria or anuria. It is commonly found in conditions leading to acute renal failure, e.g. circulatory failure from blood loss or injury and severe cases of Addison's disease and Addisonian crisis; it may occur in diabetic ketoacidosis prior to adequate treatment with insulin and intravenous solutions. Some patients with severe chronic renal failure develop hyperkalaemia especially if potassium supplements, spironolactone or potassium conserving diuretics (p. 162) are given.

Consequences of Potassium Excess. Patients with hyperkalaemia are dull and lethargic and gradually become confused. Asthenia develops and progresses to flaccid paralysis. These features are indistinguishable from those of hypokalaemia. The pulse becomes irregular and bradycardia develops from heart block of variable degree. Hyperkalaemia is of considerable clinical importance because of the danger of cardiac arrest with concentrations of plasma potassium above 7.5 mmol/l. The diagnosis is made more frequently by knowing the circumstances in which intoxication is likely to arise and confirming the suspicion by plasma potassium analysis than from any specific clinical feature. Typical electrocardiographic changes occur; these include increase in the amplitude of the T wave, atrioventricular and intraventricular conduction defects and ultimately ventricular arrest.

Treatment. It is important to prevent the occurrence of potassium intoxication in conditions associated with oliguria and anuria. The recommendations made with regard to the diet in acute renal failure (p. 497) are designed with this aim in view. When dealing with an established case of hyperkalaemia, the following measures are advised:

(*a*) Immediate restriction of foods rich in potassium (e.g. fruit juices) and in protein.

(*b*) The repair of any associated depletion of water or salt with the aim of re-establishing a normal circulation as early as possible and the correction of metabolic or respiratory acidosis by appropriate methods (pp. 167 and 170).

(*c*) The sodium or calcium loaded ionic exchange resin (Resonium A and Zeocarb) absorbs potassium in the intestine from the blood and intestinal secretions and contents. A suspension of 30 g in a small volume of water should be given by mouth 3 or 4 times per day or as required. In the event of vomiting the resin may be administered as a retention enema.

(*d*) The administration of glucose and insulin in order to encourage migration of potassium from the extracellular fluids into the cells. Ten units of soluble insulin subcutaneously and 50 g glucose by mouth should be given and may be repeated every 2 to 4 hours. The beneficial effect of this treatment is increased if $\frac{1}{2}$ to 1 litre of isotonic sodium bicarbonate is given simultaneously by intravenous injection.

(*e*) Calcium gluconate (10 per cent), 10 ml given intravenously and repeated in two to three hours, has been shown to reduce the cardiotoxic effect of potassium.

(*f*) If these methods fail or if the rise of concentration of potassium is rapid, removal of potassium by peritoneal dialysis or by haemodialysis is indicated.

Magnesium Deficiency and Intoxication

Rapid methods for determination of magnesium in body fluids now available have shown that disorders of magnesium metabolism are occasionally responsible for otherwise puzzling clinical features and are susceptible to therapeutic control.

Magnesium Deficiency. The most frequent cause of magnesium deficiency is prolonged diarrhoea or vomiting, which has been treated with parenteral fluid without magnesium supplements. It occasionally follows long continued diuretic therapy, and it is associated with chronic diarrhoea and severe undernutrition, such as occurs in kwashiorkor and the malabsorption syndrome. Aldosteronism, hyperparathyroidism and chronic alcoholism also lead to magnesium deficiency.

Clinical features are predominantly neuromuscular with tremor, choreiform movements and aimless plucking of the bedclothes. Mental depression, confusion, agitation, epileptiform convulsions and hallucinations also occur. The diagnosis should be confirmed by finding the concentration of magnesium in the plasma to be less than 0·75 mmol/l.

Magnesium deficiency is best treated parenterally; 50 mmol of magnesium chloride may be added to 1 litre of 5 per cent glucose or other isotonic solution and given over a period of 12 to 24 hours. The infusion should be repeated daily until the plasma concentration remains within the normal range.

Magnesium Intoxication. This mainly occurs in acute and chronic renal disease and contributes to the central nervous features associated with uraemia (p. 485). Its treatment is that of the primary disorder.

Water Intoxication

Healthy individuals can safely drink very large volumes of water and respond to this by a vigorous water diuresis. The capacity of the body to excrete water when given without electrolytes is dependent upon many factors which include the rate of glomerular filtration and the power of the distal tubules of the kidney to produce a dilute urine. Many patients who are ill for a variety of reasons have a restricted ability to dilute the urine when given large amounts of water. These include patients suffering from acute and chronic renal disease, severe heart failure, adrenocortical insufficiency and hepatic cirrhosis. Occasionally tumours of the lung or ovaries secrete a polypeptide with antidiuretic properties which leads to water intoxication. Post-operative subjects are also incapable of diluting the urine because of the liberation of vasopressin by the stress of the operation. In addition, a number of drugs induce water retention because of antidiuretic hormone-like effects and can lead to water intoxication. These include the oral hypoglycaemic drugs, chlorpropamide and rarely tolbutamide, drugs used in treating leukaemia, vincristine and cyclophosphamide, and also morphine.

In all these circumstances even a modest water intake reduces the plasma osmolality and the concentration of sodium and produces symptoms which are primarily those of disordered cerebral function; these include dizziness, headache, nausea and mental confusion. Severe water intoxication can produce convulsions, coma and death. Diagnosis depends upon being aware of the circumstances in which water intoxication is likely to occur and the demonstration of a plasma sodium concentration below 130 mmol/l.

Treatment consists of restricting water intake for a few days. In severe cases 100 ml 5 per cent sodium chloride solution should be given intravenously and repeated in a few hours if there is little or no response. The use of fludrocortisone is beneficial in cases of hyponatraemia due to tumours and is also indicated in Addison's disease.

Sodium and Water Accumulation

In health, the total amount of sodium in the body is kept within narrow limits in spite of great day-to-day variations in the amount ingested. Positive sodium balance with consequent accumulation of sodium in the body results from a renal excretion that is inadequate in relation to the amount ingested. The accumulation is generally accompanied by the retention of water so that the concentration of sodium in the extracellular space is usually not materially altered. When the distribution of the retained fluid is generalised, the expansion in the volume of the extracellular space does not become clinically detectable until the increase is of the order of 15 per cent.

The primary mechanisms responsible for the accumulation of water and salt which lead to oedema vary with the nature of the disease and they are discussed in the appropriate sections of this book. They include reduction in the osmotic pressure from hypoproteinaemia as occurs in the nephrotic syndrome; an increase in venous hydrostatic pressure with migration of fluid from the vascular space to the tissue spaces is an important factor in heart failure and primary renal retention of salt and water is responsible in acute proliferative glomerulonephritis. In addition several compensatory reactions occur which promote further retention of water and salt. These include a rise in the levels of circulating vasopressin and also an increased secretion of aldosterone mediated by the renin angiotensin system.

The therapeutic use of cortisone, corticotrophin, androgens or oral contraceptives with a high oestrogen content may also give rise to water and sodium retention by virtue of their action on the kidney. Other drugs which do so include carbenoxolone, phenylbutazone and many antihypertensive drugs. Some oedema is not uncommon in normal women during the premenstrual stage of the menstrual cycle, but the mechanism of this is unknown. Oedema is commonly present in normal pregnancy but is more severe and is associated with proteinuria in renal disease or pregnancy hypertension. Other disorders associated with generalised oedema include nutritional oedema and thiamin deficiency. In some diseases several mechanisms appear to be operating simultaneously. This is exemplified particularly in the oedema and ascites of hepatic cirrhosis in which portal hypertension, hypoproteinaemia and possibly salt retaining and antidiuretic hormones all contribute. It has to be admitted, however, that the knowledge of the cause of oedema in the above-mentioned diseases is far from complete.

The clinical features of water and salt accumulation depend to some extent upon the distribution of the retained fluid. These are described under the various diseases.

Principles of Treatment. These are: (a) The use of measures designed to remedy specific factors leading to the oedema, e.g. digitalis in heart failure, corticosteroids in some forms of glomerulonephritis, the intravenous administration of plasma proteins or salt-free albumin in conditions associated with hypoproteinaemia, and a high protein diet in oedema of nutritional origin, hepatic cirrhosis and the nephrotic syndrome. (b) The restriction by dietary means of the raw materials necessary for the formation of extracellular fluid, i.e. water and salt. These restrictions have largely been superseded by: (c) The excretion of salt and water by the use of effective diuretics.

Diuretic Therapy. Drugs which block reabsorption of sodium by the renal tubules increase the amount of solute particles in the tubular fluid and result in the elimination of a large volume of water. The following are the most important diuretics discussed in order of their potency.

HIGH POTENCY DIURETICS. The diuresis induced by these agents is rapid, intense and of short duration. They include frusemide, bumetanide and ethacrynic acid. They are sometimes called *loop diuretics* because their predominant action reduces the reabsorption of sodium and chloride in the ascending limb of the loop of Henle. As a result they reduce the renal concentrating power and so eliminate a greater volume of water than do other diuretics; because they deliver an increased amount of sodium to the distal tubules they also lead to increased potassium loss in the urine.

Frusemide is a sulphonamyl derivative and may be given orally (40–80 mg) or intravenously (20–40 mg). On a weight basis *bumetanide* is more potent than frusemide, comparable doses being 2 mg, but is otherwise similar in its action. Frusemide and bumetanide are drugs of great value in the treatment of severe generalised oedema and severe pulmonary oedema. They have few adverse effects but may lead to a rise in plasma urate and precipitate gout.

Ethacrynic acid represents a different chemical class of diuretic and can be given orally in doses of 50–200 mg per day. It has similar adverse effects to frusemide but in addition may induce gynaecomastia, tinnitus and deafness, especially if given in a single large intravenous dose.

MEDIUM POTENCY DIURETICS. Benzothiadiazides (thiazides, thiadiazines) were developed after attempts to find carbonic anhydrase inhibitors more potent than acetazolamide, and these drugs have two separate effects on renal function. They have a variable effect on the activity of carbonic anhydrase and so of sodium bicarbonate reabsorption in the proximal renal tubules, but their main action is to depress tubular reabsorption of sodium and chloride in the distal convoluted tubules. Potassium depletion occurs both because of the reduction of H^+ secretion and because of the delivery of increased amounts of sodium to the very distal tubular cells. Chlorothiazide was the first prototype of this group but the drugs most commonly used now are *bendrofluazide* (10 mg) and *hydrochlorothiazide* (100 mg). *Chlorthalidone* (100–200 mg) is similar in its action to chlorothiazide and its analogues but it produces a slower and more prolonged diuresis extending over 48 hours. Adverse effects of benzothiadiazides include allergic skin reactions, nausea and vomiting and blood dyscrasias. Hyperuricaemia and diabetes may be produced in susceptible patients.

LOW POTENCY DIURETICS. These consist of several agents which are not sufficiently potent by themselves but, because of other properties, are sometimes valuable when combined with more potent diuretics. *Amiloride* (20 mg) and *triamterene* (200 mg) antagonise the effects of aldosterone. Neither has a steroid structure and they do not compete for aldosterone combining sites. Their very mild naturetic effect is due to inhibition of sodium reabsorption in the distal tubule; potassium secretion is not increased and so they do not lead to potassium deficiency. *Spironolactone* (100–400 mg daily) is a specific antagonist to aldosterone and reverses the renal effect of the hormone. Its important clinical effect is the reduction in the capacity of the kidney to excrete potassium which it shares with the low potency diuretics. These diuretics should not be given with potassium supplements as dangerous hyperkalaemia may develop.

ADVERSE ELECTROLYTE EFFECTS OF DIURETIC THERAPY. *Potassium Depletion.*
High potency and benzothiadiazide diuretics produce potassium depletion, especially when given repeatedly over long periods and when combined with diets
low in sodium. Symptoms of potassium deficit may arise before satisfactory loss
of oedema has been achieved and are then superimposed upon the clinical features
of water and sodium accumulation. This state of affairs is especially prone to
develop in the treatment of severe cardiac failure and is particularly serious since
it may be responsible for increased sensitivity to digitalis, with the development of
toxic manifestations to this drug before adequate digitalisation and control of the
heart failure has been attained. In hepatic disease with oedema and ascites the
potassium depletion may seriously aggravate or precipitate the neurological
features of hepatic insufficiency. Prophylactic administration of potassium is
therefore essential when diuretics are being given frequently, e.g. on alternate
days. Between 16 and 48 mmol daily is required and given either as potassium
chloride slow tablets (8 mmol potassium each) or effervescent tablets (12 mmol).

Sodium depletion. A 'low salt syndrome' is much less common than
potassium deficiency but is more likely to occur when treatment with high potency
diureties is prolonged and when additional mechanical methods such as abdominal paracenteses are being used. These patients exhibit some of the features
of sodium depletion although they may still be oedematous. They become
apathetic and suffer from anorexia and vomiting. The circulatory characteristic of
sodium depletion is present, namely hypotension with an increase in the pulse rate.
The blood urea concentration is increased and the plasma sodium concentration is
reduced to 130 mmol/*l* or less. Such patients are usually seriously ill and, when
the oedema is cardiac in origin, may be in the last stage of their disease. In these
circumstances persistent attempts to reduce the oedema leads to further clinical
deterioration. Diuretics should be withheld and a diet unrestricted in its salt content permitted. In a few instances the intravenous administration of hypertonic
saline may be dramatically successful in relieving the symptoms of the low salt
syndrome. Two hundred ml of 5 per cent saline should be given slowly by intravenous infusion, and may be repeated after 24 hours. In the case of the
nephrotic syndrome or when oedema is severe in hepatic cirrhosis, the intravenous
administration of plasma protein is indicated (p. 484).

Diagnosis of Disturbances in Water and Electrolyte Balance

It is apparent from this summary of the consequences of body depletion of
sodium, water, potassium and magnesium and of potassium and magnesium intoxication that these disturbances present considerable diagnostic difficulty and
are not characterised by pathognomonic signs or symptoms. The apathy of
potassium depletion is indistinguishable from that of hyperkalaemia; severe
sodium depletion is attended in the majority of instances by considerable water
deficit so that these cases do not exhibit a clearly defined clinical picture. Furthermore, it is not uncommon for dual electrolytic deficits to develop simultaneously.
For example, in diabetic ketoacidosis, potassium depletion may occur in conjunction with predominant salt depletion. In addition the symptoms of lethargy,
apathy and mental confusion are common accompaniments of many diseases in
which no significant body fluid distortion exists.

It has also to be recognised that the results obtained from biochemical analysis
of blood and urine are of only limited diagnostic value. Potassium or magnesium
deficit may occur without significant alteration in their plasma concentrations,

and serious sodium depletion may develop with plasma sodium concentrations within the recognised limits of normality. A low plasma sodium may not even indicate salt depletion, and hyponatraemia is frequently seen in the late stages of malignant disease, generalised tuberculosis and more rarely in association with vasopressin secreting tumours or other causes of water intoxication.

The measurement of electrolytes in the urine without knowledge of the dietary intake is also obviously of limited value. In the majority of conditions in which there is a reduced blood or ECF volume the urinary loss of sodium is less than 10–20 mmol/l. However, the presence of larger amounts in the urine of patients who are volume-depleted strongly suggests a renal salt wasting disorder. Urinary potassium determination is also of limited value but is sometimes helpful in patients who are found unexpectedly to have hypokalaemia. Then the finding of a urinary [K^+] of more than 20 mmol/l indicates that the kidney is responsible unless extrarenal losses are of recent and sudden onset. In contrast the finding of a urinary [K^+] of less than 10 mmol/l in the presence of hypokalaemia indicates the route of the loss is extrarenal and is usually a gastrointestinal disorder.

Accurate diagnosis largely depends upon a knowledge of the conditions and diseases which may give rise to abnormalities in water and electrolyte balance. In the presence of such diseases, the suspicion that these abnormalities may exist is strengthened by the presence of the clinical features known to occur with them and possibly by the results of appropriate biochemical and electrocardiographic examinations.

By understanding the mechanism by which the economy of the fluids of the body becomes disturbed and by the intelligent use of the reparative fluids which have been described, much can be done to restore the distortions of body fluid balance wrought by disease.

Hydrogen Ion Concentration

Life is possible only if the blood is kept within a range of alkalinity, and in health a physiological hydrogen ion concentration of 36–44 nmol/l corresponding to a pH of between 7·37 and 7·45 is maintained by two widely different mechanisms which are closely integrated. Some understanding of these mechanisms is necessary to appreciate the clinical implications of acidosis and alkalosis.

The blood is alkaline because it contains bicarbonate, phosphate and proteins which are quite strong bases. It also contains carbonic acid and the [H^+] of the blood depends principally upon the ratio of the main acid component, carbonic acid and the main base bicarbonate. The concentration of carbonic acid in the plasma is determined by the partial pressure of carbon dioxide (P_{CO_2}) in the alveoli. The latter is normally about 5·3 kPa (p. 251) which gives rise to little over 1 mmol/l of carbonic acid in physical solution in the plasma. The alveolar partial pressure of carbon dioxide is itself maintained steady by the equality between its rate of production by the tissues and the rate at which ventilation eliminates it from the body. On the other hand, the concentration of bicarbonate is regulated by the tubular epithelium of the kidneys and in health is kept at about 22–24 mmol/l by the mechanism described on page 470.

A great many metabolic processes result in the production of acids and these must be eliminated from the body if the reaction of the tissue and the blood is to remain within the normal range. The route of disposal of acids depends upon whether or not they are capable of being oxidised completely to carbon dioxide and water. Carbon dioxide forms carbonic acid within the body and is eliminated as carbon dioxide by ventilation. Other acids such as acetoacetic acid or sulphuric acid which are derived from the oxidation of fatty acids or sulphur-containing proteins respectively are excreted by the kidneys. At the site of their production in the tissues and during their carriage in the blood all acids increase the hydrogen ion concentration. The extent of this increase is minimised by the stabilising power of the blood and tissues which in turn depends on the presence of the physiologically important buffers.

Carbonic acid is produced by metabolic reactions in far greater amounts than any other acid. A small part of the carbon dioxide is transported in the blood reversibly bound to haemoglobin as a carbamino compound. A greater part is converted to carbonic acid in the red blood cells which are rich in carbonic anhydrase, and is then buffered by haemoglobin when it gives its oxygen to the tissues and is converted to deoxyhaemoglobin (Fig. 5.1). The hydrogen ions of the carbonic acid are taken up by the haemoglobin in the red cells while the bicarbonate ion moves out from the red cells to the plasma in exchange for chloride ions (chloride shift). Most of the carbonic acid added to the blood therefore appears not as acid but as bicarbonate ion. When the blood passes through the lungs and the haemoglobin is reoxygenated this process is reversed and the carbon dioxide formed is expelled by ventilation.

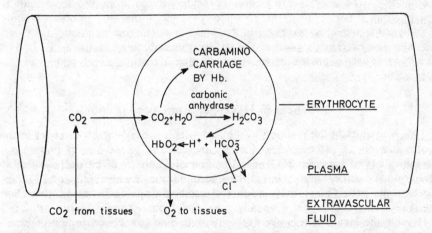

Fig. 5.1 Transport of CO_2

In health a small amount of inorganic acid is produced each day and being non-volatile requires to be excreted by the kidney. Only a small quantity of organic acid is produced in normal conditions but in diabetic ketoacidosis, for example, a large amount of acetoacetic acid is formed. The tissues and blood are buffered against these acids by a different mechanism which involves in particular the sodium bicarbonate and carbonic acid buffer system in the plasma. The addition of acid to the plasma results in a movement of the reactions in the direction indicated by the broad arrow (Fig. 5.2). As a result of this and of a similar reaction on the part of the other buffer systems, many of the hydrogen ions which would otherwise increase the acidity of the plasma are removed to form increased amounts of carbonic acid. There is a corresponding diminution in the concentration of bicarbonate ions. By this means the $[H^+]$ of the plasma rises far less than it would do if the buffers were not present. The rise in $[H^+]$ stimulates ventilation and the excess carbonic acid is removed from the body as carbon dioxide. The anion of the acid (e.g. acetoacetate) and the depleted body bicarbonate are dealt with simultaneously by the kidney. The renal tubules form carbonic acid, much of the hydrogen ion of which is used to form ammonium ions which are then excreted in the urine with the acid anion. The bicarbonate ion generated in this process is returned to the blood and reconstitutes the depleted blood buffer.

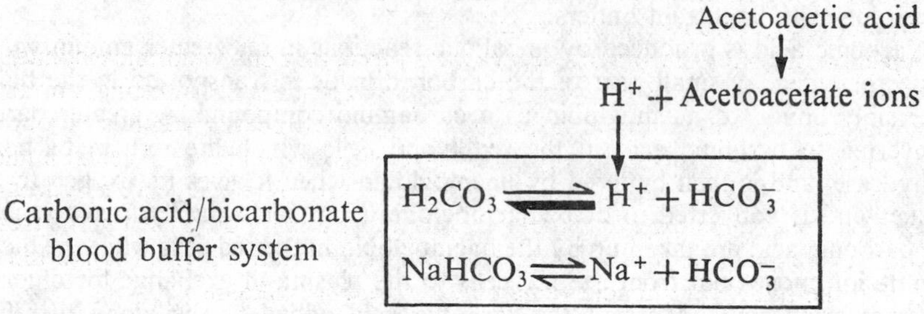

Acetoacetic acid

$\downarrow$

$H^+ +$ Acetoacetate ions

$\downarrow$

Carbonic acid/bicarbonate blood buffer system

$$H_2CO_3 \rightleftharpoons H^+ + HCO_3^-$$
$$NaHCO_3 \rightleftharpoons Na^+ + HCO_3^-$$

Fig. 5.2 Effect of acid on the blood buffer system.

These buffering and excreting mechanisms are continually in operation in response to the normal production of acids derived from the food and its metabolism. It is clear from this simplified description that the important limiting factor in the buffering power of blood is the available haemoglobin and bicarbonate. The excreting power of the kidneys is the limiting factor in the body's ability to rid itself of anions derived from inorganic and organic acids other than carbonic acid.

Disturbances in Hydrogen Ion Concentration

Abnormalities in the reaction of the body fluids are reflected in changes in the concentration of carbonic acid (i.e. $Paco_2$) and by alterations in body base, notably that of bicarbonate. The estimation of $Paco_2$ is of particular value in respiratory disorders and its use in these conditions is described on page 257. Unfortunately there is no entirely satisfactory method available for the determination of $[HCO_3^-]$. Nowadays it is usually calculated from a knowledge of $Paco_2$ and pH using the Henderson Hasselbach equation. Since the concentration of bicarbonate is itself influenced by $Paco_2$ it is common practice to express the $[HCO_3^-]$ as the concentration which would exist at a standard value of $Paco_2$ of 5·3 kPa. It is then known as standard bicarbonate and normally ranges between 22 and 26 mmol/l.

Metabolic Acidosis

Metabolic acidosis arises as a result of the production or ingestion of acids other than carbonic acid, or as a consequence of body depletion of the base bicarbonate. The condition is characterised by a rise in $[H^+]$ and a marked reduction in the concentration of bicarbonate in the plasma. The $Paco_2$ is reduced secondarily by the hyperventilation produced by stimulation of respiration; this mitigates to some extent the increased $[H^+]$ which arises from the fall in $[HCO_3^-]$.

The production of large amounts of lactic acid in vigorous exercise is probably the most common cause of acidosis and is to be regarded as physiological. Shock causes metabolic acidosis because of hypoxia of the tissues and the accumulation of organic acids, particularly lactic acid. Other important causes of acidosis are diabetic ketoacidosis and renal failure. In the former condition, β-hydroxybutyric acid and acetoacetic acid are produced in abnormally large amounts, and at a rate which is greater than the capacity of the body for their oxidation. In patients with acute or chronic renal failure, the power of the kidneys to conserve and generate bicarbonate ions and to produce and secrete hydrogen and ammonium ions is impaired and their excretion is diminished.

Depletion of body bicarbonate occurs from direct loss of sodium bicarbonate in the stools in chronic or severe acute diarrhoea or from loss of intestinal contents from fistulae or by intestinal aspiration. The therapeutic administration of acetazolamide for glaucoma may also give rise to acidosis. Acetazolamide depresses the power of the kidneys to generate bicarbonate and secrete hydrogen ions which then accumulate in the blood. Ammonium chloride is used in the treatment of severe metabolic alkalosis (p. 169); the ammonium radical is converted to urea, and the hydrochloric acid remaining reduces the alkalosis.

Consequences of Metabolic Acidosis. The most obvious consequence of acidosis is the stimulation of the respiratory centre by the abnormally high blood concentration of hydrogen ions. In severe cases the respirations become deep and rapid (Kussmaul's respiration). It is clear, however, from the list of causes given above that the clinical picture in the individual case is largely determined by the underlying condition and by the presence of other concomitant disturbances in water and salt balance. By the time acidosis is severe in diabetic ketoacidosis, considerable water and salt depletion has usually occurred. The acidosis of chronic diarrhoea is similarly associated with salt loss and especially with potassium deficit. The failure of ammonium and hydrogen ion production by the kidney in chronic nephritis, which leads to acidosis, is necessarily accompanied by abnormal loss of sodium and potassium in the urine. As in the case of disturbances in water and electrolyte balance, the diagnosis of metabolic acidosis is facilitated by an awareness of those pathological conditions in which it is likely to arise. The diagnosis should be confirmed by the determination of the concentration of bicarbonate in the blood. In acidosis of moderate degree this value is reduced to 15 m-mol/l, while concentrations below 10 mmol/l represent severe degrees of acidosis.

Treatment. Since metabolic acidosis is commonly associated with some degree of salt depletion and water deficiency, it is reasonable to correct these disturbances, in the first instance, by the administration of isotonic NaCl solution (p. 154); this is a neutral solution and by itself might be expected to have only a little influence on the reaction of the blood and tissues. In fact, provided the kidneys are not primarily diseased and provided the degree of salt and water depletion is not so severe as to impair renal function seriously, its intravenous administration is usually effective in correcting metabolic acidosis of moderate severity. Its success depends upon the capacity of the kidneys to generate bicarbonate from carbon dioxide and water and to retain this with the infused sodium, rejecting the chloride in the urine (p. 470).

In the presence of renal disease, severe acidosis and severe salt depletion giving rise to uraemia, it is unwise to depend upon the collaboration of the kidney for the alkalising effect of sodium chloride. In these circumstances, isotonic sodium bicarbonate should be given by intravenous infusion in addition to isotonic sodium chloride. The two solutions should be given in a ratio of 1 to 2 and need not be mixed. The total volume of the combined solutions required varies with the severity of the salt depletion and with the degree of acidosis. A moderately severe case of diabetic acidosis, for example, may require as much as 4–6 litres in the first 24 hours, of which 1–2 litres should be the isotonic bicarbonate solution. The latter infusion should be given for as long as there is evidence of acidosis, as determined by the estimation of the bicarbonate concentration in the blood. When this has returned to normal levels, it may be necessary to continue the intravenous infusion of isotonic sodium chloride alone. This is indicated if there is still evidence of predominant salt depletion.

In severe shock or cardiac arrest due, for example, to myocardial infarction, acidosis develops without salt depletion. In these circumstances it is best to give sodium bicarbonate in a small volume of hypertonic concentration, i.e. 200–300 ml 5 per cent solution intravenously in the course of 10 to 15 minutes.

Metabolic Alkalosis

Metabolic alkalosis arises most commonly as a result of the abnormal loss from the body of hydrochloric acid in the course of prolonged or severe vomiting. Chloride deficiency itself also leads to alkalosis by stimulating the renal tubular reabsorption of bicarbonate. More rarely alkalosis may arise from the ingestion of large amounts of sodium bicarbonate given, for example, in the treatment of peptic ulcer. This is especially likely to occur if there is associated pyloric spasm or stenosis, with vomiting. Potassium depletion also gives rise to alkalosis as this encourages the secretion of hydrogen ions by the distal renal tubules (p. 157).

Consequences of Alkalosis. The sequence of events which occurs when hydrochloric acid is lost from the body as a result of vomiting is shown in Figure 5.3. The loss of hydrogen ions in severe and continuous vomiting lowers the hydrogen ion concentration of the blood and leads to alkalosis. The effect is mitigated by an increase in the ionisation of blood carbonic acid to hydrogen and bicarbonate ions, as indicated by the broad arrow. The former tends to restore the hydrogen ion concentration towards normal, and the latter replaces the chloride in the blood which has also been lost in the gastric contents. For as long as the chloride deficiency persists increased tubular conservation of bicarbonate sustains the alkalosis.

Alkalosis of some duration is often associated with significant depression of renal function with uraemia. Protein and casts are found in the urine, and the

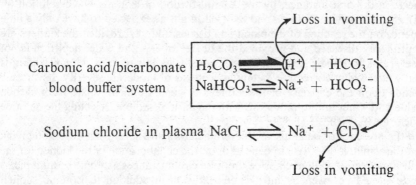

Fig. 5.3 Effect of alkalosis on the blood buffer system

diagnostic error of attributing vomiting due to pyloric stenosis to primary renal disease must be avoided. In spite of the existence of metabolic alkalosis, the urine may remain acid. There are two causes for this paradoxical aciduria. The alkalosis is frequently associated with chloride depletion, and under these circumstances an alkaline urine cannot be elaborated. Secondly, respiratory compensation for the alkalosis results in a rise in $Paco_2$ which is also known to increase renal tubular reabsorption of bicarbonate. Apathy, personality changes, delirium and stupor occur; since the patient usually suffers from associated water and potassium depletion, it is probably wrong to attribute these features solely to the effect of alkalosis. Tetany may occur spontaneously or be induced by the Trousseau manoeuvre and is due to a reduction in the concentration of plasma ionised calcium.

The diagnosis of alkalosis may be made with certainty only by estimation of the concentration of plasma bicarbonate. In moderately severe alkalosis this is elevated to 35 mmol/l. The pH of the blood is also elevated.

Treatment. In patients with mild or moderate alkalosis in whom the bicarbonate concentration is not elevated above 30 mmol/l, it is often possible to correct the abnormality by the intravenous administration of isotonic sodium chloride. This treatment is effective only if there is normal renal function. In this event the chloride is retained and excess bicarbonate in the plasma is excreted in the urine. Two to four litres may be required in the course of 24 hours.

In severe cases the administration of ammonium chloride by intravenous infusion has been found effective and is conveniently prepared in a solution which is designed also to repair the commonly associated potassium deficit. This is called the 'gastric solution'. One litre of a solution containing 63 mmol/l of sodium chloride, 17 mmol/l of potassium chloride and 70 mmol/l of ammonium chloride may be given in 4 to 6 hours and repeated as indicated by blood analysis. The use of this solution is of particular benefit in these patients who are being prepared for operation for relief of gastric outlet obstruction (p. 374) and in whom repeated daily gastric lavage is needed to prevent vomiting and reduce the size of a dilated stomach.

Ketosis without Acidosis

The excessive production of β-hydroxybutyric acid and acetoacetic acid in diabetic ketoacidosis has already been described as a cause of acidosis. Abnormal amounts of acetoacetic acid also arise in the body when the carbohydrate in the food is inadequate and increased amounts of fat are being utilised for energy. This is commonly found in cases of cyclical or severe vomiting in children, severe vomiting of pregnancy, starvation, and in postoperative vomiting. Two opposing tendencies are obviously in operation, the ketosis tending to increase, and vomiting tending to decrease the concentration of hydrogen ions in the blood. In these cases it is not uncommon, therefore, to find that metabolic alkalosis coexists with ketosis. Thus, the presence of acetoacetic acid in the urine does not necessarily imply the existence of acidosis, and the existence of metabolic acidosis is established only by the determination of the blood pH or bicarbonate concentration.

Apart from the possible need to treat concomitant acidosis or electrolyte disturbances, ketosis is best remedied by restoring the consumption of carbohydrate to normal. In cases of diabetic ketosis the administration of insulin is essential. In the other forms of ketosis this need not be given. Ample supplies of glucose should be provided; if this cannot be taken by mouth an intravenous infusion of 5 per cent glucose in water may be given. Two to 4 litres of this solution may be needed in the course of the day.

Respiratory Acidosis and Alkalosis

Respiratory acidosis arises when the effective alveolar ventilation does not keep pace with the rate of production of carbon dioxide (p. 251). As a result the $Paco_2$ and carbonic acid concentration of the blood increase, and the pH falls. The distinction between respiratory acidosis and metabolic alkalosis is usually easily made from a knowledge of the cause of the disturbance. The reaction of the arterial blood is decisive; in both the $Paco_2$ is increased, but in respiratory acidosis $[H^+]$ is increased, whereas in metabolic alkalosis the $[H^+]$ is reduced. The kidney responds to an increase in $Paco_2$ by excreting an acid urine and conserving sodium bicarbonate. The causes and consequences of respiratory acidosis are given on page 258.

Respiratory alkalosis occurs when there is excessive loss of carbonic acid by overventilation of the lungs. Most commonly this occurs in hysterical overbreathing or in overventilation during the course of assisted respiration, though it may arise also in the course of meningitis, encephalitis, salicylate intoxication, and liver failure. Tetany may ensue.

Electrolyte repair solutions play no part in the treatment of respiratory acidosis or alkalosis, and therapy should be directed to the underlying disorder. The treatment of hypercapnia is described on page 266 and that of respiratory alkalosis due to hysterical overbreathing on page 534. Tetany may be treated by an intravenous injection of 10 ml of 10 per cent calcium gluconate if necessary. The underlying causative factors should receive appropriate attention.

J. S. ROBSON

Further reading:

Black, D. A. K. (1967) Essentials of Fluid Balance. 4th edition. Oxford: Blackwell.
Lant, A. F. & Wilson, G. M. (1972) Diuretics. Ch. 23 in Renal Disease, ed. Black, D. A. K. Oxford: Blackwell.
Passmore, R. & Robson, J. S. Companion to Medical Studies. 2nd edition. Vol I (1976), Chps. 6, 31 & 35; Vol II (1973), Ch. 11. Vol. III (1974), Ch. 49. Oxford: Blackwell.
Robinson, J. R. (1975) Fundamentals of Acid Base Regulation, 5th edition. Oxford: Blackwell.

6. Diseases of the Cardiovascular System

AT all ages and in all countries, diseases of the cardiovascular system are major causes of death and disability. In communities where infection is a lesser problem than formerly, congenital heart disease now accounts for a higher proportion of deaths in infancy and is beginning to overtake rheumatic fever as a cause of heart disease in the child-bearing years. In most countries with a high standard of living, coronary and cerebral arterial disease and hypertension are responsible for more than 50 per cent of the deaths and of these at least half are due to ischaemic heart disease. Over the last century, not only have coronary attacks become more common, but now it is not unusual for men in their thirties to be admitted to a coronary care unit, particularly heavy cigarette smokers in whom arterial disease of the legs is also common. For those who breathe air polluted by smoke, pulmonary damage may lead to cardiac failure especially in men from the mid-forties onwards.

Patients present not only with breathlessness, swollen ankles and cardiac pain, which are the cardinal symptoms of heart disease, but also with major disabilities due to embolism from thrombus formed within the heart, so that the heart disease may not immediately be recognised. Patients with unexplained fever or anaemia may be found to have infective endocarditis; pericarditis may be the first manifestation of a connective tissue disorder. The presentation of cardiovascular disease is thus protean.

The Symptoms of Heart Disease

Dyspnoea. Awareness of unaccustomed breathlessness on exertion is often the first symptom of heart failure. The breathing is rapid and shallow but is generally not distinguishable by its character from that due to disease of the lungs (p. 256). The anxious patient, however, often has an intermittent sighing dyspnoea which is readily recognisable. *Orthopnoea* is the name given to breathlessness which prevents the patient lying flat. When supine there is increased work in depressing the diaphragm and, in addition, retained fluid is more likely to gravitate towards the lungs. The initial increase in venous return on first adopting the horizontal position is another factor of transient relevance. Redistribution of retained fluid towards the lungs at night may reach a critical level before a patient is awakened from sleep. When he awakens and sits up, he finds himself very breathless and often with a repetitive cough. He may struggle to the window to try to improve the situation. This *paroxysmal nocturnal dyspnoea* is an alarming experience causing tachycardia and temporary hypertension, which may make matters worse. Usually the attack subsides in a few minutes. If the breathlessness continues and the cough becomes productive of watery and often bloodstained sputum, *pulmonary oedema* has supervened. The patient sits gasping for breath. Respiration often becomes bubbly; if wheezy it is sometimes called *cardiac asthma*. The skin is cold and cyanosed and there is often intense venoconstriction which may make venepucture difficult. *Periodic breathing (Cheyne–Stokes respiration)* is common in cardiac failure but is usually detected only if special methods are used or when

it has become advanced; then there are alternating periods of apnoea and hyperpnoea due to depression of the medullary centres from decreased blood flow. It also occurs in the elderly, particularly during sleep.

Oedema is most commonly found at the ankles as its site is mainly determined
by gravity; the sacrum and thighs are areas for oedema in patients confined to
bed. Pressure with the thumb, if sustained, will displace the fluid and leave a pit.

Pain. The cardinal symptom of cardiac ischaemia is the pain known as angina
pectoris (p. 211). The pain of pericarditis is described on page 230. Precordial
catch is the name given to a stabbing pain often indicated by a finger pointing
below the left breast in anxious patients; it is momentary and sharp and quite unlike angina pectoris. Hepatic pain is felt in the epigastrium when the liver is rapidly
distended by fluid retention. Pleural pain is a feature of pulmonary infarction,
which often occurs with heart failure. Occasionally an aneurysm of the aorta or of
a grossly enlarged left atrium can cause persistent pain in the back of the chest
from pressure on the vertebrae.

Palpitation is awareness of heart beat; it is a common result of exercise or
anxiety and occurs with increased catecholamine secretion or with sympathomimetic drugs. Patients often feel the thump of an ectopic beat. Palpitation
may be the only symptom of paroxysmal tachycardia; often the patient can indicate its rate, and usually he is able to say whether the heart beat is regular as in atrial
tachycardia, or irregular as in paroxysmal atrial fibrillation.

Syncope is usually not due to heart disease. *Simple (vasovagal) syncope* results
when the venous return is not maintained, e.g. with prolonged standing, particularly when it is hot or when there is a loss of fluid, as from diarrhoea. It may
be reflex as a result of a frightening, unpleasant or painful experience. A feeling of
nausea and sometimes a failure of vision and a ringing in the ears may herald its
onset. Pallor, sweating and a slow pulse are characteristic. Syncope can also ensue when there is a rise in intrathoracic pressure sufficient to reduce the venous
return significantly, such as with the *Valsalva manoeuvre*. It may also occur with
prolonged vigorous coughing (*cough syncope*) or when elderly men strain to empty the bladder (*micturition syncope*). Syncope on standing—*postural syncope*—is
a feature in some patients with an unusually low blood pressure as in Addison's
disease. It also occurs from failure of the normal vasomotor reflexes, e.g. with
diabetic neuropathy, or, commonly nowadays, as a result of the use of some
hypotensive agents. Syncope induced by movement of the neck suggests either a
hypersensitive carotid sinus or insufficiency of the vertebro-basilar blood flow.

Cardiac causes are rare. *Exercise syncope* may occur when the cardiac output
is very much restricted with exercise, as with aortic stenosis or pulmonary
vascular obstruction. Syncope may result from certain rhythm disturbances, e.g.
Adams-Stokes attack (p. 190).

Other symptoms. Tiredness is a common complaint with severe heart failure
and with myocardial infarction. In those with valvar disease without heart failure
it should lead to a suspicion of infective endocarditis.

Nocturia is frequent and this may be accompanied by loss of ankle swelling overnight. Cough is a feature of pulmonary oedema. In severe protracted heart failure,
anorexia, nausea and vomiting are all common.

Physical Examination

While taking the history and before proceeding to the examination of the heart,
certain pertinent observations may be made. The presence should be noted of any

anaemia, obesity, breathlessness or cyanosis. Peripheral cyanosis is due to an excessive extraction of oxygen from the blood when the circulation is impaired from vasoconstriction, low cardiac output or stasis; it occurs in healthy people when the extremities are cold, and warmth abolishes it. Central cyanosis is due to oxygen undersaturation of the arterial blood from poor gaseous exchange in the lungs in such conditions as emphysema, pulmonary oedema and pneumonia or when there is a right to left shunt in congenital heart disease. If the tongue is cyanosed, it may be deduced that the cyanosis is central in origin. A combination of central and peripheral cyanosis may occur and is often seen in cardiac failure.

The temperature of the skin varies with the skin blood flow. In cardiac failure, except in those forms where the cardiac output is increased, the extremities are abnormally cold, even in an equable environment. Unduly moist palms suggest anxiety if they are cold or thyrotoxicosis if they are warm. Clubbing of the fingers occurs in cyanotic congenital heart disease and in advanced infective endocarditis. Subungual or 'splinter' haemorrhages may result from trauma; otherwise they suggest infective endocarditis. These and other observations can be made while feeling the radial pulse.

The Radial Pulse. This should be examined for rate, rhythm, volume, character of the pulse wave and condition of the vessel wall. Bradycardia (p. 182) describes a heart rate of 60 or less, and tachycardia (p. 181) a heart rate of 100 or more. In health the pulse is normally regular, but—particularly in children—a slowing of the pulse during expiration is common (sinus arrhythmia, p. 181). The other causes of irregularity are discussed on page 182. A pulse of small volume is a feature of reduced cardiac output, as in shock, major haemorrhage or massive pulmonary embolism, or with severe obstruction to blood flow at a cardiac valve. A pulse of large volume is found when there is a rapid flow of blood out of the arterial system, with peripheral vasodilation, as in fever or hyperthyroidism or with aortic regurgitation. It is also found when arterial run off is abnormally prolonged, as in complete heart block. Elevating the arm increases the run off and pulse volume—the so-called *collapsing pulse*; the sensation conveyed to the palm of the hand placed across the forearm when the arm is elevated under these circumstances has a knocking quality and is sometimes called '*muscle knock*'.

Pulsus paradoxus, a variation in volume with breathing, is an exaggerated variety of the normal and is hence misnamed. In health, arterial pulse records show that the arterial and pulse pressure fall in inspiration; with an increased intrathoracic pressure swing, as in asthma, the pulse may disappear in inspiration. Similar variation in the pulse volume is found with a sufficiently large pericardial effusion or with constrictive pericarditis. Minor degrees are best detected by allowing the pressure in a sphygmomanometer cuff to fall slowly; at the upper end the arterial (Korotkov) sounds may be audible only during expiration. Over a range of 5 mm Hg or so this is a normal finding.

In *pulsus alternans* the pulse is regular but the amplitude is large and small in alternate beats. It is also best detected with the sphygmomanometer where there may be a difference of 10 to 40 mm between the strong and weak beats. It is a sign of left ventricular failure. In aortic stenosis a notch may sometimes be felt on the upstroke of the pulse and the wave may be prolonged and of small amplitude; this is the *anacrotic pulse*. A pulse with a double peak—*pulsus bisferiens*—is suggestive of combined aortic stenosis and regurgitation.

Other Arterial Pulses. Medium-sized arteries, e.g. brachials, frequently show evidence of arterial thickening, tortuosity and undue mobility. In old age arteries lose their elasticity, and visible pulsation of the brachial arteries is often seen (locomotor brachii). These changes signify medial sclerosis, which is not, however, related to hypertension or disease of the intima; it is the last which mainly determines whether or not the arterial lumen is narrowed.

The arterial pulsation in the neck is increased in aortic regurgitation and coarctation of the aorta; in elderly patients, particularly hypertensive women, an arterial pulsation is often seen above the right clavicle due to 'kinking' of the carotid artery. A bruit heard over a major artery with the stethoscope bell is an important sign of partial obstruction. In younger hypertensive patients and in children suspected of having congenital heart disease, the radial and femoral pulse should be palpated simultaneously. With coarctation of the aorta, the femoral pulse is very seldom absent but it is of small volume and delayed after the radial pulse; measurement of the arterial pressure in the legs with a suitably large cuff shows it to be lower than in the arms.

Jugular Venous Pulse. The internal jugular veins provide a convenient manometer for the measurement of right atrial pressure. The upper level varies with respiration and can be made to rise by pressure on the abdomen. The venous pulse is distinguished from the arterial by these features and also by its less vigorous wave form, the presence of 'a' and 'v' components, a change in the upper level of filling by altering the angle of the patient, by the ability to abolish a venous pulse by light pressure at the root of the neck and the fact that a venous pulse is usually not palpable. A persistent elevation of the jugular venous pressure is one of the first signs of cardiac failure and is also found in acute pulmonary embolism and in pericardial effusion or constriction. Non-pulsatile venous distention is seen in patients with a mediastinal mass compressing the superior vena cava and is uninfluenced by pressure over the abdomen.

The jugular venous pulse normally has a presystolic or 'a' wave at the time of atrial contraction and a 'v' wave which reaches its peak immediately prior to the opening of the tricuspid valve (Fig. 6.1). Where there is abnormal resistance to right atrial discharge, as in tricuspid stenosis, or when the right ventricle is hypertrophied, the 'a' wave may be abnormally large. With tricuspid regurgitation a systolic 'cv' wave is found. Cannon waves occur in any condition in which the atrium contracts against a closed tricuspid valve, e.g. complete heart block.

Examination of the Heart. The methods employed are inspection, palpation, percussion and auscultation and at each stage the intelligent use of one of these methods often makes the deployment of the next easier. Deformities of the chest are often relevant to the function of the heart (p. 343). Enlargement of the right ventricle during the growing period may show as a prominence to the left of the sternum in children. The apical impulse may be visible in left ventricular hypertrophy and an abnormal pulsation may occasionally be seen over an area of aneurysm of the ventricle.

Systolic pulsation in the epigastrium due to aortic pulsation is common in health, particularly in those who are thin; an enlarged right ventricle, or the liver in a patient with tricuspid regurgitation, may also produce pulsation in this area. Occasionally an aneurysm of the aortic arch can be seen to move the upper sternum with each systole; when the heart is very much enlarged, as with chronic rheumatic heart disease, the whole chest may move with each beat.

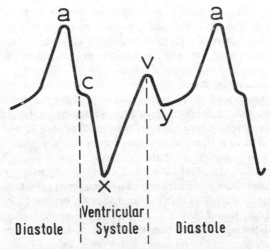

Fig. 6.1 Form of the venous pulse wave. a = atrial contraction, c = onset of ventricular contraction, v = peak pressure in right atrium immediately prior to opening of tricuspid valve, a–x = x descent, v–y = y descent.

PALPATION. The position and the quality of the cardiac apex have next to be examined. The apex beat usually lies in the fifth left intercostal space within the midclavicular line. Its position is partly dependent on the shape and size of the chest, and localisation may be impossible if there is obesity or emphysema. If the mediastinum is not displaced—e.g. by fibrosis, collapse or removal of the lung on the left side, or a pleural effusion on the right—significant displacement of the apex beat to the left is usually a reliable indication of cardiac enlargement; however, the evidence is never so good as that provided by a chest radiograph. The quality of the apex beat should also be noted. In left ventricular hypertrophy it is forceful; sharp closure of the stenosed mitral valve gives it a tapping quality. When the heart is damaged by ischaemic heart disease the apex may also be displaced to the left, usually without the apex impulse being forceful.

With right ventricular hypertrophy a pulsation may be imparted to the hand on the chest to the left of the sternum. A pulmonary artery under abnormally high pressure may cause a pulsation in the second left intercostal space beside the sternum. Closure of the semilunar valves under abnormal pressure may give a diastolic shock.

Turbulent blood flow may impart a vibration to the hand; this 'thrill' is the palpable equivalent of a loud murmur. A systolic thrill at the apex usually indicates mitral regurgitation, a diastolic thrill indicates mitral stenosis. A systolic thrill can often be felt at the lower left sternal edge with a ventricular septal defect and at the base of the heart in aortic or pulmonary stenosis. An aortic diastolic thrill is extremely rare and usually indicates rupture of an aortic valve cusp; pulmonary and tricuspid diastolic thrills are virtually unknown.

PERCUSSION is seldom used except when seeking for abnormal dullness to the right of the sternum in a patient with a suspected pericardial effusion in whom an X-ray is not available. One of the physical signs of emphysema is a loss of the normal cardiac dullness.

AUSCULTATION. It is essential to employ a satisfactory stethoscope incorporating both a diaphragm and a bell. The diaphragm, firmly pressed against the chest, preferentially conveys high-pitched sounds and murmurs, whereas the bell, lightly applied to the skin, favours the transmission of lower pitched sounds and murmurs.

Sounds. The *first heart sound* results particularly from closure of the mitral but also of the tricuspid valve. It is loudest at the apex and may be diminished in the presence of obesity or emphysema. It is accentuated by tachycardia, as in anxiety or thyrotoxicosis, and is sharp, due to abnormal closure of the mitral valve, in mitral stenosis. The first heart sound may be diminished when the valve fails to close properly with mitral regurgitation or from damage to papillary muscles by myocarditis or ischaemic heart disease. It may be obscured by the murmur of mitral regurgitation. The first heart sound is sometimes double in health, or when contraction of one ventricle is delayed as in bundle branch block.

The *second heart sound* is due to closure of the aortic and pulmonary valves and the normal timing is such that closure is synchronous in expiration and asynchronous towards full inspiration; pulmonary valve closure is then the later of the two. Accentuation of the sound of closure of the relevant semilunar valve is a feature of both systemic and pulmonary hypertension but is not a reliable sign. Similarly stenosis of either valve, particularly with calcification of the aortic valve, may impede closure so that the sound is abnormally quiet.

Delay of closure of one of the semilunar valves may result from conduction or mechanical factors. An example of the former is when aortic valve closure is delayed by left bundle branch block. This leads to reversed splitting of the second sound, whereby it is heard during expiration rather than inspiration. When pulmonary valve closure is delayed by an increased right ventricular stroke volume due to a left to right shunt through an atrial septal defect there is persistent splitting of the second heart sound.

Various added sounds may also be significant. In the young a low-pitched *third heart sound*, synchronous with left ventricular filling, is often heard at the apex. In older patients this sound is associated with abnormal ventricular filling, either from an increased volume as may occur in mitral regurgitation, or from altered left ventricular compliance, as may be found with ischaemic heart disease. A *fourth heart sound* is comparable in its genesis to the 'a' wave of the jugular venous pulse and indicates an abnormally forceful atrial discharge; it is a feature of longstanding hypertension, when left ventricular hypertrophy offers increased resistance to filling. It also results from loss of compliance of the left ventricle soon after a myocardial infarct and may be palpable. The *opening snap* is a feature of mitral stenosis with a pliant mitral valve and when found lead to a special search for the characteristic mitral diastolic murmur. The opening snap is usually even more highly pitched than the second heart sound and is best heard with the diaphragm of the stethoscope to the left of the lower sternum. An early systolic click (*ejction sound*) occurs at the time of opening of a semilunar valve in association with either hypertension or stenosis (p. 205).

Murmurs are associated with turbulent blood flow. It is a tribute to the unique design of the heart that a normal cardiac output is not associated with audible turbulence. When the cardiac output is increased, as with pregnancy or severe anaemia, the turbulent flow is usually best heard at the pulmonary valve. Murmurs also arise when blood is projected through, or leaks back through, abnormal valves; the murmurs are then usually projected in the direction of the abnormal flow. It is therefore necessary, in coming to a decision as to the cause of a murmur, to note its intensity and also where it is loudest. The murmur has also to be allocated to either systole or diastole and to the appropriate part of either. Its quality, pitch and direction of preferential conduction also need to be determined. The characteristics of the main murmurs are shown in Figures 6.20, 6.21, 6.22, 6.28, 6.30 and 6.31. As a general rule, however, a harsh murmur like a saw is almost always systolic, a fact which can be confirmed by simultaneous palpation of the carotid artery or by identifying that the murmur precedes the second heart sound, which is usually best heard at the base of the heart. The murmur of regurgitation through either of the semilunar valves is of a decrescendo blowing quality and is transmitted along the interventricular septum. Because of its quality it is easily confused with a breath sound and when seeking a quiet murmur of this type it is therefore necessary for the patient to stop breathing; it is best heard with the patient leaning forward with the breath held in expiration. The murmur of mitral stenosis, on the other hand, is low-pitched and is most likely to be heard if the bell of the stethoscope is pressed lightly at or near the apex with the patient turned half towards the left side.

Blood Pressure. The inflatable cuff of a sphygmomanometer is wrapped carefully round the upper arm with the bag over the brachial artery and is connected with a mercury or aneroid manometer. The latter is more convenient, but should be checked from time to time against a mercury column. The bell of the stethoscope is applied over the brachial artery and the cuff is inflated to a level well above that which abolishes the Korotkov sounds. The pressure in the cuff is then allowed to fall slowly and the return of the sounds is taken as the systolic pressure. As the pressure falls the sounds become louder, and then usually quite suddenly they become muffled. The point at which the sounds become muffled is usually taken as representing the diastolic pressure. When the blood pressure is to be recorded in the leg the patient should lie prone; a special large cuff should be applied to the thigh and an equivalent procedure followed with the stethoscope diaphragm placed in the popliteal fossa. The *pulse pressure* is the difference between the systolic and the diastolic pressures and it tends to be abnormally high in elderly patients with stiff arteries and in patients with conditions that give rise to an increased stroke volume. Arterial pressure may be very difficult to measure in a patient in shock or when there is beat-to-beat variation with atrial fibrillation.

The blood pressure varies throughout the day, falling to low levels during sleep and rising to high levels with anxiety. Isolated blood pressure records can therefore prove misleading, particularly in those who are unusually anxious. Sometimes this is manifest from tremor, undue sweating or tachycardia. In nervous patients repeated blood pressure readings tend to result in progressively lower figures as boredom replaces anxiety; this is, however, by no means invariable. It would be helpful if normal blood pressure could be clearly defined. This is not feasible, however, because it varies according to circumstances, particularly age. In an infant levels of 60/30 would be normal; in the 20-year-old age group, blood pressure taken at rest in most normal subjects varies between about 140/90 and 95/55. In Britain there is a tendency for blood pressure to rise with advancing years. This affects particularly the systolic pressure and is mainly due to loss of elasticity in the large arteries. In practice for a man in his third or fourth decade to have a persistent diastolic pressure of 95 or more would be unusual. It has been shown, however, that prognosis may depend as much on systolic pressure; a level persistently above 150 in this age group should be regarded as abnormal.

Electrocardiography

Electrocardiography plays an essential role in the diagnosis and investigation of heart disease. Its main value lies in the elucidation of cardiac arrhythmias and conduction defects, and in the diagnosis and location of myocardial infarction. It also provides important information about problems such as digitalis effects, electrolyte disturbances and hypertrophy of the various chambers of the heart. However, difficulties with interpretation commonly arise and the electrocardiogram (ECG) must always be viewed in the light of the clinical findings, notably such facts as blood pressure and drug therapy.

The normal resting cell is polarised as a result of an ionic gradient across the cell wall produced by the sodium pump, which reduces the intracellular and increases the extracellular sodium concentration; the reverse is true for the potassium ion. It is the potassium gradient across the cell membrane which is mainly responsible for the electrical potential difference across it.

When the membrane is electrically stimulated, the pump is inactivated. As a result, there is a sudden inrush of sodium ions, an exodus of potassium ions and the cell becomes depolarised. The sodium pump subsequently repolarises the cell but this process is slower. When an exploring electrode is so placed that the depolarisation current flows towards it there is an upright (positive) deflection; when it is flowing away the deflection is inverted (negative). The deflection recorded by the exploring electrode represents the sum total of electrical events in the heart at any one moment. As it is usual for currents to be flowing in many directions simultaneously, to a considerable extent they cancel one another.

A *unipolar lead* is recorded by connecting one electrode—the exploring electrode—to one side of a galvanometer, and the other to conjoined leads from each arm and from the left leg. The latter arrangement is called the 'central terminal'. Leads recorded in this way are known as 'voltage' or 'V' leads, and the unipolar limb leads as VR, VL and VF. The chest lead positions are shown in Figure 6.3. Augmented unipolar limb leads are usually recorded; the augmentation is 50 per cent and is obtained by removing the contribution to the central terminal of the limb where the exploring electrode is also positioned. The reader will be familiar with the arrangement of the standard leads (Lead I: left arm—right arm; Lead II: left leg—right arm; Lead III: left leg—left arm).

Normally, the impulse starts in the SA node but this cannot be detected by the ECG. The impulse then flows through the atrium producing the P wave. On reaching the AV nodal tissue, which conducts very slowly, it then goes rapidly through the left and right branches of the bundle of His to the Purkinje fibres of the ventricles. The next part of the ECG—the QRS complex—represents various components of ventricular depolarisation. The septum is first activated by the left bundle branch from left to right producing an initial upward deflection (R) in leads V1 and V2 over the right ventricle and an initial downward deflection (Q) in leads V4–V6 over the left ventricle (Figs. 6.2 and 6.3). The impulse then spreads out simultaneously through both ventricles from endocardial to epicardial surfaces. The amplitude and duration of the QRS complexes depend to some extent on the bulk of the muscle tissue through which the impulse is passing; as the left ventricle is normally much thicker than the right most of the QRS complex is due to activation of the left ventricle, causing for example an S wave in V1 and an R wave in V5. Atrial repolarisation which is occurring at the same time cannot normally be visualised. After a short period of inactivity, represented by the ST interval, repolarisation occurs producing the T wave which should normally be upright in

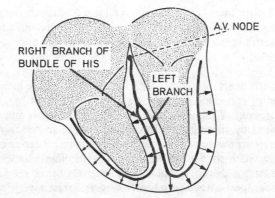

Fig. 6.2 Activation of the septum is from left to right by the left branch of the bundle of His and is followed by spread of the impulse throughout both ventricles.

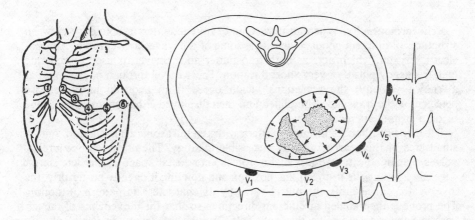

Fig. 6.3 Unipolar chest leads V1–V6 are usually recorded, in addition to standard and unipolar limb leads.

all leads except aVR and sometimes leads III and V1.

Examples of abnormal ECGs are given in the subsections of this chapter.

Other Investigative Procedures

Radiology. Radiological examination is indispensable for accurate determination of the size and shape of the heart. Individual chambers and the great vessels can also be studied (Fig. 6.19, p. 201). Characteristic configurations are often to be seen in the various forms of valvar and congenital heart disease, in syphilitic aortitis and in aneurysm of the heart and aorta. The oesophagus can be outlined by giving the patient barium emulsion to swallow and any backward enlargement of the left atrium in mitral disease can be demonstrated. Serial radiographs provide a useful record of the patient's progress.

The lung fields can also be studied. Congestion and oedema can often be shown radiologically before they can be detected clinically. Congestion is first revealed by dilated pulmonary veins; oedema by thickened septa and dilated lymphatic vessels which result in horizontal lines in the costophrenic angles. More advanced changes are a hazy opacification in the hilar region and beyond, and pleural effusion.

Screening of the heart, preferably with the aid of an image intensifier is of value in the detection of abnormal pulsations and of calcification.

Angiocardiography. The individual chambers of the heart and the great vessels may be visualised by the injection of a radio-opaque material into a vein or by catheter directly into the aorta and heart before making a series of radiographs in rapid succession. Such studies are very useful in the differentiation of various congenital cardiac lesions and of vascular from other abnormal mediastinal shadows. Coronary angiography is necessary before surgery for ischaemic heart disease.

Phonocardiography. The phonocardiograph records heart sounds and murmurs and may help to elucidate difficult problems of auscultation. It is however no substitute for auscultation.

Echocardiography. When an ultrasonic beam encounters a boundary between structures of different acoustic densities, some of the waves are reflected. A piezoelectric crystal, which acts as both transmitter and receiver, is used to generate high frequency pulses of very short duration. These travel through body tissues at a known velocity; the reflections which occur from acoustic interfaces are detected by the transducer, amplified and then displayed either on an oscilloscope or on a strip-chart recorder.

Because both bone and lung interfere with the ultrasonic transmission, only a small area of the heart is directly accessible to study. The normal procedure involves placing the transducer in the fourth intercostal space at the left sternal edge. By locating the probe in this position and pointing it directly posteriorly, the investigator can identify the mitral valve by its characteristic pattern of motion. The probe is then angled in different directions so that the movements of the left ventricle, the tricuspid valve, the aortic valve and the left atrium are displayed.

Echocardiography has proved particularly valuable in studying disorders of the mitral valve. In the normal valve, the cusps open rapidly in early diastole and quickly return towards the closed position. In mitral stenosis, the downward movement of the cusps may be well preserved but, because of the high pressure in the left atrium, the cusps are held down an abnormally long time in the left ventricular cavity—i.e. the diastolic closure rate is slow. Calcification of the mitral valve results in multiple echoes from the valve leaflets. Mitral regurgitation can be suspected by abnormal movements of the valve leaflets. Regurgitation of blood through the aortic valve produces a characteristic vibration of the anterior mitral cusp.

Echocardiography is also useful in detecting abnormalities in other forms of valve disease, pericardial effusion and most varieties of congenital heart disease.

Cardiac Catheterisation. A radio-opaque catheter can be passed from a vein into the right atrium, right ventricle and pulmonary artery; its tip can be wedged in a small pulmonary artery and thus a record of the 'pulmonary arterial wedge' or 'indirect left atrial pressure' can be obtained. A catheter may also be advanced from an artery into the aorta or left ventricle. Pressures can be recorded and the oxygen saturation of extracted blood samples estimated. Valuable information may be obtained in cases of congenital heart disease and in certain types of acquired heart disease. For example, in pulmonary hypertension the pressure in the pulmonary artery and right ventricle is increased; in pulmonary valvar stenosis the systolic pressure is higher in the right ventricle than in the pulmonary artery; in aortic valvar stenosis it is higher in the left ventricle than in the aorta. In atrial septal defect, because of the left to right shunt, the oxygen content of the blood in the right atrium is higher than that in the venae cavae; in ventricular septal defect the oxygen content of the blood in the right ventricle is higher than that in the right atrium.

If the oxygen content of blood from the pulmonary artery and brachial artery and also the oxygen consumption are known, then the cardiac output can be calculated from the Fick formula:—

$$\text{Cardiac output } (l/\text{min}) = \frac{\text{Oxygen consumption (ml/min)}}{\text{Arteriovenous oxygen difference (ml/}l)}$$

The area of a valve can be calculated if the pressure difference across it, and the forward flow throughout, are known. Likewise the volume of a shunt can be calculated from measurement of the relevant oxygen saturations, in conjunction with the oxygen uptake.

By the injection of a known quantity of a dye into a vein or directly into the heart through a catheter and estimation of its serial concentrations in an artery, the presence of a shunt can be detected and the cardiac output measured.

Disorders of Cardiac Rhythm and Conduction

The Control of Cardiac Rate. Cardiac cells have the faculty of self-excitation. The pacemaking of the heart is due to this activity and it is normally controlled by the cells with the fastest natural rate. These are usually at the sinoatrial (SA) node. The SA node has its own intrinsic rate but it is also under nervous control; vagal activity slows it and sympathetic activity accelerates it. The sinus rate may become unduly slowed with increased vagal tone, and lower centres with a faster rate may then take over the pacemaking, e.g. either the AV node—so-called junctional rhythm—or sometimes an ectopic ventricular focus. At other times the natural rate of lower centres may be increased as a result of disturbances of cellular metabolism, such as occur with electrolyte disorders and with digitalis, or as a result of cellular damage from myocardial disease. Sometimes an impulse may be unable to enter a normal pathway if it is refractory; the impulse then has to take a different course. It may arrive when the distal end of the normal pathway is no longer refractory and may then travel through it retrogradely. This short circuit, the so-called re-entry phenomenon, can lead to a rapid circus movement and is one of the causes of paroxysmal tachycardia.

Sinus Rhythms

Sinus Arrhythmia (Fig. 6.4). In breathing there is a phasic variation in the output of the two ventricles, expiration favouring left and inspiration favouring right ventricular filling. The variation in arterial pressure which results triggers baroreceptors in the carotid sinus and elsewhere and the heart rate may then slow in expiration; sinus arrhythmia is particularly common in childhood and is a normal finding.

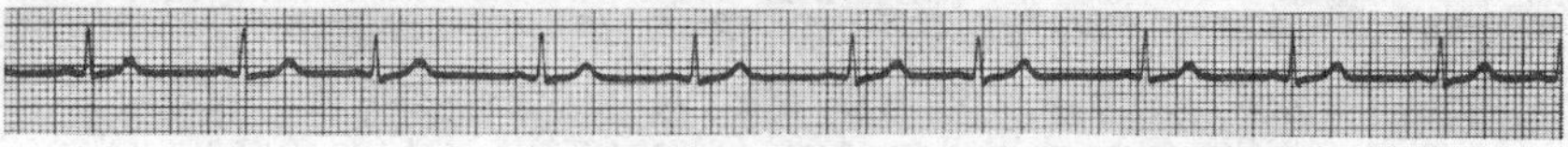

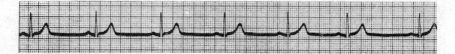

Fig. 6.4 Sinus arrhythmia. PQRST is normal but the interval between successive complexes varies.

Sinus Bradycardia (Fig. 6.5). The term is used when the sinus rate is less than 60/min and is a normal finding in many athletes. Sinus bradycardia may also be a feature of myxoedema, jaundice and raised intracranial pressure, and may occur in some patients soon after myocardial infarction. Sinus bradycardia can be caused by beta adrenergic receptor blocking drugs and by digitalis. In the *'sick sinus syndrome'* sinus bradycardia may be so extreme as to lead to syncope; in addition there may be episodes of atrial tachycardia. A cardiac pacemaker may be required for bradycardia in the sick sinus syndrome if the patient is disabled and simultaneous digoxin therapy may then be needed in those liable also to episodes of tachycardia.

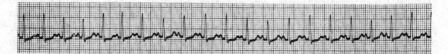

Fig. 6.5 Sinus bradycardia. The rate is 50 per min.

Sinus Tachycardia (Fig. 6.6). This is defined as a sinus rate of more than 100 and is a normal finding with exercise and anxiety. It is also a feature of fever, hyperthyroidism and acute circulatory and cardiac failure. Whatever the cause, the rate rarely exceeds 160, except in infants; the electrocardiogram is otherwise normal.

Fig. 6.6 Sinus tachycardia. The rate is about 150 per min. The QRS complexes are normal and each is preceded by a P wave.

Ectopic Rhythms

When the impulses arise elsewhere than in the SA node the rhythm is known as ectopic; it may be regular or irregular and atrial or ventricular in origin.

Atrial Ectopic Rhythms

Ectopic Beats (Atrial Extrasystoles, Atrial Premature Beats). The rhythm is basically regular, but premature beats can be heard with the stethoscope. If sufficiently premature they may produce no pulse, causing a dropped beat at the wrist. The QRS (Fig. 6.7) is normal but the P is often different because the impulse starts at an abnormal site. Atrial ectopic beats cause no symptoms other than occasionally an awareness of the irregularity and they require no treatment.

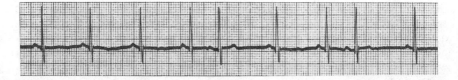

Fig. 6.7 Atrial ectopic beats. The QRS complexes of the two ectopic beats are similar to those of the normal beats and are preceded by a P wave.

Atrial Tachycardia (Fig. 6.8). Paroxysmal tachycardia may occur with a rate of between 140 and 220 as a result of a rapidly firing ectopic focus or of re-entry. This usually occurs in hearts which are otherwise normal and may last from a few seconds to a day or two when untreated. The patient is usually aware of the rapid heart rate of abrupt onset. If the heart is otherwise normal no additional symptoms occur, but some patients feel faint and others may be breathless. In prolonged attacks copious polyuria may ensue. If the heart is abnormal, cardiac pain or left ventricular failure may result. Coffee, alcohol and tobacco are all recognised as precipitating factors in some patients and anxiety may be the provoking cause in others. The last is of course a common cause of awareness of the heart beat but in anxiety alone the heart seems to beat 'strongly' rather than particularly fast.

The ECG shows a QRST of normal configuration and confirms the rapid rate. Massage of the carotid sinus on one side for a few seconds may terminate an attack. If it does not do so a sedative and retiring to bed may be all that is required; many patients then awake to find that the attack is over. Atrial tachycardia can usually be terminated by intravenous practolol or digoxin, or by DC shock. If attacks are frequent or are otherwise disabling, propranolol, digoxin or both may be helpful in reducing their frequency or in abolishing them.

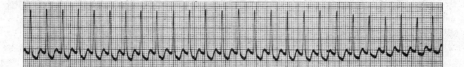

Fig. 6.8 Atrial tachycardia. The rate is 190 per min. The QRS complexes are normal.

Paroxysmal Atrial Tachycardia (PAT) with Atrioventricular Block. In this arrhythmia a rapid atrial rate (140–220/min) is also present, but it is accompanied by atrioventricular block of varying degree which controls the ventricular rate. If there is first degree block, i.e. only prolongation of the PR interval, the ventricular rate may be very rapid, and heart failure may result. Carotid sinus pressure may slow the ventricular rate by increasing the block, so that, for example, the ventricular rate may halve. With atrial tachycardia without block, carotid sinus pressure is either ineffective or stops the attack. PAT with block is the more serious because it seldom occurs in otherwise normal hearts and is frequently a manifestation of digitalis intoxication which can be lethal if digitalis is not stopped. There is nearly always intracellular hypokalaemia even if the serum potassium is normal and potassium supplements should be given. Practolol intravenously (p. 186) often restores sinus rhythm. When PAT with block occurs in those who are not taking digitalis, paradoxically as it may seem, digoxin is the treatment of choice if the ventricular rate is fast.

Atrial Flutter. The atrial rate is usually about 300/min; the underlying causes are the same as for the commoner atrial fibrillation. The majority of the impulses do not reach the ventricles and the ventricular rhythm is usually regular because of a two, three or four to one atrioventricular block. When it occurs in a patient with chronic rheumatic heart disease atrial flutter may cause cardiac failure or increase its severity.

Flutter waves can sometimes be detected at about 5/sec in the jugular venous pulse. Carotid sinus massage often increases the atrioventricular block, as from 2:1 to 3:1 for example; the pulse will then still be regular but will be slower. The ECG shows a saw-tooth appearance due to the F (flutter) waves which are usually best seen in leads II, III and aVF. Digitalis also increases the AV block, slows the ventricular rate and may either abolish the arrhythmia or change the rhythm to that of atrial fibrillation. Digitalis provides a useful prophylactic against recurrence when sinus rhythm returns; patients with mitral stenosis in particular can be protected from the rapid ventricular rate which is liable to be found with atrial flutter in the undigitalised patient.

Atrial Fibrillation. The atria, instead of having a normal organised beat, show an uncoordinated, ineffective movement when the heart is examined at thoracotomy; the baseline of the ECG (Fig. 6.9) is disturbed by so-called f (fibrillation) waves. These are obvious in atrial fibrillation of recent onset but may be almost invisible when the arrhythmia is long established, as in patients with chronic rheumatic heart disease; then the diagnosis is made by the totally irregular QRST complexes and the absence of P waves.

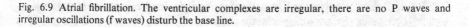

Fig. 6.9 Atrial fibrillation. The ventricular complexes are irregular, there are no P waves and irregular oscillations (f waves) disturb the base line.

Rheumatic mitral valve disease is the commonest cause of atrial fibrillation in young and middle-aged patients; ischaemic heart diseases is the usual explanation in older patients in whom thyrotoxicosis is also an important and often undetected cause. Atrial fibrillation may occur temporarily with myocardial infarction. It is rare in congenital and pulmonary heart disease and in isolated disease of the aortic valve. Sometimes it occurs with pericarditis and after thoracic operations. Atrial fibrillation may be found in the absence of any other evidence of heart disease, and then may be intermittent at first but later often permanent. Episodes of atrial fibrillation can be provoked by anxiety, alcohol and infections.

Atrial fibrillation may also cause or aggravate heart failure in those with an abnormal heart, particularly with mitral stenosis. Diastole is shortened with tachycardia and the left atrial pressure rises. The absence of the contribution of atrial systole to ventricular filling is another adverse factor. Stasis in the atrium favours the formation of thrombus and hence there is an increased danger of embolism particularly for a few days after the change of rhythm.

The pulse is totally irregular. Without digitalis the ventricular rate is usually rapid so that when the interval between heart beats is sufficiently short the ventricle may not fill enough to produce a pulse; the difference between the heart rate and the pulse rate is then called the pulse deficit. There is no 'a' to be seen in the jugular venous pulse, and in patients with mitral stenosis the presystolic murmur disappears.

Ectopic beats, if very numerous, may mimic atrial fibrillation well enough to be distinguishable only by an ECG. However, atrial fibrillation is much the more likely diagnosis if the rhythm has suddenly changed and in particular if there is evidence of thyrotoxicosis or of rheumatic heart disease. Exercise tends to eliminate ectopic beats, at least when the heart is normal.

PROGNOSIS. This varies with the cause of the arrhythmia. Atrial fibrillation can usually be abolished if thyrotoxicosis is successfully treated. Its development is a milestone on the downward path of chronic rheumatic heart disease, and is often associated with worsening of cardiac failure or the development of embolism. In the elderly, untreated atrial fibrillation is often associated with a normal ventricular rate and may be an incidental finding.

TREATMENT. Digitalis is used to reduce the ventricular rate and this alone may result in a striking improvement, particularly in patients with mitral stenosis. When atrial fibrillation persists after correction of hyperthyroidism, sinus rhythm can often be restored with DC shock. In chronic rheumatic heart disease such therapy is pointless because the arrhythmia is almost certain to return, unless mitral stenosis has been relieved by valvotomy. When atrial fibrillation develops in patients with chronic rheumatic heart disease, treatment with heparin followed by warfarin should be instituted as there is a danger of embolism at that time. There is disagreement about the value of continuing anticoagulant therapy, which has its own risks in the long term management of such patients.

Ventricular Ectopic Rhythms

Ectopic Beats (Ventricular Extrasystoles, Ventricular Premature Beats). An ectopic ventricular focus may initiate impulses which activate the ventricles prematurely as a result of ventricular escape, enhanced rate of the ectopic focus or re-entry. Ectopic beats are fairly frequent in normal people but commoner after myocardial infarction and with digitalis therapy. If an ectopic beat occurs after a normal one it may suppress the next expected normal one; when this is repetitive, coupling, or pulsus bigeminus, results.

The symptoms and signs are precisely similar to those of atrial ectopic beats from which they can be distinguished only by the ECG (Fig. 6.10). Ventricular

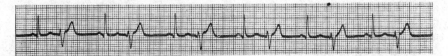

Fig. 6.10 Ventricular ectopic beats. Alternate beats have an abnormally wide QRS complex with no preceding P wave.

extrasystoles have an abnormally widened QRS complex. They are usually of little importance but in patients on digitalis therapy they may result from the drug, and the dose has often to be reduced. They may, however, be of crucial importance in myocardial infarction, for an unusually premature ventricular

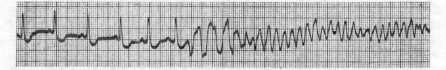

Fig. 6.11 Ventricular fibrillation. The change from sinus rhythm to ventricular fibrillation occurs when a ventricular ectopic beat falls on the T of the previous complex.

extrasystole may fall on the T of a normal beat ('R on T') and result in ventricular tachycardia or ventricular fibrillation (Fig. 6.11).

Ventricular Tachycardia (Fig. 6.12). This generally occurs in patients with serious heart disease and may constitute a clinical emergency. The ventricular rate is of the order of 140 to 220; untreated the tachycardia may last from seconds to days; it may cause heart failure or acute circulatory failure, particularly in patients with myocardial infarction.

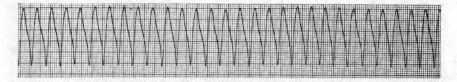

Fig. 6.12 Ventricular tachycardia. The rate is 220 per min. The complexes are broad and abnormal.

The patient may be aware of the tachycardia during an acute phase or may feel faint or become breathless. The independent atrial contractions are sometimes visible in the jugular venous pulse and are responsible for varying ventricular filling, which may be reflected in a variation in the intensity of the first heart sound and in the pulse volume. Carotid sinus pressure is ineffective.

If there is no distress urgent treatment is usually not required, but if there is, particularly immediately after myocardial infarction, lignocaine should be given intravenously (p. 192). Alternatively practolol (5 mg) may be given slowly intravenously and repeated to a total of 20 mg. Mexiletine (p. 192) may also be effective. If these measures fail DC shock should be used, unless the patient is digitilised when there would be a danger of producing ventricular fibrillation.

The prophylactic use of oral procainamide can reduce the likelihood of further episodes but should not be continued for more than 6 weeks as it is liable to produce a syndrome resembling SLE (p. 646). Some patients may require long-term prophylaxis with quinidine in a long-acting form or with oral mexiletine.

Ventricular Fibrillation. Ventricular fibrillation is the commonest immediate cause of sudden death. It is generally due to myocardial infarction but it may result from accidents such as electrocution or drowning. The ventricles have a rapid, ineffective, uncoordinated movement which produces no pulse, and the ECG (Fig. 6.11) has broad, bizarre, irregular complexes. At the onset of the attack the patient loses consciousness. Respiration ceases, the patient develops a deathly pallor and no pulse is palpable even in a large artery. Without treatment the pupils become dilated and death ceases to be potentially reversible. When this arrhythmia occurs as a complication of myocardial infarction in the coronary care unit, the immediate application of DC shock can restore sinus rhythm within seconds. Under other circumstances the circulation has to be maintained by the resuscitation procedure for cardiac arrest (p. 188). Failure of the circulation causes acidosis and sodium bicarbonate should be given intravenously (p. 167). If sinus rhythm is restored lignocaine should be given to reduce the likelihood of recurrence followed by procainamide or mexiletine orally (p. 192).

Ventricular Asystole. This is the more sinister of the two arrhythmias which cause sudden death because it is the usual one in a shocked patient with myocardial infarction and because resuscitation is so seldom successful. It can be distinguished from ventricular fibrillation only when the heart is visible or by an ECG. The treatment, if this is thought appropriate, is that for cardiac arrest, but DC shock is valueless and artificial ventricular pacing is usually either impracticable or unsuccessful.

Ventricular asystole occurs in Adams–Stokes attacks and is then self-terminating. It may also be a temporary and spontaneously reversible effect of the intravenous injection of some drugs.

Cardiac Arrest

The diagnosis of cardiac arrest is based on sudden loss of consciousness and absence of the pulse in a large artery. Resuscitation has usually to be commenced before an ECG is available to distinguish between ventricular fibrillation and ventricular asystole. The indication for resuscitation is clearest when the death has occurred as a result of an accident, as with an electric shock or from drowning, or when the cardiac arrest occurs during the course of an investigation such as cardiac catheterisation or even from an intravenous injection.

The development of the technique of closed chest cardiac massage (external cardiac massage), together with mouth-to-mouth ventilation, has improved the outlook immeasurably and now all doctors, nurses, ambulance drivers and attendants should have received instruction in this vitally important form of first aid. One of the problems in hospital practice is to determine when it is appropriate to attempt resuscitation and to ensure that such attempts are not made, with all the anxiety which they inevitably produce for other patients in the ward, when there is a great likelihood that it will be unsuccessful or that, even if successful, the quality of the life to which the patient returns may not justify the use of the procedure. Inevitably it is sometimes necessary to institute resuscitation until someone familiar with the patient's illness can make the decision as to whether the attempt should continue.

Treatment. The brain suffers irreversible damage unless some circulation of oxygenated blood can be achieved within 2 or 3 minutes. A smart blow should be given to the left of the sternum with the hand or fist, and both legs should be elevated to 90 degrees. If the heart does not start immediately, as indicated by the return of the carotid or femoral pulse, closed chest massage and mouth-to-mouth breathing should be instituted.

TECHNIQUE OF CARDIOPULMONARY RESUSCITATION. The patient is laid on his back on the floor or on boards which are put on the mattress behind the chest. The operator places his hands one on top of the other (Fig. 6.13) on the patient's lower sternum and commences forceful rhythmic compressions at the rate of

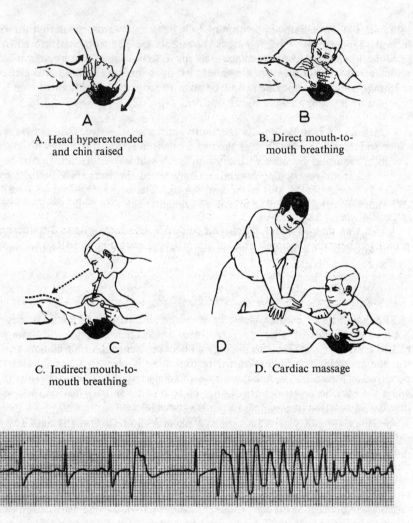

A. Head hyperextended
and chin raised

B. Direct mouth-to-
mouth breathing

C. Indirect mouth-to-
mouth breathing

D. Cardiac massage

Fig 6.13 Emergency resuscitation. The ECG shows the development of ventricular fibrillation from sinus rhythm. This is the commonest cause of cardiac arrest.

60/min. The danger of fracturing ribs is reduced if the pressure is transmitted through the ball of the hand on to the sternum. At the same time ventilation must be ensured. The head is extended and the jaw pulled forward. Mouth-to-mouth or mouth-to-nose breathing is employed until a face mask and bag are available. The lungs should be ventilated after every third or fourth compression of the sternum. Meanwhile an intravenous infusion should be set up containing sodium bicarbonate (100–150 m mol) in order to combat acidosis. Where a defibrillator is available it should be used as soon as possible, for no harm is done if the patient proves to have asystole rather than ventricular fibrillation.

The success rate is best for accidental death or for those who have had a myocardial infarction but without shock or heart failure. If it transpires that the acute circulatory failure was due to cardiac rupture following myocardial infarction, cardiac tamponade or massive pulmonary embolism, resuscitation will be almost certainly unsuccessful. Such a cause can be suspected from failure to produce a pulse and this evidence should always be sought in every patient having closed chest cardiac massage. Nowadays those who have simple syncope are increasingly at risk of overenthusiastic resuscitation measures.

Heart Block (SA and AV Block)

Sinoatrial (SA) Block. A complete cardiac cycle is missed so that a gap appears in the pulse. The electrocardiogram shows that both atrial and ventricular complexes are absent. This condition is uncommon and of little clinical importance.

Atrioventricular (AV) Block. Conduction between the atria and ventricles is impaired.

1. In *first degree heart block* (delayed AV conduction) the PR interval is prolonged beyond the upper limit of normal (0·2 sec) (Fig. 6.14).

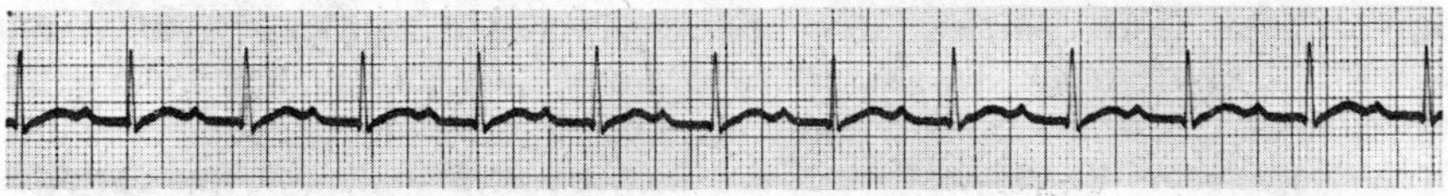

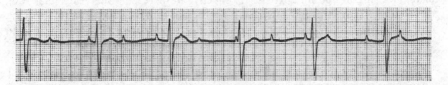

Fig. 6.14 First degree heart block. The PR interval is 0·26 sec.

2. In *second degree heart block* (partial heart block) some impulses from the atria fail to get through to the ventricles, i.e. dropped beats occur. Sometimes there is progressive lengthening of successive PR intervals followed by a dropped beat. This is known as Wenckebach's phenomenon (Fig. 6.15) and is due to progressive fatigue of the AV bundle with recovery following the rest period when the dropped beat occurs.

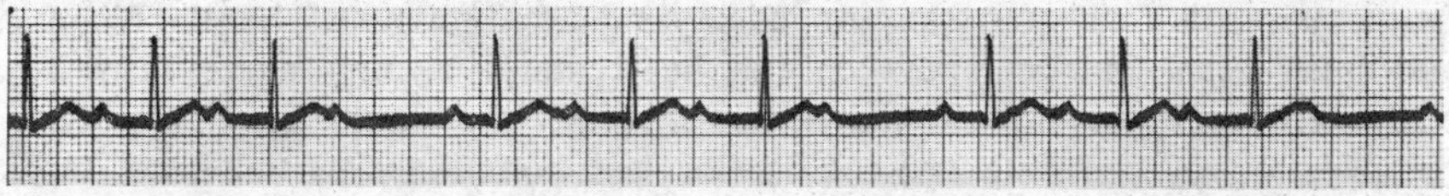

Fig. 6.15 Second degree heart block (Wenckebach's phenomenon). The first beat in the cycle has a PR of 0·28 sec; it lengthens with the next two beats and the fourth P wave is not followed by a QRS—the dropped beat.

3. In *complete heart block* no impulses from the atria reach the ventricles, which beat at their intrinsic rate of about 40 per minute (Fig. 6.16).

Fig. 6.16 Complete heart block. There is complete dissociation of atrial and ventricular complexes. The atrial rate is 70 and the ventricular rate 40 per min.

Aetiology. Depression of conductivity is most commonly due to ischaemia, fibrosis or inflammation of the AV bundle, or to vagal stimulation. Myocardial infarction is the most frequent cause of heart block which develops suddenly. Idiopathic focal fibrosis, strategically situated, is a common cause of chronic heart block, particularly in the elderly. Prolongation of the PR interval is often found in rheumatic fever and digitalis overdosage. Complete heart block may be a late manifestation of digitalis poisoning and occasionally results from a congenital maldevelopment of the bundle.

Clinical Features. *First degree heart block* can be diagnosed only by ECG. Its recognition is sometimes of help as an indication of active rheumatic carditis.

Second Degree Heart Block. When the atrial and ventricular contractions bear a simple ratio to one another such as in 2:1 and 3:1 block, the pulse is slow and regular. Change in the degree of partial heart block may give rise to sudden changes in pulse rate. The degree of block may sometimes be diagnosed by comparing the number of atrial contractions ('a' waves in the jugular pulse) with the carotid pulse. More complex ratios between atrial and ventricular contractions such as 3:2 or 4:3 block give rise to 'dropped beats'. On auscultation it can be appreciated that there has been no ventricular beat, thus distinguishing the condition from ectopic beats. Partial heart block is usually transient and may occur during an acute infection, from digitalis overdose, or from coronary heart disease.

Complete heart block should be suspected when the pulse rate is slow (30 to 40) and regular, and does not vary with exercise. There is complete dissociation between the jugular 'a' waves and the carotid pulses. There may be varying intensity of the first heart sound and audible atrial sounds. Venous 'cannon' waves (p. 174) may be seen in the neck. The pulse volume is often variable depending on whether ventricular filling has been increased by atrial contraction.

Adams–Stokes Syndrome. When cerebral blood flow ceases as a result of ventricular asystole, tachycardia or fibrillation, syncope rapidly ensues. Convulsions may occur if the heart does not begin to beat again within about 10 seconds, and death will result if asystole is prolonged beyond 2 to 3 minutes. The skin blanches and later cyanosis occurs. When the heart starts beating again there is a characteristic flush as the emptied vessels are filled with blood. The syndrome is a complication of complete heart block or less commonly partial heart block. Patients who have repeated attacks may be aware of the imminence of unconsciousness, but frequently syncope occurs without warning. Breathing may continue after the heart has stopped.

Treatment. Complete heart block in acute myocardial infarction requires treatment to prevent undue bradycardia or asystole. Isoprenaline, as an intravenous infusion (1–5 mg in 500 ml dextrose) is effective in increasing the ventricular rate, but has the disadvantage of increasing ventricular stroke work. Electrical pacing may be carried out by advancing a special electrode from a peripheral vein until its tip lies against the endocardium of the right ventricle. Its proximal end is attached externally to a pulse generator. Pacing is usually required for only a few days.

When chronic heart block is responsible for heart failure or Adams–Stokes attacks, long-acting isoprenaline may be given in a dose of 30 mg or more four times daily. More often an implanted endocardial or epicardial pacemaker is used.

Bundle Branch Block

Bundle branch block may affect either the right or the left bundle and result in delay in contraction of the right or left ventricle, respectively. Incomplete bundle branch block is the term used when the QRS complex is widened to less than 0·12 seconds. It commonly occurs when the depolarisation pathway is prolonged due to ventricular dilation as in the right bundle branch block associated with an atrial septal defect. In complete bundle branch block the QRS complex is longer than 0·12 seconds and this usually results from ischaemic disease. The condition may be recognised clinically (p. 176). Examples of the ECG abnormalities are shown in Figures 6.17 and 6.18. The treatment and prognosis are in general those of the underlying disease. Right bundle branch block may be a benign congenital condition.

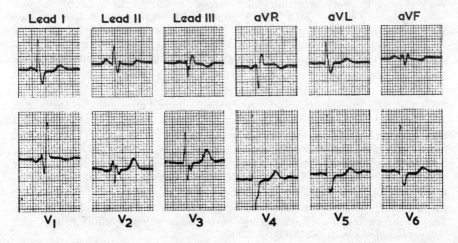

Fig. 6.17 Right bundle branch block. Note that in V1 the late secondary R wave indicates a delay in depolarisation of the right ventricle.

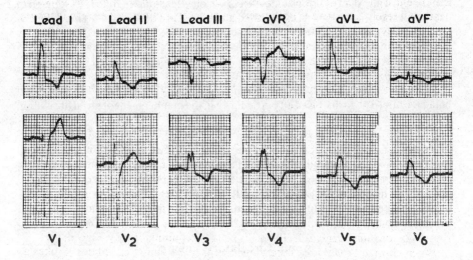

Fig. 6.18 Left bundle branch block. The wide QRS in V6 and aVL indicates a delay in depolarisation of the left ventricle.

Drugs Used in the Treatment of Arrhythmia and Bradycardia

These include drugs used to suppress or prevent ectopic rhythms, to block atrioventricular conduction, or to increase a slow heart rate.

1. *Drugs used to suppress or prevent ectopic rhythms,* whether atrial or ventricular, are thought to act mainly on the cell membrane by slowing depolarisation. Quinidine, mexiletine, lignocaine and procainamide act in this way. There may also be slowing of conduction velocity and depression of contraction amplitude. *Quinidine sulphate* is used less widely than when it was the only anti-arrhythmic available, because of its liability to cause nausea, vomiting and diarrhoea and, more importantly, because of its cardiotoxic effects, which include heart block, asystole and ventricular fibrillation. A sustained action preparation is available which is less toxic. If there are no facilities for conversion of atrial arrhythmias by electrical means quinidine may be given (0·2 g 8 hourly, rising to 0·4 g 8 hourly). When sinus rhythm is restored, a maintenance dose depending on the needs of the individual patient is used; it may be controlled by estimations of blood levels. Conversion to sinus rhythm should be monitored by ECG, watching for widening of the QRS complex, which is a warning of too great a cardiotoxic effect.

Mexiletine is effective in the management of increased ventricular excitability associated with myocardial infarction. Toxic effects include nausea and tremor. It may be given intravenously (200 mg over 5–10 minutes), or on a long-term basis (200–250 mg 6 hourly by mouth). It lacks the danger of producing an SLE-like syndrome which *procainamide hydrochloride* (500–750 mg 4 hourly) is liable to produce in the long term. Intravenous *lignocaine* is particularly useful in the coronary care unit and is given as a bolus of 5–10 ml of the 1 per cent solution, followed by an intravenous infusion of 1–2 g in 500 ml of 5 per cent glucose given at the rate of 1–2 ml per minute. Special precautions are required to ensure that this rate is not exceeded. The drug causes few side-effects, but if given too fast may cause confusion, fits, coma and respiratory depression.

Beta adrenergic receptor blocking drugs such as propranolol, oxprenolol and practolol are all of value, but the last can now be used only intravenously in the acute situation in view of the serious side-effects which occasionally follow its long-term use. Propranolol is the longest established and is used in a dose of 10–40 mg 8 hourly. Oxprenolol is similar. Side-effects are described on page 224.

Phenytoin is also effective either orally or i.v. (max 1 g, not faster than 100 mg in 5 minutes), particularly with digitalis-induced arrhythmias; its side-effects are discussed on page 224.

2. *Drugs used to depress atrioventricular conduction* are digitalis derivatives and beta blockers. The former is used particularly in the management of atrial fibrillation and the latter in thyrotoxicosis.

3. *Drugs used to increase a slow heart rate* include atropine and isoprenaline. *Atropine* (0·6–1·2 mg i.v., s.c. or i.m.) is used for sinus bradycardia with myocardial infarction. *Isoprenaline* in a long-acting form is of value in the treatment of chronic heart block in a dose of 30–60 mg 6 hourly. The patient may be aware of the 'pounding' of the heart, but in some patients it is sufficiently satisfactory in preventing Adams–Stokes attacks to spare them from the potential complications of an artificial pacemaker.

Acute Circulatory Failure

Acute circulatory failure or *shock* is the term used for a clinical state which includes pallor, sweating, hypotension and tachycardia. The most usual cause of the shock syndrome is loss of fluid from haemorrhage, severe diarrhoea or vomiting, or from exudation as a result of extensive burns. Acute circulatory failure may also occur in severe trauma and infection, e.g. bacteraemia. Shock may result from sudden failure of the heart to maintain a satisfactory circulation, as for example in myocardial infarction, and the condition is then known as *cardiogenic shock*. A sudden obstruction of the circulation, such as occurs with massive pulmonary embolism, can also cause acute circulatory failure.

When the cardiac output drops suddenly a compensatory differential alteration in the arteriolar resistances occurs which favours perfusion of the heart and brain. In some cases this may fail and oliguria and clouding of consciousness ensue. If tissue hypoxia and resultant acidosis are severe and prolonged, there may be irreversible damage to the kidneys and brain.

Treatment and Prevention. Treatment must be directed primarily at the cause and any deficiency in the blood volume corrected if possible, as for example, following haemorrhage. In order to avoid overloading the circulation, intravenous infusions must be monitored by observation of the venous pressure. As these patients have to be nursed lying flat the jugular venous pressure cannot be measured. The central venous pressure (CVP) can be measured and fluid administered through a catheter inserted along the subclavian or basilic vein to the right atrium. This procedure is particularly helpful when large or rapid infusions are required; a rise in CVP indicates an excessive load while a fall in the CVP is a useful early sign of oligaemia, e.g. from further haemorrhage.

Pain should be relieved with morphine. Heat loss should be reduced but overheating of the patient causing sweating must be avoided. Vasoconstrictor agents such as metaraminol may give an impression of benefit from their effect on blood pressure which tends to be illusory. Various other treatments have been advocated for cardiogenic shock, but with the possible exception of an ingenious pulsatile intraaortic balloon, few appear to have much to commend them.

Early recognition of the conditions likely to give rise to acute circulatory failure and prompt treatment can prevent its development in some cases. Examples of this are where haemorrhage can be stopped or where blood or fluid lost can be appropriately replaced.

Cardiac Failure

Cardiac failure is liable to develop in patients with conditions which lead to the heart having too great a load over a long period, or because the function of the heart muscle is inadequate, or from a combination of both factors. Under such circumstances a complicated derangement of cardiovascular, renal and endocrine functions can develop which includes abnormal retention of sodium and water in most cases. The increased body fluids tend to accumulate in the lungs when the left ventricle is under an abnormal load, or is itself abnormal, and then the onset of symptoms may be acute, with pulmonary oedema. Gravity is the main determinant of the site of collection of oedema when the right ventricle fails. However, because the disturbance of renal and endocrine function is common to both conditions, the terms left and right heart failure tend to be oversimplifications.

Pathophysiology. The heart may fail when overwhelmed by an excessive preload. Both ventricles may be affected when the cardiac output is increased as in hyperthyroidism, beriberi and severe chronic anaemia. Only one ventricle may be affected, e.g. the left in persistent ductus arteriosus or the right in atrial septal defect. There may be increased afterload as a result of hypertension or aortic valve obstruction. The function of the heart muscle itself may be impaired as in myocarditis or hypoxia or the myocardium may be deficient after infarction. The filling of a ventricle may be restricted by a pericardial effusion or constrictive pericarditis. Often these circumstances may be combined as in the patient with mitral stenosis who has impaired filling of the left ventricle and increased afterload of the right ventricle due to pulmonary arterial hypertension. Similarly in aortic stenosis the left ventricle has an increased afterload which may be combined with impairment of ventricular function due to the coronary blood flow being less than the hypertrophied ventricle requires.

There are, of course, compensatory responses to an extra load. In increased preloading the ventricles dilate; over the years this is a feature of a left to right shunt. When the preload develops suddenly, as with ruptured chordae of the mitral valve, there may be flooding of the lungs in the early stages, but with the passage of time the left ventricle may become able to contend with the added load. The effect of dilation is liable to be self-defeating, for the more a ventricle is stretched the greater is the amount of work required of it to eject a given quantity of blood.

In increased afterloading, as with aortic stenosis and hypertension, the left ventricle becomes hypertrophied. Ultimately the hypertrophy becomes so great that the cavity of the ventricle is reduced; the diminished compliance puts an added load on the left atrium and the nutrition of the ventricular muscle becomes impaired to such an extent that fibrosis may develop. These factors together contribute to a deterioration which reaches the stage where it is irreversible even if the valve obstruction is relieved.

After a varied length of time, impairment of myocardial contractility occurs. There may be other contributory factors, such as ventricular work wasted in expanding a myocardial aneurysm. Ultimately such effects lead to chronic congestive cardiac failure. If the situation were simply the direct effect of a failing pump, the output would be expected to fall and the upstream pressures to rise. Although this does occur the situation is made much more complicated, partly as a result of other mechanisms, such as a reduction in renal blood flow. Vasomotor controls impose a rationing system which becomes evident at first only on exercise. The needs of exercising muscles are met by reduction of blood flow to other areas, apart from the brain and heart, by appropriate differential vasoconstriction. The renal blood flow is reduced and the resultant decrease in glomerular filtration rate is a relatively minor factor in a disadvantageous retention of water and salt. Another important mechanism, which is still not understood, is a disorder of renal tubular function which is the main cause of salt and water retention. It is this process which leads to the increase of total body sodium and water, which is an almost invariable feature of heart failure of all forms. In a small proportion of patients, hyperaldosteronism is induced and is a contributory factor, but the relative inadequacy of aldosterone antagonists in improving cardiac failure helps to confirm that it is not very important. Poor tissue perfusion may also lead to migration of sodium into cells in exchange for potassium which is excreted in the urine. Reduced total body potassium therefore tends to be a feature of cardiac failure even before treatment for the failure is instituted.

In a small proportion of patients in whom the cardiac failure is due to a high metabolic demand (as in hyperthyroidism) or impairment of oxygen transfer at the periphery (as in beriberi) the heart may fail despite a cardiac output higher than in normal persons. This is known as 'high output failure'.

Fluid tends to accumulate where the transcapillary pressure is highest, namely in the lungs when there is obstruction at the mitral valve or an incompetent left ventricle, and in the legs when the right ventricle is mainly involved. However, there is no direct relationship between the height of the relevant venous pressure and the extent of transudation of fluid; for example, in the gradually increasing obstruction of the valve in mitral stenosis there are important compensatory mechanisms, such as thickening of alveolar walls and increased lymphatic drainage, which tend to protect the lungs from pulmonary oedema.

Some of the factors responsible for the development of cardiac failure are still not understood and some of the varieties of clinical presentations are still unexplained. It is best to describe the clinical syndrome found in a particular patient, e.g. pulmonary or systemic oedema or ascites, rather than to use the labels of right and left heart failure.

Clinical Features. Examination of the heart may contribute information which allows understanding of how the cardiac failure has developed, e.g. by the finding of cardiac enlargement, clinical evidence of hypertrophy of either ventricle, auscultatory evidence of valvar disease or third and fourth heart sounds.

The retention of sodium and water may show itself as oedema particularly at the ankles or, in patients confined to bed, in the sacral area or at the backs of the thighs. There may be a pleural effusion on one side or on both; sometimes there is evidence of ascites. Other clinical features are those associated with right or left atrial hypertension or restriction of cardiac output.

Right Atrial Hypertension. The jugular veins can be used as manometers to detect evidence of right atrial hypertension except in infants or in patients who are unusually fat or when the accessory muscles of respiration are in action. In infants the liver size provides the only, if rather crude, manometer of right atrial pressure.

Tricuspid regurgitation is a feature of many forms of heart failure, particularly with rheumatic heart disease and chronic cor pulmonale; the recognition of the characteristic systolic wave which often moves the ears under such circumstances in a patient reclining at 45 degrees may allow the recognition of serious heart failure by the trained eye from the end of the bed. Few physical signs are as important. Rapid distention of the liver commonly gives rise to epigastric pain and then a tender and sometimes pulsatile hepatomegaly may be found.

Left Atrial Hypertension. The most reliable evidence of left atrial hypertension is from the chest radiograph which can show dilation of the pulmonary veins of the upper lobes. If there is interstitial oedema there may be horizontal shadows in the costophrenic angles, which indicate engorgement of interlobular septa with excess fluid. With left atrial hypertension the tense pulmonary veins reduce lung compliance and are a cause of breathlessness, which is first experienced on exercise. Later the breathlessness occurs at rest. Paroxysmal nocturnal dyspnoea and pulmonary oedema may ensue (p. 171). This is liable to occur particularly when cardiac failure is due to left ventricular failure or when there is sudden reduction of mitral valve flow, as when atrial fibrillation and consequent rapid heart rate develop in a patient with mitral stenosis.

Restriction of Cardiac Output. The effects of this may be apparent at first only on effort. Syncope on exertion may be the presenting symptom, for example with aortic stenosis or pulmonary arteriolar hypertension, or occasionally when normal cardioacceleration is prevented, as in complete heart block. When the cardiac output is seriously restricted even at rest, this, combined with compensatory peripheral vasoconstriction, leads to coldness, pallor and cyanosis of the skin at the periphery. Renal and hepatic function become impaired; cachexia is common in advanced cases. The reduced limb flow is probably a factor in rendering such patients particularly liable to venous thrombosis and pulmonary embolism.

Precipitating Factors. Cardiac failure may be precipitated by atrial fibrillation, pulmonary embolism, myocardial infarction, the increased demands imposed by pregnancy, anaemia or infection, or by an increase in salt intake. The patient with cardiac failure who feels weak may take to meat extract with a high salt content which may produce disastrous effects.

Treatment. Unfortunately it is only in a small minority of patients that it is possible to eradicate the cause of the heart failure, but this possibility must not be overlooked. Thyrotoxicosis should be appropriately treated and severe anaemia should be corrected. Once medical treatment has been successfully used, surgical relief of a stenosed valve, replacement of regurgitant valves or closure of a left to right shunt may allow the patient to return to a normal life.

Reduction of the Work Load Imposed upon the Heart. In patients who are ambulant, loss of surplus weight may considerably improve the ability to exercise. Patients in severe heart failure who have not responded to medical treatment when ambulant may gain benefit from a period of complete rest in bed, as serial weight charts in the oedematous patient will show. The breathless patient may find a chair more comfortable than bed. Prolonged bed rest has its own dangers, particularly in the form of venous thrombosis. Complicating factors such as a correctable arrhythmia or infection should be treated.

Management of Salt and Water Retention. This is best treated with diuretics (p. 161). High potency diuretics such as frusemide or ethacrynic acid have a rapid action and are useful in an emergency. They are more costly than diuretics of medium potency such as bendrofluazide, which should be used for maintenance purposes. Potassium supplements must also be prescribed when diuretics are being used frequently. In resistant cases of cardiac failure an antialdosterone drug such as spironolactone (p. 162) may prove helpful.

Excessive use of high potency diuretics may lead to hyponatraemia and uraemia. In these patients the total body sodium may become dangerously low; the dose of the diuretic must be reduced and the salt intake must be unrestricted (p. 163). Hyponatraemia with persistent oedema (dilutional hyponatraemia) is characterised by an increase in total body sodium and water. The appropriate treatment is to restrict sodium, to reduce the intake of water (about 1 l/day), to continue diuretics and to give potassium supplements. The other adverse effects of diuretic therapy are described on page 163.

It is not logical to use diuretics, whose action depends on the elimination of salt and water, without also restricting the patient's salt intake, at least to some extent. The amount of salt used is largely a matter of habit and questioning will reveal that some patients are overindulgent in their use of it. A 'salt-free' diet has been described as 'not prolonging life but making it seem longer', and is not necessary except in very few patients with advanced heart failure. Most such patients can be controlled with high doses of potent diuretics (e.g. frusemide 160 mg/b.d.). Often it is useful to give the evening dose at about 5 p.m. so that the diuresis is over before bedtime.

It is seldom that serous transudates cannot be eliminated with diuretic therapy and salt restriction but occasionally aspiration of pleural effusion or ascitic fluid may be helpful.

Management of Pulmonary Oedema. This presents one of the most alarming crises that a patient can experience and provides an occasion where informed medical aid may be of dramatic benefit. By far the most effective remedy is morphine 10 to 20 mg, preferably intravenously, in a severe attack. Morphine alone transforms the situation by allaying anxiety, reducing catecholamine output and causing systemic venodilatation which allows blood to be sequestrated peripherally. Cyclizine, 50 mg, should also be injected to reduce the risk of vomiting. Morphine should not be employed in patients who are significantly hypotensive, or if there are grounds to suppose that there may be respiratory failure. Aminophylline (0·25–0·5 g i.v.), given slowly, is a useful alternative. Oxygen is helpful and an intravenous diuretic such as frusemide will make a recurrence less probable. Under dire circumstances venous occlusion cuffs on all four limbs may make a contribution though the limb blood flow is so much reduced that their benefit may be slight. Each cuff should be deflated in rotation for 5 minutes in every 15. If all these methods are ineffective venesection may be life-saving. A regular diuretic and usually digoxin should be given to prevent a recurrence.

Digitalis. After 200 years digitalis remains the most powerful inotropic drug. It increases myocardial contractility and thus reduces the diastolic cardiac volume; this in turn promotes the efficiency of cardiac contraction. The better cardiac performance is followed by an improvement in renal function so that there is a secondary diuretic effect. In addition digitalis depresses atrioventricular conduction, which is of particular value in reducing the ventricular rate. With digitalis, however, ventricular ectopic beats are common and alternate ventricular extrasystoles (pulsus bigeminus) are characteristic of over-digitalisation.

Although logic should demand that the first drug to be used in treating heart failure should be one that improves myocardial function, the difficulties in the proper administration of digitalis make it usually wiser to prescribe diuretics in the first instance. Digitalis is the most effective treatment for atrial fibrillation with a rapid ventricular rate. It is used in the treatment of paroxysmal atrial tachycardia or flutter and in the prevention of these conditions. Digitalis is contraindicated in ventricular tachycardia and usually in partial heart block because the degree of block may be increased.

Digoxin is the preparation of choice and is prescribed in an initial dose of 0·5–1 mg. When given by mouth the maximal effect is achieved in about 6 hours or, when given intravenously, in 2 hours. The dose thereafter depends on the weight of the patient. Where bioavailability is dependable, 0·25 mg once daily is usually sufficient, but some patients require double this dose. Digitalis is particularly toxic in the presence of hypokalaemia or renal failure and in the elderly. For a patient in the seventies, 0·0625 mg b.d. is often all that is required. The same preparation should be consistently employed with each patient to avoid differences in bioavailability of the glycoside in digoxin made by different pharmaceutical companies and to gain the advantages of familiarity with one preparation.

The main toxic effects consist of anorexia and nausea and the significance of these should be recognised before the onset of vomiting. Digoxin should then be omitted for 2 days and recommenced at a smaller dose. Ectopic beats, ventricular tachycardia, paroxysmal atrial tachycardia with atrioventricular block and, occasionally, complete heart block may result from digitalisation. Beta receptor blocking drugs are particularly valuable in the management of paroxysmal atrial tachycardia induced by digitalis. The adverse effects of digitalis may be precipitated by the use of diuretics and enhanced by potassium depletion.

The availability of a standard laboratory test for digoxin levels in the blood has eliminated much of the difficulty which sometimes surrounded therapy. The therapeutic range lies between 0·13 and 0·26 ng/100 ml.

Rheumatic Fever

The incidence of rheumatic fever is greatest in childhood and adolescence, 90 per cent of cases commencing between the ages of 5 and 15. In recent years the incidence in the Western world has fallen very considerably; this trend antedated the introduction of antibiotic therapy. The disease remains common in Asia, Africa and Eastern Europe. Recurrences are frequent unless prophylactic treatment is given. Mild and subclinical forms occur and about half the patients who are found to have valvar disease of the heart of rheumatic origin give no history of rheumatic fever.

Aetiology. The precise cause of rheumatic fever is unknown. However, there is much evidence that it is related to infection with Group A β-haemolytic streptococci, probably on the basis of an antigen common to the heart and the streptococcus. The disease is often preceded by tonsillitis or pharyngitis one to three weeks before. Rheumatic fever tends to occur in families but this may be due to environment rather than to heredity. It commonly affects the lower income groups and town dwellers. Poor housing and overcrowding are important factors.

Pathology. The connective tissues of the myocardium, endocardium, pericardium, synovial membranes and tendons are in particular affected. In the exudative stage there is hyperaemia, oedema of the collagen tissue and infiltration with leucocytes. The hallmark of rheumatic fever is the Aschoff nodule, which may be found in the interstitial tissues of any part of the heart, most frequently in relation to small blood vessels, particularly beneath the endocardium of the left ventricle. The mitral, and to a lesser extent, the aortic valves have pinhead-size warty vegetations. Subsequent scarring leads to the valve change of chronic rheumatic heart disease. The microscopic appearance of the Aschoff nodule is of a central area of necrosis surrounded by small round cells, histiocytes and giant cells.

Clinical Features. The onset may be sudden with pain, swelling and stiffness in one or more joints, fever, sweating and tachycardia, or it may be insidious with fatigue, malaise and loss of weight. The large joints are principally affected, e.g. knees, ankles, shoulders and wrists, but almost any joint may be involved. Characteristically there is a migrating polyarthritis, one joint improving as another becomes worse. In severe cases the joints become hot, swollen, red and very tender. The synovium and periarticular tissues are principally involved. Sterile effusions may develop. The joints become normal when the attack is over.

Fever is usual in acute attacks. Sweating may be profuse. Other accompaniments of fever, such as anorexia, furred tongue, constipation and proteinuria, are often present. Tachycardia tends to be out of proportion to the degree of fever and may persist after the latter has settled. The sleeping pulse rate will differentiate tachycardia due to anxiety or excitement, and is useful in deciding when more physical activity can be permitted.

Although pancarditis probably occurs to some extent in all cases of acute rheumatic fever, only about half of them have later evidence of chronic rheumatic heart disease. In the early stages endocarditis may be suspected from diminished intensity of the first heart sound or from the development of a systolic murmur. A transient mitral diastolic murmur may be heard (Carey Coombs murmur). Aortic regurgitation can also occur. Myocarditis may be assumed to be present if there is endocarditis or pericarditis. Its presence is also suggested by undue tachycardia, decreased intensity of the first heart sound, increasing enlargement of the heart, evidence of cardiac failure and abnormalities in the ECG (see below).

Pericarditis may be suspected as a complication when there is a recrudescence of fever with the development of malaise, restlessness and pallor. Retrosternal or precordial pain is common and pericardial friction may be heard. An effusion may develop. Characteristic changes may occur in the electrocardiogram (p. 230). Pericarditis is not in itself a serious manifestation of rheumatic fever.

Rheumatic nodules are seen far less frequently than 20 years ago because rheumatic fever is less common and less severe. They occur most often in childhood and their principal importance lies in the almost invariable association with active carditis. They are situated subcutaneously, are painless, not attached to the skin and tend to occur over bony prominences such as elbows, knees, scapulae, occiput and vertebrae or on tendons.

Erythema marginatum (erythema annulare) consists of pink patches which appear mainly on the trunk and rapidly enlarge to form irregular crescent shapes which join together to form larger areas. The margins are slightly elevated. The lesions tend to appear and disappear over a short period of time.

Chorea is described on page 734. The majority of children with Sydenham's chorea subsequently develop evidence of rheumatic valvar disease.

A polymorph leucocytosis is common in the acute stage. A raised ESR is usually present and may persist as evidence of activity of the rheumatic process when all other manifestations have subsided. In about a quarter, a group A streptococcus can be grown from the throat. A high ASO (antistreptolysin 'O') titre rising or raised to above 300 units provides evidence of recent streptococcal infection.

The chest X-ray often shows enlargement of the cardiac shadow due to dilation of the heart, a pericardial effusion or a combination of both. The commoner ECG changes are prolongation of the PR interval and abnormalities of ST segments and T waves.

Progress. Persistent rheumatic activity is suggested by the presence of fever, tachycardia, anaemia, changing cardiac signs, failure to gain weight, a raised blood sedimentation rate and abnormalities in the electrocardiogram. Activity implies progressive damage to the heart by the rheumatic process. It may be followed by a period, probably over several years, when the contraction of fibrous tissue leads to increasing deformity of the involved valves. Thereafter, unless further attacks of rheumatic fever occur, deterioration is due to the mechanical effects of valvar disease combined with myocardial damage as a sequel to the acute pancarditis. The combined effects, in varying proportion, may lead to cardiac failure.

Diagnosis. Rheumatic fever can be diagnosed if there is evidence of a recent streptococcal infection combined with two or more of the following: carditis, polyarthritis, chorea, erythema marginatum or rheumatic nodules. If only one of these is present, the diagnosis is likely if in addition there is a history of a previous attack, if there is evidence of pre-existing rheumatic valvar damage or fever, raised ESR or white blood count or prolongation of the PR interval (American Heart

Association criteria). It is necessary to distinguish rheumatic fever from other causes of arthritis (p. 638).

Treatment. *Rest in bed* is essential throughout the active stage of the disease, i.e. until symptoms and fever have subsided, the sleeping pulse rate, white count and haemoglobin level have returned to normal, and weight is being regained. Thereafter, the return to activity should be gradual. The blood sedimentation rate is a useful guide to progress.

Phenoxymethylpenicillin should be given for 7 to 10 days routinely at the start of treatment with the object of killing haemolytic streptococci in the nose and throat.

Salicylates are effective in combating fever and pain. Acetylsalicylic acid (aspirin) is preferable to sodium salicylate because it is better tolerated and has a greater analgesic effect. The daily dose of aspirin is 50 mg per kg body weight divided into 4 hourly doses, with a double dose at night to avoid waking the patient. This dosage should be continued until fever and symptoms have been controlled for at least 10 days and then gradually reduced. Should rheumatic manifestations return, larger quantities will have to be resumed. If toxic symptoms develop, the dose must be reduced and then maintained at the highest level which can be tolerated. Nausea, headache, dizziness, tinnitus and deafness are the early toxic symptoms, followed by vomiting, hyperventilation and mental symptoms. Occasionally haemorrhage may occur from hypoprothrombinaemia.

Salicylates relieve symptoms but probably do not influence the cardiac complications, or materially shorten the course of the disease. Clinical trials have shown that the combination of prednisolone with salicylates in high dosage is the most effective treatment for severe cases but has no effect on long-term results.

Convalescence in a suitable environment will be required when the active stage is over and before return to school or work. Its duration will depend on the length of the preceding illness and the presence or absence of cardiac complications.

Prevention. The problem of prophylaxis is important because there is no specific treatment for rheumatic fever and little can be done to mitigate damage to the heart which is liable to be further affected in subsequent attacks. The incidence of relapses diminishes with age; they may be largely prevented in children and adolescents by phenoxymethylpenicillin (125 mg b.d.) or sulphadimidine (0·5 g daily) if the patient is hypersensitive to pencillin. Either should be taken regularly and continued until about 20 years of age.

Diseases of the Heart Valves

The principal cause of valvar disease is rheumatic endocarditis. This most commonly affects the mitral valve, next the aortic valve, comparatively infrequently the tricuspid valve and very rarely the pulmonary valve. Syphilis may cause aortic regurgitation secondary to dilation of the aorta. Congenital lesions are responsible for most cases of pulmonary valvar disease, some cases of aortic disease and occasionally for tricuspid disease. Infective endocarditis may be superimposed on rheumatic and congenital lesions and cause further damage. Exceptionally a cusp may rupture either spontaneously or as a result of external trauma. A diseased valve may be narrowed (stenosed) or may fail to close adequately and thus permit of regurgitation of blood. The term incompetence may be used synonymously with regurgitation but the latter is preferable as a stenosed valve is obviously not 'competent'. Regurgitation may be present without structural changes in the cusps, e.g. from dilation of the mitral valve ring in left ventricular failure, the tricuspid valve ring in right ventricular failure, the pulmonary valve ring in pulmonary hypertension or the aortic valve ring in aortic aneurysm.

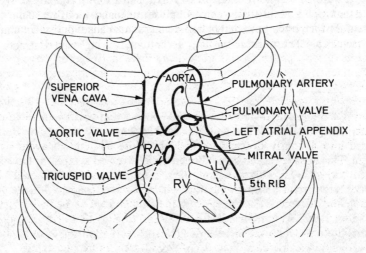

Fig. 6.19 The radiological outline of the heart and the surface projection of its valves.

Mitral Stenosis

In about half the patients there is a history of rheumatic fever or chorea. The gradual scarring process in the heart takes many years to develop fully. The commissures of the mitral valve become adherent and the chordae often become short and deformed. The mitral valve orifice is about 5 cm² in diastole in health and is reduced in severe mitral stenosis to about 1 cm². Rheumatic heart disease also includes damage to heart muscle; the more severe this is the larger the heart tends to be, and the greater the liability to atrial fibrillation and to the formation of thrombus in the left atrium. With the reduction in size of the valve orifice the cardiac output can be maintained only by a rise in left atrial, pulmonary venous and pulmonary capillary pressures with a resultant loss of lung compliance. Thickening of the alveoli and increased pulmonary arteriolar resistance and lymphatic drainage restrict the accumulation of oedema in the lungs. The right ventricle, having to work against an abnormally high pressure, becomes hypertrophied, particularly in those patients who develop disproportionate pulmonary arteriolar obstruction; this has the effect of restricting the elevation of left atrial pressure when the systemic venous return is suddenly increased, as with exercise. There may be concomitant mitral regurgitation, disease of aortic or tricuspid valves, or both.

Clinical Features. The gradual reduction in the mitral valve orifice usually produces breathlessness in about the third decade. The extra demands of pregnancy, or the loss of left atrial contraction with the onset of atrial fibrillation, are common precipitating factors and may bring on breathlessness even at rest. The elevated pulmonary vascular pressures may also cause cough and haemoptysis. Angina occurs in a few patients. Right ventricular failure is more likely to occur in the patient with a larger heart. Systemic embolism may cause a hemiplegia and is commoner in patients with atrial fibrillation.

In a proportion of patients with mitral stenosis the face may have a characteristic 'malar flush'. The specific signs, however, result from the abnormal jet through the mitral valve. The high pressure gradient at closure of the valve is responsible for the tapping quality of the apical impulse and for the loud first sound if the valve is pliant. The jet, often preceded by an opening snap, causes the murmur and often a thrill (Fig. 6.20). The murmur is usually accentuated during atrial contraction. In ear-

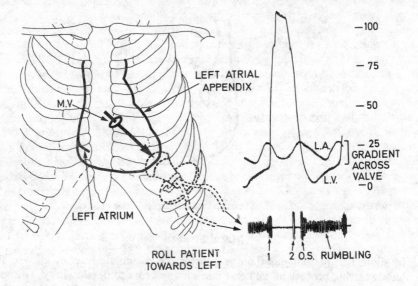

Fig. 6.20 Mitral stenosis. O.S. = opening snap.

ly and asymptomatic patients a presystolic murmur may be the only auscultatory abnormality, but in patients with symptoms the murmur usually extends from the opening snap to the first heart sound. If the valve is calcified there are usually no snaps. With accompanying mitral regurgitation there may be a pansystolic murmur.

There may be an abnormal pulsation to the left of the sternum due to right ventricular hypertrophy and pulmonary valve closure may be unusually loud. Also with pulmonary hypertension there may be a prominent 'a' in the jugular venous pulse as evidence of right atrial hypertrophy; with cardiac failure the jugular venous pressure is elevated and with accompanying tricuspid regurgitation there may be a prominent systolic venous pulse (p. 174). If the cardiac output is restricted the pulse volume may be small.

The ECG often shows the bifid P waves associated with left atrial hypertrophy or may show atrial fibrillation. There may be evidence of right ventricular hypertrophy. Enlargement of the left atrium and its appendage and of the main pulmonary trunk may be seen in the chest X-ray (Fig. 6.20). There may be horizontal shadows in the costophrenic angles to indicate engorgement of the pulmonary lymphatics. In the lateral and right anterior oblique position an enlarged left atrium causes a characteristic displacement of the barium-filled oesophagus.

The physical signs of mitral stenosis are often found before symptoms develop, or an abnormality in the cardiac outline may be noted in a routine chest radiograph. The finding of the abnormal physical signs is of particular importance in the obstetric department, since the identification of mitral disease allows appropriate decisions to be made about its management.

Treatment. When cardiac failure develops in patients with mitral stenosis the medical management is similar to that of heart failure from other causes, with the important difference that surgical relief of mitral stenosis is now a standard form of treatment. Usually operation is not advisable until symptoms develop, but it is often appropriate to recommend mitral valvotomy prophylactically at a time which avoids the slight added risk of operation during pregnancy (p. 238). Cardiac catheterisation is often used to confirm the severity of mitral stenosis by measurement of the gradient across the mitral valve, but this requires measurement of pressures in the left atrium and left ventricle, usually by transvenous puncture of the interatrial septum, and is not without risk. Echocardiography (p. 180) provides evidence as to the rigidity, calcification and rate of movement of the valve cusps and, with increasing experience, is likely to make the invasive techniques less frequently required. Mitral valvotomy may be done with a dilator introduced into the mitral valve through the left ventricle under guidance from a finger inserted into the left atrium, or under direct vision with cardiopulmonary bypass. When the operation is successful, patients can expect 5 to 10 years of benefit in most cases before the stenosis recurs. In some patients traumatic mitral regurgitation is produced and the patient may then be no better until compensatory left ventricular hypertrophy has developed. The most successful results are in the younger patients with sinus rhythm, relatively small hearts and an uncalcified valve. If there is accompanying mitral regurgitation, or the mitral valve is heavily calcified, mitral valve replacement is becoming increasingly safe and successful. Prosthetic or heterograft valves are generally used.

Mitral Regurgitation

This can result from dilation of the mitral valve ring in association with diseases involving the myocardium such as rheumatic fever, diphtheria, viral myocarditis or cardiomyopathy. It also occurs with damage to the papillary muscles, usually from infarction or from spontaneous rupture of the chordae tendinae. In the last two instances the mitral regurgitation may come on suddenly and lead to acute pulmonary oedema. The valve cusps may be damaged gradually from chronic rheumatic heart disease, in which case there is often associated mitral stenosis, and there may be abnormalities of the aortic or tricuspid valves. Mitral regurgitation may develop quickly with infective endocarditis. In old age the valve often undergoes myxomatous degeneration which may be accompanied by mitral regurgitation.

Clinical Features. The symptoms depend on how suddenly the regurgitation develops. When the valve damage is a slow process the symptoms are similar to those in mitral stenosis. In myocardial disease the mitral regurgitation exacerbates an already serious situation.

The physical signs arise from the regurgitant jet, which shows itself by an apical systolic murmur, often well heard into the left axilla and which may be accompanied by an apical systolic thrill. The abnormal valve closure is often associated also with a quiet first heart sound, and the increased forward flow through the mitral valve may give rise to a loud third heart sound or a short middiastolic murmur. The radiograph and ECG often give evidence of left atrial or left ventricular hypertrophy.

Treatment. If mitral regurgitation is due to myocardial disease, treatment, when available, is directed to the latter. When the valve disease is predominant and the symptoms severe, mitral valve replacement in good hands is now safe and reliable. Infective endocarditis should, if possible, be brought under control first with antibiotics.

Aortic Stenosis

Stenosis of the aortic valve may be a congenital fault, may arise from fusion of the valve cusps from rheumatic damage or it may be a late development from an accelerated ageing process in a congenital bicuspid aortic valve. This congenital lesion is found in 0·5 per cent of routine post mortems and accounts for a significant proportion of cases of aortic stenosis in the elderly. Rarely congenital aortic stenosis may be due to a subvalvar diaphragm or more rarely still to a supravalvar stenosis. Except in the congenital forms aortic stenosis develops slowly; the cardiac output is maintained at the expense of a gradually increasing gradient across the aortic valve. The left ventricle becomes increasingly hypertrophied and fibrotic changes may follow. The coronary blood flow may become inadequate, particularly if there is concomitant coronary atheroma. When hypertrophy involves the interventricular septum there is often reduction in the volume of the right ventricle. By these means both atria may become hypertrophied. Particularly in rheumatic heart disease there is often accompanying aortic regurgitation.

Clinical Features. The symptoms arise from restriction of the cardiac output on exercise, which may cause syncope, inadequate coronary blood flow and angina, or left ventricular failure giving rise to dyspnoea on exertion or nocturnal dyspnoea. Breathlessness does not develop until left ventricular hypertrophy fails to compensate for the obstruction and is therefore late in the disease. Sudden death is common with severe aortic stenosis.

The physical signs arise from the jet through the aortic valve (Fig. 6.21) which causes a systolic murmur and often a thrill which may be transmitted to the carotid pulse as the so-called 'carotid shudder'. The thrusting apex beat of left ventricular hypertrophy is characteristic. Left atrial hypertrophy may cause a fourth heart sound (which is not to be expected if there is concomitant mitral stenosis) and the right atrial hypertrophy an 'a' wave in the jugular venous pulse. The restricted cardiac output is often reflected in a small volume arterial pulse which rises abnormally slowly and the pulse pressure is often lower than the average for the age.

The radiographic changes are shown in Figure 6.21. Under the image intensifier calcification of the aortic valve can usually be demonstrated. The ECG shows left atrial and left ventricular hypertrophy and in advanced cases changes of the latter are gross (Fig. 6.27, p. 222).

Treatment. Unlike patients with mitral stenosis it is often necessary to recommend surgical replacement of the valve when symptoms are slight or even absent if the aortic stenosis is established to be severe. To wait too long may result in irreversible damage to the left ventricle. The valve is replaced under cardiopulmonary bypass with a prosthetic or heterograft valve. In this way left ventricular failure may be prevented and postoperatively there is usually radiographic

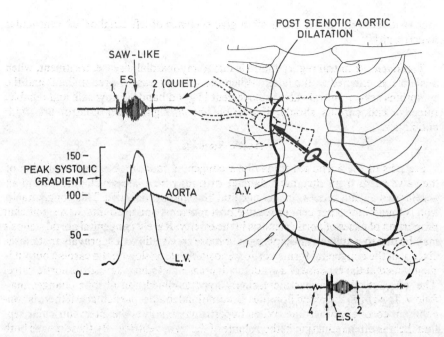

Fig. 6.21 Aortic stenosis. E.S. = ejection sound (p. 176).

and ECG evidence of reduction in the left ventricular hypertrophy. In some cases of severe congenital aortic stenosis, valvotomy may be required as an intermediate measure until an adult size valve can be inserted.

Aortic Regurgitation

This results from abnormal aortic cusps as in congenital bicuspid valves or when valves have been damaged by rheumatic heart disease or infective endocarditis. Aortic regurgitation may also be due to dilation of the first part of the aorta in cystic medionecrosis, tertiary syphilis or atheroma. When the leak is large the stroke output may be increased two- or three-fold. The major arteries are then conspicuously pulsatile; the left ventricle dilates and hypertrophies and initially compensates for the fault in the valve. The left ventricular diastolic pressure rises, at first only with exercise; the pulmonary vascular pressures then also increase and breathlessness develops.

Until the onset of breathlessness the only symptom may be an awareness of the heartbeat, particularly when lying on the left side. Often paroxysmal nocturnal dyspnoea is the first symptom. Peripheral oedema may follow. Angina may occur particularly when there is coexisting coronary atheroma or when the coronary ostia are involved in syphilitic aortitis.

The characteristic murmur is illustrated in Figure 6.22; although it is usually best heard to the left of the sternum it is sometimes louder to the right particularly with syphilitic aortitis. A thrill is very rare. When the leak is small the murmur will be heard only if the steps shown in Figure 6.22 are followed; this is of crucial importance in the early detection of infective endocarditis affecting the aortic valve. A systolic murmur due to the increased stroke volume is common and should not

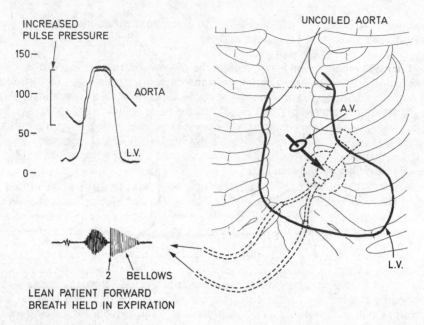

Fig. 6.22 Aortic regurgitation.

be regarded as due to accompanying stenosis without other evidence of the latter. When the leak is large the diagnosis is usually easy, with gross pulsation in the large arteries, a 'muscle knock' (p. 173), a low diastolic and an increased pulse pressure. There is usually a thrusting apex beat and often a presystolic impulse and a fourth heart sound as evidence of left atrial hypertrophy. An example of the change in the radiographic appearances is shown in Figure 6.22. The ECG usually shows left ventricular hypertrophy (Fig. 6.27, p. 222).

Replacement of the aortic valve with a prosthesis or a heterograft valve under cardiopulmonary bypass now carries a mortality of less than 5 per cent in skilled hands and is the treatment of choice if there is evidence of increasing left ventricular overload or when symptoms develop.

Tricuspid Valve Disease

Tricuspid stenosis is usually due to chronic rheumatic heart disease and is almost always accompanied by mitral stenosis and often also by aortic valve disease. The symptoms are those of the accompanying mitral valve disease, but if the tricuspid stenosis is severe there is an increased likelihood of the development of ascites and peripheral oedema. With sinus rhythm the 'a' wave in the jugular venous pulse is conspicuous and there may be presystolic hepatic pulsation. There may be a diastolic murmur similar to that heard with an atrial septal defect (Fig. 6.30, p. 234). The radiograph may show evidence of disproportionate enlargement of the right atrium; in the ECG there may be the peaked P wave of right atrial hypertrophy but more often there is atrial fibrillation.

Occasionally tricuspid valve replacement is required, but the operation is often less satisfactory than those for mitral and aortic valve disease, partly because tricuspid stenosis tends to occur in those patients who have had severe rheumatic pancarditis. There is the added difficulty in assessment because of accompanying mitral valve disease and its treatment.

Tricuspid regurgitation is common in the presence of right ventricular dilation, particularly with rheumatic heart disease and chronic cor pulmonale. Occasionally it results from rheumatic or ischaemic myocardial damage. Characteristically there is a large 'cv' wave in the jugular venous pulse which may move the ear lobes with the patient reclining at 45 degrees; systolic hepatic pulsation may also be present. With effective medical treatment these signs usually disappear except in those patients, particularly with chronic rheumatic heart disease, in whom there is organic tricuspid valve damage.

Replacement of the valve may be required in a very few patients with organic tricuspid valve damage.

Pulmonary Valve Disease

Pulmonary stenosis is usually congenital and may be isolated or part of Fallot's tetralogy (p. 236). It is recognisable from an ejection systolic murmur to the left of the upper sternum, radiating towards the left shoulder, often accompanied by a thrill which is best appreciated when the patient leans forward and breathes out. The murmur is often preceded by an ejection sound and valve closure is usually quiet. An increased right ventricular thrust, radiographic evidence of poststenotic dilation of the main pulmonary artery and ECG evidence of right ventricular hypertrophy and often right atrial hypertrophy are all to be expected if the stenosis is severe.

Some patients require pulmonary valvotomy, best done with cardiopulmonary bypass.

Pulmonary regurgitation is rare and is usually a feature of pulmonary hypertension. The Graham Steell murmur, which is characteristic, is decrescendo and heard at the left sternal edge; the distinction from aortic regurgitation can generally be made from other evidence.

Infective Endocarditis

Endocarditis may result from infection by bacteria, coxiella and fungi. In the rarer acute form the disease is fulminating, may affect normal valves and if untreated may result in death in a few days, e.g. in staphylococcal septicaemia. At the other end of the spectrum the disease is insidious and may have been present for many months before diagnosis. Abnormal valves such as bicuspid aortic, rheumatic or prosthetic valves, or various forms of congenital heart disease, e.g. ventricular septal defect or persistent ductus arteriosus, are the usual underlying lesions. Regurgitant mitral and aortic valves are the commonest to be affected. It occurs at all ages, but seldom before 20 years; it is now increasingly recognised in the elderly.

Pathology. Fibrin and platelets are deposited at the site of closure of normal valves and their absorption into the substance of the valve leads to a gradual thickening of the cusps over the years. This process is exaggerated with abnormal valves, or where an abnormal jet impinges on the endocardium, and colonisation of such deposits of fibrin and platelets by blood-borne organisms may occur.

Streptococcus viridans, a common cause of periodontal infections, is liable to enter the bloodstream at the time of a dental extraction; a history of such a procedure recently is common in subacute infective endocarditis due to this organism Staphylococci and *Streptococcus faecalis* are other causative organisms: with the latter there may be a history of urethral or pelvic surgery. *Coxiella burnetti* endocarditis is more common in, but not peculiar to, those who work with sheep or with carcases.

Affected valves develop vegetations which may be exuberant and a source of embolism; regurgitation may develop or increase due to loss of substance or perforation of a cusp. Weeks or months after the onset mycotic aneurysms may develop in systemic arteries and rupture. Normal valves, particularly the tricuspid valve, are liable to become infected in 'main-line' drug addicts. At postmortem it is common to find infarction of the spleen and the kidneys in particular. Glomerulonephritis is also found, which may be associated with an immune complex reaction (p. 43).

Clinical Features. Infective endocarditis should be suspected when a patient known to have congenital or valvular heart disease develops a fever or complains of unusual tiredness. Often, however, infective endocarditis occurs in patients whose heart disease has been hitherto unsuspected and the diagnosis is often dangerously delayed because it has not been considered. Persistent fever, often recognisable from a history of sweating at night, unexplained arterial occlusion, or the discovery of anaemia or splenomegaly may be presenting features. The disease is almost invariably fatal if untreated and now, even in treated cases, there is a high mortality. Delay in diagnosis may result in an embolic stroke, progressive valve damage, heart failure and death.

In the early stages the patient looks well but later pallor may be obvious. Other features commonly listed should nowadays be regarded as evidence of unreasonable delay in diagnosis in many instances; these include purpura and petechial haemorrhages in skin and mucous membranes and splinter haemorrhages under the fingernails which, although they occur in health, are more frequent with infective endocarditis. Osler's nodes consist of painful tender swellings at the fingertips and are rare. Clubbing is usually relatively late. The spleen is frequently just palpable. In coxiella infections the spleen and liver may be considerably enlarged, and palmar erythema is usual. Embolism may be revealed only by loss of foot pulses or may be the presenting feature with cerebral, coronary or splenic infarction. Microscopical haematuria is common. The finding of any of these features requires re-examination for hitherto unrecognised heart disease such as trivial aortic regurgitation.

Diagnosis. Elevation of the ESR is usual but not universal. Normochromic, normocytic anaemia is common. Thrombocytopenia and disturbed liver function tests, particularly elevation of the alkaline phosphatase, are usual in coxiella infections. Blood culture is the crucial procedure and should be prompt and multiple, e.g. six, preferably paired, blood cultures in the first 6 hours incubated both aerobically and anaerobically. No advantage is gained by waiting for an elevation of temperature. Fungi should normally be detected by standard methods of culture. The administration of antibiotics before taking the blood may prevent laboratory isolation of the causative organism. Q fever endocarditis can be diagnosed by showing high titres to coxiella antigens in complement fixation tests. Infective endocarditis is a disease which is easily overlooked.

Treatment. If penicillin sensitive *Streptococcus viridans* is isolated, benzyl-penicillin (3 mega units 6 hourly) should be given intramuscularly for 1 to 2 weeks, together with probenecid, to increase the blood levels. Treatment will need to be continued for 4 to 6 weeks and, as intramuscular injections are painful, it is preferable to change to oral therapy with phenoxymethyl penicillin (0·5 g 4 hourly) and probenecid, provided that antibiotic levels are then shown to be satisfactory. In *Streptococcus viridans* infection it is essential to exclude so far as possible apical dental abscesses as a cause of infection or reinfection. A tooth with evidence of an apical abscess should be extracted. For cases due to *Streptococcus faecalis*, gentamicin (80 mg 8 hourly) should be given in conjunction with the penicillin and probenecid. The dosage of gentamicin must be adjusted on the basis of the results of 'peak' and 'trough' serum gentamicin level determinations. The gentamicin should be continued for up to 4 weeks. The above regime is also suitable as initial therapy in cases in which no causative organism is found, but it may be necessary to try other antibacterial agents, e.g. co-trimoxazole or the lincomycins, if there is no response to the penicillin and gentamicin. For coxiella endocarditis there have been reports of successful therapy with combined tetracycline and lincomycin or clindamycin.

If the valve damage is extensive the valve may need to be replaced, preferably when the infection has been brought under control but sometimes as a matter of urgency, as when perforation of an aortic cusp leads to pulmonary oedema. It often proves impossible to eradicate infection from a prosthetic valve which usually needs to be replaced.

Prophylaxis. Every patient with heart disease susceptible to infective endocarditis should be warned of the absolute necessity of taking especial care of the teeth and of having antibiotic cover for dental extractions. A single dose of fortified procaine penicillin injection B.P. (300 mg procaine penicillin plus 60 mg benzyl-penicillin) given immediately before dental extraction provides both an immediate high level and persistent effect. Prolonged administration of penicillin either before or after extraction allows selection and subsequent multiplication of resistant strains and should be avoided. For other surgical procedures a 5 day course of penicillin and streptomycin (1 g 12 hourly) started 1 hour before the procedure is appropriate.

Coronary Heart Disease (Ischaemic Heart Disease)

Atheromatous disease of the coronary arteries is the most important single cause of death in the Western world. It is the commonest cause of angina pectoris and leads also to myocardial infarction and its complications, to cardiac failure and to sudden death.

The Coronary Circulation. The right coronary artery arises from the right sinus of Valsalva and passes in the right atrioventricular groove to supply the right ventricle, part of the interventricular septum and the inferior part of the left ventricle; a branch supplies the SA node. The left coronary artery arises from the left sinus and divides into an anterior descending branch, which supplies part of the septum, and the anterior and apical parts of the heart and the circumflex branch, which passes in the left atrioventricular groove and supplies the lateral and posterior surfaces of the heart. In health there are small anastomoses between the coronary arteries; these enlarge under the influence of ischaemia if the flow through a neighbouring coronary artery is compromised. With advancing years an extensive network of anastomotic vessels develops.

Aetiology. Those who have seen the major arteries at a postmortem examination conducted on natives in Africa are bound to be impressed by their normal appearance when compared with the atheromatous arteries of those who live in more prosperous countries. This is one of the findings which indicates that coronary heart disease is not an inevitable ageing process. Several factors have been implicated. A metabolic abnormality leads to deposition of cholesterol in the arterial wall; in some cases the process may be preceded by the formation of thrombus at the site. Atheromatous change is favoured by abnormalities of lipid metabolism, as in hypercholesterolaemia, which may be inherited (p. 588), and in patients with xanthomatosis or diabetes mellitus. Experimental evidence has been available for half a century showing that when rabbits are fed on a high cholesterol diet, deposition of lipids in the arterial wall is favoured. There is evidence that those races who in poverty are free of arterial disease may, if they adopt the diet of more prosperous nations, also develop their arterial diseases. These dietary factors are probably most important during the growing period.

Atherosclerosis tends also to be hastened by hereditary factors (p. 19), obesity, hypertension, lack of exercise and cigarette smoking. The attack rate is held to be higher when the calcium content of the drinking water is low. Increased intake of salt, which favours the development of hypertension, and of sugar have also been implicated. Abnormal reaction to stress is also claimed to be a factor.

Pathology. The process of reduction in the lumen of a coronary artery may be due to atheroma affecting the intima, fibrin and platelet deposition on the intima, haemorrhage under the intima, thrombosis, or to a combination of these factors. When angina develops one or more coronary arteries are usually already critically reduced in lumen or even occluded. The anterior descending coronary artery is especially vulnerable to atheroma and sudden occlusion of this vessel is particularly dangerous. In occasional cases of myocardial infarction no occlusion can be found postmortem; conversely coronary arterial occlusion may be present in patients who have had no recognisable episode of myocardial infarction and sometimes no symptoms or signs of ischaemic heart disease.

If the myocardium becomes damaged by ischaemia there may be subepicardial, subendocardial or transmural infarction. During acute infarction there is an inflammatory reaction and if the epicardial surface is affected there is usually overlying pericarditis; if the endocardial surface is affected, there may be intraventricular thrombosis. Over a period of 1 or 2 months the area damaged by infarction is replaced by fibrosis; it may ultimately become difficult to find which area was involved even at postmortem. However, the scar plays no part in the normal depolarisation of the heart so that it may often be detectable permanently from the electrocardiogram.

Angina Pectoris

Angina pectoris is the name for a clinical syndrome rather than a disease. It is likely to occur when the coronary blood flow is less than is required, and atherosclerosis is the commonest cause of this. Factors which increase requirements are any which add to ventricular preloading, such as exercise, anaemia or hyperthyroidism; additional afterload from hypertension, aortic stenosis or obstructive cardiomyopathy also demands a greater coronary blood flow. Increased tension of the ventricular wall, as occurs in dilation or hypertrophy, may reduce coronary flow. Tachycardia increases cardiac work and often brings on pain. A rapid arterial run-off during diastole reduces coronary arterial pressure and flow in aortic regurgitation.

Clinical Features. Angina pectoris is usually recognised as a sense of oppression or tightness in the middle of the chest—'like a band round the chest'—and the patient commonly places his hand or clenched fist on the sternum or both hands on the lower chest with the fingers touching at the sternum. It is usually induced by exertion, particularly out of doors, or by anxiety. Angina is likely to be worse when walking against a wind, uphill, on a cold day and particularly after meals. Some patients find that pain comes when they start walking and that later it does not return despite greater effort. Others can 'walk it off'. Some experience the pain when lying flat (*angina decubitus*), and some are awakened by it (*nocturnal angina*) particularly with 'energetic' or alarming dreams. Rarely pain may come capriciously and ECG changes occur, similar to those of acute infarction but rapidly reversible, due to coronary arterial spasm (*Prinzmetal's angina*).

The pain is often accompanied by discomfort in the arms, more commonly the left, the wrists and sometimes the hands; the patient may describe a feeling of uselessness in the limb. Angina may more rarely be epigastric or interscapular or may radiate to the neck and jaw, or occur at any of these places of reference without chest discomfort. The precipitation by effort or anxiety, and the relief within a few minutes by rest or with the use of glyceryl trinitrate, should allow the cause of the pain to be recognised. There may be accompanying breathlessness. Pain may be induced by a cardiac arrhythmia.

Physical examination is frequently negative. Aortic valve disease, particularly aortic stenosis, may cause angina. Rarely a quiet early diastolic murmur or calcification of the ascending aorta may betray syphilitic aortitis which can obstruct the coronary ostia. Evidence of atherosclerosis elsewhere should be sought, e.g. absent peripheral arterial pulses or a bruit over a major artery. Hypercholesterolaemia increases the liability to arterial disease and may then be accompanied by premature arcus senilis; there may be xanthomatous deposits on the elbows and in the tendons suggestive of a primary hyperlipidaemia.

The blood should always be examined for evidence of anaemia, and if found the anaemia should be corrected if possible; for example, some patients have been relieved of angina by the treatment of bleeding haemorrhoids. Fasting blood should also be examined for evidence of hyperlipidaemia, which can sometimes be corrected (p. 588). Conditions which increase cardiac work, e.g. hyperthyroidism or obesity, should be sought and where possible treated.

Electrocardiograms are normal in most patients at rest between attacks. In some there is evidence of established infarction. In others ischaemic changes (ST depression and T inversion) may be present or be induced by exercise. Although both 'false positive' and 'false negative' ECGs can be recorded immediately after exercise, ST depression of 2 mm or more is very much in favour of ischaemic heart disease.

Coronary arteriography is sometimes performed for diagnostic purposes and is obligatory if sugery is contemplated. There are two disadvantages: one is that coronary artery disease is common in those over 50 years even without symptoms, so that the method is useful in specifying the sites of abnormality rather than indicating the disease. The other disadvantage is that there is a mortality risk but in the best hands this is less than one in a thousand.

Differential Diagnosis. Effort angina has few significant mimics if a careful history is elicited. Musculoskeletal pains are provoked by specific movements rather than by walking. Asthma, when induced by exercise, may give a sense of tightness in the chest but lasts longer than angina and dyspnoea is more prominent. The pain of pericarditis occasionally comes only with exercise, but its other characteristics (p. 230) should help to make the distinction. Angina occurring at rest may be confused with oesophagitis, with or without a hiatus hernia, but pain due to oesophagitis usually has a burning quality and tends to be exacerbated by hot liquids and to be relieved by alkalis. A small hiatus hernia occurs in about 20 per cent of the population and certainly should not be considered to be the cause of the pain without good evidence.

Treatment. Patients usually respond to a careful explanation of the problem, which can be presented as what it is—a mismatch between coronary supply and cardiac needs. The natural process of repair by development of anastomoses should be stressed. Patients can then learn how to help themselves, e.g. by avoiding walking after meals, particularly in the cold or against a wind, and severe unaccustomed exertion. They may need encouragement and support in their endeavours to stop smoking cigarettes or to lose weight. In a few patients hyperlipoproteinaemia requires treatment by diet and other measures (p. 589).

Fresh glyceryl trinitrate (GTN 0·5 mg), allowed to dissolve under the tongue or crunched for more rapid effect and retained in the mouth, usually relieves the pain in 2 to 3 minutes and in about the same time as the onset of the slight headache which it also produces. The best use of GTN is prophylactically before exercise recognised as liable to produce pain. The good effect comes from the lowering of blood pressure and dilation of coronary vessels whose disease does not prevent this. Not more than about two per hour should be used. Patients can be reassured that GTN is not dangerous or habit forming and that it does not lose its effect. If the requirement for it increases significantly the patient should seek medical advice. The appropriate use of GTN allows exercise within the new limits set by the disability; this should be encouraged for there is evidence that exercise favours the development of collateral vessels.

The prescription of placebos, such as lactose, may bring about improvement in over 20 per cent of patients with angina. However, beta adrenergic receptor blocking drugs have been proved to be very much more effective and may make the patient symptom free. Propranolol can be prescribed initially in small doses (e.g. 10 mg 6 hourly) with progressive increments until benefit is obtained, which is often not until the resting heart rate has been significantly slowed. As much as 240 mg 6 hourly or even more may be required. A beta blocking drug should not be withdrawn abruptly because of the risks of dangerous arrhythmias and myocardial infarction. The side effects are described on page 224.

Patients who are severely disabled by angina may be dramatically improved by aorta-coronary bypass surgery, using a graft from the saphenous vein. The best surgeons have an operative mortality of as little as 1 per cent; for patients with multiple coronary arterial obstruction the operation may also improve the prognosis.

Prevention. The Joint Working Party of the Royal College of Physicians of London and the British Cardiac Society (p. 247) stressed particularly the advantage of stopping cigarette smoking in reducing the risk of coronary heart disease. This report also made general recommendations in the hope of altering the widespread habits of overeating and inadequate exercise. Only in the relatively young with established hyperlipidaemia did it recommend strict diets in which animal fat intake is reduced and butter replaced by margarines made with polyunsaturated fats, together with considerable replacement of meat with fish, and reduction in the intake of eggs and cream. There is little to suggest that there is potential benefit for those over 50 years of age who have had a heart attack by adopting diets of this kind, and many find them irksome. The advantage of controlling blood pressure is mainly in reducing the liability to stroke and renal failure rather than coronary heart disease. Oral contraceptives should preferably not be used by women in their 40s, particularly if there are other risk factors whether genetic, or from smoking, hypertension or hyperlipidaemia.

Prognosis. When prospective studies of patients with angina pectoris are sufficiently long it is recognised that the outlook is better than used to be thought. More than half live for 5 years and a third for 10 from the time of diagnosis. Spontaneous recovery, which may prove temporary, occurs in as many as a third, a fact which is useful to remember when talking to patients about their disease. Prognosis is worse in the patient who has had multiple cardiac infarcts or who has cardiac failure or who has a family history of coronary disease.

Intermediate Coronary Syndrome

Angina pectoris is the term reserved for reversible myocardial ischaemia which is generally short-lived. Myocardial infarction necessarily implies death of cardiac muscle. The terms intermediate coronary syndrome and coronary insufficiency are used to describe prolonged episodes of ischaemia without ECG evidence of infarction or enzyme evidence of myocardial necrosis and in which neither tachycardia nor hypertension appear to be responsible for the attack. Such patients are often admitted to hospital under suspicion of myocardial infarction. The fact that no evidence of infarction is found may reflect more on the inadequacies of the methods available for its diagnosis than on the disease process itself. When angina starts to develop unusually easily or to come capriciously, beta blocking drugs, rest, mild sedation and, some believe, anticoagulant therapy may reduce the risk of infarction.

Myocardial Infarction

The diagnosis of myocardial infarction was not widely made until the late 1920s, and then almost exclusively among the prosperous. More than 50 years later it is one of the commonest causes of emergency admission to hospital in affluent societies, affecting patients from all walks of life.

The illness in its mildest form may go unrecognised and only be disclosed subsequently by ECG evidence of infarction; at the other end of the spectrum there is permanent severe disability and death. At the onset of the illness sudden death, presumably from ventricular fibrillation or asystole, may occur immediately and most of the patients who die do so within the first hour before there is any possibility of being transferred to hospital. If the patient survives this most critical part of the illness, the liability to dangerous arrhythmias remains, but diminishes as each hour goes by. If the damage is sufficiently extensive the cardiac output falls and there is a wide range of consequent effects, from slight reduction in skin perfusion and blood pressure at one end to cardiogenic shock at the other. The latter, if severe and persistent, may lead to irreversible damage, e.g. from reduced perfusion in the kidneys or in other atheromatous coronary arteries causing further myocardial infarction. If the left ventricle is sufficiently damaged, upstream pressures may rise and pulmonary oedema may occur.

The *precipitating factors* leading to an episode of myocardial infarction are still imperfectly understood. In terms of blood flow the mismatch between coronary supply and myocardial demand, which is temporary and reversible in angina, may with reducing supply and/or increased demand lead to irreversible cellular damage. Myocardial infarction is particularly likely to occur in elderly patients admitted to hospital for operations of various kinds, and in many of these the coronary disease goes unrecognised until the development of the infarct.

Clinical Features. The cardinal *symptoms* are pain, breathlessness and syncope, but in addition vomiting and unaccustomed tiredness are common. The pain occurs in the same sites as for angina but is usually more severe and lasts longer. It is most often described as a tightness, heaviness or constriction in the chest. At its worst the pain is one of the most severe which can be experienced and the patient's expression and pallor may vividly convey the seriousness of the situation. Many patients are breathless and in some this is the only symptom; a few develop pulmonary oedema. Syncope may occur when the patient is upright and the blood pressure falls or from the development of a serious arrhythmia or complete heart block. Vomiting is often a feature and is commoner in the more severe cases, particularly in those with cardiogenic shock. In the first few days tiredness is a very frequent complaint. At any time after the first 12 hours or so the patient may recognise that a different pain has developed, even though it is at the same site. It is worse, or only appears, on inspiration and may be altered by a change of position. It is due to pericarditis consequent upon the infarct as is confirmed if a pericardial friction rub is heard. In rare cases the infarct may go unrecognised until endocardial thrombosis resulting from it leads to systemic embolism.

The *physical signs* may be few in a mild atack but in severe cases there is usually pallor, sweating and breathlessness. The heart rate is usually increased and with shock the pulse volume may be much reduced and the skin perfusion poor. The majority of patients admitted to hospital with a myocardial infarction have a high initial blood pressure, presumably due to the anxiety of a severe illness and the unfamiliarity of the environment. The blood pressure gradually falls over the first 3 or 4 days. In the minority who have cardiogenic shock the blood pressure is, of course, low. The jugular venous pressure is often elevated when the patient is first seen; this may be due to cardiac failure but, just as with the arterial pressure, anxiety may contribute at this stage. Examination of the heart is often relatively uninformative but the first heart sound may be quiet and a third, or more commonly a fourth heart sound, may develop. Pericardial friction is most often heard on the third or fourth day and is usually transitory. Occasionally it persists for days and exceptionally for weeks. There may be crepitations at the lung bases even after coughing as evidence of pulmonary oedema. Oliguria is common if the blood pressure is low. In many cases myocardial necrosis is associated with fever reaching a maximum on the third or fourth day and not much higher than 38°C. A leucocytosis is usually at its peak on the first day and the ESR often becomes raised. A chest X-ray may demonstrate pulmonary oedema which has been undetected clinically.

Electrocardiography. During the first few hours of the attack the infarct causes an elevation of the ST segment recorded by unipolar electrodes facing the area affected (Fig. 6.3, p. 179). When there has been anteroseptal infarction the changes are found in one or more leads from V1 to V4 (Fig. 6.23). Anterolateral infarction produces changes in leads V4 to V6, in aVL and hence also in lead I; in

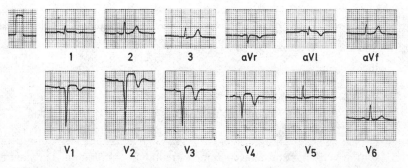

Fig. 6.23 Anteroseptal myocardial infarction. In leads V1–V4 there is ST elevation, inverted T and deep Q waves.

strictly anterior infarction the changes may be confined to leads V3 and V4. Inferior infarction is shown in lead aVF and hence in leads II and III (Fig. 6.24). Infarction of the posterior wall of the left ventricle is not recorded in standard leads by ST elevation but may be detected in V1 by ST depression.

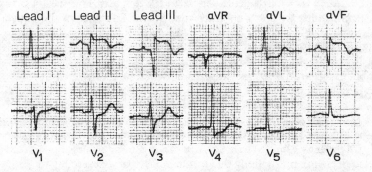

Fig. 6.24 Inferior myocardial infarction. In leads II, III and aVF there is ST elevation, inverted T and deep Q waves. In leads I, aVL and V2–V4 there is reciprocal ST depression.

The myocardial infarct, whether recent or replaced by a scar, transmits the changes of potential from within the ventricular cavity and hence produces what is sometimes called an 'electrical window'. The size of the Q and inverted T which results will depend in part on the size of this window. In established anterior infarction Q and inverted T waves are found in the anterior chest leads and in established anterolateral infarctions a prominent Q and inverted T is usually seen also in leads a VL and I (Fig. 6.25). In established inferior infarction a Q and inverted T in leads a VF, II and III are the usual pattern. With established posterior infarction Q waves are not detected in the standard leads and a tall R in VI, due to unopposed anterior depolarisation, may be the only evidence of the posterior scar (Fig. 6.26). Unipolar leads recorded from the back of the left chest may, however, also show evidence of the posterior infarction.

Often the ECG is normal in the early stages of the attack and it is a mistake to assume that this excludes myocardial infarction especially in a patient with a history strongly suggestive of the diagnosis. Although the ECG becomes abnormal in a high proportion of patients with myocardial infarction, there are a few in whom no detectable change may be found although the history, enzyme changes or other evidence may support the diagnosis.

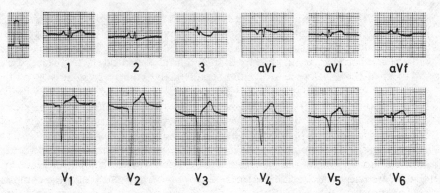

Fig. 6.25 Establish anteroseptal myocardial infarction. There is a deep Q and absent R in leads V1–V5; a Q in lead aVL indicates high lateral infarction also.

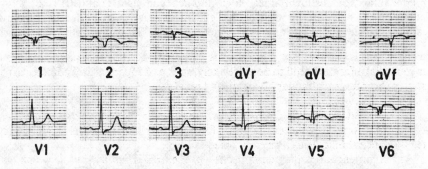

Fig. 6.26 Established posterior myocardial infarction. The depolarisation of the right ventricle is no longer opposed by the depolarisation of the back of the left ventricle ana hence there is a prominent R in the right anterior leads.

Serum Enzymes. Experimental work in dogs shows that infarction of as little as 5 per cent of the myocardium leads to a detectable rise, in the blood, of enzymes normally confined within cardiac cells and liberated as a result of myocardial necrosis. The enzymes most widely used in the detection of myocardial infarction are aspartate aminotransferase (AST), formerly known as glutamic oxaloacetic transaminase (GOT), and lactic dehydrogenase (LD). AST starts to rise about 12 hours after infarction and reaches a peak on the first or second day. LD is also liberated from haemolysed red cells and is therefore less specific. It starts to rise after 12 hours, reaches a peak after 2 or 3 days and may still be elevated for about a week; it is useful when the diagnosis is in doubt several days after a possible infarct. Serial estimations are necessary, for it is the change in enzyme levels which is of diagnostic value.

Complications. ARRHYTHMIAS. Nearly all patients with myocardial infarction have some form of arrhythmia, the minor varieties of which would be expected even in normal subjects subjected to similar monitoring.

Sinus tachycardia is the commonest and anxiety contributes to it. *Sinus bradycardia* may result in syncope; it is also a special feature of inferior myocardial infarction and may lead to ventricular escape and the development of more dangerous rhythms. *Atrial tachycardia* or *fibrillation* occur in about 15 per cent of patients; these arrhythmias may exacerbate cardiac failure or hypotension and require urgent treatment. The ventricular arrhythmias are usually even more dangerous. Patients without myocardial infarction commonly have *ventricular ectopic beats*; however, in the context of infarction if they are very frequent there is a danger of the development of more serious arrhythmias particularly when the ventricular ectopic beat coincides with a normal T wave (R on T). *Ventricular tachycardia* carries with it a high mortality. It may be difficult to distinguish electrocardiographically from the less dangerous supraventricular tachycardia with bundle branch block. *Ventricular fibrillation* appears in about 10 per cent of patients and its potential reversibility in those patients who do not have cardiogenic shock is one of the main foundations upon which the policy of acute coronary care was built. Various degrees of *atrioventricular block* are also common and of these the most sinister is the development of complete heart block in a patient with anterior myocardial infarction, for it indicates that both bundles have been involved in the infarction of the interventricular septum. Because of the extensive damage such patients usually also have cardiogenic shock.

CARDIOGENIC SHOCK (p. 193). If there is a reversible arrhythmia as an important contributory factor its correction may bring about considerable improvement. If this is not the case and shock is persistent, all the other complications of myocardial infarction tend to be more likely, such as dangerous arrhythmias, extension of the infarct, pulmonary oedema and renal failure.

OTHER COMPLICATIONS. *Cardiac failure* may occur and *pulmonary oedema* is its commonest form. Regular examination for post-tussive crepitations, oliguria or X-ray evidence should lead to its early detection.

Rarer complications include *infarction of a mitral papillary muscle* which may lead to the development of *mitral regurgitation*; occasionally this precipitates or exacerbates pulmonary oedema. *Rupture of the interventricular septum* is diagnosed by the development of the characteristic murmur of a ventricular septal defect (p. 225) and may be followed by severe hypotension and venous hypertension. *Rupture of the myocardium* may lead to cardiac tamponade (p. 230) and, if detected early, has very occasionally proved amenable to repair under cardiac bypass. *Venous thrombosis* is less common than in the days when patients with myocardial infarction were kept in bed for about 6 weeks. Venous thrombosis often first announces its presence by *pulmonary embolism*, and even a careful watch on the legs for evidence of the primary lesion will reveal only about half of them. When a thrombus forms on the endocardium of the left ventricle *systemic embolism* can occur and occlude an artery.

The *postmyocardial infarction syndrome* is due to an autoimmune reaction to necrotic myocardium and is characterised by persistent fever, pericarditis and pleurisy. If occurs a few weeks or even months after the infarct. It responds to prednisolone but may recur.

Treatment. The main needs are for the relief of pain, the prevention and treatment of arrhythmias and other complications, and the rehabilitation of the patient.

In the acute stage when the risk of dangerous or fatal arrhythmia is highest, it is desirable for most patients to be admitted, if possible, to a coronary care unit where the personnel have had special training and where monitoring and antiarrhythmic facilities are available. As prophylaxis against arrhythmia improves it may become possible to treat a higher proportion of patients at home if adequate nursing and medical supervision are available. The elderly are usually most appropriately cared for there when circumstances permit.

The patient with a severe attack is in pain and is frightened. The most effective remedies are morphine (10–20 mg s.c. or i.v.) or diamorphine (5–10 mg s.c. or i.v.) supplemented by cyclizine (50 mg i.m.) to reduce the likelihood of vomiting. The anxiety must be recognised even if it is not overt; it is essential to reassure the patient that complete recovery is the most likely outcome and that initially it is best to be where complications can most readily be treated should these arise.

During the acute phase of the illness, if there are multiple ectopic beats or particularly if there are the potentially dangerous 'R on T' extrasystoles or a ventricular tachycardia the drug of choice is lignocaine (p. 192). If lignocaine proves to be ineffective alternatives are procainamide (p. 192) or practolol (5 mg i.v. given slowly to a maximum of 25 mg) or mexiletine (p. 192). If ventricular fibrillation develops, DC shock should be used immediately without cardiac massage or artificial ventilation. Failing this the cardiac resuscitation procedure (p. 187) should be used until the defibrillator is available. Asystole is generally not amenable to treatment, but in some cases success has been achieved when resuscitation is followed by transvenous insertion of a pacemaker. Patients in shock prior to the development of asystole are very unlikely to prove amenable to resuscitation. Atrial tachycardia, flutter or fibrillation are best treated with digoxin if the ventricular rate is high. Sinus bradycardia usually does not require treatment, but if there is hypotension or ventricular escape, atropine (p. 192) should be used. In advanced heart block it is sometimes necessary to introduce a pacing catheter into the right ventricle in order to maintain a satisfactory rhythm.

Cardiogenic shock (p. 193) and cardiac failure (p. 196) are treated along the usual lines; digoxin may be prescribed unless precluded by the cardiac rhythm. Oxygen is indicated in pulmonary oedema or shock.

Anticoagulants are indicated in the treatment of venous thrombosis and pulmonary embolism (p. 245) and may be used prophylactically if the patient is at risk because of the need for prolonged immobilisation. In the latter event warfarin is given initially in a dose of 20 mg and subsequently as required to maintain the patient's prothrombin time at 2·5 times the control value. There is no convincing evidence that anticoagulants are of value in the prevention of further coronary or endocardial thrombosis.

There is pathological evidence that an infarct takes 4–6 weeks to undergo repair; it is then replaced by fibrous tissue. Accordingly it is generally thought reasonable to restrict physical activities during this period. When there are no complications the patient with a minor attack can sit in a chair within a few days, be ambulant within a week, return home in 10 days and gradually increase activity with the prospect of return to work after 6 weeks. When there are complications the regime has to be adjusted accordingly; a few patients are permanently disabled by heart failure or severe angina. The process of reassurance is essential at every stage for many patients are now recognised to be severely or even permanently incapacitated as a result of psychological rather than physical effects of a myocardial infarction. The success of restoring a patient to normal life depends very much on the attitudes of the physician. With appropriate guidance patients can be in better health after a myocardial infarction, their smoking discontinued, their obesity corrected and their life more physically active. The naturally vigorous may require restraint in the early stages but more often the anxious will need reassurance and encouragement. The spouse has often to learn to stop reminding the patient of former disability. Such efforts, however well intended, often perpetuate anxiety and restrict rehabilitation.

Ventricular aneurysm, mitral regurgitation due to papillary muscle damage and rupture of the interventricular septum are all amenable to surgical repair but preferably not earlier than 6 weeks after the infarct.

Propranolol on a long-term basis may reduce the likelihood of sudden death or recurrence of myocardial infarction over the months or years after an attack.

Prognosis. In about a quarter of all cases of myocardial infarction death occurs within the first few minutes without medical care. The mortality falls exponentially over the next few days; of those who die 60 per cent do so in the first 2 days. About 40 per cent of all affected patients die within the first month. Unfavourable features are old age, cardiogenic shock, cardiac failure, heart block and ventricular arrhythmias. Bundle branch block and high enzyme readings both indicate extensive damage. In the absence of unfavourable features the outlook is as good for those who survive ventricular fibrillation as for the others. Of those who survive an acute attack more than 80 per cent live for a further year, about 75 per cent 5 years, 50 per cent 10 years and 25 per cent 20 years. It is therefore appropriate to be reassuring to patients about their prospects. Most should be able to return to work in 2 or 3 months. Late dangerous complications include recurrence of myocardial infarction, cardiac aneurysm, cardiac rupture and pulmonary embolism.

Systemic Arterial Hypertension

The maintenance of normal blood pressure even in health is now recognised to be a process of somewhat daunting complexity. The mean arterial pressure depends principally upon the cardiac output and the arteriolar tone. The blood pressure is constantly monitored by baroreceptors and a complicated autoregulation system immediately makes adjustments to maintain blood pressure despite changes in posture, a sudden fall in venous return—as with the Valsalva manoeuvre—or to counteract the effects of exercise, heat, changes in the salt and water intake, fluid loss and other variables.

In Western civilisation the normal blood pressure gradually rises with age. Hypertension is defined arbitrarily at levels above generally accepted normals, for example, 140/90 at the age of 20 rising gradually to 170/105 at the age of 75. Hypertension is present in about 15 per cent of the population. The disorder is symptomless until complications arise so that diagnosis depends on whether there is special screening as when patients attend their doctors for other reasons. It must be emphasised that to wait for symptoms attributable to hypertension is a very inefficient method of case finding. The blood pressure depends also on the circumstances of the measurement and is higher in anxious subjects. It is insufficiently appreciated that normal individuals may develop very high blood pressure levels under stress; continuous arterial pressures recorded by miniaturised portable equipment on tape have shown blood pressures of 230/130 in 20-year-olds in oral examinations; very high levels also occur at orgasm or from straining at stool. Conversely during sleep the blood pressures may fall to less than 90/50. Many patients find medical examination very stressful. Senior physicians record significantly higher blood pressure levels than appropriately trained nurses, who to the patient appear less formidable.

Vasomotor tone is dependent on sympathetic nervous, metabolic and hormonal factors. Vasoconstriction may result from increased sympathetic activity, adrenal catecholamines and angiotensin II. Vasodilation can be produced by the kallikrein-kinin system and the prostaglandins. The most powerful vasoconstrictor is angiotensin

II, acting directly by causing contraction of arterioles, but also indirectly via the central nervous system and by increasing catecholamine release from sympathetic nerves. It also has a positive inotropic effect and leads to retention of sodium and water by the kidneys. Increased levels of renin and angiotensin II are a feature of severe essential—i.e. unexplained—hypertension, in the malignant and accelerated phases and in renovascular hypertension.

An excess of circulating aldosterone from an adrenal adenoma or from adrenocortical hyperplasia may cause hypertension. This is to be suspected from low serum potassium levels and is associated with low plasma renin activity (PRA) levels.

In about 80 to 90 per cent of patients with hypertension even the use of refined diagnostic methods will not establish a cause, and this is known as *essential hypertension*. This type of hypertension is a graded characteristic with a continuous unimodal frequency distribution with a multifactorial inheritance (p. 19); in 70 per cent of patients another member of the family is affected. Essential hypertension is especially frequent in some races, particularly American Negroes and Japanese. It is commoner where salt intake is excessive.

Systolic hypertension is a feature of the non-compliant arteries of old age. Though diastolic hypertension is usually regarded as of more sinister prognosis, it is now established that systolic hypertension found at routine examination—so-called *casual hypertension*—is of comparable prognostic importance in middle age.

Secondary hypertension. In approximately 10–20 per cent of cases of hypertension a cause can be found but only by an alert and rational approach. Its discovery is important because cure is often possible; the search is most likely to be rewarded in children and young adults.

The main causes of secondary hypertension are:

1. Coarctation of the aorta.
2. Renal disease: (a) Parenchymatous e.g. acute and chronic glomerulonephritis; pyelonephritis; systemic lupus erythematosus and polyarteritis nodosa. (b) Polycystic kidneys. (c) Renal artery stenosis.
3. Endocrine disorders and hormone therapy: (a) Phaeochromocytoma. (b) Cushing's syndrome. (c) Primary aldosteronism (Conn's syndrome). (d) Oral contraception. (e) Oestrogen therapy.
4. Pregnancy.

In hypertensive children and young adults coarctation of the aorta should be particularly suspected; it is usually easy to detect from a weak femoral pulse delayed after the radial pulse. Renal parenchymal disease, identifiable usually by urine examination, is another important cause of hypertension in this age group. Renal arterial disease and phaeochromocytomas may also be found. In the younger middle-aged subjects renal arterial and renal parenchymal disease and hypertension resulting from the use of oral contraceptives should all be considered, but phaeochromocytoma and primary aldosteronism also occur. By late middle age essential hypertension accounts for the great majority of cases but renal artery stenosis and primary aldosteronism are also found. Over the age of 50 renal artery stenosis from atheroma, and oestrogen therapy, have also to be considered as possible causes.

Clinical Features. Hypertension is frequently discovered on routine examination of apparently healthy subjects. Symptoms are generally attributable to the complications of the disease, whether from a cerebrovascular accident, from haemorrhages in the retina or visual pathways or from left ventricular failure.

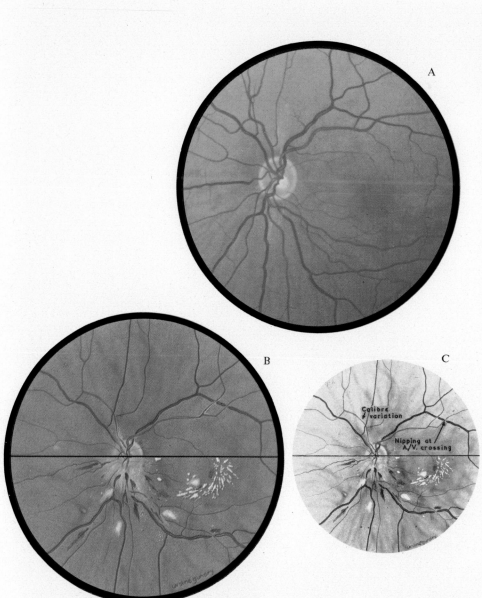

PLATE I

A, Normal retinal vessels. B, Hypertensive retinopathy. The upper half of this painting shows
the retinal blood vessels in hypertension of moderate severity. The arteriolar blood column
is narrower than normal and a central white streak ('reflex') is visible or is more prominent
than normal. Irregularity of breadth of the arteriolar blood column indicates an irregular
lumen. Veins at arterial-venous crossings are narrowed ('nipping'), partly because of pressure
by arterioles and also because opacity of the arterial wall obscures the venous blood column.
The lower half of the painting shows severe hypertensive retinopathy. Haemorrhages and
'soft' exudates are added to the abnormalities seen in the upper half and these are also more
marked. C, Key to B.

(*By permission of Professor C. I. Phillips, Department of Ophthalmology, University of Edinburgh*)

Coexisting arterial disease, causing for example angina or intermittent claudication, is also commoner than in those with normal blood pressure. Minor symptoms such as headache, dizziness, irritability, fatigue and insomnia are widespread in the population and tend to be inappropriately attributed to the hypertension when it is found. Such symptoms are commoner in patients who know that they have hypertension. The occasional patient with malignant hypertension has severe headache which is relieved by adequate treatment. Polyuria and nocturia may be due to renal failure.

Physical signs also tend to be few. Long-standing hypertension leads to left ventricular hypertrophy and may be indicated by a forceful cardiac apex displaced to the left. The hypertrophied ventricle is less compliant than a normal ventricle so that left atrial hypertrophy follows and may be inferred from a palpable and/or audible fourth heart sound. The aortic second sound is often increased. There may be an ejection sound. In the elderly with severe hypertension there may be an aortic diastolic murmur due to dilation of the aortic ring. There may be evidence of left ventricular failure from basal crepitations. However, the symptom of sudden breathlessness awakening the patient from sleep is a more reliable indication of left ventricular failure.

In the child or young adult an arterial pulsation in the neck should arouse the suspicion of coarctation of the aorta and emphasise the need to look for the other physical signs of it. In renal artery stenosis a systolic bruit may be heard in the abdomen or lumbar region over the kidney. It should be sought in young patients with severe hypertension in whom it may be due to remediable fibromuscular dysplasia of a renal artery. In older persons coexisting atheromatous disease in other arteries may be suggested by absent peripheral pulses, by a systolic bruit over a major vessel or by a 'kinked carotid' (p. 174). In polycystic disease the large kidneys are often palpable. Protein and casts in the urine are to be expected in renal parenchymal disease and in the malignant phase of essential hypertension.

Examination of the ocular fundus is crucial. In the early stages of hypertension some decrease in tortuosity and variation in calibre of the retinal arterioles becomes apparent, and at the arteriovenous crossings the thickened arteriolar wall is liable to compress the vein so that the vein appears empty at each side of it ('nipping'). Haemorrhages may occur, the most common being flame-shaped; these fade within a few weeks. Soft ('cotton wool') exudates are areas of retinal infarction resulting from occlusion of small arterioles. (Plate 1A). These indicate the onset of the malignant or accelerated phase. They also fade and leave no trace in a few weeks. Hard exudates are small, dense, whitish deposits containing lipid which may remain unaltered for months or years. Papilloedema indicates the most advanced stage of malignant hypertension and the coexistence of fibrinoid arteriolar necrosis. Early death from renal failure is likely unless prompt action is taken to maintain a lower arterial pressure.

Investigations. Evidence of left ventricular and left atrial hypertrophy may be obtained from the electrocardiogram (Fig. 6.27) and help to indicate that the hypertension is not just a temporary feature. The chest X-ray may also show left ventricular enlargement but less reliably than the physical examination and the electrocardiogram. With coarctation of the aorta there may be characteristic 'notching' of the ribs. The plasma urea or creatinine are required as a measure of renal excretory function. Estimation of plasma electrolytes is essential as hypokalaemia is an indicator of primary or secondary aldosteronism if it is not due to diuretic therapy. Measurement of plasma urate is advisable because gout is liable to

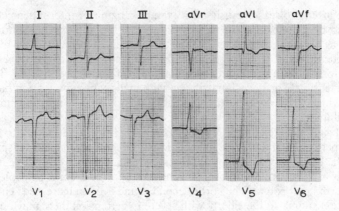

Fig. 6.27 Left ventricular hypertrophy. Note: (1) tall R waves over left ventricle (V5–6); (2) deep S waves over right ventricle (V1–2); (3) ST depression and asymmetrical inversion of T wave in leads I, aVL and V4–V6.

be produced by diuretic therapy; examination of the urine for sugar is important because hypertension and its complications are commoner in diabetics. An elevated serum cholesterol is indirectly associated with atheroma.

Radioisotope studies or excretion urography is indicated in younger patients to detect potentially remediable unilateral lesions resulting from reduced blood flow. An excretion urogram is the less reliable method but may show a delay in appearance and/or increased concentration of dye on the affected side.

Further investigation is also required for patients with manifestations suggestive of a phaeochromocytoma (p. 550) or primary aldosteronism (p. 539). In older patients routine investigation so rarely leads to radical cure that it has been proved to be uneconomical unless there is some clinical indication or unusual difficulty in treatment.

Complications. CARDIAC. The left ventricle at first maintains a normal blood flow by hypertrophy. Later the left ventricular output can no longer be maintained and cardiac failure may become manifest. Breathlessness on exercise may occur and paroxysmal nocturnal dyspnoea may be the presenting symptom in hitherto unsuspected hypertension. A fourth heart sound, and pulsus alternans, are serious signs. Atrial fibrillation sometimes occurs. Coronary artery disease is more frequent in patients with hypertension.

CEREBRAL. Cerebral ischaemia (p. 700) and cerebral haemorrhage (p. 704) are common complications. Visual disturbances occur if the optic pathways are involved in vascular lesions (Fig. 14.4, p. 671).

Hypertensive encephalopathy is an infrequent condition due to acute focal cerebral ischaemia to which cerebrovascular spasm, oedema or minor degrees of cerebral thrombosis contribute. Transient disturbances of vision or speech, paresis, paraesthesiae, disorientation, fits or loss of consciousness may occur. The blood pressure is usually very high in encephalopathy; complete recovery can be expected if it is rapidly and effectively lowered.

RENAL. The term *malignant hypertension* should be reserved for the syndrome of severe diastolic hypertension, papilloedema, retinal exudates and haemorrhages and renal failure; its importance lies in the renal arteriolar necrosis which accompanies it. Malignant hypertension occurs mainly in males in the third and fourth decades and pursues a rapidly downhill course to death from uraemia within a year unless appropriate treatment is established and maintained. Most cases of malignant hypertension before the age of 30 are caused by renal parenchymal disease. When papilloedema and renal failure suddenly develop in a person known to have essential hypertension this is described as '*accelerated hypertension*'. Papilloedema may be present temporarily during an attack of hypertensive encephalopathy or may occur in cases of transient hypertension such as with acute nephritis or pregnancy.

The Treatment of Hypertension. ESSENTIAL HYPERTENSION. When significant hypertension is discovered and found to be persistently present, it should be explained to the patient that unless the blood pressure is modified to more normal levels he is at risk of developing one of the complications of hypertension. He has to realise that once drug treatment is embarked upon it will need to be continued for life—at least in the present state of knowledge. The establishment of a good relationship between the doctor and the patient is very important. The previously asymptomatic patient who develops side-effects of treatment needs particular help: appropriate readjustment of the dose or a change of drug may restore his confidence. As with the diabetic the treatment has to be reviewed regularly; whether the supervision should be by a general practitioner, or by hospital doctors with a special interest in hypertension, depends on many factors and should be decided for the individual patient so that responsibilities are recognised.

The discovery of hypertension and the planning of management provides an opportunity to search for other factors which may add to the cardiovascular risks. Among these are heavy cigarette smoking and obesity. If the patient can stop smoking, reduce weight, and, except in severe hypertension, increase physical exercise his well-being is likely to be greater. Those who pour salt over their food in large quantities should be advised against this practice. A low salt diet, i.e. a diet containing less than $1 \cdot 0$ g per day, reduces blood pressure but it is too irksome to be of practical use. With effective drug treatment the special risks of surges of hypertension should be significantly reduced. It is customary to advise patients to 'avoid stress', but this is usually a pious hope. Spouses should be dissuaded from perpetually reminding patients of their hypertension which, with adequate treatment, may well be non-existent.

More rest may be appropriate for the patient whose life is unreasonably hectic. Rest in bed is required, and then temporarily, only for the patient with severe malignant hypertension or with heart failure or when a serious complication, such as a cerebrovascular accident, occurs.

Antihypertensive Drug Therapy. The present is a time of transition, partly as a result of knowledge of the roles of renin and angiotensin, which is still incomplete, partly as a result of new antihypertensive agents becoming available and partly because of disagreement as to whether mild hypertension (e.g. 150/95 at the age of 30) requires treatment. There is no doubt that in greater degrees of hypertension the outlook for hypertensive patients has been transformed, particularly in the reduction in the incidence of stroke, by the advent of effective antihypertensive therapy. *Pari passu* there has been a steady reduction in unwelcome side effects of treatment.

It is now known that some drugs, for example propranolol, clonidine, methyldopa and adrenergic blocking drugs have antirenin activity. This makes them particularly valuable in the treatment of hypertension with high PRA levels, such as in malignant or renovascular hypertension. In patients with essential hypertension and normal PRA levels, diuretics are commonly used; the rise in PRA levels caused by these can be opposed by a simultaneous use of a β-adrenergic blocking drug such as propranolol.

Many agents are now available but there is a growing consensus as to policy. The most logical plan is to use the smallest possible number of drugs and in the smallest possible quantities to achieve effective blood pressure control, which is usually accepted as a lying diastolic pressure of 90 or less at rest. By combining drugs when necessary it is possible to avoid the undesirable side-effects which may result from an excess of any one of them. The drug regime has to be tailored to the individual, for there is considerable variation in the side-effects with any one drug from one patient to another. The physician should not be content until the patient's blood pressure is under good control with minimal or absent side effects. Elderly patients often tolerate hypertension better than ill-judged treatment for it.

Oral diuretics, combined with moderate salt restriction, are effective in lowering blood pressure, initially by reducing blood volume, and over a longer period by reducing peripheral arteriolar resistance, probably in part by removing salt from the arterial media. They are particularly useful for minor degress of hypertension, and more specifically when total body sodium and water are increased, as with aldosteronism and renal parenchymal disease. Many have the disadvantage of causing excessive potassium loss. A cheap, long-acting thiazide diuretic together with potassium supplements, or triamterine, which conserves potassium, are both appropriate. Rapidly acting diuretics such as frusemide are less useful, unless there is accompanying cardiac or renal failure. Diuretics are also a useful adjunct to other forms of treatment.

Of the sympatholytic drugs, the *beta adrenergic receptor blocking drugs* are now the most widely used. Propranolol is effective and its reliability and relative freedom from side-effects appears to be established. The many new beta blockers include some whose use has been too brief to ensure that they are free from serious side-effects; the occasional dangers of practolol, which now preclude its oral use, took 8 years to be revealed. Propranolol is particularly valuable for its antirenin property and for the patient with labile hypertension with easily provoked anxiety, palpitation and tachycardia, or for coexisting angina pectoris. The dose has to be adjusted to the individuals needs because a large but variable proportion of the drug is destroyed in its first passage through the liver; even with equivalent blood concentration there is also a great variation in response. Often twice daily dosage will suffice, but in others high doses may be required, so that treatment initiated in a dose of 40 mg b.d. may have to be increased to as much as 160 mg q.i.d. or even more in some patients if adequate blood pressure control is to be achieved. Many patients have no side-effects, but minor gastric disturbance, undue bradycardia, persistent tiredness, bad dreams, hallucinations, cold hands, cardiac failure and bronchospasm are all recognised complications. The combination of propranolol and a diuretic usually with a potassium supplement achieves the therapeutic goal without significant side-effects in a high proportion of patients with essential hypertension. Some physicians prefer to use oxprenolol or other beta blockers.

If this proves not to be the case *other sympatholytic agents* may be effective. Clonidine, tarting with 0·1 mg t.i.d. and rising to 1 mg in total per day, has a predominantly central action. Methyldopa, starting with 250 mg t.i.d. and rising to 3 g in total per day, has both a central and peripheral action. Both may cause excessive sedation. Methyldopa may produce a haemolytic anaemia which is reversible when the drug is stopped.

The *adrenergic blocking drugs* are useful in severe hypertension but have the considerable disadvantage of causing hypotension on rising from bed and on exercise and are therefore particularly unsuitable for the elderly. Debrisoquine, starting with 10 mg t.i.d., is increased by 10 mg increments until the standing blood pressure is controlled. Bethanidine is an alternative drug which is used similarly. The adrenergic blocking drugs may cause nasal stuffiness, diarrhoea and impotence.

In severe malignant or accelerated hypertension the patient at the time of admission may have a blood pressure of the order of 300/160. This requires urgent intravenous therapy to bring it under control. For this purpose some prefer to use *diazoxide* (300–600 mg i.v. as a bolus injection) and others use *reserpine* (1–5 mg intramuscularly). Both are very effective but need to be followed by adequate oral therapy. Similar treatment is indicated in hypertensive encephalopathy.

SECONDARY HYPERTENSION. In a very small proportion of younger patients an operation to relieve stenosis of a renal artery or the removal of an ischaemic kidney may be dramatically successful in reducing blood pressure. Primary aldosteronism (p. 539) is the cause of hypertension in about 1 per cent of cases. Phaeochromocytoma (p. 550) is also a rare cause (about 1 in 200 cases). The treatment of these conditions and of other primary causes of hypertension, for example coarctation of the aorta (p. 233), is described in the appropriate section. Oral contraceptives and oestrogen therapy should be discontinued in the presence of hypertension.

Prognosis. Insurance statistics show that, in general, expectation of life is considerably reduced in those who have high blood pressure compared with those in whom the pressure is within the normal range. However, it does not follow that all who have high blood pressure necessarily have a bad prognosis. The condition is mild if the heart is not enlarged, the fundi show no abnormalities and there is no proteinuria or evidence of impaired renal function. Many such patients live a life of normal span free from related illness. Individuals with high casual readings and normal ones after a period of rest used to be regarded as having a benign condition. However, more recent evidence from prospective studies indicates that it is from such patients that an older population with serious hypertension is disproportionately drawn. On the whole, women appear to withstand hypertension better than men. Many elderly women in whom pressures are persistently of the order of 220/110 but who have no abnormalities in the optic fundi or the heart remain in good health for many years. Young men, in particular, who when first seen have high diastolic pressures together with secondary manifestations in the fundi or heart require optimal control of the blood pressure without delay. Patients with untreated malignant hypertension rarely live for more than a year. When properly administered modern treatment is effective in relieving headache, preventing or postponing complications and in prolonging life.

Treatment of hypertension continues to be difficult and necessitates much attention to detail and considerable patience on the part of both patient and doctor. Until the cause of essential hypertension is found it is too much to hope that any single drug used in its management can be entirely satisfactory; those presently available produce in some patients tolerance, undesirable side-effects or occasional unpredictable hypotension. In addition it must be remembered that once begun, treatment will almost certainly have to be continued for life. It is therefore evident that most careful consideration should be give to the issues discussed above before making the decision to administer antihypertensive drugs.

Pulmonary Arterial Hypertension

Pulmonary hypertension results from an increase in pulmonary capillary pressure, pulmonary blood flow or pulmonary vascular resistance.

Increased pulmonary capillary pressure occurs with left ventricular failure and with mitral valve disease. Pulmonary blood flow is increased with left to right shunts as in atrial and ventricular septal defects and in persistent ductus arteriosus; the hypertension is then mainly systolic. In both these groups the pulmonary hypertension is potentially reversible if the cause can be successfully treated. In some cases increased pulmonary vascular resistance may develop and be irreversible; it can also be irreversible when it results from repetitive pulmonary thromboembolism or when it arises from an unknown cause, i.e. primary pulmonary hypertension. Hypoxaemia and hypercapnia cause a reflex increase in pulmonary arterial resistance and this is one of the factors which, in the presence of respiratory failure, leads to right ventricular failure (chronic cor pulmonale).

Primary pulmonary hypertension is a rare disease of unknown aetiology which mainly affects young women. There may be a family history of the disease. Symptoms include syncope on exertion, breathlessness and sometimes angina pectoris.

There may be a left parasternal impulse either from right ventricular hypertrophy, or from an enlarged pulmonary artery, or both. If there is accompanying right atrial hypertrophy a large 'a' wave is to be expected in the jugular venous pulse. There may be an ejection sound and a loud second sound over the pulmonary valve. The ECG usually shows evidence of right atrial and right ventricular hypertrophy; in extreme pulmonary hypertension there may be tall R waves in VI and also depression of the ST segment. The radiograph may show enlargement of the pulmonary artery and its main branches.

There is no treatment and death usually occurs within a few years of diagnosis.

Pulmonary Embolism and Infarction

Pulmonary embolism occurs when a portion of thrombus in a systemic vein, or, less commonly, in the right side of the heart is discharged into the circulation. It may lodge in the pulmonary trunk and cause sudden death, or in a smaller pulmonary artery and result in pulmonary infarction. Pulmonary embolism is the commonest cause of acute respiratory illness in hospital patients in the Western world.

Aetiology. Thrombosis in the deep veins of the legs (p. 244) is the most frequent source of pulmonary embolism. As this is usually the result of stasis, embolism most often affects people who have been confined to bed. It is particularly liable to occur within ten days after a surgical operation or after childbirth. The presence of phlebothrombosis is frequently not recognised until after the embolism.

In less than 10 per cent of cases, thrombi responsible for pulmonary embolism form in the right atrium in patients with atrial fibrillation, especially if cardiac failure is present.

Clinical Features. PULMONARY EMBOLISM. With massive pulmonary embolism the patient may suddenly be seized with a sensation of great oppression in the chest and intense dyspnoea followed by cyanosis and shock. Death may occur within a few minutes, an hour or two or a day or two. Recovery is usual if the patient survives the first few hours, but there is at least a 25 per cent risk of recurrence. Pain indistinguishable from that of myocardial infarction may occur due to a combination of decreased coronary blood flow and hypoxaemia. The blood pressure falls, the jugular venous pressure rises and cardiac failure may follow in severe cases. The pulmonary second sound may be accentuated and either a third or a fourth heart sound may develop. These signs are due to a combination of right ventricular failure and a low cardiac output.

In cases of lesser severity symptoms and signs may be absent or there may be transient dyspnoea, tachycardia or syncope. Recurrent embolism may result in pulmonary hypertension which may be followed by right ventricular failure.

PULMONARY INFARCTION. The onset is sudden with either pleuritic pain or haemoptysis as the initial symptom. These two symptoms are not always present and the absence of one or even both of them does not necessarily exclude pulmonary infarction. The pain is often severe and the haemoptysis may be repeated. Other clinical features include tachycardia, dyspnoea and cyanosis. Pyrexia is usually present; in the early stages it is probably due to absorption of blood from the infarct, but later it may be due to secondary infection. A polymorphonuclear leucocytosis may be present, even in the absence of infection.

Radiological Examination. In *massive pulmonary embolism* the lung fields often appear normal but sometimes there is a hilar opacity from the blocked vessel and ischaemia distal to the embolus causes a reduction in the normal vascular markings of a lung or lobe. Pulmonary angiography is the most reliable method of diagnosing massive pulmonary embolism and should be carried out prior to urgent treatment such as embolectomy or thrombolytic therapy.

In *pulmonary infarction* there may be a pulmonary opacity or a linear scar representing the infarct. A small pleural effusion is common. The ipsilateral hemidiaphragm may be elevated. These radiological abnormalities are usually most marked at the base of one lung but are often bilateral.

Venous thrombosis is demonstrated by bilateral ascending or femoral phlebography (p. 245).

RADIO-ISOTOPE STUDIES. The intravenous injection of isotope-labelled macro-aggregated albumin can be used to delineate underperfused areas of lung not detected on a plain radiograph. This technique is of considerable value in the diagnosis of pulmonary embolism especially if combined with ventilation scanning following the inhalation of an isotope-labelled gas.

Electrocardiography. In cases of massive embolism the ECG may show a diagnostic pattern, namely right axis deviation and inversion of T waves in the right ventricular leads, abnormal displacement of the interventricular septum to the left, or the pattern of incomplete right bundle branch block. The ECG is usually normal in cases of lesser severity.

Differential Diagnosis. Massive pulmonary embolism is distinguished from myocardial infarction by the characteristic ECG and enzyme changes in the latter. Pulmonary infarction is distinguished from dry pleurisy of infective origin by the character of the sputum and the response to antibiotics.

Course and Prognosis. Massive pulmonary embolism is frequently fatal. Minor- and medium-sized emboli are much less dangerous unless they are followed by further embolisation which may itself be fatal. In retrospect it is often apparent that small 'herald' emboli have, in fact, been missed or misinterpreted. Recurrent emboli may cause chronic pulmonary hypertension and right ventricular failure. The vast majority of pulmonary infarcts resolve completely. Occasionally an infarct may become secondarily infected and result in lung abscess or empyema.

Treatment and Prevention. Heparin (10,000–15,000 units i.v.) should be administered immediately and, after a full course (p. 245), oral anticoagulants should be given in order to prevent further venous thrombosis in the legs. Thrombolytic drugs such as urokinase accelerate recovery from pulmonary embolism and are under trial; they are very expensive. Pain and apprehension should be allayed but morphine must be avoided if there is severe hypotension. Oxygen should be administered if central cyanosis is present.

Management of massive pulmonary embolism is best conducted in an area where intensive care can be provided. Occasionally a large embolus may be successfully removed from the main pulmonary artery. The chances of survival are greatest if embolectomy is carried out with the aid of cardiopulmonary bypass (p. 237). In cases of recurrent pulmonary embolism, despite anticoagulation, venous interruption may be necessary either by inserting a filter into or plicating the inferior vena cava.

An appreciation of the potential dangers of bed rest is the principal factor in the prevention of pulmonary embolism and infarction. Patients with a history of venous thrombosis and pulmonary embolism are at special risk at operation. The risk can be reduced by the use of low dose heparin, 5,000 units subcutaneously 8 hours before surgery, and 8 hourly for a few days after the operation. Alternatively 500 ml dextran 70 started preoperatively and continued 8 hourly afterwards is also effective in lowering blood viscosity and reducing platelet adhesiveness.

Diseases of the Myocardium

The myocardium is involved in most types of heart disease, but the terms myocarditis and cardiomyopathy are usually applied to those relatively uncommon forms of myocardial disease which are not the result of rheumatic fever, coronary artery disease or hypertension.

Acute Myocarditis

Aetiology. Acute myocarditis usually occurs as a complication of infections, the majority being due to the toxic effects of diphtheria, pneumonia, typhoid fever, scrub typhus fever and meningitis; it also occurs in protozoal infections such as Chagas' disease (American trypanosomiasis, p. 852) and may follow virus diseases such as influenza, poliomyelitis, infectious mononucleosis and, particularly, Coxsackie-B infections. Rheumatic myocarditis is described on page 198.

Clinical Features. Often the only evidence of myocarditis is a sinus tachycardia which is out of proportion to the severity of the infection. In more severe cases there may be a third heart sound, arrhythmias, conduction defects or acute circulatory failure.

Prognosis in most types of acute myocarditis is usually good, but it may cause death in diphtheria. In Chagas' disease, the patient usually recovers from the acute phase and after a latent period of 10 or 20 years, a chronic cardiomyopathy develops which is eventually fatal.

Treatment. There is no specific therapy for acute myocarditis; the usual forms of treatment for cardiac failure and arrhythmias should be undertaken. Prolonged rest is sometimes necessary.

Chronic Cardiomyopathies

Aetiology. In a considerable number of cases, the myocardial disease is part of a generalised disorder and the cardiac involvement may be of major or minor degree. Such disorders include haemochromatosis, sarcoidosis, amyloidosis, the muscular dystrophies, and connective tissue disorders such as systemic lupus erythematosus, scleroderma and polyarteritis. Cardiomyopathy may be associated with alcoholism and rarely with the late stages of pregnancy and the puerperium.

In the remainder there is no generalised disorder and frequently no aetiological agent can be found, although in a proportion of such cases there is a family history.

Clinical Features. The cardiomyopathies most often present in one or other of two clinical patterns: (1) The most common is '*Congestive*' with cardiomegaly and valvular regurgitation, and progressive left- and, later, right-sided cardiac failure. (2) '*Hypertrophic*' is frequently associated with such severe thickening of the interventricular septum that obstruction to outflow from the left ventricle occurs. This produces a clinical picture simulating aortic stenosis (hypertrophic obstructive cardiomyopathy). There is usually no identifiable cause although a family history is quite common.

Two rarer types of presentation are (3) a '*Restrictive*' type simulating constrictive pericarditis and (4) an '*Obliterative*' type as in endomyocardial fibrosis which is a disorder confined to humid areas of the tropics (p. 815). Fibrotic tissue and thrombus obliterate the cavities of the left and right ventricles and may lead to mitral and tricuspid regurgitation. The cause of this disorder is unknown but nutritional or infective factors may contribute.

Arrhythmias occur in all types and are a common cause of death.

Diagnosis. Cardiomyopathy should be considered whenever there is unexplained cardiomegaly or cardiac failure. The diagnosis is usually made only when the major causes of heart disease—rheumatic, hypertensive, ischaemic, thyrotoxic or congenital—have been excluded or when there is a generalised disorder of a type known to involve the heart.

Treatment. Treatment remains unsatisfactory for the majority of cases for which the cause is not known, cannot be removed or for which no specific treatment is available. A well-balanced diet is indicated in those cases in which a nutritional deficiency may be of aetiological importance and the avoidance of alcohol is essential if alcoholism is thought to be a provoking factor. Corticosteroid therapy is sometimes of value for the treatment of cardiomyopathy due to sarcoidosis or associated with connective tissue disorders.

Cardiac failure must be treated and prolonged rest is necessary in resistant cases. Beta receptor blockade or surgical resection of the hypertrophied septum is sometimes beneficial in the hypertrophic obstructive type.

Diseases of the Pericardium

Pericarditis

There are numerous causes of acute pericarditis, the commonest being myocardial infarction and Coxsackie B viral infection. Rheumatic fever and tuberculosis are also important causes but both are now rare in Britain. Pericarditis may occur as a complication of bacterial infection and of malignant disease. Other causes include uraemia, trauma and connective tissue disorders such as systemic lupus erythematosus.

Pathology. Pericarditis may be fibrinous, serous, haemorrhagic or purulent. In fibrinous pericarditis there is a fibrinous exudate on the surface which leads to varying degrees of adhesion formation and hence to obliteration of the pericardial cavity. In serous pericarditis there is in addition a serous exudate of anything from a few ml to 2 litres. The effusion is straw-coloured and often slightly turbid with a high protein content. A haemorrhagic effusion suggests a malignant origin. Purulent pericarditis is due to a pyogenic infection and the effusion is rarely large.

Clinical Features. Symptoms and signs of the underlying causative disease will often be present. The clinical features will otherwise largely depend on whether or not pericardial friction or effusion is present.

Precordial pain, which is not invariably present, may be sharp or aching in character. It may be made worse by movement, inspiration and lying flat. It is often severe in pericarditis of viral origin but is relatively uncommon in other cases, e.g. in pericarditis secondary to uraemia, myocardial infarction or malignant disease. A sensation of precordial oppression may be produced by a large pericardial effusion.

Pericardial friction is the characteristic and diagnostic sign of pericarditis. It consists of a superficial scraping, scratching sound, usually best heard to the left of the lower sternum, often localised to a small area of the precordium. It is usually loudest in systole but is often well heard also in diastole. It varies from time to time and may be transient. It may be increased by inspiration or by firm pressure with the stethoscope diaphragm.

Signs of pericardial effusion are difficult to detect until about 500 ml of fluid have accumulated. The area of cardiac dullness is increased especially to the left of the sternum. The heart sounds may become muffled.

Cardiac tamponade refers to compression of the heart by a large or rapidly increasing effusion which interferes with diastolic filling of the heart. As a result the stroke output of the heart is diminished, tachycardia occurs, the blood pressure falls, the venous pressure is increased, and the clinical picture of shock may develop. Pulsus paradoxus may occur (p. 173).

With a large effusion obliteration of the normal contours of the heart, widening of the base and diminished pulsation of the borders may be seen radiologically. Serial films may show significant changes of size over a short period of time. Echocardiography (p. 180) is helpful in detecting small effusions. The ECG in acute pericarditis shows ST elevation with upward concavity over the affected area which may be widespread. Later there is inversion of T waves; with effusion the voltage is often reduced.

Treatment, Course and Prognosis. Paracentesis of a pericardial effusion is rarely required but may have to be carried out for diagnostic purposes or to relieve severe symptoms from tamponade. The procedure is not without danger from puncture of the heart or of a coronary vessel and should be done only when strictly necessary. The needle is best inserted in the subcostal angle through the costoxiphoid notch and directed upwards, backwards, and to the left. Surgical drainage will usually be necessary if pus is found.

Treatment, course and prognosis vary with the underlying disease.

Viral pericarditis often follows an upper respiratory infection and in some cases Coxsackie virus can be isolated. Recovery usually occurs within a few weeks without after-effects but recurrences may follow and an occasional death has been reported. There is no specific treatment but corticosteroids may be helpful in accelerating recovery.

Tuberculous pericarditis may be secondary to manifest pulmonary or mediastinal tuberculosis, but the primary source may not be detectable. The disease sometimes begins with an acute febrile illness but is more commonly insidious in onset with vague malaise and low-grade fever. The subsequent course is chronic. An effusion usually develops and the pericardium may become thick and unyielding so that the heart is compressed. Pleural effusions are often associated.

The diagnosis may be confirmed by aspiration of the fluid and direct examination or culture for tubercle bacilli. Antituberculous chemotherapy is prescribed (p. 292). Aspiration must be carried out as required to relieve symptoms. Corticosteroids may prevent the development of constrictive pericarditis. In the inactive stage surgical relief may be necessary (p. 232).

Purulent pericarditis occurs rarely from direct spread from an intrathoracic infection or from a bloodstream infection, e.g. from osteomyelitis or a penetrating injury. It is now rare in Britain. Treatment is by surgical drainage and chemotherapy.

Chronic Constrictive Pericarditis

A slowly progressive fibrosis of the pericardium develops as the result of previous infection and constricts the movement of the heart, so that it cannot expand in diastole. The fibrous tissue is thick, dense and inelastic; calcification is common. The inflow of blood to the heart is impeded so that the cardiac output is diminished and the systemic venous pressure increased with resultant peripheral congestion. The heart is otherwise normal, though secondary atrophy of muscle fibres may occur.

Many cases are due to tuberculosis, and some to previous pyogenic infection; in others the cause is obscure.

Clinical Features. Symptoms depend on the degree of constriction. Unlike other types of heart disease, breathlessness is not a prominent symptom and is rarely present at rest because the lungs are often not congested. Raised jugular venous pressure is a notable feature. Enlargement of the liver and ascites occur relatively early compared with peripheral oedema.

The apex beat may be difficult to feel and a third heart sound may be heard. The pulse is rapid and of small volume; there may be pulsus paradoxus (p. 173) together with a striking 'y' descent (Fig. 6.1, p. 175). An important feature in most cases is the absence of much enlargement of the heart. This contrasts with almost all forms of cardiac failure. Atrial fibrillation occurs in about 30 per cent of cases.

Calcification of the pericardium is frequently seen, particularly in lateral or oblique X-rays. Radioscopy may show a small 'quiet' heart with diminished pulsation.

Treatment. The problem is primarily a mechanical one and surgical resection of as much as possible of the pericardium is indicated. The operation may produce dramatic relief and considerable improvement is usual, but it may take several months for maximum benefit to be obtained.

Congenital Heart Disease

The incidence of congenital cardiac abnormalities is about 1 per cent of live births. In most cases the cause of the abnormality is unknown, but some fetal defects are due to maternal infections in the early weeks of pregnancy, e.g. rubella. All degrees of severity occur. Many defects are not compatible with extrauterine life, or only for a short time. Early diagnosis is important because most types are amenable to surgical treatment. Infective endocarditis is a potential complication against which precautions must be taken.

Symptoms may be absent or consist principally of breathlessness and failure of development. Local signs vary with the anatomical lesion. Central cyanosis occurs when desaturated blood enters the systemic circulation. In the neonate the commonest cause of this is transposition of the great arteries in which the aorta derives from the right ventricle and the pulmonary artery from the left. In older children, cyanosis is usually the consequence of a septal defect combined with a severe grade of pulmonary stenosis or pulmonary vascular disease.

Persistent Ductus Arteriosus

During fetal life, before the lungs begin to function, most of the blood from the pulmonary artery passes through the ductus arteriosus into the aorta just below the origin of the left subclavian artery.

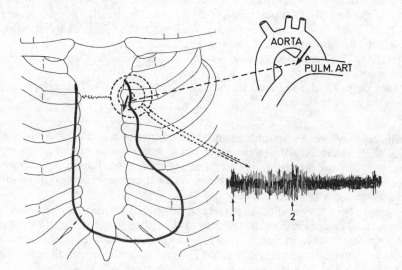

Fig. 6.28 Persistent ductus arteriosus.

Normally the ductus closes soon after birth but, for reasons which are obscure, this sometimes fails to take place. Since the pressure in the aorta is higher than that in the pulmonary artery there will be a continuous arteriovenous shunt, the volume of which depends on the size of the ductus (Fig. 6.28). As much as 50 per cent of the left ventricular output may be recirculated through the lungs with a consequent increase in the work of the heart. The condition, which may be associated with other anomalies, is much commoner in females.

There may be no relevant symptoms for many years, but if the defect is severe growth and development are retarded. In mild cases there will be no disability, but in cases of moderate severity dyspnoea on exertion and later features of cardiac failure gradually develop.

A continuous 'machinery' murmur is heard with late systolic accentuation, maximal at the second left rib near the sternum. It is frequently accompanied by a thrill.

Enlargement of the pulmonary artery, but little enlargement of the heart, may be detected radiologically. The electrocardiogram is usually normal.

In uncomplicated cases, the ductus can be divided with little risk, especially in children, and there is general agreement that this should be carried out in all cases, preferably before the child goes to school. Expectation of life is normal following successful surgical treatment. Few untreated patients live beyond the age of 40, death usually resulting from infective endocarditis or heart failure.

Coarctation of the Aorta

Narrowing of the aorta occurs in the region where the ductus arteriosus joins the aorta, i.e. just below the origin of the left subclavian artery (Fig. 6.29). The condition is more common in males.

Symptoms are often absent. Headaches and cardiac symptoms may occur from hypertension in the upper part of the body and occasionally weakness or cramps in the legs may result from decreased circulation in the lower part of the body.

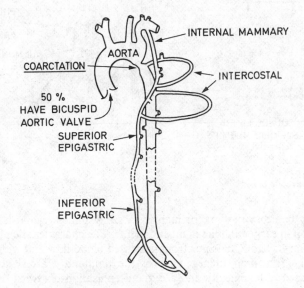

Fig. 6.29 Coarctation of the aorta.

The blood pressure is raised in the arms but is normal or low in the legs. Unduly large arterial pulsations may be visible in the neck. The femoral pulses are weak and delayed after the radial. A systolic murmur is often present over the sternum but is usually loudest over the coarctation posteriorly. Evidence of collateral circulation is present in the older child and adult. Dilated, tortuous vessels exhibiting arterial pulsation may be visible or palpable around the scapulae or in the posterior intercostal spaces, especially if the patient bends forward.

Radiological examination in early childhood is often normal but at a later age may show changes in the contour of the aorta and notching of the under surface of the ribs from tortuous loops of enlarged intercostal arteries. The electrocardiogram may show left ventricular hypertrophy.

The constricted portion of the aorta can be resected and the divided ends of the aorta anastomosed. In untreated severe cases, death may occur from left ventricular failure, rupture of the aorta, cerebral haemorrhage or infection of the bicuspid aortic valve which is often also present.

Atrial Septal Defect

Atrial septal defect is more common in females. Since the normal right ventricle is much more compliant than the left, a large volume of blood shunts through this defect from left to right atrium and thence to the right ventricle and pulmonary arteries (Fig. 6.30). As a result there is gradual enlargement of the right side of the heart and of the pulmonary artery and its main branches. In time, the pressure in the right side of the heart may increase until the shunt is reversed.

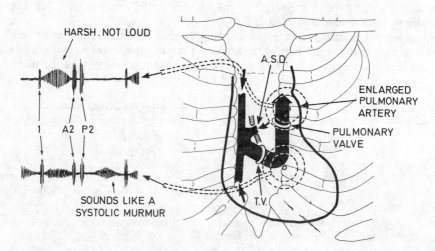

Fig. 6.30 Atrial septal defect.

There may be no symptoms for many years. Dyspnoea, cyanosis and cardiac failure develop in early adult life in most patients. The characteristic physical signs are a pulmonary systolic murmur from increased blood flow and wide splitting of the second heart sound. Enlargement of the pulmonary artery and its main branches is seen radiologically and a dynamic pulsation observed on the screen ('hilar dance'). The right ventricular enlargement can also be seen and may be reflected in the electrocardiogram. Incomplete right bundle branch block is common.

Surgical closure of a large defect should be carried out, preferably before the age of 10 years, following which the expectation of life is probably normal. Most patients used to die from cardiac failure.

Ventricular Septal Defect

Since the pressure in the left ventricle is higher than that in the right ventricle, the shunt is normally from left to right (Fig. 6.31).

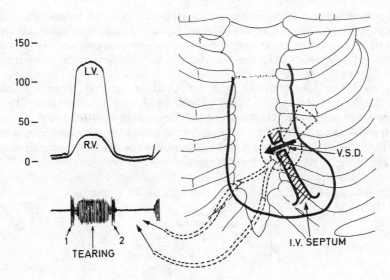

Fig. 6.31 Ventricular septal defect.

Usually there are no relevant symptoms. The characteristic signs are a harsh systolic murmur and thrill maximal in the fourth intercostal space to the left of the sternum. In many cases the defect is not sufficiently large to embarrass the circulation. In some a large additional load causes left ventricular failure. In a few, severe pulmonary hypertension develops and the shunt reverses.

Radiological and electrocardiographic examinations are normal except in the more severe cases when the heart is enlarged.

The defect can be repaired by open heart surgery. This is not necessary for small defects and is dangerous if there is a severe pulmonary hypertension. Surgical treatment is curative if carried out before the heart is much enlarged. Otherwise prognosis depends on the size of the defect.

Pulmonary Stenosis

Pulmonary stenosis may occur as an isolated anomaly in which case there is no cyanosis, or in association with an atrial or ventricular septal defect in which case there may or may not be cyanosis depending on the relative pressures on the two sides of the defect. Stenosis may occur at the level of the pulmonary valve or in the infundibular region of the right ventricle.

Pulmonary Stenosis with Closed Interventricular Septum. In many cases the stenosis is mild. In severe cases there may be dyspnoea, fatigue or, occasionally, syncope. The characteristic signs are a harsh systolic murmur and thrill, maximal in the second intercostal space to the left of the sternum. The pulmonary second sound is diminished. The pulmonary artery is usually dilated beyond the stenosis. The right ventricle is hypertrophied. There may be an associated atrial septal defect.

In mild cases, no treatment is necessary. When the stenosis is severe, pulmonary valvotomy should be carried out as sudden death or progressive cardiac failure otherwise occur.

Pulmonary Stenosis with Ventricular Septal Defect (Fallot's Tetralogy). This is the most common form of cyanotic congenital heart disease in children or adults. The tetralogy comprises pulmonary stenosis, ventricular septal defect, dextroposition of the aorta which overrides this defect and right ventricular hypertrophy (Fig. 6.32).

Dyspnoea and fatigue are the principal symptoms and the child characteristically assumes the squatting position after exercise. The principal signs are: central cyanosis and clubbing of the fingers; a loud systolic murmur, and often a thrill, maximal to the left of the upper sternum; soft pulmonary component of the second sound; enlargement of the right side of the heart; absence of the normal pulmonary artery curve on radiological examination.

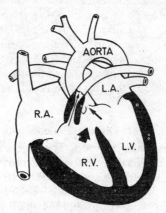

Fig. 6.32 Fallot's tetralogy.

In infancy a palliative operation in the form of an anastomosis can be made either between the left or right pulmonary artery and the corresponding subclavian artery (Blalock's operation) or between the pulmonary artery and the aorta thereby increasing the blood supply to the lungs. Later total correction can be carried out. This abolishes symptoms and restores life expectancy in most cases. Without surgical treatment few patients reach adult life.

Surgery and the Heart

The Surgical Treatment of Heart Disease. Surgery is playing an increasingly important part in the management of heart disease; it is now possible, for example, to correct most types of congenital heart disease and to alleviate many cases of rheumatic and ischaemic heart disease.

Some operations, such as mitral valvotomy and the correction of coarctation, can be performed under normal circulatory conditions with blood continuing to flow through the heart. Most procedures, however, require an open heart so that the circulation must be temporarily occluded (open-heart surgery). In such cases, adequate time for intracardiac surgery can be obtained by the use of an extracorporeal circulation (bypass surgery). With this technique, venous blood is drained from the great veins into a reservoir and is then passed through an oxygenator before being pumped back into the aorta. The heart can then be stopped for several hours whilst an adequate circulation is maintained to the other vital organs. The mortality of bypass surgery should be less than 1 per cent but patients subjected to this procedure are at risk from several hazards, including cerebral air embolism, trauma to the blood from the pump oxygenator and electrolyte and acid-base disturbances. The lungs may become abnormally rigid in the postoperative phase and pulmonary infection is common.

In certain types of disorder, such as patent ductus arteriosus and atrial septal defect, complete correction can be achieved by ligation or suture. In other cases, for example some instances of ventricular septal defect and coarctation of the aorta, prosthetic materials may be needed to effect the repair. In some forms of valve disease, such as pure mitral stenosis, a satisfactory result may be obtained by a simple plastic operation. In others, the valve must be replaced either by a prosthesis or a graft. Although results on the whole are satisfactory with prosthetic valves, they are liable to lead to complications which include thromboembolism and haemolysis. Because of the risk of thrombosis, patients with prosthetic valves are usually kept on long-term anticoagulant therapy. Grafts may be of human origin (homograft) or of animal origin (heterograft). When such grafts are used, the risks of haemolysis and thrombosis are slight but the operation is technically more difficult and the long-term results remain uncertain.

Surgery in Patients with Heart Disease. Patients with heart disease undergoing surgery are at risk from the anaesthetic and from the surgery itself. Skilled anaesthesia is particularly important and an appropriate anaesthetic should be chosen to take account of the nature of the cardiac abnormality and operation being undertaken. Thus, induction may be dangerous particularly when intravenous barbiturates are used; a fall in blood pressure is particularly undesirable.

On the whole, patients with heart disease tolerate surgery remarkably well. Exceptions to this rule are patients with recent myocardial infarction and those who have cardiac or respiratory failure. Only in exceptional circumstances should patients be operated on within 3 months of a coronary occlusion; cardiac and respiratory failure should be brought under control before operation if possible. If heart block is present, a temporary or permanent pacemaker electrode should be inserted prior to surgery.

Hypertension is usually not a contraindication to surgery, but it is necessary for the anaesthetist to be aware of what antihypertensive therapy is being used as excessive hypotension may result from such drugs as adrenergic blocking agents.

In some patients it is better to defer surgery until the heart disease has been corrected or ameliorated. Thus, elective general surgery should be deferred until after mitral valvotomy, if this is indicated. On the other hand, if the cardiac surgery required necessitates long-term anticoagulants it may be preferable to undertake general surgery first.

Heart Disease in Pregnancy

Pregnancy leads to increases of blood volume and cardiac output of up to 50 per cent. In the early weeks of pregnancy, this is probably mainly a consequence of endocrine activity. Subsequently, the increasing demands of the fetus and the arteriovenous shunt in the uterus are the main contributory factors. These changes produce characteristic physical signs. The extremities feel warm and the pulse is of large volume. Tachycardia is present and there may be a rise in venous pressure. The arterial diastolic pressure is lower than in the non-pregnant state because of vasodilation. The heart may be slightly enlarged and may be displaced outwards because of the high diaphragm. A pulmonary systolic murmur due to high flow is usual and there may also be a physiological third heart sound.

The increased load on the heart often provokes or worsens symptoms in patients with heart disease. These do not usually occur before about the 12th week and tend to become maximal from the 24th week onwards. The main symptom of heart disease in pregnancy is breathlessness but oedema may also occur. Angina is very unusual. However, symptoms are a poor guide to the severity of the heart disease as some patients are totally asymptomatic until they develop acute pulmonary oedema in late pregnancy or shortly after delivery.

The commonest major form of heart disease encountered in pregnancy is mitral stenosis; other valvular lesions are not uncommon but seldom give rise to problems. Pregnancy should be deferred in patients with severe mitral stenosis, but it is usually safe after valvotomy has been performed. If a patient with advanced mitral stenosis does become pregnant, either valvotomy or termination should be carried out before the 16th week. With less serious degrees of mitral stenosis and with other forms of heart disease, pregnancy can be allowed to continue and in most cases is uncomplicated. However, if objective evidence of deterioration is taking place, bed rest must be enforced, combined if necessary with digitalis and diuretics. With careful management, even those with advanced heart disease can be carried successfully through pregnancy and delivery.

Patients with congenital heart disease are being seen with increasing frequency during pregnancy, but usually the lesion has been corrected before the pregnancy has occurred. In most cases, no problems arise but pregnancy is a formidable hazard in those who have pulmonary vascular disease in association with congenital heart disease. Maternal mortality may be as high as 25 per cent or more and it is usually wise to terminate the pregnancy early.

DISEASES OF ARTERIES

For clinical purposes it is convenient to classify arterial disease under the general headings of degenerative, inflammatory and vasospastic causes.

Degenerative Arterial Disease

Arteriosclerosis

Arteriosclerosis is a term which in the past has been applied rather indiscriminately to various unrelated forms of arterial disease. Its retention is justified only if it is confined to the degenerative changes which are part of the normal ageing process and which affect the whole arterial tree.

Medial or Mönckeberg's sclerosis is the name given to degenerative changes which occur in old age in the muscular coats of medium sized arteries such as the radial. Calcification of the media is the characteristic change and accounts for the 'pipe stem' arteries so commonly palpable in the elderly and of no clinical significance. Since the medium and large vessels are mainly affected and their lumina are not greatly reduced in size, clinical features are usually absent.

Atherosclerosis

Atherosclerosis is a condition which principally affects the aorta, large arteries and certain medium-sized vessels, particularly the coronary and cerebral arteries. It becomes increasingly common as age advances, but it is not an inevitable concomitant of ageing, and there is a great variation in its extent and severity. Although often associated with and accelerated by hypertension, atherosclerosis may be advanced even in the presence of a normal blood pressure. It may also occur in response to a persistent elevation of pressure in the pulmonary arteries.

The basic atheromatous lesion is the plaque, the most important constituents of which are cholesterol and other lipids which may be free in the intimal tissues or inside cells. At a later stage the plaque becomes sclerosed and calcified. Thrombosis is liable to occur on the surface of the plaque, particularly if it ulcerates. Embolism is frequent.

Atherosclerosis Obliterans

This condition affects males more commonly than females and usually after the age of 50. It is particularly common in diabetics and in heavy cigarette smokers. Atherosclerosis is rarely seen in the upper limbs.

Clinical Features. The principal symptoms which follow impairment of blood supply to the extremities are (1) pain, which occurs on exercise (intermittent claudication) and (2) cold extremities. Although the pathological changes are usually present in both lower limbs, symptoms commonly present first on one side.

Intermittent claudication appears on walking and is rapidly relieved by rest. It most commonly occurs in the calf and causes the patient to limp or stop. Pain occurs at rest with severe ischaemia. Pain which is relieved by elevation of the part suggests venous obstruction, and pain which is relieved by dependency suggests gross arterial obstruction.

Ischaemia may lead to dryness, scaling and inelasticity of the skin, loss of hair and brittle nails. There may be a change of colour of the skin, delay in the return of colour after blanching with light finger pressure, ulceration or gangrene. Where gross lesions are present in one limb, the lower temperature is appreciable to the touch. If the ischaemic limb is first raised 75 degrees above the horizontal, it will blanch more quickly than normal. If then placed in the dependent position, there will be delay in flushing and in venous filling.

Loss of pulsation of one or more peripheral arteries is a common and important feature of arterial disease; bruits may be heard over the larger arteries if they are partially obstructed.

Patients seldom die from peripheral vascular disease but frequently succumb to myocardial infarction.

Investigation. A plain X-ray will show any calcification. This is especially common in Mönckeberg's sclerosis but does not necessarily indicate that the arterial lumen is significantly narrowed. Intra-arterial injection of a radio-opaque dye will show the site of vascular occlusion and the extent of any collateral circulation. Where there are good facilities for arteriography, reactive hyperaemia and oscillometry are now little used. Research techniques include the use of ultrasonic blood flow detectors, clearance measurements using isotopes and electromagnetic metering.

Treatment. Until the pathogenesis of atherosclerosis has been clearly established and until specific measures are discovered which are accepted as being effective for its prevention and cure, the treatment of peripheral vascular disease must continue to be unsatisfactory. Diabetes or obesity may require attention. Smoking should be forbidden.

Cold should be avoided and suitable woollen clothing worn, especially on the limbs. The application of heat to the affected limb is harmful because it raises the local metabolism but does not increase the inflow of blood to the ischaemic area. Pain at rest may be reduced by raising the head of the bed or by lowering the limb below the horizontal and keeping it cool.

Protection against trauma and the early treatment of sepsis are most important. Fungal infection between the toes should be treated. Detailed instructions on the care of the feet and nails must be given. The feet should be kept scrupulously clean, carefully dried after washing, especially between the toes, and dusting powder containing zinc oxide and salicylic acid applied. Nails should be cut carefully and corns pared with caution. It is wise to employ the services of a chiropodist. Socks and shoes should be well fitting. Even the slightest abrasion should be taken seriously and medical advice sought. Dressings to keep the part dry are required for any breach of surface.

Regular exercise encourages the development of collateral vessels. Patients should not be alarmed by the development of pain and they should be encouraged to believe that with exercise and the stopping of smoking improvement is expected and that the occurrence of gangrene is improbable.

Buerger-Allen exercises should be carried out three or four times daily. The legs are raised and supported 45 degrees above the horizontal for one minute (or until blanched), then lowered over the side of the bed or couch for a minute until thoroughly pink. While still dependent the feet are dorsiflexed and plantarflexed alternately and the toes are moved repeatedly for two minutes. This cycle is repeated four to six times. Vasodilators are not recommended as they act by dilating normal vessels elsewhere and may divert blood from the affected site.

Areas of gangrene should be kept clean and dry until a clear line of demarcation appears. Thereafter surgical treatment will be required. Sympathectomy may be of value when the limb is cold or rest pain is present but it seldom helps claudication. Direct arterial surgery is indicated for disabling claudication, rest pain or gangrene provided the vessels are shown to be suitable by arteriography.

Sudden Occlusion of a Major Artery

This may result from thrombosis or embolism. The limb becomes painful, cold, numb and pale, and pulses distal to the block are absent. The outcome depends on the collateral circulation and on subsequent treatment. Pain should be relieved and the limb kept at rest and exposed to room temperature. The other limbs and body should be kept warm and reflex vasodilation encouraged by an electric blanket or hot-water bottles applied to the trunk.

Embolectomy should be considered whenever a major artery (for example, brachial or femoral) is occluded; the early intervention of a surgeon skilled in this field is important. The Fogerty balloon-tipped catheter is especially valuable. It is introduced by arteriotomy, the tip is pushed beyond the thrombus, the balloon inflated and the catheter withdrawn thus extracting the thrombus. Heparin should be given intravenously (p. 245). Amputation for gangrene may be necessary.

Atherosclerosis and Aneurysm Formation

Atherosclerosis is frequently present in the aorta but seldom affects its function. It may, however, be responsible for aneurysms of any part of this vessel. An aneurysm in the ascending portion is usually due to tertiary syphilis and may cause pain because of erosion of the ribs or sternum; a pulsating mass may occasionally be visible. An aneurysm of the arch of the aorta may produce wheezing or hoarseness from its effect on the trachea or recurrent laryngeal nerves. Aneurysms of the abdominal aorta are generally due to atherosclerosis; their rupture leads usually to sudden death. The results of resection and replacement with a graft are improving and operation is therefore more frequently performed.

Dissecting Aneurysm of the Aorta

In this condition a tear occurs through the intima secondary to degeneration of the media. As a result blood makes its way in a split in the media to form a new channel. Death usually occurs from rupture through the adventitia into the pericardium or elsewhere. Some patients are hypertensive. In women it may occur peripartum.

Dissecting aneurysm may also occur in *Marfan's syndrome* in which there is loss of elastic fibres in the media as part of a generalised disorder of connective tissue; long thin extremities and subluxation of the lens are other characteristics.

The onset of dissection is sudden with severe, tearing, chest pain which often radiates into the neck, abdomen, legs or back of the chest. It may be precipitated by exertion and may simulate myocardial infarction. Neurological features may result from occlusion of branches of the aorta supplying the spinal cord. One or more of the peripheral pulses may be obliterated.

Diagnosis is suggested by the sudden onset of the characteristic pain and the absence of the ECG and enzyme abnormalities of myocardial infarction unless the dissection includes a coronary artery. The chest radiograph may be helpful in showing a broadened mediastinum due to widening of the aorta.

In the initial stages the blood pressure, if high, should be lowered by antihypertensive drugs to normal levels. Surgical treatment is usually necessary later.

Inflammatory Arterial Disease

The principal types of inflammatory arterial disease are syphilitic aortitis, polyarteritis, thromboangiitis obliterans, cranial (giant cell) arteritis and Takayasu's syndrome (pulseless disease).

Syphilitic Aortitis

Syphilitic aortitis is much rarer in Britain than it was 30 years ago but is still important in many parts of the world. There is often a latent period of 15 to 20 years following infection before clinical manifestations are evident in the cardiovascular system. Neurosyphilis infrequently coexists.

Pathology. The disease begins just above the aortic valve cusps. In the adventitia there is infiltration of lymphocytes and plasma cells round the vasa vasorum, which are obliterated by intimal proliferation. Elastic tissue is gradually replaced by fibrous tissue and this leads to dilation of the aorta. Proliferation of the intima occurs and may involve the mouths of the coronary arteries leading to myocardial ischaemia, or spread along the valve cusps which become thickened, everted and incompetent.

Clinical Features. Syphilitic aortitis occurs most frequently between the ages of 40 and 55. The diagnosis is difficult in the early uncomplicated stages. Suspicions may be aroused by an aortic systolic murmur, together with accentuation of the second sound. Later there is aortic regurgitation similar to that of rheumatic origin but the diastolic murmur radiates more commonly to the right of the sternum. Dilation and calcification of the ascending aorta may be demonstrated by radiological examination. The diagnosis is confirmed by serological tests.

Treatment. If adequate antisyphilitic therapy is given in the early stages of the infection cardiovascular manifestations in later life are prevented. Treatment of syphilitic aortitis consists of a course of procaine penicillin, i.e. 600 mg daily for 10 days. If cardiac failure is present this should first be controlled. Surgical treatment may be indicated for aortic regurgitation or aneurysm.

Thromboangiitis Obliterans

This uncommon condition, known also as *Buerger's disease*, is of obscure origin. It usually begins before the age of 40 and is almost confined to males. Cigarette smoking is an important aetiological factor. The lower limbs are principally affected. The wall of the artery is infiltrated with polymorphs and the lumen may be obstructed by clot. The adjacent vein is often involved.

The symptoms and signs are essentially those of diminished blood supply to the limb; persistent pain in a cold, cyanosed toe is often the presenting complaint. This is followed by intermittent claudication and rest pain. In the leg, atrophic changes and finally gangrene may develop. Involvement of the veins may cause recurrent thrombophlebitis.

There is no specific treatment but it is essential that cigarette smoking is stopped.

Polyarteritis

This is an uncommon condition of unknown aetiology, most often seen in men between the ages of 20 and 50. In some patients it appears to be due to hypersensitivity to serum or to drugs such as penicillin or sulphonamides. The characteristic lesions consist of multiple nodules on the smaller arteries. The vessel wall is infiltrated by polymorphs and necrosis follows with resultant aneurysmal dilation. Thrombosis may occur.

Clinical features such as fever, tachycardia, wasting, sweating and generalised pain are accompanied by local manifestations of ischaemia in various parts of the body. The vessels of the kidney, gastrointestinal tract, heart, peripheral nerves and skin are particularly affected giving rise to such varied manifestations as haematuria, abdominal pain, angina, pericarditis, peripheral neuropathy, subcutaneous nodules or localised oedema. Involvement of the lungs may cause asthma. There may be leucocytosis or eosinophilia. Hypertension is usual at some stage.

The course is usually progressive but mild cases may recover. There is no curative treatment, but corticosteroids are worthy of trial. Administered before vascular damage is too extensive, they may produce a remarkable remission. The outlook in more advanced cases is less hopeful. The fibrosis which follows healing of the vascular lesions may be sufficiently extensive to lead to myocardial infarction or renal failure.

Cranial Arteritis

Cranial or *giant cell arteritis* is a panarteritis of medium-sized vessels. It is a distinct clinical entity in which the striking finding is tender, thickened cranial arteries. The cause of the disease is unknown. It is related to polymalgia rheumatica (p. 648).

The vessel wall is infiltrated by mononuclear cells, plasma cells and giant cells. Thrombosis may occur. The vessels of the scalp, particularly the temporal arteries, are usually affected but other arteries may also be involved, for example those of the retinae and brain, and the condition may be widespread throughout the body.

Intense headache and sometimes blindness are prominent features. Other manifestations include fever, pain and stiffness of hips and shoulders, weakness and loss of weight. It affects elderly persons, and usually ends in recovery after several months. Cranial arteritis responds promptly to prednisolone which may also prevent blindness.

Takayasu's Syndrome

This disorder, known also as *pulseless disease* and the *aortic arch syndrome*, is rare except in some communities, e.g. Japan. It predominantly affects young females. An arteritis of unknown origin involves the aortic arch with narrowing of its major branches. The pulses are diminished or absent in the upper extremities, neck and head. Headache, syncope, visual disturbance and muscular wasting may occur. The prognosis is poor but corticosteroids are sometimes of value.

Vasospastic Disorders
Raynaud's Disease

Raynaud's disease is the name given to a peripheral vascular disturbance consisting of spasmodic contraction of the digital arteries, which is precipitated by cold, emotion and by other causative factors mentioned below. Primary Raynaud's disease is commonest in young women and is an exaggerated physiological response to cold. The term 'secondary Raynaud's disease or phenomenon' is used to describe the disorder which occurs from (i) pressure of a cervical rib, (ii) obliterative arterial disease, (iii) certain occupations in which the arms and hands are exposed to vibrations from pneumatic drills, polishing tools, etc. or (iv) occasionally from cold agglutinins and cryoglobulins. It may also occur in disorders of connective tissue, especially scleroderma.

In the early, uncomplicated stages, there are no pathological changes. Later obliterating endarteritis may occur and result in thrombosis in the lumen leading to ischaemic changes in the skin of the digits and nails, superficial necrosis and finally gangrene.

Clinical Manifestations. Symptoms are usually bilateral and fingers are more affected than toes. Numbness, tingling and burning are more prominent than pain. Sensitivity to cold may be extreme and disabling.

Colour changes usually consist of three phases: pallor, cyanosis and redness. If the limb is bloodless it will be pale. If blood flow is sluggish excessive deoxygenation results in cyanosis. Redness is a rebound phenomenon due to reactive hyperaemia which may follow the vasospasm.

Treatment. Any primary disease should be treated if possible. Protection from cold is obviously indicated. Vasodilator drugs may be tried, but the results are very disappointing. In severe cases, sympathectomy, to remove vasomotor tone, should be considered; the long-term results are poor in the arms but fairly good in the legs. Cigarette smoking should be stopped.

DISEASES OF VEINS

Venous Thrombosis

A distinction may be made between *thrombophlebitis* when the endothelium is injured by inflammation, and *phlebothrombosis* when thrombosis is the primary disturbance. The latter is the more common condition and carries a much greater risk of pulmonary embolism.

Aetiology. The following factors are of importance:

1. *Slowing or Obstruction of the Blood Stream.* This may result from rest in bed, particularly if a pillow is placed under the knees, especially in the elderly or from unduly prolonged sitting, e.g. in journeys by air. Cardiac failure also leads to slowing of the circulation.

2. *Injury to the Vein.* This may be due to trauma and may follow accidents, operations, childbirth, intravenous infusions or injections.

3. *Increased Coagulability of the Blood.* Many factors may disturb the dynamic equilibrium which normally exists between coagulation and fibrinolysis, notably an increase in platelet adhesiveness. This may occur for example in malignant disease or with the use of oral contraceptives. An increased liability to thrombosis also occurs in dehydration and polycythaemia due to an increase in the blood viscosity.

Pathology. At first the thrombus consists mainly of dense layers of platelets and fibrin; later it is a loose, friable, jelly-like mass of fibrin and red cells which readily becomes detached to form an embolus. After a few days inflammatory changes occur in the wall of the vein. The thrombus may undergo lysis or organisation.

Venous thrombosis is most common in the lower limbs, particularly in the venous sinuses of the soleus muscle in the calf and in the femoral and iliac veins. It is much less frequent in the upper limb but the axillary vein may be involved as a complication of trauma, neoplasm or radiotherapy. Superficial thrombophlebitis most commonly occurs in the saphenous vein more particularly if there are associated varicosities.

Suppurative thrombophlebitis is a rare but very serious condition usually involving the veins of the pelvis following sepsis.

Clinical Features. The patient may complain of pain in the calf but the process is often silent and undiagnosed. An unexplained slight pyrexia may be the only warning. If the lumen of a main vein is occluded, there is dilation of the superficial veins, a slight rise in the skin temperature of the leg, the affected leg is often abnormally pink and there may be oedema at the ankle. In extensive occlusive iliofemoral thrombosis the whole lower limb is swollen and white if the collateral channels remain patent. If the collaterals are also occluded, the leg is blue—a pregangrenous condition. In contrast there may be no signs in the presence of an extensive non-occlusive, potentially lethal thrombus. Pulmonary embolism is frequently the first clinical manifestation of venous thrombosis.

Diagnosis. The most certain way of establishing the diagnosis is by phlebography. The veins from the ankle to the inguinal ligament can be demonstrated by ascending lower limb phlebography—a relatively straightforward procedure. Percutaneous iliofemoral phlebography may also be required. Other techniques which are of value, though not available generally, are the uptake of ^{123}I labelled fibrinogen and ultrasound. The former is used for the early detection of thrombosis, for example post-operatively. Ultrasound is used to assess the patency of deep veins in patients who present with a swollen leg or with pulmonary embolism.

Prevention. Efforts must chiefly be directed to the avoidance of venous stasis. This is easiest in surgical patients when the period of risk can be defined. Almost all post-operative thromboses begin during or within 72 hours of operation. Early ambulation should be encouraged after surgery and medical illnesses. This means more than simply transferring the patient from lying in bed to sitting in a chair. Active exercises should be prescribed and at other times the leg should be elevated. A graduated elastic support should be worn if the patient is at particular risk. If confinement to bed is unavoidable, the patient should be encouraged to move the lower limbs frequently. In hospital, exercises can be organised under the supervision of a physiotherapist. Faulty posture in bed must be corrected, constricting bandages avoided and cardiac failure and dehydration should receive attention.

For patients at particular risk other prophylactic measures include low dose subcutaneous heparin or intravenous dextran 70 (p. 228).

Treatment. The aim of treatment is to prevent propagation of thrombus and pulmonary embolism, damage to the valves of the vein and chronic venous insufficiency. These objectives are usually best achieved by heparin. The role of oral anticoagulants is to prevent recurrences by longer term treatment.

Unless there is an obvious contraindication, such as active peptic ulceration or a bleeding surface as after prostatectomy, treatment is initiated with heparin and continued with warfarin. Heparin is preferably given for 7–10 days by intravenous infusion or, ideally, by an infusion pump in a dose of 25,000–40,000 units daily controlled by a clotting time of twice or thrice normal. Alternatively, 10,000 units may be given every 6 hours by intravenous injection. If bleeding occurs, it usually stops when heparin is withdrawn. Protamine sulphate (10–30 mg i.v.) is a specific antidote to heparin but is rarely required.

For longer term treatment warfarin is preferable to phenindione as hypersensitivity reactions are common with the latter. A single dose of 20–40 mg is given and the prothrombin time measured on the third day, the aim being a value of 2–2½ times that of a control. The maintenance dose of warfarin varies from 1 to 10 mg daily. The oral anticoagulant should be continued for at least one month and for six months if there has been swelling of the legs. The risk of haemorrhage is increased as control is difficult if there is liver disease, or if the patient is also taking phenylbutazone, indomethacin, salicylates, clofibrate or antibiotics. The abrupt withdrawal of phenobarbitone is also dangerous as this drug promotes enzyme induction (p. 633). Vitamin K_1 (10–20 mg i.v.) is the specific antidote for warfarin overdosage.

Thrombolytic therapy with streptokinase is expensive but can be considered for iliofemoral thrombosis. Thrombectomy may occasionally be required for a recent non-occlusive thrombosis at this site.

The legs should be elevated to 15 degrees and physiotherapy commenced after 48 hours. Straining at stool often causes separation of venous thrombi and should be avoided.

The venous flow is accelerated by the support of graduated elastic hose but care must be taken to avoid a constricting effect by the hose rolling up. The ambulant woman should wear elastic support tights and for men knee-length elastic hose is best. Support of this kind will probably be necessary permanently after a severe thrombosis to control chronic venous insufficiency.

Superficial thrombophlebitis usually responds to an elastic support and phenylbutazone (200 mg t.i.d. for 6 days). There may be complicating deep venous thrombosis, particularly if the proximal saphenous vein is involved. Then anticoagulants will be required.

Prospects in Cardiology

Advances in diagnosis proceed fast. The antenatal recognition of those fetal abnormalities which carry a high risk of concomitant heart disease will allow for the first time a reduction in the incidence of congenital heart disease by therapeutic abortion. Transvenous cardiac biopsy is now acceptably safe and provides tissue for microscopic and ultramicroscopic examination and is likely to prove increasingly useful. The second generation of echocardiographic equipment offers a gradual partial replacement of invasive methods of investigation which cause anxiety. and discomfort to the patient and are not without risk. Imaging by radioisotopes is still at an early stage but already allows information to be obtained about differential myocardial blood flow, for example, which cannot be obtained in other ways. So far computerised axial tomography is too slow a process for the heart. The value of the 24 hour portable ECG monitor is already established and much can be anticipated of its use, particularly where computerised analysis of the records is available.

Studies in cardiac metabolism and pharmacokinetics are steadily improving the understanding of myocardial function. Beta adrenergic receptor blocking drugs, perhaps the greatest advance in cardiac therapy since digitalis, are being put to new uses. Their success however has led to the market being flooded with new preparations; time will show whether they have adverse effects.

Coronary bypass surgery offers improved vascularisation of the heart and usually a low mortality and good symptomatic benefit. Enthusiasm for it is such that in 1975 an estimated 40,000 operations for aorta-coronary saphenous vein bypass were performed in the United States. Doubt remains about the effect of such procedures on the prognosis and about the fate of both grafted and native vessels. Multicentre controlled trials should clarify the position but their value may be restricted by variation in surgical skills at the different centres. Experience gained in this field, in valve replacement and in heart transplantation has led to technical advances whereby the cardiac surgeon will be contributing still more to therapy, for example where an abnormal pathway is responsible for paroxysmal tachycardia which cannot be managed with drugs, in infective endocarditis and following myocardial infarction. The belated recognition of the fact that after a myocardial infarct and cardiac surgery many patients fail to return to normal activity for psychological rather than physical reasons has led to a new active interest in rehabilitation which is likely to pay further dividends.

The epidemic proportions of premature arterial disease remains a considerable enigma despite the identification of several risk factors and remains the principal present-day challenge to further investigation. The solution of the problem and the discovery of how to prevent atheroma will undoubtedly be achieved, and when it is and when atheroma can be prevented, it is possible to look forward to a striking reduction in the incidence of heart disease.

D. G. JULIAN
M. B. MATTHEWS

Further reading

Goldman, M. J. (1973) *Principles of Clinical Electrocardiography*. 8th edition. Los Altos, California: Lange. A standard textbook for reference purposes.

Holling, H. E. (1972) *Peripheral Vascular Diseases*. Philadelphia: Lippincott.

Hurst, J. W. (1974) *The Heart*. 3rd edition. New York: McGraw-Hill.

Julian, D. G. (1973) *Cardiology*. 2nd edition. London: Baillière & Tindall. An introduction to cardiology for the non-specialist.

Matthews, M. B. (1976) Examination of the cardiovascular system. In *Clinical Examination*. 4th edition, editor, Macleod, J. Edinburgh: Churchill Livingstone.

Report of a Joint Working Party of the Royal College of Physicians of London and the British Cardiac Society (1976) Prevention of coronary heart disease. *Journal of the Royal College of Physicians*, **10**, 213.—The latest British recommendations by an expert committee: considers all the risk factors.

7. Diseases of the Respiratory System

Anatomy

The *upper respiratory tract*, which includes the nose, nasopharynx and larynx, is lined by vascular mucous membrane. The rich blood supply ensures that the inspired air enters the lungs at body temperature and fully saturated with water vapour. The whole respiratory epithelium down to the terminal bronchioles is equipped with cilia, which, aided by the layer of sticky mucus covering them, have the important function of trapping foreign particles and bacteria, and propelling them towards the pharynx. They contribute to the prevention of respiratory infection.

The maxillary, frontal, ethmoidal and sphenoidal *nasal sinuses* communicate with the nasopharynx by narrow openings and are frequently involved in upper respiratory infections. Adequate drainage of infected sinuses is often prevented by inflammatory oedema of the mucosa lining their narrow openings: as a result, resolution of sinus infection is often slow and sometimes incomplete.

The *larynx*, in addition to being the organ of voice production, has the function of preventing particles larger than can be dealt with by the cilia from reaching the lower respiratory tract. This it does by means of the *cough reflex*. The larynx is often involved in disease, particularly infection. It is sometimes obstructed by oedema or exudate, or by an impacted foreign body. *Laryngeal paralysis* (p. 308) is usually due to a lesion of the recurrent laryngeal branch of the vagus nerve. As the left recurrent laryngeal nerve runs part of its course within the thoracic cavity, in close proximity to the aortic arch and the left pulmonary hilum, a bronchial carcinoma in the left hilar region and, less frequently, an aortic aneurysm may cause paralysis of the left vocal cord. Paralysis of the right vocal cord is rare, most cases being due to an aneurysm of the right subclavian artery.

The *trachea* begins at the cricoid cartilage and ends at the level of the sternal angle by bifurcation into the two *main bronchi*. The trachea is usually palpable in the suprasternal notch, where in normal subjects it is exactly in the midline. Deviation of the trachea to either side, in the absence of a local lesion in the neck, is a valuable indication of displacement of the upper mediastinum.

The *right main bronchus* is more vertical than the left, with the result that a foreign body entering the trachea is more likely to lodge in that bronchus or one of its divisions than the left. The right main bronchus first gives off from its lateral wall the *upper lobe bronchus* and then from its anterior wall the *middle lobe bronchus*, after which it continues as the *lower lobe bronchus*. The *left main bronchus* gives off the *upper lobe bronchus* from its lateral wall and continues as the *lower lobe bronchus*. The tongue-shaped part of the left upper lobe corresponding to the middle lobe on the right side is supplied by a large branch of the left upper lobe bronchus, named the *lingular bronchus* by reason of the shape of the part of lung which it supplies. The anatomical position of these bronchi is shown diagrammatically in Figure 7.1.

The three lobar bronchi on the right side and the two on the left divide and subdivide like the branches of a tree (the term 'bronchial tree' is in common use) until the respiratory bronchioles are reached. Each respiratory bronchiole communicates with a cluster of alveoli, and the 'bronchopulmonary lobule' so constituted is the basic structure of all lung tissue. The alveoli are tiny air vesicles bounded by a single layer of flattened epithelial cells which are in direct contact with the pulmonary capillaries. Exchange of the respiratory gases, oxygen and carbon dioxide, takes place between the air in the alveoli and the blood in the pulmonary capillaries.

The *right lung* differs from the left in having three lobes instead of two. The *left lung* is divided into *upper* and *lower lobes* by the *oblique fissure* which extends from the junction of the fourth or fifth rib with the vertebral column behind to the sixth costochondral junction in front, crossing the midaxillary line at the level of the fifth rib. As the posterior end of the fissure is at a much higher level than its anterior end, the upper lobe, as well as being *above* the lower lobe, is also largely in front of it. It therefore follows that upper lobe lesions produce physical signs mainly on the front of the chest and lower lobe lesions on the back.

On the *right* side the oblique fissure corresponds in position to that on the left, but the lung above it is divided into *upper* and *middle lobes* by the *transverse fissure*, which runs laterally in a horizontal direction from the junction of the fourth costal cartilage with the sternum to join the oblique fissure at the level of the fifth rib in the midaxillary line. The middle lobe is thus situated behind the lower part of the anterior chest wall.

Each lobe is composed of two or more *bronchopulmonary segments*, which represent the portions of lung tissue supplied by the main branches of each lobar bronchus.

In many diseases, e.g. pneumococcal pneumonia, collapse and lung abscess, the lesion is typically confined to a single lobe or segment. A knowledge of pulmonary anatomy, when applied to the interpretation of radiographs, is thus of value in determining the nature of the lesion as well as its situation.

Each lung is closely invested with *visceral pleura*. *Parietal pleura* lines the chest wall, mediastinum and diaphragm, and is continuous with the visceral pleura at the pulmonary hilum. In health the two pleural layers are separated only by a thin film of lymph, but between them there is a negative (subatmospheric) pressure. This results from the natural tendency of the lung to recoil towards the hilum, a property given to it by the rich supply of elastic fibres in the bronchi, blood vessels and lung parenchyma.

If a communication develops with the atmosphere as, for example, with a penetrating wound of the chest wall or from the rupture of an emphysematous bulla, the negative intrapleural pressure draws air between the pleural layers and the potential intrapleural space becomes a real one. There is then said to be a *pneumothorax*. When the space is created by the presence of clear fluid there is said to be a *pleural effusion* or a *hydrothorax*; by pus, an *empyema*; by blood, a *haemothorax*; by both clear fluid and air, a *hydropneumothorax*; by both pus and air, a *pyopneumothorax*; and by both blood and air, a *haemopneumothorax*.

When the pleural space contains air or fluid the elastic recoil of the underlying lung is to some extent released and the lung shrinks towards the hilum, this shrinkage being referred to as *pulmonary collapse*. The larger the amount of air or fluid between the pleural layers the more marked is the degree of pulmonary collapse and the greater the impairment of function of the collapsed lung. If the quantity of air or fluid is very large it causes displacement of the mediastinum towards the opposite side, with the result that function of the opposite lung is also impaired. A gross degree of mediastinal displacement may, in addition, embarrass

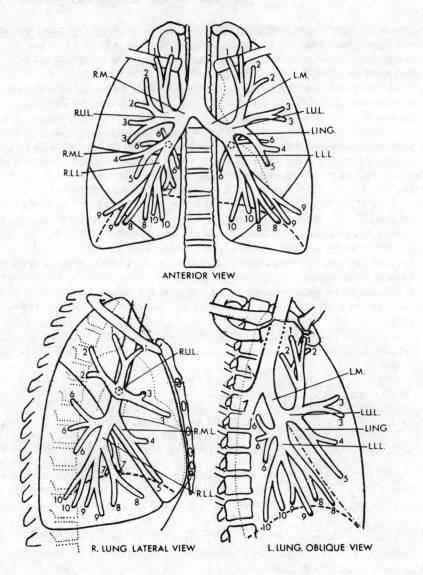

ANTERIOR VIEW

R. LUNG LATERAL VIEW   L. LUNG. OBLIQUE VIEW

Key to Fig. 7.1

Major Bronchi

R.M.	Right main bronchus.	L.M.	Left main bronchus.
R.U.L.	Right upper lobe bronchus.	L.U.L.	Left upper lobe bronchus.
R.M.L.	Right middle lobe bronchus.	LING.	Lingular bronchus.
R.L.L.	Right lower lobe bronchus.	L.L.L.	Left lower lobe bronchus.

Segmental Bronchi[1]

Right upper lobe.	1. Apical.	2. Posterior.	3. Anterior.
Right middle lobe.	4. Lateral.	5. Medial.	
Right lower lobe.	6. Apical.	7. Medial basal (cardiac).	8. Anterior basal.
	9. Lateral basal.	10. Posterior basal.	

the action of the heart. Mediastinal displacement is recognised clinically by alteration in position of the trachea and of the cardiac apex beat.

Collapse of the lung may also occur without air or fluid in the pleural space as a result of bronchial obstruction (p. 318).

The anatomy of the *mediastinum* has an important bearing on the diagnosis of intrathoracic disease, particularly tumours and aneurysms. These lesions are liable to involve mediastinal structures and, as a result, certain readily recognisable symptoms, physical signs and radiological abnormalities may be produced. The structures involved and the abnormality produced in each case are discussed in the section on mediastinal tumours (p. 325).

Physiology

Knowledge of the normal processes of respiration is of value in understanding the effects of disease of the lungs and airways, and is of great importance in therapy. Oxygen therapy, the treatment of ventilatory failure and much of the treatment of chronic bronchitis and asthma have a rational basis in applied respiratory physiology.

The aspects of the physiology of respiration which merit special attention are:

1. *Ventilation*, which includes (a) the mechanical processes of inspiration and expiration and (b) the control of ventilation at a level appropriate to metabolic needs.
2. *Perfusion* of the lungs by the output of the right ventricle.
3. *Distribution* of ventilation and perfusion within the lungs.
4. *Diffusion* of oxygen and carbon dioxide between the terminal airways, the alveoli and the pulmonary capillary blood.

In a typical normal adult at rest the normal pulmonary blood flow of 5 *l*/min carries 11 mmol/min (250 ml/min) of oxygen from the lungs to the tissues and normal ventilation of about 6 *l*/min carries 9 mmol/min (200 ml/min) of carbon dioxide out of the body. The pressures of oxygen and carbon dioxide in the arterial blood are closely controlled. The normal range of Po_2 is 11–13 kPa (83–98 mm Hg) and of Pco_2 4·8–6 kPa (36–45 mm Hg). Observation of changes in these pressures in disease is of importance in assessing the nature and severity of any disturbance of lung function (p. 257).

Left upper lobe.	1. Apical.	2. Posterior.	3. Anterior.
Lingula.	4. Superior.	5. Inferior.	
Left lower lobe.[2]	6. Apical.	8. Anterior basal.	9. Lateral basal.
	10. Posterior basal.		

[1] The names of the segmental bronchi are not included in the text but are given here for future reference, numbered according to international agreement.
[2] There is no medial basal bronchus on the left side.

Fig. 7.1 The anatomy of the bronchi.

The oblique view of the left bronchi is shown in preference to the lateral view because at bronchography (p. 262) the right bronchi are normally outlined first and a lateral view of the left bronchi cannot then be obtained. The oblique view, which must be taken instead, has the additional advantage of showing the disposition of the left bronchi more clearly.

Ventilation

The respiratory muscles, in ventilating the lungs, do mechanical work of two kinds, elastic and non-elastic. The first is performed against elastic forces in the lungs and chest wall which together tend to bring the chest to the position it occupies at the end of a normal expiration. Movement of the chest from this position of equilibrium involves the performance of elastic work and the storage of kinetic energy which is later available for non-elastic work during the return to the resting position. This second kind of work is largely expended in overcoming the resistance of the airways to the inspiratory and expiratory flow of air and to a smaller extent in displacing soft and inelastic tissues.

During quiet breathing inspiration is 'active' and expiration 'passive'. Inspiration against abnormal resistance (whether elastic or non-elastic) may bring accessory muscles such as the sternomastoids and scaleni into play; expiration, if forced or performed against abnormal airway resistance, is accomplished with the aid of the accessory muscles of expiration, chiefly those of the abdominal wall.

Elastic work is increased when the lungs are made more rigid (less compliant) by pulmonary oedema or fibrosis or when the chest wall is made more unyielding by ankylosing spondylitis or severe kyphoscoliosis. Rapid shallow breathing is often observed in these conditions. Non-elastic work is increased by rapid breathing and by conditions causing airway obstruction such as asthma, chronic bronchitis, emphysema and tumours of major bronchi. The metabolic cost of breathing is normally low: an increase in ventilation of 1 l/min raises oxygen uptake by about 45 μmol/min (1 ml/min) at most. In disease, this figure may rise to as much as 450 μmol (10 ml) oxygen per min per l/min increase in ventilation. Under such circumstances breathing accounts for an important fraction of metabolic oxygen uptake.

Not all the volume of the inspired ventilation takes part in gas exchange in the lungs. Some of each breath ventilates the conducting airways down to the respiratory bronchioles, which constitute the 'anatomical' dead space; because of maldistribution (see below) some of each breath is wasted in ventilating underperfused parts of the lungs. The proportion of wasted ventilation in each breath (physiological dead space: tidal volume ratio, Vd/Vt) is normally one-fifth to one-third, but may be much increased, sometimes to as much as two-thirds, in disease. The volume which remains takes part in gas exchange and constitutes the alveolar ventilation, which is normally about 5 l/min at rest. It follows that if the proportion of wasted ventilation is greater than normal a greater total ventilation is needed to achieve normal alveolar ventilation.

Normally, alveolar ventilation is closely matched to the excretion of carbon dioxide and this matching is reflected in a normal level of arterial P_{CO_2}. If alveolar ventilation is reduced in proportion to carbon dioxide excretion, the arterial P_{CO_2} must rise (hypercapnia), and if alveolar ventilation becomes excessive, the arterial P_{CO_2} will fall (hypocapnia). Indeed, the arterial P_{CO_2} reflects alveolar ventilation and the production of carbon dioxide just as the blood urea concentration reflects renal urea clearance and the metabolic production of urea.

Generalised alveolar underventilation is most commonly found as a late result of chronic bronchitis and emphysema. It also occurs if respiration is depressed by narcotics, anaesthetics or intracranial disease. It may ensue when the respiratory muscles are paralysed or when gross deformity of the chest wall limits thoracic or diaphragmatic movement, as in kyphoscoliosis. Lowering of the arterial P_{O_2} (hypoxaemia) is an inevitable result of alveolar underventilation when air is breathed. Giving oxygen will correct this, but the hypercapnia is corrected only when alveolar ventilation is improved.

Alveolar overventilation occurs in asthma of mild or moderate severity, in interstitial lung disease, in pulmonary vascular disease (e.g. pulmonary embolism), in salicylate overdosage, as a result of pontine lesions, or from anxiety or hysteria. It is often a prominent manifestation of metabolic acidosis (p. 116).

CONTROL OF BREATHING

Rhythmical discharges originating in the reticular substance of the brain stem provide the basis for co-ordinated respiratory movements; it is convenient to use the term 'respiratory centre' for the neurones involved in breathing, but the distribution and organisation of these neurones is highly complex. Normal breathing is modified by afferent impulses from many sources, which are best considered in two groups:

1. Those arising within the central nervous system and from receptors other than chemoreceptors ('neural stimuli').
2. Those arising from chemoreceptors sensitive to the composition of blood or cerebrospinal fluid ('chemical stimuli').

Afferent impulses of the first group mediate (a) the changes in rate and depth of breathing which may be consciously induced for short periods, (b) the central neurogenic hyperventilation which occurs in certain lesions of the pons and midbrain, (c) the respiratory depression associated with medullary compression and (d) the respiratory stimulation which originates in limb receptors, as in exercise. These impulses may also arise from receptors in muscles and joints in the chest wall, and from pulmonary receptors sensitive to stretch, bronchial irritation and pulmonary capillary distension. Pulmonary inflation and deflation (Hering-Breuer) reflexes are present in the newborn, but are weak in adults except under general anaesthesia.

The second group of afferent impulses arises in chemosensitive cells located in the carotid and aortic bodies (peripheral chemoreceptors) and intracranially (central chemoreceptors). In animals central chemosensitive areas are located on the ventrolateral surface of the medulla, but in man their situation is uncertain.

Ventilation is increased when the peripheral chemoreceptors are stimulated by arterial hypoxia; at rest, the stimulus is not strong unless arterial Po_2 is below 8 kPa (60 mm Hg), and becomes powerful at about 4 kPa (30 mm Hg). The peripheral chemoreceptors are also stimulated by an increase in the hydrogen-ion activity of arterial blood. Central chemoreceptors are stimulated by an increase in the hydrogen-ion activity of cerebrospinal fluid (CSF). A rise in Pco_2 of the arterial blood is accompanied by increasing acidity of both blood and CSF and therefore stimulates both central and peripheral chemoreceptors. For this reason, inhalation of carbon dioxide is one of the strongest known respiratory stimulants. In the presence of mild or moderate hypoxia its effect is increased, but severe hypoxia acts as a central depressant, as in asphyxia. Pyrexia increases the sensitivity of the respiratory centre; all sedative drugs, particularly opiates, depress it.

In some patients with chronic bronchitis the normal sensitivity to increased arterial Pco_2 is greatly reduced. In such patients chronic alveolar underventilation occurs and relief of the concurrent hypoxaemia may, by removing one of the remaining stimuli to breathing, be followed by worsening of the hypercapnia.

Distribution of Gas and Blood in the Lungs

Gas exchange in the lungs is inefficient unless alveolar ventilation is distributed uniformly to different parts of the lungs and is matched by uniform distribution of blood flow. The composition of blood leaving an individual alveolus depends on the composition of the mixed venous blood entering the pulmonary capillaries and the ratio between the ventilation of and blood flow around the alveolus. The possible Values of this ventilation: perfusion ratio ($\dot{V}A/\dot{Q}$) lie between infinity (ventilation but no perfusion) and zero (perfusion but no ventilation). Thus areas of lung with $\dot{V}A/\dot{Q} = \infty$ behave as dead space, giving rise to wasted ventilation, while areas with $\dot{V}A/\dot{Q} = 0$ behave as a physiological right-to-left shunt or venous admixture effect, giving rise to wasted perfusion.

The number of alveoli in the lung and the possible range of ventilation : perfusion ratios is so large that it has become conventional to treat the lungs *as if* they were made up of three compartments:

(a) a compartment normally ventilated and perfused,
(b) physiological dead space, contributed to by all alveoli whose $\dot{V}A/\dot{Q}$ exceeds unity, and including the anatomical dead space,
(c) physiological shunt, contributed to by all alveoli with $\dot{V}A/\dot{Q}$ less than unity, and including the small anatomical or 'true' right-to-left shunts through such pathways as bronchial-pulmonary venous anastomoses.

It follows that if the range of ventilation : perfusion ratios found in the lungs is wider than normal the physiological dead space and physiological shunt will be larger than normal and gas exchange will become less efficient.

Even in the normal lung, distribution of ventilation and perfusion is imperfect. In the erect posture, gravity affects distribution of both ventilation and blood flow, causing regional $\dot{V}A/\dot{Q}$ to be increased at the apices and reduced at the bases of the lungs. In most forms of lung disease, distribution of ventilation and perfusion is further impaired, and it is easy to visualise how pathological mechanisms may have this effect. For example, distribution of ventilation may be impaired by

(a) bronchial or bronchiolar obstruction (tumour, secretions, mucosal oedema, bronchoconstriction),
(b) destruction of elastic tissue (as in emphysema),
(c) pulmonary collapse, consolidation, fibrosis or oedema,
(d) chest wall deformities.

Blood flow is reduced or abolished by pulmonary embolism or thrombosis or by obliteration of areas of the pulmonary capillary bed by necrosis or fibrosis.

The consequences of maldistribution are twofold. First, as has been shown above, an increase in physiological dead space means that a greater total ventilation is needed to achieve a given alveolar ventilation. Secondly, any increase in physiological shunt causes arterial hypoxaemia. Any tendency to hypercapnia due to perfusion of alveoli with low $\dot{V}A/\dot{Q}$ ratios can be compensated for by overventilation of alveoli with high $\dot{V}A/\dot{Q}$ ratios. This preserves a normal or low arterial P_{CO_2}, but the arterial hypoxaemia is little affected. Maldistribution, with areas of low $\dot{V}A/\dot{Q}$ ratio, is therefore the most important single cause of hypoxaemia in disease, and is found in a wide variety of conditions. Fortunately, administration of oxygen raises the alveolar P_{O_2}, even in poorly ventilated alveoli, and corrects the hypoxaemia.

Diffusion of Gases in the Lungs

Oxygen and carbon dioxide move by molecular diffusion in the gas phase along the terminal airways and alveoli, and are also exchanged across the alveolar membrane by diffusion in the liquid phase from a site of higher to one of lower partial pressure. It might be expected that if the alveolar wall became thickened, as in so-called interstitial lung disease, diffusion of gases, particularly of oxygen, would be impaired. However, most conditions which might be expected to have this effect can also give rise to maldistribution of ventilation and blood flow, and analysis suggests that the effect on distribution is usually the chief cause of hypoxaemia in these conditions.

If the area available for gas exchange is reduced (e.g. in emphysema) or if, because of maldistribution, the effective area is reduced, the ability of the lung to transfer gases will also diminish. Such a reduction may not be significant at rest, but may limit the amount of oxygen which can be taken up during exercise and may become a cause of hypoxaemia under these circumstances. It can be corrected by administration of oxygen.

The overall ability of the lung to transfer gases can be readily measured by relating the uptake of carbon monoxide to the alveolar CO pressure when a very weak mixture of the gas is breathed. By this method, values for *gas transfer factor* or *diffusing capacity* of the lung are obtained. The name *gas transfer factor* is preferable, since 'diffusing capacity' carries the implication that diffusion itself is being measured, whereas in fact the measurement is affected by other factors, such as maldistribution.

Common Manifestations of Respiratory Disease

1. **Cough.** This is the most frequent of all respiratory symptoms. It may be short, painful and half-suppressed, as when dry pleurisy accompanies pneumonia. It may be loose and readily productive of sputum, as in bronchiectasis, or paroxysmal, ineffectual and exhausting, as in some cases of chronic bronchitis and asthma. It is usually an early symptom in bronchial carcinoma but may be a relatively late development in pulmonary tuberculosis. Generally it is worse at night or on waking. Often it is aggravated by changes in temperature or weather. The explosive character of a normal cough is lost when laryngeal paralysis is present ('bovine cough'). It is accompanied by stridor (p. 257) in whooping-cough and in the presence of laryngeal or tracheal obstruction.

2. **Sputum.** Purulent sputum is due to bacterial infection in the respiratory tract and is typically seen in acute bronchitis, infective exacerbations of chronic bronchitis, bacterial pneumonia, bronchiectasis and lung abscess. In the last two conditions the sputum may be copious and is sometimes foetid. Mucoid sputum is due to oversecretion of bronchial mucus. It is frequently present in chronic bronchitis and bronchial asthma. In early cases of pulmonary tuberculosis the sputum is mucoid but in advanced cases it is usually purulent.

3. **Haemoptysis.** Haemoptysis of all grades of severity may occur, from slight streaking of the sputum with blood, which is a common symptom in acute and chronic bronchitis, to a massive haemorrhage. Frank haemoptysis, however small, must always be regarded as of potentially serious significance and demands the fullest investigation. Bronchial carcinoma, pulmonary infarction, bronchiectasis, pulmonary tuberculosis and mitral stenosis are the most common causes.

4. **Chest Pain.** Broadly speaking there are two types of chest pain associated with respiratory disease:

(*a*) Central retrosternal pain of a sore, 'scratchy' character made worse by coughing, but not by deep breathing, and usually caused by tracheitis.

(*b*) Lateral chest pain, usually in the pectoral or axillary regions but sometimes in the back, of a sharp, stabbing character, made worse by deep breathing and coughing, and caused by inflammation of the pleura.

The second type of pain, which is referred to as *pleural pain*, is of greater clinical importance than the first and is a common symptom in respiratory disease. The pain is thought to be due to stretching of the inflamed parietal pleura (the visceral pleura is insensitive to painful stimuli) and, as would be expected, it is maximal at the end of inspiration. Patients with pleural pain try to minimise it by taking shallow breaths and by suppressing cough as much as possible. The pain is referred to the area of skin supplied by the same spinal nerves as those supplying the inflamed area of pleura. Usually it is referred to the chest wall, but when the pleura lining the diaphragm is inflamed it may be referred to the cutaneous distribution of the supraclavicular nerves which have the same spinal roots (third and fourth cervical) as the phrenic nerve. Pain in the front and top of the shoulder is thus characteristic of diaphragmatic pleurisy. Pleural pain may also be referred to the anterior abdominal wall, where it may be difficult to distinguish from the pain of an acute abdominal emergency.

A *pleural rub*, which is a common physical sign in dry pleurisy, is due to the rubbing together of pleural surfaces roughed by fibrinous exudate. The effusion of fluid between the layers of the pleura diminishes pain by reducing the movement of the chest wall and abolishes the pleural rub by separating the pleural surfaces.

5. **Dyspnoea.** It has been said that breathing is the only involuntary act which is carried out by voluntary muscle, and this is normally so. Dyspnoea is a subjective sensation in which the effort of breathing reaches consciousness, usually under circumstances in which a normal person would not be aware of his breathing at all. It should be distinguished from *hyperpnoea*, where the volume of ventilation is increased, but no abnormal sensation is felt, and *tachypnoea*, an excessive respiratory rate.

Dyspnoea occurs as a symptom in a wide variety of diseases, and no single theory can adequately explain why it occurs. In conditions where airways resistance is high, such as asthma or chronic bronchitis, the increased mechanical work needed to achieve a given volume of ventilation may account for it. A similar explanation may be given for dyspnoea in diseases causing lung stiffness, such as fibrosing alveolitis, with the added factor that the hypoxaemia which occurs readily during exercise in such diseases may still further increase the drive to breathe. This explanation is less satisfactory for the dyspnoea of heart disease, and still less so for the dyspnoea found in anaemia, where both the lungs and the arterial oxygen pressure are normal. It has been suggested that the sensation arises from 'inappropriateness' between the amount of breathing which the patient feels is needed for a given task and the amount he has in fact to produce—a feeling comparable to that experienced when picking up what seems to be an ordinary rubber ball and finding it is filled with lead. This throws some light on the nature of the sensation, but still leaves its cause obscure.

In mild heart or lung disease, dyspnoea is noticeable only on effort, and the presence of dyspnoea at rest is an indication that the disease is severe or advanced. In conditions such as chronic bronchitis, much of the respiratory reserve may have been lost before a sedentary patient complains of dyspnoea, and measurements of ventilatory capacity show that irreversible airway obstruction is already established. Complaints of dyspnoea should therefore be taken seriously, for although the symptom is commonly found in anxiety states, it also may occur early in diseases such as pulmonary thrombo-embolism or interstitial lung disease at a stage when abnormalities may not be apparent clinically or radiologically. Tests of pulmonary function and objective assessment of exercise capacity are then of value.

6. **Wheeze.** In all forms of generalised obstructive airway disease, particularly bronchial asthma, wheeze is usually a conspicuous symptom. It is a musical sound heard best during expiration, and is associated with numerous rhonchi on auscultation. *Stridor*, on the other hand, occurs when one of the major airways (larynx, trachea or main bronchus) is obstructed. It is a crowing sound heard best during inspiration, and is associated with a persistent low-pitched rhonchus audible all over the chest.

7. **Hypoxaemia.** Hypoxaemia is present if either the pressure or content of oxygen in arterial blood is reduced, and if severe enough may result in visible central cyanosis. The normal arterial Po_2 is over 12 kPa (90 mm Hg) at the age of 20, and falls to around 11 kPa (82 mm Hg) at 60. Above this age a further fall in Po_2 of up to 1·3 kPa (10 mm Hg) occurs on recumbency because of closure of airways in the dependent regions of the lungs. The most frequent and important cause of hypoxaemia in respiratory disease is the presence in the lungs of areas where the distribution of ventilation and perfusion is disturbed and where ventilation is low in relation to perfusion. Hypoxaemia also inevitably results from alveolar under-ventilation (which increases alveolar and arterial Pco_2) or if an atmosphere poor in oxygen is breathed, as at high altitudes. Impairment of diffusion across the alveolar wall may cause hypoxaemia during exercise, but is hardly ever an important factor at rest. The hypoxaemia due to all these causes is reversed by giving oxygen (p. 264). Hypoxaemia due to congenital heart disease (p. 232) or vascular anomalies, with shunting of blood from the right to the left of the circulation past the lungs, is never entirely reversed by oxygen. Hypoxaemia also occurs if the oxygen capacity of the blood is reduced, as in anaemia or carbon monoxide poisoning.

8. **Hypercapnia.** Hypercapnia is present if the pressure of carbon dioxide in the arterial blood ($Paco_2$) exceeds the normal limits (4·8–6·0 kPa or 36–45 mm Hg at rest). Clinically significant hypercapnia occurs when the $Paco_2$ exceeds 7 kPa (52 mm Hg). As has been seen, the finding of a raised $Paco_2$ implies that alveolar ventilation is inadequate in relation to the carbon dioxide production of the body; the causes of hypercapnia are therefore those of alveolar underventilation. Alveoli in which the ventilation:perfusion ratio is low also contribute to hypercapnia.

The finding of hypercapnia also implies either that the normal sensitivity of the respiratory centre to carbon dioxide has been reduced, or that mechanical limitation prevents a normally responsive centre from maintaining adequate alveolar ventilation.

Clinical features suggestive of hypercapnia include peripheral vasodilatation, with warm extremities and bounding pulses, sweating, muscle twitching, headache, drowsiness, coma, retinal venous distension and, rarely, papilloedema.

Unfortunately, none of these signs is specific and the diagnosis must be made by measurement of the pressure of carbon dioxide in arterial or mixed venous blood.

Hypercapnia has three consequences of clinical importance: (*a*) it aggravates hypoxaemia by lowering the pressure of oxygen in the alveolar gas, (*b*) when acute, it increases the arterial hydrogen ion concentration (respiratory acidosis), although renal retention of bicarbonate tends to compensate for this over a period of hours or days (p. 170), and (*c*) when of a severe degree ($Paco_2 > 11$ kPa or 82 mm Hg), it induces drowsiness, which may proceed to coma.

9. **Respiratory Failure.** Respiratory failure is said to occur when the normal pressures of oxygen and carbon dioxide in the blood are no longer maintained. For practical purposes, this means the finding of either a Pao_2 of less than 8 kPa (60 mm Hg) or a $Paco_2$ of more than 7 kPa (52 mm Hg).

It follows that two varieties of respiratory failure can be recognised. In so-called Type 1 respiratory failure the $Paco_2$ is normal or low, but Pao_2 is reduced. Type 2 respiratory failure, in which the $Paco_2$ is elevated and the Pao_2 is reduced, is often termed 'ventilatory failure'. The mechanisms responsible for the hypoxaemia in each type have already been discussed (p. 257), but it must be stressed once more that the finding of hypercapnia means that the normal mechanisms controlling breathing have been upset.

The causes of Type 1 respiratory failure are many, and include any of the pathological causes of maldistribution of ventilation and perfusion in the lungs (p. 254). Among the most important are bronchial asthma, pneumonia, pulmonary collapse, pulmonary oedema, fibrosing and allergic alveolitis, myocardial infarction and shock.

The most common pulmonary cause of ventilatory failure is chronic bronchitis, particularly when complicated by acute respiratory infection. Other causes include respiratory paralysis (p. 723), deformities of the chest such as severe kyphoscoliosis, and depression of the respiratory centre, particularly by narcotic or sedative drugs.

The treatment of Type 1 respiratory failure, in which hypoxaemia is not accompanied by hypercapnia, must always include oxygen, which can be given without strict control of the inspired concentration. In addition, treatment appropriate to the particular cause of the failure must be given. Treatment of ventilatory failure is discussed on page 266.

10. **Clubbing of the Fingers and Toes.** The cause of clubbing, which is most readily recognised in the fingers, is not known but it is frequently found in patients with certain types of respiratory disease, notably lung cancer, chronic intrathoracic suppuration and fibrosing alveolitis. It does not occur in chronic bronchitis or emphysema unless there is accompanying pulmonary suppuration or if the patient has developed a tumour, nor in pulmonary tuberculosis except in advanced cases.

Clubbing also occurs in certain other conditions. It is usually present in infective endocarditis and cyanotic congenital heart disease; it is found occasionally in Crohn's disease, malabsorption syndrome and cirrhosis of the liver, and rarely in healthy subjects as a familial trait. The earliest indication of finger clubbing is an abnormal degree of fluctuation at the bases of the nails. With more advanced clubbing there is, in addition, an increase in the curvature of the nails and bulbous swelling of the finger tips.

The Investigation of Respiratory Disease

In most respiratory diseases a reasonably accurate diagnosis can be made from the history and physical examination alone, but in several important conditions, notably pulmonary tuberculosis and bronchial carcinoma, these methods are in-adequate and the diagnosis can be confirmed or excluded only by more specialised procedures such as radiological, bacteriological or endoscopic examination. In taking the history, particular enquiry must always be made about symptoms such as cough, sputum, haemoptysis, pain, breathlessness, wheeze and nasal discharge. The patient must also be asked about any previous respiratory illness, about any family history of tuberculosis and about any occupational exposure to dust.

Physical Examination

Before the chest itself is examined the temperature should be taken, and a note made of the rate and character of breathing, the type and severity of any cough and the amount and character of the sputum. In addition, particular care must be taken to determine whether or not there is cyanosis, clubbing of the fingers or enlargement of the supraclavicular lymph nodes, these features being of special significance in respiratory disease.

The upper respiratory tract should be examined next, with particular regard to nasal discharge or obstruction, oral sepsis, and infection or enlargement of the tonsils. The presence of hoarseness or a 'bovine' cough would draw attention to the need for laryngoscopic examination (p. 262). The chest wall should then be carefully inspected for soft tissue abnormalities such as cutaneous lesions, sub-cutaneous swellings (including lumps in the breast) and bulging or indrawing of in-tercostal spaces, and for skeletal abnormalities such as an increase in the antero-posterior diameter of the chest relative to its lateral diameter. The position of the trachea and of the apex beat should be noted and the chest expansion measured. Rib movement, vocal fremitus and the percussion note should be compared in equivalent positions on the two sides of the chest. The terms used to describe the various types of percussion note are: hyper-resonant, normal, impaired, dull and stony dull. At auscultation, attention should be directed in turn to the breath sounds, added sounds and vocal resonance.

Breath Sounds. The following terms are used: vesicular, vesicular with prolonged expiration, diminished vesicular, absent breath sounds, high-pitched bronchial ('tubular'), low-pitched bronchial (including 'amphoric') breath sounds.

Added Sounds
(i) *Rhonchi* are produced by narrowing of the lumen of the bronchi by spasm of bronchial muscle, swelling of bronchial mucosa or tenacious mucus adherent to bronchial walls. Rhonchi may be high-pitched, medium-pitched or low-pitched, according to the size of the bronchi in which the sounds are produced.

(ii) *Crepitations* are usually produced by secretion lying within alveoli, bronchi or pulmonary cavities. They may be fine, medium or coarse in quality, and may either disappear or become more numerous after coughing. Crackling cre-pitations, unaltered by coughing, are a feature of interstitial lung disease (p. 328).

(iii) *Pleural rub* is a diagnostic sign of pleural inflammation. It is a grating or creaking sound, unaltered by coughing, audible during both inspiration and expiration.

Vocal Resonance. The following terms are used: normal, increased, diminished or absent vocal resonance, aegophony, whispering pectoriloquy.

THE INTERPRETATION OF PHYSICAL SIGNS

Certain groups of physical signs are typically associated with certain pathological changes in the lungs and pleura. Such changes are not necessarily specific for one particular disease. For example, consolidation may occur in pneumonia or tuberculosis, and fluid may be present in the pleural space in tuberculous pleurisy, empyema or congestive cardiac failure. Each group of physical signs should therefore be correlated with the gross pathological lesion by which the signs are produced rather than with any specific disease, the diagnosis of which depends on an analysis of all the clinical and other evidence.

The physical signs of the more common lesions are shown on Table 7.1

SPECIAL METHODS OF INVESTIGATION

1. Radiological Examination of the Chest. Although radiological examination of the chest is widely employed as a primary diagnostic measure it should not be regarded as a short-cut to diagnosis. It may, however, provide:

(*a*) Evidence of a lesion within the thorax too small to be detected by physical examination or which because of its nature or situation does not give rise to abnormal physical signs, e.g. early tuberculosis or tumour.

(*b*) A more accurate assessment of the size and position of pulmonary, pleural and mediastinal lesions than can be obtained from physical examination. Lateral as well as postero-anterior radiographs are necessary for this purpose.

(*c*) More accurate information about the nature of the lesions than can be obtained from physical examination. *Tomography* is of particular value in this respect as it provides better definition of intrathoracic lesions, and facilitates the recognition of features such as cavitation, calcification and bronchial obstruction.

(*d*) Accurate information regarding the size, shape and position of the heart.

(*e*) Information regarding the position and function of the diaphragm, which can be observed radiologically by the technique of radioscopy.

(*f*) Evidence of disease or injury affecting the bony structures of the thorax.

It is important to remember that in some diseases, such as bronchitis and asthma, the chest radiograph may be normal.

Radioisotope scanning is of particular value in pulmonary infarction (p. 227).

2. Bacteriological and Cytological Examination

(*a*) SPUTUM. Bacteriological examination of the sputum seldom provides conclusive diagnostic information except when tubercle bacilli are isolated. The findings in other circumstances must be interpreted in conjunction with the results of clinical and, if necessary, radiological examination.

Cytological examination, by demonstrating cancer cells in the sputum, may enable a diagnosis of bronchial carcinoma to be made.

(*b*) PLEURAL FLUID. This should always be examined cytologically and bacteriologically. A special search should be made for tubercle bacilli if the fluid is serous and for pyogenic organisms and tubercle bacilli if it is purulent. When malignant disease is suspected, especially if the fluid is blood-stained, it should also be examined histologically for cancer cells.

Table 7.1   Summary of typical physical signs in the more common respiratory diseases

Pathological Process	Movement of Chest Wall	Mediastinal Displacement	Percussion Note	Breath Sounds	Vocal Resonance	Accompaniments
Consolidation as in lobar pneumonia	Reduced on side affected	None	Dull	High-pitched bronchial	Increased (with aegophony) Whispering pectoriloquy	Fine crepitations early Coarse crepitations later
Collapse due to obstruction of major bronchus	Reduced on side affected	Towards lesion	Dull	Diminished or absent	Reduced or absent	None
Collapse due to peripheral bronchial obstruction	Reduced on side affected	Towards lesion	Dull	High-pitched bronchial	Increased (with aegophony) Whispering pectoriloquy	None early— coarse crepitations later
Localised fibrosis and/or bronchiectasis	Slightly reduced on side affected	Towards lesion	Impaired	Low-pitched bronchial	Increased	Coarse crepitations
Cavitation (typical signs only when cavity is large and linked with bronchus)	Slightly reduced on side affected	None, or towards lesion	Impaired	'Amphoric' bronchial	Increased Whispering pectoriloquy	Coarse crepitations
Pleural effusion Empyema	Reduced or absent (depending on size) on side affected	Towards opposite side	Stony dull	Diminished or absent (occasionally high-pitched bronchial)	Reduced or absent (occasionally increased with aegophony)	Pleural rub in some cases (above effusion)
Pneumothorax	Reduced or absent (depending on size) on side affected	Towards opposite side	Normal or hyper-resonant	Diminished or absent (occasionally faint high-pitched bronchial)	Reduced or absent	Tinkling crepitations when fluid present
Bronchitis: Acute Chronic	Normal or symmetrically diminished	None	Normal	Vesicular with prolonged expiration	Normal	Rhonchi, usually with some coarse crepitations
Bronchial asthma	Symmetrically diminished	None	Normal	Vesicular with prolonged expiration	Normal or diminished	Rhonchi, mainly expiratory and high-pitched
Diffuse lobular pneumonia	Symmetrically diminished	None	May be impaired	Usually harsh vesicular with prolonged expiration	Normal	Rhonchi and coarse crepitations
Diffuse pulmonary emphysema	Symmetrically diminished	None	Normal	Diminished vesicular with prolonged expiration	Normal or reduced	Rhonchi and coarse crepitations from associated bronchitis
Interstitial lung disease	Symmetrically diminished	None	Normal	Harsh vesicular with prolonged expiration	Usually increased	Crackling crepitations uninfluenced by coughing

(From *Clinical Examination*, 4th ed. 1976. Macleod, J. Edinburgh: Churchill Livingstone.)

3. **Serological Examination.** This may be of value in the diagnosis of virus infections (p. 268) and some allergic disorders (p. 307).

4. **Haematological Examination.** Estimation of the total and differential leucocyte count may help to distinguish pyogenic infection from tuberculous or viral infection.

5. **Skin Tests.** The tuberculin test (p. 287) and Kveim test (p. 329) may be of value in the diagnosis of tuberculosis and sarcoidosis respectively. Skin sensitivity tests (p. 302) are useful in the investigation of allergic diseases.

6. **Laryngoscopy.** The larynx is inspected either by means of a mirror placed in front of the uvula (*indirect* laryngoscopy) or through an illuminated metal tube (*direct* laryngoscopy).

7. **Bronchoscopy.** The trachea and larger bronchi are inspected by a bronchoscope of either the rigid or the fibreoptic type. Tissue can be removed for histological examination (bronchial biopsy). The range of vision with the rigid instrument extends to the origins of all segmental bronchi but more peripheral lesions can be detected with the fibreoptic bronchoscope.

8. **Bronchography.** The bronchi are outlined by contrast medium instilled into the trachea, and chest radiographs (bronchograms) are then taken.

9. **Lymph Node Biopsy.** Histological examination of an enlarged lymph node removed from the neck or axilla, or from the mediastinum by the technique of *mediastinoscopy*, may provide a firm diagnosis in conditions such as bronchial carcinoma, tuberculosis, reticulosis and sarcoidosis.

10. **Pleural Biopsy.** In patients with pleural effusion it is possible to obtain a specimen of parietal pleura suitable for histological examination by means of Abrams' pleural biopsy 'punch'. This procedure is simple and safe, and may be of considerable value in determining the cause of a pleural effusion.
   If it is unsuccessful, the pleural surfaces can be inspected with a thoracoscope inserted through an intercostal space, and if a pleural lesion is seen, a biopsy can be performed under telescopic vision.

11. **Lung Biopsy.** When a diagnosis cannot be made in any other way it may be necessary to obtain a specimen of lung tissue for histological examination either by formal thoracotomy, by needle biopsy through the chest wall or by transbronchial lung biopsy via a fibreoptic bronchoscope.

12. **Tests of Pulmonary Function.** Many of the procedures mentioned above are of great assistance in arriving at a pathological diagnosis, but investigations of a different type are necessary to determine the effects of disease on pulmonary function and to assess the response to therapy (p. 302). Disturbances of the mechanical properties of the lungs, of ventilation, of control of breathing, of the distribution of ventilation and perfusion within the lungs and of diffusing capacity can all be measured. Some of the tests require a high degree of skill and elaborate apparatus, but others are simple routine procedures which can be undertaken by any doctor without special training.

(*a*) ESTIMATION OF VENTILATORY CAPACITY. The patient is asked to take in as deep a breath as possible and then expel it as hard and as fast as possible. If the forced expiration is made into a recording spirometer of low resistance and low inertia, the *forced expiratory volume* in the standard time of 1 second (FEV_1) can be measured; if the forced expiration is continued till no more gas can be expelled, the *forced vital capacity* (FVC) is measured. The ratio of these two volumes may be expressed as a percentage (FEV/FVC %); normal people can expel between 80 and 65 per cent of the FVC in 1 second, depending on age and sex.

In diseases which cause narrowing of the airways during expiration, such as asthma and chronic bronchitis, the FEV/FVC % is reduced, sometimes to 40 per cent or less. This is due to a greater reduction in FEV than in FVC, and this type of ventilatory defect is called '*obstructive*'. In diseases such as interstitial lung disease or ankylosing spondylitis, which make the lungs or chest wall more rigid, FEV and FVC are reduced in the same proportion and FEV/FVC % is normal, as the airways are relatively unaffected. This is called a '*restrictive*' ventilatory defect. Discovery of airways obstruction is an indication to repeat the spirometric measurements after a bronchodilator drug (p. 302) has been given; reversibility of airways obstruction is found in asthma and in some patients with chronic bronchitis.

During forced expiration, the *peak expiratory flow* (PEF) can be measured by apparatus which is simpler and cheaper than the average spirometer. PEF is reduced in conditions causing airways obstruction, and is a good indicator of the severity of the obstruction. The measurement has therefore become popular in clinical practice because of its speed and simplicity. PEF is little affected by conditions causing a restrictive type of ventilatory defect, and is therefore of no value in diagnosing or assessing them.

Even if no apparatus other than a watch and stethoscope is available, forced expiration can still be used to assess ventilatory capacity. Normal people can empty their chest from full inspiration in 4 seconds or less. Prolongation of the *forced expiratory time* (FET) to more than 6 seconds indicates airways obstruction and a reduction in FEV/FVC % to less than 50 per cent. The end-point of FET is detected by placing the chest-piece of a stethoscope over the trachea in the suprasternal notch.

(*b*) ANALYSIS OF ARTERIAL BLOOD. Apparatus for arterial blood-gas analysis is now available in most hospitals, but the estimations require skill. Knowledge of the $Paco_2$ provides the answer to the question, 'Is the patient breathing enough?', and is of particular value in the management of ventilatory failure (p. 266). If the arterial hydrogen ion concentration (activity) or pH and the $Paco_2$ are known, it is often possible to deduce the type of any disturbance of acid:base balance (p. 270) which may be present. Knowledge of the Pao_2 or arterial oxygen saturation allows accurate assessment of hypoxaemia (p. 257) and of the effects of oxygen therapy (p. 264).

These simple measurements are thus of value in distinguishing between some types of respiratory disorder, as well as in providing an index of their severity. Serial measurements are valuable in following changes in pulmonary function, whether occurring spontaneously or in response to treatment.

The Treatment of Respiratory Disease

Infection

Bacterial Infection. The chemotherapy of bacterial infection of the bronchi, lungs and pleura will be described in the sections on individual diseases. Certain general principles are, however, applicable to all cases.

Before any treatment is started a specimen of sputum, a laryngeal swab (if there is no sputum) or a specimen of pleural fluid should be sent for bacteriological examination.

In acute bacterial infections it is usually necessary to begin chemotherapy before the results of bacteriological examination are available. The choice of antibiotic in these circumstances is based on clinical impressions of the nature and severity of the illness.

If a clinical diagnosis of acute bronchitis, pneumonia or empyema is made and the patient is not seriously ill or if the acute infection is a complication of chronic bronchitis, asthma or bronchiectasis, ampicillin should be given initially. If the patient is gravely ill and there is any reason to suspect infection with *Staph. pyogenes*, an antibiotic to which that organism is unlikely to be resistant, e.g. cloxacillin must be added.

As soon as the results of bacteriological examination and sensitivity tests are received, modifications in antibiotic therapy can be made, if necessary.

Factors which interfere with the response to antibiotics must be corrected, e.g. an empyema must be aspirated or drained, and bronchiectatic cavities and lung abscesses must be kept dry by postural drainage.

Viral Infection. The viruses which infect the respiratory tract are uninfluenced by chemotherapy, but secondary bacterial infection, which occurs in many cases, often requires treatment with an appropriate antibiotic. Infection caused by small bacteria, such as coxiella, mycoplasma and chlamydia, usually responds to tetracycline.

Fungal Infection. The treatment of respiratory diseases caused by fungi is described on page 299.

Oxygen Therapy

Oxygen is present in the air at a concentration of 21 per cent and at sea level the pressure of oxygen in inspired tracheal air is almost 20 kPa (150 mm Hg). Arterial blood of normal haemoglobin concentration contains about 9 mmol oxygen per litre (20 ml/100 ml); at a Pao_2 of 13·5 kPa (100 mm Hg) 135 μmol oxygen per litre (0·3 ml/100 ml) are dissolved in the plasma (i.e. a solubility of 10 μmol/kPa) and the rest is bound to haemoglobin.

Therapeutic Indications. The objectives of oxygen therapy are (1) to overcome the reduced pressure and quantity of oxygen in the blood found in hypoxaemia, and (2) to increase the quantity of oxygen carried in solution in the plasma even when the haemoglobin is fully saturated. The causes of hypoxaemia have already been discussed (p. 257). Raising the alveolar Po_2 by administration of oxygen overcomes the hypoxaemia consequent upon a high alveolar Pco_2; when the oxygen pressure is raised in alveoli which are poorly ventilated but perfused, the blood perfusing them becomes fully saturated and the hypoxaemia due to maldistribution of ventilation and perfusion is overcome. A raised alveolar Po_2 will also correct hypoxaemia caused by limitation of diffusing capacity.

The cause of hypoxaemia least susceptible to oxygen therapy is right-to-left shunting, either through circulatory channels by-passing the lungs, or through parts of the lungs in which the alveoli are completely unventilated and thus inaccessible to inspired oxygen. The increased amounts of dissolved oxygen carried by blood which has perfused alveoli with a high Po_2 can saturate the haemoglobin in small quantities of shunted blood; persistence of cyanosis when pure oxygen is breathed indicates that the shunt is larger than 20 per cent of the cardiac output. This accounts for the observation that the cyanosis of congenital heart disease is not relieved by oxygen.

In anaemia or in heart failure the arterial blood may be normally saturated with oxygen when air is breathed, but the delivery of oxygen to the tissues is reduced. In these conditions oxygen therapy may benefit seriously ill patients by increasing the amount of dissolved oxygen in the blood. In carbon monoxide poisoning (p. 809) high pressures of oxygen favour the dissociation of carboxyhaemoglobin; such pressures may be achieved in hyperbaric chambers in which oxygen is breathed at a pressure of two atmospheres, or by inhalation of as high a concentration of oxygen as possible at atmospheric pressure.

Adverse Effects. Pure oxygen is both irritant and toxic if it is inhaled for more than a few hours. Premature infants develop retrolental fibroplasia if exposed to excessive concentrations of oxygen. Normal subjects notice cough and bronchial irritation, and in patients ventilated with high concentrations of oxygen for several days pulmonary oedema and consolidation ('white lung') may occur. If such patients require oxygen it is important to give, whenever possible, an inspired concentration which corrects hypoxaemia but does not exceed 60 to 70 per cent.

Technique of Oxygen Administration. Hypoxaemia is such a common consequence of respiratory diseases that oxygen may well be the most frequently prescribed 'drug' used in their treatment. It is important that prescriptions for oxygen should be in writing, and that flow rates or concentrations should be clearly specified. Administration of oxygen should be continuous; there is now no place for deliberate intermittent oxygen therapy, though continuous therapy may prove hard to maintain in confused or restless patients. The risk of fire should never be forgotten when any concentration of oxygen above atmospheric is given, and special precautions are needed in hyperbaric chambers.

Oxygen masks are of two types: 1. Those which are designed to produce a high concentration of O_2 in the inspired air. Examples of this type of mask are the Polymask (British Oxygen Co. Ltd.) and the M.C. mask (Medical and Industrial Equipment Ltd.), both of which deliver about 60 per cent O_2 when the flow rate is 4–6 l per min.

2. Those which are designed to produce slight O_2 enrichment of the inspired air and do not permit the rebreathing of expired CO_2. Examples of this type of mask are the Edinburgh mask (British Oxygen Co. Ltd.) and the Ventimask (Vickers Limited Medical Group). With the Edinburgh mask adjustments of the O_2 flow rate can provide inspired O_2 concentrations at any level between 23 and 35 per cent. The Ventimask is available in three models, which deliver 24, 28 and 35 per cent O_2 respectively.

Nasal Cannulae. Double nasal cannulae fit comfortably into the nostrils. Their main advantages are that they do not permit rebreathing of CO_2 and do not interfere with eating, drinking and the wearing of spectacles. The inspired O_2 concentration they provide is somewhat unpredictable, but an O_2 flow rate of 2 l/min. will usually raise it to about 30 per cent. They are of particular value if oxygen is administered for long periods.

Oxygen Tent. This is cumbersome, hampers nursing and physiotherapy and provides an extremely variable O_2 concentration because of leaks and repeated access by attendants. It has a place in the treatment of children but its use in adults has now been abandoned.

Humidification. When Polymasks or M.C. masks are used, the oxygen must be humidified, either by passing it over the surface of warm water in an electrically heated canister (East-Radcliffe humidifier) or through a nebuliser. This is not necessary with Edinburgh masks, Ventimasks or nasal cannulae, as a high proportion of atmospheric air is mixed with the oxygen in these devices.

Treatment of Ventilatory Failure

1. **Acute Ventilatory Failure.** A clear airway is essential. In conscious patients this can often be secured and maintained by determined efforts to encourage expectoration, every 15 minutes or so at first, under the strict supervision of a doctor, nurse or physiotherapist. If this policy fails, and particularly if the patient has become confused or unconscious, a cuffed endotracheal tube should be inserted through the mouth or nose under general anaesthesia, and connected to a mechanical ventilator. At frequent intervals the trachea and bronchi should be cleared of secretions by aspiration through a soft catheter. Most patients are intolerant of artificial ventilation in the early stages and require heavy sedation with opiates. The endotracheal tube can be left in place for 3 or 4 days while treatment is continued. Some patients recover adequate spontaneous ventilation before the tube is due to be removed, but others require tracheostomy to allow tracheobronchial aspiration and mechanical ventilation to be continued for a longer period. These intensive methods of resuscitation are contraindicated in patients who have had severe respiratory disability for several months before the onset of ventilatory failure. Bronchoscopic aspiration may be of value as an initial measure to clear the airways of secretion, and if the patient can thereafter cough effectively tracheal intubation may not be required.

During mechanical ventilation through an endotracheal tube the depressant effect of a high Pao_2 on respiration can be ignored, and there is no objection to ventilating the patient with a high concentration (up to 60 per cent) of O_2. When artificial ventilation is stopped, however, or in cases where it has not been employed, increasing hypercapnia is a potential hazard of O_2 administration, and the concentration of O_2 in the inspired air should initially be kept below 30 per cent by using a Ventimask, an Edinburgh mask or a double nasal cannula (p. 265). It is seldom necessary or desirable to increase the inspired O_2 concentration above this level. When O_2, even in a concentration of 30 per cent or less, is being administered to patients with acute ventilatory failure, the Pao_2, $Paco_2$ and hydrogen-ion concentration or pH should be measured at regular intervals. An indwelling cannula in the brachial or radial artery can conveniently and safely be used for obtaining blood samples. If a steady increase in $Paco_2$ is accompanied by clinical deterioration and/or by a rise in hydrogen-ion concentration above 60 nmol/litre (fall in pH below 7·25 units), this is another indication for artificial ventilation, either short-term via an endotracheal tube or long-term via a tracheostomy tube. The disturbances in Pao_2, $Paco_2$ and pH can usually be corrected within 24 hours, but it may be several days before the patient is capable of maintaining a sufficiently high level of alveolar ventilation to allow him to dispense with mechanical assistance.

In all cases respiratory infection should be treated (p. 264). Water and electrolyte balance should be maintained, by intravenous infusion if necessary, as dehydration increases the viscosity of bronchial mucus and makes it difficult to dislodge.

Analeptic drugs have a limited but useful place in treatment. Nikethamide (2–4 ml of a 25 per cent solution 1 to 2 hourly) or doxapram (infusions of up to 3 mg/min.) given intravenously for 24 hours, may successfully tide the patient over a period of underventilation and obviate the need for protracted intubation or tracheostomy, particularly if bronchial secretions are not present in large amounts. Although analeptic drugs seldom produce sustained stimulation of respiration, they may improve the level of consciousness and thus restore effective expectoration. Should sedation be necessary, diazepam is probably the drug least liable to depress respiration.

2. **Chronic Ventilatory Failure.** Many patients with progressive respiratory disease eventually enter a state in which Pao_2 and $Paco_2$ never return to normal. In such patients, attempts to increase ventilation by orally administered drugs (such as the carbonic anhydrase inhibitor, dichlorphenamide) are sometimes advocated. However, there is no clear evidence that such treatment is beneficial and there is a possibility of doing harm. At present, therefore, treatment should be directed to the prevention of acute respiratory infections, the relief of airways obstruction and the management of right ventricular failure. In chronic ventilatory failure a worthwhile increase in exercise tolerance has been shown to result from the use of light, portable oxygen equipment. The provision of such equipment for all patients who could derive benefit from it presents a formidable problem. However, patients confined to their homes may be helped by the intermittent use of low concentrations of oxygen obtained from a static supply; it must be admitted that such benefit may often be psychological rather than physical. The potential benefits of continuous low-concentration oxygen therapy in the home are still under investigation.

Symptomatic Treatment in Respiratory Disease

Cough, when productive of sputum, should be encouraged and not suppressed. Those who are physically weak should be exhorted at regular intervals to clear their bronchi of secretion. Those with bronchiectasis or lung abscess should practise postural drainage, and those with tenacious sputum should be given hot drinks and inhalations of either steam or nebulised water to help them to bring it up more easily.

Unproductive, distressing cough should be suppressed. Demulcent lozenges are occasionally effective, but many patients require antitussive drugs, especially if sleep is disturbed by coughing. The two most effective preparations, suitable for general use in bronchitis, pneumonia, bronchial carcinoma and pulmonary tuberculosis, are pholcodine linctus (B.P.C.), and methadone linctus (B.P.C.), each given in a dose of 5–10 ml.

Airways obstruction in bronchitis and asthma is treated by bronchodilator drugs (p. 303) and in some cases by corticosteroids given by mouth or by inhalation (p. 304).

Chest Pain. Pleural pain can usually be relieved by the application of a rubber hot-water bottle or by an electric heating pad to the chest wall, supplemented by an analgesic and, if necessary, by an antitussive drug. Mild analgesics, such as acetylsalicylic acid, or codeine compound tablets (B.P.C.), are adequate in most cases but a few patients may require pethidine, 50–100 mg by mouth or intramuscular injection, or even morphine, 10–15 mg subcutaneously. Opiates must, however, be avoided in patients with poor respiratory function and in those who have difficulty in coughing up sputum.

The pain of acute tracheitis usually responds to the application of heat to the front of the chest, combined with inhalations of steam medicated with benzoin (p. 272). Pain due to invasion of the chest wall by a malignant tumour, if not relieved by radiotherapy, usually demands a powerful analgesic such as pethidine or morphine, given by injection. In advanced cases these drugs may become ineffective and neurosurgical measures may be required for the relief of intractable pain.

INFECTIONS OF THE RESPIRATORY SYSTEM

Infections of the respiratory tract may be caused by large and small bacteria, by viruses and by fungi. 'Small' bacteria include coxiella causing Q-fever, mycoplasma causing pneumonia, and chlamydia causing psittacosis and ornithosis. The patterns of illness produced by small bacteria and viruses are summarised in Table 7.2, page 270. Pulmonary tuberculosis and diseases caused by fungi are described in separate sections.

The number of viruses known to cause respiratory infection is continually increasing. They are universally distributed, of high infectivity and thus of great economic importance. The early diagnosis of viral infection is difficult because the excretion of some viruses is of short duration and the organisms die rapidly unless laboratory examination is undertaken quickly. Nasal and pharyngeal washings give a higher yield than throat swabs. Enteroviruses may be isolated from faeces over a longer period. Viral isolations are made on tissue cultures in various media including eggs and monkey kidney. More frequently a retrospective diagnosis is made from serological studies by neutralisation or complement-fixation tests. Serum specimens should be taken at the beginning of the illness and 10 to 14 days later. A four-fold rise in titre suggests a recent infection. Fluorescent antibody tests or electron microscopy may provide more rapid diagnosis in the future.

Acute Coryza (Common Cold)

Aetiology. The early features are produced by primary infection of the nose and nasopharynx by a number of viruses (Table 7.2, p. 270), especially the rhinoviruses. Subsequent bacterial infection by *Strept. pneumoniae*, *H. influenzae* or staphylococci is usual. Immunity is short-lived and is specific for each virus.

Clinical Features. The onset is usually sudden with a tickling sensation in the nose accompanied by sneezing. The throat often feels dry and sore, the head feels 'stuffed', the eyes smart and there is a profuse watery nasal discharge. These symptoms last for 1 to 2 days, after which, with secondary infection, the secretion becomes thick and purulent, and impedes nasal breathing.

Coryza may be complicated by sinusitis when there is usually more systemic upset. Headache is often present and may be severe, and there may be pain or discomfort over the face. Localised tenderness on palpation over the maxillary and frontal sinuses may be elicited. Sinus infection is liable to become chronic, particularly in the maxillary sinuses, causing persistent purulent discharge from the front and back of the nose, often accompanied by nasal obstruction and headaches.

Other complications are infections of the lower respiratory tract, catarrh of the auditory tubes causing deafness, and otitis media, causing fever and aural pain.

Frequent attacks of sneezing and watery rhinorrhoea, without systemic upset, suggest nasal allergy (p. 299) rather than viral infection.

Treatment. The congestion and excessive secretion of the nasal mucous membrane may be reduced by the periodic use of 1 per cent ephedrine in normal saline either sprayed or dropped into the nose. Steam medicated with benzoin inhalation or menthol and benzoin inhalation, 1 teaspoonful to 1 pint of boiling water, is beneficial, especially if the nasal sinuses are involved or there is obstruction of the auditory tubes. Antibiotic therapy is required only for the treatment of complications.

The spread of coryza to others can be reduced by voluntary isolation of patients for 2 to 3 days during the early, highly infectious stage.

Pharyngoconjunctival Fever

The pharyngeal syndrome, which is sometimes accompanied by conjunctivitis particularly amongst schoolchildren in spring and summer and in holiday camps, may be caused by several viruses (Table 7.2, p. 270) especially adenoviruses. *Herpangina* may occur in infections with Coxsackie A viruses.

Conjunctivitis may be the first symptom, but sore throat is the dominant feature and may be slight or severe. The pharynx, tonsils and adenoids become inflamed and yellow exudate may be present. Cervical lymph nodes are enlarged and tender. The degree of constitutional symptoms—shivering, malaise, anorexia, headache and fever—is variable. In herpangina, typical vesicles, which may become punched-out ulcers, are present on the fauces. Acute streptococcal sore throat may be clinically indistinguishable from pharyngoconjunctival fever, but *Strept. pyogenes* will be isolated from such cases. Infectious mononucleosis (p. 615) may also be difficult to differentiate from the pharyngeal syndrome in the early stages.

Treatment. Antibiotics are unnecessary. Gargles are often prescribed but are ineffective. Lozenges containing local anaesthetic, e.g. benzocaine compound lozenges are helpful when the throat is painful. A mild analgesic such as codeine compound tablets relieves systemic symptoms.

Acute Laryngotracheobronchitis

This illness, which is particularly serious in very young children because of the small calibre of their airways, may be caused by several viruses (Table 7.2). Superinfection with bacteria, especially *Strept. pyogenes* and staphylococci, may occur. The mucosa is intensely inflamed, the secretions are extremely tenacious and fibrinous casts of the bronchi may form.

The initial symptoms may be those of the common cold (p. 268). These are followed by severe and sometimes violent cough which may be paroxysmal, accompanied by dyspnoea and stridor ('croup'), contraction of accessory muscles and indrawing of intercostal spaces. The child may be cyanosed, and asphyxia may occur if appropriate treatment is not given.

Treatment. Warm humid air should be supplied by means of a steam kettle or

Table 7.2   Respiratory disorders caused by viruses, chlamydia, Mycoplasma and Coxiella

Aetiological Agent	Clinical Syndrome (Excluding Pneumonia)	Pneumonia
Adenoviruses	Acute coryza Pharyngoconjunctival fever Acute laryngitis	Occasional epidemics: cold agglutinins present
Coxsackie virus	Pharyngoconjunctival fever Herpangina	
Echoviruses	Acute coryza Pharyngoconjunctival fever	
Influenza virus A, B, (C)	Epidemic influenza Acute laryngotracheobronchitis (croup)	Primary rare: usually secondary infection with bacteria
Parainfluenza virus	Acute coryza Acute laryngotracheobronchitis (croup)	Primary rare: usually secondary infection with bacteria
Respiratory syncytial (RS) virus	Acute coryza Acute laryngotracheobronchitis (croup)	May cause severe and sometimes fatal bronchiolitis and pneumonia in infants
Rhinoviruses	Acute coryza	
Measles	Described on p. 81	Primary rare: usually secondary infection with bacteria
Chickenpox	Described on p. 84	Usually primary viral pneumonia: almost exclusively in adults
Chlamydia (psittacosis-ornithosis)		Primary pneumonia
Mycoplasma pneumoniae		Commonly in young adults: epidemics in institutions
Coxiella burneti (Q-fever)		Primary pneumonia

tent. Clearing of secretions is of the utmost importance, and bronchoscopy and tracheostomy may be required as life-saving measures. As bacterial superinfection is often present, an antibiotic should be given. Attention to adequate hydration is also important and oxygen therapy may be necessary.

Influenza

Influenza is a specific acute illness caused by a group of myoxviruses. It occurs in epidemics, and occasionally pandemics, often explosive in nature.

Aetiology. Three types of virus are described, A, B and C. Influenza A is responsible for the pandemics which occur from time to time. At least four strains have been identified and the so-called 'Asian' strain has been responsible for recent epidemics. Influenza B is usually associated with smaller and less virulent epidemics. The C virus is found only rarely. The immunity which follows is type-specific and of short duration. This causes problems in securing effective immunisation.

Clinical Features. The incubation period is 1 or 2 days. The illness starts suddenly with malaise, headache, pain in the back and limbs, anorexia and sometimes nausea and vomiting. Pyrexia to 39°C (102°F) remits for 2 or 3 days, with chills and shivering but seldom rigors. The face is flushed, conjunctivae suffused and fauces hyperaemic with prominent lymphoid follicles. The pulse is rapid. There is often leucopenia ($2 \cdot 0$–$4 \cdot 0 \times 10^9/l$). There may be a harsh unproductive cough, without physical signs over the lungs. At this stage the case is indistinguishable clinically from a severe upper respiratory infection due to other respiratory viruses. The disease may spread rapidly throughout a household or institution.

During epidemics the diagnosis is usually easy. Most sporadic cases are identifiable only as respiratory virus infections unless the virus is isolated or serological tests for specific antibodies are positive.

Course and Complications. In many cases no further symptoms develop and recovery ensues within 3 to 5 days. The disease may, however, be complicated by tracheitis, bronchitis, bronchiolitis and lobular pneumonia. Secondary bacterial invasion by *Strept. pneumoniae*, *H. influenzae* and occasionally *Staph. pyogenes* causes these complications.

Toxic *cardiomyopathy* may cause sudden death, especially when there is pre-existing cardiac disease. *Encephalitis* and *postinfluenzal demyelinating encephalopathy* are rare complications. *Postinfluenzal asthenia* and *depression* are common, often marked, and may last for a week or two.

Treatment and Prevention. The patient should be kept in bed until the fever has subsided. A mild analgesic usually relieves the headache and backache. A linctus containing pholcodine or methadone (p. 267) may be used to suppress unproductive cough. The treatment of complications such as bronchitis (p. 272) and pneumonia (p. 281) is dealt with later.

Immunity is type-specific and if the antigenic constitution of an epidemic can be detected early, a specific vaccine may give about 70 per cent protection. Annual winter vaccination is recommended for patients suffering from chronic pulmonary, cardiac or renal disease.

Acute Catarrhal Laryngitis

Acute catarrhal laryngitis usually occurs either as a complication of coryza or as a manifestation of one of the infectious fevers, e.g. measles. It may also be caused by the inhalation of irritant gases. The laryngeal mucous membrane is swollen, congested and coated with mucus. Microscopically it is infiltrated with inflammatory cells. Rarely, in children, there may be a membranous exudate resembling diphtheria.

The throat is dry and sore. The voice is at first hoarse and then reduced to a whisper. Speaking may be painful. There is an irritating, nonproductive cough, but the general upset is usually mild. In children the small laryngeal opening may be obstructed by viscid secretion and spasm, giving rise to 'croup' (p. 269).

Acute laryngitis usually clears up in a few days, but if frequently repeated it may predispose to chronic laryngitis. Downward spread of the infection may cause tracheitis, bronchitis, or even pneumonia.

Treatment. The patient must be put to bed in a warm room and, to rest the larynx, he must not raise his voice above a whisper and must not smoke. Inhalations of medicated steam should be given 3 or 4 times a day, along with a linctus containing pholcodine or methadone (p. 267).

Acute Bronchitis

Aetiology. This condition is an acute inflammation of the trachea and bronchi caused by pyogenic organisms such as *Strept. pneumoniae*, *H. influenzae* and, rarely, *Staph. pyogenes*. Infection by these organisms is a common sequel to coryza, influenza, measles and whooping-cough, and is particularly prone to develop in patients with chronic bronchitis.

Other factors predisposing to the development of infection include cold, damp, foggy and dusty atmospheres, and cigarette smoking.

Clinical Features. The first symptom is an irritating, unproductive cough accompanied by upper retrosternal discomfort or pain caused by tracheitis. When the bronchi become involved there is also a sensation of tightness in the chest, and dyspnoea with wheezing respiration may be present. Respiratory distress may be particularly severe when acute bronchitis complicates chronic bronchitis and emphysema. The sputum is at first scanty, mucoid, viscid and difficult to bring up, and occasionally may be streaked with blood. A day or two later it becomes mucopurulent and more copious. As the infection extends down the bronchial tree there is a general febrile disturbance, with a temperature of 38–39°C (100–103°F) and a neutrophil leucocytosis. In the vast majority of cases recovery takes place gradually over the next 4 to 8 days without the patient ever becoming seriously ill. Occasionally the dyspnoea and general symptoms increase in severity, cyanosis appears, and if the infection reaches the smallest bronchi and bronchioles ('bronchiolitis') the condition becomes indistinguishable from lobular pneumonia.

Tracheitis without bronchitis produces no abnormal physical signs. In bronchitis there is no impairment of chest wall movement or percussion note. The breath sounds are vesicular, or vesicular with prolonged expiration, and are accompanied by *bilateral* rhonchi and, occasionally, coarse crepitations.

The disease is usually mild and of short duration, the patient recovering within a few days if a suitable antibiotic is given. In severe cases it lasts longer, especially if bronchiolitis and lobular pneumonia develop.

Treatment. The patient should be confined to bed and tetracycline or ampicillin, 250–500 mg 4 times daily, given by mouth. Co-trimoxazole, a combination of trimethoprim and sulphamethoxazole, is equally effective in a dose of 2 tablets twice daily. In the early stages, when cough is painful and unproductive, the tough viscid secretion should be loosened by the inhalation 3 or 4 times a day of steam medicated with benzoin or menthol. A steam kettle or steam tent is more suitable for children. The cough should be controlled at night by the use of a sedative linctus containing pholcodine or methadone (p. 267). If symptoms or signs of airways obstruction are present a bronchodilator drug (p. 303) may be of some value. Oxygen (p. 264) is seldom required in uncomplicated acute bronchitis.

The Pneumonias

Pneumonia is the term used to describe inflammation of the lung. There are many different kinds of pneumonia, some common, others rare. Aetiologically they can be divided into the specific pneumonias, in which the disease is caused by a specific pathogenic organism, and the aspiration pneumonias, in which some abnormality of the respiratory system predisposes to the invasion of the lung by organisms of relatively low virulence. As the term implies, infection generally reaches the alveoli by aspiration from other parts of the respiratory tract. *H. influenzae*, some types of *Strept. pneumoniae* and certain of the bacteria forming the flora of the upper respiratory tract and mouth are the organisms most frequently cultured from the sputum.

In some types of specific and aspiration pneumonia, destruction of lung tissue by the inflammatory process, a high incidence of abscess formation and the subsequent development of pulmonary fibrosis and bronchiectasis are prominent features. The term *'suppurative pneumonia'* has been applied to this group of cases and this condition merits separate description (p. 279).

The Specific Pneumonias

This group may be further subdivided into pneumonias caused by (1) 'large' bacteria, and (2) viruses and 'small' bacteria.

Large bacteria known to produce specific types of pneumonia are *Strept. pneumoniae*, *Staph. pyogenes*, *Klebsiella pneumoniae*, *H. influenzae*, *Mycobacterium tuberculosis*, *Yersinia pestis* and *Y. tularensis*.

Many viruses, including those described in Table 7.2 (p. 270), may produce a specific pneumonia, as may small bacteria such as *Coxiella burneti* (Q-fever), *Mycoplasma pneumoniae* and *Chlamydia* of the ornithosis (psittacosis) group.

Pneumonia due to the pneumococcus still constitutes the largest proportion of all specific pneumonias and will be described in detail. Shorter accounts will be given of the other types.

PNEUMOCOCCAL PNEUMONIA

(*Syn.: Acute Lobar Pneumonia*)

Pneumococcal pneumonia is characterised by homogeneous consolidation of one or more lobes or segments. The disease occurs at all ages but most frequently in early and middle adult life. The highest incidence is in winter. It is usually a sporadic disease, the mode of spread being by droplet infection.

Pathology. The pneumonic process usually affects only one lobe or segment but the infection may spread to other lobes or segments in the same or opposite lung. There is associated inflammation of the overlying pleura. The affected lobes or segments undergo consolidation in which there is exudation of fibrin, red blood cells and later white blood cells into the alveoli. Resolution is achieved first by liquefaction of the exudate by macrophages and then by its absorption or expectoration. Resolution is usually complete: fibrosis and bronchiectasis seldom follow this type of pneumonia.

Clinical Features. The onset is sudden, with rigor, or with vomiting or a convulsion in children. The temperature rises in a few hours to 39–40°C (102–104°F). Malaise, loss of appetite, headache, and aching pains in the body and limbs accompany the pyrexia. Localised pain of pleural type (p. 256) develops at an early stage in the illness. It is generally referred to the chest wall but may on occasion be referred to the shoulder or to the abdominal wall. There is a short, painful cough, dry at first but later productive of tenacious sputum which is often rust-coloured and occasionally frankly blood-stained. Respiration is rapid (30 to 40 per minute in adults, 50 to 60 in children), shallow and painful. The pulse is rapid, the skin is hot and dry, the face is flushed, and central cyanosis may be observed in severe cases. Herpes labialis is often present. A marked neutrophil leucocytosis, 15·0–30·0 × 10⁹/*l*, is characteristic. *Strept. pneumonia* can usually be isolated from the sputum, and a positive blood culture may be obtained in severe cases.

Physical Signs in the Chest. For the first 24 to 48 hours of the illness there is diminution of respiratory movement, slight impairment of the percussion note, and often a pleural rub on the affected side. At a variable time after the onset, generally within 2 days, signs of consolidation appear (p. 261), the breath sounds being of the high-pitched bronchial type. When resolution begins, numerous coarse crepitations are heard, indicating liquefaction of the exudate. If a sterile or purulent effusion develops, the physical signs of fluid in the pleural space are usually found, but often bronchial breath sounds persist and the presence of an effusion may be suspected only from the stony dullness on percussion.

Radiological Examination. This shows a homogeneous opacity localised to the affected lobe or segment, appearing within 12 to 18 hours of the onset of the illness. Radiological examination is particularly helpful when the diagnosis is in doubt or if a complication such as empyema is suspected.

Course. Most cases respond promptly to chemotherapy and within a week the patient is well again. Delayed recovery suggests either that some complication has developed (e.g. empyema) or that the diagnosis of pneumococcal pneumonia is incorrect.

Occasionally in old or debilitated persons the response to treatment is unsatisfactory. The symptoms rapidly become worse, there is increasing weakness, dyspnoea, cyanosis and delirium, and death takes place within a few days from hypoxia or peripheral circulatory failure. A fatal outcome is more liable to occur if there has been a delay in starting specific treatment.

Complications. 1. PULMONARY. *Delayed resolution.* In most cases the abnormal physical signs disappear within 2 weeks and the radiological opacity within 4 weeks. Although resolution is occasionally delayed for longer periods, particularly in patients with massive pneumonic consolidation, such delay is often due to the presence of some underlying lesion such as bronchial carcinoma. This possibility must always be kept in mind when a pneumonia is slow to resolve.

2. PLEURAL. Spread of the infection to the pleura may occur with the development of a sterile *pleural effusion* (p. 336) or *empyema* (p. 337).

3. CARDIOVASCULAR. (*a*) *Circulatory failure* (p. 192). (*b*) Acute pneumococcal *pericarditis* and *endocarditis* (rare).

4. NEUROLOGICAL. (*a*) *Meningism.* This is not uncommon in children, and lumbar puncture may be required to distinguish it from meningitis (p. 714). (*b*) Pneumococcal *meningitis* (rare).

Differential Diagnosis. The following conditions may be difficult to distinguish from pneumococcal pneumonia:
1. *Other types of acute specific and aspiration pneumonia* (pp. 275–281).
2. *Pulmonary infarction* (p. 226), in which pyrexia is less marked and is un-

influenced by antibiotics, frank haemoptysis is common, cough is inconspicuous and the site of origin of the embolus can often be identified.

3. *Tuberculous pleurisy with effusion*, in which the correct diagnosis can usually be suspected from the insidious onset, the virtual absence of cough and sputum, the physical signs of pleural effusion, the absence of leucocytosis, the failure of the pyrexia to respond to antibiotics, the radiological findings and the aspiration of serous fluid, in which lymphocytes predominate, from the pleural space.

4. *Pulmonary tuberculosis*, acute cases of which may simulate pneumonia. The patient is, however, seldom as acutely ill as in pneumococcal pneumonia; it is uncommon for the respiratory rate to be markedly increased and the white blood count is seldom above $12 \cdot 0 \times 10^9/l$. The diagnosis can usually be made by radiological examination, and the isolation of tubercle bacilli from the sputum puts it beyond doubt.

5. *Inflammatory conditions below the diaphragm*, such as cholecystitis, perforated duodenal ulcer, acute appendicitis, subphrenic abscess, generalised peritonitis and hepatic amoebiasis, may occasionally be mistaken for pneumococcal pneumonia. A carefully taken history is one of the most valuable means of determining the site and nature of the primary disease. A high temperature and a rapid respiratory rate favour a diagnosis of pneumonia, whereas tenderness of the abdominal wall suggests that the primary lesion is below the diaphragm. Sometimes radiological examination of the chest is necessary before the presence of pneumonia can be confirmed or excluded.

Treatment and Prognosis. The treatment of pneumonia is described on page 281. The prognosis depends on the virulence of the infecting pneumococcus, the age of the patient (the mortality rises above the age of 60), the general state of health (the mortality is increased when pneumonia complicates other serious disease or develops in a chronic alcoholic), and the stage of the illness at which specific treatment is instituted. The prognosis is less favourable in the absence of a brisk temperature response or when there is a poor leucocytosis, marked cyanosis, delirium or acute circulatory failure, or extension of pneumonia to other lobes.

OTHER TYPES OF SPECIFIC PNEUMONIA

1. **Staphylococcal Pneumonia.** Pneumonia due to *Staph. pyogenes* may occur either as a primary respiratory infection or as a blood-borne infection from a staphylococcal lesion elsewhere in the body, e.g. osteomyelitis. The second condition is essentially one of pyaemic abscess formation in the lungs. Unless an empyema is produced by rupture of an abscess into the pleura, the pulmonary lesions may pass unnoticed, overshadowed by the severe general illness.

Primary staphylococcal pneumonia, although it occurs much less frequently than pneumococcal pneumonia, is a relatively common illness, especially as a complication of influenza. It may present as a lobar or segmental pneumonia, which may be difficult to distinguish clinically from a severe pneumococcal infection, or as a suppurative pneumonia (p. 279) with multiple lung abscesses which may persist as thin-walled cysts after the acute infection has subsided. Culture of the sputum yields a growth of coagulase-positive staphylococci which are frequently resistant to penicillin, streptomycin, tetracycline and co-trimoxazole. At the present time few strains of staphylococci causing pneumonia are resistant to erythromycin, cloxacillin, cephaloridine or sodium fusidate, but this relatively favourable situation may alter if these drugs are prescribed on a larger scale.

2. **Klebsiella Pneumonia (Friedländer's Pneumonia).** Pneumonia due to *Klebsiella pneumoniae* is a rare disease. There is usually massive consolidation and excavation of one or more lobes, the upper lobes being most often involved, with profound systemic disturbance, the expectoration of large amounts of purulent, sometimes chocolate-coloured, sputum and a high mortality. The diagnosis is made by the radiological appearances and the isolation of the causative organism from the sputum. Streptomycin plus chloramphenicol is the first choice in antibiotic therapy, modified according to the results of sensitivity tests.

3. **Tuberculous Pneumonia** (p. 289), **Plague** (p. 866) and **Tularaemia** (p. 868).

4. **Pneumonia Caused by Viruses and Small Bacteria.** A distinctive form of pneumonia may be produced by certain viruses, and by small bacteria which exhibit a similar pathogenicity to lung tissue (Table 7.2, p. 270). The clinical picture differs from that of the bacterial pneumonias in that fever and toxaemia usually precede the respiratory symptoms by several days. Severe headache, malaise and anorexia are characteristic features in the early stages. The physical signs in the chest, if there are any, appear later and are seldom gross. The existence of a pulmonary lesion may not be recognised unless a radiograph is taken. The spleen may be palpable in the first week. The white blood count is generally normal and the pyrexia does not respond to penicillin. If facilities for virological investigation are available the diagnosis can often be confirmed by isolation of the causal organism or by serological tests.

The disease is usually self-limiting. The pyrexia subsides by lysis after 5 to 10 days, and complete recovery and radiographic resolution follow, the latter sometimes being slow. Very rarely, death takes place from widespread extension of the pneumonia or from viral encephalitis.

The *influenza*, *parainfluenza* and *measles* viruses rarely produce a specific pneumonia. The pneumonia caused by *chickenpox* virus, however, is usually characteristic. The radiograph shows numerous miliary nodular shadows which may eventually calcify. It occurs almost exclusively in adults. The *adenoviruses* cause occasional mild epidemics of specific pneumonia, cold agglutinins being present in many cases.

Respiratory syncytial virus is the most important respiratory pathogen of early childhood, especially in the first 2 months of life. This is because it causes bronchiolitis and pneumonia and carries an important risk of mortality in this age group. The infant is fevered, and cough, wheezy respiration and occasionally an erythematous rash are prominent features. The virus is not susceptible to any known antibiotic, and immunisation is ineffective.

Psittacosis (parrot-fever) and *ornithosis* are caused by *Chlamydia*. These used to be regarded as viruses but have in fact the structural and biochemical properties of bacteria and rickettsiae. The diseases are primarily infections of birds and are transmitted to humans by inhalation of dust containing faeces from infected birds. The pneumonia caused by these organisms, which are susceptible to tetracyclines, is occasionally extensive and associated with severe toxaemia.

Mycoplasma pneumoniae is a pleomorphic bacterium capable of passing through a filter. It is susceptible to tetracyclines though a few strains are sensitive only to erythromycin. Cold agglutinins can be demonstrated in a high proportion of cases. Antibodies can be detected and haemagglutination and complement-fixation tests are available for diagnosis. Outbreaks of pneumonia caused by this organism are common in barracks and institutions. Most cases occur in children and young adults.

Coxiella (*Rickettsia*) *burneti* is the organism responsible for *Q-fever*. The usual sources of infection are cattle and sheep. Endocarditis may be present as well as pneumonia in this disease. The diagnosis is made by examining specimens of serum at an interval of 2 weeks.

The Aspiration Pneumonias

Aetiology. This group, sometimes described as the 'non-specific' pneumonias, comprises a large number of different conditions, their common features being the absence of any specific pathogenic organism in the sputum and the existence of some abnormality of the respiratory system which predisposes to the invasion of the lung by relatively avirulent organisms derived from the upper respiratory tract or from the mouth, e.g. streptococci, certain types of pneumococci, *H. influenzae*, Vincent's spirochaetes and fusiform bacilli.

Infection may reach the lungs in various ways. Pus may be aspirated from an infected nasal sinus, or septic matter may be inhaled during tonsillectomy or dental extraction under general anaesthesia. Vomitus or the contents of a dilated oesophagus may enter the larynx during general anaesthesia, coma or even sleep. Infected secretion in the bronchi and pus from bronchiectatic cavities or from a lung abscess may also be carried into the alveoli by the air stream or by gravity.

Ineffective coughing caused by postoperative or post-traumatic thoracic or abdominal pain, by debility or immobility, or by laryngeal paralysis may also predispose to the development of aspiration pneumonia.

Bronchial obstruction, partial or complete, as for example by a carcinoma, is another potential cause of aspiration pneumonia, as it allows infection derived from the upper air passages to become established in the inadequately ventilated portion of lung beyond the obstruction.

There are *four* types of aspiration pneumonia with fairly well-defined clinical and pathological features: (1) acute lobular pneumonia, (2) benign aspiration pneumonia, (3) hypostatic pneumonia, and (4) postoperative pneumonia.

1. ACUTE LOBULAR PNEUMONIA

(Syn.: Acute Bronchopneumonia)

This type of pneumonia is invariably preceded by bronchial infection, which accounts for the widespread, lobular distribution of the lesions. It occurs most frequently in children and in elderly people. In children it is often a complication of measles or whooping-cough, in adults of acute bronchitis or influenza. It is particularly common in patients with chronic bronchitis and emphysema.

Pathology. There is acute inflammation of the bronchi, especially the terminal bronchioles, which are filled with pus. Collapse and consolidation of the associated groups of alveoli follow. The lesions are distributed bilaterally in small patches which tend to become larger by confluence and are often more extensive in the lower lobes. The alveolar exudate consists of neutrophil leucocytes with a small amount of fibrin. There is interstitial oedema and cellular proliferation in the alveolar walls, and compensatory emphysema around the collapsed alveoli. Resolution of lobular pneumonia may be incomplete, and in such cases pulmonary fibrosis and bronchiectasis are common sequelae.

Clinical Features. The patient first exhibits for 2 or 3 days the clinical features of acute bronchitis and then, as lobular pneumonia develops, the temperature rises to a higher level, the pulse and respiratory rates increase, and dyspnoea and central cyanosis appear. There is generally a severe cough with purulent sputum. Pleural pain is relatively uncommon and herpes labialis is seldom present, in contrast to pneumococcal pneumonia.

During the early stages the physical signs are those of acute bronchitis but crepitations later become more numerous. In many cases no signs of consolidation can be detected, but these may develop when lobular lesions coalesce and radiological examination shows mottled opacities in both lung fields, chiefly in the lower zones. Blood examination shows a neutrophil leucocytosis.

Course and Complications. The disease is of more insidious onset and tends to run a more protracted course than pneumococcal pneumonia (7 to 10 days). Incomplete resolution may lead to bronchiectasis, but the number of patients developing this complication has fallen dramatically since antibiotics became available. The mortality is higher at the extremes of life, especially if the disease supervenes on chronic bronchitis and emphysema, chronic nephritis or heart disease.

Treatment and Prevention. The treatment of pneumonia is discussed on page 281. The incidence of lobular pneumonia can be reduced by careful attention to apparently benign upper respiratory infections such as coryza and acute bronchitis, especially when they occur at the extremes of life and in patients with chronic bronchitis. Measures to prevent whooping-cough and measles, and adequate treatment of those diseases, are also important in prophylaxis.

2. BENIGN ASPIRATION PNEUMONIA

This type of pneumonia is due to the aspiration of infective secretion into the lungs during the course of an upper respiratory infection such as coryza or sinusitis. It is thus often associated with segmental pulmonary collapse. The organisms causing the pneumonia, being derived from the upper respiratory tract, are generally of low virulence and the degree of systemic disturbance is usually slight. In fact, the symptoms are often no more severe than would be expected with an uncomplicated upper respiratory infection and the existence of a pneumonia may be discovered only by radiological examination. As a rule, however, the condition manifests itself by cough, purulent sputum, low-grade pyrexia and sometimes pleural pain, in association with a frank upper respiratory infection. Localised coarse crepitations are often the only abnormal physical signs. A neutrophil leucocytosis is usually present. The radiological lesions are typically. unilateral, the characteristic appearance being a mottled opacity involving a single lobe or segment, which in some cases may be collapsed.

The condition is liable to be confused with viral pneumonia, but the coexistent upper respiratory infection and the minimal systemic upset are useful distinguishing features. Pulmonary tuberculosis may be erroneously diagnosed on the basis of a single radiograph. Re-examination 10 to 14 days later, following treatment with an antibiotic, will resolve the diagnosis as recovery is generally rapid in aspiration pneumonia.

3. HYPOSTATIC PNEUMONIA

This type of aspiration pneumonia occurs in elderly or debilitated people and is a common cause of death. These patients, being physically weak and immobilised in bed, have difficulty in expectorating bronchial mucus and the alveolar transudate which tends to form as a result of hypostatic pulmonary congestion. These secretions gravitate to the bases of the lungs where infection, usually with upper respiratory commensal organisms, frequently supervenes. The lobular pneumonia which results is a relatively mild process but is sufficient to cause death in patients enfeebled by old age, heart failure or toxaemia.

The onset of symptoms in hypostatic pneumonia is insidious, often almost imperceptible at first. A slight cough accompanied by an increase in pulse and respiration rates is usually the earliest manifestation. Pyrexia and leucocytosis may occur but are seldom marked. Physical signs in the chest are usually bilateral and confined to the lower lobes. Frank signs of consolidation may be present, but numerous coarse crepitations at both lung bases without signs of consolidation are a more common finding. Once the condition is established it pursues a rapidly fatal course, usually with little apparent discomfort to the patient.

Preventive measures are all-important. Elderly people should not be confined to bed unless this is absolutely necessary. Patients who have to be kept in bed should have their position changed frequently and be given deep-breathing exercises.

4. POSTOPERATIVE PNEUMONIA

Primarily this condition is not pneumonia but pulmonary collapse due to obstruction of a large bronchus by viscid secretion which cannot be expectorated owing to postoperative pain. Infection may occur secondarily with the production of an aspiration pneumonia. The condition is more fully described on page 322.

Suppurative Pneumonia

(Including Pulmonary Abscess)

Suppurative pneumonia is the term used to describe a form of pneumonic consolidation in which there is destruction of lung parenchyma by the inflammatory process. Although abscess formation is a characteristic histological feature of suppurative pneumonia, it is usual to restrict the term 'pulmonary abscess' to lesions in which there is a fairly large localised collection of pus, or a cavity lined by chronic inflammatory tissue, from which pus has been evacuated.

Aetiology. Suppurative pneumonia and pulmonary abscess may be produced by infection of previously healthy lung tissue with *Staph. pyogenes* or *Klebsiella pneumoniae*. These are, in effect, specific bacterial pneumonias associated with pulmonary suppuration.

More frequently, suppurative pneumonia and pulmonary abscess are forms of aspiration pneumonia. They may develop after the inhalation of septic material during operations on the nose, mouth or throat under general anaesthesia, or of vomitus during anaesthesia or coma. In such circumstances gross oral sepsis is an important predisposing factor. Bacterial infection of a pulmonary infarct or of a collapsed lobe may also produce a suppurative pneumonia or a pulmonary abscess. The organisms isolated from the sputum may include *Strept. pneumoniae*, *Staph. pyogenes*, *Strept. pyogenes*, *H. influenzae* and, in a few cases, anaerobic streptococci and other anaerobes such as Vincent's spirochaetes and fusiform bacilli. In some cases, however, no pathogens can be isolated, particularly when antibiotics have been given.

Pathology. Descriptions have already been given of staphylococcal pneumonia (p. 275) and of klebsiella pneumonia (p. 276). When suppurative pneumonia follows the inhalation of infective material from the upper air passages, it is more often unilateral than bilateral, and is usually situated in the axillary part of either upper lobe or in the apex of a lower lobe, these being the most dependent areas when the patient is lying on his side or on his back respectively. In other cases the site depends on the nature and situation of the primary pathological lesion. For example, when the abscess is secondary to bronchial obstruction by a carcinoma its site is determined by the position of the tumour in the bronchial tree.

In suppurative pneumonia destruction of lung parenchyma leads to pulmonary fibrosis and bronchiectasis (p. 316). Usually the suppurative process is localised but occasionally it spreads by direct continuity until a whole lung is irreparably damaged. Abscesses, when present, may be single or multiple. Occasionally they may become very large as a result of inflation caused by a 'check valve' mechanism at the junction of the cavity and the draining bronchus.

Clinical Features. These depend to a large extent on the pathogenesis of the lesion. The onset of the illness may be either insidious or acute, but cough with purulent sputum, usually large in amount, sometimes foetid and occasionally blood-stained, is present from an early stage. There is high, remittent pyrexia with shivering and sweating, and a neutrophil leucocytosis in the region of $15 \cdot 0 - 25 \cdot 0 \times 10^9/l$. Pleural pain is common and clubbing of the fingers may develop as early as 10 to 14 days after the onset of the illness. Progressive deterioration in general health with marked loss of weight ensues if the patient remains untreated. The rupture of a large localised abscess into a bronchus can be assumed when a large quantity of pus is suddenly expectorated. Such an incident is often preceded by blood-staining of the sputum and followed by remission of the pyrexia.

Physical signs in the chest also depend on the nature of the primary pathological process. Signs of consolidation (p. 261) are the most frequent finding. Frank signs of cavitation are rarely found. A pleural rub is often present.

Radiological Examination. There may be a homogeneous lobar or segmental opacity consistent with consolidation or collapse. Alternatively, if the lesions are of lobular distribution, multiple coarse, mottled opacities may be found. A large homogeneous opacity, which may later cavitate and show a fluid level within it, is the characteristic finding when a frank pulmonary abscess is present.

Diagnosis. This cannot be considered complete unless the primary aetiological factor or factors are identified. Sputum should be sent for bacteriological examination, and if a pathogenic organism is isolated its sensitivity to the various antibiotics should be determined.

Suppurative pneumonia must be distinguished from:

1. Pulmonary tuberculosis, by examination of the sputum for tubercle bacilli.
2. Bronchial carcinoma, by bronchoscopy.

Pulmonary abscess must be distinguished from:

1. Pulmonary tuberculosis with cavitation, by examination of the sputum for tubercle bacilli.
2. A cavitated malignant growth, by the radiological appearances and, if necessary, by bronchoscopy.
3. Empyema, which gives the physical signs of fluid in the pleural space and from which pus can be obtained by paracentesis.

Course and Prognosis. In most cases there is a good response to antibacterial therapy, and although residual fibrosis and bronchiectasis are common sequelae, these seldom give rise to serious morbidity. Empyema (p. 337) may complicate the acute phase of the disease.

Prevention. Every precaution should be taken during operations on the mouth, nose and throat to prevent the inhalation of blood, tonsillar fragments, etc. Oral sepsis should be eradicated, especially if a general anaesthetic is contemplated.

Actinomycosis

Formerly included amongst the fungal diseases, this is now regarded as a bacterial infection. It is caused by *Actinomyces israeli*, an anaerobic organism, which exists as a commensal in the mouth. It presumably gains access to the lungs by aspiration, and may produce a widespread suppurative lobular pneumonia. Empyema, often bilateral and associated with persistent chest wall sinuses, may develop later, or occasionally *de novo*.

The Treatment of Pneumonia

1. **Chemotherapy.** The principles governing the specific treatment of bacterial infections of the respiratory tract have already been stated (p. 264). When a clinical diagnosis of pneumonia is made, provided the patient is not gravely ill, the initial treatment should consist of ampicillin, 500 mg four times daily, or co-trimoxazole, 2 tablets twice daily. Patients who are gravely ill and in whom a staphylococcal infection is suspected should receive, in addition to ampicillin or co-trimoxazole, an antibiotic to which the organism is unlikely to be resistant, e.g. cloxacillin, 500 mg 6 hourly by mouth or 250 mg 6 hourly by intramuscular injection, or lincomycin, 500 mg 6 hourly by mouth.

(a) If *Strept. pneumoniae*, *Strept. pyogenes* or an anaerobic streptococcus is isolated, or no pathogenic organisms are reported on culture, and the patient appears to be making satisfactory clinical progress, treatment with ampicillin or co-trimoxazole should be continued, but the dose of ampicillin can be reduced to 250 mg 6 hourly.

(b) If *Staph. pyogenes* is isolated, treatment must be modified in accordance with the results of sensitivity tests. Resistance to penicillin may be due to the production of pencillinase, and such infections can usually be controlled by a combination of benzylpenicillin (600 mg twice daily i.m.) and oral or intra-muscular cloxacillin (250–500 mg four times daily). In other cases lincomycin (500 mg 8 hourly), sodium fusidate (500 mg 8 hourly) or cephalexin (500 mg 6 hourly) by mouth, or gentamicin (80 mg thrice daily) by intramuscular injection, may be indicated. There may be an advantage in combining two of these drugs.

(c) If *Klebs. pneumoniae* is isolated, sensitivity tests will indicate which drug is likely to prove most effective. Those to which this organism is most frequently sensitive are gentamicin, chloramphenicol, ampicillin and co-trimoxazole.

(d) If *Actinomyces israeli* is isolated, benzylpenicillin is given by intramuscular injection in a dose of 5 g daily for up to 6 weeks.

(e) If bacteriological examination is uninformative and a virus pneumonia is suspected, it is advisable to give an antibiotic to prevent or control secondary bacterial infection. In these circumstances tetracycline is the drug of choice as it is effective against organisms such as *Coxiella burneti, Mycoplasma pneumoniae* and *Chlamydia*. A dose of 500 mg four times daily is recommended.

(f) If recovery is progressing satisfactorily, the isolation of an organism showing *in vitro* resistance to the antibiotic in use is not necessarily an indication for a change in treatment. If, however, the patient is not improving and is still febrile when such an organism is isolated, an appropriate change in antibiotic is imperative.

The impulse to substitute another antibiotic, *where there is no bacteriological indication for doing so*, should be resisted. The failure of patients to respond to treatment may be due to a complicating factor such as pleural infection, tuberculosis or bronchial obstruction by a tumour, and these conditions must be carefully excluded before the antibiotic is changed.

(g) No definite rule can be laid down for the *duration* of chemotherapy. In most cases of uncomplicated pneumococcal pneumonia a 7-day course of treatment is usually adequate but this may have to be extended if the response to treatment is slow. In staphylococcal and klebsiella pneumonia, and in other forms of suppurative pneumonia, chemotherapy should be continued for a minimum of 2 weeks and should not be stopped until the causative organism has been eliminated from the sputum.

2. **General Measures.** The usual regimen of treatment for an acute infection should be instituted. If respiratory distress is marked the patient should be propped up comfortably with pillows or a backrest.

Cough, when distressing and unproductive, should be controlled by the measures described on page 267. When secretions are present in the bronchi the patient should be firmly encouraged to cough them up, even if the effort to do so causes pleural pain. In these circumstances a mild analgesic (p. 267) and the support of a nurse's hand on the painful side of the chest may relieve the distress of coughing. Postural drainage is of value if the sputum is difficult to bring up, particularly if it is copious, as in suppurative pneumonia, or when pneumonia complicates bronchiectasis.

Pleural pain should be treated with local heat and analgesics (p. 267). It is, however, dangerous to prescribe morphine if even a mild degree of ventilatory insufficiency is present, and the safest policy is not to use this drug at all in the treatment of pneumonia.

Hypoxia demands oxygen therapy (p. 264).

Delirium, which in the early stages is caused mainly by the high temperature, and later by cerebral hypoxia, may have to be controlled by sedation. The safest drug to use is diazepam, 5–10 mg, by intramuscular injection.

Peripheral circulatory failure occurring in the course of pneumonia is seldom reversible once it has become established. Fluid replacement with intravenous plasma or dextran, monitored by measurements of central venous pressure, is essential, and massive doses of intravenous hydrocortisone (3 g per day or more) may be of some value. The administration of pressor agents, such as metaraminol hydrogen tartrate (Aramine) by intramuscular injection or by continuous intravenous infusion, may do more harm than good.

Abscess formation. Suppurative pneumonia is not in itself a reason for any departure from standard antibiotic policy. When an abscess cavity is present, however, it must be kept empty by regular postural drainage. Medical treatment is almost invariably successful and surgical measures nowadays are seldom required. In occasional instances, however, a large abscess may have to be dra:..ed externally or residual bronchiectasis resected.

Tuberculosis

Although tuberculosis is a problem of rapidly diminishing proportions in Western Europe and North America, it remains, in the words of a World Health Organisation report, 'the most important specific communicable disease in the world'. As the disease decreases in frequency there is a tendency for tuberculosis to be overlooked in differential diagnosis.

Aetiology. The fact that tuberculosis is a specific infective disease was first proved by Koch's discovery of the tubercle bacillus in 1882. Three types of mycobacteria are responsible for the disease in man: (*a*) the *human* type—now responsible for almost all infections in man, (*b*) the *bovine* type—endemic in cattle, but very rarely responsible for disease in man, and (*c*) the *atypical* or *opportunistic* mycobacteria. The clinical importance of the last group of organisms lies in their ability to cause infection in cervical lymph nodes in children and, rarely, pulmonary disease in adults, when treatment may be a problem because the mycobacteria are primarily resistant to many drugs.

Entry of the tubercle bacillus into the body by the alimentary or respiratory tract is not necessarily followed by a clinical illness, the development of which is dependent on several other factors:

1. *Natural resistance.* Susceptibility to tuberculosis is not inherited in the strict sense of the word, but the fact that certain races, such as Africans and Indians, and even certain regional groups, such as the inhabitants of the Western Isles of Scotland and of Ireland, are more prone to develop tuberculosis suggests that natural resistance varies from race to race and even from region to region. The natural resistance of a community tends to rise as the period of exposure to tuberculosis increases.

2. *Acquired immunity.* The nature and effects of acquired immunity in tuberculosis are not fully understood. It has, however, been proved that if a person contracts and recovers from a primary tuberculous infection (p. 286) he is less likely to develop active tuberculosis on subsequent exposure to the tubercle bacillus than a patient who has not previously been infected. The use of a vaccine containing an attenuated bovine bacillus (Bacille Calmette Guérin—BCG) to induce a controlled and innocuous primary infection is based on this observation.

3. *Allergy.* After the primary infection has become established the tissues react to the tubercle bacillus in a way that differs from their initial reaction. This altered response or allergy, takes the form of hypersensitivity to tuberculin, a complex protein constituent of the tubercle bacillus, and can be recognised by the finding of a positive tuberculin reaction (p. 287). This is a cell-mediated hypersensitivity (p. 43).

4. *Age and Sex.* In Europe and America, tuberculosis used to affect predominantly the young people in the community and especially the young female. There has been a radical change in the age and sex incidence. Whereas 20 years ago, only 20 per cent of notifications came from patients over 45 years of age, nowadays 60 per cent of

patients are over 45 years of age, males predominating. This change is important in case-finding.

5. *Standard of living.* The prevalence of tuberculosis diminishes as social and economic conditions improve. Poor housing with associated over-crowding increases the risk of massive infection or reinfection occurring if one of the occupants suffers from open tuberculosis. The precise role of diet is uncertain, but gross deficiency of protein and vitamins commonly found in the developing countries in Asia and Africa may be an important aetiological factor.

6. *Conditions Affecting Individual Patients.* Diabetes mellitus, gastrectomy and congenital heart disease all predispose to the development of tuberculosis, as does treatment with corticosteroids or immunosuppressant drugs. Pregnancy may have an unfavourable influence on the course of untreated pulmonary tuberculosis but has no adverse effect on patients under correct supervision and treatment.

Pathology. The characteristic lesion of tuberculosis is the *tubercle*. This consists of a microscopic nodular collection of epithelioid cells surrounded by zones of lymphocytes and fibroblasts. There may be giant cells and a few bacilli in the centre. Adjacent tubercles enlarge and coalesce at an early stage, and this is followed by central necrosis or 'caseation' which may advance rapidly with widespread tissue destruction. The lesions tend to heal by fibrosis and calcification, but destructive and reparative processes frequently coexist.

The initial 'primary' tuberculous infection usually occurs in the lung but occasionally in the tonsil or in the alimentary tract, especially the ileocaecal region. The primary infection differs from later infections in that the primary focus in lung, tonsil or bowel is almost invariably accompanied by a caseous lesion in the regional lymph nodes, i.e. in the mediastinal, cervical or mesenteric groups respectively.

In most people the primary infection and the associated lymph node lesion heal and calcify. In a few, healing (particularly of the lymph node lesion) is incomplete and surviving tubercle bacilli may under certain circumstances, such as a lowering of the general health or an alteration of the balance between allergy and immunity, be discharged into the blood stream. Such patients may in consequence develop tuberculous lesions elsewhere in the body. The most common sites for '*haematogenous*' *lesions* of this kind are the lungs, bones, joints and kidneys. Such lesions may develop months or even years after the primary infection.

The primary infection may in some cases fail to heal. A primary pulmonary lesion, particularly when it occurs during adolescence or early adult life, may lead to progressive pulmonary tuberculosis. A tuberculous mediastinal lymph node, in children especially, may compress a lobar or segmental bronchus (rarely a main bronchus) and produce pulmonary collapse. Occasionally the node may ulcerate through the bronchial wall and discharge caseous material into the lumen, with the production of acute tuberculous lesions in the related lobe or segment. Infection may also be carried by lymphatics from tuberculous mediastinal glands to the pleura or pericardium with the production of *tuberculous pleurisy* or *pericarditis*. Comparable complications may occur when the primary lesion is in the tonsil or gut, e.g. '*cold abscess*' of the neck or tuberculous *peritonitis*.

Rarely, a caseous tuberculous focus either at the site of the primary infection or, more commonly, in an associated lymph node ruptures into a vein and produces acute dissemination of the disease throughout the body, a condition known as *acute miliary tuberculosis. Tuberculous meningitis* often accompanies this condition.

Progressive pulmonary tuberculosis may develop directly from a primary lesion or it may occur later, following reactivation of an incompletely healed primary focus in the lung or as a result of haematogenous dissemination from an unhealed lymph node lesion. Alternatively it may be the result of reinfection from an outside source after the primary focus has healed completely. All these forms of pulmonary tuberculosis, although differing in pathogenesis, have similar pathological features and can be grouped together under the term *postprimary pulmonary tuberculosis*. The characteristic pathological feature of this condition is the *tuberculous cavity*, which forms when the caseated and liquefied centre of a tuberculous pulmonary lesion is discharged into a bronchus.

Extension of the infection to the pleura either by direct or lymphatic spread causes *tuberculous pleurisy*, which is sometimes accompanied by effusion and is occasionally followed by the development of a *tuberculous empyema*. Blood-borne dissemination to other organs of the body is uncommon in postprimary pulmonary tuberculosis.

Clinical Features. There are two groups of clinical features in tuberculosis:

1. Those due to the systemic effects of the disease, which include lassitude and malaise, impairment of appetite, loss of weight, anaemia, sweating especially during sleep, pyrexia and tachycardia. The pyrexia is usually most marked in the late afternoon or evening and sometimes occurs only at these times. The absence of constitutional symptoms does not necessarily mean that the disease is inactive.

2. Those caused by the local effects of the tuberculous lesions, which are summarised below according to anatomical site.

Lungs and bronchi: cough, sputum, haemoptysis, dyspnoea.

Pleura: pleural pain, dyspnoea due to pleural effusion.

Larynx: hoarseness, with dysphagia at a later stage from involvement of pharynx.

Tongue: ulceration (rare).

Intestine: diarrhoea, malabsorption or intestinal obstruction.

Peritoneum: ascites, attacks of intestinal obstruction due to plastic peritonitis.

Pericardium: pericardial effusion, constrictive pericarditis later.

Kidneys and bladder: haematuria, increased frequency of micturition. (These are relatively late developments, early renal lesions being symptomless.)

Epididymo-orchitis: painless swelling, sinus formation later.

Fallopian tubes: salpingitis, tubal abscess, infertility.

Brain: tuberculoma with or without focal neurological signs.

Meninges: symptoms and signs of meningitis.

Lymph nodes: enlargement of nodes, often with 'cold' abscess and sinus formation later.

Adrenal glands: symptoms and signs of Addison's disease.

Bones and joints: osteitis, synovitis, 'cold' abscesses.

Skin: lupus vulgaris, erythema nodosum.

Eyes: phlyctenular keratoconjunctivitis, iridocyclitis, choroiditis.

In the sections which follow an account is given of those manifestations of tuberculosis which involve the lungs, namely primary pulmonary tuberculosis, acute miliary tuberculosis and postprimary pulmonary tuberculosis. Tuberculous pleurisy is described on page 335. For information regarding other manifestations of tuberculosis the reader should refer to the appropriate sections of the book. The treatment and prevention of tuberculosis are dealt with on pages 292–297.

Primary Pulmonary Tuberculosis

The pathological features of this type of tuberculosis have already been described (p. 284). The primary infection usually occurs in childhood but is sometimes delayed until adult life. A history of contact with a case of active pulmonary tuberculosis is obtained in many instances.

Clinical Features. 1. In the vast majority of cases the primary infection produces no symptoms or signs and passes unnoticed unless routine radiological examination of the chest happens to be carried out at the appropriate time or serial tuberculin tests show conversion from negative to positive. Such close observation is seldom undertaken unless there is a particular liability to tuberculous infection, e.g. in children or nurses exposed to open cases of tuberculosis.

2. In a few cases the primary infection produces a febrile illness. It is generally mild and lasts for no more than 7 to 14 days, but it may be accompanied by other systemic features of tuberculous infection. It is unusual for gross focal symptoms or signs to develop in an uncomplicated case, but a slight dry cough is occasionally present. The leucocyte count is usually normal but the erythrocyte sedimentation rate is invariably raised.

3. The primary infection may be accompanied by *erythema nodosum*. This condition is characterised by bluish-red, raised, tender cutaneous lesions on the shins and, less commonly, on the thighs, and is associated in some cases with pyrexia and polyarthralgia. The lesions of erythema nodosum do not exhibit the histological features of tuberculosis and tubercle bacilli cannot be isolated from them. They are thus assumed to be non-specific focal manifestations of allergy. Erythema nodosum may, however, be the first clinical indication of a tuberculous infection. In such cases the tuberculin reaction (p. 287) is always strongly positive and evidence of primary tuberculosis can usually be detected on the chest radiograph.

Erythema nodosum may be seen in conditions other than primary tuberculosis, e.g. sarcoidosis, streptococcal infections and, rarely, following the administration of a sulphonamide drug. It may also occur as an isolated phenomenon without apparent cause. In countries where tuberculosis is no longer prevalent, sarcoidosis (p. 328) is the condition with which erythema nodosum is most frequently associated. In such cases the tuberculin reaction is negative or only weakly positive and the chest radiograph usually shows *bilateral* enlargement of the hilar lymph nodes without at this stage any pulmonary abnormalities.

4. Occasionally the primary pulmonary infection pursues a progressive course (p. 284). Symptoms and signs due to its complications may appear either during the course of the initial illness or after a latent interval of weeks or months. Such complications include dry pleurisy or pleural effusion (p. 335), lobar or segmental collapse (p. 321), acute miliary tuberculosis (p. 288), tuberculous meningitis (p. 715), and postprimary pulmonary tuberculosis (p. 289).

Diagnosis. The three most valuable diagnostic investigations in primary pulmonary tuberculosis are:

1. *Radiological examination of the chest.* In children this usually shows unilateral enlargement of the hilar lymph nodes and demonstrates the primary intrapulmonary lesion if it is large enough to be visible radiologically. In adolescents and young adults the lymph nodes component of the primary complex is usually

less conspicuous than in children and the pulmonary lesion more prominent. Complications such as pleural effusion, collapse and acute pneumonic tuberculosis may be superimposed.

2. *Tuberculin test*. With the Mantoux technique a solution of Old Tuberculin or purified protein derivative (PPD) tuberculin is injected intradermally on the flexor aspect of the forearm. The test is regarded as positive if, 2 to 4 days after injection, there is a reaction consisting of a raised area of inflammatory oedema not less than 5 mm in diameter, with surrounding erythema. The test is regarded as negative if there is no reaction or if there is an immediate (non-specific) reaction which disappears completely within 48 hours. The test should first be carried out with 1 tuberculin unit (TU) in 0·1 ml of normal saline. If there is no reaction it should be repeated with 10 TU in the same volume of saline. In order to obtain accurate results it is essential to use freshly prepared dilutions of tuberculin.

Differential tuberculin testing with antigens prepared from other mycobacteria, e.g. PPD-A (*M. avium*) or PPD-Y (*M. kansasii*) is often a satisfactory method of distinguishing atypical mycobacterial infection from tuberculosis.

The significance of the tuberculin test in relation to tuberculous infection has already been discussed (p. 203). The younger the patient the greater the diagnostic significance of a positive test. A repeatedly negative test over a period of 6 weeks from the onset of symptoms practically rules out a diagnosis of tuberculosis except in the elderly, after acute exanthemata, and in miliary tuberculosis and tuberculous meningitis.

Tuberculin testing is an essential part of the examination of the family contacts of cases of tuberculosis. Apart from its value as a diagnostic measure it indicates which of the contacts should be vaccinated with BCG. When large numbers are being tested, particularly children, the *Heaf multiple puncture tuberculin test* is preferable to the Mantoux technique as it is more rapidly performed and is less painful. For this test a solution containing 100,000 TU of PPD tuberculin per ml, to which adrenaline has been added, should be used. These tests may be read from the third to the seventh day and four grades of positivity are recognised.

Grade I—At least four discrete papules.
       II—The papules coalesce to form a ring.
     III—The area encircled by the papules is completely indurated.
     IV—Any reaction which is greater than III, including central necrosis.

Reaction in grades III and IV indicates infection with mammalian tubercle bacilli and a grade I reaction usually indicates infection with atypical tubercle bacilli. The significance of a grade II reaction is uncertain. The *tuberculin tine test* is performed with a disposable unit thus avoiding any risk of transmitting hepatitis. The unit has four prongs or 'tines' 2 mm in length mounted on a disc, the tines having been coated with Old Tuberculin.

3. *Bacteriological examination*. Sputum is seldom available in cases of primary pulmonary tuberculosis, but tubercle bacilli can sometimes be isolated by culture of fasting gastric juice or of secretion obtained by swabbing the larynx. At least three specimens should be examined. The isolation of tubercle bacilli is absolute proof of the diagnosis, but a negative result does not exclude it.

Primary pulmonary tuberculosis must be distinguished from other febrile illnesses such as influenza and infectious mononucleosis, from acute respiratory infections such as acute bronchitis and pneumonia, and from other causes of hilar lymph node enlargement such as the lymphomas (p. 622) and sarcoidosis (p. 328).

Prognosis. Since primary pulmonary tuberculosis and its complications respond satisfactorily to antituberculosis chemotherapy (p. 292), which should be given in every case, the prognosis is excellent.

Miliary Tuberculosis

The pathogenesis of this condition has already been discussed. Hitherto it has occurred chiefly in children and young adults. With the changing age-structure of tuberculosis in many countries it is now affecting persons in older age groups in whom it takes the form of an insidious illness—the so-called 'cryptic' type—which is often difficult to diagnose. Before the introduction of chemotherapy the disease was invariably fatal but most cases now recover completely.

Clinical Features. The disease may start suddenly or may be preceded by a few weeks of vague ill-health. In children and young adults the systemic disturbance rapidly becomes profound. In particular there is high remittent or intermittent pyrexia with drenching sweats during sleep, marked tachycardia, loss of weight and usually progressive anaemia. Cough and dyspnoea are occasionally present. There may be no abnormal physical signs in the lungs, although widespread fine crepitations are not infrequently heard at some stage of the disease. The liver is often enlarged and the spleen often palpable and sometimes tender. Choroidal tubercles may be visible in the fundus on ophthalmoscopy but are rarely present in miliary disease affecting the elderly. Leucocytosis is usually absent or slight and the erythrocyte sedimentation rate variable. If chemotherapy is not given the patient's condition deteriorates rapidly and death takes place from exhaustion or from tuberculous meningitis within 4 to 8 weeks.

The 'cryptic' form of the disease occurs in older age groups, particularly females. General malaise and eventual exhaustion, loss of weight, and anaemia are common presenting features. Respiratory symptoms are rare, and the characteristic miliary shadows are absent. Choroidal tubercles are never observed in this form of the disease. A variety of specific blood disorders—neutropenia, pancytopenia and leukaemoid reaction—may be found. The clinical features are often so non-specific that the diagnosis is frequently made only at autopsy.

Diagnosis. The clinical diagnosis of acute miliary tuberculosis can be made with certainty only when radiological examination of the chest shows the characteristic fine, 'miliary' mottling symmetrically distributed throughout both lung fields or when choroidal tubercles are seen. These changes take a few weeks to develop but the diagnosis can often be suspected at an earlier stage by the symptoms, progressive clinical deterioration, persistent pyrexia and splenomegaly. Bacteriological confirmation should be sought by culture of sputum, urine or bone-marrow. In difficult cases, liver biopsy may be diagnostic. Although the tuberculin reaction (p. 287) is usually positive, a negative result does not always exclude acute miliary tuberculosis, as tuberculin sensitivity is occasionally depressed in the acute phase of the illness. In 'cryptic' cases, a therapeutic test of chemotherapy with ethambutol and isoniazid (p. 292) is essential as death is inevitable if treatment is not given.

Acute miliary tuberculosis must be distinguished from other causes of severe pyrexia without obvious localising symptoms or signs, such as enteric fever (p. 67), infective endocarditis (p. 207), staphylococcal septicaemia (p. 63), empyema

(p. 337), subphrenic abscess (p. 403), acute pulmonary tuberculosis (below) and the lymphomas (p. 622).

Prognosis. Antituberculosis chemotherapy (p. 292) has reduced the mortality of miliary tuberculosis from 100 per cent to less than 5 per cent. The cause of death is often tuberculous meningitis, although many patients who develop this complication make a complete recovery, provided there has been no delay in starting treatment.

Postprimary Pulmonary Tuberculosis

Most of the morbidity and mortality from tuberculosis is caused by this form of the disease. Although in developing countries it is most prevalent in adolescence and early adult life, the majority of cases in Western Europe and North America now occur in middle-aged and elderly subjects, particularly males.

The lesions are most frequently situated in the upper lobes. Another common site is the apex of a lower lobe. The disease is often bilateral; usually it starts in one lung and spreads via the bronchi to the other; less commonly it develops in both lungs at the same time. Occasionally, when the disease takes an acute form, the initial lesion is pneumonic or bronchopneumonic.

Clinical Features. The onset of postprimary pulmonary tuberculosis is usually insidious, with the gradual development of general symptoms or of cough and sputum. Sometimes a dramatic incident such as a haemoptysis, an attack of pleurisy or a spontaneous pneumothorax marks the onset of the disease, but the diagnosis is now frequently made by radiography before any symptoms have appeared.

The local respiratory symptoms which may occur during the course of postprimary pulmonary tuberculosis are the following. *Cough,* which may be one of the earliest symptoms or which may not be troublesome until a late stage. Its absence does *not* exclude a diagnosis of pulmonary tuberculosis. *Sputum,* like cough, may not become a prominent feature until the disease has reached an advanced stage. It is usually mucoid at first but later becomes purulent. It is rarely foetid. *Haemoptysis,* in the early stages, is due to the erosion of a small vessel in a caseating lesion and the bleeding is usually slight. In the late stages it originates from a large vessel in the wall of a cavity and the haemorrhage may be large, occasionally fatal. *Dyspnoea on exertion* is usually a late symptom, but may develop acutely when due to a spontaneous pneumothorax or to a rapidly developing pleural effusion. *Pleural pain* is usually due to dry pleurisy but occasionally to spontaneous pneumothorax.

Physical Signs. In the early stages none may be elicited, but despite this an extensive lesion may be visible radiologically. The earliest physical signs consist of a few medium or coarse crepitations, usually situated over one or other lung apex posteriorly. These crepitations may be present only after coughing.

As the disease advances the percussion note over the site of the lesion loses its normal resonance and there is a change in the character of the breath sounds, which may become either diminished in intensity or harsh vesicular with prolonged expiration. The crepitations become more numerous and more coarse. Ultimately the physical signs of consolidation, cavitation and fibrosis may appear (p. 261). Pleurisy, with or without effusion, and spontaneous pneumothorax may modify the pulmonary signs.

Radiological Examination. This is of paramount importance for diagnosis in the early stages before physical signs appear and for assessment of the extent and progress of the disease. The earliest radiological change is an ill-defined opacity or opacities, usually situated in one of the upper lobes. In more advanced cases opacities are larger and more widespread, and may be bilateral. Occasionally there is a dense, homogeneous shadow involving a whole lobe ('pneumonic tuberculosis').

An area or areas of translucency within the opacities indicates cavitation. Very large cavities may be visible in some cases. If there is progress towards healing the opacities shrink, become more clearly defined, and may later show calcification. When fibrosis is marked the trachea and heart shadow are displaced towards the side of the lesion.

In any case of tuberculosis it is common for lesions at different stages of development to coexist. Thus in one area there may be cavitation, in a second evidence of fibrosis and in a third an opacity due to recent disease.

The presence of cavitation in an untreated case usually indicates that the disease is active. When cavitation is absent, however, it may sometimes be difficult to assess the activity of a tuberculous lesion from a single radiograph. Observation of the lesion over a period of time will be necessary in doubtful cases.

The radiological appearances of pleural effusion and pneumothorax, which may accompany those of pulmonary tuberculosis, are described on pages 334 and 341.

Diagnosis. The symptoms and signs suggesting a diagnosis of tuberculosis have already been stated. The grounds on which pulmonary tuberculosis should be suspected are:

1. Unexplained cough persisting for more than three weeks.
2. Haemoptysis.
3. Pleural pain not associated with an acute illness.
4. Spontaneous pneumothorax (although most cases are *not* tuberculous).
5. Unexplained tiredness or loss of weight, even in the absence of respiratory symptoms.

The presence of any of these symptoms demands immediate radiological examination of the lungs and, if any abnormality is found, the examination of at least three specimens of sputum for tubercle bacilli.

When bacilli are numerous, the diagnosis can readily be made by microscopical examination of sputum smears stained by the Ziehl-Neelsen method, but culture of sputum (or of fasting gastric juice or laryngeal swabs, if no sputum can be obtained) is essential for the isolation of bacilli present in small numbers and for the detection of drug resistance (p. 295). Cultural methods are thus of great practical value and should be used in the examination of every specimen, if facilities permit.

The conditions with which pulmonary tuberculosis may be confused include pneumonia, bronchial carcinoma, bronchiectasis, chronic bronchitis, infective endocarditis, diabetes mellitus and thyrotoxicosis.

In the vast majority of cases the diagnosis of pulmonary tuberculosis can be made with certainty by radiological examination of the chest, bacteriological examination of the sputum for tubercle bacilli, or a combination of the two. In some cases it is necessary to carry out further radiological examination after a course of treatment with an antibiotic in order to exclude an acute inflammatory cause for an abnormal shadow.

Pulmonary tuberculosis must be regarded as active and requiring treatment if one or more of the following features is present:

1. Local or general symptoms, particularly haemoptysis or pleural pain.
2. A radiological opacity known or suspected to be of recent development, or one which has increased in extent during a period of observation.
3. Radiological evidence of cavitation.
4. Tubercle bacilli isolated from sputum, gastric juice, or laryngeal swabs.

Complications
1. *Pleurisy with or without effusion.* This common complication is described on pages 333–336.
2. *Spontaneous pneumothorax.* This may be due to rupture of a tuberculous lesion into the pleural space (p. 339).
3. *Tuberculous empyema or pyopneumothorax* (p. 337). This may complicate spontaneous pneumothorax.
4. *Tuberculous laryngitis.* This usually occurs as a complication of advanced pulmonary disease.
5. *Tuberculous enteritis.* This is practically confined to advanced cases. It is due to the swallowing of heavily infected sputum.
6. *Ischiorectal abscess and fistula-in-ano.* The abscess forms as a result of tubercle bacilli passing through an abrasion in the rectal mucosa. Secondary pyogenic infection invariably occurs, and a fistula may form when the abscess is incised or if it ruptures spontaneously.
7. *Dissemination of tuberculosis via the blood stream* is very unusual in post-primary pulmonary tuberculosis, but may occur in advanced cases with the production of renal tuberculosis or tuberculous meningitis.
8. *Ventilatory failure* (p. 258) and *right ventricular failure* (p. 195) are important late complications if extensive areas of lung tissue are destroyed by tuberculosis or were resected when surgery was the only effective treatment. Although the tuberculous infection itself can be controlled, the residual pulmonary damage and the fibrosis and emphysema with which it is invariably associated may leave the patient seriously disabled by exertional dyspnoea.
9. *Secondary infection* of a healed cavity with fungi such as *Aspergillus fumigatus* may lead to the development of a mycetoma (p. 298). Occasionally the rupture of a large blood vessel in the wall of a pulmonary cavity or a dilated bronchus may result in a massive or even fatal haemoptysis long after the tuberculous infection has been eradicated.

Prognosis. With the advent of effective chemotherapy there has been a remarkable decline in the mortality from pulmonary tuberculosis. Provided the tubercle bacilli are not initially drug-resistant and chemotherapy is used correctly, a fatal outcome is extremely uncommon, even if the disease has reached an advanced stage when it is first recognised. The advent of new effective antituberculosis drugs has also improved the outlook for those patients whose bacilli are resistant to two or three drugs. The serious late complications of ventilatory failure and secondary infection with pyogenic bacteria or fungi can all be prevented if pulmonary tuberculosis is diagnosed at a reasonably early stage and is efficiently treated.

The Treatment of Tuberculosis

General Principles

1. *Antituberculosis chemotherapy* is by far the most important measure in the treatment of all forms of tuberculosis and should be given to every patient with active disease.

2. *Rest* is unimportant except in a few specific circumstances. The current practice is to keep patients in bed only until acute symptoms have subsided. The majority of patients are ambulant throughout treatment, many of them remaining at work. Immobilisation is of course necessary in certain forms of skeletal tuberculosis.

3. *Isolation* of patients who are excreting tubercle bacilli and who are therefore potentially infectious has always been an important principle. The observation made in Madras that the frequency of disease amongst contacts was not greater whether the patient was treated at home or in a sanatorium has led to the adoption of a policy whereby patients, even those who are sputum-positive on microscopy, are treated wholly as out-patients. However, many authorities still prefer to isolate patients from contact with young children. Hospitalisation for an initial period of treatment, as distinct from isolation, may be recommended for patients who cannot be relied upon to adhere to the regimen advised and for those with difficult therapeutic problems.

4. *Surgical treatment* such as pulmonary resection, nephrectomy or removal of superficial lymph nodes is now rarely required. However, an irreparably damaged kidney should be removed and drainage of an abscess from tuberculous lymph nodes or of an empyema may be necessary. Early surgical treatment of tuberculosis of the spine ensures stability and prevents deformity.

Chemotherapy

Effective treatment of tuberculosis demands not only a detailed knowledge of the drugs used but also of the most appropriate treatment regimen for the individual patient.

Drugs. In Britain, five drugs—rifampicin, isoniazid, ethambutol, streptomycin and sodium aminosalicylate (PAS)—are normally considered in the initial treatment of tuberculosis. Thiacetazone, which is cheap, is widely used in developing countries. Pyrazinamide is particularly useful in the treatment of tuberculous meningitis because it diffuses well into the cerebrospinal fluid. Apart from a few minor variations in dose and duration of treatment (pp. 294 and 295) the policy governing the use of antituberculosis drugs is the same for all manifestations of the disease.

The drugs should be used in the following once daily doses:

Rifampicin	Children	10–20 mg/kg
	Adults weighing less than 50 kg	450 mg
	Adults weighing more than 50 kg	600 mg
	Intermittent regimen	600–1,200 mg
Isoniazid	Children	3 mg/kg
	Adults	200–300 mg
	Intermittent regimen	15 mg/kg*
	Miliary/meningitis	10–12 mg/kg*

Ethambutol†	Initial 8 weeks in short-course regimen	25 mg/kg
	Other daily regimens	15 mg/kg
	Intermittent regimen	90 mg/kg
Streptomycin sulphate	Children	30 mg/kg
	Adults under 40 years and weighing more than 45 kg	1 g
	Adults 40–60 years or weighing less than 45 kg	0·75 g
	Adults over 60 years or in patients with renal failure	According to serum levels
	Intermittent regimens	0·75–1 g
Sodium amino-salicylate (PAS)†	Children	300 mg/kg
	Adults	10–12 g
	Intermittent regimen	10–12 g
Pyrazinamide	Daily	30 mg/kg (max 2·5 g)
	Intermittent regimen	90 mg/kg
Thiacetazone	Children	2 mg/kg
	Adults	150 mg

* Plus pyridoxine 10 mg to prevent peripheral neuropathy (p. 137).

† In patients with renal failure the doses of ethambutol and PAS given may also need to be determined according to serum levels.

SIDE-EFFECTS. In choosing a suitable drug regimen for individual patients it is important to bear in mind those side-effects which are particularly liable to cause serious chronic disability, such as vestibular disturbance due to streptomycin and optic neuritis due to ethambutol. Streptomycin must be prescribed with caution in the middle aged and elderly, who find difficulty in compensating for vestibular disturbance. Even in the relatively low dose recommended for ethambutol, a few patients develop optic neuritis and a proportion of them are left with a permanent visual defect. This potential hazard must be taken into consideration whenever ethambutol is prescribed. Patients should be instructed to test their own visual acuity daily.

Streptomycin and PAS, and occasionally isoniazid, ethambutol and rifampicin, may produce a hypersensitivity reaction, consisting of pyrexia and an erythematous skin eruption, which usually develops 2 to 4 weeks after treatment is started.

Rifampicin is a potent liver enzyme inducer (p. 426) and should be used with appropriate caution when the following drugs are prescribed: oestrogens (e.g. oral contraception), anticoagulants, corticosteroids and digoxin. It should, if possible, be avoided in patients with liver disease.

The principal side-effects are:

Streptomycin: vestibular disturbance (see above); hypersensitivity (see above); deafness (rare).

PAS: hypersensitivity (see above); anorexia, nausea, vomiting, diarrhoea (common); goitre and hypothyroidism (rare); hepatitis, usually associated with hypersensitivity (rare); intestinal malabsorption (rare); hypokalaemia (rare); haemolytic anaemia (rare).

Isoniazid: hypersensitivity (occasionally, see above); polyneuropathy (rare); lack of mental concentration (rare).

Ethambutol: optic neuritis (see above); hypersensitivity (occasionally, see above).

Rifampicin: drug interaction (see above); hypersensitivity (occasionally, see above); hepatitis (rare); purpura (rare); fever, respiratory, cutaneous and abdominal syndromes (intermittent regimens only).

Thiacetazone: nausea, vomiting, anaemia (rare); leucopenia (rare).

REGIMENS. The following regimens are now considered to be optimal in the treatment of tuberculosis, those containing rifampicin having the advantage that the period of treatment can be shortened to nine months:

1. An *initial* phase lasting eight weeks:

Rifampicin 450–600 mg *plus* ethambutol 25 mg/kg *plus* isoniazid 200–300 mg *or* rifampicin 450–600 mg *plus* streptomycin 0.75–1 g *plus* isoniazid 200–300 mg *or* streptomycin 0·75–1 g *plus* PAS 10 g *plus* isoniazid 200–300 mg followed by:

2. *A continuation phase* in which an unsupervised oral or a fully supervised regimen may be selected. Oral regimens include a combination of isoniazid with rifampicin, ethambutol (15 mg/kg) or PAS. In young children, PAS is to be preferred to ethambutol because of difficulty in the early identification of ocular toxicity in this age group. Rifampicin, which colours the urine pinkish-orange, should be administered about half an hour before breakfast.

Isoniazid and rifampicin may be prescribed together (Rimactazid, Rifinah), as may isoniazid and ethambutol (Mynah). Isoniazid and PAS are dispensed together in the following forms:

Sodium aminosalicylate and Isoniazid cachets, B.P.C., 4 cachets twice daily.

Pasinah D (Wander), 2 cachets daily.

Inapasade S.Q. (Smith and Nephew), 1 packet daily.

Alternatively a supervised regimen may be given twice weekly at 3- and 4-day intervals in the following doses:

Streptomycin sulphate 1 g by intramuscular injection.

Isoniazid 15 mg/kg body weight by mouth.

Pyridoxine 10 mg to prevent peripheral neuropathy.

This type of chemotherapy is particularly valuable for uncooperative patients, as treatment can be wholly supervised, the tablets being administered at the same time as the injections.

Inexpensive Treatment Regimens. In developing countries it will usually be impossible for economic reasons to adhere to the recommended chemotherapeutic regimens. The following inexpensive forms of treatment are reasonably effective if administered for 12 months:

(*a*) Streptomycin (1 g) by intramuscular injection *plus* isoniazid (15 mg/kg) by mouth plus pyridoxine (10 mg) on 2 days per week. This is 90 to 95 per cent effective: if 1 or preferably 2 months of daily treatment with streptomycin, PAS and isoniazid can be afforded as initial treatment, the effectiveness of this regimen is nearly 100 per cent.

(*b*) Isoniazid (300 mg) plus thiacetazone (150 mg) given in a single daily dose by mouth is extremely cheap, and is about 80 to 85 per cent effective.

Response to Treatment. If the bacilli at the start of treatment are fully sensitive to the drugs in use it is most unusual, even in advanced cases, for cultures of sputum, gastric washings, laryngeal swabs or urine to remain positive for longer than 6 months. Where facilities for sensitivity testing do not exist, reliance must be placed on smear examination.

Persistence of a positive sputum culture after 6 months' treatment suggests that drug resistance has occurred. Alternatively, failure may have been due to irregular treatment. Chemical tests to detect the presence of PAS, isoniazid and rifampicin in urine are available.

Duration of Treatment. If the regimen includes rifampicin throughout, the duration of treatment for all forms of the disease is 9 months. In regimens which do *not* include rifampicin throughout, the recommended duration of treatment remains 12 months for primary lesions, miliary tuberculosis, pleural effusion, and minimal pulmonary tuberculosis; 18 months for advanced pulmonary tuberculosis and for genitourinary, lymph node and skeletal tuberculosis.

Drug-resistant Tubercle Bacilli. The treatment of patients infected with drug-resistant tubercle bacilli presents a problem requiring specialised knowledge for its solution. Additional drugs available for the treatment of such cases are:

Capreomycin	0·75–1 g	intramuscularly
Ethionamide	0·75–1 g	
Prothionamide	0·75–1 g	given in a single
Pyrazinamide	30 mg/kg	oral dose daily
Cycloserine	0·75–1 g	

Corticosteroid Drugs

These agents suppress the inflammatory reaction excited by the tubercle bacillus and by interfering with tissue defence mechanisms may promote a rapid dissemination of infection throughout the body. If, however, a corticosteroid drug is given in conjunction with effective antituberculosis chemotherapy it may exert a favourable influence on the course of the disease by reducing the severity both of the local inflammatory reaction and of the associated systemic disturbance. In acute cases of pulmonary tuberculosis such treatment will rapidly relieve pyrexia and will often produce a dramatic improvement in the radiological appearances. The effect is temporary and ceases when the corticosteroid drug is withdrawn, but it may save the lives of patients with fulminating tuberculous infection by enabling them to survive until antituberculosis chemotherapy has had time to exert its influence. Prednisolone is given in a dose of 20 mg daily for about 3 months.

Corticosteroid drugs in combination with chemotherapy may also be of value in tuberculous pleural and pericardial effusion, tuberculous disease of intrathoracic or superficial lymph nodes, tuberculosis involving the eye and particularly in tuberculous meningitis. Whenever there is evidence of ureteric obstruction in genitourinary tuberculosis, corticosteroids should be administered in addition to chemotherapy, for such treatment significantly reduces the need for surgical treatment.

Symptomatic Treatment

Haemoptysis. A sedative may be given to allay anxiety, e.g. diazepam. Morphine, which depresses the cough reflex, may have the effect of allowing blood clot to accumulate in the bronchi and should seldom be prescribed. Haemoptysis nearly always stops spontaneously, and reassurance to this effect lessens the strains of what, to the patient and his relatives, is a most alarming experience.

If the haemorrhage is very severe a blood transfusion should be given and, if respiratory obstruction develops, the blood must be removed from the bronchi by aspiration through a bronchoscope. Control of the bleeding by surgical measures is occasionally required.

Pleural pain due to dry pleurisy or spontaneous pneumothorax and *cough* are treated as described on page 267. *Fever and sweating* usually subside soon after chemotherapy is started. When persistent and excessive they should be treated by repeated tepid sponging. *Hoarseness* is usually due to tuberculous laryngitis, which responds rapidly to specific chemotherapy provided the organism is not drug-resistant. Severe and continuous *diarrhoea* in a patient with pulmonary tuberculosis is usually due to tuberculous enteritis. In most cases it can be rapidly controlled by chemotherapy. It must be remembered, however, that diarrhoea may also be caused by PAS.

The Prevention of Tuberculosis

Mortality rates are no longer considered very important in the assessment of the success of control measures because of the very low rates now existing in some countries and the inaccuracy of certification in the many countries where tuberculosis remains a major problem. The frequency of tuberculous meningitis is, however, a crude yardstick of the progress being made towards eradication. *Notification rates* are of limited value because of the adoption of varying standards, but the annual recording of the number of smear-positive patients with pulmonary tuberculosis is a useful indication of the efficiency of preventive measures. Another useful parameter is the *tuberculin index*, i.e. the percentage of positive reactors to tuberculin at a standard age, e.g. 5 or 13 years. It is important to assess the possible influence of the prevalence of atypical bacteria in the community and of BCG vaccination policy on the tuberculin index. It is also useful to assess periodically the percentage of patients who on initial diagnosis are found to excrete drug-resistant tubercle bacilli.

The following control measures are important in the achievement of the goal of eradication of the disease.

1. **Improvement in socio-economic conditions** mainly in respect of adequate housing, ventilation and nutrition may still be the most important control measure of all.

2. **Case-finding.** (*a*) *Mass radiography* is an expensive method of case-finding and should now be used exclusively in a selective manner concentrating on the following specific groups:

High Incidence Groups	Danger Groups
Symptom groups (GP referrals)	Individuals in contact with children
Persons in prisons, borstals and mental hospitals	Barmen and waitresses
Elderly men especially those in lodging houses	Bus conductors
Immigrants to Britain, especially from Asia	Hairdressers
Diabetics, postgastrectomy patients	Doctors, dentists and nurses

Open access to mass radiography for general practitioners and minimum waiting time for patients are essential for success. Mobile units are often employed to visit a locality in which several cases have occurred over a short period or when a highly infectious patient may have spread the disease widely in a community.

(b) *Sputum-smear examination* is an important and inexpensive method of case-finding in developing countries. The provision of a microscope and the training of a health worker in the examination of smears can be readily undertaken.

(c) *Contact examination* achieves a high yield in case-finding. Efforts should be concentrated on the immediate examination of household contacts of sputum-smear positive patients especially amongst contacts under 25 years of age.

3. **Chemotherapy.** The proper use of appropriate chemotherapy regimens makes a significant contribution to tuberculosis control by the rapid elimination of sources of infection.

4. **Isolation.** Isolation of patients is rarely considered necessary nowadays except where very young children are at risk, provided the source case is being properly treated by chemotherapy.

5. **BCG Vaccination.** This is carried out by the administration of freeze-dried vaccine, reconstituted at the time of use, by the intradermal route ($0 \cdot 1$ ml) injected at the junction of the upper and middle thirds of the upper arm. The multiple puncture method (40 needles) is less commonly used. Complications such as local abscess formation and enlargement of regional lymph nodes are very rare. BCG vaccine should not be give in the presence of immunodeficiency. The duration of protection is about 3 to 7 years. Vaccination reduces the incidence of pulmonary tuberculosis in young adults by 80 per cent and eliminates the risk of serious disseminated disease—miliary tuberculosis and tuberculous meningitis.

Policy in relation to BCG vaccination in a community depends upon the size of the problem locally. If the infection rate is very low (1 per cent or less) vaccination is inappropriate on the grounds of cost and the fact that BCG interferes with the diagnostic value of the tuberculin test in such a situation. Where there are many positive tuberculin reactors, as occur in communities with low living standards, the vaccination of the newborn is usually indicated. Where infection rates are falling to low levels, vaccination at puberty may be appropriate.

6. **Chemoprophylaxis.** The concept of administering chemotherapy to individuals in order to try to prevent the development of tuberculosis is adopted in different communities with varying degrees of enthusiasm. Chemoprophylaxis, using isoniazid (5 mg/kg by mouth) daily for 1 year, is indicated in: (a) tuberculin positive children under 3 years of age, as this is a vulnerable group in respect of miliary tuberculosis and tuberculous meningitis; (b) individuals who have recently become tuberculin-positive; (c) patients on immunosuppressive drugs.

Chemoprophylaxis may be considered in: (a) tuberculin-positive adolescents with a high level of tuberculin sensitivity; (b) minimal tuberculous lesions of doubtful activity; (c) infants of highly infectious parents, when isoniazid-resistant BCG vaccine may be administered, isoniazid chemoprophylaxis being given for 6 weeks thereafter to prevent infection until vaccination exerts its protective effects. effects.

7. **Elimination of Bovine Infection.** Although bovine infection is extremely rare nowadays, constant vigilance will be required to ensure that it remains so.

Respiratory Diseases Caused by Fungi

Most fungi encountered by man are harmless saprophytes, but some species may in certain circumstances infect human tissues or promote damaging allergic reactions.

The term *mycosis* is applied to disease caused by fungal infection. Predisposing factors include metabolic disorders, such as diabetes mellitus, toxic states such as chronic alcoholism, diseases such as leukaemia and myelomatosis in which immunological responses are disturbed, treatment with corticosteroids, immunosuppressive drugs and X-ray therapy. Local factors, such as tissue damage by suppuration or necrosis and the elimination of the competitive influence of a normal bacterial flora by antibiotics, may also facilitate fungal infection.

Allergic reactions to fungi may cause bronchial asthma (*A. fumigatus* and *Cladosporium herbarum*), pulmonary eosinophilia (*A. fumigatus*) or allergic alveolitis (*Micropolyspora faeni, Thermoactinomyces vulgaris, Coniosporium corticale* and *Aspergillus clavatus*). These conditions are described in the following section on allergic diseases of the respiratory tract.

The diagnosis of a pulmonary mycosis is usually made by mycological examination of the sputum, supported by serological tests for precipitating antibodies, and in some instances by skin sensitivity tests.

Aspergillosis. This is the most common respiratory mycosis in Britain. Inhaled air-borne spores of *Aspergillus fumigatus* lodge and germinate in pulmonary cysts or bullae, 'healed' tuberculous cavities, dilated bronchi, or pulmonary infarcts. In most cases the fungal infection remains localised to the site of the original lesion, but occasionally, when resistance is low, it may extend into adjacent normal lung tissue, or via the bronchi into the opposite lung, with the production of extensive pulmonary necrosis and grave systemic disturbance (*necrotising pulmonary aspergillosis*).

When a pre-existing pulmonary cavity is infected by *A. fumigatus*, a large spherical mass of fungal mycelium may form within the cavity, producing on X-ray examination a tumour-like opacity to which the term *mycetoma* or *aspergilloma* is applied. This type of lesion can readily be distinguished from a peripheral bronchial carcinoma by the presence of a crescent of air between the mycelial mass and the cavity wall. An aspergilloma usually produces no specific symptoms, but is occasionally responsible for recurrent haemoptysis.

Whenever mycelium is present in large quantities in a pulmonary cavity, or in any other lesion, precipitating antibodies can be detected in the serum by means of a gel diffusion test, using an antigen derived from *A. fumigatus*. This test is of considerable diagnostic value.

Candidiasis. Occasionally, in debilitated subjects oral thrush (p. 355) extends downwards into the respiratory tract, with the production of bronchial or pulmonary candidiasis.

Other Pulmonary Mycoses. These, all of which are rare, include nocardiosis, cryptococcosis (p. 923), mucormycosis, blastomycosis (p. 923) and sporotrichosis (p. 923). Only the first three of these conditions have been encountered in Britain. In a somewhat different category are histoplasmosis (p. 919) and coccidioidomycosis (p. 924), which are endemic in certain areas of North America and

Africa, and produce local or systemic granulomatous lesions resembling tuberculosis.

Treatment of the Pulmonary Mycoses. This is difficult and unsatisfactory. The administration of antibacterial drugs should be stopped, and antifungal agents substituted. Nystatin and natamycin by inhalation may control the more superficial respiratory mycoses involving the trachea and bronchi. For grave pulmonary infections amphotericin B, a potent but highly toxic antifungal agent, may have to be given intravenously in a dose of 0·25 mg per kg body weight on alternate days, increasing gradually to 1 mg per kg over the course of 1 to 2 weeks if side-effects permit. Surgical resection of a mycetoma may have to be considered if severe haemoptysis occurs.

ALLERGIC DISEASES

Many types of particle suspended in the atmosphere possess antigenic properties, and are capable of stimulating the production of specific antibody when inhaled (p. 30). Further exposure to antigen of an individual 'sensitised' in this way may provoke an allergic reaction which causes pathological changes and disturbances of function in the tissue where the reaction occurs. Three types of allergic response are concerned in the production of respiratory disease. The Type I or anaphylactic response (p. 38), mediated by reaginic antibody (immunoglobulin IgE), is associated with an immediate hypersensitivity reaction, the clinical manifestations of which include allergic rhinitis and bronchial asthma. The Type III or Arthus-type response, mediated by precipitating antibody (immunoglobulin IgG), is associated with a late hypersensitivity reaction which may contribute to the production of allergic alveolitis. Both Type I and Type III responses may be concerned in the production of some forms of pulmonary eosinophilia, such as allergic bronchopulmonary aspergillosis. Type IV or tuberculin-type allergic responses, which are cell-mediated and do not involve circulating antibody, are usually associated with delayed hypersensitivity reactions in conditions such as tuberculosis, but may be concerned in predominantly Type III reactions, such as allergic alveolitis.

Ingested antigens, or drugs acting as haptens, such as aspirin and PAS, occasionally produce allergic respiratory disorders, such as bronchial asthma and pulmonary eosinophilia, and auto-antigens may have a similar role in conditions such as polyarteritis and systemic lupus erythematosus.

In this chapter, allergic rhinitis, bronchial asthma, pulmonary eosinophilia and allergic alveolitis will be described in some detail, but for a description of other forms of allergic disorder the reader should refer to Chapter 2.

Allergic Rhinitis

This is a disorder in which there are episodes of nasal congestion, watery nasal discharge and sneezing. It may be *seasonal* or *perennial*.

Aetiology. Allergic rhinitis is due to a Type I antigen-antibody reaction in the nasal mucosa. The antigens concerned in the seasonal form of the disorder are pollens from grasses, flowers, weeds or trees. Grass pollen is responsible for *hay fever*, the most common type of seasonal allergic rhinitis in Britain, and this disorder is at its peak between May and July.

Perennial allergic rhinitis may be a specific reaction to antigens derived from house dust, fungal spores or animal dander, but similar symptoms can be caused by physical or chemical irritants, such as pungent odours or fumes, including strong perfumes, cold air and dry atmospheres. In this context the term 'allergic' is a misnomer.

Clinical Features. In the seasonal type there are frequent sudden attacks of sneezing, with profuse watery nasal discharge and nasal obstruction. These attacks last for a few hours, and are often accompanied by smarting and watering of the eyes and conjunctival injection. In the perennial type the symptoms are similar, but more continuous and generally less severe.

Diagnosis. In seasonal allergic rhinitis the diagnosis is usually obvious because the attacks occur only during the pollen season. In the perennial type it may be more difficult, because the symptoms may initially be indistinguishable from those of coryza. In coryza, however, the subsequent appearance of pus in the nasal discharge usually makes the diagnosis clear.

In seasonal allergic rhinitis skin sensitivity tests or nasal provocation tests with the relevant antigen are usually positive, and are thus of diagnostic value, but these tests are less useful in perennial rhinitis, and may be completely negative.

The symptoms of both types of allergic rhinitis, particularly the seasonal type, can usually be controlled by drugs, and in some cases the condition subsides spontaneously. It is more a serious inconvenience than a disease.

Treatment. The following symptomatic measures, singly or in combination, are usually effective in both seasonal and perennial allergic rhinitis:

1. An antihistamine drug, such as chlorpheniramine maleate, 4–8 mg thrice daily, but in some cases this causes intolerable drowsiness.
2. A decongestant nasal spray, e.g. 1 per cent solution of ephedrine hydrochloride in saline.
3. Sodium cromoglycate nasal spray, 10 mg into each nostril 6 times daily.
4. Beclomethasone dipropionate nasal spray, one metered dose of 50 μg into each nostril 4 times daily.

Patients failing to respond to these measures may obtain symptomatic relief from weekly intramuscular injections of 0·5–1 mg of tetracosactrin zinc, but this form of treatment should be reserved for those patients whose symptoms are very severe and interfere seriously with business and social activities.

Prevention. In the seasonal type an attempt should be made to avoid exposure to pollen, or at least reduce it to a minimum, for example by avoiding country districts and keeping indoors as much as possible, with the windows closed, during the pollen season. Some patients with hay fever may benefit from preseasonal hyposensitisation with a grass pollen extract. The prevention of perennial rhinitis consists of avoiding, as far as possible, exposure to any identifiable aetiological factors. Specific hyposensitisation is probably of little value.

Bronchial Asthma

Bronchial asthma is characterised by paroxysms of dyspnoea accompanied by wheezing, resulting from temporary narrowing of the bronchi by muscle spasm, mucosal swelling or viscid secretion. The bronchial narrowing interferes with pulmonary ventilation and increases the work of breathing by raising the resistance to air flow within the bronchi. Being more marked during expiration it also causes air to be 'trapped' in the lungs. The narrowed bronchi can no longer be effectively cleared of mucus by the act of coughing, and obstruction of many of the smaller bronchi by inspissated and often very tenacious secretion adds to the respiratory embarrassment. In fatal cases this is usually the most conspicuous finding at autopsy.

Aetiology. Asthma may begin at any age, but in most cases it starts either in childhood or in middle age. 'Early onset' asthma is slightly more common in males, and 'late onset' asthma in females. 'Early onset' asthma occurs in atopic individuals, i.e. those who readily form reaginic antibodies to commonly encountered allergens (p. 38). Such individuals can be identified by skin sensitivity tests (p. 302), which give positive reactions with a wide range of common allergens. They often suffer from other allergic disorders, such as allergic rhinitis and eczema, and a family history of these disorders and of 'early onset' asthma is common. It is unusual for a single allergen to be the sole cause of asthma, and clinical experience indicates that many different allergens are implicated in almost every case, although the importance of each of them may vary from time to time. 'Late onset' asthma generally occurs in non-atopic individuals, and it would appear that external allergens play no part in the production of this form of the disease, to which the term 'intrinsic asthma' is sometimes applied.

The allergens responsible for asthma in atopic individuals generally enter the bronchi with the inspired air, and are derived from organic material, such as pollen, mite-containing house dust, feathers, animal dander and fungal spores. Previous exposure to these agents will have stimulated the formation of reaginic antibody (the immunoglobulin IgE), and a Type I antigen-antibody reaction in the bronchi may follow further exposure to specific allergen. This releases pharmacologically active substances, such as histamine, bradykinin, slow-reacting substance (SRS-A) and serotonin, which provoke bronchial constriction and an inflammatory reaction of allergic type in the bronchial mucosa. Much less frequently, similar effects may be produced by ingested allergens derived from certain foods, such as fish, eggs, milk, yeasts and wheat, which presumably reach the bronchi via the blood stream. Ingested non-protein substances, particularly drugs, of which aspirin is a notable example, occasionally cause asthma by forming haptens.

It is possible that a Type III allergic reaction may also be implicated in the pathogenesis of bronchial asthma, particularly where antigens derived from fungi, such as *A. fumigatus*, are concerned.

Regardless of whether asthma occurs in atopic or non-atopic individuals, the symptoms are often aggravated by non-specific factors, such as bronchial irritation caused by tobacco smoke, dust, acrid fumes and cold air, bacterial infection in the respiratory tract, and emotional stress. Strenuous exertion can also provoke an asthmatic attack in predisposed individuals, particularly children.

Clinical Features. Bronchial asthma may be either *episodic* or *chronic*, and although there is a good deal of overlap between these two syndromes, the distinction is clinically useful, particularly in terms of prognosis and management. In general, atopic individuals tend to develop episodic asthma, and non-atopic individuals chronic asthma.

In typical cases of episodic asthma the paroxysms, which may occur at any hour of the day or night, are of sudden onset, but may be preceded by a feeling of tightness in the chest. The dyspnoea, which may be intense, is chiefly expirtory in character. Expiration becomes a conscious and exhausting effort, in contrast to inspiration which is short and gasping. The patient adopts an upright position, fixing the shoulder-girdle to assist the accessory muscles of expiration. Wheezing, chiefly expiratory, is heard, and there may be an unproductive cough which aggravates the dyspnoea. In severe attacks there is tachycardia, pulsus paradoxus, and central cyanosis.

The attack may end abruptly within an hour or two, sometimes with the coughing up of tough viscid sputum, but a less intense degree of expiratory wheeze may persist for many hours or even for several days before subsiding gradually. The term *status asthmaticus* describes a state of intense asthma which persists for many hours or days. The sputum, usually scanty, may contain numerous eosinophil leucocytes and, occasionally, gelatinous casts of small bronchi. In most cases there is an increase in the number of eosinophil leucocytes in the blood.

In *chronic asthma* the paroxysmal character of the symptoms is usually less conspicuous, the chief clinical features being continuous wheeze and breathlessness on exertion. Cough and mucoid sputum, with recurrent episodes of frank respiratory infection, are common in this type of asthma, and may be due to associated chronic bronchitis.

Physical Signs in the Chest. 1. During a paroxysm the chest is held near the position of full inspiration. The percussion note may be hyper-resonant. The breath sounds, which are obscured by numerous high-pitched musical rhonchi, are vesicular in character with prolonged expiration. In very severe asthma airflow may be insufficient to produce rhonchi, and a 'silent chest' in such patients is an ominous sign.

2. Between paroxysms there are usually no abnormal physical signs except in patients with chronic asthma, who are seldom without rhonchi. Severe asthma starting in childhood usually causes a 'pigeon chest' deformity.

Radiological Examination. In uncomplicated bronchial asthma the chest radiograph is normal. In long-standing cases the signs of emphysema may be present, and the lateral view may demonstrate a 'pigeon chest' deformity. Occasionally, when a bronchus is obstructed by tenacious mucus, there is an opacity caused by lobar or segmental collapse.

Pulmonary Funtion Tests. Measurements of the forced expiratory volume in 1 second (FEV_1) and forced vital capacity (FVC) or of the peak expiratory flow rate (PEFR) provide a fairly reliable indication of the degree of airway obstruction (p. 263), and can also be used to determine whether and to what extent it can be relieved by bronchodilator drugs or corticosteroids. Such tests thus have an important place in the diagnosis and treatment of bronchial asthma. Measurements of arterial blood gas pressures (Pao_2 and $Paco_2$) are indispensable to the management of patients with status asthmaticus (p. 303).

Skin Sensitivity Tests. A tiny prick is made in the skin through a drop of a specially prepared solution of the substance to be tested, and a positive reaction is indicated by the development of a wheal and flare, which begins to appear within a few minutes. Tests are usually performed with solution of common substances known to possess antigenic properties. It is seldom possible with these tests to identify one particular substance as the cause of asthma in an individual case, and their chief value is to distinguish atopic from non-atopic subjects.

Differential Diagnosis. Bronchial asthma seldom presents problems in diagnosis, except at the beginning, when it may be difficult to distinguish from left ventricular failure (p. 195) and tracheal obstruction (p. 310). Chronic asthma and chronic bronchitis often coexist, but a good response to bronchodilator drugs or corticosteroids suggests that asthma is the predominant condition.

Course and Prognosis. The prognosis of the individual attack is good, except in severe status asthmaticus where there is occasionally a fatal outcome. Spontaneous recovery is fairly common in episodic asthma, particularly in children, but rare in chronic asthma, which often causes permanent pulmonary damage. Seasonal fluctuations occur in both types of asthma. Atopic subjects with episodic asthma are usually worse in the summer, when they are more heavily exposed to antigens, while chronic asthmatics are usually worse in the winter months because of their increased liability to bacterial infection.

Treatment

1. MANAGEMENT OF AN ASTHMATIC ATTACK. The patient should be allowed to take up the position which he finds most comfortable, either propped up in bed or sitting in a chair. If central cyanosis is present, oxygen should be administered with a 28 per cent Ventimask or an Edinburgh mask (p. 265). Although a higher inspired oxygen concentration is more effective and usually safe in most patients with asthma, it should be deferred in a severe case until after the patient has been admitted to hospital. A β_2-adrenergic receptor stimulant, salbutamol or terbutaline, should be given by inhalation. For maximum bronchodilatation 2 doses ('puffs') should be inhaled at a time, the second 5 minutes after the first. The relief obtained usually lasts for 3 to 4 hours. It is seldom profitable, and possibly unsafe, to repeat the inhalation within this period. Isoprenaline, which is also available for inhalation from a pressurised dispenser, has a more pronounced action on cardiac β-receptors than the other two drugs, and is potentially more dangerous in the presence of hypoxia. It should therefore not be used in the treatment of asthma. Salbutamol (4 mg) or terbutaline (5 mg) by mouth may control mild attacks of asthma but are less effective than the much smaller doses given by inhalation.

When an attack of asthma fails to respond to the inhalation of a salbutamol or terbutaline aerosol, one of these two drugs should be injected subcutaneously or intramuscularly in a dose of 0·5 mg or aminophylline injected slowly intravenously in a dose of 250–500 mg in 10–20 ml of sterile water. Adrenaline by subcutaneous injection is not recommended because, unlike salbutamol and terbutaline, it does not have a selective action on bronchial β-adrenoreceptors and, by stimulating α-adrenoreceptors, may even have a mild bronchoconstrictor effect in some cases.

If there is not a rapid response to treatment with bronchodilator drugs, prednisolone should be given by mouth in a dose of 15 mg 6 hourly on the first day, 10 mg 6 hourly on the second, and 5 mg 6 hourly for the next 5 days. Patients who are gravely ill should receive 100 mg of prednisolone by mouth in the first 12 hours, along with hydrocortisone hemisuccinate intravenously in a dose of 200 mg every 2 hours until the attack begins to subside. During this critical period the airways obstruction can often be relieved by a 0·5 per cent salbutamol aerosol in 40 per cent oxygen administered by intermittent positive-pressure ventilation (using a Bennett or Bird ventilator with a tightly fitting face mask) for 3 minutes every 1–2 hours. Alternatively, salbutamol may be given intravenously in a dose of 100–300 μg every 1–2 hours, or by continuous intravenous infusion. Hypoxia must be treated with the highest concentration of oxygen consistent with the maintenance of a normal or subnormal $Paco_2$ and arterial hydrogen ion concentration. Dehydration, which increases the viscosity of the sputum, and metabolic acidosis must be corrected. If the patient's condition continues to deteriorate, and particularly if the $Paco_2$ rises above 7 kPa (52 mm Hg), intermittent positive-pressure ventilation through a cuffed tube inserted into the trachea through the mouth or nose (p. 266) should be instituted.

Unless the patient is being artificially ventilated, hypnotics should be used with caution and opiates must never be given. Diazepam, 5–10 mg intramuscularly, is possibly the safest drug to use in these circumstances, but is not devoid of risk in hypoxic patients. As status asthmaticus is often complicated by respiratory infection, which may not always be readily recognisable in the early stages, a suitable antibiotic (p. 272) should be administered in every case.

The usual procedure after the patient begins to recover is to continue treatment with prednisolone in diminishing dosage for 10 to 14 days. Corticosteroids have, however, only a temporary suppressive effect, and asthma frequently recurs a few weeks or even a few days after treatment is stopped.

2. TREATMENT OF CHRONIC ASTHMA. Patients who have frequent recurrences of episodic bronchial asthma and those with chronic asthma present a special problem in management, as many of them are incapacitated for prolonged periods by breathlessness on exertion. In some cases the symptoms can be kept in check by bronchodilator drugs given by inhalation as often as necessary. Oral treatment with drugs such as salbutamol (4 mg), terbutaline (5 mg), ephedrine (30 mg) or choline theophyllinate (200 mg) 4 times daily is less effective and often causes side-effects. Severe chronic asthma responds only transiently to these measures, and many such patients require regular treatment with corticosteroids by mouth or by inhalation. Before this is started, however, it is advisable to confirm, by serial recordings of FEV, that a short (7-day) course of prednisolone by mouth produces significant improvement. If a satisfactory response is recorded, and the symptoms are not particularly severe, asthma can often be adequately controlled by a topical corticosteroid preparation, such as beclomethasone dipropionate, administered by inhalation from a pressurised dispenser in 2 metered doses of 50 μg 4 times daily. Since very little of this small dose of corticosteroid will be absorbed from the bronchial mucosa, systemic side-effects seldom occur but oropharyngeal candidiasis may be a troublesome local complication. If this form of treatment is not effective, it will have to be supplemented by oral prednisolone in a dose of up to 10 mg per day. In such cases the risk of serious side-effects must be weighed against the dangers of uncontrolled asthma and the degree of disability for which it is responsible. The regular administration of sodium cromoglycate (p. 305) is an effective prophylactic measure in some cases of chronic asthma.

3. MANAGEMENT OF FACTORS OF AETIOLOGICAL IMPORTANCE

(a) Allergy. The patient should try to avoid allergens which may be contributing to the production of his asthma. This may not be difficult when the allergy is to substances such as animal dander, feathers, articles of diet or drugs, but it is virtually impossible in the case of ubiquitous allergens such as pollens or fungal spores. Efforts can, however, be made to reduce the amount of dust in bedrooms occupied by patients who are sensitive to allergens present in house dust. Vacuum cleaning of mattresses is particularly useful, as dust from this source contains large numbers of mites (*Dermatophagoides pteronyssinus*) which contribute significantly to the antigenicity of house dust.

Hyposensitisation (p. 300) with extracts of antigenic substances is of little or no value, except in the case of grass pollen allergy, which can sometimes be controlled in this way by using preparations of mixed grass pollens.

Antihistamine drugs are of no value in the prevention of bronchial asthma, but sodium cromoglycate, which is believed to act by preventing the release of bronchoconstrictor substances from mast cells in the bronchial wall, has a useful prophylactic effect in about 40 per cent of all asthmatics. Even better results are obtained in atopic subjects, particularly children. A dose of 20 mg four times daily by inhalation (in the form of a dry powder) should be given initially, but a smaller maintenance dose is adequate in many cases.

(*b*) *Respiratory Infection.* Where the attacks of asthma are clearly related to bacterial infection they can sometimes be prevented if the infection is controlled promptly by an antibiotic.

(*c*) *Exertion.* Exercise-induced asthma can often be prevented by the inhalation of a bronchodilator aerosol a few minutes previously, or by regular treatment with sodium cromoglycate.

(*d*) *Emotional Disturbance.* Sedation is indicated if emotional stress appears to be present. For this purpose diazepam in a dose of 5–10 mg thrice daily is usually adequate. An attempt should be made to deal with causes of friction and anxiety. This can usually best be done by the family doctor, but the assistance of a psychiatrist may be required in some cases.

4. BREATHING AND POSTURAL EXERCISES. The main purpose of these exercises is to prevent chest deformity and defective posture, which are prone to develop in all patients with asthma, especially children.

Pulmonary Eosinophilia

This term is applied to a rather heterogeneous group of conditions which have two features in common—an increase in the number of circulating eosinophil leucocytes and transient radiographic opacities in the lungs. These conditions can be classified as follows:

1. Eosinophilic pneumonia (Löffler's syndrome).
2. Tropical pulmonary eosinophilia.
3. Asthmatic pulmonary eosinophilia (including allergic broncho-pulmonary aspergillosis).
4. Polyarteritis.

Eosinophilic Pneumonia. This may be the result of an allergic reaction in the lung to various foreign proteins and to certain drugs presumably acting as haptens. In tropical countries the antigen is usually derived from helminth larvae, including ascaris and schistosomes, as they migrate through the lungs, but in temperate regions the antigenic agent is usually a drug, such as PAS, nitrofurantoin or a sulphonamide. A mild degree of pyrexia and a slight cough are often the only clinical abnormalities, radiographic examination shows transient pulmonary opacities, and the eosinophil count in the blood is slightly or moderately increased ($0.5–1.5 \times 10^9/l$). Treatment consists of eradicating the parasitic infection or withdrawing the offending drug.

Rarely, extensive eosinophilic pneumonia may occur in the absence of any identifiable aetiological factor. These patients usually require corticosteroid therapy.

Tropical Pulmonary Eosinophilia. This condition occurs in many tropical regions, and is thought to be an allergic reaction to microfilariae (*Dirofilaria* or *Brugia pahangi*) in the lungs, which show numerous focal collections of eosinophil leucocytes and a few giant cells. There is a persistent cough with or without asthma, pyrexia, miliary shadowing on the chest radiograph and a marked degree of eosinophilia in the blood. The illness usually responds to treatment with diethylcarbamazine.

Asthmatic Pulmonary Eosinophilia. This condition is due in most cases (estimates vary between 50 and 90 per cent) to combined Type I and Type III allergic reactions (p. 38) in the bronchi and lungs to the fungus *Aspergillus fumigatus*. The allergens responsible for the other cases have not yet been identified. The condition is invariably associated with chronic asthma, and the eosinophil count in the blood is usually between $0.5–1.5 \times 10^9/l$. The pulmonary lesions are of two types: (1) segmental or subsegmental (occasionally lobar) collapse caused by occlusion of the related bronchus by a mucinous cast coated with eosinophils, which often contains fungal hyphae, and (2) areas of pulmonary infiltration in which the alveolar spaces and alveolar walls contain numerous eosinophils, and varying numbers of lymphocytes and plasma cells. The first type of lesion is more common than the second. The radiographic appearances reflect the pathological changes—absorption collapse of a segment, or of a larger or smaller bronchopulmonary unit, in the first type, and an ill defined pulmonary opacity in the second. These lesions may recur at intervals for many years, anywhere in the lungs, but more often involving the upper lobes. Bronchiectasis frequently develops in collapsed bronchopulmonary segments.

When allergic bronchopulmonary aspergillosis is responsible for the pulmonary eosinophilia, the diagnosis can usually be made by mycological examination of the sputum or of a bronchial cast, combined with skin sensitivity tests and serological tests. In most cases *A. fumigatus* can readily be isolated on culture. An extract from this fungus gives a positive skin reaction (in which there may be 'immediate' and 'late' components), and a positive gel diffusion test (which indicates the presence of precipitating antibody).

Treatment of this condition can be very difficult. Efforts to eliminate the fungus from the respiratory tract by regular inhalations of natamycin (p. 299) seldom succeed. Corticosteroids may relieve the asthma, and at the same time prevent recurrent pulmonary infiltrations and the formation of new bronchial casts. If established casts cannot be dislodged by postural drainage they should be extracted through a bronchoscope. Failure to deal effectively with these casts is an important factor in the production of bronchiectasis.

Polyarteritis. This disease may present with respiratory symptoms, including asthma, recurrent pulmonary opacities on radiological examination, and a moderate increase in the eosinophil count. Other organs are usually involved at a later stage. The condition is described on page 242.

Allergic Alveolitis

In this condition the inhalation of certain types of organic dust produces a diffuse allergic reaction in the walls of the alveoli and bronchioles. There is a cellular exudate consisting of polymorphs, lymphocytes and plasma cells, and small epithelioid granulomata may also be seen. These changes cause decreased pulmonary compliance and ventilation : perfusion inequalities. They are presumably also responsible for the widespread coarse crepitations heard on auscultation, and for the diffuse micronodular shadowing seen on the chest radiograph. Precipitating antibodies in the serum against the relevant antigens would seem to indicate that allergic alveolitis is a Type III immune reaction, but the finding of small pulmonary granulomata suggests that a Type IV immune reaction may also be implicated (p. 43).

Some of the agents which produce allergic alveolitis, the source of these agents, and the names applied to the resulting diseases are shown in Table 7.3. The term *extrinsic* allergic alveolitis is sometimes applied to this group of diseases, to indicate that the antigen is of external origin. If patients with this disorder continue to expose themselves to the relevant antigen for long periods, they may eventually develop permanent pulmonary damage with severe respiratory disabillity.

Table 7.3 Types and causes of extrinsic allergic alveolitis

Agent	Source	Disease
Micropolyspora faeni	Mouldy hay	Farmer's lung
Thermophilic actinomycetes	Compost	Mushroom worker's lung
	Mouldy sugar cane fibre	Bagassosis
Aspergillus clavatus	Malting barley	Maltworker's lung
Coniosporium corticale	Bark of maple trees	Maple bark disease
Avian protein in pigeon and budgerigar droppings	Pigeon loft or bird cage	Bird fancier's lung
Proteolytic enzyme derived from *Bacillus subtilis*	Air-borne dust in factory making 'biological' washing powder	Terminology undecided

Allergic alveolitis should be suspected when a person regularly exposed to a heavy concentration of organic dust complains, a few hours after re-exposure to the same dust, of general malaise, dry cough and dyspnoea without wheeze. If the cause of these symptoms is not appreciated, and further exposure to the dust hazard permitted, they are likely to become continuous, and in some cases very severe. At this stage the patient may be febrile, cyanosed and dyspnoeic at rest, coarse crepitations (but no rhonchi) can be heard all over the chest and a chest radiograph may show diffuse micronodular shadowing. The FEV_1 and FVC are both reduced, but the FEV_1/FVC ratio is normal—indicating a restrictive ventilatory defect without airways obstruction. The Pao_2 is reduced, and the $Paco_2$ is slightly subnormal as a result of overventilation.

The diagnosis of allergic alveolitis is confirmed serologically by a positive precipitin test and, if necessary, by a positive provocation test, in which the inhalation of an aerosol containing the relevant antigen is followed after 3 to 6 hours by pyrexia and a reduction in FVC, often associated with a recurrence of symptoms.

Mild forms of allergic alveolitis rapidly subside when exposure to the dust ceases. In severe cases a corticosteroid preparation should be given for 3 to 4 weeks, starting with 40–60 mg of prednisolone per day. Severely hypoxic patients may require oxygen in high concentration (60 per cent).

DISEASES OF THE LARYNX, TRACHEA AND BRONCHI

Acute infections of the larynx have already been described (p. 271). Other common disorders of the larynx include chronic laryngitis, laryngeal tuberculosis (p. 285), laryngeal paralysis and laryngeal obstruction. Tumours of the larynx are relatively common, but for information on these conditions the reader should refer to a textbook of diseases of the ear, nose and throat.

Chronic Laryngitis

Chronic laryngitis occurs as a result of repeated attacks of acute laryngitis, excessive use of the voice, especially in dusty atmospheres, e.g. in auctioneers, heavy tobacco smoking, mouth breathing from nasal obstruction and chronic nasal and oral sepsis.

The surface of the mucous membrane is dry and covered with small papillary projections. The vocal cords are thickened and opaque. Microscopically the submucosa is infiltrated with chronic inflammatory cells. The chief symptom is hoarseness and the voice may be lost. There is irritation of the throat and spasmodic cough with a little mucoid sputum. The disease pursues a chronic course frequently uninfluenced by treatment, and in long-standing cases the voice is often permanently impaired.

As chronic and progressive hoarseness may also be caused by tuberculosis and tumours of the larynx and by laryngeal paralysis, these conditions must be considered in the differential diagnosis if the hoarseness does not improve within a few weeks. In some cases a chest radiograph may bring to light unsuspected pulmonary tuberculosis or a bronchial carcinoma. If no such abnormality is found the patient should be referred to a specialist for laryngoscopic examination.

Treatment. The voice must be rested completely. This is particularly important in the case of public speakers. Smoking should be prohibited. Some benefit may be obtained from frequent inhalations of steam medicated with benzoin or menthol. Predisposing conditions must be remedied.

Laryngeal Paralysis

Aetiology. Laryngeal paralysis may be organic or functional.
Organic paralysis is due to interference with the motor nerve supply of the larynx and may be caused by:
1. Lesions of the brain stem, e.g. bulbar paralysis due to vascular lesions, motor neurone disease or poliomyelitis.
2. Toxic and infective lesions of the vagus nerve or its recurrent laryngeal branch.
3. Interruption of the recurrent laryngeal nerve, or of the vagus trunk above the origin of that nerve, by tumour, aneurysm or trauma (p. 683). This is the most common way in which laryngeal paralysis is produced. The paralysis is nearly always unilateral and, by reason of the intrathoracic course of the left recurrent laryngeal nerve, usually left-sided. Accidental division of one or both recurrent

laryngeal nerves is one of the hazards of thyroidectomy.

Functional paralysis of the larynx occurs as a manifestation of hysteria.

Clinical Features

1. *Hoarseness* always accompanies laryngeal paralysis whatever its cause. Paralysis of organic origin is seldom reversible, but when only one vocal cord is affected the hoarseness may improve or even disappear after a few weeks as a result of a compensatory adjustment whereby the unparalysed cord crosses the mid-line and approximates with the paralysed cord on phonation.

2. *'Bovine' cough*, which is a characteristic feature of organic laryngeal paralysis, results from the loss of the explosive phase of normal coughing consequent upon the failure of the cords to close the glottis. The difficulty in bringing up sputum which some of these patients experience can be explained on the same basis. 'Bovine' cough does not occur with hysterical paralysis.

3. *Dyspnoea* and *stridor* are occasionally present but are seldom severe except with bilateral laryngeal paralysis of organic origin.

4. *Laryngoscopy* is necessary to establish the diagnosis of laryngeal paralysis with certainty. The paralysed cord lies in the so-called 'cadaveric' position, midway between abduction and adduction. In hysterical paralysis only adduction of the cords, a voluntary movement, is affected.

Treatment. The treatment is that of the underlying disease. The psychological basis for hysteria should be determined and, if possible, adjusted. In bilateral paralysis of organic origin the passage of an endotracheal tube or even tracheostomy may be required for the relief of laryngeal obstruction (below). Eventually, in these cases, it may be necessary to perform a plastic operation on the larynx in order to secure permanent restoration of the airway.

Laryngeal Obstruction

Aetiology. The laryngeal opening (glottis) may be obstructed by (1) inflammatory or allergic oedema or exudate, (2) spasm of the laryngeal muscles, (3) inhaled foreign body, (4) inhaled vomitus in an unconscious patient, (5) tumours of the larynx, (6) bilateral vocal cord paralysis and (7) fixation of both cords in advanced rheumatoid arthritis. Laryngeal obstruction is more liable to occur in children than in adults because of the smaller size of the glottis.

Clinical Features. These depend on whether the obstruction is complete or incomplete and on the rapidity of its onset.

Sudden complete laryngeal obstruction by a foreign body produces the clinical picture of acute asphyxia—violent but ineffective inspiratory efforts with indrawing of the intercostal spaces and the unsupported lower ribs, accompanied by deep cyanosis. Unrelieved, the condition progresses rapidly to coma, and death ensues within 5 to 10 minutes. When, as in most cases, the obstruction is incomplete at first, the main clinical features are progressive dyspnoea and cyanosis, stridor and indrawing of the intercostal spaces and lower ribs on both sides. The great danger in these cases is that the obstruction may at any time become complete and result in sudden death.

Treatment. Transient attacks of laryngeal obstruction due to exudate and spasm, which may occur with acute laryngitis in children (p. 269) and with whooping-cough, are potentially dangerous but can usually be relieved by the inhalation of steam.

Laryngeal obstruction from all other causes carries a high mortality and demands prompt treatment. The following measures may have to be employed:

1. *The relief of obstruction by mechanical means.* When a foreign body is known to be the cause of the obstruction it can often be dislodged by turning the patient head downwards and thumping the back vigorously. In other circumstances the nature of the obstruction should be ascertained whenever possible by direct laryngoscopy, which may also permit the removal of a foreign body or the insertion of a tube past the obstruction into the trachea.

Tracheostomy must be performed without delay if these procedures fail to relieve the obstruction, but except in dire emergencies the operation should be performed in the operating theatre by a surgeon.

2. *Treatment of the cause.* In cases of diphtheria, antitoxin should be administered and for other infections the appropriate antibiotic should be given. In angioneurotic oedema the patient should receive adrenaline, 0·5–1·0 ml of 1 : 1,000 solution subcutaneously, and hydrocortisone hemisuccinate, 100 mg intravenously. It must be remembered that these remedies take time to act and that tracheostomy may be required in the intervening period.

Diseases of the Trachea

Acute tracheitis is a common complication of viral and bacterial infection of the upper respiratory tract, and is usually associated with acute bronchitis. Other primary disorders of the trachea are rare.

Tracheal Obstruction. Intrinsic benign and malignant tumours may produce tracheal obstruction, but external compression by enlarged mediastinal lymph nodes containing metastatic deposits from a bronchial carcinoma is a much more common cause. Rarely, the trachea may be compressed by an aneurysm of the aortic arch, or in children by tuberculous mediastinal lymph nodes. Tracheal stricture is an occasional complication of tracheostomy.

Stridor (p. 257) can be detected in every patient with severe tracheal obstruction. Endoscopic examination of the trachea should be undertaken without delay in these patients to determine the degree of obstruction and its nature. Localised tumours of the trachea can be resected, but reconstruction of the resected segment may present complex technical problems. Radiotherapy or the administration of cytotoxic drugs may temporarily relieve compression by malignant lymph nodes. Tracheal strictures can sometimes be dilated, but may have to be resected.

Tracheo-oesophageal fistula. This may be present in newborn infants as a congenital abnormality. In adults, it is usually due to malignant lesions in the mediastinum, such as carcinoma or malignant lymphoma, eroding both the trachea and oesophagus, to produce a communication between them. Swallowed liquids enter the trachea and bronchi through the fistula, and provoke a 'spluttering' cough. Surgical closure of a congenital fistula, if undertaken promptly, is usually successful, but malignant fistulae are incurable, and death from overwhelming pulmonary infection rapidly supervenes.

Chronic Obstructive Airways Disease

Although chronic bronchitis and emphysema are pathologically distinct, they frequently co-exist, and it may then be difficult or impossible to determine the relative importance of each condition in the individual case. Generalised airways obstruction is a prominent feature of both diseases. In chronic bronchitis it is chiefly due to swelling of the bronchial mucosa and the accumulation of tenacious mucus within the air passages. In emphysema, on the other hand, the main factor in the production of airways obstruction is extramural bronchial compression and collapse caused by overdistended alveoli in which air has been 'trapped' during expiration. This phenomenon is aggravated by chronic bronchitis and bronchopulmonary infection.

Chronic bronchitis and emphysema are often grouped together under the heading of 'chronic obstructive airways disease', and can be regarded as forming a spectrum, with 'pure' chronic bronchitis at one end and 'pure' emphysema at the other. For descriptive purposes, however, it is convenient to deal with them separately, with emphasis on their similarities and differences, and on the relationships which frequently exist between them.

Chronic Bronchitis

Aetiology. Chronic bronchitis is the name given to the clinical syndrome which many individuals develop in response to the long-continued action of various types of irritant on the bronchial mucosa. The most important of these is tobacco smoke, but they also include dust, smoke and fumes, occurring as specific occupational hazards or as part of a general atmospheric pollution in industrial cities and towns. Infection is sometimes a precipitating factor in the onset of chronic bronchitis, but its main role is in aggravating the established condition. Exposure to dampness, to sudden changes in temperature and to fog may also be responsible for exacerbations of chronic bronchitis.

The disorder occurs most commonly in middle and late adult life. More males are affected than females and there may be a familial predisposition. As might be expected, it is more common in smokers than in non-smokers, and in urban than in rural dwellers.

On culture of the sputum *Strept. pneumoniae* and *H. influenzae* are isolated in most cases. These organisms become more numerous during acute exacerbations.

Pathology. In all cases there is overactivity of the mucus-secreting glands and goblet cells in the bronchi and bronchioles. The vast excess of mucus so produced coats the bronchial walls and clogs the bronchioles. Mucosal oedema further reduces the calibre of the air passages and as the degree of obstruction is greater during expiration air is 'trapped' in the alveoli. With the passage of time the alveoli become permanently overdistended and there is extensive rupture of their walls. These changes, which constitute one form of 'emphysema', are more fully discussed on page 313.

Clinical Features. The disease usually starts with repeated attacks of 'winter cough', which show a steady increase in severity and duration with successive years, until cough is present all the year round. Wheeze, dyspnoea and tightness in the chest are common complaints, especially in the morning before the bronchial secretions are cleared, often with difficulty, by coughing. The sputum may be scanty, tenacious, mucoid, and occasionally streaked with blood, or copious and watery. A frankly purulent sputum is indicative of bacterial infection, which supervenes from time to time in most cases of chronic bronchitis.

Dyspnoea in chronic bronchitis is caused by airways obstruction, and is aggravated by infection or by an increase in mucosal oedema which may be produced by cigarette smoking and by adverse atmospheric conditions.

Variable numbers of inspiratory and expiratory rhonchi, mainly low and medium pitched, are present in most cases of chronic bronchitis and there may also be some coarse crepitations. Physical signs attributable to emphysema (p. 261) coexist in some cases.

Radiological Examination. Chronic bronchitis produces no characteristic abnormality in the radiograph, but bronchography shows various irregularities of bronchial calibre, outline and branching. The features of emphysema (p. 314) may be prominent in some cases.

Pulmonary Function Tests

1. The forced expiratory volume in 1 second (FEV_1) is reduced, and the ratio of FEV_1 to forced vital capacity (FVC) is also subnormal. In advanced cases of emphysema the FEV_1 may be less than 1 l, and the FEV/FVC ratio may be as low as 30 per cent. Such changes are common to all forms of obstructive airway disease (p. 263).

2. Because of 'air trapping' and alveolar distension the residual volume of the lungs is increased at the expense of vital capacity.

3. As the distribution of ventilation and perfusion within the lungs becomes disturbed (p. 254), the Pao_2 falls below normal.

4. In the later stages, when generalised alveolar underventilation supervenes, often following an infective exacerbation of chronic bronchitis, there is a further fall in Pao_2 and a rise in $Paco_2$ accompanied by respiratory acidosis (p. 170).

Course and Prognosis. Chronic bronchitis is usually a progressive disease, punctuated by acute exacerbations and remissions, and eventually causing ventilatory and cardiac failure (p. 315). Some patients die within 5 years of the onset of symptoms, while others survive for 20 to 30 years, with gradually diminishing respiratory reserve.

Treatment. 1. *Bronchial irritation* must be reduced to a minimum. If a tobacco smoker, the patient should be urged to give up the habit completely and permanently. Dusty and smoke-laden atmospheres should be avoided. This may require a change of occupation or environment, often involving a reduction of income. Most patients find it difficult to accept this advice, but in a condition as potentially serious as chronic bronchitis it is important to point out that if exposure to dust or smoke continues the patient may become totally incapacitated long before he reaches retiring age.

2. *Respiratory infection* must be promptly controlled, as it aggravates dyspnoea and may precipitate ventilatory failure. The patient should be instructed to observe the colour of his sputum every morning, and if it becomes purulent he should be given tetracycline or ampicillin in a dose of 250 mg four times daily or co-trimoxazole, 2 tablets twice daily, for 5 to 7 days. Intelligent patients can be provided with a stock of antibiotic tablets, and permitted to start a course of treatment on their own initiative when the need arises.

As the vast majority of bacterial infections in chronic bronchitis are caused by *Strept. pneumoniae* or *H. influenzae*, bacteriological examination of sputum is essential only when the response to standard treatment is unsatisfactory, and the sputum remains purulent. In that event a change of antibiotic, guided by the results of bacterial sensitivity tests, will be indicated. If *Staph. pyogenes* is isolated, antibiotics such as cloxacillin or sodium fusidate (p. 93) will be required.

Continuous suppressive treatment with tetracycline or ampicillin, given throughout the winter or even throughout the year, is not advised, since it is apt to promote the emergence of a drug-resistant respiratory tract flora, and may merely add to the therapeutic problems.

3. *Symptomatic measures* may be required to control unproductive cough during the night, to enable sputum to be coughed up more easily and to relieve breathlessness and wheeze. Nocturnal unproductive cough will often be less troublesome if the patient sleeps in a heated bedroom, but pholcodine or methadone (p. 267) may be required to control it. A hot drink or the inhalation of steam helps to liquefy sputum and make it easier to bring up. So-called expectorant cough mixtures are of little or no value. Measures for the relief of asthmatic symptoms are described on page 304.

4. *Ventilatory failure* must be promptly treated (p. 266).

Prevention. The abandonment of tobacco smoking and the prompt treatment of acute respiratory infections are the most important preventive measures. The control of atmospheric pollution in urban areas and the increased use of measures to prevent the inhalation of dust by industrial workers would also help to reduce the prevalence of chronic bronchitis.

Emphysema

The word 'emphysema' means 'inflation' in the sense of unnatural distension with air, and this phenomenon, thus defined, can occur anywhere in the body. Air may, for example, enter the mediastinum (*mediastinal emphysema*) following the rupture of overdistended alveoli into the interstitial tissues of the lung in patients with severe bronchial asthma, or following rupture of the oesophagus. If a very large amount of air escapes rapidly into the mediastinum, it may produce cardiac tamponade (p. 230), but in most cases it tracks harmlessly upwards into the soft tissues of the neck, where it imparts a characteristic crackling sensation to the palpating fingers (*subcutaneous emphysema*). Penetrating wounds of the chest wall may also cause subcutaneous emphysema, and when a spontaneous pneumothorax is treated by pleural decompression with an intercostal tube (p. 341), widespread subcutaneous emphysema is an occasional complication, which is alarming but not serious.

Pulmonary Emphysema

The term 'pulmonary emphysema' covers a wide variety of pathological processes, ranging from overdistension of otherwise normal alveoli in conditions such as bronchial asthma (p. 300), obstructive emphysema (p. 320) and compensatory emphysema (p. 319) to the widespread disruption of the alveolar walls which occurs in the more serious forms of pulmonary emphysema. There is a close association between the latter and chronic bronchitis, but the physical signs and radiological changes attributable to 'emphysema' may be more conspicuous in some cases of chronic bronchitis than in others. Chronic bronchitis and emphysema can both cause severe pulmonary damage, but it is of a different type in the two conditions. In emphysema generalised destruction of the alveolar walls ('panacinar' emphysema) is the dominant lesion. Where emphysema occurs along with a major component of chronic bronchitis, it is usually 'centrilobular' or 'centriacinar', and principally affects these alveoli which are most closely related to the respiratory bronchioles. Although these two types of emphysema develop in different ways, factors such as bacterial infection, alveolar overdistension and distortion of the airways may eventually blur their distinctive features. The predominance of either chronic bronchitis or emphysema may, however, be sufficiently clear-cut to produce two separately identifiable syndromes (Table 7.4). In the chronic bronchitis syndrome, ventilatory capacity is fairly well preserved, but severe hypoxia and hypercapnia, pulmonary hypertension and right ventricular failure occur at an early stage (the 'blue bloater'). In the emphysema syndrome, on the other hand, grave impairment of ventilatory capacity and disabling exertional dyspnoea may antedate by many years the manifestations of respiratory and cardiac failure (the 'pink puffer'). A mixed syndrome of chronic bronchitis and emphysema is, however, much more commonly seen than either of the two individual syndromes.

Emphysema in young adults, mainly affecting the lower lobes, may be associated with genetically determined α_1-antitrypsin deficiency in the serum.

Clinical Features. Most patients with pulmonary emphysema complain of exertional dyspnoea, but since other causes of airways obstruction, such as chronic bronchitis and bronchial asthma, often co-exist, it is seldom possible to assess the contribution of emphysema *per se* to the production of this symptom. In patients with chronic bronchitis and emphysema there is a progressive increase in respiratory disability, but the tempo of deterioration varies widely from one case to another. For example, in patients with a relatively minor component of chronic bronchitis the exertional dyspnoea increases slowly over a period of several years, but the course of the disease tends to be more rapid where chronic bronchitis is a dominant feature. Other important differences between these two contrasting forms of chronic bronchitis and emphysema are shown in Table 7.4.

The *physical signs* which may be observed in emphysema are summarised in Table 7.1 (p. 261). Other clinical abnormalities recorded in this condition (many of which are due to chronic airway obstruction) include (1) a reduction in the length of the trachea palpable above the sternal notch, (2) tracheal descent with inspiration, (3) contraction of the sternomastoid and scalene muscles on inspiration, (4) excavation of the suprasternal and supraclavicular fossae during inspiration, (5) jugular venous filling during expiration, (6) indrawing of the costal margins during inspiration, and (7) an increase in the anteroposterior diameter of the chest relative to the lateral diameter.

Radiological Features. A firm diagnosis of emphysema cannot be made by radiological examination alone, but the following abnormalities suggest that it may be present: 1. Unusually translucent lung fields, with loss of peripheral vascular markings. 2. Bullae (p. 316). 3. A low flat diaphragm, which moves poorly on fluoroscopy (2 cm or less). 4. Abnormal prominence of the pulmonary arterial shadows at both hila.

Abnormalities caused by pulmonary infection ('inflammatory shadowing') may also be present, especially in patients with an important degree of chronic bronchitis. In the late stages, when pulmonary hypertension and right ventricular failure supervene, there is enlargement of the main pulmonary artery, the right ventricle and the right atrium.

Pulmonary Function Tests. See page 262.

Table 7.4 Chronic bronchitis and emphysema

	Predominant Abnormality	
	Chronic Bronchitis	Emphysema
Appearance	Blue and bloated	Pink and puffing
Age	Middle-aged	Elderly
Build	Thick-set	Slender
Degree of bronchitis	Severe	Mild
Episodes of bacterial infection	Frequent	Occasional
Duration of exertional dyspnoea	Fairly short (2–5 years)	Long (5–20 years)
Degree of exertional dyspnoea	Variable but seldom severe	Slowly progressive but eventually severe
Central cyanosis	Moderate or severe	Slight or absent
Rhonchi	Numerous	Few
Pao_2	Markedly reduced (8–4 kPa or 60–30 mm Hg)	Slightly reduced at rest (8 kPa or 60 mm Hg)
$Paco_2$	Always increased (7–12 kPa or 50–90 mm Hg)	Normal or slightly increased (5·5–7 kPa or 40–50 mm Hg)
Residual volume	Moderately increased	Markedly increased
Gas transfer factor (Tco)	Usually normal	Usually decreased
X-ray chest	'Emphysema' slight or absent 'Inflammatory shadowing' often present	'Emphysema' marked 'Inflammatory shadowing' slight or absent
ECG	Pattern of right ventricular hypertrophy relatively common	Usually normal
Right ventricular failure	Early	Late

Differential Diagnosis. It is important to exclude unrelated or remediable causes of dyspnoea in patients suspected of having emphysema. These are (1) *left-sided cardiac failure* due to hypertension or to valvular or ischaemic heart disease, in which crepitations from pulmonary oedema may be wrongly ascribed to bronchitis; (2) *spontaneous pneumothorax*, the physical signs of which may pass unnoticed in the presence of emphysema; and (3) *giant bullae*, which may be the main cause of dyspnoea in a patient with only a mild or moderate degree of emphysema. In order to exclude these conditions, radiological examination should be undertaken whenever an emphysematous patient experiences a rapid increase in dyspnoea.

Bronchial carcinoma, pneumoconiosis and *pulmonary tuberculosis* can be excluded by radiography and bacteriological examination. *Pneumoconiosis* confers certain pension rights, and in any suspected case a detailed occupational history should always be taken.

Complications. 1. *Ventilatory failure* (p. 258); *secondary polycythaemia* (p. 613).

2. *Pulmonary hypertension* and *right ventricular failure* are the inevitable end-results of chronic bronchitis and emphysema. The increase in pulmonary arterial pressure is due to vasoconstriction mediated by the effect of hypoxia on pulmonary arterioles and ultimately to destruction of the pulmonary vascular bed. As hypoxia is aggravated by any increase in the degree of airway obstruction, bacterial infection in the respiratory tract, oedema of the bronchial mucosa,

oversecretion of bronchial mucus and spasm of the bronchial muscles (which can all cause hypoxia) are liable to increase the pulmonary arterial pressure and precipitate right ventricular failure. Conversely, effective treatment of these causes of hypoxia, combined with oxygen therapy (p. 264) and diuretics (p. 161) may relieve pulmonary hypertension and cardiac failure, at least for a time.

3. *Pulmonary bullae*, single or multiple, large or small, may develop in emphysematous lung tissue, regardless of the primary pathology. Bullae are inflated thin-walled spaces created by rupture of the alveolar walls. They are usually situated subpleurally, and are commonly found along the anterior borders of the lungs. A small bulla may rupture, causing *spontaneous pneumothorax*. In other circumstances bullae may increase progressively in size, and eventually become so large that they interfere seriously with pulmonary ventilation.

Treatment. There is no specific remedy for emphysema, but the patient may benefit considerably from the treatment of associated chronic bronchitis (p. 312), and ventilatory failure (p. 266), which is a common complication. Obesity must be prevented or corrected, as excess weight is an intolerable burden on the reduced cardiorespiratory reserve. Breathing exercises of the traditional type, encouraging the patient to force air out of his lungs, are of no value; indeed, by increasing air trapping, they may even be harmful. If physiotherapy in emphysema has any purpose at all, it should be to induce relaxation of the cervical muscles and to show the patient how to exhale slowly and steadily through pursed lips. The surgical ablation of giant bullae, where this is feasible, may allow relatively normal lung tissue compressed by the bullae to re-expand and this may bring about a dramatic improvement in pulmonary function.

Bronchiectasis

Aetiology and Pathogenesis. Bronchiectasis, which is the term used to describe abnormal dilatation of the bronchi, may be produced in different ways:

1. When pulmonary collapse follows obstruction of groups of *small* bronchi by secretion, the shrinkage of the affected portion of lung exerts outward traction on the walls of the medium-sized bronchi, which become dilated. Bronchiectasis arising in this way may be reversible if the obstructed bronchi can be cleared of secretion before the walls of the dilated bronchi are seriously damaged by infection. When the bronchial obstruction is itself the result of severe bronchopulmonary infection the bronchiectasis is liable to become permanent. Damage to the deeper layers of the bronchial walls, such as occurs in all types of suppurative pneumonia and lung abscess, and in some cases of pulmonary tuberculosis and acute lobular pneumonia, is much more important in this respect than the relatively superficial lesions of acute bronchitis.

2. Bronchiectasis may be due to bronchial distension resulting from the accumulation of pus beyond a lesion obstructing a major bronchus, such as a bronchial carcinoma, a tuberculous hilar lymph node or an inhaled foreign body.

3. In cystic fibrosis (p. 388) recurrent infection and chronic obstruction by viscid mucus are both factors in causing bronchiectasis.

4. Rarely, it may be the result of congenital maldevelopment of the bronchi.

Because of the many different causes of bronchiectasis no precise age incidence can be stated. When it occurs following acute pulmonary infections or secondary to obstruction of a bronchus by tuberculous lymph nodes (the two most common causes), the disease usually starts in childhood but may not produce severe symptoms until some years later.

Pathology. The bronchial dilatations may be cylindrical, fusiform or saccular in type. Although bronchiectasis may involve any part of the lungs, depending on the site of the primary pathological process, the lower lobes are more frequently affected than the upper and middle. In addition, the more efficient drainage by gravity of the upper lobes renders bronchiectasis there less liable to produce serious symptoms than when it involves the lower lobes. The bronchiectatic cavities may be lined by granulation tissue, squamous epithelium or normal ciliated epithelium, depending on the degree of infection present. There may also be inflammatory changes in the deeper layers of the bronchial walls and chronic inflammatory and fibrotic changes in the surrounding lung tissue.

Clinical Features. Three groups of clinical features occur in bronchiectasis:

1. *Those due to the accumulation of pus in the bronchiectatic cavities:*

(a) *Chronic cough*, usually worse in the mornings and often induced by changes in posture.

(b) *Purulent sputum*, which in advanced cases is copious and sometimes foetid.

2. *Those due to inflammatory changes in the surrounding lung tissue and pleura:*

(a) *Febrile episodes*, commonly ascribed to influenza or pneumonia, which often follow an upper respiratory infection and usually last for a few days but occasionally for weeks. Malaise, shivering and sleep sweating accompany the pyrexia; there is an increase in the amount of cough and sputum and a neutrophil leucocytosis is usually present.

(b) *Dry pleurisy*, which frequently accompanies the febrile episodes.

(c) *Empyema*, which is an occasional complication of bronchiectasis.

When chronic suppuration, either in the bronchi or in the lungs, is a marked feature it causes a decline in the patient's general health, with lassitude, anorexia, loss of weight, sleep sweating and clubbing of the fingers and toes. In many cases, however, symptoms are slight, consisting merely of recurrent episodes of cough and purulent sputum with no symptoms in the intervening periods and no deterioration in general health.

3. *Haemoptysis*, caused by bleeding from thin-walled anastomotic vessels connecting the pulmonary and bronchial arteries, and situated in the walls of the bronchiectatic cavities. It ranges in amount from blood-stained sputum to massive haemorrhage. It may be present in association with the first two groups of symptoms, but recurrent haemoptysis may also occur as an isolated symptom in the absence of cough and sputum ('dry' bronchiectasis).

Physical Signs in the Chest. These may be unilateral or bilateral and are usually basal. If the bronchiectatic cavities are dry and there is no collapse, there may be *no* abnormal physical signs. If a large amount of secretion is present, numerous coarse crepitations are heard over the affected areas. When collapse is present the character of the physical signs depends on whether or not the major bronchi in the collapsed lobe are patent. The signs found in both circumstances are described on page 261.

Radiological Examination. In ordinary radiographs the dilated bronchi themselves may not be visible, but radiological changes may be produced by associated pulmonary inflammation or collapse. A diagnosis of bronchiectasis can be made with certainty only by bronchographic examination.

Diagnosis. When bronchograms are available the diagnosis of bronchiectasis is self-evident, but other conditions, notably chronic bronchitis and active pulmonary tuberculosis, may coexist. It is of particular importance, when surgical treatment for bronchiectasis is contemplated, to consider whether the symptoms may not be principally due to chronic bronchitis. This should always be suspected when dyspnoea, wheeze and rhonchi are prominent features.

Bacteriological examination of the sputum is necessary in every case to exclude tuberculosis and to identify other pathogenic bacteria.

Course and Prognosis. With antibiotic therapy the prognosis, even in advanced cases, has greatly improved and the incidence of complications such as pneumonia, empyema, cerebral abscess and amyloidosis has fallen considerably.

Treatment. *Postural Drainage.* The purpose of this measure is to keep the dilated bronchi emptied of secretion. Efficiently performed it is of great value both in reducing the amount of cough and sputum and in preventing the 'toxaemia' caused by associated bronchopulmonary infection. In its simplest form, postural drainage consists of adopting a position in which the lobe to be drained is uppermost, so as to allow secretions in the dilated bronchi to gravitate towards the trachea, from which they can readily be cleared by vigorous coughing. The optimum duration and frequency of postural drainage depends on the amount of sputum, but 5 to 10 minutes once or twice daily is adequate in most cases.

Chemotherapy. The policy governing the use of antibiotics in bronchiectasis is the same as that in chronic bronchitis.

Surgical Treatment. If surgical treatment is being considered, it is essential to obtain bronchograms demonstrating exactly the extent of the bronchiectasis. For this purpose the bronchi of all segments of *both* lungs must be outlined with a radio-opaque contrast medium. Pulmonary function should also be assessed.

The use of antibiotics has greatly reduced the need for surgical treatment. Unfortunately many of the cases in which medical treatment has been unsuccessful are also unsuitable for surgical treatment either because the bronchiectasis is too extensive or because most of the symptoms are due to coexisting chronic bronchitis. Emphysema of even moderate severity is a contraindication to surgical treatment, as the increase in exertional dyspnoea which inevitably results is more distressing to the patient than the symptoms of bronchiectasis. The most favourable cases for surgery are children and young adults in whom the bronchiectasis is confined to a single lobe or part of a lobe. Lobar or segmental resection in these patients is a highly satisfactory operation, carrying little risk.

Other Measures. Chronic sepsis in the nose, mouth and pharynx should be treated, and anaemia should be corrected.

Prevention. As bronchiectasis commonly starts in childhood following measles, whooping-cough or a primary tuberculous infection, it is essential that these conditions receive adequate treatment. The early recognition and treatment of bronchial obstruction is particularly important in this respect.

Bronchial Obstruction

Aetiology. The lesions most likely to obstruct a large bronchus are:

1. Tumours, e.g. bronchial carcinoma (p. 322) or adenoma (p. 325).
2. Enlarged tracheobronchial lymph nodes, malignant or tuberculous.

3. Inhaled foreign bodies.
4. Bronchial casts or plugs, consisting of inspissated mucus or blood clot.
5. Collections of mucus or mucopus retained in the bronchi as a result of ineffective expectoration.

Rare causes of bronchial obstruction include congenital bronchial atresia, fibrous bronchial stricture (often post-tuberculous), aortic aneurysm, giant left atrium and pericardial effusion.

Clinical Features. The manifestations of obstruction of a large bronchus depend on whether the obstruction is complete or partial, on secondary infection and on the effect on pulmonary function. The clinical features also vary with the cause of the obstruction.

1. COMPLETE OBSTRUCTION. When a large bronchus is completely obstructed, the air in the lung, lobe or segment it supplies is absorbed, the alveolar spaces close, and the affected portion of lung tissue contracts and becomes solid (*absorption collapse*). The percussion note over the collapsed lung or lobe is dull, the breath sounds are diminished or absent, and radiological examination shows displacement of the trachea and/or heart shadow towards the side of the lesion, elevation of the diaphragm on the same side and a dense pulmonary opacity of characteristic size, shape and position (Fig. 7.2). If the collapse involves a smaller portion of lung (e.g. the right middle lobe or a bronchopulmonary segment), displacement of the mediastinum may not occur, and abnormal physical signs may be difficult to detect, but a characteristic radiographic opacity will be present. The radiological features of pulmonary collapse are shown in Figure 7.3. Semisolid material, such as mucus, mucopus or blood clot, obstructing a large bronchus is apt to fragment, and portions of it may then be aspirated into the peripheral bronchi, leaving the larger bronchus clear. The diminished or absent breath sounds are then replaced by bronchial breath sounds, but the other clinical and radiological abnormalities do not change.

2. PARTIAL OBSTRUCTION. If a large bronchus is partially obstructed, a situation occasionally arises in which there is less resistance to air flow through the narrowed bronchus during inspiration than during expiration, when the obstruc-

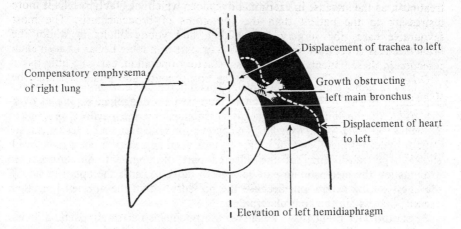

Compensatory emphysema of right lung

Displacement of trachea to left

Growth obstructing left main bronchus

Displacement of heart to left

Elevation of left hemidiaphragm

Fig. 7.2 The effects on neighbouring structures of collapse of the left lung.

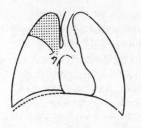
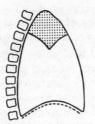
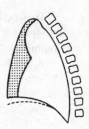

RIGHT UPPER LOBE   LEFT UPPER LOBE

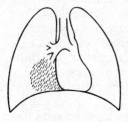
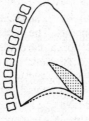
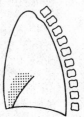

RIGHT MIDDLE LOBE   LINGULA

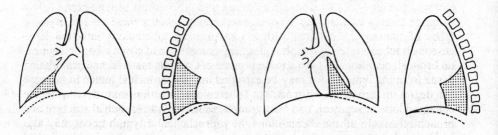

RIGHT LOWER LOBE   LEFT LOWER LOBE

Fig. 7.3 Radiological features of pulmonary collapse caused by bronchial obstruction. The dotted line represents the normal position of the diaphragm.

tion may become temporarily complete. This differential between inspiratory and expiratory airway resistance, which is increased by coughing, results in over-distension of the lung, lobe or segment supplied by the partially obstructed bronchus (*obstructive emphysema*). The percussion note over such a lesion is resonant or hyper-resonant, and the breath sounds are diminished. A chest radiograph shows hypertranslucency of the affected part of lung, and on fluoroscopic examination the mediastinum can be seen to move towards the opposite side of the chest during expiration, because the pressure within the affected lung then exceeds that within the contralateral lung.

3. SECONDARY INFECTION. Whenever a bronchus is narrowed, bacterial infection of the lung tissue it supplies is virtually inevitable, and this may occur even when the degree of obstruction is insufficient to cause pulmonary collapse. This

explains why pneumonia may be the first clinical manifestation of bronchial carcinoma. The infection is usually of low virulence, but in some cases severe pulmonary suppuration may occur, with empyema as a further complication.

4. PULMONARY FUNCTION. Bronchial obstruction impairs pulmonary function, but this is unlikely to produce symptoms unless a main or lobar bronchus is involved, or if the patient's overall pulmonary function is so poor that obstruction of a smaller bronchus critically diminishes the respiratory reserve. Sudden occlusion of a main or lobar bronchus by mucus or mucopus occurring as a postoperative complication may cause severe dyspnoea and hypoxia.

5. CLINICAL FEATURES RELATED TO THE CAUSE OF THE OBSTRUCTION.

(i) *Tumours.* Bronchial obstruction by a carcinoma usually produces pulmonary collapse at an early stage and seldom causes obstructive emphysema. Pulmonary infection is common, and this may be complicated by empyema. The degree of exertional dyspnoea produced by a bronchial carcinoma is directly related to the size of the obstructed bronchus. The rate of growth of a bronchial adenoma is much less rapid than that of a carcinoma. Complete bronchial obstruction and pulmonary collapse are therefore later developments in the presence of an adenoma, and obstructive emphysema, caused by partial bronchial obstruction, may be observed during the intervening period.

(ii) *Enlarged Tracheobronchial Lymph Nodes.* By compressing or invading the bronchial wall, enlarged lymph nodes may produce the same clinical manifestations of bronchial obstruction as a tumour within the lumen, and in bronchial carcinoma both types of lesion may co-exist. Bronchial obstruction by enlarged lymph nodes in Hodgkin's disease and other forms of lymphoma is less common than in bronchial carcinoma, presumably because these are less invasive types of tumour. In children with severe primary tuberculous infection large caseous tracheobronchial lymph nodes may compress and erode lobar or segmental bronchi, occasionally even a main bronchus. Caseous material and granulation tissue from the lymph node may be extruded into the bronchial lumen to increase the degree of bronchial obstruction. Tuberculous infection may develop in the collapsed lobe or segment, and later complications include bronchial stricture and bronchiectasis. In all these conditions the supraclavicular lymph nodes may also be involved, and biopsy of one of these nodes may provide a positive histological diagnosis of tumour, lymphoma or tuberculosis.

(iii) *Foreign Bodies.* An inhaled foreign body generally lodges in the right main, intermediate or lower bronchus, as these bronchi are almost directly in line with the trachea. Children inhale foreign bodies more often than adults. These include nuts (usually peanuts), peas, beans and small pieces of metallic or plastic toys. Adults, on the other hand, are more likely to inhale fragments of tooth during extractions under general anaesthesia, and pieces of mutton or rabbit bone. When a foreign body becomes impacted in a bronchus, it first produces, after an initial episode of choking, either obstructive emphysema or absorption collapse, and a persistent low-pitched rhonchus may be audible all over the chest. Within a few days pathogenic bacteria, carried into the respiratory tract with the foreign body, give rise to a suppurative pneumonia in the collapsed lobe. The patient at this stage often has a high temperature, cough productive of purulent sputum, and pleural pain. On clinical examination there may be a pleural rub and physical signs of either pulmonary collapse or consolidation. Radiological examination shows either obstructive emphysema or collapse and/or pneumonic consolidation of the lobe or lobes supplied by the obstructed bronchus. A radio-opaque foreign body may be visible on the film.

(iv) *Bronchial Casts or Plugs*. These may consist of either inspissated mucus or blood clot. Plugs of mucus may cause bronchial obstruction in patients with asthma or allergic bronchial aspergillosis (p. 306). Secondary bacterial infection of the collapsed lung may occur, but is seldom severe. Bronchial obstruction by blood clot frequently follows severe haemoptysis, but as this complication is usually recognised and treated at an early stage, secondary bacterial infection of collapsed lung tissue seldom occurs.

(v) *Retained Secretions*. A main, lobar or segmental bronchus may be obstructed by retained mucus or mucopus when a patient is unable to cough effectively because of chest pain, muscular weakness or general debility. Pulmonary collapse following an upper abdominal or thoracic operation, or an injury to the chest wall, is due to this type of bronchial obstruction. Secondary bacterial infection of the collapsed lung tissue supervenes at an early stage.

Diagnosis and Treatment of Bronchial Obstruction. The cause of the bronchial obstruction can be discovered by bronchoscopic examination, and in the case of tumour and tuberculosis histological confirmation of the diagnosis can usually be obtained by bronchial biopsy. Foreign bodies can be extracted by bronchoscopy or bronchotomy. If bronchial casts, plugs or secretions cannot be dislodged by postural coughing, they should be removed through a bronchoscope. In other forms of bronchial obstruction the treatment is that of the primary condition.

Postoperative pulmonary collapse can usually be prevented by forbidding patients to smoke for 3 weeks prior to operation, by vigorous pre- and postoperative breathing exercises, and by regularly supervised coughing during the immediate postoperative period.

INTRATHORACIC TUMOURS
Tumours of Bronchus and Lung

Bronchial carcinoma is by far the most common malignant pulmonary tumour. Benign tumours are rare. A primary carcinoma in any organ, but particularly in breast, kidney, uterus, ovary, testis, thyroid or in lung itself, may give rise to pulmonary metastatic deposits, as may an osteogenic or melanotic sarcoma.

Bronchial Carcinoma

Bronchial carcinoma accounts for almost 40 per cent of all male deaths from malignant disease. It is five times more common in men than in women, and occurs most frequently between the ages of 50 and 75. Cigarette smoking is responsible for most cases of bronchial carcinoma, and the increased risk is directly proportional to the amount smoked. For example, the death rate from the disease in heavy cigarette smokers is 30 times that in non-smokers. The death rate is slightly higher in urban than in rural dwellers, presumably because of atmospheric pollution. There is also a higher incidence in certain occupations (p. 332).

Pathology. The tumour, which may be a squamous or small cell (oat cell) carcinoma or, occasionally, an adenocarcinoma, arises from bronchial epithelium or mucous glands and at an early stage may occlude the bronchial lumen. It also invades the deeper layers of the bronchial wall and the surrounding lung tissue. When the tumour obstructs a major bronchus it causes pulmonary collapse and infection (p. 319). A tumour arising from a peripheral bronchus may attain a very large size without producing a significant degree of collapse. A tumour of this type may undergo central necrosis and cavitation.

The tumour may involve the pleura either directly or by lymphatic spread, causing a pleural effusion which is often blood-stained. It may also invade the chest wall and cause severe pain by irritation of the intercostal nerves or the brachial plexus. The tumour or its lymph node metastases may extend into the mediastinum, involving the phrenic and recurrent laryngeal nerves, the sympathetic trunk, the superior vena cava, the pericardium and myocardium, the trachea and the oesophagus.

Lymphatic spread may occur to the supraclavicular ('scalene') lymph nodes as well as to the mediastinal lymph nodes and pleura. Blood-borne metastases occur most commonly in liver, bone, brain, suprarenals, skin and kidneys. Even a small primary tumour may cause widespread metastases.

Clinical Features. The onset is usually insidious. Cough is the most common early symptom. The amount and character of the sputum depend on the degree of secondary infection present. Repeated slight haemoptysis is a common and characteristic feature. Dyspnoea may occur early when a lobe or lung is collapsed, but in other circumstances is a late symptom unless the patient is coincidentally suffering from chronic bronchitis and emphysema. Pulmonary infection beyond an obstructing tumour gives rise to pneumonia which is unusually slow to respond to treatment. Pleural pain is a frequent symptom and may be due either to infective pleurisy or to malignant invasion of the pleura. A small pleural effusion in a patient with a bronchial carcinoma is often due to infection but a massive blood-stained effusion is almost invariably due to invasion of pleura by tumour. Pain in the chest wall or in an upper limb with a nerve root distribution may be present if the tumour involves intercostal nerves or the brachial plexus. An apical bronchial carcinoma may cause Horner's syndrome (p. 684). Rib destruction often accompanies these nerve lesions.

The symptoms and signs which may occur when the tumour invades the mediastinum are described in the section on mediastinal tumours (p. 325).

Occasionally the presenting symptom is due to a metastatic deposit, e.g. headache, fits or personality change (cerebral metastasis), pathological fracture (skeletal metastasis), haematuria (renal metastasis), skin nodules, usually tender (cutaneous metastases). Clubbing of the fingers is often seen and a few patients present the features of hypertrophic pulmonary osteoarthropathy, peripheral neuropathy (p. 750), or cerebellar degeneration, none of these manifestations necessarily being related to the presence of metastatic tumour. Rarely an oat-cell carcinoma may act as an ectopic source of adrenocorticotrophic, antidiuretic or other hormone, and the patient may present with symptoms and signs of endocrine dysfunction. Lassitude, anorexia and loss of weight are *late* symptoms except when pulmonary suppuration is an early development.

Physical Signs in the Chest. Depend on the size of the tumour, but even more on the nature and extent of its secondary effects on lung and pleura.

In the early stages a tumour may cause no abnormal physical signs. A tumour obstructing a large bronchus produces the physical signs of collapse or obstructive emphysema (p. 320). A massive tumour may give rise to signs resembling those of a pleural effusion. Involvement of the pleura either by infection or by tumour may produce signs of dry pleurisy or of a pleural effusion.

Radiological Examination. A bronchial carcinoma may produce (i) a dense, irregular, hilar opacity, (ii) a dense, fairly well circumscribed, peripheral pulmonary opacity, usually large when first discovered, sometimes irregularly cavitated or (iii) an opacity consistent with collapse of a whole lung, a lobe or a segment which may be associated with a hilar opacity due to the tumour itself.

In some cases radiological examination may also show a pleural effusion (indicating either infection or secondary tumour in the pleura), broadening of the mediastinal shadow (due to lymph node metastases), osteolytic lesions of the ribs (indicating either direct invasion by tumour or blood-borne metastases) or unilateral diaphragmatic paralysis (indicating involvement of the phrenic nerve). A paralysed hemidiaphragm is usually raised and on radioscopic examination moves 'paradoxically' when the patient sniffs, i.e. it moves upwards instead of downwards.

Bronchoscopy (p. 262). Inspection of the intrabronchial portion of the tumour and removal of tissue for histological examination is possible in over 60 per cent of cases. In this way the diagnosis can be established with certainty, often at an early and curable stage. Bronchoscopic examination may also indicate the extent of the tumour, which has an important bearing on the patient's suitability for surgical treatment.

Diagnosis. The diagnosis of bronchial carcinoma should be considered in all middle-aged or elderly persons, particularly cigarette smokers, who complain of respiratory symptoms of recent onset which do not clear up completely within a period of 2 weeks, particularly if haemoptysis or pleural pain is present. Radiological examination should be carried out in all such cases, followed by bronchoscopy whenever the radiological appearances are at all suggestive of tumour. A normal chest radiograph does not exclude a diagnosis of bronchial carcinoma in a patient presenting with haemoptysis, and bronchoscopy is indicated in these cases also. Examination of the sputum for malignant cells is a valuable diagnostic measure when practised by a pathologist with special interest and experience in this procedure, but in other circumstances the results can be seriously misleading.

The differential diagnosis includes chronic bronchitis, bronchiectasis, slowly resolving pneumonia, lung abscess, pulmonary tuberculosis, aspergilloma (p. 298), primary mediastinal tumour and metastatic pulmonary tumour. Sputum examination is essential in all cases to exclude tuberculosis. It should not be forgotten that tuberculosis and carcinoma may coexist.

Treatment and Prognosis. Unless surgical treatment is practicable the average period of survival after the diagnosis is made is less than 1 year. Resection of the lung (pneumonectomy) or, in selected cases, of the lobe containing the tumour (lobectomy) offers the best prospect of survival. The operation can be performed only on the small number of cases (about 20 per cent) in which the tumour is discovered at an early and relatively localised stage and pulmonary function is adequate. The tumour is liable to recur even after an apparently satisfactory operation, and only 30 per cent of such patients survive for more than 5 years. Early diagnosis provides slightly better results, but the prognosis depends to an even greater extent on the histological type of tumour and on the presence or absence of metastatic deposits in the hilar lymph nodes. The outlook is particularly unfavourable when the tumour is an oat-cell carcinoma.

Small tumours can occasionally be eradicated by X-ray therapy, but this form of treatment is more often used to relieve distressing complications such as superior vena caval obstruction, recurrent haemoptysis and pain caused by chest wall invasion or by skeletal metastatic deposits. Obstruction of the trachea and main bronchi can also be relieved temporarily by irradiation, but as the latter may initially produce tumour swelling and a dangerous increase in the degree of obstruction, a cytotoxic drug, e.g. mustine hydrochloride intravenously, should be given first. Cytotoxic drugs, given alone, are in general less effective than radiotherapy for palliative treatment, except in malignant pleural effusion.

Bronchial Adenoma

This is an uncommon tumour occurring in a younger age group than carcinoma and affecting females as often as males. Although classified as a benign tumour it possesses some of the properties of a malignant growth and may eventually give rise to metastases. A bronchial adenoma of the 'carcinoid' type may secrete 5-hydroxytryptamine or a related substance, and give rise to the carcinoid syndrome (p. 405). The usual pathological lesion is a small, vascular tumour within the bronchial lumen with a large encapsulated extrabronchial extension.

The main clinical features, which may have a duration of several years, are recurrent haemoptysis, due to the vascularity of the tumour, recurrent pulmonary infection resulting from bronchial obstruction and, in rare cases, the carcinoid syndrome. The physical signs most frequently found are those of collapse. The diagnosis from bronchial carcinoma can be made only by bronchoscopy and histological examination of a portion of the tumour.

Treatment consists of resection of the pulmonary lobe or segment containing the tumour along with the bronchus from which it arises.

Secondary Tumours of the Lung

Blood-borne metastatic deposits in the lungs may be derived from malignant disease almost anywhere in the body. The usual sites of the primary tumour have already been stated (p. 322). The secondary deposits are usually multiple and bilateral. Haemoptysis occurs in some cases but often there are no respiratory symptoms and the diagnosis is made by radiological examination.

Extensive infiltration of the pulmonary lymphatics by tumour may develop in patients with carcinoma of breast, stomach, pancreas or bronchus. This condition, known as *pulmonary lymphatic carcinomatosis*, causes severe and rapidly progressive dyspnoea.

Tumours of the Mediastinum

Classification. *Tumours of the lymph nodes*, e.g. secondary carcinoma, usually from bronchus or breast; lymphomas, including Hodgkin's disease; leukaemia.

Thymic tumours, e.g. malignant thymoma.

Connective tissue tumours, e.g. fibroma, lipoma (benign); sarcoma (malignant).

Neural tumours, e.g. neurofibroma.

Developmental tumours and cysts, e.g. teratoma; dermoid, bronchogenic and pleuro-pericardial cysts.

Other lesions presenting as mediastinal tumours, e.g. aortic aneurysm, aneurysmal dilatation of left atrium, intrathoracic goitre, sarcoidosis involving lymph nodes.

Pathology and Clinical Features. BENIGN TUMOURS. The conditions in this category include neural tumours, teratoma, developmental cysts and intrathoracic goitre. All of them are rare. The effects produced by a benign tumour are related mainly to its size, and symptoms are present only when it compresses vital structures. The diagnosis of benign tumour is usually made by chance, when radiological examination of the chest is undertaken for some other reasons. Many of the cases are found by mass radiography. It a tumour becomes very large it may cause dyspnoea by compression of lung tissue, or occasionally by narrowing the trachea. A benign tumour in the upper part of the thorax occasionally compresses the superior vena cava (see below). Invasion of mediastinal structures, bronchi or lungs never occurs.

MALIGNANT TUMOURS. Included in this category are mediastinal lymph node metastases, malignant lymphomas, leukaemia, malignant thymic tumours and mediastinal sarcoma. Aortic and innominate aneurysms have invasive features resembling those of malignant mediastinal tumours. All these conditions, except lymph node metastases, are uncommon.

The distinguishing feature of this group of tumours is their power to invade as well as to compress mediastinal structures, bronchi and lungs. As a result of this property even a small malignant tumour can produce symptoms, although as a rule the tumour has attained a considerable size before this happens.

The structures which may be invaded or compressed and the symptoms and signs produced in each case are:

(a) *Trachea:* dyspnoea, stridor, brassy cough.

(b) *Main bronchus:* pulmonary collapse, dyspnoea.

(c) *Oesophagus:* dysphagia.

(d) *Phrenic nerve:* diaphragmatic paralysis (p. 324).

(e) *Left recurrent laryngeal nerve:* paralysis of left vocal cord, hoarseness.

(f) *Sympathetic trunk:* Horner's syndrome (p. 684).

(g) *Pericardium:* pericarditis, either *dry* with pericardial rub, or *with effusion*.

(h) *Superior vena cava:* oedema and cyanosis of head and neck, and sometimes of upper limbs also, with distension of external jugular veins and dilated anastomotic veins on anterior chest wall and in axillary regions.

Radiological Examination. A *benign mediastinal tumour* generally appears as a large, round, sharply circumscribed opacity, situated mainly in the mediastinum but often encroaching on one or both lung fields.

A *malignant mediastinal tumour* seldom has a clearly defined margin and often presents as a general broadening of the mediastinal shadow.

Diagnosis. The only common mediastinal tumour is that produced by lymph node metastases from a bronchial carcinoma. An aortic aneurysm and an intrathoracic goitre can often be recognised from the other clinical features, and leukaemia from the blood picture, and a diagnosis of sarcoidosis or of malignant lymphoma can often be made from biopsy of a superficial lymph node. The known radiosensitivity of the lymphomas is sometimes used as a diagnostic test, rapid shrinkage of the tumour following radiotherapy being a typical feature.

As bronchial carcinoma is such a common primary cause of mediastinal tumour, bronchoscopy should be carried out in all cases. If enlarged mediastinal lymph nodes are suspected one of these can be removed for histological examination by the technique of mediastinoscopy (p. 262). In some cases, however, an exact diagnosis cannot be made without surgical exploration of the chest and removal of the tumour or a portion of it for histological examination.

Treatment. *Benign Mediastinal Tumours.* These should be removed surgically as soon as they are discovered because (*a*) they tend to produce symptoms sooner or later and (*b*) some of them, particularly cysts, may become infected while others, especially neural tumours, may undergo malignant change. The operative mortality is very small.

Malignant Mediastinal Tumours. In the malignant lymphomas, leukaemia and malignant thymoma, radiotherapy often produces a remarkable clinical improvement by reducing the size of the tumour. The improvement, although only temporary, may last for months or even years. Lymph node metastases from bronchial carcinoma sometimes respond fairly well to radiotherapy and complications such as superior vena caval and tracheal obstruction can often be relieved in this way.

INTERSTITIAL LUNG DISEASE

This term is applied to a group of pulmonary diseases which have the following features in common:

1. Thickening of the alveolar walls by oedema, cellular exudate or fibrosis.
2. Increased stiffness of the lungs (reduced compliance), associated with exertional dyspnoea.
3. Mal distribution of pulmonary ventilation and perfusion and a gas diffusion defect leading to hypoxia, hyperventilation and hypocapnia.

Aetiology. Interstitial lung disease is caused by several aetiologically distinct pathological processes, but these all give rise to similar symptoms, physical signs, radiological changes and disturbances of pulmonary function. They are thus worthy of collective consideration. The most frequently recognised causes of interstitial lung disease are:

1. Chronic pulmonary odema, e.g. secondary to mitral valve disease (p. 201).
2. Allergic alveolitis (p. 307).
3. Fibrosing alveolitis associated with the connective tissue disorders or of unknown aetiology (cryptogenic fibrosing alveolitis).
4. Pulmonary damage following radiotherapy to thorax.
5. Sarcoidosis (p. 328), asbestosis (p. 322), and idiopathic pulmonary haemosiderosis (p. 328).

Although the cardinal features of all forms of interstitial lung disease are similar, these conditions differ considerably in other respects, including aetiology and extrapulmonary manifestations.

Fibrosing Alveolitis

This condition exemplifies many of the typical features of interstitial lung disease. It may be a manifestation of one of the connective tissue disorders, such as rheumatoid disease, systemic lupus erythematosus or systemic sclerosis, or it may occur as an isolated pulmonary abnormality, possibly auto-allergic in origin. Progressive exertional dyspnoea is usually the presenting symptom, often accompanied by a persistent dry cough. In most cases there is gross clubbing of the fingers and toes. Chest expansion is poor, but hyperventilation is always a striking feature. Numerous bilateral coarse crackling crepitations are audible on auscultation. Radiologically, there are diffuse pulmonary opacities, the diaphragm is high and the lungs appear small. The FEV_1 and FVC are reduced proportionately, the carbon monoxide transfer factor is low, and arterial blood-gas studies show hypoxia and hypocapnia. The diagnosis can usually be made with confidence from these findings, but should in doubtful cases be confirmed by lung biopsy. Serological tests for antinuclear and rheumatoid factors may be positive, even in cases without evidence of connective tissue disorder. The rate of progression of the pulmonary changes varies considerably, from death within a few months to survival with minimal symptoms for many years. Treatment with corticosteroids is effective in perhaps 30 per cent of the acute cases, but not in the others. It may have to be maintained for several years, or even for life.

HONEYCOMB LUNG. The radiological phenomenon of 'honeycomb lung', in which diffuse pulmonary shadowing is interspersed with small, thick-walled cystic translucencies, may be observed in some cases of interstitial lung disease, but it may also be a characteristic feature of certain rare diseases, such as histiocytosis X and tuberous sclerosis. Honeycomb lung, whatever its cause, is associated with an increased incidence of spontaneous pneumothorax, and eventually produces respiratory failure, pulmonary hypertension and right ventricular failure.

Idiopathic Pulmonary Haemosiderosis

This is a rare disease of unknown cause, in which spontaneous haemorrhage into the lungs causes recurrent episodes of pyrexia, haemoptysis and iron-deficiency anaemia. With every incident, red blood cells in large numbers are extravasated into the interstitial tissues of the lungs, where haemosiderin released from macrophages stimulates fibroblastic activity. If the patient survives the acute haemorrhagic episodes, the interstitial fibrosis may eventually cause respiratory failure and pulmonary hypertension. Pulmonary haemosiderosis may also be associated with acute glomerulonephritis (Goodpasture's syndrome, p. 478).

During the acute episodes widespread coarse crepitations are present, and diffuse stippled shadowing, chiefly involving the mid-zones of both lung fields, is seen on the chest radiograph. In the later stages the clinical and radiographic abnormalities may be indistinguishable from those of fibrosing alveolitis.

Sarcoidosis

Sarcoidosis is a systemic granulomatous disease of unknown cause. Apart from the absence of caseation and tubercle bacilli, the lesions are histologically similar to tuberculous follicles, but there is no convincing evidence to support the view that the disease is caused by any of the mycobacteria. Chronic beryllium poisoning produces a disease which mimics sarcoidosis both pathologically and clinically, but exposure to beryllium is extremely uncommon and few cases of sarcoidosis can be caused in this way. Histological changes resembling those of sarcoidosis are occasionally seen in individual organs, such as lymph nodes, in conditions such as carcinoma, reticulosis and fungal infections, but these localised 'sarcoid reactions' are not associated with systemic sarcoidosis.

Pathology. The mediastinal and superficial lymph nodes, lungs, liver, spleen, skin, eyes, parotid glands and phalangeal bones are most frequently involved. The characteristic histological feature consists of non-caseating epithelioid follicles. These lesions usually resolve spontaneously but in some cases they stimulate the production of fibrous tissue, which may have grave effects on local structure and function. The disease is seldom fatal, and then only when it affects vital organs such as the lungs, the heart or the central nervous system. An increase in serum calcium, which is rare, may produce renal calcinosis and uraemia.

Clinical Features. Sarcoidosis may present in a subacute or a chronic form. Subacute sarcoidosis is usually a benign and self-limiting disorder, spontaneous resolution occuring within 2 years in most cases. One of its most common manifestations is bilateral and often symmetrical enlargement of the hilar lymph nodes. The paratracheal lymph nodes may also be involved. Erythema nodosum, pyrexia and polyarthralgia may be present at the outset. Later, transient pulmonary changes may be seen on radiological examination in addition to the lymph node enlargement. Other cases of subacute sarcoidosis may present with bilateral parotid swelling or iritis, which often persist for several weeks. Neurological manifestations, which are uncommon, include arachnoiditis, cranial nerve lesions and polyneuropathy.

Chronic sarcoidosis is a more serious condition, which is less likely to resolve spontaneously and is more liable to cause permanent damage to the structures it involves. Chronic pulmonary sarcoidosis may lead to the development of interstitial fibrosis, pulmonary hypertension and cor pulmonale. The vital capacity and carbon monoxide transfer factor (p. 255) are the most useful indices of impairment of lung function in this disease. Myocardial sarcoidosis may produce arrhythmias and cardiac failure. The commonest ocular lesion is bilateral chronic iritis which, if untreated, may cause blindness. Various types of skin lesion may be seen, such as cutaneous 'sarcoids' (reddish-brown papules) or lupus pernio (raised purple plaques, usually on the face, resembling chilblains). Cystic lesions may develop in the phalangeal bones of the hands or feet.

Diagnosis. In most cases skin sensitivity to tuberculin is depressed or absent, and the Mantoux reaction (p. 287) is therefore a useful 'screening' test, a strongly positive reaction to 1 TU virtually excluding sarcoidosis. Although the diagnosis can often be made with a fair measure of confidence from the clinical and radiological features and the tuberculin test, it should, if possible, be confirmed histologically by biopsy of a superficial lymph node or of a skin lesion, when these are present. The Kveim test is also a useful diagnostic procedure, provided a potent antigen can be obtained from human sarcoid tissue. The antigen (0·1 ml) is injected intradermally and when the test is positive a small nodule develops about 4 weeks later, biopsy of which reveals typical sarcoid follicles.

Treatment. As subacute sarcoidosis usually resolves spontaneously treatment is seldom required, but occasionally patients with persistent erythema nodosum, pyrexia, parotid swelling or iridocyclitis may have to be given oral corticosteroid drugs for a short period. Patients with chronic sarcoidosis, particularly if it involves the lungs, eyes or other vital organs, are much more likely to require treatment with corticosteroids, which may have to be continued for several years. The dose should be kept to the minimum required to suppress the manifestations of the disease. Some physicians who believe that sarcoidosis is a form of tuberculosis advise that antituberculosis chemotherapy should be given at the same time, but this is probably unnecessary.

OCCUPATIONAL LUNG DISEASES

In certain occupations the inhalation of dusts, fumes or other noxious substances may give rise to specific pathological changes in the lungs. The nature of each substance, the occupation in which the hazard occurs, the description of each disease and the pathological changes produced in the lungs are summarised in Table 7.5.

Table 7.5   Causes and effects of occupational lung disease

Cause	Occupation	Description of Disease	Pathological Changes in Lungs
Mineral dusts:			
Coal dust	Coal mining	Coal-worker's pneumo-coniosis	
Silica	Gold mining Iron and steel industries (metal casting) Metal grinding Stone dressing Pottery	Silicosis	Focal and interstitial fibrosis Centrilobular emphysema Progressive massive fibrosis
Asbestos	Manufacture of fireproof and insulating materials	Asbestosis	Asbestos bodies Interstitial fibrosis Bronchial carcinoma Pleural mesothelioma
Iron oxide	Arc welding	Siderosis	Mineral deposition only
Tin dioxide	Tin ore mining	Stannosis	
Beryllium	Aircraft and atomic energy industries	Berylliosis	Granulomata Interstitial fibrosis
Organic dusts:			
Cotton, flax or hemp dust	Textile industries	Byssinosis	Acute bronchiolitis Bronchoconstriction
Fungal spores from mouldy hay, straw or grain, mushroom compost, bagasse, etc.	Agriculture and related industries	Farmer's lung Maltworker's lung Mushroom worker's lung Bagassosis	Extrinsic allergic alveolitis
Gases and fumes:			
Irritant gases (ammonia, chlorine, phosgene, sulphur dioxide and trioxide)	Various industries (accidental exposure)		Acute pulmonary oedema
Toluene di-isocyanate	Plastic and rubber industries		Bronchial asthma
Cadmium	Welding and electroplating		Chronic bronchitis and emphysema

In many forms of respiratory disease it is most important to take a detailed occupational history and not to rest content with recording the current occupation. It must also be emphasised that in many types of pneumoconiosis a long period of exposure to dust is required before radiological changes appear and these may precede symptoms by several years. The regulations relating to compensation in Britain are set out in the Department of Health and Social Security report of 1973 on pneumoconiosis and byssinosis. New industrial processes are constantly being introduced and it is necessary to remain alert to the possibility that they may be associated with new occupational lung diseases.

Diseases Caused by Mineral Dusts (Pneumoconiosis)

The dust particles, after inhalation, are conveyed by macrophages from the bronchial mucosa to minute foci of lymphoid tissue throughout the lungs. There the irritation produced by solution of the particles in tissue fluid may initiate widespread pulmonary fibrosis. The fibrogenic capacity of mineral dusts vary, silica being markedly fibrogenic whereas iron is almost inert. The most important types of pneumoconiosis are coal-worker's pneumoconiosis, silicosis and asbestosis.

Coal-worker's Pneumoconiosis

The disease results from prolonged inhalation of coal dust. For clinical purposes—and for certification—the condition is subdivided into simple pneumoconiosis and progressive massive fibrosis. It must be emphasised that for certification purposes in Britain the diagnosis rests at present on radiological, and not clinical, features.

Simple Coal-worker's Pneumoconiosis. This is categorised radiologically into 3 grades, depending on the size and extent of the nodulation present. It does not progress if the miner leaves the industry.

Progressive Massive Fibrosis. In this form of the disease, large dense masses, single or multiple, occur mainly in the upper lobes. These may be irregular in shape and may cavitate. This type of disease may be complicated very rarely by tuberculosis. It may be disabling and may shorten life expectancy. This form of the disease progresses even after the miner leaves the industry.

Antinuclear factor is present in the serum of about 15 per cent of patients with coal-worker's pneumoconiosis. Rheumatoid factor is present in some patients—so-called *Caplan's syndrome*—in which rheumatoid arthritis coexists with rounded fibrotic nodules 0·5 to 5 cm in diameter, mainly in the periphery of the lung fields. This syndrome may also occur in other types of pneumoconiosis.

Clinical Features. Cough and sputum due to associated chronic bronchitis are frequently present. The sputum may be black. Progressive breathlessness on exertion occurs in the later stages, and ventilatory and right ventricular failure supervene as terminal events. There may be no abnormal physical signs in the chest, but where present, they are those of chronic obstructive airways disease.

Silicosis

This disease is becoming much more rare as the standards of industrial hygiene improve. It is caused by the inhalation of fine free crystalline silicon dioxide (silica) dust or quartz particles. It occurs in the following occupations: mining of coal, tin, gold and other minerals; quarrying, mining and dressing of sandstone and granite; the pottery and ceramics industry; the manufacture of silica bricks and abrasive soaps; iron and steel foundrymen; sand blasting, metal grinding and boiler scaling.

Silica is a very fibrogenic dust and causes the development of hard nodules which coalesce as the disease progresses. Tuberculosis may modify the silicotic process, and caseation and calcification may occur. The radiological features are similar to those seen in coal-worker's pneumoconiosis though the changes tend to be more marked in the upper zones. The hilar shadows may be enlarged and 'eggshell' calcification in the hilar lymph nodes is a distinctive feature. The disease progresses even when exposure to dust ceases. The sufferer should be removed from the offending environment immediately.

Clinical features are similar to those described in coal-worker's pneumoconiosis.

Asbestos-related Diseases of the Lungs and Pleura

The main types of asbestos are chrysotile, which accounts for 90 per cent of the world's production, and crocidolite (blue asbestos). Exposure occurs in the following occupations: mining and milling of the material; manufacturing processes involving asbestos; pipe lagging and spraying of limpet asbestos; demolition workers, including those who may work alongside them, e.g. joiners, painters and electricians.

Three forms of disease related to inhalation of asbestos are recognised—calcified pleural plaques, progressive pulmonary fibrosis and malignant disease of pleura and peritoneum.

Pleural plaques are best seen in the early stages on oblique films. They are most commonly found on the diaphragm and anterolaterally.

Progressive pulmonary fibrosis is characterised by increasing shortness of breath on exertion and cough, by the presence of clubbing of the fingers and dry crepitations at the bases and anterolaterally, and by typical radiological and physiological abnormalities. The radiological abnormalities are usually confined to the lower two-thirds of the lung fields and consist of mottled shadows with some streaky opacities and sometimes 'honeycombing'. The cardiac silhouette becomes shaggy in outline. The most important physiological abnormalities are a reduced carbon monoxide transfer factor (p. 255) and a restrictive ventilatory defect (p. 263). Ventilatory and right ventricular failure eventually supervene. The incidence of bronchial carcinoma is much increased, about ten-fold, in persons suffering from asbestosis.

Mesothelioma of the pleura is usually linked with exposure, often relatively trivial, to blue asbestos. The patient frequently presents with an ache in the chest. A pleural effusion develops and this causes breathlessness. The effusion may be blood-stained. The diagnosis is often difficult to confirm on pleural biopsy and even at thoracoscopy.

Diagnosis of asbestosis is based on evidence of exposure, clubbing of fingers, characteristic crepitations, typical radiological features, and the physiological abnormalities of restrictive lung disease. Lung biopsy may be required to confirm the diagnosis, but is not without risk and should not be carried out solely for the purpose of allowing the British patient to claim Industrial Injuries Benefit.

Treatment and Prevention of Pneumoconiosis. No specific treatment is available. In the later stages treatment is required for associated conditions such as chronic bronchitis and ventilatory failure, pulmonary tuberculosis or malignant pleural effusion.

Improvement of standards of industrial hygiene are now enforced by law in many countries; such measures as wearing respirators, damping dust and efficient ventilation systems are already proving effective in a number of industries.

Diseases Caused by Organic Dusts

In *byssinosis* the initial lesion is an acute bronchiolitis, associated with symptoms and signs of generalised airway obstruction which tend to be worse after week-end breaks, but eventually become continuous. There is no radiological abnormality. Recovery usually follows removal from exposure to the dust hazard.

All the other diseases caused by organic dusts are forms of *extrinsic allergic alveolitis*, which have already been fully described (p. 307).

Pulmonary Fibrosis

There are three main types of pulmonary fibrosis:

1. *Replacement fibrosis*, in which the fibrous tissue replaces lung parenchyma damaged by infection or by some other destructive process (e.g. infarction). Fibrosis of this type is a common feature of pulmonary tuberculosis and of all types of pulmonary suppuration (p. 279), and is often associated with bronchiectasis.

2. *Focal fibrosis*, which is a common manifestation of pneumoconiosis.

3. *Interstitial fibrosis*, which is the end-result of interstitial lung disease (p. 327).

If pulmonary fibrosis is extensive, it will cause exertional dyspnoea and hypoxia, and this is more likely to be the case in the focal and interstitial fibrosis than in replacement fibrosis. On the other hand, the physical signs and radiological changes will usually be more conspicuous in replacement fibrosis, which generally produces gross localised abnormalities.

Pulmonary fibrosis cannot usefully be discussed as a single entity, and the reader is therefore referred to its various causes.

DISEASES OF THE PLEURA AND CHEST WALL

Fibrinous ('Dry') Pleurisy

This term is used to describe cases of pleurisy at the stage of fibrinous exudation when there is no significant degree of effusion. It is usually secondary to bacterial infection in the underlying lung, but may also occur in association with a virus infection (Coxsackie B), which primarily involves the intercostal muscles and is known as '*Bornholm disease*'. Dry pleurisy is a common feature of pulmonary infarction, and may be an early manifestation of pleural invasion by a pulmonary tumour or of pulmonary tuberculosis.

Clinical Features. The characteristic symptom of dry pleurisy is *pleural pain*. On examination, rib movement is restricted and the breath sounds, though vesicular, may be diminished on the affected side. A *pleural rub* is heard in a high proportion of cases. In all cases the rub is increased by deep breathing and is never heard when the patient is holding his breath except near the pericardium, where a so-called *pleuropericardial rub* may be heard. In the acute stage of dry pleurisy, respiration may be so painful that the limited range of movement of the chest wall may be insufficient to produce an audible rub.

The other clinical features depend on the nature of the lesion causing the pleurisy. Depending on the cause, complete clinical recovery may ensue or an effusion may develop, either serous or purulent.

Diagnosis. 'Dry pleurisy' is not a complete diagnosis. An attempt should always be made to find a primary cause. Radiological examination must therefore be performed in every case. A negative radiograph does not necessarily exclude a pulmonary cause for the pleurisy. A preceding history of a few days' cough, purulent sputum and pyrexia is presumptive evidence of a pulmonary infection which may not have been severe enough to produce a radiographic abnormality or which may have resolved before the film was taken.

Dry pleurisy must be distinguished from intercostal myalgia (pleurodynia), fractured rib, costochondritis, herpes zoster, spontaneous pneumothorax and acute upper abdominal disease.

Treatment. The primary cause of the pleurisy must be treated. The symptomatic treatment of pleural pain is described on page 267.

Pleural Effusion

This term, by general consent, is applied only to serous effusion. The condition of purulent effusion or empyema is described separately on page 337. The passive transudation of fluid into the pleural cavity (*hydrothorax*) occurs in cardiac failure, nephrotic syndrome, advanced cirrhosis of the liver and severe malnutrition.

The most common causes of pleural effusion are pneumonia, tuberculosis, malignant disease and pulmonary infarction. Pleural effusion, often bilateral, may also be a manifestation of systemic lupus erythematosus, rheumatoid disease and malignant lymphomas. Inflammatory lesions below the diaphragm, such as subphrenic abscess and pancreatitis, occasionally produce a pleural effusion.

Clinical Features. The symptoms and signs of dry pleurisy often precede the development of effusion, but the onset in other cases may be insidious, with little or no pleural pain. Pyrexia occurs in most cases, whatever the primary cause, but is more severe in the presence of infection, and more protracted when the infection is tuberculous.

The principal symptom related to the effusion itself is dyspnoea. The severity of the dyspnoea depends on the size of the effusion and on the rate at which it accumulates. The physical signs in the chest are those of fluid in the pleural space.

Radiological Examination shows a dense uniform opacity in the lower and lateral parts of the hemithorax shading off above and medially into translucent lung. When the effusion is loculated, e.g. in an interlobar fissure, a localised opacity is seen.

Diagnosis. The presence of a pleural effusion can usually be recognised from the physical signs, but in some cases it may not be suspected until radiological examination is carried out. Absolute proof that an effusion is present can be obtained only by the aspiration of fluid. A needle should be inserted through an intercostal space over the area of maximum dullness on percussion or, ideally, at the site of maximum radiological opacity as shown by postero-anterior and lateral films or by fluoroscopy. At least 50 ml of fluid should be withdrawn, 20 ml or more being placed in a sterile container for bacteriological examination, 20 ml in a citrated container for cytological examination and 10 ml in a chemically clean container for biochemical examination.

Failure to obtain fluid in a suspected case of pleural effusion may be due to faulty localisation, but if aspiration with a wide-bore needle at various sites is repeatedly unsuccessful, it is unlikely that a significant amount is present. The clinical features and radiological appearances should then be reviewed with four possibilities in mind: pneumonia, pulmonary infarction, pulmonary collapse and pleural thickening.

Pleural thickening, fibrinous or fibrous, which may follow a pleural effusion, produces similar physical signs except that the mediastinum is either central or displaced *towards* the side of the lesion. Thickening of the pleura can often be recognised by a sensation of resistance transmitted from the point of the needle to the hand manipulating the aspirating syringe when the pleura is penetrated.

Many investigations, apart from diagnostic aspiration, may be required to determine the primary cause of a pleural effusion. Estimation of the total and differential leucocyte count in the peripheral blood and examination of the sputum for tubercle bacilli should never be omitted. Radiological examination of the chest may disclose underlying pulmonary disease and indicate its nature. If the lung is obscured by a massive effusion a large volume of fluid should be removed before the film is taken. Pleural biopsy (p. 262) may provide a histological diagnosis in effusions due to tuberculosis or malignant disease. Other investigations which may help to determine the cause of a pleural effusion include bronchoscopy, biopsy of a scalene lymph node, thoracoscopy and serological tests for antinuclear and rheumatoid factors.

Tuberculous Pleural Effusion

This type of effusion may develop in the course of postprimary pulmonary tuberculosis, but most cases occur in the absence of recognisable pulmonary disease. The pleural infection is always secondary to tuberculosis elsewhere, usually in the underlying lung or in the mediastinal lymph nodes, reaching the pleura by direct extension, by lymphatic spread or, occasionally, by haematogenous dissemination. When a pleural effusion occurs in the absence of radiologically apparent pulmonary disease it is usually the sequel to a primary tuberculous infection 3 to 6 months previously. In these cases, which commonly occur in adolescence or early adult life, and less frequently in childhood, the pleural infection is presumably derived either from a minute subpleural primary pulmonary focus or by lymphatic spread from caseous mediastinal lymph nodes. Although a pleural effusion of this type cannot occur in the absence of tubercle bacilli, the number of bacilli may be small and the disproportionately severe pleural reaction may be due mainly to hypersensitivity of the pleural tissues to tuberculoprotein which develops after the primary tuberculous infection (p. 286).

The onset of a tuberculous pleural effusion may in some cases be sudden, with severe pleural pain preceding the physical signs of effusion for several days. In others the only complaints may be of vague ill-health and loss of weight for a period of weeks or even months before the effusion is discovered. In untreated cases, pyrexia of a remittent type, rising to 39°C (101–103°F) is generally present for the first 3 to 6 weeks of the illness, and sleep sweats are a common feature. The patient, however, never appears as seriously ill as one with acute pneumonia. There is usually a considerable degree of tachycardia, but the respiration rate is not markedly increased and dyspnoea at rest is present only if the effusion is very large. Unless frank pulmonary tuberculosis coexists, cough is not a prominent symptom and tubercle bacilli can seldom be isolated from sputum or laryngeal swabs. These tests, however, should be performed in all cases, in conjunction with radiological examination of the chest, to determine whether or not there is an active tuberculous lesion in the lungs.

The total white blood count, which is usually within normal limits in tuberculous pleural effusion, is often a useful diagnostic aid in the early stages of the illness when the differential diagnosis from pneumonia may be difficult.

The pleural fluid in tuberculous effusions is amber or straw-coloured, with a specific gravity of 1·016 or more and a total protein content of over 40 g/l. It usually clots on standing. The cells, which are relatively few, are chiefly lymphocytes. The fluid is sterile on ordinary methods of culture, but tubercle bacilli can often be isolated on culture. In such cases the sensitivity of the organism to antituberculosis drugs (p. 287) should always be ascertained.

Normal lung fields on radiological examination with negative bacteriological findings in sputum and pleural fluid do *not* exclude tuberculosis as the cause of the effusion, and in young adults a tuberculous aetiology should be assumed unless the tuberculin reaction (p. 287) is negative or some other cause can be clearly established. Now that a simple and effective method of pleural biopsy is available (p. 262) it is possible in many cases to confirm the diagnosis of tuberculous pleurisy histologically and by examining stained sections for acid-fast bacilli.

Treatment. The patient should be kept in bed until the pyrexia has subsided. Antituberculosis chemotherapy (p. 292) should be started as soon as the diagnosis is made. As much pleural fluid as can be obtained should be aspirated with a large syringe and needle every 3 to 4 days until the effusion ceases to reaccumulate. Very rapid absorption of pleural fluid can usually be obtained by giving a corticosteroid drug such as prednisolone by mouth, in addition to antituberculosis chemotherapy. The patient can be allowed to resume work a few weeks after he starts to get up and no restrictions need be placed on his activities.

Postpneumonic Serous Pleural Effusion

A serous pleural effusion may be a complication of any type of pneumonia, but is particularly common with pneumococcal pneumonia. The effusion is usually small and, apart occasionally from a slight recrudescence of pyrexia, seldom produces clinical features distinct from those of the pneumonia itself. The pleural fluid is clear, amber or straw-coloured, the cells it contains are predominantly neutrophil leucocytes, and it is usually sterile on culture. In a few cases the effusion becomes purulent: such an outcome was common before the advent of specific treatment.

A serous effusion can safely be regarded as 'postpneumonic', and therefore non-tuberculous, only if there is a preceding history typical of pneumonia, a neutrophil leucocytosis in the blood of over $12·0 \times 10^9/l$ and a predominance of these cells in the pleural fluid.

Treatment. Specific treatment for the pneumonia should be continued until after the pyrexia subsides, and the effusion should be aspirated every 2 or 3 days until it stops reaccumulating. This usually occurs within 7 to 10 days and if it takes longer the diagnosis should be reviewed, with particular regard to the possibilities of empyema and tuberculous pleural effusion.

Malignant Pleural Effusion

The most common cause of pleural effusion over the age of 40 is malignant disease. A malignant effusion is usually secondary to a bronchial carcinoma or to a primary tumour elsewhere. A primary pleural tumour (mesothelioma) may be due to exposure to asbestos (p. 332). Pleural effusion, often bilateral, may occur in patients with lymphomas. A malignant pleural effusion is usually large, and dyspnoea is an early and prominent symptom. Pyrexia may be present but is not as common as with effusions of inflammatory origin.

The pleural fluid may be serous or blood-stained. Clumps of malignant cells may be found by special staining methods.

In some cases bronchoscopy demonstrates a primary bronchial growth. In females the breasts should previously have been examined with care in order to exclude a primary tumour there. When bronchoscopy is negative and the primary tumour is thought to be extrapulmonary, the stomach, kidneys and pelvic organs should be investigated. In most cases, especially if a primary lesion cannot be located, an attempt should be made to obtain histological confirmation of the diagnosis by pleural biopsy (p. 262).

Treatment. Malignant disease of the pleura is incurable, but reaccumulation of fluid, which causes severe dyspnoea and demands frequent pleural aspiration, can often be prevented by treatment aimed at obliterating the pleural space. The method most frequently employed is to inject 20 mg of mustine hydrochloride in 60 ml of normal saline into the effusion, which is then drained by aspiration or through an intercostal tube 24 hours later. By this time the visceral and parietal surfaces are acutely inflamed, and tend to adhere when the lung re-expands. Although mustine, a cytotoxic drug, may produce some necrosis of tumour cells on the pleural surfaces it is of value in the treatment of malignant pleural effusion chiefly or entirely because it is a chemical irritant, and other substances with similar properties (p. 342) may be equally effective.

Empyema Thoracis

This is the term used to describe the presence of pus in the pleural space. The pus may be as thin as serous fluid, or so thick that it is difficult to aspirate through even a wide-bore needle. Microscopically, neutrophil leucocytes are present in large numbers. The causative organism may or may not be isolated from the pus. An empyema may involve the whole pleural space ('total' empyema) or only part of it ('loculated' or 'encysted' empyema). It is almost invariably unilateral.

Aetiology. Empyema is always secondary to infection in a neighbouring structure, usually the lung. The principal infections liable to produce empyema are the bacterial pneumonias and tuberculosis. Other causes of empyema are infection of a haemothorax and rupture of a subphrenic abscess through the diaphragm. Empyema has become a relatively rare disease because pulmonary infection can now be so readily controlled by antibacterial therapy.

Pathology. Both layers of pleura are covered with a thick, shaggy, inflammatory exudate. In the course of time the exudate becomes converted into fibrous tissue which may encase the collapsed lung so rigidly that it cannot re-expand when the pus is removed by aspiration or by an external drainage operation. The pus in the pleural space is often under considerable pressure and if the condition is not adequately treated it may rupture into a bronchus, from which it is expectorated, or through an intercostal space with the formation of a subcutaneous abscess or sinus. When an empyema ruptures into a bronchus, a bronchopleural fistula is produced. This allows air to enter the pleural space, and a pyopneumothorax is formed.

The only way in which an empyema can heal is by apposition of the visceral and parietal layers of the pleura with obliteration of the empyema space by organisation of the intervening exudate. This cannot occur unless re-expansion of the collapsed lung is secured *at an early stage* by removal of all the pus from the pleural space. Re-expansion of the lung cannot take place if, through delay in treatment or inadequate drainage, the visceral pleura becomes grossly thickened and rigid, if the pleural layers are kept apart by air entering the pleura through a bronchopleural fistula, or if disease in the lung itself, such as bronchiectasis, bronchial carcinoma or pulmonary tuberculosis, renders it incapable of re-expansion. In all these circumstances an empyema tends to become chronic and healing may not take place without recourse to major thoracic surgery.

Clinical Features. Empyema should be suspected in patients with pulmonary infection if there is a recurrence of pyrexia which fails to respond or responds only partially to the continued administration of a suitable antibiotic. In other cases the illness produced by the primary infective lesion may be so slight that it passes unrecognised and the first definite clinical features are due to the empyema itself.

In the fully developed case two separate groups of clinical features are found:

Systemic features: (*a*) Pyrexia, usually high and remittent but sometimes slight. (*b*) Rigors, sweating, malaise, anorexia and loss of weight. (*c*) Neutrophil leucocytosis in the blood.

Local features: (*a*) *Dyspnoea*, when the empyema is large. (*b*) *Pleural pain*, usually confined to the initial stage of the illness. (*c*) *Cough and purulent sputum*, usually related to the primary lung disease, but occasionally caused by the rupture of an empyema into a bronchus.

Physical Signs in the Chest. An empyema usually produces the typical signs of fluid in the pleural space (p. 261), but occasionally, as with a serous effusion, the breath sounds may be bronchial instead of diminished or absent. In these cases, however, the presence of fluid can usually be suspected from the 'stony' dullness of the percussion note. A small localised empyema, particularly when situated in an interlobar fissure, may produce no abnormal physical signs.

Radiological Examination. The appearances are indistinguishable from those of serous pleural effusion (p. 334). When air is present in addition to pus (pyopneumothorax), a horizontal 'fluid level' marks the junction of the fluid and the air if the film is taken in the erect position.

Diagnosis. Although the clinical features suggest the diagnosis in most cases, final confirmation of the presence of an empyema depends on the aspiration of pus. A wide-bore needle should be inserted through an intercostal space over the area of maximal dullness on percussion. Whenever possible the position of the empyema should have previously been confirmed by posteroanterior and lateral radiographs. Bacteriological examination of the pus may help to determine the cause of the empyema.

In postpneumonic cases where intensive treatment with antibiotics has been given the pus is frequently sterile. The distinction between tuberculous and nontuberculous cases can usually be made from the radiological changes in the lungs or by the isolation of tubercle bacilli from pus or sputum.

Course and Prognosis. With early drainage and antibiotic therapy most patients with acute empyema quickly recover. Chronic empyema, on the other hand, causes general ill-health, recurrent episodes of pyrexia, clubbing of the fingers and, in severe cases, amyloid disease, and always requires surgical treatment. With specific chemotherapy tuberculous empyema is no longer a serious condition, but complete recovery may take some months.

Treatment. NON-TUBERCULOUS EMPYEMA

1. *Acute.* When the patient is acutely ill, and the pus is thin in consistence:
(*a*) An intercostal tube should be inserted into the most dependent part of the pleural space and connected to a water seal drainage system (p. 341).
(*b*) An antibiotic to which the organism causing the empyema is sensitive should be given by intramuscular injection or by mouth.

If treatment is started early enough, and the organisms are drug-sensitive, an empyema can often be aborted by these measures. If, however, the intercostal tube is not providing adequate drainage, which is apt to happen when the pus thickens and clots, a short segment of rib should be resected, the empyema cavity cleared of pus and clot, and a wide-bore tube inserted.

2. *Chronic.* If the diagnosis is made before any drainage procedure is carried out, it may be feasible to resect the empyema sac *in toto*, provided the patient is fairly fit and the underlying lung is healthy. If open drainage has been performed, and re-expansion of the lung is prevented by gross thickening of the visceral pleura, 'decortication' may be required. This procedure will allow the lung to re-expand and obliterate the pleural space. Few patients nowadays need to be left with a permanent pleural drain, but this may be unavoidable when respiratory function is poor, or if the underlying lung is badly damaged and the patient is unfit for a major pulmonary resection.

TUBERCULOUS EMPYEMA. Antituberculosis chemotherapy (p. 292) should be started immediately, and the pus in the pleural space should be aspirated through a wide-bore needle until it ceases to reaccumulate. In many cases no other treatment is necessary, but surgical measures are occasionally required to ablate the residual space.

Spontaneous Pneumothorax

Aetiology. The two chief causes of spontaneous pneumothorax are:

1. Rupture of a subpleural emphysematous bulla or of the pulmonary end of a pleural adhesion.
2. Rupture of a subpleural tuberculous focus into the pleural space.

In Britain the first cause is very much more common than the second. Active pulmonary tuberculosis is, in fact, responsible for very few cases of spontaneous pneumothorax, a finding which is in sharp contrast with the experience of 50 years ago.

Certain other conditions such as staphylococcal lung abscess, pulmonary infarction and bronchial carcinoma may, in rare instances, give rise to spontaneous pneumothorax. As with tuberculosis, the pneumothorax results from the rupture of a pulmonary lesion situated close to the pleural surface.

Pathology. There are three types of spontaneous pneumothorax:

1. *Closed* (Fig. 7.4A). The communication between pleura and lung seals off as the lung collapses, and does not reopen. In this type of case the air is gradually absorbed and the lung re-expands.

2. *Open* (Fig. 7.4B). The communication is generally with a bronchus (bronchopleural fistula) and does not seal off when the lung collapses. The air pressure in the pleural space thus approximates to atmospheric pressure on both inspiration and expiration and the lung cannot re-expand. Moreover, the large bronchial communication facilitates the transmission of infection from the air passages into the pleural space and empyema is a common complication.

3. *Valvular* (Fig. 7.4C). The communication between pleura and lung persists but is small and acts as a one-way valve which allows air to enter the pleura during inspiration but prevents it from escaping during expiration. Very large amounts of air may be 'trapped' in the pleural space during bouts of coughing and the intrapleural pressure may rise to well above atmospheric level. This results not only in complete collapse of the underlying lung but also in gross mediastinal dis-

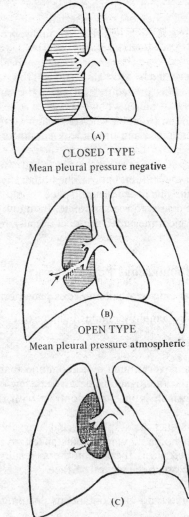

(A)

CLOSED TYPE

Mean pleural pressure **negative**

(B)

OPEN TYPE

Mean pleural pressure **atmospheric**

(C)

VALVULAR (TENSION) TYPE

Mean pleural pressure **positive**

Fig. 7.4 The mechanisms of spontaneous pneumothorax

placement towards the opposite side with compression of the opposite lung. This type of pneumothorax is usually referred to as a 'tension pneumothorax'.

Clinical Features. The onset is usually sudden, with pain or a feeling of 'tightness' on the affected side of the chest, which may be aggravated by deep inspiration. The patient then becomes increasingly breathless and in severe cases central cyanosis may be present. The physical signs in the chest are those of air in the pleural space (p. 261). When the pneumothorax is small and localised there may be no abnormal signs, and the condition may be revealed only by radiological examination.

Closed spontaneous pneumothorax. Dyspnoea, which is seldom severe, gradually abates over the course of a few days. Progressive spontaneous absorption of the air takes place and re-expansion of the lung is complete between 2 and 6 weeks later, depending on the initial size of the pneumothorax. Pleural infection is uncommon in this type of pneumothorax.

Open spontaneous pneumothorax is usually of tuberculous origin. The onset is similar to that of the closed type, but the dyspnoea, although it is not rapidly progressive, does not improve and within a few days the appearance of pyrexia and systemic disturbance, accompanied by physical and radiological signs of air and fluid in the pleural space, indicate the development of a pyopneumothorax. In tuberculous cases acid-fast bacilli can be isolated from the pleural fluid.

Valvular pneumothorax ('tension pneumothorax') produces the most dramatic clinical picture of all. The dyspnoea is rapidly progressive from the start and is accompanied by central cyanosis. The patient may die from asphyxia within a few minutes, but usually the course of events is less rapid and medical attention can be obtained in time to avert a fatal outcome.

Recurrent spontaneous pneumothorax is not uncommon, especially in patients with emphysematous bullae. Subsequent incidents are usually on the same side as the first but may also occur on the opposite side.

Radiological Examination shows the sharp edge of the collapsed lung, and between this and the chest wall there is complete translucency with no lung markings. The degree of pulmonary collapse varies from case to case.

Diagnosis. The diagnosis of spontaneous pneumothorax can usually be made on the history and physical signs but should, whenever possible, be confirmed by radiological examination. This also shows the size of the pneumothorax and the degree of mediastinal displacement, and gives information regarding the presence or absence of pleural fluid and underlying pulmonary disease. Bacteriological examination of sputum and of pleural fluid, if present, is of great importance in distinguishing tuberculous from non-tuberculous cases.

Treatment

1. *Closed Spontaneous Pneumothorax.* When the pneumothorax is small and the patient is only slightly dyspnoeic no treatment is required but observation should be continued until re-expansion of the lung is complete. If, however, the pneumothorax is large and causing moderate or severe dyspnoea, it is essential to employ more active measures. Immediate and complete re-expansion of the lung can be obtained by inserting a catheter into the pleural cavity through an intercostal space and connecting it to a water-seal drainage system (Fig. 7.5) or a non-

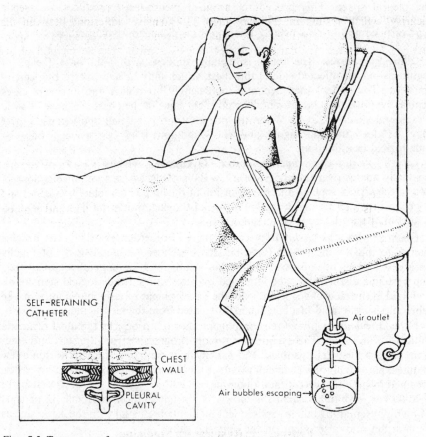

Fig. 7.5 Treatment of spontaneous pneumothorax by pleural intubation and 'water-seal' decompression. The water-seal allows air to leave the pleural space but prevents it from re-entering. This reduces the intrapleural pressure and promotes re-expansion of the lung. The insert shows the position of the self-retaining (Malecot) catheter in the pleural space.

return (Heimlich) valve. The catheter is left in place for 5 or 6 days. This form of treatment considerably shortens the period of incapacity.

If a tuberculous aetiology is suspected, specific chemotherapy (p. 292) should be started immediately. If a pleural effusion develops, the fluid may be drained through the catheter by suitable posturing or aspirated with a needle and syringe.

2. *Open Spontaneous Pneumothorax.* There is a frank bronchopleural fistula, and pleural infection rapidly supervenes. Such cases are seldom amenable to medical treatment and, whether tuberculous or non-tuberculous, should be referred to a thoracic surgeon for treatment of the resulting pyopneumothorax.

3. *Tension Pneumothorax.* This constitutes an acute medical emergency. An intercostal catheter should be inserted at once and connected to a water-seal drainage system, as shown in Figure 7.5. Symptomatic relief is immediate and dramatic. If suitable equipment for this procedure is not at hand a wide-bore needle should be used instead. This should be attached to a length of tubing, the end of which should be placed under water in a bottle or basin.

4. *Recurrent spontaneous pneumothrax*, unilateral or bilateral, is first treated by the introduction of an irritant substance, such as an emulsion of kaolin, into

the pleural space. This procedure (artificial pleurodesis) produces an aseptic pleurisy, which results in the formation of extensive adhesions between the parietal and visceral surfaces, and usually prevents further episodes of spontaneous pneumothorax. Parietal pleurectomy is a more reliable method of artificial pleurodesis, but involves a major thoracic operation.

Deformities of the Chest Wall

An increase in the anteroposterior diameter of the chest relative to the lateral diameter is a common feature of emphysema, but only the most severe forms of this abnormality merit the description of 'barrel chest'. *Pectus carinatum* ('pigeon chest') is seen in patients who have suffered from severe obstructive airways disease (chronic bronchitis or asthma) since early childhood. *Pectus excavatum* ('funnel chest') is a condition in which the body of the sternum, often only its lower end, is curved backwards. The heart is displaced to the left, and may be compressed between the sternum and vertebral column, but only very rarely is this associated with disturbance of cardiac function. It may, however, restrict chest expansion and reduce the vital capacity. The impairment of cardiac or pulmonary function is seldom sufficiently severe to warrant surgical correction, but this may be indicated for cosmetic reasons.

Severe *thoracic kyphoscoliosis* causes ventilation : perfusion imbalance in the lungs and pulmonary underventilation. Patients with this type of chest deformity later develop ventilatory failure, pulmonary hypertension and right ventricular failure, and many die before the age of 50. The tempo of deterioration is often accelerated by bacterial infection in the bronchi and lungs. The prognosis in these cases can be improved only by early surgical correction of the spinal deformity. Ventilatory failure may also occur in ankylosing spondylitis, particularly if there is any interference with the function of the diaphragm.

Prospects in Respiratory Medicine

Advances in immunology, immunopathology and immunopharmacology have already opened the way to a clearer understanding of the nature of certain respiratory diseases, notably bronchial asthma, pulmonary eosinophilia and extrinsic allergic alveolitis. These same disciplines may in time help to elucidate the pathogenesis of conditions such as cryptogenic fibrosing alveolitis, some types of occupational lung disease and even bronchial carcinoma. Immunology also has a further contribution to make in the field of respiratory infection. Until recently research effort was concentrated mainly on the pathogenic properties of microorganisms, but with increasing awareness of the importance of the host reaction there is now a growing interest in methods of investigating the integrity of the various mechanisms, local and systemic, which protect the lungs against both acute and chronic infection by bacteria, viruses and fungi.

New non-invasive techniques are becoming available for the diagnosis of localised pulmonary lesions and of diseases which cause abnormalities of ventilation and perfusion, such as emphysema and pulmonary thromboembolism. These techniques, which include computerised axial tomographic scanning and new methods of radioisotope scanning, are still in an early stage of development, but when fully exploited are certain to revolutionise the investigation of respiratory disease. On a more mundane level further improvement can be expected in the technique of bronchoscopy and of bronchial and pulmonary biopsy.

The empirical treatment of respiratory disease has recently seen many important advances, particularly in regard to antibiotics, bronchodilator drugs and corticosteroids. Efforts to discover drugs or other forms of treatment which can influence the basic causes of allergic and malignant disease and of chronic bronchopulmonary infection have so far met with only limited success, but this situation is bound to change when we have more precise knowledge of the pathogenesis of these diseases.

I. W. B. GRANT
N. W. HORNE
G. J. R. McHARDY

Further reading:

Cotes, J. E. (1975) *Lung Function: Assessment and Application in Medicine.* 3rd edition. Oxford: Blackwell.

Crofton, J. & Douglas, A. C. (1975) *Respiratory Diseases.* 2nd edition. Oxford: Blackwell.

Grant, I. W. B. (1971) Examination of the respiratory system. In *Clinical Examination.* 4th edition, ed. by Macleod, J. Edinburgh: Churchill Livingstone.

Ross, J. D. & Horne, N. W. (1976) *Modern Drug Treatment in Tuberculosis.* 6th edition. London: Chest, Heart and Stroke Association.

Scottish Home and Health Department and Scottish Health Services Council (1969) *Uses and Dangers of Oxygen Therapy.* Edinburgh: HMSO.

8. Diseases of the Alimentary Tract and Pancreas

Functions and Examination of the Alimentary Tract

THE alimentary tract is a coordinated structure with the function of ingesting and absorbing nutrients and excreting unabsorbed and waste products. It should not be regarded as a series of separate organs since the role of each component is closely related to that of other parts of the tract. Its operation may be considered under the following headings:

(1) *Controlling and Coordinating Mechanisms*. The autonomic nervous system and hormones, including gastrin, secretin and cholecystokinin-pancreozymin, control and coordinate motility and secretion.

(2) *Motility*. The carefully controlled motility of the tract is responsible for the orderly progression of nutrients through the system so that the stage of digestion and absorption is appropriate to a given region of the tract.

(3) *Secretion*. The secretion of enzymes and detergents enables protein, carbohydrate and fat to be digested prior to absorption. The secretion of electrolytes provides the correct pH for each stage of digestion.

(4) *Absorption*. The absorptive system consists of specialised cells, together with a portal venous system and lymphatics.

(5) *Defence Mechanisms*. These are necessary to protect the mucosa from its own digestive enzymes and from the bacterial population to which it is exposed. These mechanisms include a rapid turnover of the epithelial cells, the production of mucus and a specialised immunological system.

1. The Controlling and Coordinating Mechanisms

The smooth muscle and the secretory cells of the gastrointestinal tract are richly supplied by the autonomic nervous system. Preganglionic parasympathetic fibres of the vagi synapse with the parasympathetic motor neurones of the enteric plexuses. Sympathetic fibres run in the splanchnic nerves to make contact with the plexuses and the smooth muscle cells. The plexuses are situated at different levels in the bowel wall—subserous, myenteric, submucosal and mucosal—each varying in density from organ to organ. In general, the parasympathetic system is excitatory and the sympathetic inhibitory but there is also evidence for nonadrenergic inhibitory nerves. This nervous system exerts an effect on the contraction of the smooth muscle cells and on the secretion of enzymes, electrolytes and hormones by the mucosa. It is assisted in its control by sensory nerves in the mucosa and in the gut wall which respond to chemical stimuli and to stretch, and by the enteric hormones. Since these are released in response to food in the upper gastrointestinal tract, it is logical that they should modify nervous control so as to affect the progression of nutrients as well as stimulate secretions. The hormone gastrin is released from the antral mucosa initially in response to vagal stimulation; it then acts on the body of the stomach to produce acid and pepsin to digest the protein. As with the stomach, exocrine pancreatic secretion is stimulated partly through nervous and partly through hormonal mechanisms.

The nervous mechanisms operate through the vagus and prime the acinar cells to secrete in response to the hormones secretin and cholecystokinin-pancreozymin.

2. Motility

Apart from the striated muscle in the upper oesophagus, smooth muscle is responsible for the motility of the gastrointestinal tract. The smooth muscle produces 'slow waves' which are conducted over long distances. These do not result in contraction but they enable contractions in different areas to be coordinated.

Oesophagus. The upper oesophageal sphincter is formed by the striated cricopharyngeus muscle which exerts constant tone to keep the sphincter closed except during swallowing. Once the upper oesophageal sphincter relaxes, peristalsis sweeps along the length of the body of the oesophagus, but occasionally, even in the normal oesophagus, the contractions are not coordinated. In the disorder of diffuse spasm these uncoordinated contractions predominate. The lowest few centimetres of the oesophagus form the lower oesophageal sphincter. This has a high resting tension which prevents reflux of gastric contents into the oesophagus. Normally the sphincter relaxes when the peristaltic wave arrives but the characteristic feature in achalasia is that it fails to do so. The sphincter is controlled by nervous and hormonal mechanisms. It is supplied by the symphathetic and parasympathetic systems both of which may cause contraction.

Stomach. When the swallowed food arrives in the stomach, the normal tonic contraction of the stomach is inhibited, probably by means of a centrally mediated vagal reflex. This is termed receptive relaxation so that a large increase in volume is accompanied by only a small rise in pressure within the lumen. The gastric slow wave controls the frequency and direction of antral peristalsis which is responsible for the thorough mixing of the gastric contents and their progressive emptying into the duodenum. Several mechanisms exist to prevent the duodenum receiving more nutrient than it can deal with. Chemoreceptors for fat and acid and osmoreceptors in the duodenal mucosa control gastric emptying by means of local reflexes and by regulating the secretion of secretin and cholecystokinin-pancreozymin. Approximately half of a semisolid meal has left the stomach in about 30 minutes.

Small Intestine. Here also coordination is due to the slow wave in the longitudinal muscle fibres. It is the pacemaker which dictates the times at which any given segment of the gut can contract. The frequency of the slow wave in the duodenum is greater than in the ileum, thus enabling the proximal bowel to override more distal areas. By this means contractions are coordinated both to mix and propel the small bowel content so that all nutrients can be exposed to the absorptive cells. It is thought that the myenteric plexus and the enteric hormones determine the local response to the slow wave so that contraction may or may not occur depending on the state of affairs in the lumen at any one time.

Colon. Motility here is poorly understood. There is probably a slow wave but it is not known how it coordinates contractions. Observation of the colon suggests two main types of contraction occur which may be associated with two different functions. Firstly, there is segmentation which consists of contraction rings forming and disappearing over long periods of time: these produce a slow mixing of faeces but no propulsion, thus facilitating the absorption of water and electrolytes. Secondly, propulsion occurs through 'mass movement', a peristaltic wave which occurs several times a day. This action carries out the second function of the colon, namely the elimination of faeces. All activity in the colon is increased after eating, and defaecation is more likely to occur at this time. The enteric hormones may be responsible for this activity. Finally, in diarrhoea the colon is quiet whereas in constipation the activity of the colon is greater than normal. This is explained on the basis that the main activity in the colon, segmentation, causes mixing only and is responsible for the resistance to flow along the lumen.

3. Secretion

The production of secretions for the digestion of nutrients is under nervous and hormonal control.

Gastric Secretion. In response to the sight or smell of food, the vagus stimulates acid and pepsin secretion by a direct effect on the parietal and peptic cells. It also initiates the release of gastrin from the antrum. More sustained output of this hormone is produced by a rise in pH and by ingested protein. Gastrin then enters the bloodstream and acts on the body of the stomach to produce acid and pepsin to digest the protein. It may stimulate acid secretion through the release of histamine as a mediator. Mechanisms are also required to turn off gastric secretion once digestion within the stomach is complete. These are largely the same as those which slow gastric emptying, i.e. the release of the enteric hormones secretin and cholecystokinin-pancreozymin and also the presence of a low pH in the gastric antrum which inhibits the further release of gastrin.

Pancreatic Secretion, Bile and Intestinal Secretions. Acid, fat and hypertonic solutions in the duodenum release the hormones secretin and cholecystokinin-pancreozymin from the duodenal mucosa into the bloodstream. Secretin stimulates the acinar cells of the pancreas to produce bicarbonate which neutralises the gastric acid and provides a neutral pH for the activity of the pancreatic enzymes, lipase, amylase and trypsin. These are produced in response to cholecystokinin-pancreozymin, which also causes contraction of the gall bladder so that an adequate supply of bile salts reaches the intestine at a time when fat has to be digested. The enteric hormones are also responsible for the secretion, by the mucosa of the small intestine, of succus entericus which contains bicarbonate and additional enzymes.

4. The Absorptive System

To increase the surface area for absorption in the small intestine the mucosa is formed into villi and the surface of the absorptive cells is specialised in the form of microvilli which possess a multitude of enzyme systems for the final stages of digestion of nutrients followed by their absorption. In coeliac disease the surface area of the small intestine is reduced because of the absence of villi, and malabsorbtion results.

Under normal circumstances nutrients are transported from the absorptive cell by the lymphatic system (for example fat and fat soluble vitamins) or by the portal venous system (amino acids and hexoses).

The absorptive system is discussed in more detail on page 390.

5. Defence Mechanisms

Cell Turnover. The epithelial cells of the gastrointestinal tract are constantly renewed so that, for example, the epithelial surface of the small intestine is replaced every 48 hours. The desquamated cells are digested and their products reabsorbed. In the intestine, cellular turnover has been shown to be slower than normal in germ-free animals and it can be argued that this turnover is to some extent a protective mechanism. Drugs such as phenylbutazone slow down cell turnover in the stomach and predispose to peptic ulceration.

Production of Mucus. Mucus producing cells are present at all levels of the gastrointestinal tract. Mucus may provide a protective covering for the mucosa and when its composition is altered, for example by corticosteroids, peptic ulceration may occur.

Immunological System. The lamina propria of the stomach and intestines contains many lymphocytes and plasma cells. Some of these cells synthesise secretory IgA which is resistant to digestion by intestinal enzymes and has a role in protecting mucosal surfaces from bacterial invasion. It is thus of particular importance in the small intestine where bacterial colonisation is deleterious.

The Symptoms of Alimentary Disease

Pain is often the most important symptom of gastrointestinal disease. It must be analysed in relation to its main site, radiation, character, severity, duration, frequency, times of occurrence, aggravating and relieving factors and any associated phenomena. The characteristics of abdominal pain are often diagnostic, for example in peptic ulceration and acute appendicitis. *Loss of appetite* (anorexia) may have a local cause such as carcinoma of the stomach but may also be a feature of debilitating disease or of a psychological disturbance. *Vomiting* may occur in diseases of the stomach or small intestine, peritonitis, appendicitis, or cholecystitis. Numerous other conditions may also be responsible, for example meningitis, uraemia, migraine, drugs such as digoxin or morphine and, in the child, infection. The type, timing and related features of the vomiting are important diagnostically. Sudden vomiting without preceding nausea may be due to direct stimulation of the vomiting centre in the medulla and thus be an indication of intracranial disease. Vomiting in the morning may be due to pregnancy or alcoholism. Vomiting of large quantities of food and secretions late in the day or night indicates gastric outlet obstruction. Vomiting which relieves pain is often due to a peptic ulcer. The complaint of persistent vomiting without loss of weight is nearly always indicative of a psychological disturbance. *Heartburn* is a burning retrosternal sensation due to reflux oesophagitis as in a sliding hiatus hernia. *Regurgitation* is the appearance of previously swallowed food in the mouth without warning. It usually has an acid or bitter taste because of the presence of gastric juice but not in patients with obstruction in the oesophagus. *Dysphagia*, i.e. difficulty in swallowing, is discussed on page 357. *Flatulence* is often due to excessive swallowing of air (*aerophagy*) which in turn may be due to anxiety. Under normal circumstances a small amount of air is swallowed with food, drink and saliva. Some of this gas may be expelled as a belch. The remainder passes into the intestine. Some will be absorbed but most, particularly the nitrogen, will be expelled per rectum. A plain X-ray of the abdomen shows that gas is normally present in the stomach and colon but that very little is seen in the small intestine. *Constipation* and *diarrhoea* are sometimes difficult to define. In Britain fewer than 10 per cent of people have less than one bowel motion per day and only 1 per cent have a bowel movement less frequently than 3 times a week. These latter should be regarded as constipated. In addition, if the stool is hard and difficult to pass the patient should be regarded as constipated whatever the frequency of bowel movement. In contrast, less than 1 per cent of the population have more than three bowel movements daily and this should be regarded as abnormal, particularly if the stool is not formed. When the stool is liquid or semi-formed it must be regarded as abnormal whatever the frequency of bowel movement. The diet in Western countries is low in roughage; where a high residue diet is usual, more than three bowel movements daily may be normal. An explanation must be found for any change in bowel habits which were previously regular. *Loss of weight* may be due to a reduced intake of food because of anorexia, nausea or vomiting, to malabsorption of nutrients or to the loss of protein from a diseased bowel as in ulcerative colitis. Carcinoma is the commonest alimentary cause of loss of weight. Occasionally there may be abnormal gain in weight as in some patients with duodenal ulceration who eat to relieve pain.

Examination of the Abdomen

The mouth and throat are always examined either before or after the abdomen. Particular points to look for are the state of the teeth, the presence of infection in the mouth, throat or fauces, evidence of vitamin deficiency (p. 354) and tumours of the tongue and lips. The abdomen is examined systematically by inspection, palpation, percussion and auscultation and the rectum by digital examination.

Investigation of the Gastrointestinal Tract

Radiological Examination

Plain Films. On the plain X-ray it is possible to see the normal soft tissue shadows due to the liver, spleen and kidneys and also abnormal shadows. Gas in the intestine acts as a contrast medium so that the distribution of the bowel within the abdomen can be assessed. In obstruction there may be an excessive amount of gas and fluid in the bowel above the obstruction and films with the patient erect will demonstrate fluid levels. Finally, areas of opacification due to stones or to calcification in the liver, pancreas, cysts or blood vessels may provide important diagnostic information. A chest X-ray is helpful in delineating the diaphragmatic areas and any subphrenic collections of gas or fluid. Pulmonary lesions from which pain may be referred to the abdomen can also be identified.

Barium Studies. These will demonstrate a break in the continuity of the outline of the organ, abnormalities in the appearance of the mucosa and disorders of motility. Preparation of the patient for each examination should always be undertaken so that mucosal detail will not be obscured by contents. For studies of the upper gastrointestinal tract, the patient is fasted and in addition, if pyloric stenosis is suspected, the stomach is washed out to remove food debris. For barium enema studies, the colon should be cleared of faeces by means of laxatives and in some cases by bowel washout prior to examination.

The Barium Swallow and Meal Examination. The oesophagus is studied whilst barium is being swallowed. This may demonstrate a disorder of motility, filling defects caused by tumours or varices, a stricture, a diverticulum or a hiatus hernia.

The mucosa of the stomach can be examined by using a small amount of barium together with the introduction of gas—a double contrast study. More usually, the stomach is filled with a larger volume of barium and the contour examined carefully with varying rotation of the patient. The fundus is examined with the patient supine. Ulcers are seen as projections beyond the normal outline while tumours cause filling defects in the barium shadow. Various manoeuvres may be necessary to demonstrate a hiatus hernia including the placing of the patient prone over a bolster or supine with the left side raised. Finally, direct observation of the motility of the stomach may indicate an inert area which might be caused by infiltrative disease such as carcinoma. The duodenal cap is also examined by observing the mucosal pattern which may demonstrate folds radiating from an ulcer and by observing the contours of the cap when it is completely filled with barium.

Hypotonic duodenography is a method of outlining the duodenum after the administration of an antispasmodic. A double contrast picture is obtained with a mixture of barium and gas to show mucosal changes, as in carcinoma of the ampulla of Vater, and indentations, as might be caused by a pancreatic tumour.

The Follow-through Examination. When disease of the small intestine is suspected, barium administered as part of the meal examination is observed during its passage through the small intestine and X-rays are taken at intervals. The outline of the barium may indicate structural abnormalities such as diverticula or strictures. When there is malabsorption, the barium may clump and flocculate in the excessive amount of fluid present within the lumen.

Barium Enema. This procedure is uncomfortable and sometimes exhausting, particularly in the elderly or in those with cardiac disease in whom an arrythmia may be induced. Barium alone or, for double contrast examination, barium and air, is run into the bowel through a self-retaining catheter. X-rays are taken with the whole colon filled with barium in order to see any filling defects or diverticula. In some patients barium will reflux into the terminal ileum which can be outlined. Then the patient empties the bowel and further X-rays are taken which show the texture of the mucosa coated by the small amount of remaining barium.

Cautionary Note. Exposure to X-rays in the early months of pregnancy may upset normal development of the fetus and be responsible for deformity or still birth. These risks apply not only to radiographic examination of the abdomen such as barium enema but also to procedures such as excretion urography and X-rays of the lumbar spine and pelvis. Inadvertent irradiation in the first few weeks of pregnancy can be avoided by restricting radiological examination of the lower abdomen in women at risk to the 10 days immediately following the onset of the last menstrual period—'the 10 day rule'.

Radioisotope Studies. In the pancreatic scan, 75 selenomethionine is used. This aminoacid is taken up by the pancreatic acinar cells and used in the same way as methionine for the synthesis of pancreatic enzymes. Unfortunately selenomethionine is also taken up by the liver and in greater concentration. This makes a pancreatic scan difficult to interpret and a significant proportion of false negative and false positive results occur in the diagnosis of pancreatic tumours and pancreatitis. The procedure is also costly.

Endoscopy

With fibreoptic instruments it is not difficult to examine the whole of the oesophagus, stomach, duodenum and colon. Two bundles of many thousands of fine glass fibres are contained in the instrument's shaft. One bundle carries light to the tip of the instrument in order to illuminate the organ being examined whilst the other can transmit an image back to the observer. The fibre bundles are flexible so that the whole shaft can be bent and easily passed into the upper gastrointestinal tract or colon. The shaft of the instrument also carries controls so that the tip of the instrument can be moved, and channels through which air or forceps can be passed to insufflate the organ or to take a biopsy from the mucosa.

Rigid instruments are used to examine the rectum and lower pelvic colon (sigmoidoscope) and occasionally the oesophagus (oesophagoscope).

Examination of the Upper Alimentary Tract. It is usual to carry out the procedure with the patient under sedation, often as an out-patient. After a 12-hour fast the patient is sedated and the pharynx is anaesthetised with a xylocaine spray or lozenge. The instrument is passed with the assistance of the patient in swallowing and the procedure, whilst uncomfortable, should be no more so than any other intubation. Possible complications are perforation of the oesophagus whilst passing the instrument or during biopsy, and the inhalation of secretions. Fortunately these are rare with flexible fibreoptic instruments.

Oesophagoscopy. This is always carried out when there is dysphagia or when the barium swallow suggests that a tumour or a stricture is present. Relative indications include suspected oesophagitis, varices or a motility disorder.

Gastroscopy. This is indicated so that a biopsy can be taken when a gastric ulcer which may be malignant has been demonstrated on barium studies. Healing of the ulcer may be assessed by further gastroscopy. Other suspicious areas on the barium study can be seen and biopsies taken. Gastroscopy is nearly always necessary in the assessment of patients with symptoms after gastric surgery because the appearances are difficult to assess radiologically.

Duodenoscopy. This is indicated in the investigation of the patient suspected of having duodenal ulceration.

At most examinations it is usual to examine the oesophagus, stomach and duodenal cap with the same instrument. This is because the presence of one lesion does not exclude another and double lesions are common, e.g. hiatus hernia and duodenal ulcer. Upper alimentary endoscopy is also carried out as an emergency procedure on patients with haematemesis and melaena, once the stomach has been cleared of blood and clot by gastric lavage. It is also invaluable in patients with radiologically negative dyspepsia since an abnormality is often found which could not have been identified otherwise.

Endoscopic Retrograde Cholangio-Pancreatography (ERCP) is a special application of fibreoptic endoscopy. At duodenoscopy the ampulla of Vater is cannulated with a fine bore catheter passed through the shaft of the instrument and radio-opaque dye is injected into the biliary and pancreatic ducts. The procedure is of great value in patients suspected of having pancreatic disease since distortion or obstruction of the ductal system may confirm a diagnosis of chronic pancreatitis or pancreatic carcinoma. Obstruction or distortion of the common bile duct by a stone or a tumour can also be demonstrated.

Examination of the Lower Alimentary Tract. *Proctoscopy and Sigmoidoscopy.* These are simple procedures which should always be carried out in patients with symptoms referable to the lower bowel or anus. Both terms are inaccurate since proctoscopy visualises the anal canal and only 2–3 cm of the rectum, and sigmoidoscopy examines the rectum and the lower few centimetres of the pelvic colon. It is usual to carry out the procedures without preparation but if the rectum contains faeces, then endoscopy is repeated after the bowel has been emptied. The examination is carried out with the patient in the knee–elbow position, or on the left side with the knees drawn up. Digital examination of the rectum should always precede endoscopy and the instruments should be warmed and well lubricated. Proctoscopy is used for the demonstration and injection of haemorrhoids. Sigmoidoscopy is necessary for the diagnosis of polyps, cancer of the rectum, ulcerative proctitis and Crohn's disease of the large bowel. Biopsy of the mucosa or lesion is also taken. Sigmoidoscopy is carried out under anaesthesia when there is a painful condition of the anus such as a fissure; it should be avoided in fulminating ulcerative colitis because of the danger of perforation.

Colonoscopy. The flexible colonoscope allows examination of the whole colon but the procedure is time-consuming and occasionally difficult. The bowel must be carefully prepared over several days, first with laxatives and then by lavage so that no faecal material remains. The procedure is the only alternative to laparotomy in patients who on barium enema examination, show changes which could be due to carcinoma.

Biopsy and Cytology

Biopsy of lesions is an essential part of each endoscopic procedure and biopsy of an apparently normal mucosa can also provide important diagnostic information. Apart from rectal biopsies the only problem with biopsies taken at endoscopy is their small size which makes interpretation by the pathologist difficult.

Biopsy of the Small Intestine. This is indicated if malabsorbtion is suspected and is carried out by means of the Crosby capsule. After an overnight fast the capsule is passed into the jejunum attached to a stiff radio-opaque catheter and the biopsy is taken just distal to the duodenojejunal flexure. Suction via the catheter draws mucosa into a small port on the side of the instrument. The negative pressure which develops within the capsule also fires the knife which severs the mucosa. The intubation and biopsy are completed in about one hour. Bleeding occurs occasionally and for this reason biopsies should not be carried out unless the platelet count and prothrombin time are normal. Another rare complication is perforation of the intestine. The biopsy specimens are inspected under the dissecting microscope immediately after removal from the capsule.

Cytological Studies. These are not widely used in gastroenterology because the cytological appearances are difficult to interpret and require the services of an expert cytologist. However, gastric cytology can be an accurate method for the diagnosis of gastric cancer. The patient is fasted for 12 hours, a nasogastric tube is passed into the stomach and a vigorous lavage with saline is carried out. The fluid is aspirated, centrifuged and the sediment is spread on to slides for examination by the pathologist.

Secretory Studies

The Pentagastrin Test. The acid output is measured in response to gastric stimulant, pentagastrin, a synthetic pentapeptide which exerts the biological effects of gastrin. Preparation consists of an overnight fast. A barium meal examination should not be performed on the day before the test because some barium might remain in the stomach. Anticholinergic drugs must be stopped for at least 48 hours since they will suppress acid secretion. A soft, radio-opaque tube is passed through the nose or mouth and its tip is positioned by fluoroscopy at the middle of the greater curvature of the stomach. The patient is placed supine and tilted slightly to the left. The fasting contents are aspirated and their volume measured and then the secretions are collected continuously for one hour. This is termed the 'basal acid output'. Then pentagastrin is given subcutaneously in a dose of 6 μg/kg body weight and the secretions are collected for a further hour. The acid output in this hour is termed the 'maximum acid output'. Acid outputs are calculated from the volume of secretion and the concentration of acid as assessed by titration to pH 7.

The pentagastrin test is helpful because: (a) an increased volume of fasting juice is often an indication of obstruction of the gastric outlet; (b) a very high basal acid output may indicate that the patient has the Zollinger–Ellison syndrome (p. 376); (c) in patients with peptic ulcer, the level of the acid output may influence the choice of operation; (d) the presence of achlorhydria can be demonstrated. Achlorhydria means absence of hydrochloric acid in the gastric juice; it is said to occur when the pH of the gastric juice does not fall below 6 after stimulation with pentagastrin.

The Insulin Test. This test is used after gastric surgery to indicate the completeness of vagotomy. The preparation and procedure are similar to those described above but the gastric stimulant is soluble insulin which is given intravenously. The resulting hypoglycaemia stimulates the vagal centres and gastric acid is secreted if the vagal innervation of the stomach has not been completely divided.

Pancreatic Function Tests. These are described on page 384.

Bacteriological Studies

The malabsorption syndrome may be due occasionally to the overgrowth of bacteria (p. 396). When this is suspected, secretion can be obtained for bacteriological studies by passing a fine sterile tube into the upper small intestine. A mercury bag attached to the tip of the tube ensures that the tube moves rapidly to the correct site. The patient should not be receiving antibiotics.

Motility Studies

The barium meal gives a rough idea of the motility of the oesophagus, stomach and small intestine. On occasion cineradiology may be used and this is particularly helpful in the analysis of dysphagia.

Motility can be studied more accurately by measuring the pressure changes in the lumen of the organ but only in the case of the oesophagus is this of diagnostic value. Fine open ended tubes are passed into the stomach and pressures are transmitted to transducers and measured at intervals whilst the tube is gradually withdrawn with the patient swallowing. The procedure may be of value in establishing the relationship between chest pain and abnormal oesophageal contractions, for the diagnosis of motility disorders of the oesophagus and in determining the position of the oesophageal sphincter when there is a hiatus hernia. Motility studies are also helpful in disorders of the large bowel, e.g. diverticular disease.

Examination of the Stool

In malabsorption the stool may be pale and frothy, in the irritable bowel syndrome it may be like pellets or ribbon with or without mucus. In mild ulcerative disease of the colon there may be flecks of blood in the mucus. Inspection of the stool is sufficient to diagnose fresh bleeding from the lower alimentary tract while the loss of over 60 ml of blood from a site proximal to the ascending colon will produce a black tarry stool.

In order to detect small amounts of blood it is necessary to use a chemical test for haematin. Specimens obtained on the finger-stall at rectal examination can readily be examined.

Microscopic examination is of value particularly in distinguishing amoebic dysentery and other parasitic diseases and in pancreatic insufficiency.

DISEASES OF THE MOUTH

The mouth acts as a receptacle in which food can be broken down into small particles during mastication. Into the mouth flows the saliva which is secreted in response to the sight, taste and smell of food, and also to the act of chewing. Saliva has several functions. It facilitates speech, moistens the food and lubricates the process of swallowing. By its solvent action on the foodstuffs, it enables tasting to take place. It also contains an enzyme ptyalin which is concerned in the digestion of polysaccharides to disaccharides.

Disorders of the Teeth

The reduction of food to a soft pulp by efficient mastication is an important prerequisite to good digestion. It is essential therefore to determine whether the patient has an adequate number of teeth, and whether those that are present are directly in apposition in the lower and upper jaw. If dentures are used, they must be comfortable, otherwise they may be worn only for the sake of appearances, and removed at mealtimes. Oral sepsis is not only an unpleasant social condition, but it may also predispose to disease. Respiratory infection may result from the inhalation of septic material or micro-organisms from the mouth, and bacteraemia may have its source in dental disease such as ulcerative stomatitis or a periapical abscess. Bacteraemia from these sources is particularly liable to occur after dental manipulation and may cause endocarditis in patients with valvular disease of the heart; for this reason such patients should always be given prophylactic antibiotics both before and after dental extraction (p. 209). All patients should be advised to consult a dentist regularly in order to conserve the teeth and to prevent or treat foci of infection in the mouth.

Stomatitis

Stomatitis, or inflammation of the mouth, is of several varieties; it may involve the gums (gingivitis), the lips (cheilosis), or the angles of the mouth (angular stomatitis).

Non-specific gingivitis and stomatitis. The mouth harbours a dense population of commensal micro-organisms. Normally, this microbial population is controlled by a reasonable standard of oral hygiene; if this is neglected the bacterial population may proliferate on the cervical margins of the teeth and cause gingivitis or a more generalised stomatitis. Non-specific gingivitis and stomatitis may also occur when resistance to the commensal population is altered by febrile illness, wasting diseases, or blood dyscrasias. It occurs particularly when the mouth is not cleaned regularly. The gums are swollen and painful and the mucous membrane is reddened. In those patients with severe illness, the mouth should be washed repeatedly. In otherwise healthy people, non-specific gingivitis may be treated and controlled by proper oral hygiene and if necessary by dental procedures such as scaling and polishing. The anti-convulsant drug phenytoin may cause hypertrophic gingivitis, in which the gums becomes swollen and encroach on the teeth.

Stomatitis due to Deficiency of Nutritional Factors. This may arise directly from an insufficient intake or indirectly as a result of impaired absorption of vitamins, especially niacin, riboflavin, folic acid, and cyanocobalamin. Stomatitis may also be caused by long-standing iron deficiency. When the deficiency is acute and severe, the tongue is red, raw and painful. When the deficiency is chronic and less severe the tongue appears moist and unduly clean because of atrophy of the papillae. Angular stomatitis often accompanies glossitis, especially in the case of severe iron deficiency. Severe vitamin C deficiency is characterised by gingivitis so that the gums become swollen and spongy and bleed readily if the patient is not edentulous.

Ulcerative Stomatitis (Vincent's infection). This occurs mainly in adults in conditions associated with malnutrition and poor dental hygiene; it is not commonly seen nowadays in Britain. Ulcers with ragged necrotic margins occur especially on the gums, but may involve the palate, the lips, or the inner aspects of the cheeks; the ulcers are covered by a grey slough surrounded by an erythematous margin. A stained smear shows many spirochaetes and fusiform bacilli; these organisms are present in small numbers in the normal commensal population of the mouth and the condition may be regarded as an endogenous infection due to proliferation of the organisms because of some alteration in host resistance. The condition is infectious, so that the patient's food vessels and cutlery should be sterilised. The acute phase responds to local treatment with metronidazole in a dose of 200 mg three times per day for 4 days, or to penicillin. Necrosis of the gums may occur, so that when the acute phase has been controlled it is most important that proper dental treatment is undertaken; surgical correction of the deformities resulting from tissue necrosis may be necessary.

Candidiasis. The fungus *Candida albicans* is a normal commensal in the mouth but it may proliferate to cause thrush in babies, the aged and particularly in debilitated patients. Thrush is also common in those receiving corticosteroids, immunosuppressive therapy or prolonged treatment with antibiotics, especially tetracycline. White sloughs covering areas of superficial ulceration appear on the tongue and buccal mucosa and they enlarge and coalesce to form an easily detached membrane; there is little surrounding inflammation. In severe infection, the lower pharynx and oesophagus may be affected, causing dysphagia, or the fungus may spread to the lungs. Candidiasis may be treated by painting the oral cavity with 1 per cent aqueous solution of gentian violet, three times a day for 4 days or a suspension or lozenges containing 500,000 units of nystatin should be retained in the mouth for as long as possible, and should be given four times daily for at least 4 days.

Aphthous Stomatitis. This is a common condition which is characterised by the development of one or more ulcers in the mouth; the lesion begins as a small vesicle which then develops into a shallow or occasionally a deep ulcer. The ulcers are often multiple, and may occur in crops. Apart from the fact that the condition may follow periods of emotional stress, the aetiology is unknown. Aphthous stomatitis may occur in association with various gastrointestinal disorders such as ulcerative colitis, but more commonly there is no obvious physical disease. The condition is extremely painful and does not readily respond to therapy. In general, treatment should be limited to the local application of tincture of benzoin paint to relieve pain. Secondary infection may be controlled by the use of a 2 per cent chlortetracycline mouthwash for not more than 7 days. Some patients may gain relief by sucking pellets of 2·5 mg hydrocortisone or local anaesthetic.

Allergic Stomatitis. Stomatitis can also result from an allergic reaction to certain chemicals as in toothpaste, dentures or mint sweets, or to antibiotics especially if they have been used locally. It may also occur in angio-oedema.

Metals such as bismuth, mercury, gold or arsenic may rarely cause stomatitis. A characteristic blue-black line may be seen where the gum margins adjoin the teeth in lead poisoning. Treatment of the stomatitis consists of removing the patient from exposure to the metallic poisons, or stopping their administration.

Skin diseases such as lichen planus, pemphigus, and erythema multiforme involve the mouth and sometimes do so before being seen on the skin.

Disorders of the Tongue

In health the tongue is moist with only a slight white fur on the dorsum. The papillae are readily seen. Mouth breathing causes a dry tongue, but otherwise dryness of the tongue is an indication of dehydration. The tongue may be coated with a whitish-yellow fur in persons who smoke excessively but in general, the presence of fur on the tongue has little clinical significance.

Glossitis. Acute or more usually chronic glossitis, may be a prominent feature of stomatitis resulting from nutritional deficiency (p. 354).

Ulceration may occur in association with various forms of stomatitis, or as a result of trauma from the sharp edges of damaged teeth, badly fitting dentures or biting during epileptic fits.

In all cases of chronic ulceration of the tongue it is essential to exclude a carcinoma and if any doubt exists biopsy should be carried out.

Syphilis may occur as a primary chancre, in the secondary stage as 'mucous patches', or in the tertiary stage as painless gummatous ulcers.

Leukoplakia is a chronic affection characterised by the presence of white, firm, smooth patches beginning at the side of the tongue and later spreading over the dorsum. In the early stages the tongue is not painful but later the patches are split by fissures with resultant pain and tenderness. The importance of leukoplakia is that it may precede the development of carcinoma, and a biopsy of such lesions should always be undertaken.

Psychogenic Pain. The patient complains of a persistently painful tongue but the tongue is normal on inspection and the pain has no relation to substances such as vinegar or hot liquids as occurs with a true glossitis. The psychological origin of these symptoms is usually obscure and the complaint amounts virtually to a delusion. The symptom is often intractable.

Disorders of the Salivary Glands

Excessive salivary secretion may be a response to irritation or inflammation in the mouth, e.g. oral sepsis, or it may develop reflexly as in trigeminal neuralgia; it is an important symptom in oesophageal obstruction. An increased amount of saliva may be secreted in post-encephalitic parkinsonism. Certain drugs, such as potassium iodide and the heavy metals, are excreted in the saliva and may cause an increased secretion. Symptomatic treatment consists of the administration of drugs such as atropine which inhibit parasympathetic action.

Xerostomia. Deficient secretion of saliva is most commonly associated with acute febrile conditions and states of marked dehydration. Xerostomia is one of the features of Sjögren's syndrome (p. 645). Anticholinergic drugs also depress salivary excretion.

Parotitis. Inflammation of the parotid glands may be due to the virus of mumps or to bacterial infection of the glands. The latter tends to develop during severe febrile illnesses and after major abdominal operations if adequate attention is not given to oral hygiene and to the prevention of dehydration and toxaemia. Its treatment consists of the parenteral administration of penicillin and surgical drainage if abscess formation has occurred.

Enlargement of the parotid glands may be found in patients with sarcoidosis.

Salivary Calculi. These occur occasionally in the submandibular gland or its duct. They cause pain and swelling brought on by eating. Infection of the gland is a complication. Stones in the duct can be felt in the floor of the mouth and can be removed by incision over the duct. Stones in the body of the gland may require excision of the gland.

Tumours. The only common tumour is the mixed salivary tumour which presents as a slow, painless enlargement of one parotid gland. The tumour shows a variable degree of malignancy and is treated by excision.

DISEASES OF THE OESOPHAGUS

Dysphagia

Since the only function of the oesophagus is the transmission of food from mouth to stomach, most diseases of the oesophagus and its adjacent structures cause difficulty in swallowing (dysphagia).

Causes of Dysphagia. 1. PAINFUL DISEASES of the mouth and pharynx, e.g. stomatitis, tonsillitis, tuberculous laryngitis or retropharyngeal abscess, produce dysphagia, the cause of which is usually apparent.

2. NEUROLOGICAL DISTURBANCES of deglutition, e.g. as a result of bulbar and pseudobulbar paralysis, diphtheritic neuritis or myasthenia gravis, or disorders of oesophageal motility, as in achalasia and oesophageal spasm, are not uncommon. 'Dysphagia' also occurs in association with psychological stress, e.g. globus hystericus (p. 419).

3. EXTRINSIC COMPRESSION of the oesophagus, as from a goire or an aortic aneurysm; or from enlarged mediastinal lymph nodes, secondary to a lymphoma or to a carcinoma of the breast or bronchus.

Dysphagia from such causes is rarely a presenting symptom and the underlying cause is usually apparent.

4. INTRINSIC DISEASE OF THE OESOPHAGUS:
(a) *Congenital Abnormalities.* Atresia, the upper oesophagus ending blindly at

about the level of the tracheal bifurcation, occurs occasionally requiring urgent surgery in the newborn. A short oesophagus with hernia and stricture can occur as congenital abnormalities, though most examples are probably due to acquired disease.

(b) *Ulceration.* Oesophagitis is most commonly due to reflux of gastric contents through a sphincter made incompetent by a sliding hiatus hernia. There is acid-pepsin digestion of the oesophageal mucosa immediately above the hernia, with ulceration, spasm and eventual stricture formation.

Oesophagitis and stricture are occasionally caused by the ingestion, accidental or otherwise, of corrosives such as bleach or caustic soda.

(c) *Sideropenic Dysphagia (Plummer Vinson Syndrome).* This form of dysphagia is mostly seen in middle-aged or elderly women and is associated with iron deficiency anaemia, glossitis, diminished gastric secretion, and perhaps koilonychia and splenic enlargement. There is degeneration and atrophy of the epithelium of tongue, pharynx, oesophagus and stomach. The actual cause of the dysphagia is believed to be spasm at the entrance to the oesophagus. At this site, a film or fold of degenerating epithelial cells—the 'postcricoid web'—may be demonstrable radiographically or endoscopically. The dysphagia is to solids rather than to liquids, is intermittent, and may therefore mistakenly be thought to by hysterical. The dilation associated with diagnostic endoscopy is often sufficient to relieve symptoms.

(d) *Systemic sclerosis* (p. 648) is a rare cause of dysphagia.

(e) *Tumour.* Carcinoma of the oesophagus or of the cardia of the stomach is the usual cause of dysphagia in elderly patients with no preceding history of indigestion or heartburn.

Investigation. The exclusion of malignant disease is essential in the investigation of any patient who complains of dysphagia. Barium swallow and oesophagoscopy are required. Where the disorder appears to be one of function rather than structure, as for example in achalasia or systemic sclerosis, then manometry can give valuable additional information.

Oesophageal Hiatus Hernia and Reflux Oesophagitis

Normally once food has been propelled into the stomach it does not reflux into the oesophagus. The mechanism of the valvular junction between oesophagus and stomach is not clearly understood. In part it may depend on the presence of a physiological sphincter in the lower oesophagus and in part also on the angle of entry of the oesophagus into the stomach. When the latter is altered, as in herniation of the oesophagogastric junction through the oesophageal hiatus in the diaphragm, there may be reflux of gastric content into the oesophagus despite the physiological sphincter. If reflux continues over any lengthy period, the exposure of the lower oesophageal mucosa to the irritant effects of gastric juice results in oesophagitis. Occasionally such reflux takes place in the absence of a demonstrable hiatus hernia.

Hiatus hernia is most frequent in middle-aged and elderly women probably because of the weakening of the diaphragmatic muscle that occurs with ageing. An increase in intra-abdominal pressure, as a result of pregnancy or obesity, promotes the development of a hiatus hernia.

Paraoesophageal or 'Rolling' Hiatus Hernia

Here a knuckle of stomach herniates alongside the oesophagus through the hiatus. The lower oesophageal sphincter remains below the diaphragm and competent even in extreme cases when most of the stomach rotates to follow the herniated knuckle into the chest. Often there are no symptoms but a big hernia in the posterior mediastinum may lead to cardiac arrhythmias and breathlessness. Occasionally symptoms become acute because of obstruction, distension and even gangrene of the herniated portion of stomach and then surgery may be required urgently. In a few patients, and as a planned procedure, surgical repair of the hernia may be required if the disability is severe.

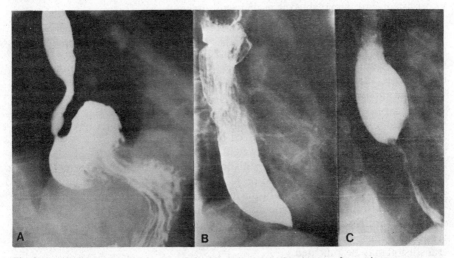

Fig. 8.1 A. Sliding hiatus hernia. B. Achalasia of cardia. C. Carcinoma of oesophagus.

Oesophagogastric or 'Sliding' Hiatus Hernia

In this variety, the oesophagogastric junction herniates into the thorax and there is free gastric reflux. This is the common form of hiatus hernia (Fig. 8.1).

Clinical Features. Heartburn is the characteristic symptom of reflux oesophagitis. It is a deeply placed 'burning' pain, felt retro-sternally and brought on by bending, stooping or by the exertion of lifting or straining with consequent increase in intra-abdominal pressure. It may also occur on lying down at night. It wakens the patient who finds that he can gain relief by sitting up, or by taking food or alkali. When severe, some patients find it more comfortable to spend the night in an easy chair. No other pain produced in the alimentary tract is so closely linked to change of posture as that of reflux oesophagitis.

The nocturnal pain of reflux oesophagitis, awakening the patient from sleep, can be confused with the hunger pain of duodenal ulcer. Posture has no effect on the latter, which comes on later in the night, but some patients suffer both types of pain because duodenal ulcer and hiatus hernia may coexist. Confusion here is of less import than in the case of coronary artery disease (p. 212). The management and particularly the prognosis of duodenal ulcer and hiatus hernia are similar, whereas a patient mistakenly thought to have heart disease may suffer needless restriction.

Once a stricture has developed, the oesophagitis becomes less acute and the pain diminishes or disappears, because the narrowing tends to protect the oesophagus from reflux. For a time the patient believes cure to be imminent, but he is disillusioned when he discovers that swallowing becomes increasingly difficult.

Unless they give rise to significant reflux, to oesophagitis or to dysphagia, many hiatus hernias remain symptomless. Some patients may present with severe anaemia due to blood loss from the inflamed oesophagus and of those who do, about one-third have no other symptom. Oesophagitis should therefore be sought in persistent and unexplained iron deficient anaemia.

Occasionally there is frank bleeding due to the development of an ulcer in the herniated portion of stomach and this may at times require emergency treatment. Confirmation of the diagnosis of hiatus hernia depends on radiological examination with barium, and oesophagoscopy is necessary to diagnose the presence of oesophagitis; oesophagoscopy will also exclude the presence of other lesions in the vicinity of the hernia, such as a small gastric carcinoma or an ulcer.

Treatment. The majority of patients with reflux oesophagitis have relatively mild symptoms which can be controlled by medical treatment. The most important single measure is reduction of weight in patients with obesity. Meals should be small and well masticated. Women should avoid wearing tight garments. The head of the bed should be elevated on blocks and the patient should be taught to sleep in a semi-upright position. In the acute stage, an ulcer regime with antacids particularly last thing at night should be recommended. Cimetidine (p. 369) may be used in severe cases. During the day, stooping and bending should be avoided. Anaemia will usually respond to oral iron, although where there is severe blood loss, transfusion may be indicated.

Persistent oesophagitis and stricture formation are indications for surgery. This includes repair of the hernia and reconstitution of the valve mechanism. An acid reducing procedure (p. 370) is carried out at the same time if there is a concomitant duodenal ulcer. Stricture will usually respond to these measures, supplemented by bouginage in the post-operative period; if it does not, resection is occasionally required.

Diverticulum of Oesophagus

Traction Diverticulum is most commonly situated in the anterior wall of the oesophagus just below the level of the tracheal bifurcation. It is due to chronic inflammation, usually tuberculous, in related lymph nodes. By the time the diverticulum is discovered, often accidentally during barium swallow, the disease in the lymph nodes has healed. It is seldom that the diverticulum itself causes symptoms and surgical treatment is rarely necessary.

Pharyngeal Pouch. This diverticulum develops at the site of the inferior constrictor of the pharynx. It begins as a posterior bulge of mucosa which enlarges to form a sac that extends downwards and to the left between oesophagus and cervical spine. The fully-formed sac causes dysphagia due to displacement forwards of the oesophagus. There is swelling and gurgling in the neck on swallowing. The patient may present with recurrent attacks of stridor or inhalation of contents of the sac may lead to pneumonia.

The condition is seen almost exclusively in middle-aged subjects. For long it was thought to be due to a congenital weakness between the two components of the inferior pharyngeal constrictor, but its late onset and the fact that dysphagia precedes the formation of the pouch indicate that the condition is the result of muscle incoordination.

Treatment is surgical, a one-stage resection of the pouch with careful suture of its neck being carried out after preliminary cleansing and under antibiotic cover. The danger is leakage or contamination with consequent mediastinitis.

In Edinburgh, pharyngeal pouch is remembered as the affliction of Lord Jeffrey (1773–1850), a Scottish judge and wit who, in these days before surgery, emptied his pouch with a specially designed silver spoon.

Achalasia of the Cardia

Although apparently confined to the lower end where there is failure of the sphincter to relax, this is in fact a motility disorder of the whole oesophagus which shows progressive atony and dilatation. The cause is probably a failure of nerve conduction due to diminution in the number of ganglion cells. In South America, Chagas' disease—an infection with a trypanosome—produces similar changes (p. 852). Achalasia is also known, less appropriately, as *cardiospasm*.

Clinical Features. The dysphagia of achalasia is insidious and at first amounts to little more than a slowness in swallowing which the patient may accept as normal and not seek medical advice. With increasing dysphagia, the site of obstruction is felt to be behind the lower end of the sternum. Until a later stage the patient continues to eat food of reasonable variety and amount, the excess accumulating in the capacious non-contractile oesophagus. Putrefaction of the retained residue leads to halitosis, while inhalation may occur silently at night to cause recurrent pulmonary infection. There is progressive loss of weight.

Investigation. A chest X-ray may be sufficient to show an enlarged oesophageal outline, perhaps with a fluid level behind the heart shadow. A barium swallow shows the dilated atonic oesophagus coming to a smooth pointed termination (Fig. 8.1). There is absence of the usual gas shadow in the fundus of the stomach. While the appearances are typical, they are not diagnostic because they can be mimicked by a carcinoma at the lower end of the oesophagus or in the cardiac portion of the stomach. Treated or untreated, patients with achalasia have an increased liability to carcinoma of the oesophagus which makes initial endoscopy essential and periodic review after treatment desirable.

Oesophagoscopy should always be carried out. Usually cleansing of the oesophagus is required with mechanical removal of the larger retained food fragments, and this may involve repeated lavage, aspiration and oesophagoscopy. Once the oesophagus is clean, its wall can be inspected, its termination studied, bougies passed and biopsies taken.

Motility studies are of value in establishing the diagnosis and in determining the extent and severity of the lesion.

Treatment. Treatment may be by dilatation or cardiomyotomy. When the choice is dilatation, a bougie is passed through the lower end of the oesophagus and a distensible bag guided through the narrowed segment. Using water pressure, the bag is forcibly distended in order to split the circular muscle fibres of the oesophagus. A single dilatation may cure the patient. If not, it can be repeated.

Failure of hydrostatic dilatation or inability to introduce the bougie or dilator are indications for operation, which takes the form of cardiomyotomy (Heller's operation). Here the muscle at the lower end of the oesophagus and for some distance above and below is slit to expose but not to penetrate the mucosa. The operation can be performed through the chest or the abdomen and is relatively effective and safe, even in the elderly. Both procedures may be followed immediately by reflux oesophagitis or oesophageal perforation.

Diffuse Spasm of the Oesophagus

Like achalasia, diffuse spasm is probably caused by a disorder of the oesophageal nerve cells. Often there is hypertrophy of the muscle wall of the oesophagus.

The main symptom is pain precipitated by eating or by emotional stress. The pain is retrosternal and there may be radiation to the back, neck or arms, thus making the differential diagnosis from coronary artery disease difficult. The pain may or may not be accompanied by dysphagia. The diagnosis is established by barium swallow which shows a hold-up of barium in the oesophagus due to multiple uncoordinated contractions. The appearance resembles a 'corkscrew'. Manometry confirms the lack of a coordinated peristaltic wave.

Treatment involves education in eating in a relaxed atmosphere with adequate mastication. Nitroglycerine may relieve pain. Since most patients are over the age of 60, the physician has to persist with medical management but in the occasional younger patient, an extended cardiomyotomy may be required.

Carcinoma of the Oesophagus

Carcinoma of the oesophagus occurs mainly in men and at a later age than other cancers. It has some association with smoking, the consumption of spices and spirits, and with achalasia. No other tumour has such a wide geographical variation in incidence; it is common, for example, in parts of Southern Africa.

In the Western Hemisphere, the most frequent site of carcinoma is the lower third of the oesophagus; it is less common in the middle third and least common in the upper third. The lesion is usually ulcerative in form, and it extends circumferentially and longitudinally in the wall of the oesophagus. Direct invasion of surrounding structures and involvement of related lymph nodes is common by the time of diagnosis. Histologically the growth is squamous celled. Where an adenocarcinoma is found, it has probably spread from the stomach to invade the lower oesophagus. Rarely primary adenocarcinoma of the oesophagus occurs and is presumed to originate in submucosal glandular elements.

Clinical Features. Progressive dysphagia is typical. It starts with the 'sticking' of solid food, at first intermittently and then regularly and proceeds to difficulty with semisolids and eventually with liquids. There is discomfort, not amounting to pain at the site of the obstruction which is usually well localised by the patient. The development of symptoms occupies some months so that by the time the patient first attends, weight loss is already a feature and there may be metastases in lymph nodes, liver and related structures in the mediastinum.

Investigation. Obstruction and an irregular narrowing of the oesophagus, seen at barium swallow, are highly suggestive of the diagnosis. At the lower end it may not be possible to distinguish between carcinoma of the oesophagus and achalasia of the cardia. Oesophagitis and a benign stricture may also simulate carcinoma and the differentiation is rendered more difficult when a hiatus hernia is present.

Oesophagoscopy should always be carried out and provides an opportunity of removing tissue for histological examination. Repeated biopsy may be required to obtain positive confirmation of the diagnosis, and this is particularly so when stricture formation prevents further insertion of the oesophagoscope or the biopsy forceps. In these circumstances, the passage of a brush through the narrowed area and examination of dislodged cells is of value.

Treatment. The choice lies between palliation and radical treatment. The chances of cure seldom exceed 10 per cent. In squamous carcinoma, particularly of the upper and middle thirds, high voltage radiotherapy is the treatment of choice in those centres possessing the necessary facilities. Otherwise, and with tumours of the lower third, oesophagogastrectomy offers the best hope. There is the possibility that a combined approach of surgery with preoperative radiotherapy may lead to an enhanced survival rate.

Extensive tumours that are unsuitable for radical surgery or for intensive radiotherapy are treated palliatively, occasionally by bypass surgery, but more often by intubation. This allows liquids to be taken and is effective in relieving the patient of that most distressing problem—the inability to swallow saliva.

Gastrostomy as a palliative measure offers no relief to the patient, fails to prolong his survival and is therefore not advisable.

DISEASES OF THE STOMACH AND DUODENUM

Peptic Ulcer

In the Western Hemisphere, peptic ulcer is one of the commonest diseases of the alimentary tract. It affects particularly the working years of a patient's life and its social implications are therefore considerable.

Aetiology. The term 'peptic ulcer' refers to an ulcer found in the lower end of the oesophagus, the stomach, the duodenum, in the small intestine after surgical anastomosis to the stomach, or rarely at the junction of a Meckel's diverticulum with the small intestine. Although the immediate cause of peptic ulceration is digestion of the mucosa by acid and pepsin of the gastric juice, the sequence of events that leads to the development of the ulcer are unknown. Digestion by acid–pepsin cannot be the only factor involved, since ulcers do not develop in some normal people who secrete acid and pepsin in substantial amounts. The problem is aptly stated in the question, 'Why does the stomach not digest itself?' The answer must be that the normal stomach is capable of resisting digestion by its own secretions, so that the problem of ulcer aetiology may be written: *Acid plus pepsin versus mucosal resistance.*

Theoretically, peptic ulceration may result if gastric secretion is increased on the one hand, or if the resistance of the mucosa is reduced on the other; it is convenient to consider the factors believed to be involved in the development of chronic peptic ulcers according to how they may alter either side of the balance. Both local mechanisms and general or constitutional factors are associated with the development of peptic ulcer. These are:

Gastric Hypersecretion. The evidence that ulcers occur only in the presence of acid and pepsin is very strong. Peptic ulceration has never been found in patients with pernicious anaemia, and it is very doubtful if a benign chronic ulcer ever occurs in association with achlorhydria. On the other hand, severe intractable peptic ulcer occurs in patients with the Zollinger Ellison syndrome (p. 376), which is characterised by very high rates of gastric secretion. Moreover, patients with duodenal ulcer considered as a group secrete about twice as much acid as do normal individuals, and the duodenal ulcer heals when gastric hypersecretion is reduced by vagotomy. However, gastric hypersecretion does not occur in all patients with duodenal ulcer.

It is in patients with gastric ulcer that factors influencing mucosal resistance must be considered:

Mucus and Cellular Turnover. Alkaline mucus is the first line of defence. The ability of the superficial layer of cells to prevent the entry of hydrogen ions into the mucosa has led to the concept of a 'gastric mucosal barrier'. The barrier may be breached by drugs such as aspirin or by bile.

Aspirin. When aspirin is in solution at a pH below 3·5 it is undissociated and fat-soluble so that it is absorbed through the lipoprotein membrane of the surface epithelial cells. During absorption it damages the membrane thus disrupting the gastric mucosal barrier. Aspirin has been shown to be an important epidemiological factor in gastric ulcer in Australia and this may also be so in other countries with a high consumption of aspirin. There is also a relationship between aspirin ingestion and acute bleeding from the upper gastrointestinal tract (p. 370).

Bile Reflux. Reflux of bile and other secretions into the stomach occurs more frequently in patients with gastric ulcers than in normal individuals or in patients with duodenal ulcers, due presumably to an abnormal pyloric sphincter. Whatever the mechanism, the increased concentration of bile salts in the stomach interferes with the integrity of the gastric mucosa, thus predisposing to the development of gastritis and ulceration.

Inflammatory Change. Gastritis, which may be both extensive and severe, commonly occurs in patients with gastric ulcer and, although there is no certain evidence, it seems likely that the gastritis in fact precedes the development of the ulcer; if so, the inflammatory change may well predispose to the development of ulceration by lowering the resistance of the mucosa to digestion.

Blood Supply. One of the classical theories of ulcer formation is that the resistance of the mucosa to digestion is reduced as a result of impaired blood supply; such impairment could occur as a result of venous or arterial thrombosis, or because of 'shunting' of blood within the mucosa. It is possible that these mechanisms play a role in the development of 'stress' ulceration.

Stress. There is an undoubted association between the development of acute ulcers in the stomach or duodenum and physical or mental trauma or surgical operations; similarly there is little doubt that acute anxiety is a significant factor in precipitating ulcer recurrences and sometimes ulcer complications such as haemorrhage or perforation.

Heredity. There is no doubt that peptic ulcer tends to occur in families, and the tendency tends to run true to type, so that the children of parents with duodenal ulcer develop duodenal ulcer, and likewise for gastric ulcer. A strong family history is frequently found in patients who develop ulcer in childhood or adolescence. Heritability is estimated on page 19.

Sex Incidence. There are obvious differences in both the incidence and behaviour of peptic ulcer. Earlier this century duodenal ulcer occurred 5 to 10 times more often in men than in women and perforation occurred 20 times more often in men. Now these ratios have been reduced to 3 : 1 and 4 : 1. Although these effects may be due to differences in the life pattern of men and women, there are grounds for supposing that the female sex hormones in some way protect against peptic ulcer. During pregnancy active ulcers are virtually unknown; ulcer symptoms which remit during pregnancy commonly recur soon afterwards. The incidence of ulcer symptoms and complications increases sharply in women at about the menopause. The sex difference in the incidence and behaviour of gastric ulcer is much less than for duodenal ulcer.

Environmental Factors. There are marked variations in the incidence of gastric and duodenal ulcer between different countries, and even between different parts of the same country—for example, the proportion of duodenal ulcer to gastric ulcer is very much higher in Scotland than it is in London. There are also differences in the incidence of ulcer as between social classes so that duodenal ulcers tend to be evenly distributed throughout the entire population, while gastric ulcer occurs more commonly in the lower socio-economic classes.

Seasonal Factors. There are strong seasonal factors which can be shown to influence the incidence of ulcer symptoms and mortality rates; in Britain, ulcer mortality is at its lowest in August and September and begins to rise in October, with a further exacerbation of ulcer symptoms in the Spring. The cause is unknown.

Pathology. Ulcers occurring in the stomach and duodenum may be acute or chronic, the difference being that a chronic ulcer penetrates the muscularis mucosae, whereas an acute ulcer or an erosion does not. Chronic ulcers occur with remarkable regularity in certain sites: in the stomach on the lesser curvature just above the angulus or less frequently at or near the pylorus, while duodenal ulcers occur within 1 cm of the pylorus on the anterior or posterior wall. Acute lesions are frequently multiple, and are less regularly distributed. Benign ulcers occur only rarely on the greater curvature or on the anterior wall of the stomach.

Clinical Features. While there are good grounds for believing that gastric and duodenal ulcers are different diseases with different aetiology and natural history, it is convenient to describe the general features of 'peptic ulcer' as inclusive of both, noting differences where they occur.

Peptic ulcer may present in different ways. The commonest is chronic, episodic pain extending over months or years. However, the ulcer may come to attention as an acute episode with bleeding or perforation, with little or no previous history. Occasionally the patient presents with the symptoms of gastric outlet obstruction, having had negligible trouble previously.

Pain is the characteristic symptom of peptic ulcer, and it has three notable features—sharp localisation to the epigastrium, relationship to food, and periodicity. Ulcer pain is typically referred to the epigastrium, in the midline or to the right; wherever it occurs, it is usually sharply localised so that the patient can point to the site, 'the pointing sign'. Occasionally ulcer pain is not clearly localised; it may be referred diffusely in the epigastrium, the lower chest or to the back in the interscapular region in the fifth to eighth thoracic segments. Pain referred to the interscapular area, especially if it is a new feature, suggests the possibility that the ulcer has penetrated posteriorly, involving structures such as the pancreas. The description of the pain is not especially helpful, although patients commonly describe it as gnawing or burning. Pain varies considerably in severity, and it is sometimes helpful to ask the patient to qualify the symptom as 'pain' or as 'discomfort' as a measure of its intensity.

Most patients recognise a relationship of the pain to food, although the relationship varies between patients, and in the same patient from time to time. Duodenal ulcer pain tends to occur between meal times, so that the patient may describe it as 'hunger' pain, which is characteristically relieved by food. A notable feature of duodenal ulcer is pain awakening the patient from sleep 2 to 3 hours after retiring. The pain of gastric ulcer occurs less regularly; it frequently occurs within an hour of eating, is less often relieved by food, and it rarely occurs at night. Besides the characteristic relief obtained after eating, ulcer pain is almost invariably relieved by antacids, by vomiting and by bed rest in hospital.

Ulcer pain is characteristically episodic occurring regularly each day for days or weeks at a time, then disappearing, to recur weeks or months later. Between attacks, the patient feels perfectly well, and may eat and drink with impunity. Bouts of pain may at first last only a day or so at a time, and occur only once or twice a year. As the natural history evolves, however, episodes begin to last longer and occur more frequently, so that in severe cases remissions of pain may be short-lived and pain or discomfort becomes more or less persistent. The cause for these relapses is difficult to establish. Seasonal factors may be operative, sometimes psychological stress may be blamed, sometimes dietary indiscretion, and sometimes alcoholic excess. Most commonly, no reason can be found for the relapse.

Pain is sometimes absent or so slight as to be dismissed by the patient. Such individuals may complain of other symptoms such as a feeling of 'distension' in the epigastrium or a poorly defined sense of unease after eating. Other complaints include episodic nausea and sometimes anorexia, as well as heartburn or waterbrash. Nausea, anorexia, vomiting and weight loss occur more frequently in gastric ulcer than in duodenal ulcer. Vomiting in ulcer patients almost always relieves pain and when it is persistent may result in weight loss. This helps to distinguish it from vomiting of psychological origin, in which weight is usually maintained. Persistent vomiting in an ulcer subject usually indicates some degree of gastric outflow obstruction, whether due to spasm or organic narrowing of the gastric outlet. In such patients, vomiting is usually copious, so that the patient is 'surprised' at the volume; the patient often recognises food eaten twelve or more hours previously, and he is aware of the unpleasant smell of the vomitus. Although there is no constant change in bowel rhythm during an ulcer relapse, some patients are aware of constipation or diarrhoea when dyspepsia reappears.

Physical Signs. The only physical sign that may be present is 'the pointing sign' which, when accompanied by localised tenderness, is practically diagnostic of an ulcer. However, tenderness may be completely absent. In patients with gastric outlet obstruction, the stomach may be visibly distended, a succussion splash may be present, and gastric peristalsis may be seen.

Investigation. The diagnosis of peptic ulcer can usually be made from the characteristic history, but it requires confirmation by barium meal examination (Fig. 8.2) or endoscopy. In some patients the peptic ulcer may present with bleeding, perforation or even pyloric stenosis with few or no previous symptoms. The patient with troublesome dyspepsia, in whom barium meal examination is negative, presents difficulties. Some of these patients will be found to have an ulcer at endoscopy and indeed some may be found to have an early carcinoma. Some clinical judgement has to be exercised in order to distinguish between dyspepsia of psychological origin and that due to organic lesions which have not been detected

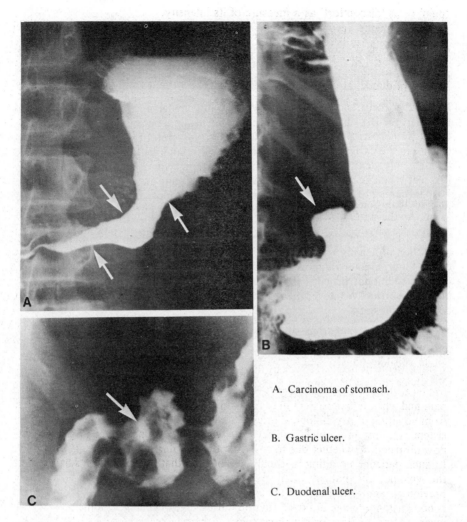

A. Carcinoma of stomach.

B. Gastric ulcer.

C. Duodenal ulcer.

Fig. 8.2

radiologically. In general, the history in the former is more diffuse, the symptoms rarely as clear cut, the pain poorly localised, and there are no sharply defined tender areas. Positive evidence of a psychological abnormality can usually be obtained. It is a good rule that patients who develop dyspepsia for the first time in middle age should be examined endoscopically if the X-ray is negative. Probably all patients with gastric ulcer should be examined endoscopically and biopsies taken to exclude a carcinoma. This procedure is also indicated if the physician has any doubt about the nature of the disorder.

Treatment. There are three objectives in the management of peptic ulcer, namely, the alleviation of symptoms, the healing of the ulcer and the prevention of its recurrence. While there are effective methods for relieving symptoms, few drugs accelerate ulcer healing and there is no means of preventing ulcer recurrence or of altering the natural tendency of ulcer symptoms to remit and relapse. A major problem in interpreting the effectiveness of any particular treatment is the fact that ulcer symptoms do not necessarily reflect ulcer activity. Relief of symptoms can occur in a few days, whereas healing may take weeks. Thus the relief of symptoms, which is naturally the main concern of the patient, does not necessarily mean that the ulcer has healed; some ulcers may persist for many months without any further recurrence of pain, and without any change in size. The more chronic the ulcer, the less chance there is of obtaining healing, because the tissues are distorted by fibrosis. It seems a reasonable aim, therefore, to try to produce ulcer healing in the early stages, in the hope of preventing irreversible changes. Unfortunately this ideal is difficult to attain for economic reasons since the patient is frequently unable to take sufficient time off work, and in any case admission to hospital cannot be offered to all patients with an active ulcer, but has to be reserved for patients with complications such as stenosis, bleeding or intractable pain.

REST. The single most effective measure for the relief of ulcer pain and the promotion of healing is bed-rest. This may be undertaken at home under the care of the family doctor or more effectively in hospital; undoubtedly rest in hospital confers additional benefit, possibly because of the release from domestic and business worries. Whatever the reason, pain usually disappears after a few days of bed-rest in hospital.

DIET, ALCOHOL AND TOBACCO. It is usually said that a suitable diet for ulcer patients should be mechanically and chemically non-irritating and should consist of small frequent meals. However, there is little experimental evidence to support this advice. It has been shown, for example, that hourly feedings of milk provoke more acid secretion in the stomach than does the ordinary routine of three meals a day, and there is no evidence that the rate of ulcer healing can be accelerated by the traditional bland ulcer diet. Indeed, persistence with such diets may be harmful since they may lead to suboptimal intake of vitamin C. Nevertheless, when symptoms are severe, the patient usually obtains relief from frequent feeds. The patient should avoid foods or alcohol which exacerbate symptoms. There is good evidence to show that stopping smoking accelerates the healing of gastric ulcers, and it is likely that this also applies to duodenal ulcers. Thus tobacco smoking should be prohibited.

DRUGS. *Antacids*. Ulcer pain is relieved by antacids. The effectiveness of an antacid is limited by the rate at which it leaves the stomach, so that a dose of an antacid theoretically sufficient to neutralise the gastric acid secreted over many hours in fact does so for less than an hour. Therefore the most effective antacids are those with the quickest neutralising capacity. Sodium bicarbonate is perhaps the most effective of all, but because it can be absorbed it may produce alkalosis; however, this rarely occurs except with excessive dosage, or with vomiting, or when renal disease is present. Accordingly, non-absorbable antacids are usually prescribed, although they do not give such rapid relief because of their slower rate of neutralisation. Calcium carbonate leads to constipation and hypercalcaemia and it may also stimulate further acid secretion once its neutralising effect is spent. Magnesium compounds cause diarrhoea. They should not be given to patients with renal failure because the small amount of magnesium which is absorbed cannot be excreted and magnesium toxicity can develop. Aluminium antacids cause constipation and they also prevent the absorption of broad spectrum antibiotics.

However, where pain is severe, antacids should be given frequently, e.g. hourly. In the less acute phase, this dose of antacid is best given 1 hour after each meal. For the ambulant patient with minor discomfort, antacid preparations in tablet form are more convenient; they may be carried in the pocket, and chewed or sucked whenever pain occurs. The diarrhoea caused by magnesium salts and the constipation produced by calcium salts or aluminium hydroxide can be prevented by a suitable mixture of the two groups of antacids, the exact proportions depending on the individual patient.

Histamine H_2-receptor Antagonists. It has long been known that the stimulating effect of histamine on gastric secretion could not be blocked by the standard antihistaminics. This led to the idea that there might be a second type of histamine receptor situated on, or near, the parietal cells. The possibility of blocking this second type of receptor and so reducing gastric secretion led to the development of the group of drugs known as the histamine H_2-receptor antagonists. Whereas earlier preparations depressed the bone marrow, the newer drug cimetidine is safe and does not appear to have significant side-effects. The results of clinical trials establish that cimetidine promotes the healing of duodenal ulcers, and probably gastric ulcers also. The dosage is 200 mg t.i.d. with meals and 400 mg at bedtime for 4–6 weeks. Cimetidine may prove to be the treatment of choice for uncomplicated duodenal ulcer.

Anticholinergics. Drugs of the anticholinergic group inhibit vagal stimulation, thereby reducing gastric secretion and motility. All drugs of this class exert a general anticholinergic effect, so that salivary secretion is reduced, intraocular pressure is raised, and constipation and urinary retention may occur. Many such drugs have been synthesised with the object of increasing the desired effect on the stomach and of reducing unwanted side-effects, but there is no good evidence that any one preparation is better than another in this respect. Of the drugs available, propantheline (15 mg) and poldine methylsulphate (2–6 mg) are perhaps best. The dose is that which just avoids side-effects; the drug is taken three or four times a day and the amount is gradually increased until tolerance is established. Doubling the dose to be taken at night is useful in preventing the occurrence of nocturnal pain. Large doses of anticholinergics cannot be tolerated by ambulant patients because of the blurring of vision; they are not well-tolerated by the elderly, and they are contraindicated in patients with glaucoma, prostatism, gastric retention or reflux oesophagitis.

Liquorice Derivatives. It has been shown that carbenoxolone sodium accelerates the healing of gastric ulcers in ambulant patients. The evidence that it exerts a beneficial effect on duodenal ulcer is not convincing. The drug is given in an initial dose of 100 mg t.i.d. for 2 weeks, the dose then being reduced to 50 mg q.i.d. for 2 months. Carbenoxolone may cause sodium and water retention, potassium depletion and hypertension; these side-effects are an indication for terminating treatment with carbenoxolone. It should be prescribed only when the patient can be properly supervised and is contraindicated when the patient is elderly or where there is hypertension or a previous history of heart failure.

Other Drugs. Psychological stress may precipitate a relapse and ulcer symptoms in turn may lead to further anxiety. Thus tranquillisers such as diazepam are useful in controlling anxiety or as an adjunct to bed rest.

Many other drugs have been recommended for the treatment of peptic ulcers but there is no firm evidence that they alleviate symptoms or promote healing.

SURGICAL TREATMENT. This has much to offer the patient with intractable peptic ulceration. It can relieve severe or persistent symptoms and prevent complications. While in many cases the assessment of the patient's disability is straightforward, in patients in whom anxiety or depression is present, the decision becomes difficult. Elective surgery should be considered in the following circumstances:

1. When an ulcer has failed to heal, and symptoms persist or recur so as to interfere with the enjoyment of life, or reduce the capacity to work. The indications for surgery are strengthened if the ulcer has developed in adolescence or young adult life, if there is a strong family history, or if there has been a previous complication such as haemorrhage or perforation.

2. When there is an ulcer which has produced gastric outlet obstruction, or an hour-glass stomach because of fibrosis.

3. When there is a gastric ulcer the nature of which is uncertain or which has failed to heal in three months.

4. In a recurrent ulcer following previous gastric surgery.

There is no single, ideal operation suitable for all ulcers and all patients. For a gastric ulcer, the operation of choice is partial gastrectomy preferably with a Billroth I anastomosis, in which the ulcer itself and the ulcer-bearing area of the stomach is resected (Fig. 8.3). For duodenal ulcer the acid secretory capacity of the stomach may be reduced by partial gastrectomy preferably with a Polya (Billroth II) anastomosis or by vagotomy which eliminates nervous stimulation of gastric secretion. (Fig. 8.3). At truncal vagotomy the main nerves are divided and thereafter gastric emptying may be retarded so that truncal vagotomy has to be combined with a drainage operation such as pyloroplasty or gastroenterostomy. One of these procedures is also required in selective vagotomy in which vagal innervation to the small intestine, pancreas and biliary tree is preserved. The newer operation of proximal gastric (highly selective) vagotomy is now used in some centres. The aim of this operation is to denervate the acid-producing area of the stomach while leaving intact the vagal supply to the antrum and pylorus. A drainage procedure is not required.

Vagotomy is preferred to partial gastrectomy because of the lesser mortality and lower incidence of long-term complications. The choice of operation may be guided to some extent by measurement of the secretory capacity of the stomach. When the acid output is very high, some surgeons prefer to combine partial gastrectomy with vagotomy in order to ensure that gastric secretion is sufficiently reduced. At the other end of the scale, gastroenterostomy alone without vagotomy may be considered in patients with a low acid output.

It should be re-emphasised that relief of symptoms is the objective in elective surgery for a peptic ulcer and while it is important that the patient should not be overpersuaded to accept operation, it must also be remembered that much unnecessary suffering can be imposed on patients by denying surgery when medical management has failed.

Complications. The common complications of peptic ulcer are haemorrhage, perforation and obstruction. Ulcer-cancer is discussed on page 382.

Gastroduodenal Haemorrhage

Bleeding as judged by a positive test for occult blood in the stools can be detected at some time or another in most cases of peptic ulcer. Gastroduodenal haemorrhage as a complication is taken to mean bleeding of sufficient severity as

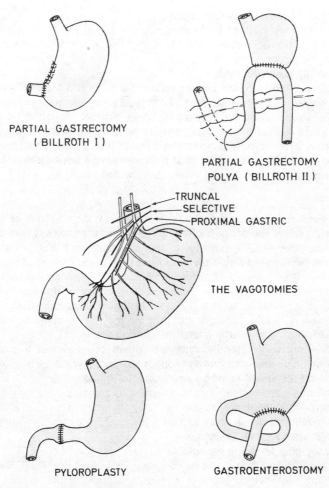

PARTIAL GASTRECTOMY
(BILLROTH I)

PARTIAL GASTRECTOMY
POLYA (BILLROTH II)

TRUNCAL
SELECTIVE
PROXIMAL GASTRIC

THE VAGOTOMIES

PYLOROPLASTY

GASTROENTEROSTOMY

Fig. 8.3 Operations for peptic ulceration

to cause symptoms on its own account. It is a serious complication of peptic ulcer, carrying a mortality of the order of 10 per cent, so that all patients with a history of significant blood loss within the previous 48 hours should be admitted to hospital.

Aetiology. The common causes are, (1) chronic duodenal ulcer, (2) 'acute' gastric ulcer or gastric erosions, (3) chronic gastric ulcer, (4) carcinoma of the stomach, and (5) portal hypertension causing oesophageal varices. In Britain the first three account for about 90 per cent of the cases.

Acute ulcers range from minute erosions to shallow ulcers about 2–4 cm in diameter and involving only the mucosa; erosions may occur singly, in small groups, or in severe cases may be so numerous as to be virtually confluent causing an acute erosive gastritis. They are difficult to demonstrate radiologically; a positive diagnosis requires direct inspection by endoscopy. Salicylates are the commonest cause of haematemesis associated with acute erosions, the majority of patients giving a history of aspirin ingestion within the previous 48 hours. In some cases the erosions are related to the consumption of alcohol or a combination of alcohol and aspirin; other causes include drugs such as phenylbutazone. Bleeding from an acute ulcer or erosion may follow burns, head injury, systemic infection or stress (especially postoperative).

Bleeding from oesophageal varices secondary to portal hypertension can be extremely severe and demands special measures for its management. It is a relatively infrequent cause of haematemesis in Britain, though it occurs more frequently in the United States; even in those patients, however, bleeding may be due to an associated acute or chronic ulcer, rather than from the varices. Bleeding from peptic oesophagitis is usually mild but more severe haemorrhage may result from lacerations of the cardia due to repeated vomiting (Mallory–Weiss syndrome).

Clinical Features. Haemorrhage manifests itself by the vomiting of blood (i.e. *haematemesis*) or by the passage of altered blood in the stools (i.e. *melaena*). A frank haematemesis usually indicates a large bleed whereas melaena alone often indicates that bleeding is slow. If the blood has been in the stomach for any length of time, it becomes partially digested and appears brown and granular in the vomit—so-called 'coffee grounds'. Blood passing through the intestinal canal is also altered in appearance, so that the stool becomes black and sticky; however, in severe bleeding, transit through the intestine may be so rapid that the blood passed per rectum may be little altered in appearance.

Whatever the cause of the bleeding the patient complains of weakness, and faintness sometimes amounting to syncope, nausea or sweating; these symptoms are followed by the actual vomiting or passage of blood.

On examination, the patient is pale, sweating and anxious. He may be restless or disorientated because of cerebral anoxia. The pulse rate will be raised and the blood pressure may fall. These signs may be absent in the young patient in whom compensatory mechanisms are more effective.

The haemoglobin level will not alter until haemodilution occurs, and this may not take place for some hours, nor be complete for some days. There is no simple laboratory procedure which will give a reliable estimate of the amount of blood loss until haemodilution is complete, so that in ordinary circumstances the assessment of the degree or rate of bleeding depends on clinical judgement; serial recording of the pulse rate and blood pressure gives some indication, but for a more accurate assessment in patients who continue to bleed, measurement of central venous pressure is necessary. This and endoscopy are discussed below.

Treatment and Further Investigation. The patient should be put to bed, and blood taken for haemoglobin estimation, packed cell volume and blood grouping. A half-hourly chart of blood pressure and pulse rate is begun. An intravenous drip must be set up in case further haemorrhage occurs, and a naso-gastric tube should be passed into the stomach. The patient is usually restless and anxious, but this may be due as much to cerebral anoxia as it is to fright. Sedation should be given and drugs such as diazepam are to be preferred to morphine which may itself cause vomiting. A blood transfusion is indicated if the pulse rate is faster than 100 per minute or the systolic pressure lower than 100 mm Hg. It is important that every patient is transfused adequately, because cerebral anoxia may lead to restlessness or even delirium, and if it is sufficiently prolonged cerebral thrombosis may develop in the elderly. Similarly, the coronary blood supply may be compromised leading to angina or even myocardial infarction. Prolonged hypotension may result in acute renal failure and permanent renal damage. The danger from overtransfusion is heart failure; in the elderly, especially in those presenting with severe bleeding or those likely to have continued bleeding, the safest guide is measurement of the central venous pressure (p. 193). The hourly or half-hourly aspiration of stomach contents by means of the nasogastric tube is also useful in detecting further bleeding.

The next step in management is to decide the further investigation of the patient in consultation with a surgical colleague. The importance of doing so early cannot be overemphasised; although the immediate situation may not give rise to anxiety, the surgeon should see the patient at the earliest opportunity in case there is recurrent haemorrhage. The cause of the bleeding should be established as soon as shock has been corrected. Endoscopy is the procedure of choice since, in contrast to a barium study, it can demonstrate erosions and in the event of more than one lesion being present, it can demonstrate which one is bleeding. Subsequent management is determined largely by the age of the patient, the severity of the haemorrhage, the site or cause of the bleeding, and recurrent bleeding. There are no absolute criteria governing the decision to operate, and again each case has to be considered on its merits. As a general rule emergency surgery should be advised in any patient over 50 who has had severe bleeding, or is known to have a chronic ulcer, or who bleeds again after admission. On the other hand, if the patient can be shown to be bleeding from acute erosions, medical therapy including cimetidine (p. 369) can be continued much longer.

Opinions differ as to the choice of operation. In general, partial gastrectomy (Bilroth I) is the operation of choice for a chronic gastric ulcer, whereas in duodenal ulcer the lesion may be exposed by an incision at the pylorus, occluded by sutures and a pyloroplasty and vagotomy performed (Fig. 8.3).

Prognosis. Approximately 10 per cent of patients admitted to hospital with acute gastrointestinal haemorrhage will die. Patients over the age of 60, those with chronic ulcers, particularly gastric ones, and those patients who have a large bleed as evidenced by haematemesis have an increased chance of dying. Patients with recurrent bleeding in hospital and those who undergo surgery where shock is uncorrected also have a poorer prognosis.

Patients with a chronic ulcer are likely to bleed again months or years later; in such patients, elective surgery for the ulcer should be considered, after they have recovered from the initial bleed.

Acute Perforation of a Peptic Ulcer

When free perforation occurs, the contents of the stomach escape into the peritoneal cavity. If perforation occurs without loss of contents, as in the accidental perforation of the empty stomach at gastroscopy, few symptoms are produced and the accident may even pass unnoticed. It follows that the symptoms of perforation are those of peritonitis, and they are in proportion to the extent of peritoneal soiling. Occasionally the symptoms of perforation appear and rapidly subside; presumably the perforation has then closed spontaneously, or more commonly the ulcer has perforated locally into an area confined by adhesions to adjacent structures. Perforation occurs more commonly in duodenal than in gastric ulcers, and usually in ulcers on the anterior wall. About one-quarter of all perforations occur in acute ulcers.

Clinical Features. Although perforation may be the first sign of ulcer, usually there is a history of dyspepsia. The most striking symptom is sudden, severe pain, the onset of which may be so incisive that the patient can time it to a minute. The pain is usually intense, and its distribution follows the spread of the gastric contents over the peritoneum. Thus, initially the pain may be referred to the upper abdomen, but very quickly it becomes generalised; shoulder tip pain may occur as a result of irritation of the diaphragm. The pain is accompanied by the signs of shock and shallow respiration due to limitation of diaphragmatic movements. The abdomen is held immobile, and there is generalised board-like rigidity; intestinal sounds are absent, and liver dullness to percussion may decrease due to the presence of gas under the diaphragm. Vomiting is common. After some hours, the symptoms improve, though the abdominal rigidity remains. This period of improvement may deceive the clinician examining the patient for the first time; after this temporary improvement, manifestations of general peritonitis follow the initial peritoneal irritation and the patient's condition deteriorates.

A plain film of the abdomen in the erect position may help to establish the diagnosis since free gas within the peritoneal cavity, if in sufficient amount, will show as a translucent crescent between the liver and diaphragm.

Treatment. After initial treatment of the patient for shock, the acute perforation should be treated surgically either by simple closure, or occasionally in the case of perforation of a chronic ulcer by closure combined with vagotomy and drainage. More than half the patients who have a simple closure will eventually require a further elective operation for recurrence of ulcer symptoms, and for this reason some surgeons recommend a definitive procedure for the ulcer at the time of operation.

Prognosis. Acute perforation carries a mortality of about 5 per cent, but the outlook depends on the degree of peritoneal soiling, and therefore on the size of the perforation and the amount of stomach contents released into the peritoneum. The time interval elapsing between the onset of perforation and the time of operation also determines the outcome—the longer the delay, the greater the risk of death from peritonitis.

Gastric Outlet Obstruction

An ulcer in the region of the pylorus may result in fibrosis leading to the complication of gastric outlet obstruction. This may be due to actual organic narrowing from scar tissue or to oedema or spasm produced by the ulcer; frequently it is a combination of all three. Long-standing obstruction may lead to severe 'retention' gastritis, or even to secondary gastric ulcer.

In addition to chronic duodenal ulcer, or benign gastric ulcer at or near the pylorus, gastric outlet obstruction may be caused by carcinoma of the antrum and by a rare condition known as *adult hypertrophic pyloric stenosis*. The syndrome of gastric outlet obstruction is loosely described as *'pyloric stenosis'*, even when the cause is chronic duodenal ulcer, and the stenosis is distal to the pylorus; thus in 'pyloric' obstruction due to duodenal stenosis, the pylorus itself may be seen radiologically to be greatly dilated.

Clinical Features. Most commonly the condition is due to a chronic duodenal ulcer, so that there will be a preceding history of dyspepsia. When there is no such history, a patient with gastric outlet obstruction is likely to have a pyloric carcinoma. When there has been an ulcer, the symptoms of dyspepsia change, so that vomiting becomes a prominent feature, and nausea replaces normal appetite. Vomiting produces such striking relief that a patient may even start to eat or prepare food immediately after the stomach has been emptied. If the obstruction progresses, the stomach dilates and accommodates large volumes so that eventually surprisingly large amounts of gastric content may be vomited. Articles of food which have been eaten 24 hours previously may be recognised in the vomit. An earlier symptom is a sense of repletion soon after eating: the patient feels satisfied and full up after taking a relatively small amount of food. The vomit of pyloric obstruction is characteristically foul-smelling and free of bile. The loss of gastric contents results in water and electrolyte depletion. The blood urea may be raised because of dehydration. Alkalosis develops if large amounts of hydrochloric acid are lost, as occurs particularly in obstruction due to duodenal ulcer.

Physical examination shows evidence of wasting and dehydration, and there may be signs of tetany (p. 533). Splashing may be elicited four hours or more after the last meal or drink, and sometimes the patient is aware of it himself. In normal persons splashing occurs for less than an hour after meals because gastric emptying is rapid. Visible gastric peristalsis is the sign of greatest value in pyloric obstruction and the abdomen should be inspected for its presence. If the patient takes a fluid diet with large amounts of milk, the signs of obstruction may be masked and nutrition may be maintained, even resulting in obesity.

Investigation. The diagnosis can be confirmed by *aspiration of the stomach*. A volume in excess of 100 ml after fasting or 200 ml four hours after a meal is suggestive; if the aspirate contains food residue, or is foul, the diagnosis is certain. However, a fine bore nasogastric tube may become blocked by debris, giving a false impression of normality; if in doubt a wide stomach tube should be used. If a large gastric residue persists after several days treatment, barium meal examination is unlikely to be helpful and the patient should be prepared for surgery.

The radiological signs are (1) an increase in the fasting residue of the stomach, (2) dilatation of the stomach with or without excessive peristalsis, (3) a lesion at or near the pylorus, and (4) delayed gastric emptying.

Endoscopy may demonstrate the cause of the obstruction and its degree.

Treatment. The stomach is washed out to remove all food debris and then aspirated 2 to 4 hourly for 3 to 4 days at which point, if the volume of aspirate has decreased, it may be possible to allow fluids by mouth. Dehydration and electrolyte disturbance must be corrected by intravenous fluids. In the first 24 hours 4 litres of isotonic saline are given and thereafter the daily requirement is based on the volume of aspirate together with other body losses. Potassium, 80 mmol/day, is given in the infusion. Where obstruction is not severe a homogenised diet may be prescribed. A multivitamin preparation should be given by injection to all but the mildest cases.

The majority of patients will be greatly improved by these methods; the volume of the gastric aspirate steadily declines, and emptying of the stomach returns to near normal. It is then necessary to consider the timing of an operation such as gastroenterostomy or gastrectomy. Operation should not be too long deferred. If obstruction persists, with no improvement after 5 to 7 days, nothing is gained by procrastination, and indeed the patient may deteriorate because of electrolyte imbalance. Relief of obstruction by medical means should be seen as an opportunity to complete investigation and to render the patient as fit as possible for subsequent elective surgery.

Zollinger–Ellison Syndrome

This is a rare disorder in which severe peptic ulceration and marked gastric hypersecretion are associated with a tumour of the islets of the pancreas. The tumour cells secrete large amounts of the hormone gastrin into the circulation; this in turn stimulates the parietal cells excessively, resulting in hypersecretion. The acid output of the stomach may be so great that the 'acid tide' may reach the upper small intestine, reducing the luminal pH to 2 or less; at this pH pancreatic lipase is inactivated and bile salts may be precipitated, resulting in diarrhoea and steatorrhoea. Excessive gastric secretion is almost invariable, giving large volumes on aspiration under 'basal' conditions. A characteristic feature is that the administration of an exogenous stimulus such as histamine or pentagastrin does not increase the secretory rate much above resting or 'basal' values, since the stomach is already continuously secreting at or near maximal rates because of the high levels of endogenous gastrin in the circulation.

The ulcers are often very large and may occur in unusual sites such as the jejunum or the oesophagus. The history is usually short and bleeding and perforation are common. The syndrome may present in the form of severe recurrent ulceration following a standard operation for peptic ulcer, the underlying cause not having been recognised at the time of operation.

The diagnosis should be suspected in all patients with unusual or severe peptic ulceration, especially if the barium meal examination shows abnormally coarse gastric mucosal folds, and may be confirmed by finding very high levels of gastrin in the circulation. Medical treatment is ineffective. Theoretically the condition should be cured by removing the pancreatic tumour, but this is not usually possible because of its diffuse nature or the presence of metastases. In these circumstances, a total gastrectomy is the treatment of choice, since any procedure which leaves functioning parietal cells in the stomach will lead to recurrent ulceration.

Complications following Operations on the Stomach

Although most operations carried out for the relief of peptic ulcer are successful, 10 per cent of patients will develop complications months or years afterwards. Some of these complications such as anaemia and nutritional impairment develop insidiously, so that patients who have had an operation on the stomach should be seen at least once yearly for review. Only the late complications of gastric operation are considered here.

Recurrent Ulcer

As a general rule, recurrence of ulceration after surgery for duodenal ulcer implies failure to reduce the secretory capacity of the stomach to a level which is safe. A *jejunal ulcer* may develop, just distal to the jejuno-gastric anastomosis after partial gastrectomy or after gastroenterostomy; since the jejunal mucosa is more susceptible to acid-pepsin digestion than the mucosa of the stomach or duodenum, the level of acid secretion at which jejunal ulceration may develop is lower than that found in unoperated duodenal ulcer. After an inadequate vagotomy, a jejunal ulcer may occur if the vagotomy has been combined with a gastroenterostomy, or the original duodenal ulcer may recur if the vagotomy has been combined with pyloroplasty.

Clinical Features and Investigation. After months or years of freedom following the operation, ulcer pain recurs. The symptoms are much the same as they were prior to operation; in the case of a jejunal ulcer the relationship to food is not so clear cut and pain may be referred to the midline or to the left. Occasionally a jejunal ulcer will come to light because of a melaena or unexplained anaemia of recent onset, or more rarely because of a perforation. Recurrent ulcers of the jejunum and duodenum are difficult to demonstrate by X-ray examination. In the case of a jejunal ulcer, only 'jejunitis' or coarsening of the jejunal mucosa may be seen instead of an ulcer niche. It may be impossible to distinguish a recurrent duodenal ulcer from the deformity that is inevitably produced by pyloroplasty. In both instances, however, it may be possible to see the ulcer at endoscopy. Gastric secretion tests are helpful, since it is unusual to find a jejunal ulcer where the maximal acid output is low. After vagotomy an insulin test of gastric secretion will show whether or not vagal section has been complete.

A rare but serious complication of a jejunal ulcer is a *gastro-jejuno-colic fistula*, due to perforation of the jejunal ulcer into the colon. Flow is from colon to jejunum, and this leads to bacterial contamination of the upper intestine with resultant diarrhoea, malabsorption and consequent weight loss. The fistula is best demonstrated by a barium enema examination. The clinical condition of the patient may deteriorate very rapidly, so that urgent operation is often necessary.

Treatment. In general, the symptoms of jejunal or recurrent duodenal ulceration cannot be controlled by medical treatment; for this reason, and because of the enhanced risk of bleeding or perforation, further surgery is usually advised. When ulcer recurrence is due to an incomplete vagotomy, unless a major nerve trunk is found at laparotomy, an antrectomy or limited gastrectomy is the wisest procedure; in the case of a jejunal ulcer occurring after partial gastrectomy, a vagotomy is indicated rather than revision of the gastrectomy alone.

Suture Ulcer

Jejunal ulcer is to be distinguished from an ulcer which appears on the anastomosis. The latter is due to the presence of non-absorbable sutures such as silk which erode into the lumen and can be seen as knots or lengths of material on gastroscopy. Unlike jejunal ulcers, suture ulcers are not necessarily associated with high acid outputs; however, they are similarly unresponsive to medical management, and usually require further operation in the form of a local resection and reconstruction of the anastomosis. Occasionally a single suture can be removed endoscopically.

Recurrent Gastric Ulcer

An ulcer in the body of the stomach away from the anastomosis may also occur. This usually develops in association with gastric stasis, and surgical relief of the obstruction may be required to attain healing.

Biliary Gastritis

This results from a reflux of bile into the stomach. On endoscopy the mucosa is often red and bleeding. The patient complains of loss of appetite, nausea and epigastric discomfort sometimes brought on by eating, hot drinks or the taking of alcohol. The physician may suspect the development of carcinoma. Patients are reassured that they have not developed another ulcer. They are advised to stop smoking and drinking alcohol and to take frequent small dry meals. Additional measures include metoclopramide monohydrochloride, 10 mg q.i.d. before meals. Revisional surgery may be required when these measures fail and especially if there is any suggestion of a mechanical cause for bile reflux into the stomach.

Postcibal Syndromes

After any operation on the stomach, a number of patients will complain of symptoms after eating a meal and these may be classified as follows:

1. **The Small Stomach Syndrome.** About 50 per cent of patients feel distended and uncomfortable during and after a meal. After gastrectomy, the belief is that the remnant cannot readily accommodate the volume of the meal. The same symptom may occur after vagotomy and drainage; then interference with the mechanisms regulating accommodation–relaxation of the intact stomach is presumed to be responsible. Although these symptoms tend to lessen with time, a few patients restrict their food intake more or less permanently because of these symptoms and this, rather than malabsorption, may account for their failure to gain weight.

2. **Food Intolerance.** Approximately 5 per cent of patients find that they are no longer able to eat such foods as eggs, milk or tomatoes.

3. **Dumping Syndrome.** The symptoms consist of a feeling of intense drowsiness coupled with muscular weakness which may be described as 'tiredness' or 'fatigue'; there may be flushing and palpitations in addition. The sensation of weakness may be so intense that the patient finds it necessary to lie down. These symptoms usually develop immediately after a meal, and particularly after hot sweet foods such as milk puddings, and liquids such as cocoa. The pathogenesis of these symptoms is still uncertain, but they are probably related to the rapid emptying of the stomach contents which are 'dumped' into the jejunum. This in turn may produce movement of fluid from the extracellular compartment into the bowel lumen, and to a reduction in plasma volume; these or other factors may cause release of vaso-active substances into the circulation causing peripheral vasodilatation. Whatever the mechanisms, clinical experience shows that this train of symptoms disappears with time in the majority of patients as they become adapted to the stimuli which produce them and learn what foods to avoid.

TREATMENT. The patient should be given an explanation of his symptoms and advice concerning his eating habits. Avoidance of hot fluids like soup or strong sweet tea may prevent attacks. Meals should be of small bulk and eaten dry, and fluids taken between meal times. If it is found that a large meal is the chief offender, it may be eaten at the end of the day when the patient has the opportunity of resting afterwards. Treatment with anticholinergics to delay emptying, or propranolol 20–40 mg before meals to reduce the circulatory symptoms, may be worth a trial. If symptoms are severe and persistent, it may be necessary to advise further surgical treatment.

4. **Hypoglycaemia.** Symptoms of weakness, tremor and faintness, associated with a hungry or empty sensation in the epigastrium, may develop between 1 and 2 hours after a meal. These symptoms are due to hypoglycaemia and can be prevented by taking glucose at the appropriate time or, better still, by eating ample amounts of meat or fat at the two main meals. This measure may slow the emptying rate of the stomach and hence reduce the tendency to hypoglycaemia. Elderly patients who are subject to these attacks may have to be warned of the dangers of driving a car; similarly, patients in dangerous occupations such as steel erecting may have to seek other employment.

Anaemia

Anaemia is a common sequel to operations on the stomach, particularly partial gastrectomy. It occurs more frequently in women, in up to 50 per cent, even after vagotomy. Anaemia is due to inadequate absorption of iron, or to recurrent minor blood loss from gastritis or oesophagitis. Its incidence increases in the first 10 years as the stores of body iron are exhausted. Its occurrence is a measure of the degree of postoperative supervision, because it is preventable by and responds to the administration of iron. Megaloblastic anaemia is comparatively rare and responds promptly to vitamin B_{12}.

Postoperative Diarrhoea

Diarrhoea may occur after any operation on the stomach, but especially after vagotomy. Most patients report some looseness of the stools following vagotomy, but this may be no inconvenience to the patient, and indeed is often welcomed. Moderate or severe diarrhoea occurs in about 10 per cent. This is characteristically episodic, several watery stools being passed daily for several days, to be followed by constipation or by normal bowel habit. A striking feature is the sense of urgency associated with the diarrhoea; defaecation may be precipitate, and the patient becomes worried because of the fear of soiling himself.

Treatment is difficult, since the diarrhoea is unpredictable in occurrence. The usual symptomatic measures should be tried, such as codeine and the patient advised to take a substantial dose when diarrhoea occurs. If vagotomy has produced a marked depression of acid secretion, the diarrhoea may be associated with bacterial colonisation in the small intestine; it is then worth trying a short course of tetracycline in order to alter the bacterial flora. If there is an associated steatorrhoea the cause should be sought and corrected if possible. If no cause is found a low-fat diet is indicated.

Nutritional Impairment and Osteomalacia

In a small proportion of patients there is some nutritional impairment following gastric surgery, and this increases with the extent of any resection. Severe weight loss is its most common manifestation. There may also be malabsorption with steatorrhoea and osteomalacia which may develop for the first time 15 to 20 years after partial gastrectomy, and may present as bone pain or as a pathological fracture.

Gastritis

Gastritis signifies an acute or chronic inflammation of the stomach. Our knowledge of the changes that occur in the gastric mucosa has been obtained in three ways: (1) by direct observation of the gastric mucosa in patients with gastrostomies, as in the famous cases of Alexis St Martin observed by Beaumont over a century ago, and the more recent subject Tom; (2) by gastroscopic observation; and (3) by histological examination of specimens removed at operation, biopsy or autopsy.

There is poor agreement between these different approaches, so that the classification of gastritis is difficult. If histological specimens are examined, it is very rare to find a normal stomach completely free from any signs of inflammation. In this sense 'gastritis' is almost an invariable finding in adults. However, there are gross departures from this 'normal' state of affairs, even if they do not give rise to symptoms. For these reasons the condition is best defined in histological terms as acute or chronic gastritis.

Acute Gastritis

The commonest form of acute inflammation of the gastric mucosa is that caused by the ingestion of irritant materials such as alcohol or drugs, e.g. aspirin and phenylbutazone. Acute gastritis may also occur during the course of specific infection such as diphtheria or influenza; a particularly severe variety may occur during the course of septicaemia. Bile is also irritant to the stomach and may cause an acute gastritis as a complication of gastric surgery.

Macroscopically, there is engorgement of the mucosa with swelling, patches of adherent mucus and sometimes small erosions. Microscopically, there is hyperaemia, infiltration with inflammatory cells, and desquamation of the superficial layer. In his original observations on Alexis St Martin, Beaumont noticed the considerable degree of inflammation that might occur in the stomach without symptoms. This finding has been repeatedly confirmed, suggesting that the gastric mucosa is a relatively insensitive tissue.

Clinical Features. The symptoms associated with acute inflammation of the stomach are anorexia, nausea, epigastric ache and heartburn; since the superficial layers of the gastric mucosa can regenerate within 72 hours, it seems unlikely that a single attack or even several attacks of acute gastritis could lead to permanent histological change in the stomach. Presumably for the same reason, the symptoms of acute gastritis are short-lived.

Gastritis cannot be diagnosed with certainty by radiological examination. At gastroscopy, the mucosa is reddened, swollen, easily damaged and friable.

Any inflammatory process is likely to decrease the acid output by depressing the activity of the parietal cells, and also by increasing the secretion of the alkaline non-parietal component. Acid secretion tends to recover after the inflammation has subsided.

Treatment. A patient who consumes alcohol to excess should obviously cease doing so and the symptoms will disappear in a few days, though it may be longer before the gastric mucosa returns to normal. Similarly, the gastritis associated with specific fevers disappears as infection subsides. The treatment of biliary gastritis is dealt with on page 378.

Chronic Gastritis

Two stages are recognised, according to the severity of the histological changes. In *chronic superficial gastritis* there is infiltration of the mucosa with plasma cells, eosinophils and neutrophils, and there is some atrophy of the superficial parts of the glands. In *chronic atrophic gastritis* there is more extensive inflammatory cell infiltration, with marked atrophy of the glandular structures, and a great diminution in the specific secretory cells.

Chronic gastritis is found in association with gastric ulcer and gastric carcinoma. It occurs invariably in pernicious anaemia, and also in some patients with thyroiditis and Addison's disease; in these patients it is believed that the atrophic changes are due to an autoimmune process, this concept being supported by histological evidence of lymphocytic and plasma cell infiltration, and the presence of circulating antibodies to the gastric mucosa and to other tissues.

Clinical Features. It is very doubtful whether atrophic gastritis can produce gastrointestinal symptoms. Its existence is usually suspected only because of an associated anaemia or diminished or absent secretion of acid or intrinsic factor.

Severe chronic gastritis may be diagnosed on barium meal examination, because the mucosal folds are smaller than normal and reduced in number or even completely absent as in pernicious anaemia. These appearances may be confirmed at gastroscopy when, in addition, the submucous plexus of veins may be seen through the thin mucosa. These atrophic appearances are constantly present in pernicious anaemia, and they are often seen in localised patches in patients with gastric ulcer and gastric carcinoma. The diagnosis can be confirmed by biopsy.

Treatment. No method is known for stimulating the mucosa to regenerate.

Carcinoma of the Stomach

Carcinoma of the stomach is one of the commonest malignant tumours of the gastrointestinal tract, although its incidence varies considerably in different parts of the world—for example, the tumour is frequent in Japan and relatively uncommon in the U.S.A. These variations have been attributed to environmental factors, such as trace elements in water, or differences in methods of food preparation: the incidence of gastric cancer in Japanese immigrants to America is much less than it is in Japan. Patients with pernicious anaemia have a 10 per cent chance of developing gastric cancer and this increased risk may extend to achlorhydria from other causes, including gastric surgery.

Pathology. Almost 70 per cent of all gastric cancers occur at the pylorus or in the antrum; the lesion does not spread to the duodenum. Such growths may produce symptoms of obstruction to the gastric outlet. Lesions of the body of the stomach often involve the greater curvature and produce a fungating ulcerating mass. Least common is a diffuse infiltrating lesion spreading throughout the body of the stomach and producing the so-called leather-bottle stomach. These are the descriptions of advanced cancer. In the early stages, when the carcinoma is confined to the mucosa, the lesion may be represented only by a depressed area with obliteration or distortion of the mucosal folds, by irregular ulceration on an elevated base, or by a small polypoid lesion. Such changes can be seen and a biopsy taken during gastroscopy at a stage when the cancer is potentially curable by resection. The tumour is generally an adenocarcinoma and spreads by direct extension through the stomach wall, by lymphatic permeation and by embolism via the portal vein to the liver and thence to the systemic bloodstream.

Gastric carcinoma may present as a malignant ulcer, and whether it is then the result of malignant transformation of a benign ulcer is debatable. Most authorities believe that chronic peptic ulcer rarely becomes malignant, and that malignant ulcers, however long they have been present, have always been malignant. Whatever the truth of the matter the problem in the individual case is to decide whether a given ulcer is benign or malignant.

Clinical Features. Loss of appetite, slight nausea and discomfort after meals occurring for the first time in middle age should always arouse suspicion. If the diagnosis is to be made early, then such patients require careful investigation. Early curable cancer may be missed at radiological examination or appearances may be misinterpreted; thus the only method of establishing a positive diagnosis is by gastroscopy and biopsies of suspicious areas. Unfortunately the majority of patients have advanced gastric carcinoma before they seek advice. In some there have been no symptoms; in others symptoms have been present for 6 months or even a year. Dyspepsia, which is at first vague, becomes troublesome with increasing anorexia and nausea, discomfort or pain, vomiting and weight loss. There may be cachexia and pallor, a mass may be palpable or peristalsis visible. The abdomen may be distended by ascites from peritoneal metastases. Sometimes it is the presence of metastases in the liver, pelvis or supraclavicular region which first brings the patient to the physician.

Carcinoma of the stomach should always be considered as a cause of unexplained iron deficiency anaemia in the middle-aged person or as an uncommon cause of haematemesis or melaena. Tumours at the cardia may cause dysphagia, and tumours at the gastric outlet may cause vomiting. In the infiltrating type of tumour, diarrhoea may occur because of rapid emptying from the stomach.

Radiological Examination. The commonest appearance is a filling defect in the antrum or body of the stomach (Fig. 8.2). If obstruction to the gastric outlet is present, it may not be possible to determine whether the lesion is benign or malignant until the stomach is aspirated and washed out. It may be difficult, if not impossible, to distinguish a malignant from a benign gastric ulcer; when doubt exists, and it commonly does, gastroscopy and biopsy should be performed. An early cancer may cause little more than distortion of the mucosal pattern which may be misinterpreted or go unobserved. A double contrast barium meal (p. 349) may overcome this difficulty. In the rare diffuse infiltrating scirrhous carcinoma, the radiograph is that of a rigid tube through which the barium pours rapidly into the intestine. If dysphagia is the presenting symptom, a lesion in the cardia will probably be found, but symptomless lesions in this area can be very easily missed.

Other Investigation. Gastroscopy and biopsy should always be carried out when X-ray examination leaves any room for doubt. Exfoliative cytology will confirm the diagnosis of cancer of the stomach if the stomach washings contain obvious malignant cells (p. 352). Secretory studies may show diminished secretion of acid, but this is not of diagnostic value. Examination of the blood may show hypochromic anaemia, with an elevated ESR. Finally, if these investigations are equivocal, laparotomy should be advised.

Treatment. The only curative treatment is gastrectomy, but it is usually only at laparotomy that the possibility of resection can be decided. Only about one-third of patients coming to operation are found to have tumours capable of removal; in the remainder it is possible to perform only a palliative procedure. This is worthwhile if pyloric obstruction is present, even if there are secondary deposits; such an operation relieves the distressing vomiting and gives the patient some comfort. A total gastrectomy may be required for tumours involving the upper part of the stomach. Careful preoperative treatment is essential; this may require the restoration of fluid and electrolyte balance and the correction of anaemia, while every effort should be made to improve nutrition, if necessary by an elemental diet or intravenous feeding.

Prognosis. The prognosis in carcinoma of the stomach is very poor and has shown little improvement in the last 40 years. The overall 5 year survival rate is probably not more than 5 per cent. Of all patients with cancer of the stomach, only a small percentage find their way to hospital; of these about two-thirds are fit for operation, and radical removal is possible in about half of those who come to surgery. Among those who survive an apparently successful resection, the 5 year survival rate is in the region of 20 per cent. Pending an entirely new approach to the problem, the only means currently available by which the prognosis can be improved is the detection of gastric cancer when it is at a curable stage; this requires a vigorous approach to the problem of dyspepsia in the middle-aged, including careful radiological and endoscopic examination and the critical follow-up of doubtful abnormalities.

Malignant Ascites

Carcinoma of the stomach may be associated with the exudation of fluid into the peritoneal cavity. This follows the deposition of malignant cells on the peritoneal surface and is a sign of gross spread of the disease. The fluid is rich in protein and its sediment contains malignant cells which may be identifiable on microscopy. Other tumours which may be associated with malignant ascites include carcinoma of the colon and carcinoma of the ovary.

Treatment is palliative. Relief of abdominal distension can be obtained by paracentesis, while instillation of antimitotic agents such as methotrexate may slow the rate of re-accumulation.

DISEASES OF THE PANCREAS

The pancreas is a gland producing exocrine secretions which play important roles in digestion and also endocrine secretions concerned with the regulation of carbohydrate metabolism. The exocrine tissue, composed of tubulo-acinar glands of serous cells forms almost the entire mass of the gland. The exocrine secretion (the pancreatic juice) is discharged into the intestine through the pancreatic duct, which usually enters the duodenum together with the common bile duct at the sphincter of Oddi; in about 10 per cent of individuals, however, the main outflow of the pancreatic juice reaches the duodenum by a separate duct.

The endocrine tissue is composed of specialised cells collected together in the small islets of Langerhans scattered throughout the gland, and accounts for only 1 per cent of the mass of the pancreas. The endocrine secretions include insulin, which is produced by the beta cells of the islets, and glucagon which is produced by the alpha cells; the functions of both are discussed in the chapter on diabetes mellitus.

Pancreatic juice is an alkaline secretion (pH 7·5–8·5) which is isotonic with plasma, the main cations being sodium and potassium while the main anion is bicarbonate. It contains enzymes which digest carbohydrate, fat and protein, the main ones being amylase, lipase and trypsin. These enzymes are elaborated by the serous cells of the pancreatic acini, and they are secreted in parallel concentrations; they all require an alkaline medium for optimal efficiency, so that theoretically digestion may be impaired if the bicarbonate content of the pancreatic juice is reduced.

Exocrine pancreatic secretion is stimulated partly through nervous and partly through hormonal mechanisms (p. 347), and a maximum flow is reached between two and three hours after a meal; in all, about 1 litre is secreted daily.

Investigation of the Pancreas

The pancreas is difficult to investigate. It is relatively inaccessible to direct methods of study and it cannot easily be examined by radiographic techniques.

Radiological Examination. A plain film of the abdomen may show calcification in the pancreas, and in acute pancreatitis there is often evidence of ileus in the duodenum and jejunum. A barium meal may show distortion of the mucosal folds of the duodenum or displacement of the stomach when the pancreas is enlarged by inflammation, cysts or tumours. An intravenous cholangiogram may show narrowing or distortion of the common bile duct due to neoplastic or inflammatory changes in the head of the pancreas.

Radioisotope studies following an intravenous injection of 75 selenomethionine (p. 350) may reveal defects of uptake that suggest destruction of acinar tissue due to tumour or chronic inflammation.

Selective arteriography of the coeliac and superior mesenteric arteries can show distortion and compression of vessels from some tumours, or may outline the abnormal vascular pattern of others.

Pancreatograms can be obtained during operation by cannulation of the duct and injection of contrast material. In expert hands retrograde pancreatograms can be made using fibreoptic duodenoscopy (ERCP p. 351).

Tests of Exocrine Pancreatic Function. DIRECT TESTS. Pancreatic function is tested by passing tubes into the stomach and duodenum under radiological control. The gastric juice is aspirated throughout the test so that it does not mix with the pancreatic secretions. Secretin and pancreozymin are given by intravenous injection and the pancreatic secretions are collected for one hour. Measurements are made of the volume of secretion, the bicarbonate concentration and the concentration of amylase or trypsin.

In pancreatic insufficiency low volumes of secretion may be obtained with reduction in the concentration and output of bicarbonate and enzymes. The test is also of use in excluding pancreatic disease as a cause of malabsorption. In patients with carcinoma of the pancreas, the duodenal aspirate may contain blood and cytological examination may reveal exfoliated malignant cells. Fibreoptic duodenoscopy may allow the direct collection of pancreatic secretion for cytological examination. The value of these tests is limited because of the technical difficulties involved and because early disease of the pancreas may not be detected.

INDIRECT TESTS. When pancreatic insufficiency is severe, the digestion of fat and protein is impaired and microscopy of the stool reveals abundant fat globules (steatorrhoea) and undigested meat fibres (creatorrhoea). This simple examination may be enough to detect pancreatic insufficiency in childhood but it is of less value in adults because fat globules and undigested meat fibres may be present in the stools of any patient with intestinal hurry. Steatorrhoea and creatorrhoea may be confirmed by chemical analysis of the faeces.

Tests of Endocrine Pancreatic Function. A diabetic response to a glucose tolerance test in steatorrhoea suggest a pancreatic cause for the malabsorption of fat. When carcinoma of the pancreas is suspected, an abnormal glucose tolerance test is a frequent and valuable finding in a condition difficult to diagnose.

Acute Pancreatitis

This is a serious disorder which arises from digestion of the pancreas by its own enzymes. It may proceed to haemorrhagic necrosis of pancreatic tissue with the formation of a local or generalised peritonitis. The disease is most common between the fourth and seventh decades with an equal sex incidence.

The exact mechanism which initiates the destruction of the pancreatic tissue has not been established. The frequent association between biliary tract disease and acute pancreatitis has given rise to the widely accepted theory that an obstruction at the sphincter of Oddi due to a gall-stone, oedema or spasm allows a reflux of bile along the pancreatic duct. This causes an activation of the enzymes trypsin and lipase leading to autodigestion of the pancreatic blood vessels and parenchyma. Although in only a small proportion of cases can a stone be found at operation or post-mortem, a bile-stained pancreas is seen in many cases of acute pancreatitis and a common terminal channel for both the bile and pancreatic ducts is usually present in fatal cases. It seems unlikely that infection plays an initial role as cultures made in early cases are usually sterile. Once the process has started, however, oedema, haemorrhage and fat necrosis may continue, with destruction of much of the pancreas, with the liberation of a serosanguineous exudate into the peritoneal cavity, including the lesser sac, and with the chemical splitting of fat deposits in the omentum and mesentery. In Britain about 60 per cent of cases appear to be associated with underlying biliary disease and an increasing number—over 20 per cent—with a history of alcoholic excess. The exact mechanism by which alcohol causes pancreatitis is unknown. In some countries, particularly the U.S.A. and South Africa, alcohol is a much more common cause of pancreatitis than in Britain. In a small proportion of cases, acute pancreatitis may result from obstruction of the pancreatic duct due to carcinoma. Occasionally it occurs after abdominal trauma or surgery, and rarely as a complication of mumps, hyperparathyroidism, pregnancy or hypothermia.

Clinical Features. The onset is sudden with agonising pain in the epigastrium or right hypochondrium. It often occurs within 12 to 24 hours following the consumption of alcohol or a large meal. The pain is usually persistent and radiates most frequently through to the back, to either shoulder, or to one of the iliac fossae before spreading to involve the whole abdomen. Nausea and vomiting are frequent. In severe cases profound shock soon supervenes; occasionally the patient may present with shock and without pain. In milder cases moderate fever occurs, and slight jaundice may develop, especially in cases with gall-stones.

Despite the severity of the pain, there may be little or no guarding of the abdominal muscles at first. Later the upper abdomen becomes tender and rigid as peritoneal irritation increases and the initial shock passes off.

Investigation. A most important point in the diagnosis of acute pancreatitis is for the practitioner to remember it as one of the causes of severe abdominal pain. About one-third of cases are proven for the first time at laparotomy, having been diagnosed as perforated peptic ulcer, acute intestinal obstruction or acute appendicitis. The condition may also simulate acute cholecystitis (with which it may coexist), and myocardial infarction. In the early stage of an acute case the determination of the serum amylase is of great diagnostic importance. Within the first few hours levels may be found in excess of 750 Somogyi units/100 ml (normal < 100 units/100 ml). Such amylase estimates are useful only in the early stages of the acute disease since the concentration may be normal in mild cases and subsiding cases. Moreover the issue may be confused because moderate elevation of the serum amylase may occur in other conditions such as perforated peptic ulcer and intestinal obstruction. The high serum amylase is short-lived because of rapid renal excretion. It follows that amylase measured in a 24-hour collection of urine may provide the diagnosis when serum levels are normal. A persistently raised serum amylase suggests the formation of a pseudocyst.

Biochemical findings may be helpful in the detection and monitoring of some complications. Hyperglycaemia is common in the first two days and hypocalcaemia may occur five to eight days after the attack because calcium is sequestered into the area of pancreatic necrosis.

A plain film of the abdomen may show evidence of ileus (p. 384), and barium meal and hypotonic duodenography often demonstrate oedema and displacement of the duodenum.

Treatment. When the diagnosis of acute pancreatitis can be established with certainty, the present tendency is to avoid operation in favour of conservative treatment. However, laparotomy is imperative if diagnostic uncertainty exists. Once the diagnosis is confirmed, the abdomen is closed without any definitive procedure being performed unless there is associated disease in the biliary tract.

Medical management consists of measures to combat shock, to relieve pain, to suppress pancreatic secretion and to prevent infection.

In the stage of shock, intravenous isotonic saline (1 to 2 l) is given initially followed by up to 4 l of plasma in the first 24 hours. In severe cases part of the requirement is given as blood. Total fluid replacement is assessed by the measurement of central venous pressure, haematocrit and urine output. The initial treatment of shock is followed by continuous parenteral electrolyte therapy until the ileus has resolved.

Intravenous injections of calcium may be required if hypocalcaemia develops and blood sugar should be monitored regularly so that developing diabetes can be treated promptly.

For the relief of pain, repeated injections of methadone (10 mg) or pethidine (100 mg) should be given. If pain is very severe, hypodermic injections of morphine (10–20 mg) may be required, but this drug, and pethidine to a lesser degree, may have the undesirable effect of causing spasm of the sphincter of Oddi. Nasogastric suction is instituted as a treatment for ileus. In addition it reduces the amount of acid entering the duodenum so that the stimulus for the production of secretin is greatly decreased.

Antibiotics may be administered with the object of preventing secondary bacterial infection of the damaged tissues. Corticosteroids have no specific place in the treatment of acute pancreatitis. Good results have been claimed for aprotinin, which inhibits proteolytic enzymes, and for glucagon, which suppresses pancreatic secretion and increases splanchic blood flow. Further studies of the use of both are required.

Complications. Haemorrhage into the gastrointestinal tract because of digestion of the duodenal wall, or obstruction of the duodenum by the swollen pancreatic head may necessitate emergency surgery. At a later stage surgery may be necessary for residual abscess, pseudocyst, or disease of the biliary tract.

Prognosis. About 20 per cent of patients die from the attack, nearly all the deaths occurring in those with haemorrhagic pancreatitis. Of those patients recovering only a minority experience recurrent episodes or insidiously develop chronic pancreatitis, whereas the chronic alcoholic who continues to drink and the person with untreated biliary disease will suffer recurrent attacks.

Chronic Pancreatitis

This condition is due either to the laying down of excessive fibrous tissue in the pancreas as the result of recurrent inflammatory changes or to atrophy of acinar tissue following obstruction of a main duct. It may follow repeated attacks of acute or subacute pancreatitis or be associated with chronic inflammation of the biliary tract. It may occur following the penetration of a chronic duodenal ulcer into the pancreas. In many cases some cause of obstruction of the main pancreatic duct is found, including traumatic stricture, ampullary papilloma and stone. In these conditions when fibrosis is present, it is most marked between the lobules of epithelial cells, and whereas the acinar tissue is destroyed, the islet cells are spared for a long time. Pancreatic fibrosis of an intralobular type may occur in haemochromatosis with replacement of the parenchyma and early atrophy of the islet tissue.

Clinical Features. These depend on the nature of the associated primary disease, the amount of destruction of the acinar and islet tissue and the degree of obstruction of the common bile duct caused by the fibrotic and sometimes enlarged head of the pancreas. Chronic pancreatitis most commonly occurs in males in the fifth and sixth decades and many of these are alcoholics.

Pancreatic pain may be so characteristic that the diagnosis may be suggested on the history alone. It may be located in the epigastrium or in the right or left subcostal areas. The characteristic feature, however, is radiation of pain to the back, relieved by crouching forward or by lying prone; sometimes the patient kneels crouching on the bed or leans forward over a chair to obtain relief. This type of pain occurs in a proportion of patients, but if such a description is elicited, a pancreatic cause should always be suspected. Characteristically the episodes of pain occur on the day after an occasion of alcoholic excess.

Diabetes is common and may be the presenting feature. The occasional patient presents with malabsorption and marked weight loss; there is chronic diarrhoea with an excess of fat and undigested muscle fibres in the stools. Symptoms may also result from complications such as jaundice or duodenal obstruction caused by enlargement of the pancreas.

Investigation. In a small proportion of cases of chronic pancreatitis the plain film of the abdomen shows calcification in the duct system or throughout the gland. The barium meal or hypotonic duodenography may show deformity of the duodenal cap as a result of oedema, and flattening and rigidity of the medial wall of the duodenum. Retrograde pancreatography during duodenoscopy has proved valuable in making a diagnosis in patients with unexplained abdominal pain. Pancreatic insufficiency may be suggested if steatorrhoea and an excessive output of faecal nitrogen are present on chemical analysis of the faeces collected over a period of five days. The diagnosis of pancreatic insufficiency is virtually certain if steatorrhoea is associated with a diabetic type of glucose tolerance curve, especially if xylose absorption is normal (p. 391). Serum amylase estimations are of little value in the diagnosis of chronic pancreatitis. Pancreatic function tests often demonstrate a low volume of secretion and reduced concentration of amylase and bicarbonate. The uptake in an isotope scan is poor and patchy or absent in advanced disease. Tests to demonstrate an increased salt content of sweat will be required if cystic fibrosis is suspected.

Treatment. It is imperative that the patient stops drinking alcohol and remains abstinent permanently. The diet should have a moderately low fat content. If steatorrhoea is present the fat should be reduced to about 45 g daily and pancreatic extracts should be taken both between and with meals.

Insulin is required when, as is often the case, diabetes mellitus supervenes, and is necessary to allow the patient to continue to have sufficient carbohydrate to compensate for the decreased calorie intake associated with fat restriction.

Surgery should be contemplated for the relief of intractable pain. Drainage of the pancreatic duct into the small bowel, removal of part or most of the pancreas, or sphincterotomy are the most usual procedures. The ultimate result is so dependent on the patient's ability to give up alcohol that operation is not worth while in the patient who cannot do so. The indication for surgery is stronger when cysts and the possibility of cancer of the pancreas are present. The best results are obtained in those patients who are shown to have stones in the bile ducts or stenosis of the ampulla of Vater. Correction of these abnormalities will result in recovery of pancreatic function and the relief of symptoms.

Cystic Fibrosis of the Pancreas

This is an autosomal recessive disease characterised by generalised dysfunction of all exocrine glands, including those which secrete mucus. Blockage by viscid secretion causes cystic changes in the pancreas and also bronchiectasis.

Clinical Features. Frequently cystic fibrosis presents with repeated attacks of respiratory infection in early life. Defective pancreatic enzymes give rise to malabsorption of fat and bulky, foamy and foul-smelling stools. The child is often poorly nourished. Bronchiectasis, pulmonary fibrosis and, ultimately, right ventricular failure may ensue.

The diagnosis is established by the finding of an increase in the concentration of sodium in sweat to above 80 mmol/*l*.

Treatment and Prognosis. Both the child and the parents require long-term support. The treatment of pancreatic insufficiency is dicussed above. Antibiotic therapy, adapted to the sensitivity of the organism and supplemented with physiotherapy, requires careful supervision. In the newborn, small intestinal obstruction from tenacious meconium may require surgical treatment.

Until the advent of antibiotics the prognosis was very poor and most children dies before puberty. However, with skilled medical treatment, an increasing number of patients are surviving into adult life. Genetic advice should be made available to the parents (p. 21).

Pancreatic Cysts

A *pancreatic pseudocyst* may occur about three weeks after the onset of acute pancreatitis or follow trauma to the pancreas. Usually the cyst occupies the lesser sac and displaces the stomach. It may cause obstruction particularly of the duodenum. On examination there is a smooth tender mass in the upper abdomen. The diagnosis is made on this examination, a persistent leucocytosis and raised serum amylase; a mass may be seen on plain X-ray or defined by ultrasound scanning. Barium meal examination may show displacement of the stomach. Pseudocysts which fail to resolve spontaneously within six weeks are treated surgically by drainage into the stomach or small intestine.

Intrapancreatic or retention cysts are usually small and multiple and are found in chronic pancreatitis. These cysts may cause abdominal pain but the diagnosis is difficult to make except by retrograde pancreatography. Symptomatic cysts are treated surgically.

Occasionally a cyst is secondary to carcinoma.

Tumours of the Pancreas

Carcinoma is the main tumour of the pancreas and it arises from the acinar epithelium of from the ampulla (cholangiocarcinoma, p. 466). Adenomas arise from the islets of Langerhans and are rare tumours.

Carcinoma of the Pancreas

This is an adenocarcinoma of scirrhous nature and in two-thirds there is involvement of the head of the gland. It tends to spread early to neighbouring structures and to the liver. The condition is more common in males than in females, and occurs most frequently between the ages of 55 and 70 years.

Clinical Features. Epigastric pain, which is one of the earliest and most significant symptoms, may occasionally be absent throughout the course of the disease. The pain is variable in type but is characteristically dull and boring and radiates through to the back. It is often intensified by food and by lying supine, especially at night. It may be relieved by crouching forward. Vague dyspeptic symptoms are common and include anorexia, nausea, discomfort and sometimes vomiting. These symptoms may be the only manifestations until metastases occur.

Other clinical features depend largely on the site of the growth. In the majority of cases with involvement of the head of the pancreas jaundice is the presenting feature and may be painless and progressive. A large firm liver eventually develops. An abdominal mass is present in one-quarter of all patients and occasionally a distended gall-bladder is palpable or ascites can be detected. Jaundice may not appear at all in cases where the lesion affects mainly the body and tail of the pancreas. The symptoms of diabetes mellitus may occasionally be the presenting feature in this disease.

Carcinoma of the pancreas is a rapidly progressive emaciating disease especially in cases in which the head is involved, when death usually occurs within six months of the onset of obstructive jaundice.

Investigation. Radiological examination by barium meal or hypotonic duodenography may show distortion of the duodenal wall in carcinoma arising from the head of the pancreas and a forward displacement of the stomach in lesions of the body, but by then the tumour is almost certainly inoperable. Intraveous cholangiography in the absence of jaundice may reveal distortion of the common bile duct. In ampullary carcinoma fluctuating jaundice is common, and blood may be aspirated from the duodenum and be detected on testing the stool. Pancreatic function tests should be carried out and where facilities for exfoliative cytology are available the duodenal aspirate should be examined for malignant cells. In all cases where the symptoms are suggestive or where the cause of obstructive jaundice cannot be firmly established, exploratory laparotomy should be advised. Unless this is done, those cases of stone in the common bile duct in which pain is not a prominent feature may be erroneously diagnosed as carcinoma.

Endoscopy and scanning are discussed on pages 351 and 350.

Treatment. This is by surgical means. In carcinoma of the pancreas radical surgery is rarely possible, but a bypass may be fashioned to relieve the obstructive jaundice. Such patients, however, rarely live more than one year. In early cases of ampullary carcinoma a cure may be achieved by excision of the duodenum and head of the pancreas.

Islet-cell Tumours

A benign adenoma may arise rarely from the beta cells of the islets and produce hyperinsulinism with attacks of spontaneous hypoglycaemia (p. 573). Even more rare are tumours, usually malignant, from other islet cells which elaborate polypeptides, e.g. gastrin or allied substances, the secretion of which into the blood causes a variety of syndromes. The most common is the Zollinger-Ellison syndrome (p. 376). The treatment of these conditions is by removal of the adenoma where possible.

DISEASES OF THE SMALL INTESTINE

Malabsorption

A number of disorders result in malabsorption of one or more of the essential nutrients, electrolytes, minerals or vitamins. Some or all of the following features may ensue: diarrhoea, abdominal pain and distension, loss of weight, anaemia, or other evidence of specific deficiency. However, some patients complain only of vague ill-health, and the diagnosis may not be made for many years.

The sequence followed in this section is first to review the basic processes of absorption and the means of testing them. Then the ways in which the processes of absorption can be deranged are discussed. Finally, the clinical presentation and treatment of malabsorption in general and then of specific disorders are described.

Absorption and Tests of Absorption

Fat Absorption. This takes place predominantly in the duodenum and upper jejunum. Dietary fat occurs largely in the form of insoluble long-chain triglycerides. These are emulsified mechanically in the stomach and by detergents (mainly bile) in the small intestine. Then pancreatic lipase hydrolyses the triglycerides to monoglyceride and fatty acids. Pancreatic bicarbonate is required to maintain the optimum pH for this hydrolysis and for the next step in fat absorption, the solubilisation of the monoglycerides and fatty acids by bile acids. This consists of their incorporation into micelles which orientate the fatty acid and monoglyceride in such a way that they can be presented to the intestinal mucosal cell for absorption. Once in the absorptive cell, the monoglycerides and fatty acids are reformed (re-esterified) into triglycerides which then coalesce into chylomicrons. The chylomicron passes out of the cell to be transported by the lymphatic system into the blood (p. 424).

TEST OF FAT ABSORPTION. Fat excretion in the stool is measured over a 5-day period, whilst the patient is receiving a normal diet (which contains less than 100 g fat per day). The upper limit of normal for faecal fat excretion is 7 g per day and any value above this constitutes steatorrhoea.

The fat-soluble vitamins A, D and K are absorbed in the same way as dietary fat and measurement of their absorption can be used as an indirect assessment of fat absorption. For example, the plasma vitamin A level can be measured after oral administration of retinol for two or three days.

Carbohydrate Absorption. Carbohydrate in the diet is in the form of starch (60 per cent), lactose (10 per cent) and sucrose (30 per cent). These are digested to glucose, galactose and fructose. Glucose and galactose are absorbed into the cell by active transport mechanisms, the process requiring sodium ions and energy. The fructose molecule is too large to move across the cell membrane by simple diffusion and it is thought that it must be facilitated by a carrier.

TESTS OF CARBOHYDRATE ABSORPTION. *The glucose tolerance test* (p. 562) is sometimes used and the absence of a rise in blood sugar can indicate malabsorption, but there are so many variables that the test is difficult to interpret in the context of absorption.

In the *xylose absorption test*, 25 g of d-xylose are given orally after an overnight fast. Only a small proportion is metabolised within the body and 5–8 g should be excreted in the urine over the next 5 hours.

In the *lactose tolerance test*, 50 g of lactose are given orally and blood glucose levels are measured as in the glucose tolerance test. Normally this disaccharide is broken down by intestinal lactase to glucose and galactose which are absorbed so that blood glucose levels rise. If the enzyme lactase is deficient in the intestinal mucosa, there may be no rise in blood glucose and the patient may complain of colic and diarrhoea because the unabsorbed lactose acts as an osmotic agent in the gut being broken down by colonic bacteria.

Protein Absorption. Initial hydrolysis of dietary protein molecules is performed by gastric pepsin and pancreatic enzymes. Further hydrolysis of peptides takes place at the brush border and a mixture of peptides and amino acids is absorbed into the cell. A large amount of protein, other than dietary, enters the lumen of the gastrointestinal tract each day, derived from various secretions, desquamated cells and the exudation of plasma proteins. These proteins are absorbed by the same mechanisms as dietary protein.

TESTS OF PROTEIN ABSORPTION. Measurement of the amount of nitrogen in the stool provides a very crude estimate of the above processes. Stools are collected for 3 to 5 days and no more than 2·5 g of nitrogen per day should be excreted.

An excessive loss of nitrogen in the stool can result from the loss of albumin and other plasma proteins into the lumen of the tract. This is termed *protein losing enteropathy* and it can be detected by labelling serum proteins with radioactive chromium and measuring radioactivity in the stool.

A low serum albumin level in the absence of hepatic or renal disease may indictate protein malabsorption or protein losing enteropathy.

Folate Absorption. Folate is absorbed throughout the small intestine by an active transport process. In tests of folate absorption a large quantity of folic acid is given to saturate body stores, then a test dose is given orally. Folate is then measured in the blood or urine by microbiological assay. Some tests make use of radioactive folic acid.

Vitamin B_{12} Absorption. Dietary vitamin B_{12} binds to intrinsic factor in the stomach and proceeds along the intestine in this bound form to be absorbed from the terminal ileum. In the *Schilling test* the fasting patient is given a small dose (1 μg) of radioactive vitamin B_{12}. Two hours later a large dose (1,000 μg) of non-radioactive B_{12} is given by injection and the urine is collected for 24 hours. The injected vitamin B_{12} saturates the plasma so that in a normal subject more than 16 per cent of the absorbed radioactive vitamin B_{12} is excreted in the urine. A normal result is also obtained if intrinsic factor is given together with radioactive vitamin B_{12} to a patient with Addisonian pernicious anaemia but not in patients in whom there is malabsorption of vitamin B_{12} due to disease of the terminal ileum.

Absorption of Other Substances. Calcium is absorbed in the upper small intestine by an active mechanism which requires vitamin D. Iron is also absorbed by the proximal small intestine in an ionic form and as haem. Suitable diagnostic tests of the absorption of these substances are not available but the degree of absorption can be inferred from the serum levels. For example, a low serum iron level may indicate malabsorption if there is no evidence of blood loss or inadequate intake. Similarly a low serum calcium level may indicate vitamin D deficiency due to malabsorption.

Causes of Malabsorption

1. **Disorders of Intraluminal Digestion.** Here there is an insufficiency of a digestive enzyme or detergent within the lumen. The main feature is steatorrhoea with deficiency of fat soluble vitamins. Since the intestinal mucosal cells are normal, there is no impairment of absorption of other substances less dependent on intraluminal digestion, e.g. carbohydrate, protein, vitamin B_{12}, folate and iron.

(*a*) PANCREATIC INSUFFICIENCY. A deficiency of pancreatic lipase causes malabsorption of fat, for example, in chronic pancreatitis, cystic fibrosis and carcinoma of the pancreas.

(*b*) DEFICIENCY OF BILE ACIDS. This may occur in two circumstances:

(i) *Interruption of the Enterohepatic Circulation of Bile Acids.* When there is disease or resection of the terminal ileum, as in Crohn's disease, bile acids cannot be reabsorbed (p. 425). Instead they pass into the colon and are lost in the faeces.

Whilst in the colon they interfere with water and electrolyte absorption and this results in diarrhoea. The loss of bile acids cannot be compensated for by the liver synthesising more bile acids. There is therefore an inadequate concentration of bile acid in the upper jejunum and micelles cannot be formed.

(ii) *Colonisation of the Small Bowel by Bacteria.* The upper part of the small intestine is practically sterile under normal conditions. If a large number of bacteria are present (p. 396) then some of these bacteria may deconjugate bile acids, i.e. the glycine or taurine is split from the molecule. The deconjugated bile acids are inefficient in micelle formation and so steatorrhoea results.

Colonisation can affect other aspects of the intraluminal phase. For example, bacteria can utilise amino acids which are about to be absorbed and they may also take up vitamin B_{12} so that it is unavailable for absorption.

(c) DISTURBANCES OF GASTRIC FUNCTION. After gastric surgery it is possible for the correct enzymes, detergents and electrolytes to be delivered into the intestinal lumen and yet malabsorption may occur. This is because gastric emptying is no longer co-ordinated with the correct stage of digestion. For example, after gastroenterostomy or a Polya partial gastrectomy, bile and pancreatic juice may be delivered after food from the stomach has already passed down the efferent loop.

2. **Disorders of Transport in the Mucosal Cell.** In these disorders, the intraluminal digestive phase is normal, but the absorptive cells are not, because of:

(a) *Generalised disorders* such as coeliac disease, tropical sprue, giardiasis and extensive Crohn's disease. In these conditions, because the mucosa is damaged, it is usual to find widespread disturbances of absorption involving, for example, xylose, folate, vitamin B_{12}, iron, calcium and amino acids in addition to steatorrhoea.

(b) *Specific Disorders.* Here the mucosa looks normal but a specific substance is malabsorbed because of the absence of a particular enzyme. Thus there may be malabsorption of lactose because of an insufficiency of lactase in the mucosa. Another example is the malabsorption of vitamin B_{12} because of a lack of intrinsic factor in pernicious anaemia.

3. **Disorders of Transport from the Mucosal Cell.** These are rare and result from the blockage of the lymphatic system which is responsible for the transfer of chylomicrons from the absorptive cell to the systemic circulation. This may occur in abdominal lymphoma or in the rare condition of primary lymphangiectasia in which the mesenteric lymphatic system is abnormal.

Clinical Features and Diagnosis of Malabsorption

The patient can present in various ways. In severe forms there may be general malnutrition, with loss of weight and energy and a slow deterioration in health or, in a child, a failure to grow and thrive. Abdominal distension is often a striking feature. *Steatorrhoea* may be the presenting symptom. The patient complains of diarrhoea, with the passage of loose, pale, bulky and offensive stools which float on water, so that to cleanse the toilet-pan may require several flushes from the cistern. This difficulty is almost pathognomonic of steatorrhoea. The patient may have an anaemia which is the direct consequence of a deficiency of iron, cyanocobalamin or of folate. Haemorrhagic phenomena due to a deficiency of vitamin K may be an occasional presenting feature. Tetany may occur as a result of hypocalcaemia. The features of rickets or osteomalacia and various other disorders due to deficiency of vitamins may be noted, such as sore tongue, angular stomatitis and dry and atrophic skin. Oedema may occur as a consequence of hypoalbuminaemia. In other patients, malabsorption may be suspected because of gastric surgery or intestinal resection. In patients with mild malabsorption, there may be no disturbance of bowel function and the condition may be diagnosed only after investigation for non-specific abdominal complaints or anaemia.

The diagnosis may be suspected as a result of a barium follow-through examination in a patient with abdominal symptoms. The small intestine shows dilated loops with flocculation and segmentation of barium (Fig. 8.4).

Malabsorption is confirmed by the tests of absorption which may also provide a clue as to the basic cause of the disorder. For example, malabsorption of several substances is likely when there is a generalised disorder of the absorptive cells.

Biopsy of the small intestine (p. 352) may be normal, which excludes coeliac disease, or it may show subtotal villous atrophy, which is diagnostic of coeliac disease. Partial villous atrophy can occur in a variety of disorders, such as tropical sprue, Crohn's disease and in mild cases of coeliac disease. If the intestinal biopsy is normal, other investigations may be necessary to provide the diagnosis—for example, pancreatic function tests (p. 384) or the culture of intestinal aspirates for bacteria.

Treatment of Malabsorption

A gluten-free diet must be prescribed in coeliac disease. Pancreatic insufficiency is treated by pancreatic supplements (p. 388). Insufficiency of bile salts should not be treated with oral bile salts because these would pass into the colon, interfere with salt and water absorption, and so worsen the diarrhoea. The effect of the endogenous bile salts on the colon is counteracted by giving the binding agent cholestyramine in a dose of up to 12 g per day. In addition, a low fat diet should be given because cholestyramine will not correct the steatorrhoea.

In severe forms of malabsorptive disease, it may be necessary to treat dehydration and electrolyte deficiency by intravenous infusions.

Replacement therapy is often necessary for those patients with anaemia, bone disease or coagulation defects. Folic acid and iron supplements are given orally and vitamin B_{12} by a monthly injection. Vitamin D and calcium supplements may be required. Calcium is normally given as gluconate or lactate by mouth, but when there is tetany 10 ml of 10 per cent calcium gluconate is given slowly intravenously. Glossitis and cheilosis are indications for the administration of vitamin B complex.

The Principal Disorders Causing Malabsorption

Coeliac Disease

Coeliac disease is characterised by an abnormal mucosa in the small intestine which results in the malabsorption of several nutrients. In most cases the abnormality is due to gluten, a protein contained in wheat and rye flour. The toxic agent is gliadin, a polypeptide component of gluten. In some way as yet unexplained it damages the mucosa of the small intestine in susceptible individuals.

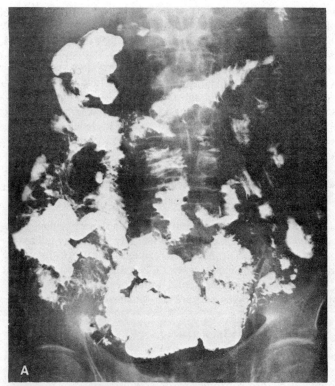

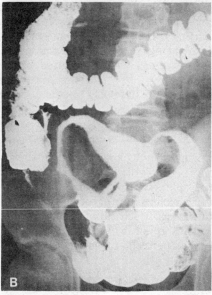

A. Malabsorption. Note dilated loops, segmentation and flocculation.

B. Crohn's disease. Note narrowed segments.

Fig. 8.4

Clinical Features. Gluten-induced enteropathy usually begins in the first three years of life. The child ceases to thrive and becomes fractious and irritable, the stools become voluminous and pale and as the disorder progresses growth is retarded, iron deficiency anaemia develops, and the abdomen becomes distended. On the other hand, the disorder may manifest itself for the first time in adult life. In adults, the presenting symptoms range from those of a mild anaemia and listlessness of long duration, to a florid malabsorptive state developing rapidly over a period of weeks or months. The commonest features are diarrhoea, weight loss and anaemia, the anaemia being usually due to combined deficiency of folic acid and iron. Gluten-induced enteropathy appears to predispose to the development of lymphomas and other forms of malignancy in the alimentary tract; colicky abdominal pain and unexpected weight loss in a previously well-controlled patient with malabsorption should arouse suspicion of these complications.

Treatment. A gluten-free diet must be given for many years or for life. This can result in histological improvement in the intestinal mucosa and improvement in absorption. If a small amount of gluten remains in the diet, the patient may fail to respond, and so the patient is given strict diet sheets and recipes for the use of gluten-free flour. A booklet produced by the Coeliac Society (P.O. Box 181, London) is of great value in this regard. In patients who fail to respond it may be necessary to use corticosteroids. Mineral and vitamin supplements are also given when indicated.

Lactose Intolerance

This disorder is being seen more often in Britain because immigrant Asian and African races have insufficient lactase in the mucosa of the small intestine to digest the large amounts of lactose consumed in this country.

The patient complains of abdominal discomfort, colic and diarrhoea after the ingestion of milk or milk products. The symptoms can be reproduced by the lactose tolerance test (p. 391) and the condition responds to the reduction of lactose in the diet.

Bacterial Colonisation of the Small Intestine

The effects of this proliferation have been discussed on page 393. The presentation is with anaemia due to vitamin B_{12} deficiency or with diarrhoea and nutritional deficiencies. The diagnosis depends on the radiological demonstration of a lesion causing stasis in the intestine; these include jejunal diverticula, a long afferent ('blind') loop after gastrectomy or gastroenterostomy, Crohn's disease, stricture formation and subacute obstruction. Other causes are a fistula between colon and small intestine or disordered peristalsis in the small intestine such as may occur in scleroderma.

Culture of jejunal aspirate supports the diagnosis, which is confirmed by the correction of steatorrhoea and vitamin B_{12} malabsorption by the administration of broad spectrum antibiotics. Occasionally surgical correction of an abnormality may be required.

Crohn's Disease

This disease is characterised by localised areas of non-specific, granulomatous inflammation of the bowel. It was formerly termed regional ileitis, since it was considered to be a disease confined to the terminal ileum. However, the eponymous designation 'Crohn's disease' is preferable since it is now known that it can affect the alimentary tract from the mouth to the anus, the sites most commonly involved being, in order of frequency, terminal ileum, terminal ileum and right side of colon, colon alone, ileum and jejunum. The disease may occur at any age, but most commonly between the ages of 20 and 40; it affects both sexes equally. In its chronic form, it is a debilitating disease which often interferes profoundly with a patient's life requiring repeated admission to hospital for medical and surgical treatment.

Aetiology. The cause is unknown. No specific organism has been identified from the bowel content, the bowel wall or the regional lymph nodes. One of the histological characteristics of the disease is the presence of granulomas composed of collections of epithelioid and giant cells. These granulomas closely resemble those found both in tuberculosis and sarcoidosis, thus raising the possibility that the three diseases are related. However, Crohn's disease can be sharply distinguished from tuberculosis because of the absence of caseation in the affected areas. Although the histological differentiation from sarcoidosis is more difficult, it is now accepted that these diseases are not related, since the clinical course is so different. Like sarcoidosis, however, patients with Crohn's disease show deficiences in delayed hypersensitivity. A current hypothesis is that Crohn's disease is the consequence of an abnormal immune response in the gut wall to an unidentified antigen. Crohn's disease, ankylosing spondylitis and ulcerative colitis all occur more commonly than might be expected amongst the families of patients with Crohn's disease, suggesting that all three diseases share a common but incomplete genetic basis.

Pathology. Although the disease may affect any part of the alimentary canal, the terminal ileum is most often involved. Macroscopically, the bowel is engorged and oedematous so that the lumen is markedly narrowed, sometimes enough to produce obstruction; the mucosa is oedematous, showing a 'cobble-stone' pattern with linear ulceration and fissuring. Characteristically, these changes are patchy; even when a relatively short segment of bowel is affected, it can be seen that the inflammatory process is interrupted by islands of normal mucosa occurring in the diseased area, the change from normal mucosa to the affected part being abrupt. The lesions may be discontinuous over a length of the bowel, a small lesion separated in this way from a major area of involvement being referred to as a 'skip' lesion. The affected lymph nodes are enlarged and the mesentery thickened. Microscopically, inflammatory change involves all coats of the bowel wall. All grades of inflammation may be seen and characteristically there is oedema and hyperplasia of the lymphoid follicles. Granulomas are seen in about 50 per cent of cases. Another feature is the presence of deep clefts or fissures opening on to the mucosal surface and sometimes passing through the entire thickness of the bowel wall. These clefts are responsible for the fistula formation which is such a characteristic feature of the disease; fistulae may develop between adjacent loops of bowel or between affected segments of bowel and the bladder, uterus or vagina, or may present as a faecal fistula through an abdominal incision as a complication of surgical treatment.

Clinical Features. The clinical features vary and depend in part on the site and extent of the bowel affected; many other diseases may be mimicked. Crohn's disease may present acutely with features indistinguishable from acute appendicitis. At laparotomy the terminal ileum is red and oedematous and provided the abdomen is closed without resection the prognosis is relatively good.

In the chronic form of the disease, pain is the commonest symptom and may be due either to peritoneal involvement, obstruction or both. Since the terminal ileum and right side of the colon are most commonly affected, this type of pain occurs most frequently in the right lower quadrant and it may be associated with local tenderness or guarding. A mass is palpable by abdominal and frequently by rectal examination. This consists of inflamed loops of bowel bound together, possibly including an abscess, and may be of any size. Colicky pain suggests obstruction, and may be associated with nausea and vomiting and excessive borborygmi. Indeed, recurrent episodes of colic due to attacks of subacute obstruction are a prominent feature in the life history of a patient with Crohn's disease; however, severe acute obstruction is uncommon.

Malabsorption occurs for a variety of reasons in Crohn's disease. The enterohepatic bile salt circulation may be interrupted by disease or resection of the ileum. Other areas of the small intestine may be involved, thus reducing the surface area for absorption. Strictures and fistulae may lead to bacterial colonisation of the small intestine. The inflamed mucosa may allow plasma proteins to be lost so that there is a protein losing enteropathy.

Diarrhoea is frequent, but is rarely so marked as in ulcerative colitis. The stools may be formed or loose, and rarely contain frank blood, mucus or pus unless the colon is involved. A diagnostic feature, when present, is the occurrence of anal lesions such as oedematous skin tags or perianal abscesses and fistulae; they are more common when the colon is affected.

Weight loss is frequent and most patients have a low-grade fever and moderate anaemia. Clubbing of the fingers may be present. A number of other manifestations may occur, including arthritis, ankylosing spondylitis, iritis, aphthous stomatitis and erythema nodosum; the relationship between these disorders and the bowel is not clear. Abnormal liver function tests are relatively common, while renal complications include hydronephrosis due to involvement of the right ureter in an inflammatory mass.

Radiological Examination. Barium meal and follow-through examination may show alteration of the mucosal pattern, deep ulceration or the pathognomonic 'string sign' due to marked narrowing of a segment of affected bowel (Fig. 8.4). The lesions tend to be discontinuous along the length of the bowel. A barium enema should be carried out since the disease may affect the small bowel and the colon simultaneously. In about 50 per cent of cases, the caecum will show radiological abnormalities. In some instances there will be segmental areas of deep ulceration or stricture formation elsewhere in the colon, and occasionally the entire colon is involved so that the radiological appearances may be indistinguishable from ulcerative colitis.

Other Investigation. Pus cells and red blood corpuscles may be found on microscopic examination of the faeces, but culture of the stool yields no specific organism. Moderate anaemia is usually present because of blood loss, while protein loss from the inflamed, ulcerated mucosa may cause hypoproteinaemia. Vitamin B_{12} absorption is likely to be impaired if there is extensive disease of the terminal ileum, and this can be confirmed by an abnormal Schilling test (p. 392). The diagnosis may be confirmed either by rectal biopsy or by excision of perianal skin tags; a rectal biopsy will sometimes show the characteristic granulomatous lesions although the mucosa appears normal to the naked eye.

Differential Diagnosis. The symptoms, signs and radiological findings are usually sufficient to suggest a lesion in the lower part of the small bowel. The other common diseases in this part of the intestinal tract are appendicitis or an appendix abscess and carcinoma of the caecum. In the acute phase, it may be impossible to distinguish between these possibilities, so that a laparotomy may be necessary. In patients with a chronic illness, the diagnosis may be established by further investigation—for instance, a barium enema examination or by biopsy of the rectum or perianal skin lesions. Although tuberculosis of the ileo-caecal region is becoming rare in Britain it may occur in the immigrant population and should be borne in mind because of the possibility of cure. Ileo-caecal tuberculosis usually occurs in association with an obvious pulmonary lesion so that the diagnosis is suggested by the chest X-ray; however, it can sometimes occur in patients in whom the primary lung lesion is minimal and has been overlooked. A 'negative' tuberculin test is common in patients with Crohn's disease and excludes an active tuberculous process. Sometimes no conclusive proof of Crohn's disease is obtained, and the diagnosis can only be presumptive; such patients should be kept under observation until the natural history of the illness declares itself.

Treatment. Crohn's disease is a chronic condition with remissions and relapses over many years. There is no known cure at present and treatment is largely a matter of managing particular problems as they arise and improving the general condition of the patient.

General Measures. A low residue diet will reduce the frequency of intestinal colic, while diarrhoea may be reduced by the use of codeine, 30 mg four times daily. When the terminal ileum is extensively diseased or has been resected, cholestyramine will reduce the diarrhoea due to the cathartic effect of the unabsorbed bile salts on the colon; hydroxocobalamin should be given to such patients for life since vitamin B_{12} will not be absorbed.

Malabsorption with steatorrhoea may occur in patients with extensive involvement of the small intestine, contributing to weight loss and inanition. A low fat diet is then required and a course of oral antibiotics if bacterial colonisation of the upper intestine is suspected. Supplements of iron, folic acid, calcium, vitamins and electrolytes, especially potassium, may also be necessary. Hypoproteinaemia may require plasma or blood infusions in addition to a high protein diet.

An elemental (no residue) diet will relieve the symptoms of partial obstruction and will restore nutrition. It is useful also in preoperative preparation, particularly for patients with external fistulas.

Drugs. Corticosteroids may induce remission in patients with active disease. Prednisolone should be given in a dose of 40–60 mg daily in divided doses for 1 or 2 weeks depending on response, and the dose gradually reduced thereafter to 10–20 mg daily for 4 to 6 weeks and then withdrawn. Every effort should be made to stop the drug, but in the occasional case this may be difficult because of early relapse when the dose is reduced. In these circumstances, the effect of sulphasalazine (2–4 g daily) is worth a trial, much as it is used in ulcerative colitis (p. 410). In contrast to colitis, oral antibiotics may be of some benefit, and a course of ampicillin, 1–2 g daily for 4 to 6 weeks can be tried, especially in patients with mild disease or in those not responding to prednisolone. Treatment with immunosuppressant drugs has been used with variable success in patients unresponsive to other forms of therapy.

Surgical Treatment. Although attacks of subacute obstruction can usually be managed conservatively by intestinal decompression and intravenous feeding (p.

401), operation may be necessary if attacks occur frequently. Surgery may also be required because of abscess or fistula formation, the principal alternatives being resection of the diseased segment or a bypass procedure. With localised disease, resection yields better results than bypass, but with extensive disease massive resection may result in malabsorption. Recurrence of the disease is always a danger, and therefore as much bowel as possible should be preserved. Resection nevertheless is indicated for the management of intestinal, vesical and vaginal fistulae. When the colon is extensively involved a total proctocolectomy as in ulcerative colitis may be the procedure of choice, though less extensive resection, for example a hemicolectomy, may suffice for localised disease.

Intestinal Obstruction

Intestinal obstruction may be complete or incomplete, acute or chronic, intermittent or continuous. The most important point to decide is whether the obstruction is *simple* or associated with *strangulation*. The latter occurs when there is interference with the blood supply to the intestine, as when the bowel is trapped or twisted. Urgent relief is required if the dangers of gangrene, perforation and peritonitis are to be avoided.

Causes. Obstruction may be mechanical, when the lumen of the bowel is blocked, or paralytic, when the propulsive power of the bowel is lost. In general the former type will require surgical relief, while the latter may respond to conservative measures, but the distinction is not always clear cut. Sometimes the mechanically obstructed bowel becomes exhausted and non-contractile, or it perforates at the site of the obstruction or proximally, the resultant peritonitis being responsible for paralysis of the adjacent bowel loops.

Mechanical Obstruction. At all ages adhesions and hernias are common causes of obstruction. In the young, intussusception is a frequent cause, while in the elderly, volvulus, tumours of the large bowel and diverticular disease account for a large proportion of cases. Impaction of faeces in the rectum presents with the picture of intestinal obstruction in the aged or bedridden patient. It is important to remember that acute appendicitis can mimic intestinal obstruction.

Paralytic obstruction or ileus occurs temporarily after any abdominal operation and is a feature of shock, spinal injury and hypotension. Commonly it is due to peritonitis.

Fluid and Electrolyte Changes. In obstruction of the upper small bowel, fluids and electrolytes are lost because of vomiting. When the obstruction is lower down, there is stagnation in the distended bowel loops, normal absorption from the gut is interrupted, and the body is deprived of fluid even in the absence of vomiting.

Biochemically, there is haemoconcentration with loss of water and electrolytes, particularly chloride, sodium and potassium. Elderly patients may develop secondary renal failure and this will add to the electrolyte imbalance. A vicious circle develops as increasing obstruction raises the tension in the bowel and further diminishes absorption; then increasing electrolyte imbalance interferes with intestinal peristalsis rendering the obstruction more complete. Recovery is heralded by diuresis, signifying return of peristalsis and re-absorption of fluid from the lumen of the bowel.

Clinical Features. *Pain.* In mechanical obstruction this is colicky and often originates at or about the site of the obstruction. Episodes of pain are accompanied by loud borborygmi. The advent of constant severe pain is indicative of strangulation. Paralytic obstruction is associated with a dull constant pain in an abdomen which is ominously silent.

Vomiting. This is copious in high obstructions and may be late or absent in obstructions of low small bowel or large bowel. The effortless trickle of foul-smelling fluid from the corner of the mouth of the lethargic patient is seen in untreated paralytic ileus, whereas in mechanical obstruction vomiting is projectile and intermittent.

Distension. This may be absent or confined to some loops of the bowel which can be seen in the thin patient as ridges across the abdomen forming the so-called ladder pattern. Diffuse distension is late and often indicative of a large bowel obstruction.

Bowel movements. In complete obstruction neither faeces nor flatus is passed. In high obstructions, the bowels may continue to move unaided or with enemas because of residual contents below the obstruction, while in large bowel obstruction, spurious diarrhoea may be due to an out-going of faecal-stained mucus.

Physical Examination. The diagnosis of obstruction and its cause can usually be made on physical examination alone. The hernial orifices should be palpated for the presence of a tender irreducible swelling. In fat patients particular care must be taken to check the femoral regions.

The presence of scars from previous abdominal operations is noted. Distension, particularly of individual loops, is significant. A distended caecum may be both seen and felt in thin patients and immediately points to a large bowel cause. Tenderness anywhere in the abdomen is suggestive of peritoneal irritation and bowel strangulation. A palpable mass is associated with large bowel tumours and diverticular disease. A transient mass, felt perhaps during bouts of colic, indicates intussusception. Classically bowel sounds are increased and tinkling in mechanical obstructions, but in advanced cases they are infrequent and auscultation must be prolonged to detect the occasional tinkle. In paralytic ileus sounds are virtually absent.

Rectal examination usually reveals an empty ballooned rectum. In low obstructions there may be some blood and mucus. Obstruction due to carcinoma of the rectum is rare.

In cases of doubt, and for confirmation of the diagnosis, serial measurements of abdominal girth will detect progressive abdominal distension. A diagnostic enema will confirm the presence of obstruction, particularly if repeated washouts yield neither flatus nor faeces.

Radiological Examination. Plain films of the abdomen, taken in the erect and supine positions, are most informative. The presence of fluid levels on the erect film, and of gas-distended loops on both films, indicate not only the diagnosis but also the site and probable cause of the obstruction. Where the completeness of the obstruction is in doubt, serial films can be compared for any change in the gas patterns. Barium examination should be avoided lest it makes the obstruction worse.

Treatment. If intestinal obstruction is suspected, the opinion of a surgeon should be sought, even if non-operative measures are to be used.

The mainstays of treatment are decompression by gastrointestinal suction, the intravenous replacement of fluids and electrolytes, and operative relief of the obstruction. Urgent surgery is indicated for an irreducible hernia and where there is strangulation. Correction of electrolyte deficiency must extend into the postoperative period, but in most cases of sudden onset the electrolyte upset is not marked.

In cases of more gradual development where there is a possibility that the obstruction can be relieved even temporarily, and in paralytic ileus, conservative measures assume greatest importance. Passage of a nasogastric tube in an ill and nauseated patient requires skill and patience. Once in place, continuous suction with an electric pump, with periodic checks with a syringe to confirm that the tube is patent, will achieve upper intestinal decompression, and is as effective as intestinal intubation.

Intravenous infusion may require to be prolonged and biochemical estimations may be frequent, so that the veins should be treated with care. Frequent change of the site of infusion, using a fine needle of the butterfly type originally developed for scalp veins or infusion into the subclavian vein will reduce the incidence of phlebitis. Where there has been blood loss, as in carcinoma of the bowel and diverticular disease, blood transfusion is required. Throughout conservative management, accurate fluid balance charts should be kept.

Peritonitis

Peritonitis is the reaction of the peritoneum to an irritant. Usually this is the result of infection, although sometimes the irritation is chemical at least initially, as when bile or duodenal contents leak into the peritoneal cavity. Appendicitis is one of the commonest causes of peritonitis and *Esch. coli* is the organism usually responsible.

Infection or chemical irritation cause the peritoneum to become congested and oedematous. There is an outpouring of fluid rich in antibodies and protein and containing large quantities of leucocytes. Dilution and destruction of the irritant is accompanied by its localisation by the formation of adhesions. Failure of these defence mechanisms is characterised by spread of the infection and by septicaemia and toxaemia. There is still a distressingly high mortality from generalised peritonitis.

Acute Peritonitis

In perforations, the onset is sudden, with severe abdominal pain, tenderness, rigidity and shock. The patient lies immobile, the respirations are short and grunting and the abdomen is retracted and motionless. These initial severe features then gradually decrease; the patient passes into a stage where he appears to have improved, and the diagnosis can be missed. Then, as paralytic ileus develops and fluid collects in the peritoneal cavity, there is increasing distension, the rigidity lessens, the tenderness remains and toxicity develops.

When peritonitis is secondary to inflammation of a viscus, such as appendicitis, the initial signs are those of the underlying disease, later to be replaced by the features of peritonitis. In advanced cases, only the history of onset remains to point to the probable cause.

Treatment. Established peritonitis is treated by removal of the contaminating source when it is due to such conditions as appendicitis or perforation of the bowel or gall bladder. Drainage of the abdomen, intravenous replacement of fluids and electrolytes, parenteral administration of wide spectrum antibiotics and the treatment of the concomitant ileus by naso-gastric suction form the basis of conservative and supportive management.

While the treatment of peritonitis is that of the cause, the ideal is its prevention. Thus acute appendicitis should be diagnosed before perforation and perforated peptic ulcer should be operated upon before the stage of chemical peritonitis is past.

Prognosis. General peritonitis may resolve completely, but often it localises to form an abscess at the primary site, in the subphrenic region or in the pelvis. Persistence of fever, or continued elevation of pulse rate, white blood count and ESR, should lead to efforts to locate such residual infections.

Pelvic Abscess

Usually resulting from localisation of a general peritonitis, a pelvic abscess forms in the lowest part of the peritoneal cavity, in front of the rectum. The abscess may irritate the bladder causing frequency of micturition or the bowel causing diarrhoea with the passage of mucus and a feeling of incomplete emptying. It is evident on rectal or vaginal examination as a tender mass.

Treatment is conservative as outlined above with, in addition, hot baths and douches. Discharge of the abscess rectally or vaginally is followed by rapid recovery.

Subphrenic Abscess

Localisation of pus between diaphragm and liver on the right side, or between the diaphragm and the liver, spleen and stomach on the left, is a complication of peritonitis most commonly due to perforation of the stomach, duodenum or gall-bladder or to operation on these organs.

There are signs of persistent infection; there may be dullness at the base of the lung and tenderness and slight oedema over the lower ribs posteriorly. Diagnosis is aided by X-ray of the diaphragmatic region which may show elevation of the diaphragm, a fluid level below it or changes in the lung above. Treatment is by surgical drainage.

Tuberculous Peritonitis

Although this condition is now rare in Britain, it is still relatively common in the Middle East, Africa and Asia. It is secondary to a tuberculous focus in the abdomen, usually in a mesenteric lymph node and it is characterised by wasting, malaise and abdominal distension. The abdomen contains fluid rich in protein from which tubercle bacilli may be cultured. Masses caused by matted omentum and loops of bowel may be palpable.

In the adult, the condition may be confused with advanced malignant disease and an unnecessarily hopeless prognosis given. Confirmation of the diagnosis may in some cases require laparotomy. The response to antituberculous chemotherapy (p. 292) is good and often dramatic.

Acute Appendicitis

Though this condition is rightly regarded as surgical, it is of such importance as one of the most common causes of the 'acute abdomen' that it should be discussed in a textbook of medicine.

Aetiology. The disease occurs in both sexes and though it may develop at any age it is more common in young people. It is presumed that the rapid increase in the frequency of acute appendicitis since the turn of the century is connected with change in dietetic habits to a highly processed, low residue diet and a general adoption of a more sedentary existence. Acute appendicitis is usually obstructive, the lumen of the appendix being narrowed by swelling of lymphoid tissue in its wall, or by stricture from previous inflammation. Obstruction is made complete by impaction of a retained faecolith. Infection and distension lead to gangrene, perforation and peritonitis.

Clinical Features. The classical history is of the sudden onset of vague central abdominal pain followed in a few hours by shift of the pain to the right iliac fossa, where it becomes localised to McBurney's point, situated one-third of the distance along a line from the anterior superior iliac spine to the umbilicus. There is nausea and general malaise. There may be vomiting, but this is seldom severe and is often absent. In the early stages there is little elevation of temperature, so that rigors and a high temperature make the diagnosis of appendicitis unlikely. The pulse rate is increased, the tongue is furred and the breath foul.

Locally there is tenderness and guarding in the right iliac fossa, progressing to rigidity as peritonitis develops. Rectal examination should always be carried out, because it may disclose tenderness to the right.

The 'classical' history and findings account for less than 50 per cent of cases. The inflamed appendix may simulate many other diseases of the abdomen. In addition to pain, the patient may present with diarrhoea, with urinary symptoms, or with gynaecological complaints. On occasion acute cholecystitis or perforated peptic ulcer may be mimicked.

Differential Diagnosis. In children and adolescents *non-specific mesenteric lymphadenitis* may resemble appendicitis. This condition is probably due to a virus. It is characterised by vague abdominal pain, slight fever and a doughy sensation on palpation. There is ill-defined tenderness in the right iliac fossa. The distinction from appendicitis may be difficult and if in doubt it is safer to operate; otherwise treatment is conservative, recovery taking place gradually over a few weeks.

Formerly a diagnosis of *chronic appendicitis* was made, often in young women, to cover a multitude of chronic or recurring abdominal pains. Removal of the appendix failed to give relief because these patients were suffering from conditions such as the irritable bowel syndrome or dysmenorrhoea. Rarely chronic appendicitis is found in children in association with thread-worm infestation.

Treatment. The diseased appendix should be removed as early in the acute stage as possible. Attempts to temporise in the belief that mild forms of appendicitis can be distinguished from severe are dangerous, because the condition is notoriously deceptive. When there is obvious peritonitis, vigorous treatment with an antibiotic such as ampicillin given intramuscularly is indicated from the time of the operation.

A conservative policy is allowable only when a clearly defined appendix mass is present, without generalised abdominal signs. Once the mass has subsided, probably within 2 to 3 weeks, the appendix should be removed. Not all patients presenting with an appendix mass require antibiotics. Some need no more than rest, restriction of diet and the avoidance of purgatives. Others in whom there is more marked local tenderness, with low grade fever and general malaise, benefit from ampicillin given orally.

Tumours of the Small Intestine

Tumours of the small intestine are rare, although there is some evidence that lymphoma is more likely to develop in patients who have gluten-induced enteropathy. Simple tumours such as polyps and leiomyomas may cause chronic anaemia or intussusception or may be found unexpectedly in the course of radiological investigation or laparotomy.

Carcinoid Tumours

These arise from argentaffin cells and are usually seen in the appendix or ileum, although they may occur anywhere in the alimentary tract. Carcinoid tumours produce a variety of substances including 5-hydroxytryptamine. When they originate in the small bowel, they may be multiple and usually spread to mesenteric glands and to the liver. The local effects of obstruction then take second place to the general effects of flushing, diarrhoea and borborygmi brought about by the high levels of 5-hydroxytryptamine coming in part from the tumour, but mainly from its metastases. These systemic manifestations—the *carcinoid syndrome*—thus indicate spread of the disease, in spite of which long-term survival is possible.

Treatment. The primary tumour and associated lymphatic and visceral metastases should be removed whenever possible with the aim of reducing the total volume of secreting tumour. Hepatic lobectomy can be considered when spread appears localised to one lobe. Drugs for the control of flushing are generally unhelpful but diarrhoea can be reduced by parachlorophenylalanine.

DISEASES OF THE LARGE INTESTINE

The main functions of the large bowel are the removal of water from the intestinal contents, the storage of faeces, and their evacuation at controlled intervals. Continence depends on training, on the function of a sphincter mechanism in the anal canal and on rectal sensation whereby the need to defaecate is appreciated.

The anal canal is sensitive to pain and touch, as is well demonstrated by the severe pain occasioned by fissures and inflamed piles. The rectum is insensitive to painful stimuli, so that the injection of a sclerosing agent for the treatment of haemorrhoids is painless. Rectal 'sensation' applies to an ability to appreciate distension and contraction.

In addition to clinical examination, including digital examination of the rectum, endoscopy (p. 351), stool examination (p. 353) and radiological investigation (p. 350) are all important aids to diagnosis.

Ulcerative Colitis

Apart from the bacillary and amoebic dysenteries and tuberculous enterocolitis, there are certain non-specific chronic inflammatory bowel diseases which are associated with ulceration of the colon. One of these is Crohn's disease which may affect both the large and the small bowel; the other, commoner disease affecting the colon, is ulcerative colitis.

Aetiology. The aetiology of ulcerative colitis is not known. It is not due to simple infection, no specific organism having been identified from the faeces or the bowel wall. It is possible, however, that the disease is due to an abnormal immune response to faecal bacteria, since there is some evidence to suggest that antibodies formed to certain strains of *Esch. coli* may act as autoantigens to the colonic mucosa. Further evidence in favour of an autoimmune process is the detection of anticolon antibodies in the serum of some patients with colitis. It has been suggested that hypersensitivity to certain foods, especially milk, may be a causative factor, and in practice temporary withdrawal of milk from the diet appears to improve diarrhoea in a few patients. However, the deleterious effects of milk in these patients could be due to lactose intolerance because of the development of secondary alactasia (p. 396) rather than to specific allergy to milk protein. Some authorities believe that psychological disturbances are responsible and claim that patients with colitis have a particular personality structure characterised by traits such as undue dependence on others, extreme sensitivity to personal slight and obsessive tendencies. It seems probable, however, that these traits are largely due to the disease process itself, since they disappear or greatly improve during a remission; indeed, one of the most rewarding effects of successful treatment is the remarkable improvement that may occur in the psychological well-being of the patient. Moreover, similar psychological features occur in patients with severe long-standing diarrhoea due to specific causes such as dysentery; nevertheless the patient and his physician may relate the attack or exacerbation to a recent stressful event. A familial tendency is suggested by the increased incidence of the disease amongst relatives of patients and by the association between ulcerative colitis, ankylosing spondylitis and Crohn's disease (p. 397).

Pathology. The rectum is always involved and the inflammatory process may be limited to this organ (proctitis). From the rectum the disease may spread to involve the distal colon (distal colitis) or the entire colon (total colitis). Whatever the extent of the disease, the inflammatory change is continuous throughout the affected part, in contrast to the patchy changes that occur in Crohn's disease of the colon. In the early stages the mucosa is swollen and reddened, and punctate bleeding points may be seen. As the disease progresses, ulceration involves the colon; the ulcers may be superficial or may penetrate deeply, spreading longitudinally beneath the mucosa. In severe disease the mucosa may slough in parts to expose granulation tissue; the mucosa that remains becomes oedematous, hyperplastic and raised, giving the appearance of pseudo-polyposis. In acute fulminant disease the bowel, especially the transverse colon, may be greatly dilated and the bowel wall becomes thin like paper and may rupture. In long-standing disease, the colon is shortened and generally narrowed with a lack of haustrations.

Microscopically, in contrast to Crohn's disease, the disease is characteristically confined to the mucosa which shows varying degrees of inflammatory change. In early colitis there is an increase in blood vessels and polymorphs and the lamina propria is oedematous. There may be collections of polymorphs in the lumen of the crypts which are termed 'crypt abscesses'. These may progress to destruction of the mucosa which is replaced by granulation tissue. Finally, on healing, the mucosa has a reduced number of crypts.

Clinical Features. The disease occurs most commonly between the ages of 20 and 40 years, but is seen at all ages. The clinical features and the management are largely determined by the extent to which the colon is involved, the severity of the inflammatory process, and the duration of the disease.

The principal symptom is diarrhoea with loose bloody stools containing mucus; defaecation is often accompanied by pain or lower abdominal discomfort, although severe pain is uncommon. Tenesmus may occur because of proctitis. Tenderness may be present on palpation of the colon, especially in the left iliac fossa; when peritoneal irritation is present, it signifies that the serosa is involved in the inflammatory process.

In severe ulcerative colitis, there is exhausting diarrhoea, fever, tachycardia and signs of dehydration. Toxic dilatation represents the most severe form. There is tachycardia, a high swinging temperature and abdominal distension. Untreated, the patient dies as a result of colonic perforation.

There is also a chronic stage of the disease in which the bowel is permanently damaged as a result of fibrosis. The colon in such cases behaves as a rigid tube incapable of absorbing fluid properly or of acting as a faecal reservoir. There is no toxaemia, but the patient lives in chronic ill-health and with persistent diarrhoea.

When the disease is confined to the rectum, the symptoms may be trivial if the inflammation is mild and consist of loose motions and perhaps blood-streaking of the stool. However, a severe proctitis will give tenesmus, frequent small and loose stools, together with bleeding per rectum, but systemic disturbance is absent. Paradoxically in distal colitis there may be constipation, with hard scybalous faeces and marked faecal retention on the right side of the colon.

Occasionally relapse can be associated with a period of emotional stress or intercurrent infection. There is no special risk during pregnancy, when indeed it is usual for the disease to remit; however, the disease may relapse early in the puerperium and if it does the attack is nearly always severe.

The patient is often anaemic and there may be leucocytosis and a raised ESR. In severe cases there are electrolyte disturbances and protein loss from the colon may lead to hypoalbuminaemia. Sometimes the liver function tests are abnormal. The stool is cultured for pathogenic bacteria and a search is made for amoebae to exclude an infective cause for the colitis. Proctitis can occasionally be due to gonorrhoea. Blood cultures are required if septicaemia is suspected.

Sigmoidoscopy. Although the diagnosis may be suggested by the history, sigmoidoscopy is essential for confirmation in most cases, but should not be performed in toxic dilatation which is diagnosed from the history, examination and straight X-ray of the abdomen.

The appearances of the mucosa depend on the severity of the disease. In proctocolitis of any severity, the mucosa appears engorged and hyperaemic and the normal vascular pattern is obliterated. In severe disease spontaneous bleeding will be seen; in less severe cases the mucosa appears intact, and bleeds only when it is gently rubbed, while in mild cases the only abnormality may be the absence of the normal vascular pattern.

Rectal biopsy is carried out to confirm the diagnosis and to exclude other causes of proctitis, such as Crohn's disease.

Radiological Examination. While sigmoidoscopy confirms the diagnosis of ulcerative colitis, a barium enema examination demonstrates its extent. If only the rectum is affected, no abnormalities may be seen. When the disease is more extensive or severe, the various changes described under pathology can be seen, for example, shortening and narrowing of the colon and ulceration of the mucosa (Fig. 8.5). Often there is undermining of the mucosa ('collar-stud' ulcer), and the formation of pseudopolypi.

Barium enema examination should not be attempted in patients with severe colitis because of the risk of perforation. In these cases, plain films of the abdomen may allow a positive diagnosis to be made, since the colon will usually contain sufficient air to outline an abnormal mucosal pattern.

Complications. *Intestinal Stricture.* In the chronic forms of the disease, stricture may occur at any level in the colon, but usually in the anal canal.

Carcinoma of the Colon. Carcinoma of the colon develops much more often in patients with long-standing ulcerative colitis than it does in the normal population, the risk being related to the duration, extent and age at onset of the disease. The risk increases greatly after the disease has been present for 10 years or more. It is greatest in patients with total colitis who develop the disease under the age of 20 years; in this group the risk of cancer of the colon is about 40 times greater than it is in a comparable normal population.

Systemic Complications. These include arthropathy affecting principally the large joints, ankylosing spondylitis, aphthous stomatitis and skin lesions such as erythema nodosum and, rarely but significantly, pyoderma gangrenosum. Cholangitis, hepatitis and septicaemia may also occur. These complications are most common in advanced cases.

Treatment. Admission to hospital is required for patients with severe bowel symptoms, especially when there are general disturbances such as weight loss, anaemia, fever or tachycardia. Such patients may require intense supportive treatment until the disease remits or as a preparation for surgery. The measures should include correction of dehydration and electrolyte deficiencies, especially hypokalaemia, blood and plasma infusions to correct anaemia and hypoproteinaemia, and a high protein, low residue diet. Blood cultures should always be taken initially and be repeated throughout the course of the illness if fever persists. Gram-negative bacteria are the commonest organisms involved; if septicaemia is suspected parenteral administration of broad spectrum antibiotics is necessary. However, antibiotics have no special place in the primary management of ulcerative colitis. Moniliasis of the mouth and upper pharynx is common, especially in severely ill patients on corticosteroids, so the mouth should be inspected regularly and swabs taken for culture if moniliasis is suspected. Treatment is with gentian violet and nystatin (p. 355).

There is no satisfactory drug for controlling diarrhoea. Codeine phosphate, 30–60 mg 3 to 6 hourly, is of some value, alternatively, an anticholinergic such as propantheline may be prescribed. However, all these drugs should probably be avoided in severely ill patients since they may precipitate an attack of toxic dilatation.

Almost all patients with severe colitis show some anxiety and agitation and may benefit from tranquillisers.

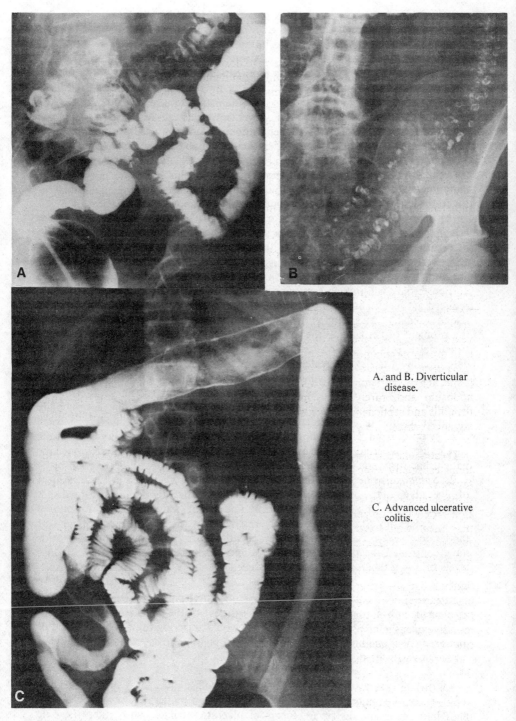

A. and B. Diverticular disease.

C. Advanced ulcerative colitis.

Fig. 8.5

ANTI-INFLAMMATORY DRUGS. 1. *Corticosteroids*. Although there is no specific treatment for ulcerative colitis, the introduction of corticosteroids and corticotrophin has greatly improved the outlook.

(*a*) *Local Treatment.* When the disease is confined to the distal colon or the rectum, symptoms may be limited to moderate diarrhoea (three or four stools per day) with the passage of blood from time to time, while general health is maintained. Such patients may be treated by administration of corticosteroids as suppositories when there is local rectal involvement, or as self-administered enemas if the distal colon is involved. The preparations commonly used are prednisolone-21-phosphate or betamethasone, and both are available in disposable enema form. The patient is taught to administer the enema himself, twice daily, retaining the material for as long as possible; suppositories may be inserted twice or three times daily for the treatment of proctitis. Either form of treatment may be continued for several weeks, the duration being judged by the sigmoidoscopic appearances.

(*b*) *Systemic Treatment.* Of the various corticosteroids available prednisone or prednisolone are the preparations most commonly used. These are given in doses of between 20–60 mg daily by mouth for 3 to 6 weeks depending on response. The usual contraindications to the use of these drugs must be observed (p. 549) and supplements of potassium salts should be given (p. 163). Used in this way, the corticosteroids will induce remission in the majority of patients, the dose being reduced at weekly intervals as improvement takes place. The corticosteroids give rise to a sense of well-being in the patient and in addition improve appetite, so that the problem of persuading the patient to eat sufficient food is often solved. The beneficial effects of corticosteroid therapy have been established as a result of careful clinical trials; the evidence suggests that they are more effective in a first attack of ulcerative colitis, whereas corticotrophin may be more beneficial in the treatment of relapse. A long-acting form of corticotrophin (e.g. tetracosactrin zinc phosphate complex) should be used, and given in doses of the order of 1 mg daily by intramuscular or subcutaneous injection. This dosage is continued for a week after symptoms have remitted and it is then reduced at weekly intervals as in the case of corticosteroids. For convenience prednisolone may be substituted once the patient has responded adequately.

2. *Sulphasalazine*. This sulphonamide derivative is also used in the treatment of ulcerative colitis, but is less effective than the corticosteroids. It has the disadvantage of causing nausea, vomiting and rashes; occasionally it induces blood dyscrasias. Its use is generally restricted to the management of mild or moderately severe colitis and in the prevention of relapses once corticosteroids have controlled the disease; under these circumstances it is prescribed at dose levels of 3–4 g daily, the dose being reduced gradually depending on response.

IMMUNOSUPPRESSIVE THERAPY. Because ulcerative colitis has been shown to be associated with autoimmune reactions, treatment of the disease by immunosuppressive drugs such as azathioprine (p. 49) would seem logical. Such a method of management is still under trial and it is not yet possible to say whether the advantages outweigh the disadvantages.

SURGICAL TREATMENT. If the appropriate medical measures are carried out assiduously, the majority of patients with proctitis or moderately severe colitis will pass into remission. In severe forms of ulcerative colitis, where there is toxic dilatation of the colon or perforation and in the occasional patient with severe haemorrhage, emergency surgical treatment is required. Usually it takes the form of colectomy with ileostomy, the rectum and distal colon being removed at a later stage when the crisis is over.

Acute ulcerative colitis which fails to respond to medical treatment, or which relapses in spite of adequate treatment, is an indication for proctocolectomy. This is also indicated in chronic forms, where the disease burns out but leaves a permanently damaged bowel, perhaps with stricture formation. Long-standing disease, particularly when the onset has been in childhood, carries a risk of carcinoma and accordingly total bowel involvement, with activity extending over more than 10 years, should lead to surgery.

At all stages of the disease, the timing of and preparation for surgery are important and require a joint medical and surgical approach. In emergency situations, intensive pre-operative replacement of blood, fluid and electrolytes is needed and operation is performed as soon as the patient is fit to withstand surgery. In less urgent situations, the moment for surgery depends on the degree of improvement in the patient's general condition to be expected from preoperative medical measures. The aim is to get the patient into the best possible condition, the art being to avoid the need to operate in a deteriorating position.

Operation usually implies total proctocolectomy with a permanent ileostomy. Whenever possible, in addition to a full explanation of ileostomy and its management, with a demonstration of the actual appliance to be used, the patient should have the opportunity before operation of meeting someone with an established ileostomy. Modern surgical techniques and the range of ileostomy appliances available make for easy management of the stoma and allow the patient to live an almost normal life with little restriction of physical activity. To be kept in touch with advances in techniques of ileostomy care, he should join an ileostomy association or be enrolled in a stoma therapy clinic.

Prognosis. It is extremely difficult to give a prognosis in ulcerative colitis. The extent of involvement of the colon is an important consideration, the outlook being very much better, for example, if only the rectum is involved. The immediate death rate in patients with fulminating disease, however treated, is not less than 40 per cent, and it is high also in patients developing an attack over the age of 60. In general, the overall mortality from ulcerative colitis is of the order of 10 per cent, but this figure can be very greatly reduced when the patient is treated by those with special experience of the disease. Thus, the mortality from total proctocolectomy done during a remission by an experienced surgeon is about 2 per cent, whereas mortality for proctocolectomy done as an emergency procedure is 10 per cent in the best hands, and may be 20 per cent or 30 per cent in those with little experience of the disease. Attention has been drawn to the risk of carcinoma in long standing cases.

Diverticular Disease

Though diverticula occur throughout the gastrointestinal tract, they are most common in the large bowel. The presence of diverticula is known as *diverticulosis*; when they are inflamed the condition is known as *diverticulitis*. Such inflammation occurs almost exclusively in colonic diverticula. Because it is often difficult to separate the two conditions on clinical or radiological evidence, they are grouped together under the term 'diverticular disease'.

Aetiology. In diverticulosis the muscular coat of the bowel is often greatly thickened, suggesting that the diverticula have formed as a result of increased intracolonic pressure. Manometric measurements support this view. It can be shown that pressure in the bowel is high and that there is an area of spasm or failure to relax at the pelvirectal junction. Epidemiological evidence suggests that dietary factors may be at least partly responsible. Diverticulosis is rare in areas of the world such as Africa and Asia where the usual diet is one of high residue; by contrast the incidence is increasing in Western countries where natural fibre is removed from the diet in the processes of food refining. Moreover there is evidence that intracolonic pressures vary with the bulk of the faecal residue, a high faecal residue being associated with a low intraluminal pressure and vice versa.

Diverticulosis occurs especially in middle-aged or elderly subjects and affects males and females equally.

Pathology. The pelvic colon is most commonly involved. Its muscle wall is thickened but the diverticula themselves are pouchings of the mucosa and have no muscle coat. It is not clear how they become inflamed. Radiological examination frequently shows the presence of a faecolith in a diverticulum, and it may be that faeces collect because of the inability of the diverticulum to contract. An area of inflammation may develop in the diverticulum and whilst this may resolve, it may become acute with perforation, local abscess formation, fistula and peritonitis. When there are repeated attacks of diverticulitis, the bowel wall becomes progressively thickened with narrowing of the lumen leading eventually to large bowel obstruction.

Clinical Features. Pain or discomfort felt in the left iliac fossa is a common complaint and there may be associated local tenderness. Acute diverticulitis can give rise to severe pain, guarding and rigidity on the left side, the signs of peritonitis and obstruction being combined. Change of bowel habit, either of increasing constipation or constipation alternating with diarrhoea, is frequent. This is the most important symptom of colonic disease and can occur with any lesion. By middle age, bowel habits are firmly established and a definite alteration usually betokens organic disease in the colon such as carcinoma or diverticulitis and always calls for investigation. Another presentation is with severe rectal bleeding as the first sign of diverticular disease.

In the chronic forms, there may be symptoms of subacute obstruction with increasing abdominal distension, borborygmi and colicky pain. Urinary frequency and dysuria may be present. Occasionally a fistula to the bladder gives rise to pneumaturia and faecal contamination of the urine.

On examination, the thickened tender colon may be palpable in the left iliac fossa. A mass may be present in those patients who have developed diverticulitis, with or without abscess.

Rectal examination and sigmoidoscopy are of no value in making the diagnosis of diverticular disease, but are essential to exclude cancer of the rectum and pelvirectal junction. Both conditions may coexist in an age group which is liable to both, or one may mimic the other to the extent that even at operation the true diagnosis is uncertain.

Radiological Examination. Diverticulosis produces a characteristic picture in which the sacs are outlined as pouchings from the main contour of the gut (Fig. 8.5). If a faecolith is present in the diverticulum, the barium partially surrounds it in a crescentic fashion. When a barium enema is evacuated, barium is frequently left behind in the diverticula which are clearly outlined. If diverticulitis is present, there will be narrowing, rigidity and lack of normal haustration of a segment of colon. Whether or not there are diverticula present, the main diagnostic difficulty is to distinguish the appearances from those of carcinoma and the distinction may be impossible.

Treatment. Asymptomatic diverticulosis is common, is often found accidentally and requires no treatment. Patients who have mild or moderate symptoms will be relieved by regulation of the bowel. A diet with plenty of roughage in the form of vegetables, fruit, or bran is usually sufficient. If not, a bulk laxative such as methylcellulose should be used. Purgatives should be avoided.

During an attack of acute diverticulitis, bed rest, antibiotics, fluids intravenously and orally, or even cessation of feeding and nasogastric suction may be required. Most severe attacks subside spontaneously but a few require emergency surgery which will probably be confined to a temporary defunctioning proximal colostomy, to be followed later by local resection. An emergency partial colectomy may be required for acute bleeding.

Elective surgery is indicated, after recovery from an acute attack, in patients who develop obstructive features, who have complications such as fistula and those in whom the possibility of carcinoma cannot be excluded. The treatment of choice is resection of the involved segment of pelvic colon with primary anastomosis.

A few patients fail to respond adequately to medical treatment and of these some will be considered for surgery. This may take the form of resection, or of myotomy of the pelvic colon loop. In patients without advanced fibrotic changes the latter procedure gives good results but its long term efficacy has still to be established.

Carcinoma of the Colon and Rectum

In Britain, carcinoma of the large intestine is the most common malignant tumour of the alimentary tract. In contrast it is rare in Africa and Asia. It is a disease of advancing years, affecting males more than females.

Aetiology. The only diseases known to be clearly associated with cancer are long-standing ulcerative colitis and familial multiple polyposis. There is no established association between carcinoma and diverticular disease. The variation in incidence of the disease between different countries has led to speculation that dietary factors and differences in bacterial content of the bowel may be involved.

Pathology. In two-thirds of patients, cancer of the large bowel occurs in the left colon or rectum. Multiple tumours are present in 2 per cent of cases. Macroscopically the tumour may be proliferative and fungating, ulcerative and infiltrating, polypoidal or encircling as a 'string' stricture.

Spread occurs directly in and through the bowel wall, by lymphatics and by the bloodstream through both portal and systemic circulations. Colon carcinoma is capable of direct implantation on exposed surfaces, such as a suture line or area of trauma in the bowel. The liver is the organ most commonly involved in metastases.

Clinical Features. Symptoms vary depending on the site of the carcinoma. In tumours of the left colon, obstruction is early. Tumours of the right colon present with anaemia, cachexia and alteration of bowel habit, but obstruction is late because of the relatively fluid nature of the bowel contents. As a consequence left-sided tumours tend to be diagnosed earlier.

Change in bowel habit, anaemia, weight loss and sometimes excessive borborygmi, abdominal distension and colicky pains indicating subacute obstruction, all point to a large bowel tumour. Some, however, are relatively symptomless until the patient presents as an emergency with obstruction.

Carcinoma of the rectum causes early bleeding with mucus discharge and later a feeling of incomplete emptying of the bowel. Obstruction is a feature of tumours of the pelvirectal junction but not the rectum proper, which is capacious and distensible.

The findings on physical examination range from no obvious abnormality to the signs of advanced malignancy. The majority of rectal tumours can be palpated on rectal examination. Fresh blood in the stool should always suggest the possibility of a tumour of the rectum or pelvic colon. Occult blood is found in the stool if an ulcerating lesion is present higher in the colon.

Endoscopy. More than 50 per cent of malignant tumours of the large bowel occur in a part accessible to direct inspection with the sigmoidoscope, i.e. the rectum and the lower pelvic colon. With the colonoscope the whole left side of the bowel at least can be inspected, thus bringing into range 75 per cent of all tumours. Endoscopy therefore should always be carried out. The whole or part of a growth may be seen and a biopsy specimen removed. Even when direct vision is impossible, there may be blood and mucus in the lumen. In rectal carcinoma histological proof should always be obtained before resection.

Radiological Examination. Barium enema is a more useful method of examination for diseases of the colon than the 'follow-through' of a barium meal, though the latter may be helpful for examination of the ascending colon. The caecum and the rectum are difficult to examine radiologically and diagnosis in the former may depend on laparotomy, while in the latter reliance should be placed on endoscopy. The usual radiological appearances of a carcinoma are either those of a stricture or a filling defect in the barium outline (Fig. 8.6).

Treatment. The treatment of choice is resection of the tumour as a one-stage procedure. If there is no colonic obstruction, or if it can be overcome by enemata, time should be spent in preparing the bowel by washouts and antibiotics. Any anaemia should be corrected by preoperative transfusion.

Carcinoma of the rectum will almost always require total removal of the rectum with permanent colostomy and for this the patient requires pre-operative introduction to colostomy and its management (p. 411).

In general the outlook of surgery for carcinoma of the large bowel is good, but success depends on early diagnosis and operation before spread has occurred and before obstruction renders the surgeon's task more complicated. The possibility of carcinoma must be considered when anyone of middle age presents with rectal bleeding, change of bowel habit or anaemia.

Serial estimations of CEA levels (p. 50) may lead to the earlier detection of recurrence after operation.

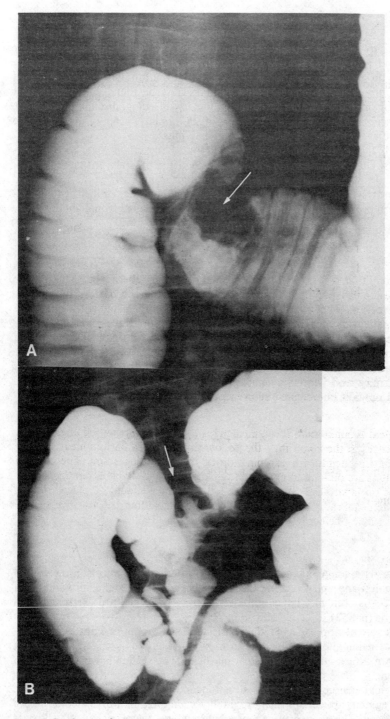

Fig. 8.6 Carcinoma of colon. A. Filling defect in transverse colon. B. Stricture in pelvic colon.

Benign Tumours of the Large Intestine

Only polyps are found with any frequency. These tumours may be single or multiple and are most commonly found in the left side of the colon. They are round and on a stalk, which may lengthen so that the tumour can move up and down the lumen of the bowel. These tumours may be found coincidentally at operation or on barium enema, or they may cause bleeding, discharge of mucus, or intussusception. Occasionally, because of its mobility, a polyp may prolapse through the anus to appear as a red cherry-like mass.

Although they are primarily benign, polyps of the colon may become carcinomatous. The malignant change may not extend into the stalk, so that removal of the polyp and stalk may suffice. It follows that polyps should be treated seriously and removed and that the stalk as well as the polyp itself should be examined histologically. In general polyps of more than 1 cm in diameter are probably malignant.

Multiple Polyposis

In this condition, transmitted by autosomal dominant inheritance, there may be thousands of small polyps diffusely scattered over the mucosal surface of the colon and rectum. They appear at adolescence and turn malignant in about 15 years, the patient often dying from carcinomatosis before the age of 40. The disease can be recognised by routine examination from adolescence onwards of members of affected families. Prevention of carcinoma means removal of the colon and rectum with permanent ileostomy, although symptomless members of the family may find ileorectal anastomosis with diathermy removal of rectal polyps and periodic surveillance more acceptable.

Megacolon

Megacolon is a condition characterised by dilatation of the colon and obstinate constipation. The disease may be separated into two groups, congenital or Hirschsprung's disease proper, and acquired megacolon.

Hirschsprung's Disease

The cause is a congenital absence of the myenteric nerve plexus in the wall of the pelvic colon and upper rectum. Occasionally the defect extends proximally. A similar defect is seen in Chagas' disease where the ganglia are destroyed by a trypanosome (p. 852).

Boys are often more affected than girls and symptoms of constipation, abdominal distension and vomiting date from birth. They may come in attacks, but even between attacks there is persistent pot-belly. The rectum is empty on digital examination.

Radiological examination with small amounts of barium show a small rectum, a narrow segment above and then proximally wide dilatation of the colon full of retained faeces. The diagnosis can be confirmed by rectal biopsy of sufficient thickness to include muscle of the bowel wall.

Treatment is by excision of the abnormal segment of colon and rectum.

Acquired Megacolon

In this group of cases, there is no defined aetiology and no defined age-group. Some are examples of a milder, short segment form of Hirschsprung's disease. Others are associated with an endocrine disturbance as in cretinism.

Radiologically, acquired megacolon usually shows no narrowed segment, the dilatation instead extending down to the anus. The rectum is full of faeces.

Most cases can be managed conservatively, by treatment of the cause where identifiable, by high residue diets, laxatives and perhaps colonic washouts. In a few patients colon resection has been used as a last resort in the relief of obstinate constipation.

Infections of the Alimentary Tract

Infections of the mouth due to thrush and other organisms are discussed on page 354, and gastroenteritis caused by bacterial food poisoning on page 69. Epidemics of acute but transient gastroenteritis may be caused by Echo, Coxsackie and other viruses. Usually identification of the viral nature of the infection is not possible and diagnosis is presumptive when no bacterial cause has been demonstrated.

The small intestine is involved in typhoid and paratyphoid fevers (p. 67), cholera (p. 862), staphylococcal enterocolitis (p. 63), tuberculosis (p. 285), giardiasis (p. 845), strongyloidiasis (p. 909) and ancylostomiasis (p. 907).

The principal infections involving the large intestine are bacillary dysentery (p. 72) and amoebic dysentery (p. 382).

Treatment. Bacterial resistance is readily induced by the indiscriminate use of antimicrobial agents in infections of the gut, many of which are not of bacterial aetiology. Specific therapy is usually not required in bacillary dysentery due to shigella and in gastroenteritis due to *Esch. coli*. When it is indicated by the presence of systemic upset, local knowledge of sensitivity is important as resistance may have been acquired to one or more of the antibacterial agents commonly used in that area. Most forms of food poisoning due to salmonella similarly do not require specific chemotherapy but more severe attacks may be associated with bacteraemia and must be treated, usually with ampicillin.

Abdominal infection complicating surgical or gynaecological operations and diverticulitis are commonly caused by *bacteroides fragilis* for which the lincomycins are the antibiotics of choice. Prophylactic antibiotics should not be given to cover 'clean' surgery as there is no evidence that they are beneficial.

Travellers' Diarrhoea

A short attack of diarrhoea commonly affects travellers, especially in the tropics. The attack is usually acute, with watery stools and sometimes vomiting. It lasts 2 to 5 days and is self-limiting. Enterotoxigenic *Esch. coli* has been implicated in some attacks. Specific antimicrobial treatment is not indicated but fluid balance should be maintained by adequate drinking or, rarely, intravenous fluids. Symptoms may be controlled by oral codeine phosphate 60 mg or diphenoxylate hydrochloride (Lomotil) 2·5 mg every 6 hours. If diarrhoea persists stools should be examined microscopically for *Giardia lamblia* and *Entamoeba histolytica*, and cultured for salmonella and shigella. Persistence of mild diarrhoea after travel is a feature of giardiasis (p. 845) and amoebiasis (p. 842).

Vascular Disorders of the Alimentary Tract

Vascular disorders of the alimentary tract usually occur in elderly patients with other evidence of degenerative arterial changes or in patients with heart disease or arrhythmias.

Occlusion of the Superior Mesenteric Artery

Sudden severe abdominal pain, vomiting and watery diarrhoea form the classical triad of initial symptoms in this condition. The cause is either thrombosis of the superior mesenteric artery secondary to atherosclerosis, or embolism often associated with atrial fibrillation.

Clinical diagnosis is difficult and tends to be delayed until gangrene of the bowel and peritonitis have developed. By then the outcome is almost always fatal. Early diagnosis is facilitated by emergency aortography to outline the origin and course of the superior mesenteric artery. Diagnosis in the first few hours offers the possibility of restoration of the blood supply to the bowel by embolectomy, end-arterectomy or arterial bypass.

Occlusion of the Inferior Mesenteric Artery

Atheroma with secondary thrombosis or embolism lodging in the inferior mesenteric artery imperils the viability of the pelvic and descending colon.

The clinical picture is less severe than that of occlusion of the superior mesenteric artery. Diagnosis may be made at laparotomy for what is thought to be diverticular disease or volvulus, and treatment is left hemicolectomy.

Chronic Ischaemia

With the greater use of angiography, the symptoms of chronic ischaemia of the bowel are becoming recognised. Pain, brought on by meals (abdominal angina) malabsorption, disturbance of bowel function and stricture formation are some of the modes of presentation. In the large bowel, in the region of the splenic flexure where superior and inferior mesenteric blood flows anastomose, ischaemic stricture is most commonly seen and may be first recognised in a barium enema.

Ischaemic colitis may be acute or chronic, widespread or localised. In approximately 50 per cent of older patients no underlying cause is detected, although in patients under the age of 50, a predisposing factor is usually identifiable.

Unless gangrene develops, treatment is conservative in the acute stage, by drip, suction, bed rest and antibiotics.

Psychogenic Disorders

Disorders of the digestive system due to psychological factors are common and they may mimic organic disease. Stress may be associated with a symptom such as dyspepsia ('indigestion'), abdominal discomfort or diarrhoea. It is known both from direct and indirect observations that gastrointestinal functions such as gastric secretion, alimentary motility and blood flow can alter with change in emotion.

Patients with anxiety states may develop a wide range of alimentary symptoms such as dryness of the mouth, a feeling of a lump in the throat (globus hystericus), anorexia, nausea, vomiting, abdominal discomfort, aerophagy with belching, abdominal pain, diarrhoea or constipation. Patients with a depressive illness may have similar complaints, notably anorexia, a bad taste in the mouth, nausea and vomiting especially in the morning, and constipation. Any or all of these symptoms may be due to organic disease and it should never be forgotten that the patient with an anxiety or depressive illness may also have an organic lesion such as peptic ulceration or alimentary carcinoma.

A careful history will usually identify complaints of psychological origin; pain of this type may have no discernible pattern with no clear time or food relationships and the patient often has difficulty in describing it. The more bizarre the description, the less likely is the symptom to be organic in origin. The history will usually also provide evidence of a psychological disturbance.

Occasionally the physical examination will reveal a manifestation of anxiety such as inappropriate sweating or tachycardia. If abdominal tenderness is elicited, this is often quite disproportionate both to the patient's physical well-being and to his complaint.

Globus Hystericus

Some patients complain of a feeling of a lump in the pharynx, frequently described as difficulty in swallowing. On questioning, however, it becomes clear that the sensation actually occurs between meals, rather than during the act of swallowing so that there is no true dysphagia. The symptom occurs most frequently in tense, anxious individuals, and is probably related to a heightened awareness of the act of swallowing saliva. Before accepting that the symptom is psychological in origin it is necessary to exclude a structural lesion in the upper pharynx by barium examination and if necessary by endoscopy. Occasionally sideropenic dysphagia will be responsible for the symptom (p. 358).

Psychogenic Dyspepsia

This term is used to describe a condition in which epigastric discomfort, a feeling of undue satiety after eating, occasional anorexia, nausea or vomiting and a complaint of excessive 'wind' are associated with psychoneurotic features such as anxiety, irritability, or a feeling of tension. Other somatic symptoms include attacks of sweating or tachycardia, or a sense of weakness. Sometimes the principal feature is pain and the history may bear superficial resemblance to that obtained in peptic ulcer; however the pain is diffuse rather than localised, is often described in bizarre terms, and has no relationship to food or time. The symptoms may have been present for months or years. The diagnosis can often be suspected both because the symptoms are not compatible with organic disease and because of evidence of psychoneurosis. However, organic disease should be excluded by appropriate investigations and frequently symptoms are relieved after the reassurance that barium meal or endoscopy is negative. The extent to which investigation should be carried out is a matter for clinical judgement. For example, the early symptoms of an organic lesion such as peptic ulcer may themselves precipitate a mild anxiety state which in turn overshadows the original symptoms; the early symptoms of a gastric carcinoma are characteristically vague, and dyspepsia in the middle-aged should never be attributed to neurosis without full investigation. On the other hand unnecessary investigation may consolidate the psychological difficulties of inadequate, overdependent personalities, some of whom, consciously or unconsciously, may be manipulating the doctor.

Treatment. The exclusion of organic disease is an important part of the management because it allows the physician to reassure the patient with confidence. The psychological origin of the symptoms should be explained to the patient. Frequently, such patients recognise that they have a 'weak' stomach which bears the brunt of recurrent stress, but they may come to a doctor for reassurance from time to time. Sometimes a patient with obsessive tendencies discovers some private ritual or diet to which he attaches great importance. Provided such a diet is harmless and does not exclude essential foodstuffs it can be left unaltered.

Psychogenic Vomiting

This is not an uncommon manifestation of anxiety states and it occurs usually on wakening, or immediately after breakfast; only rarely does it occur later in the day. It is probably a reaction to awakening and facing up to the worries of everyday life; in the young it can occur as a school phobia. There may be retching alone or the vomiting of gastric secretions or food. Although psychogenic vomiting may occur regularly over long periods, there is little or no weight loss and this is of value in distinguishing it from vomiting due to organic disease of the alimentary tract. Early morning vomiting also occurs in pregnancy and depression.

It is essential in all cases to assess and, if possible, alleviate the underlying psychological disturbance. Tranquillisers and antiemetic drugs have only a secondary part to play.

The Irritable Bowel Syndrome

One of the commonest disorders of the alimentary tract is that of long-standing colonic dysfunction associated with abdominal pain and for which no organic cause can be found. Bowel habit is disturbed by diarrhoea or constipation occurring alone, or alternating. This irritable bowel syndrome is also known as *spastic colon* and *idiopathic diarrhoea*.

Aetiology. Manometric studies from the distal colon have shown various patterns. When constipation and pain are the predominant symptoms, intraluminal pressure is usually increased and there is an increased frequency of pressure waves, whereas motor activity is often reduced in patients with painless diarrhoea. These changes are not constant, and may not be detectable when the patient is symptom-free. Motility studies are not of value for diagnostic purposes.

Several factors may be involved in causation. Psychological disturbances, especially anxiety, are frequent; patients with the irritable bowel syndrome are often tense, conscientious individuals who worry excessively about family or financial affairs. Many relate the onset of their symptoms to an attack of infective diarrhoea. Some patients seem obsessed with bowel function and have taken purgatives constantly to ensure regular defaecation.

Clinical Features. The syndrome occurs more commonly in women, usually between the ages of 20 and 40 years. The commonest symptom is abdominal pain, occurring in attacks and referred to the left or right iliac fossa or to the hypogastrium; it may be continuous or colicky, diffuse or localised and is rarely severe. It is generally relieved by defaecation and is sometimes provoked by food. In some patients pain is associated solely with constipation, the stools being hard and pellet-like and accompanied by mucus. In other patients occasional bouts of diarrhoea are interspersed by periods of constipation when purgatives may be taken which precipitate another episode of diarrhoea, leading to a vicious cycle. Some patients complain of intermittent painless diarrhoea, passing several loose or watery stools daily during an attack. Diarrhoea occurs characteristically during the morning, either before or immediately after breakfast and it almost never occurs during the night. Defaecation is often precipitate especially after meals, presumably due to an exaggerated gastrocolic reflex.

Other symptoms include abdominal distension, especially after meals and an awareness of intestinal peristalsis ('rumblings') or audible borborygmi. Nausea, anorexia and complaints of tiredness and weakness occur, especially during attacks of diarrhoea. Vomiting is uncommon.

The patient may appear tense and anxious, but seems well otherwise. Abdominal tenderness is common, especially over the right or left parts of the colon, and the pelvic colon may be contracted and pencil-thin on palpation in the left iliac fossa. There is no evidence of peritoneal irritation. About one-third of patients show the scar of an appendicectomy or have had a gynaecological operation. Characteristically the same symptoms have continued since the operation.

Investigation. Although the diagnosis is usually suggested by the history alone, organic bowel disease has to be excluded, especially in patients developing symptoms for the first time over the age of 40 years. Rectal examination is normal and the rectum is usually empty. Sigmoidoscopy is essential to exclude an organic lesion of the distal colon. The mucosa appears normal in the irritable bowel syndrome but the colon may show marked motor activity, contracting and relaxing quite unlike the normal inert bowel. Barium enema examination is necessary principally to exclude organic disease; there are no diagnostic radiological features. There is no anaemia and ESR is normal. In patients whose principal complaint is painless diarrhoea, the possibility of lactose intolerance (p. 396) or mild hyperthyroidism (p. 516) should not be overlooked.

Treatment. The patient must first be reassured on the basis of the normal findings on examination and investigation, as anxiety may precipitate or aggravate the condition and there is sometimes an underlying fear of cancer. A simple explanation of the physiological basis for the symptoms often leads at least to a temporary improvement. In patients with persistent or troublesome symptoms, measures designed to modify the intestinal dysmotility are required. For constipation and pain, the patient should be encouraged to increase the roughage content of the diet and one of the hydrophilic colloids should be prescribed in a dose sufficient to ensure a normal bowel movement. It is important that the patient should stop laxatives. Pain may be relieved by an anticholinergic drug such as dicyclomine thrice daily. As an alternative mebeverine hydrochloride which has a direct effect on smooth muscle, causing it to relax may be prescribed in a dose of 100 mg four times a day. For patients with painless diarrhoea, improvement is commonly obtained with some dietary restriction, particularly the avoidance of fresh fruits and salads. Diarrhoea is treated with an anticholinergic four times a day with a larger dose first thing in the morning since symptoms are often worse at this time. Codeine phosphate and diphenoxylate are useful drugs which act quickly and can be carried by the patient to use in an emergency or they can be taken before any event which is known to precipitate diarrhoea.

Prospects in Alimentary Disease

The past decade has seen major advances in the accurate diagnosis of gastrointestinal disease mainly because of the advent of fibreoptic endoscopy and improved radiological techniques. Now, research in gastroenterology offers the prospect of an increased understanding of many conditions and their more effective treatment.

Several newly recognised hormones produced in the gastrointestinal tract are being studied and it seems possible that their imbalance may be important in such conditions as peptic ulcer and reflux oesophagitis. In the latter condition the hormonal and nervous control of the lower oesophageal sphincter may be at fault and in the future we may be disregarding the hiatus hernia and stimulating the sphincter pharmacologically to prevent reflux. The discovery of two different pharmacological agents—the prostaglandins and the histamine H_2-receptor antagonists—which reduce gastric acid secretion, offers new prospects in the management of peptic ulceration. The histamine H_2-receptor antagonists, in particular, exert powerful effects in reducing gastric acid secretion. They have been shown to cause duodenal ulcers to heal and their further development and use may well reduce the number of patients who require surgery. In those who fail to respond to medical management, there is already a tendency to perform less radical forms of gastric surgery. In this respect, the early results of highly selective vagotomy are very promising.

The immunological system of the gastrointestinal tract is another focus of interest. Further knowledge of its role is expected to help us understand and treat coeliac disease, ulcerative colitis and perhaps Crohn's disease.

Epidemiological studies have drawn attention to the associations between diet and many disorders of the gastrointestinal tract. The incidence of diverticular disease and appendicitis may be reduced by a high roughage diet and there is also circumstantial evidence to link cancer of the colon with the refined and low roughage diet of 'Westernised' society. In other cancers of the alimentary tract, particularly cancer of the oesophagus, certain ingestants seem to be of importance. Thus there is the prospect of developments in preventive medicine by appropriate dietary advice for the individual and for the community.

G. P. CREAN
D. J. C. SHARMAN
W. P. SMALL

Further reading:

Clinics in Gastroenterology. London: Saunders.—A series of specialist volumes consisting of three numbers annually and each dealing with a specific disorder of the alimentary tract. Recommended for selective reading and as a reference library to current practice.

Cummack, D. H. (1969) *Gastrointestinal X-ray Diagnosis.*—Edinburgh: Churchill Livingstone.—A comprehensive atlas of gastrointestinal lesions with informative legends and concise text.

French, E. B. (1976) Examination of the Alimentary System. In *Clinical Examination*. 4th edition, editor, Macleod, J. Edinburgh: Churchill Livingstone.—Complementary to this chapter and designed to be read in conjunction with it.

Sleisenger, M. H. & Fordtran, J. S. (1973) *Gastrointestinal Disease*. London: Saunders.—The most complete single volume reference text presently available. Contains extensive bibliographies to each chapter.

9. Diseases of the Liver and Biliary Tract

THE LIVER

Anatomy

Structure. The liver is the largest organ in the body, weighing 1200–1500 g. It has right and left lobes separated by the falciform ligament anteriorly, the fissure of the ligamentum teres inferiorly and the fissure of the ligamentum venosum posteriorly. The right lobe is the larger; it contains the quadrate lobe on the anteromedial part of the inferior surface and the caudate lobe on the medial part of the posterior surface. The left lobe is relatively larger in infancy and contributes to the protuberant abdomen at that age.

Histologically, the liver is divided into lobules based on a central vein, peripheral portal tracts, and between these a regular network of sinusoids. The central veins are tributaries of the hepatic veins which drain to the inferior vena cava; the portal tracts contain branches of the hepatic artery, the portal vein, lymphatics and the bile ducts; the sinusoids are channels, lined by endothelial and phagocytic (Kupffer) cells, which receive blood separately from the hepatic arterial and portal venous systems and convey it to the central veins. The liver cells (hepatocytes) themselves are arranged in single-cell sheets which lie between the sinusoids, separating them from one another. Between the liver cells and the sinusoidal cells is the space of Disse which contains fluid draining to the lymphatics in the portal tracts. Individual hepatocytes either line the space of Disse or abut on other liver cells; electron microscopically, the part of the membrane lining the space of Disse has irregular microvilli, while a part of the membrane adjacent to other liver cells helps to form the lining of the bile canaliculi, and here regular microvilli project into the canalicular lumen. These bile canaliculi form networks between the hepatocytes conveying bile towards the terminal bile ducts which link the intralobular bile canaliculi to the larger interlobular bile ducts in the portal tracts.

Blood Supply. The liver has an arterial and a venous blood supply and total blood flow is normally about 1,500 ml/min. The arterial supply is by the hepatic artery, a branch of the coeliac axis, which enters the liver in the porta hepatis and is distributed throughout the liver via the portal tracts. Its precise terminal distribution is uncertain, but most of its blood enters the sinusoids directly. In man, the hepatic artery supplies about 35 per cent of the total liver blood flow and about 50 per cent of its total oxygen supply. The portal vein drains its blood from the alimentary tract, spleen, pancreas and gall bladder. It also enters the liver in the porta hepatis, is distributed throughout the liver via the portal tracts and empties its blood into the sinusoids. The oxygen content of portal blood varies and is lowest during digestion.

Clinical Aspects. The upper border of the liver extends from the fifth rib medial to the right midclavicular line to the sixth rib in the left midclavicular line. Its lower margin crosses the epigastrium midway between the xiphisternum and the umbilicus. As the liver descends 1–3 cm in inspiration, it can normally be palpated in adults below the right costal margin during deep inspiration. Heavy percussion from above and light percussion from below in the right midclavicular line helps to determine liver size; percussion is of greatest value in revealing a small liver. Auscultation over the liver may reveal a rub due to tumour or perihepatitis, a venous hum between the xiphisternum and umbilicus due to portal hypertension, or, rarely, an arterial bruit due to hepatoma or acute alcoholic hepatitis.

Liver-cell Functions

Liver cells carry out a wide variety of metabolic functions facilitated by the rich blood supply derived from the gut as well as the systemic circulation and by the intimate contact between hepatocytes and blood due to the highly permeable sinusoidal lining. All hepatocytes appear capable of performing the many functions of the liver.

Carbohydrate Metabolism. The liver is the most important organ for maintenance of normal blood glucose concentration. It can convert glucose, fructose, galactose, glycerol, certain amino-acid residues, and 2- and 3-carbon compounds such as lactate, pyruvate and oxaloacetate to glucose or to glycogen. When exogenous carbohydrate is not available, the blood glucose concentration is maintained by endogenous glucose production, 90 per cent of which is derived from the liver by glycogenolysis or gluconeogenesis.

Glycogen stores become exhausted within about 24 hours of fasting, after which further glucose is provided directly by gluconeogenesis. Extrahepatic factors such as insulin, adrenaline, thyroxine, cortisol and glucagon profoundly affect carbohydrate metabolism in the liver.

Protein Metabolism. The synthesis of many proteins and their export into the blood is a major liver function. Indeed, all the plasma albumin and most of its globulins, other than the gammaglobulins, are made there. Globulins made in the liver, often exclusively, include coagluation factors I (fibrinogen), II (prothrombin), V, VII, IX and X, many of the components of the complement system, transport proteins such as transferrin, the haptoglobins and proteins with no certain physiological function such as caeruloplasmin, α_2-macroglobulin, and α_1-antitrypsin. Alpha-fetoprotein is made normally in substantial amounts only prior to and shortly after birth (p. 432). The result of this extensive synthetic activity is that the electrophoretic pattern of the plasma proteins is largely determined by liver function. The liver is also an important site of amino-acid deamination prior to their interconversion and oxidation. Urea synthesis from the amino groups released by this process occurs solely in the liver.

Lipid Metabolism. Dietary triglyceride enters the blood in chylomicrons (p. 390) and, aided by plasma lipoprotein lipase, is taken up by a number of tissues, particularly the liver. There the triglyceride is broken down to 2-carbon fragments which may be used in many metabolic processes. Free (nonesterified) fatty acids, liberated from the fat stores into the blood, are also taken up by the liver and used similarly. Among these processes is the synthesis of new lipid molecules—triglyceride, phospholipid and cholesterol—which are combined with specific apoproteins to form lipoproteins which are released into the blood. These lipoproteins include the very low density (pre-β) lipoproteins, which transport triglyceride as a source of energy to muscles and other tissues, or to the fat depots for storage, and the low density (β) and high density (α) lipoproteins the functions of which are uncertain. In biliary obstruction of any severity the serum lipid concentration increases, largely due to the formation of an abnormal lipoprotein known as lipoprotein X.

The liver synthesises more cholesterol than any other organ in the body. In addition to its incorporation into lipoproteins, cholesterol is used to make bile acids. Much cholesterol is excreted into the bile.

Bilirubin. This is produced from the ferroporphyrin haem after removal of its iron component. Most (80 per cent) is derived from haemoglobin breakdown by reticuloendothelial cells in the liver, spleen and bone marrow, the rest being formed by catabolism of other haem-containing proteins, particularly enzymes (e.g. cytochromes, peroxidases, and catalase) and myoglobin. This unconjugated bilirubin is not water-soluble and is carried in the plasma bound to albumin; consequently, it does not pass into the urine. In the liver bilirubin is transported into the hepatocytes, conjugated with glucuronic acid in the microsomes to form predominantly bilirubin diglucuronide, mainly through the action of the enzyme glucuronyl transferase, and excreted by active transport into the bile. Only water-soluble bilirubin diglucuronide enters the bile.

Conjugated bilirubin is not absorbed in the small intestine. Bacteria in the terminal ileum and colon, however, reduce it to a group of tetrapyrrolic substances. Most of these (stercobilinogen) are excreted in the stool (100–200 mg/day). Some are absorbed from the gut and pass to the liver where most are re-excreted in the bile; a small amount (4 mg/day) passes through the liver and is excreted in the urine where it is known as urobilinogen. Urobilinogen and its oxidation product urobilin in the urine are identical, respectively, with stercobilinogen and its oxidation product stercobilin, in the faeces.

Bile Acids. Cholic and chenodeoxycholic acids, the primary bile acids, are produced in the liver from cholesterol. They are conjugated with glycine or taurine and secreted into the bile in which they reach the duodenum. Most (95 per cent) of the bile acids are reabsorbed into the portal blood at specific sites in the terminal ileum; they pass to the liver and are re-excreted in the bile. Small amounts reach the colon and are metabolised by the colonic bacteria. Deconjugation and changes in the structure of the primary bile acids themselves occur, resulting in the production of secondary bile acids, deoxycholic acid from cholic acid, and lithocholic acid from chenodeoxycholic acid. Most of the secondary bile acids are excreted in the faeces. However, small amounts are absorbed, reach the liver where they are conjugated with glycine or taurine, and are excreted in the bile. Bile, therefore, contains two primary bile acids—cholic and chenodeoxycholic—and two secondary bile acids—deoxycholic and lithocholic. This *enterohepatic circulation* allows large amounts of bile acid to be delivered to the intestine daily from a relatively small total bile acid pool owing to frequent recycling through the bowel. Synthesis of new bile acid compensates only for that lost in the faeces. The hepatic capacity for bile acid synthesis is limited, and large losses from the bowel cannot be replaced.

Bile acids, as they enter bile, combine to form micelles (p. 390). In the small intestine, provided the bile acid concentration remains sufficient to maintain the micellar state, this greatly increases the efficiency of fat absorption. Insufficiency of bile acids results in poor absorption of dietary fat and fat-soluble vitamins, notably D and K. Such deficiency may result from impaired synthesis in chronic liver disease, biliary obstruction, small intestinal overgrowth of bacteria capable of deconjugating and dehydroxylating bile acids, and loss of bile acids into the colon in disease of the terminal ileum or after its resection. In this last instance, the bile acids interfere with colonic water and electrolyte metabolism causing diarrhoea, while their absence from the small intestine results in steatorrhoea.

Vitamin Metabolism. Some vitamins are stored in the liver. These include vitamins A, D, K, B_{12} and folate. In addition, vitamin K is required by hepatocytes for production of coagulation factors II, VII, IX and X. Metabolic reactions in the liver involving vitamins include conversion of tryptophan to nicotinic acid (p. 133), phosphorylation of thiamin (p. 128), and 25-hydroxylation of vitamin D (p. 118).

Hormone Metabolism. Many hormones are metabolised and inactivated, including steroid hormones such as cortisol and oestrogens, thyroxine, and vasopressin. Some of the metabolic products, e.g. those of oestrogen, are excreted in the bile.

Drug Metabolism. The liver is quantitatively the most important organ for this function. Most drugs metabolised are fat-soluble and their conversion into water-soluble substances makes them suitable for excretion in bile or urine. These conversions are carried out by enzyme systems of low specificity located in the microsomes. Two types of reaction usually occur; first, oxidation, reduction, or hydroxylation reactions, and second, conjugation reactions in which glucuronides are usually produced. Methylation, acetylation, sulphation and amino-acid conjugation may also occur. The pharmacological results of drug metabolism vary. Barbiturates undergo oxidation with loss of activity; cyclophosphamide is metabolised from an inactive substance to an active alkylating agent; phenylbutazone is oxidised to another active agent, oxyphenbutazone; and codeine is converted in part to morphine. Conjugation, as occurs with salicylates, paracetamol and morphine, almost always causes loss of activity. Acetylation of sulphonamides makes drugs less soluble and therefore potentially more harmful. When two drugs are metabolised by the same microsomal enzymes, each retards the metabolism of the other, leading to prolongation of drug action and the danger of overdosage. This is an example of one mechanism for an undesirable drug interaction in therapy.

The action of many drugs is determined largely by their speed of metabolism in the microsomal enzyme system, the activity of which may be altered by dietary and hormonal factors. In particular, microsomal enzyme activity may be greatly increased by certain drugs they themselves metabolise, an effect referred to as *enzyme induction* and thought to be due to an increase in enzyme protein which disappears rapidly when the drug is withdrawn. Drugs producing this effect—'inducing agents'—are many and include barbiturates, phenylbutazone and phenytoin. Enzyme induction has important therapeutic consequences, for an enzyme inducer such as a barbiturate may increase the required dose of another drug, such as warfarin; if only the inducing drug is then stopped, bleeding from overdosage of the anticoagulant may occur.

The liver metabolises about 90 per cent of all alcohol (ethanol) ingested, the rest being excreted by the lungs and kidneys. It is oxidised via acetaldehyde to acetate with the eventual formation of carbon dioxide. These reactions are carried out mainly by alcohol dehydrogenase, a mitochondrial enzyme, and the microsomal ethanol oxidising system. The latter, like other microsomal enzyme systems, may be induced by drugs, including alcohol itself, and this may in part account for increased alcohol tolerance in drinkers and for their resistance to the action of microsomally metabolised drugs. Conversely, the effects of alcohol may be enhanced when a microsomally metabolised drug is taken concomitantly; this is a very important example of drug interaction.

In liver disease, drug metabolism may be impaired, and care is needed to avoid overdosage, particularly with sedative drugs. The extent to which individual drugs are metabolised in an altered manner is very variable and cannot be predicted. Special care should, therefore, be taken whenever hepatic damage is present, particularly where there is evidence of severe liver damage, such as ascites, encephalopathy, hypoalbuminaemia, or a prolonged prothrombin time.

Reticuloendothelial Function

Approximately 20 per cent of the hepatic cell mass is due to reticuloendothelial cells, including the Kupffer cells. Effete red cells are broken down by these cells. The Kupffer cells also have important but poorly understood immunological functions. Antigens from the gut normally gain repeated access to the body. They are carried in the portal blood to the liver where the Kupffer cells phagocytose them and prevent their eliciting immunological responses. Kupffer cells are also very efficient at removing immune complexes from the blood. The liver, therefore, is able to prevent undesirable immunological reactions.

Liver Function Tests

The term 'liver function tests' refers to a group of biochemical investigations useful in confirming that the liver is diseased, in indicating whether hepatic cells (parenchymal liver disease) or the biliary tree (obstructive or cholestatic liver disease) is primarily involved, in giving an indication of the extent of liver damage and in assessing progress. The term is misleading in that many of the investigations do not measure liver functions and most liver functions are not tested in clinical practice; however, the term has become generally accepted. Liver function tests are variably abnormal in patients with liver disease and therefore a group of tests is usually done. It is important to realise that there are no patterns of abnormality indicative of specific diagnoses and that normality of all the commonly used tests does not prove that the liver is normal.

Bilirubin. The normal serum bilirubin concentration is 4–18 μmol/l (0·2–1·0 mg/100 ml) and for practical purposes it is all unconjugated. Hyperbilirubinaemia may be due to increased bilirubin production, as in haemolysis. In such cases, the bilirubin concentration rarely exceeds 85 μmol/l (5 mg/100 ml) and is of the unconjugated type. Other tests of liver function are normal in uncomplicated cases. In Gilbert's syndrome (p. 436), the biochemical findings are similar though without accompanying evidence of overt haemolysis. In such patients, where liver function tests show an 'isolated' hyperbilirubinaemia, estimates of unconjugated and conjugated bilirubin are useful in indicating the likely diagnosis. In parenchymal liver disease the serum bilirubin concentration varies widely depending on the severity of liver injury, whether the disease is acute or chronic and the stage in the evolution of the disease. Very high concentrations of bilirubin occur most frequently in biliary tract obstruction, with sustained high levels where this is due to malignant disease and more fluctuating levels where obstruction is caused by gallstones. In all forms of jaundice, the serum bilirubin concentration gives an accurate measure of the depth of jaundice; repeated estimations may be useful in following the progress of disease.

Simple, sensitive, inexpensive tablet and dipstick tests for bilirubin in the urine are available and useful. Unconjugated bilirubin is bound to albumin in the blood and does not pass into the urine. Conjugated bilirubin is not detectable in the urine of normal persons. Consequently, bilirubinuria detected by these tests implies a conjugated hyperbilirubinaemia and points to hepatobiliary disease. Conversely, absence of bilirubinuria in a jaundiced patient suggests haemolysis or a congenital non-haemolytic hyperbilirubinaemia such as Gilbert's syndrome.

Urobilinogen. A simple test in the form of a dipstick (Urobilistix) is available to detect excessive urobilinogenuria. There is normally a diurnal variation in the urinary output of urobilinogen, maximal excretion occurring in the afternoon when tests are best performed. Since it is readily oxidised to urobilin on exposure to air at room temperature, only fresh urine samples should be used. Excess urinary urobilinogen occurs in haemolytic diseases owing to increased bilirubin excretion leading to increased urobilinogen formation; in these patients bilirubinuria is not present. Any cause of hepatic parenchymal dysfunction—viral hepatitis, cirrhosis, malignancy, partial biliary obstruction, pyrexia or cardiac failure—will reduce the biliary re-excretion of urobilinogen and increase its excretion in the urine; bilirubinuria may or may not be present. In viral hepatitis, urobilinogenuria occurs early in the illness, disappears at the height of the jaundiced phase owing to biliary obstruction, and reappears early in recovery as obstruction is relieved. In cholestatic jaundice, absence of urinary urobilinogen for over a week indicates complete biliary obstruction.

Enzymes. Liver cells contain many enzymes which may be released into the blood in various pathological processes. Measurement of the activity of these enzymes in the blood may give evidence of the existence of hepatocellular disease and of its general nature. In practice, maximum information may be obtained by measuring the activity of relatively few enzymes. It must be remembered in interpreting the results of these tests that none of the enzymes usually measured is specific to the liver and alternative sources should be considered, particularly where abnormalities have been found incidentally in patients with minimal or no other evidence of liver disease.

TRANSFERASES. The two important enzymes in this group are aspartate amino transferase, AST (previously known as glutamic oxaloacetic transaminase, GOT) and alanine aminotransferase, ALT (glutamic pyruvic transaminase, GPT); both are present in the cytosol of the hepatocytes, the latter also being found in the mitochondria. Normal serum contains low enzyme activity (5–40 i.u./l) the source of which is unknown. Irrespective of the cause, whenever liver cells are damaged or killed the enzymes are liberated into the blood; this is therefore a test of the integrity of the liver cells. The highest activities are found following any form of acute liver damage; in viral hepatitis there is generally increased activity even in the prodromal phase, maximal levels of 10 to 100 times the normal value usually being reached in the jaundiced phase after which activity falls rapidly. Equally high activity may occur in acute hepatitis due to drugs, in acute circulatory failure and in exacerbations of chronic active hepatitis. Most patients (80 per cent) with infectious mononucleosis also have an acute hepatitis (few [10 per cent] become jaundiced) with serum transferase activity raised 2 to 10 times. Serum transferase activity rarely rises more than five-fold in acute alcoholic hepatitis. Patients with cirrhosis may show modest elevations of serum transferase. In obstructive jaundice activity may rise up to four-fold but rarely more unless cholangitis is present.

Increased serum transferase activity is a very sensitive index of hepatic damage. Neither enzyme is specific to the liver, but as alanine aminotransferase is found there in much higher concentration than in other organs, increases in its activity indicate more specifically that hepatic damage is present. These enzymes are of principal value in the diagnosis of acute hepatitis and in differentiating hepatocellular from obstructive jaundice. Their estimation is of no prognostic value in either acute or chronic liver disease.

ALKALINE PHOSPHATASE. This enzyme occurs in almost all tissues; in liver cells it is situated principally in the canalicular and sinusoidal membranes. Normal serum contains alkaline phosphatase activity (40–100 i.u./l) derived mainly from bone and liver, and to a lesser extent intestine; in pregnancy additional activity of placental origin is found. When hepatocytes are damaged relatively little alkaline phosphatase is liberated into the blood, most probably coming from cells which are killed. In hepatocellular disease, either acute or chronic, alkaline phosphatase does not usually exceed 250 i.u./l. When the biliary tract is obstructed at any level, new alkaline phosphatase is synthesised in the hepatocyte membrane much of which escapes into the blood. A greatly increased blood alkaline phosphatase activity is, therefore, the main indicator of biliary obstruction though it does not give any information regarding the site of that obstruction. The alkaline phosphatase activity has no prognostic significance in liver disease.

Sometimes a raised blood alkaline phosphatase activity may be found incidentally and may be the sole abnormality. In such cases hepatobiliary disease may be present, but it is important to ensure that the alkaline phosphatase does not have an extrahepatic origin before investigating the liver further. This may be done by electrophoretic separation of the isoenzymes of alkaline phosphatase. Bone is the main alternative origin of a raised serum alkaline phosphatase: it results from increased osteoblastic activity, such as occurs in adolescents, when it may reach 250 i.u./l, in Paget's disease, rickets, hyperparathyroidism, and in metastatic tumour in bone. Myelomatosis, though affecting bone extensively, is not associated with much bone repair and the blood alkaline phosphatase is not usually raised. During pregnancy, alkaline phosphatase of placental origin may increase the serum activity to 250 i.u./l.

OTHER ENZYMES. Measurement of the serum activity of numerous enzymes has been advocated in the investigation of liver disease. These include $5'$ nucleotidase, a membrane-bound enzyme the activity of which, like alkaline phosphatase, rises especially in biliary obstruction, and γ-glutamyl transpeptidase, a microsomal enzyme, the activity of which rises in many liver diseases and in response to drugs, including alcohol, which induce microsomal enzymes. In practice, however, the transferases and alkaline phosphatases usually give all the information needed.

Plasma Proteins. *Albumin* is made solely in the liver and its production is impaired by severe parenchymal damage. In chronic liver disease, especially cirrhosis, the serum albumin concentration is frequently below normal (35–45 g/l), reflecting the clinical state and indicating impaired hepatic synthetic capacity; serial readings offer some guide to prognosis. Low serum albumin concentrations in patients with ascites may be partly dilutional, and other non-hepatic factors contributing to hypoalbuminaemia include malnutrition and fever. Serum albumin has a long half-life (20–26 days) and consequently changes in concentration occur slowly. Thus, even in severe acute hepatitis, the serum albumin remains normal unless the illness continues for many weeks.

Globulins. It is characteristic of chronic liver disease that hyperglobulinaemia (> 30 g/l) occurs in addition to hypoalbuminaemia and it may be found irrespective of changes in the serum albumin concentration in prolonged viral hepatitis or active chronic hepatitis. Once established, hyperglobulinaemia tends to persist in most patients with cirrhosis. It represents a reaction of the reticuloendothelial system in general and does not directly reflect liver cell damage. The causes of hyperglobulinaemia are not fully understood; increases in gammaglobulins are prominent and probably reflect an increased activity of the immune system, to which many factors may contribute; in those with hypoalbuminaemia it may represent a response to a reduced colloid osmotic pressure in the plasma. Individual immunoglobulins are variably increased IgG mainly in active chronic hepatitis and cryptogenic cirrhosis, IgA mainly in alcoholic liver disease and IgM in primary biliary cirrhosis. Variations, however, are frequent so that Ig measurements are not of much diagnostic value.

Plasma Protein Electrophoresis. Various changes occur in the electrophoretic pattern of the plasma proteins in cirrhosis. The commonest are a decreased albumin and an increased gammaglobulin peak. There is some relation between certain electrophoretic patterns and particular forms of liver disease, but this is not precise enough to be of great diagnostic value. Monoclonal gammopathy occurs rarely but does not have any clear diagnostic or prognostic implication.

Coagulation Factors. Severe liver damage impairs the production of several coagulation factors. This is most readily detected by the one stage prothrombin time which depends, among other things, on coagulation factors II, VII and X of liver origin. As the plasma concentration of these factors has to fall to very low levels before the prothrombin time becomes abnormal, prolongation in chronic liver disease indicates severe liver dysfunction. Furthermore, as the normal plasma half-life of these factors is short (5–72 hours), prothrombin time changes occur relatively quickly after liver damage and abnormalities are found in severe acute hepatitis. Indeed, in acute hepatitis, such as viral hepatitis, the prothrombin time is a most valuable prognostic guide; an abnormal value indicates severe damage and an increasing prothrombin time indicates a progressively worse prognosis.

Vitamin K is required for coagulation factor production by the liver, and deficiency of this should be corrected by giving vitamin K_1 (10 mg) parenterally. This is particularly important in patients with biliary obstruction in whom vitamin K is not absorbed. A prothrombin test must be done in all such cases and any abnormality corrected prior to surgery.

Bromsulphthalein (BSP) Excretion. When injected intravenously, BSP is rapidly bound to albumin; little (2 per cent) is excreted in the urine and the rest is taken up by the liver, conjugated partially with glutathione and excreted into the bile.

Estimation of its clearance from the blood is a sensitive test of liver function. However, the effectiveness of the tests mentioned above, the misleading results with BSP in old, febrile, or hypoalbuminaemic patients, the fact that it is invalid in the presence of jaundice and the occasional hypersensitivity reaction which may even be fatal, make BSP excretion a test with limited applicability. It is of particular value in the diagnosis of the rare Dubin-Johnson syndrome (p. 437); blood concentrations of BSP are measured 45 minutes and 2 hours after injection, a higher value at 2 hours confirming the diagnosis.

Other Investigations in Liver Disease

Hepatitis B Surface Antigen (HBsAg). The HBsAg (Australia, serum hepatitis, or hepatitis-associated antigen) is located on capsular material of the hepatitis B (serum hepatitis) virus. Recently, very sensitive haemagglutination and radioimmunoassay methods have been developed for its detection in addition to previously available electrophoretic methods. It is a reliable marker of the hepatitis B virus and its discovery in blood implies infection of the patient with that virus. In acute type B hepatitis, the HBsAg appears in the blood late in the incubation period or in the prodromal phase of the illness; it may be present for only a few days, disappearing even before jaundice occurs, usually lasts for 3 to 4 weeks, or may persist for up to 3 months from the onset of disease. In patients suspected of having viral hepatitis, therefore, it should be sought as soon as possible. In about 5 per cent of patients with type B hepatitis, the HBsAg does not disappear from the blood and continues to be present for a long time, possibly permanently. These patients, then, develop a chronic type B hepatitis virus infection and, while the long-term outcome for most is unknown, some develop chronic hepatitis and occasionally cirrhosis. Patients with chronic hepatitis or cirrhosis may also have the HBsAg in the blood, and in these the hepatitis B virus is considered to be the cause of the disease. The proportion of patients with acute viral hepatitis, chronic hepatitis, and cirrhosis with the HBsAg shows great geographic variation, the highest proportion being found in tropical and Mediterranean countries. The antigen may also be found in patients with hepatoma, though as yet the relation of the hepatitis B virus to this disease is less certain.

Some individuals without a history of acute hepatitis and lacking any clinical evidence of liver disease may be long-term carriers of the hepatitis B virus as evidenced by a positive HBsAg test. This occurs in 0·1 per cent of healthy European and North American people, but much more frequently (3–15 per cent) in those in tropical countries. Certain patients with poor immune responses may also develop this condition; it occurs especially in Hodgkin's disease and other lymphomas, in those on immunosuppressive drugs, in patients on long-term dialysis and in institutionalised patients with mongolism. These persons may or may not have clinical, biochemical, or histological evidence of liver disease but their blood and other body fluids are potentially infectious.

Autoantibodies. Three autoantibodies in the blood are important in liver disease: antinuclear antibody, smooth muscle antibody and antimitochondrial antibody. None is absolutely specific to liver disease; antinuclear and antimitochondrial antibodies occur in connective tissue diseases and in autoimmune diseases, including various thyroid disorders and pernicious anaemia, while smooth muscle antibody has been reported in infectious mononucleosis and in a variety of malignant diseases. In liver disease, smooth muscle antibody, and to a lesser extent antinuclear antibody, may occur transiently and at low titre in acute viral hepatitis.

The autoantibodies are, however, more important in chronic liver disease where they are often present for long periods of time and at relatively high titres. They are found particularly in active chronic hepatitis, cryptogenic cirrhosis and primary biliary cirrhosis. In a patient with chronic liver disease, the presence of one or more of the autoantibodies indicates the likelihood of one or other of these disorders, the differential diagnosis being made on other clinical and laboratory evidence. In a patient with cholestasis, the antimitochondrial antibody is of particular value in indicating that primary biliary cirrhosis is present. Antimitochondrial antibody occurs in primary biliary cirrhosis in 90 per cent of cases and in less than 1 per cent of patients with obstruction of the large biliary ducts. An antimicrosomal antibody has also been described which may become important in certain forms of active chronic hepatitis. None of the autoantibodies damages liver tissue, and they are therefore unlikely to have aetiological importance.

Alpha-fetoprotein. This alpha-globulin is made by the fetal liver, production falling to very low levels a few weeks after birth. The reappearance of alpha-fetoprotein in substantial amounts in adult life is almost always due to a hepatoma, though rarely it may be associated with an embryonal tumour of the testis or with a carcinoma derived from foregut epithelium, especially the stomach. Electrophoretic tests are positive for alpha-fetoprotein in about 30 per cent of patients with hepatoma in Europe and North America, and in up to about 70 per cent of those in Africa and Asia. Recently, sensitive radioimmunoassays have shown that slightly increased serum alpha-fetoprotein concentrations, not detectable by electrophoresis, may also occur in non-malignant liver disease, particularly acute viral hepatitis and active chronic hepatitis. In viral hepatitis this may indicate hepatocyte proliferation; its implication in chronic non-malignant liver disease is unknown. A rising level, however, suggests hepatoma.

Caeruloplasmin. This is a copper-containing serum alpha-globulin produced by the liver. It is of value in the diagnosis of Wilson's disease (p. 732) in which serum caeruloplasmin is not detectable or is present at low concentration. Low levels may also occur in fulminant hepatic failure and in other advanced and severe chronic liver diseases, as well as in protein-losing enteropathy and malabsorption.

Serum Iron, Iron-binding Capacity, and Ferritin. In liver disease, measurement of the serum iron and iron-binding capacity may indicate that haemochromatosis is present. In this condition the serum iron is increased and the serum iron-binding capacity is over 80 per cent saturated with iron. Such findings are not, however, diagnostic and further investigations are necessary to confirm the diagnosis (p. 456). Recently, the serum ferritin concentration has been shown to reflect the total amount of iron in the body; high values are found in haemochromatosis. Both the serum iron and iron-binding capacity and the serum ferritin concentration can be used to follow the effect of venesection therapy in this disease.

Alpha$_1$-antitrypsin deficiency, detectable by absence of the α_1 peak on serum protein electrophoresis, is a well-established cause of liver disease in infancy and childhood. Rarely it occurs in adult liver disease.

Investigative Procedures in Liver Disease

Liver Biopsy. Liver biopsy is a simple and safe procedure in the hands of an experienced clinician. It is carried out with a special needle, usually through an intercostal space, using local analgesia. It requires a co-operative patient who will stop breathing when the biopsy is actually taken. The bleeding and coagulation mechanisms must be intact as indicated by a prothrombin time not more than 3 sec longer than the control value and a platelet count above 100,000/dl. After the procedure, the patient remains in bed for 24 hours, regular pulse and blood pressure measurements must be recorded and blood for transfusion (2 units) should be available. The main complications are abdominal and/or shoulder pain, bleeding and, rarely, biliary peritonitis which usually occurs when there is obstruction of a large bile duct.

Biopsy yields only a tiny sample of liver and consequently the best results are obtained in patients with diffuse liver disease. The procedure is essential in the diagnosis of chronic hepatitis and in separating its persistent and aggressive forms. It is also important in establishing a diagnosis of cirrhosis in which it may indicate a cause such as alcohol abuse or the iron overload of haemochromatosis. In cholestasis it may suggest obstruction of a large bile duct or give evidence of a disease of the smaller bile ducts or liver cells such as primary biliary cirrhosis. It is not usually required in acute hepatitis in which the diagnosis can normally be made on other grounds; it may be needed, however, in atypical cases. Localised disease, particularly malignancy, is less accurately diagnosed unless the site of disease is first identified by some other method. Operative liver biopsy may sometimes be valuable as in the staging of patients with lymphoma.

Peritoneoscopy. This can be performed under local analgesia or general anaesthesia and involves the creation of a pneumoperitoneum. An excellent view is obtained of the anterior and superior surfaces of the liver as well as some of its inferior aspect and the gall bladder. The spleen, the prominent blood vessels of portal hypertension, and evidence of peritoneal disease may also be seen. Biopsies can be taken directly from diseased areas which is especially valuable in focal disorders. The main contraindications are coagulation abnormalities, marked ascites and previous surgery which may have caused adhesions.

Scanning. Radioisotopes or ultrasound are used to scan the liver and spleen. Radioisotope scans are more widely used at present. They are most commonly performed with material taken up by the reticuloendothelial cells (e.g. technetium sulphur colloid) though more specialised radiopharmaceuticals are also available. Radioisotope scanning is most useful in detecting focal liver disease such as tumours, cysts, or abscesses though more diffuse disease such as cirrhosis can be recognised. As a hepatic lesion must exceed 2 cm in diameter to be detected, a normal liver scan cannot exclude liver disease. Furthermore, abnormalities are not specific for particular diseases; when the scan has localised the lesion, other methods must be used to confirm its nature. Ultrasound scanning is valuable in differentiating tumour deposits from abscesses or cysts as this method can show that a lesion is solid or that it contains fluid. Ultrasound is being used increasingly for other purposes, such as the detection of dilated obstructed bile ducts and gallstones; it may become more important in future.

Radiology. Specialised radiological techniques may be useful in investigating the liver. Angiography can define the site and nature of localised lesions and is valuable in planning hepatic surgery. Splenoportography, mesenteric angiography and direct portography via the umbilical vein may all be used to investigate the portal venous system in portal hypertension prior to the surgical creation of portasystemic shunts. The portal venous pressure can be measured at splenoportography or direct portography, as well as by catheterising the hepatic veins, as the wedged hepatic venous pressure closely reflects the portal venous pressure in cirrhosis. Hepatic venography can be used to identify hepatic venous obstruction.

Paracentesis. Analysis of ascites may give valuable information. In cirrhosis, the fluid is clear, the protein content usually below 30 g/l, and in the absence of infection there are less than 300 cells/dl. Ascitic protein concentrations above 30 g/l occur in peritoneal infection, especially tuberculosis, peritoneal tumour, hepatic venous obstruction and ascites associated with pancreatic disease. Amylase activity is high in ascites caused by pancreatitis. The presence of infection, such as tuberculosis, can be determined by bacteriological examination of ascitic fluid.

Jaundice

Jaundice is a clinical term referring to the yellow appearance of the skin and mucous membranes resulting from an increased bilirubin concentration in the body fluids. It is detectable when the serum bilirubin concentration exceeds 50 μmol/l (3 mg/100 ml); less marked hyperbilirubinaemia is called 'latent' jaundice. Internal tissues are also stained except the brain as bilirubin does not pass the blood-brain barrier other than in the immediate neonatal period. Pathological mechanisms giving rise to jaundice fall into three groups: haemolytic, hepatocellular and obstructive or cholestatic.

Haemolytic Jaundice

This results from an increased rate of destruction of red blood cells causing the production of more bilirubin. As a healthy liver can excrete a bilirubin load six times greater than normal before unconjugated bilirubin accumulates in the plasma, jaundice due to haemolysis is usually mild. Exceptions to this occur in the newborn when the hepatic bilirubin transport mechanism is immature and in patients with liver disease. Haemolysis may be due to intrinsic defects of the red blood cell or to various extracorpuscular factors (p. 597).

Clinical Features. Certain findings are common to all types of haemolytic jaundice. It is mild; the serum bilirubin is dominantly unconjugated (<15 per cent conjugated) and rarely exceeds 85 μmol/l (5 mg/100 ml). In some patients hyperbilirubinaemia is insufficient to cause jaundice. Bilirubin cannot be detected in the urine. Most patients have splenomegaly due to excessive activity of the reticuloendothelial system or congestion of the red pulp and also reticulocytosis and anaemia. The degree of anaemia depends on the severity of haemolysis and on the ability of the bone marrow to increase production of red blood cells. Increased bilirubin excretion leads to more stercobilinogen and stercobilin in the stools, which are therefore not pale, and to increased urobilinogen in the urine as more of this substance is absorbed from the gut. The urine rapidly becomes deep yellow on standing due to urobilin formation. Other tests of liver function are normal.

Hepatocellular Jaundice

Hepatocellular jaundice results from inability of the liver to transport bilirubin into the bile as a result of liver cell damage. Bilirubin transport across the hepatocytes may be impaired at any point between uptake of unconjugated bilirubin into the cells and transport of conjugated bilirubin into the canaliculi. In addition, swelling of cells and oedema resulting from the disease itself may cause obstruction of the intrahepatic biliary tree. In hepatocellular jaundice the concentrations in the blood of both unconjugated and conjugated bilirubin increase, perhaps because of the variable way in which bilirubin transport is disturbed.

Acute parenchymeal liver diseases, usually due to the hepatitis A or B virus (p. 439) or to toxins, usually drugs or alcohol (p. 438), are common causes. Immature bilirubin transport mechanisms in the newborn, especially in prematurity, and congenital defects in bilirubin transport (p. 436) are very specific metabolic defects in the liver cell causing jaundice.

The clinical features vary depending on the underlying diseases. Jaundice ranges from mild to very severe.

Obstructive Jaundice

Obstruction to the excretion of bilirubin anywhere between the biliary canaliculus and the ampulla of Vater may cause jaundice. As a result, the concentrations of both unconjugated bilirubin reaching the liver cells and conjugated bilirubin, unable to enter the canaliculi, increase in the blood.

CAUSES. The criterion for classifying obstructive jaundice used to be whether or not it was amenable to surgical treatment. The terms 'surgical' and 'medical' obstructive jaundice fail to focus thought on particular disease sites, while the terms 'extrahepatic' (surgical) and 'intrahepatic' (medical) obscure the possibility that an obstruction to a large duct inside the liver is occasionally amenable to surgical treatment. Consequently, the terms used here are 'large (bile) duct obstruction' and 'small (bile) duct obstruction'.

Large Duct Obstruction. The most common causes are impaction of a gallstone in the common bile duct and carcinoma of the head of the pancreas. Other causes include carcinomas of the ampulla of Vater or bile duct, strictures of the bile duct usually the result of previous surgery, metastatic tumours impinging on the bile ducts, sclerosing cholangitis and, very rarely, involvement of the common bile duct by a duodenal ulcer.

Small Duct Obstruction. Widespread small duct obstruction is required to produce jaundice, and there are many causes of this including secondary carcinoma. Particularly important are drugs (p. 437), including alcohol, which may have their main effect either on the liver cells or on the bile ducts. Other conditions causing obstruction are often primary diseases of the liver cells which also involve the small bile ducts, particularly the biliary canaliculi whose walls are formed by the hepatocytes; such conditions include the cholestatic episodes which may occur in viral hepatitis, active chronic hepatitis, or cirrhosis and the cholestasis of pregnancy. Cholestasis, sometimes with deep jaundice, may also occur for unknown reasons following surgery, in severe bacterial infections and in Hodgkin's disease. Diseases involving the smaller interlobular ducts and the ductules include primary biliary cirrhosis and the pericholangitis of ulcerative colitis.

Clinical Features. Apart from the manifestations of the causative disease, these include jaundice itself which, if prolonged and severe, may give the skin a greenish appearance, pale or clay-coloured stools due to deficiency of bilirubin and to steatorrhoea and dark urine due to the renal excretion of conjugated bilirubin.

In some patients there is generalised pruritus, anorexia, or a metallic taste in the mouth. Upper abdominal pain occurs particularly in large duct obstruction by a gallstone or pancreatic carcinoma. Fever, sometimes with rigors, suggests cholangitis, which occurs most often with gall-stone obstruction. A palpable gall-bladder strongly suggests large-duct obstruction by a carcinoma, usually of the pancreas. The absence of this does not exclude a neoplasm. A very large and irregular liver indicates hepatic neoplasm. In prolonged obstructive jaundice, xanthomatous skin lesions, especially on the upper eyelids, occasionally appear as well as features due to secondary intestinal malabsorption; these latter include weight loss, a haemorrhagic tendency (vitamin K deficiency) and pain due to bone disease (calcium and vitamin D deficiency). In long-standing cases, clinical and biochemical evidence of hepatocellular dysfunction occurs.

Congenital Non-haemolytic Hyperbilirubinaemia

With the exception of Gilbert's syndrome, the congenital abnormalities of bilirubin transport are very rare. In adults they all have an excellent prognosis, need no treatment and are clinically important only because they may be mistaken for more serious liver disease.

Gilbert's Syndrome. This is usually first recognised in adolescents or young adults. It is almost certainly a condition of varied aetiology and in some cases may be inherited as an autosomal dominant with low penetrance. Gilbert's syndrone generally presents as mild jaundice, usually noticed incidentally or occasionally following viral hepatitis from which there has been an otherwise complete recovery, or is found incidentally with other diseases or from biochemical investigations. Many patients have no symptoms; others suffer episodes of malaise, anorexia and upper abdominal pain, the last occasionally severe, with increase in the jaundice. These episodes may be related to infection, fatigue or fasting. Apart from the presence of mild jaundice, examination is normal. Investigations show unconjugated hyperbilirubinaemia, generally below 100 μmol/l (6 mg/100 ml), with no abnormality of other liver function tests. No bilirubin or excess of urobilinogen is found in the urine. The haemoglobin, red blood cell count, red blood cell indices, reticulocyte count and the serum haptoglobin concentration are normal, giving no evidence of overt haemolysis. Special investigations show that the red blood cell survival is reduced slightly in some patients, but not sufficiently to cause the hyperbilirubinaemia. Liver biopsy is normal, though in the absence of a history suggesting liver disease a biopsy is not necessary.

The main cause of the unconjugated hyperbilirubinaemia is a reduced ability to conjugate bilirubin consequent on a deficiency of glucuronyl transferase; in some cases uptake of unconjugated bilirubin from the plasma may also be impaired. Glucuronyl transferase activity may be increased by the inducing agent phenobarbitone (60 mg thrice daily) which can be used if necessary to diminish jaundice and to ameliorate any other symptoms.

Crigler-Najjar Syndrome. This autosomal-recessive condition, which is due to deficiency of glucuronyl transferase, is very rare. It is now known to occur in two forms. In the Crigler-Najjar syndrome (type I), there is complete absence of glucuronyl transferase from the liver. It causes severe unconjugated hyperbilirubinaemia and kernicterus in the newborn leading to early death, though a few patients have survived to adulthood. The less severe condition (type II), due to partial deficiency of the enzyme, does not cause kernicterus and patients usually survive to adult life.

Dubin-Johnson Syndrome. This condition is also very rare, occurs in young adults, is autosomal recessive and is caused by a reduced ability to transport organic anions, such as bilirubin glucuronide, into the biliary canaliculi. It causes malaise and variable mild jaundice apart from which examination is normal. The serum bilirubin is raised and conjugated in type. Additional organic anions which are poorly transported include BSP, which can be used to diagnose the condition (p. 430), and the contrast agents for biliary radiology so that the gall bladder, though normal, is frequently visualised poorly or not at all on cholecystography. Liver biopsy shows a characteristic dark pigment related to melanin in the centrilobular cells. The prognosis for these patients is excellent as it is also for those with an even rarer variant known as *Rotor syndrome* in which there is no hepatic pigment.

Effect of Drugs on Bilirubin Metabolism

Numerous drugs and chemicals affect bilirubin metabolism, and these should be kept in mind as possible causative factors in patients with jaundice. In normal adults drugs interfering with bilirubin disposal produce only mild hyperbilirubinaemia, sometimes without jaundice, but more marked jaundice may occur where the ability to metabolise bilirubin is impaired. This occurs in the newborn, where hyperbilirubinaemia may become sufficient to cause kernicterus (p. 733), in those with congenital non-haemolytic hyperbilirubinaemia and in patients with chronic liver diseases such as cirrhosis. This type of hyperbilirubinaemia disappears readily when the drug is stopped.

The main sites at which drugs may interfere with bilirubin metabolism are shown in Table 9.1. Sulphonamides and salicylates displace unconjugated bilirubin from the binding sites on serum albumin; given to a newborn child with haemolytic disease or to the mother in late pregnancy, they may precipitate the development of kernicterus without increasing the serum bilirubin. Drugs which raise the serum bilirubin may increase either its unconjugated or conjugated forms depending on whether they act prior to or at the stage of conjugation or thereafter. Unconjugated hyperbilirubinaemia occurs when drugs produce haemolysis, im-

Table 9.1 Sites of action of some drugs *reducing* the plasma protein binding of bilirubin or its uptake, transport, conjugation or excretion by hepatocytes

	Site of action		
Plasma	Hepatocyte		
Protein binding	Uptake and transport	Conjugation*	Excretion into canaliculus
Sulphonamides	Rifampicin	Novobiocin	Sulphadiazine
Salicylates	Filix mas		Oral contraceptives
	Cholecystographic media		Methyltestosterone
			Anabolic steroids (C-17α alkyl substituted testosterones)
Unconjugated bilirubin		Conjugated bilirubin	

* Phenobarbitone *increases* conjugation of bilirubin.

pair transport from the plasma to the conjugating site or reduce conjugation itself. Conjugated hyperbilirubinaemia occurs when transport of conjugated bilirubin into the biliary canaliculus is impaired; drugs which do this also reduce BSP transport and increase BSP retention in the blood. Inducing agents, such as phenobarbitone can increase the capacity of the liver to conjugate bilirubin so that patients on long-term treatment with such agents, e.g. epileptics, tend to have low serum bilirubin concentrations.

Oral Contraceptives. These agents often contain an oestrogen capable of causing cholestasis and a progestogen. Occasionally they cause jaundice, almost always within the first three cycles. The serum bilirubin often exceeds 170 μmol/l (10 mg/100 ml) and the alkaline phophatase activity is high indicating cholestasis. The reaction is a complex one, however, as the serum transferase activity is also moderately increased and liver biopsy shows some hepatocellular damage in addition to cholestasis. Those who develop jaundice due to oral contraceptives frequently also develop cholestasis of pregnancy and both conditions may reflect an unusual hepatic reaction to a steroid agent. This may have a genetic basis as both conditions show a similar geographic distribution.

Acute Parenchymal Disease of the Liver

Aetiology. In acute parenchymal liver disease (acute hepatitis) there is a sudden episode of widespread damage in which variable numbers of hepatocytes undergo necrosis. These episodes are due largely to infective or toxic agents.

Infections. The most important infective causes are the hepatitis A and B viruses. Cytomegalovirus, Epstein-Barr virus and yellow fever virus occasionally cause clinically apparent acute hepatitis. Other viruses, however, have been implicated only rarely. Less frequently non-viral agents such as *Leptospira icterohaemorrhagiae* (Weil's disease), *Toxoplasma gondii* (toxoplasmosis) and *Coxiella burneti* (Q fever) may cause acute hepatitis. Hepatic damage can also occur in severe extrahepatic infections, especially with septicaemia; this is not due to infective agents reaching the liver.

Toxic Substances. Most substances causing acute hepatitis are drugs. How often an individual drug is responsible depends on the frequency with which it is used and in what proportion of cases hepatic damage occurs. Usually, liver damage caused by drugs is due to idiosyncratic reactions (i.e. reactions occurring in a few individuals who become hypersensitive in a broad sense to the drug); among the drugs more commonly responsible are: chlorpromazine and other phenothiazines, phenelzine and other monoamine oxidase inhibitors, imipramine, amitryptiline, erythromycin, isoniazid, rifampicin (and occasionally other antituberculous drugs), halothane, methyldopa, phenylbutazone, indomethacin, chlorpropamide and thiouracil. Liver damage due to drugs is reported increasingly, and any drug should be suspected. A few drugs cause liver damage in all people in a dose-related manner. These include tetracycline, especially in pregnancy or in those with renal dysfunction, and paracetamol which is often used in self-poisoning.

Potent liver poisons include carbon tetrachloride and yellow phosphorus. Where there are strict rules regarding their use, damage due to these agents is rare. Occasionally severe liver damage from eating poisonous fungi (*Amanita phalloides*) occurs. Alcohol is by far the most important liver toxin; in addition to chronic liver damage it may produce acute alcoholic hepatitis.

Other conditions. Rarely, severe fatty degeneration of the liver of unknown cause may be encountered, for example in pregnancy.

Pathology. Viral hepatitis and most drug-induced hepatitis show similar hepatic lesions. Cell damage throughout the liver is the dominant abnormality, though individual lobules are variably affected. Most damage occurs in the centrilobular areas where it may be enough to cause some collapse of the reticulin framework, especially around the central veins. Damaged hepatocytes have a swollen granular appearance, while dead ones become shrunken and deeply stained, sometimes losing their nuclei to form eosinophilic Councilman bodies; these bodies, originally described in yellow fever, suggest acute hepatitis. The lobules may be infiltrated with mononuclear cells, especially in the centrilobular areas. Polymorphonuclear leucocytes and fatty change are not seen. The portal tracts are enlarged with a predominantly mononuclear cell infiltrate. More severe damage is accompanied by collapse of the reticulin framework, particularly between the central veins and portal tracts which become linked to one another; this is known as bridging or subacute hepatic necrosis. Very severe damage results in destruction of whole lobules (massive necrosis) and is the lesion underlying fulminant hepatic failure. In occasional cases cholestasis is very prominent.

In some patients, the main histological abnormality is fatty change. This occurs in damage due to carbon tetrachloride, yellow phosphorus and a number of other direct toxins as well as in the acute fatty liver of pregnancy. The changes are most marked in fatal cases.

Viral Hepatitis

Viral hepatitis is almost always caused by one of two agents specific to humans giving rise to illnesses which are similar in their clinical and pathological features. Both frequently also cause asymptomatic infections.

Acute Type A Hepatitis

(Infectious, Epidemic, Short Incubation Hepatitis)

Aetiology. Type A hepatitis is due to a virus for which there is no generally available method of culture. It is highly infectious and is usually spread by human faeces entering the body via the oral route directly or indirectly. Infected persons may excrete virus in the faeces for up to 3 weeks before the onset of jaundice and for about 2 weeks thereafter. Children are most commonly affected and conditions of overcrowding and poor sanitation facilitate spread. In occasional outbreaks, water, milk and shellfish have been the vehicles of transmission. Though faeces is the usual source, other body constituents may also spread disease; the hepatitis may, for example, be spread by blood transfusion. The sources in the community appear to be persons incubating or suffering from the disease; a carrier state, analogous to that for hepatitis B virus, has not been identified. The incubation period of type A hepatitis is 30 to 45 days (range 15 to 110 days).

Pathology. The disease is generalised with involvement of the gastrointestinal tract, heart, pancreas, spleen, etc., but the main lesion is in the liver (see above).

Clinical Features. In the case of average severity, prodromal symptoms precede the development of jaundice by a period of from a few days to 2 weeks. They are the usual manifestations of an acute infectious disease, and include chills, headache and malaise. Gastrointestinal symptoms may be prominent; anorexia and distaste for cigarettes are common and early complaints, and nausea, vomiting and diarrhoea may follow. A non-colicky upper abdominal pain occurs as a result of stretching of the peritoneum over the liver as the organ enlarges; the pain is severe in some patients. Physical signs are scanty in the initial stages; the liver is usually tender, though not readily palpable. Tender enlarged cervical lymph nodes may be found and splenomegaly may occur, particularly in children.

The appearance of bile in the urine and a yellow tint to the sclerae herald the onset of jaundice. As the element of obstruction to the biliary canaliculi develops, the jaundice deepens, the stools become paler and the urine darker, while the liver becomes more easily palpable. At this time the appetite often improves and gastrointestinal symptoms diminish in intensity. Thereafter the jaundice usually recedes, the stools and urine regain their normal colour, the liver enlargement regresses and, in the course of 3 to 6 weeks the great majority of cases gradually recover. Milder cases occur or the disease may run a non-icteric course which is recognised by the association of vague gastrointestinal complaints or malaise with biochemical evidence of hepatic dysfunction.

Laboratory Data. A raised serum transferase activity, even before jaundice develops, is the most striking abnormality. The serum bilirubin reflects the degree of jaundice, the alkaline phosphatase activity rarely exceeds 250 μmol/l (30 K.A. units/100 ml) unless marked cholestasis develops and the albumin concentration is normal. The prothrombin time is increased in severe cases and in these circumstances is a good guide to prognosis. Bilirubinuria is an early finding, occurring in the prodromal phase and usually continuing into the convalescent period. Urobilinogenuria appears just before jaundice, disappears at the the height of the jaundice owing to intrahepatic cholestasis and reappears early in convalescence as a sign of recovery. Mild proteinuria may be present. The white cell count is normal or low in uncomplicated cases, sometimes with a relative lymphocytosis; this is of some value in differentiation from Weil's disease (p. 79). The hepatitis B antigen is not found.

Course and Prognosis. Almost all patients make a full recovery. During convalescence a small proportion relapse with a return of symptoms and signs; in these cases the relapse almost always subsides spontaneously. More frequently, the serum transferase activity increases without any return of clinical illness; these asymptomatic 'biochemical' relapses also subside spontaneously. Either from the onset or during the course of the illness, more severe jaundice of a clinically and biochemically obstructive type may develop and it may follow a prolonged course. Liver biopsy shows the features of hepatitis with prominent cholestasis and no evidence of chronic liver damage. This clinical syndrome is known as *cholestatic viral hepatitis* and, though it may continue for many months, the prognosis is good.

Following clinical and biochemical recovery, debility for 2 to 3 months is common. Sometimes, particularly in anxious patients, there may be prolonged malaise, anorexia, nausea and right hypochondrial discomfort without clinical, biochemical or histological evidence of liver disease. This syndrome, which may be exacerbated by too frequent clinical and biochemical assessment, is known as the *posthepatitis syndrome*; liver disease is not present and it should be treated by reassurance.

Chronic liver disease, though rare, may occasionally occur. Some patients develop persistent hepatitis (p. 449), while others who have suffered a severe and prolonged acute illness may go on to develop cirrhosis within a few months or years (posthepatitic cirrhosis). Active chronic hepatitis (p. 449) may also occur, but in these cases it is possible that the initial acute illness was, in fact, the first manifestation of active chronic hepatitis itself. A proportion of patients found to have cirrhosis give a history of jaundice many years before from which recovery was apparently complete; any relation between the two conditions in such cases is doubtful as patients with cirrhosis of known aetiology may give just such a history.

Death from acute type A hepatitis is very uncommon. In young adults, the mortality is around 0·2 per cent. With increasing age, however, the frequency of severe episodes and death increases so that over the age of 60 years mortality reaches about 3 per cent. Evidence regarding mortality during pregnancy is conflicting; most reports suggesting an increased mortality derive from countries in which the standard of living is low where factors such as poor nutrition may be important. In Europe and North America the mortality in pregnant women is probably not increased. Virtually all who die of the acute illness do so after developing fulminant hepatic failure (p. 443). Rarely, pancytopenia may complicate viral hepatitis, occurring some months after recovery.

Differential diagnosis is discussed on page 444.

Treatment. There is no specific therapy; general measures applicable to all forms of acute hepatitis are discussed on page 445. Although for many years patients have been treated in general medical wards without cross-infection occurring, indicating that isolation is not essential, precautions for preventing the spread of enteric infections are advisable.

Prevention. The most effective measures are to improve social conditions, particularly overcrowded and unhygienic situations. In sporadic cases prevention of disease in contacts cannot be achieved as the patient is infectious during the incubation and prodromal stages. However, once the disease is recognised, contacts may be protected by gammaglobulin, especially those at particular risk such as close contacts, the elderly, those with other major disease and perhaps pregnant women. Persons travelling to endemic areas may be protected by gammaglobulin for about 6 months. A vaccine against type A hepatitis virus is not available.

Acute Type B Hepatitis

(Serum, Post-transfusion, Long Incubation Hepatitis)

Aetiology. Type B hepatitis is due to a virus which cannot yet be grown but which can be transmitted to certain primates, such as the chimpanzee, in which it may replicate. The virus and an excess of its capsular materal circulate in the blood where it can be identified by its HBsAg. Blood and certain blood products are the main sources of infection. Only those blood products subjected to pasteurisation (albumin solutions, γ-globulin fraction) can be regarded as wholly free of risk. Spread may follow transfusion of infected blood or blood products or injections with contaminated needles, a mode of spread most common among parenteral ('mainline') drug abusers who share needles. Tattooing may also spread this disease as needles are reused frequently. In the past, vaccines to measles, mumps and yellow fever, using human serum, have transmitted infection.

The ability to identify the hepatitis B virus by the HBsAg has led to the realisation that some patients thought to have sporadic type A hepatitis actually have sporadic type B hepatitis and that in these cases the usual parenteral modes of spread have not occurred. Infected serum can transmit disease orally and the discovery of the HBsAg in other body fluids, such as saliva, urine, semen and vaginal secretions, suggests many alternative modes of spread. Currently, close personal contact seems necessary and sexual intercourse, especially in male homosexuals, may be an important route of transmission. Finally, the virus may be spread from mother to child; the exact mechanisms whereby this occurs are not certain, but transmission at or soon after birth seems more likely than transplacental spread. Humans are the only source of the hepatitis B virus; in addition to those incubating or suffering from the disease, some asymptomatic individuals carry the virus in the blood over long periods, perhaps for life (p. 431). The incubation period of type B hepatitis is 60 to 120 days (range 30 to 210 days). A negative test for the HBs antigen in the blood does not exclude type B hepatitis.

Pathology. The pathology is as for type A hepatitis (p. 439).

Clinical Features. The clinical features are as in type A hepatitis, though type B hepatitis tends to be a more severe disease. In its post-transfusion form, it obviously tends to occur in older people and in those with serious underlying disease. Transient rashes, including urticaria, may occur and arthralgia is common. Though these can occur in type A hepatitis, they are much more suggestive of type B hepatitis. Arthritis strongly suggests type B hepatitis. Even in previously healthy people, the virus persists in some 5 per cent of cases (p. 431).

Course and Prognosis. This is very similar to that for type A hepatitis; however type B hepatitis tends to be a more severe disease. In about 5 per cent of cases chronic hepatitis B carriage follows the acute clinical episode. The mortality in type B hepatitis is higher depending on the virulence of the virus, age of the patient and the underlying disease; it may then reach 30 per cent.

Chronic Asymptomatic Carriers. Some otherwise healthy people with no history of hepatitis may be long-term carriers of the hepatitis B virus. Most have no clinical evidence of liver disease and, in many, liver function tests are normal. Although the prognosis of this condition is uncertain, the virus may be carried for many years without severe chronic liver damage occurring. Those without clinical or biochemical evidence of liver disease need not be investigated further; those with persistent biochemical abnormalities should be investigated by biopsy as those with active chronic hepatitis may benefit from therapy (p. 450). Although chronic asymptomatic carriers may transmit hepatitis, their degree of infectivity is fairly low, especially when liver function tests are normal. Precautions to avoid transmission are needed when these patients undergo medical or dental treatment.

Treatment and Prevention. No specific treatment is available. Supportive therapy is described on page 445.

Post-transfusion type B hepatitis can be largely prevented by scrupulous blood transfusion technique, by eliminating donors with a history of jaundice and by screening all blood for the HBsAg, especially by using highly sensitive methods. These precautions will not, however, eliminate post-transfusion hepatitis as the laboratory tests are not infallible and as the condition may be caused by other than the hepatitis B virus. Pooled dried plasma has proved a potent source of hepatitis which can be virtually eliminated by limiting the pool size to 10 donors. Sterile needles and syringes should always be used and if disposable equipment is not available these should be autoclaved for 20 minutes at 120°C. Washing in 2 per cent carbolic acid and boiling in water for 20 minutes is an acceptable emergency procedure.

Standard gammaglobulin is of no value in the prevention of type B hepatitis. Recently, however, gammaglobulin prepared from the blood of persons with HBs antibody has been shown to prevent this disease. Where available it should be given to persons without HBsAg or its antibody in their blood within a week of exposure to infected blood in circumstances likely to cause infection; these include accidental needle puncture, gross personal contamination with infected blood or exposure to infected blood in the presence of cuts and grazes.

Fulminant Hepatic Failure

(Acute Massive Liver Necrosis)

Fulminant hepatic failure is a rare syndrome in which hepatic encephalopathy, characterised by mental changes progressing from confusion to stupor and coma, results from sudden severe impairment of hepatic function. The syndrome is defined further as occurring within 8 weeks of onset of the precipitating illness in the absence of evidence of pre-existing liver disease to distinguish it from those instances in which hepatic encephalopathy represents a deterioration in an on-going chronic liver disease.

Aetiology. Acute viral hepatitis, either type A or type B, is the commonest cause. Drugs are the next most frequent cause (p. 438). Rarely, it may occur in pregnancy (acute fatty liver of pregnancy), in Weil's disease, following surgical shock or from poisons such as carbon tetrachloride.

Pathology. Extensive parenchymal necrosis is the most obvious lesion (p. 439). In fatal cases, less than 30 per cent of the liver cells appear viable histologically and often few such cells are seen. Severe fatty degeneration is characteristic of some causes of this syndrome.

Clinical Features. Cerebral disturbance (encephalopathy) is the cardinal manifestation of fulminant hepatic failure. Its cause is unknown, but is thought to be due to toxic substances, including ammonia, fatty acids and nitrogenous substances; these last may act as false neurotransmitters. The earliest features are reduced alertness and poor concentration progressing though behaviour abnormalities including restlessness, aggressive outbursts and mania, to drowsiness and coma. Confusion, disorientation, inversion of sleep rhythm, slurred speech, yawning, hiccoughing and, in the late stages, convulsions may occur. More general symptoms include weakness, nausea, and vomiting. Right hypochondrial pain is only an occasional feature.

Examination shows jaundice which develops rapidly and is usually deep in fatal cases though, rarely, death may occur before it develops. Fetor hepaticus, a sweet musty odour to the breath, may be present and is said to be due to methyl mercaptan. A flapping 'hepatic' tremor of the extended hands is characteristic. The liver may be enlarged initially, but later becomes impalpable. Hepatic dullness on percussion may disappear indicating much shrinkage and a bad prognosis. Splenomegaly is uncommon and never prominent. Ascites and oedema occur in a few patients surviving a week or more. Purpura and overt bleeding such as melaena reflect severe haemostatic disturbance. Neurological examination may show chorea, muscle spasticity and extensor plantar responses. Other features include fever, sweating, hypotension, tachycardia, hyperventilation and renal failure.

Laboratory Data. The serum bilirubin concentration reflects the degree of jaundice. Initially, serum transferase activity is very high (>30 fold increase), but with progression of damage activity falls; this investigation has diagnostic but not prognostic significance. Alkaline phosphatase activity is variable. Serum albumin concentration remains normal unless the course is prolonged. Increased serum and urine amino acids are characteristic but are not generally measured. The prothrombin time rapidly becomes prolonged as coagulation factor synthesis fails; this is the laboratory test of greatest prognostic value, a progressive and marked prolongation being a very bad prognostic sign. White blood cell counts vary, leucocytosis occurring even in the absence of infection. The urine contains protein, bilirubin and urobilinogen. Investigations required for the detection of complications are discussed on page 432.

Course and Progress. The progress of fulminant hepatic failure is closely related to the encephalopathy. When only minor signs are present and drowsiness is not prominent some two-thirds of patients survive. Once the patient is comatose only 10 to 20 per cent survive. The prognosis is worse with increasing age and perhaps when due to certain agents such as halothane. In fatal cases, death usually occurs within a week. Life-threatening complications, some amenable to conservative therapy, may arise in the course of the illness. These include profound hypoglycaemia, cerebral oedema, respiratory failure, hypothermia, bacterial infections, bleeding due to coagulation disorders, pancreatitis and renal failure with severe oliguria. Electrolyte disturbances, particularly hyponatraemia, hypokalaemia and alkalosis, may also occur. The great majority of those who recover from fulminant hepatic failure regain normal hepatic structure and function.

Treatment. There is no specific therapy. Supportive measures are described on page 445.

Differential Diagnosis of Acute Parenchymal Disease of the Liver

Most patients with acute parenchymal liver disease are suffering from viral hepatitis. This diagnosis depends on the clinical features described above, a history of contact with a jaundiced person or of transfusion, injection, or damage to the skin when handling blood within an appropriate incubation period, the results of liver function tests, and tests for the HBsAg. The possibility of drug-induced hepatitis should always be considered, the diagnosis depending on exposure to the drug within a period not more than 2 weeks prior to the onset of symptoms with no other detectable cause for the illness. In the preicteric phase there may be confusion with other acute generalised infections, acute abdominal emergencies when pain is present, or gastroenteritis. Especially in young persons, there may be confusion with *infectious mononucleosis* in which sore throat, lymphadenopathy and splenomegaly are prominent, atypical blood lymphocytosis is present, and the Paul-Bunnell test generally positive; in this disease abnormal liver function tests are common and jaundice may occur. *Cytomegalovirus infection* should be considered in those with poor immune responses who have received blood transfusion; a specific antibody response occurs, virus may be isolated from the urine, and giant-cells and intranuclear inclusions found on liver biopsy.

Weil's disease may cause severe jaundice and usually occurs in persons exposed to rats such as sewer workers, agricultural workers and miners. In contrast to viral hepatitis, there is a polymorphonuclear leucocytosis and protein, blood and casts are found in the urine. The diagnosis is made by demonstrating a rise in specific antibodies, and leptospires may be isolated from the blood or urine (p. 80).

A most difficult problem is to differentiate jaundice due to viral hepatitis from that due to *large-duct biliary obstruction* usually caused by a stone or a neoplasm. This is particularly so when an episode of viral hepatitis becomes prolonged and obstructive features develop. Clinically, a patient over 40 years old, previous attacks of abdominal pain, the gradual onset of fluctuant or progressive jaundice, marked pruritus, weight loss and right upper quadrant abdominal pain or a palpable gall-bladder indicate a large duct obstruction. Leucocytosis or a positive test for blood in the stool also suggest large-duct obstruction. Liver function tests are of greatest value at an early stage; in viral hepatitis serum alkaline phosphatase does not usually exceed 150 units/l (30 KA units/100 ml) and serum transferase activity almost always exceeds 100 units/l, while in biliary obstruction the reverse usually obtains. This laboratory differentiation becomes less clear as the disease progresses, however, and in biliary obstruction cholangitis may increase serum transferase activity. A plain X-ray of the abdomen may show gallstones, though only 10 per cent of these are radio-opaque, and hypotonic duodenography (p. 350) may reveal an obstructing lesion arising from the head of the pancreas or ampulla of Vater. Oral cholecystography and intravenous cholangiography are of no value in these jaundiced patients; however, the biliary tract may be demonstrated by either transhepatic cholangiography or endoscopic retrograde cholangiopancreatography (p. 351). Liver biopsy may also be useful in revealing hepatitis or features of large bile-duct obstruction. The HBsAg and the antimitochondrial antibody must always be sought. Where viral hepatitis is a possibility, laparotomy should be avoided as these patients withstand anaesthesia and surgery poorly.

Treatment of Acute Parenchymal Disease of the Liver

Aetiological Factors. In most cases nothing can be done to eliminate the cause of the disease. It is important to detect drug-induced acute hepatitis so that the drug may be stopped and the patient warned to avoid its use in future. Penicillin, given early, is effective in Weil's disease (p. 80).

Bed Rest. When symptoms are marked bed rest should be advised, the patient rising to the toilet if desired. Thereafter, the younger patient may be up and about taking care only to avoid exhaustion. For those in whom the risks of hepatitis may be greater, bed rest should be empirically prolonged until symptoms and signs have disappeared and liver function tests have returned substantially towards normal. These patients include those over 50 years, the pregnant, and those with other major disease.

Diet. A good general diet containing some 3,000 kcal daily is desirable. Initially, owing to anorexia and nausea, this may not be tolerated, in which case a light diet supplemented by fruit drinks and glucose is usually acceptable. The content of the diet should be dictated largely by the patient's wishes; however, a good protein intake should be encouraged.

Drugs. Corticosteroids have been advocated in viral hepatitis. Current evidence, however, is that they do not increase recovery and that they may cause serious side-effects. In general, therefore, they should not be used. On the other hand, in patients with marked malaise, anorexia or vomiting they may cause rapid regression of symptoms with return of appetite. In this small group of patients prednisolone may be given provided the HBsAg test is negative as there is some evidence that corticosteroids may lead to chronic HBs antigenaemia. The dose is reduced rapidly from 20 mg daily as symptoms remit. Drugs metabolised in the liver should be avoided where possible, a principle applying especially to sedative and hypnotic agents. Alcohol must be avoided during the illness and should not be taken in the ensuing 6 months. Oral contraceptives may be resumed after clinical and biochemical recovery has occurred.

Fulminant Hepatic Failure. The development of hepatic encephalopathy greatly alters management. There is no specific treatment but certain measures should be instituted as soon as possible once cerebral changes occur. The patient's life is sustained in the hope that hepatic regeneration will occur spontaneously. There should be close observation so that steps may be taken quickly to correct complications as they occur. Encephalopathy is treated by withdrawing all nitrogen intake, by reducing the nitrogen-producing colonic flora with neomycin, 1 g orally 6 hourly and by increasing faecal output with lactulose 15 ml orally twice or thrice daily. If tests for stool blood are positive the colon should be washed out. Electroencephalography may be used to follow the course of the encephalopathy. Sedative drugs must be used with very great care, restlessness and excitement being best controlled, if necessary, with diazepam 5 mg intravenously.

Calories are provided as glucose 300 g daily either orally, if necessary by nasogastric tube, or into a large central vein as a 10–20 per cent solution (0·6–1·2 mol/*l*). Fluid and electrolyte therapy depends on maintenance of accurate fluid balance records and on daily measures of serum urea, sodium, potassium and bicarbonate. Saline must be used cautiously to avoid sodium overload and potassium deficiency, which occurs readily, should be corrected. The blood-glucose should be measured 6 hourly in the severe phase as potentially fatal hypoglycaemia often occurs; its treatment may require large amounts of glucose.

As these patients have poor vasomotor control, early detection of bleeding and rapid correction of blood volume by transfusion is required. This is facilitated by regular recordings of pulse, blood pressure and if possible central venous pressure. Impaired haemostasis leads to bleeding, particularly from the gastrointestinal tract. Intramuscular injections are best avoided. The development of a bleeding tendency is detected by regular haemoglobin, platelet count, prothrombin time and faecal occult blood measurements. Treatment may require fresh frozen plasma, coagulation concentrates and platelet. Cimetidine may prevent gastrointestinal bleeding.

Infection is common and serious. As fever and leucocytosis may result solely from the liver disease itself, these are no guide and regular blood, urine, and throat cultures and chest X-ray should be carried out. Prophylactic antibiotics should not be used; if infection is strongly suspected they may be given once specimens have been taken for culture. A suitable regime is the use of parenteral gentamycin and lincomycin.

A close watch on the respiration is needed as initial hyperpnoea may rapidly become apnoea, requiring tracheostomy and assisted ventilation. Renal failure, revealed by a rising blood urea, may eventually require dialysis. The temperature must be measured 4 hourly as hypothermia can follow central loss of temperature control. Unexplained continuing coma may be due to cerebral oedema even in the absence of papilloedema; treatment with parenteral dexamethasone, 4 mg 6 hourly, can be given. This condition requires intensive patient care, access to varied specialised help, and a hospital with great technical resources.

Many special treatments have been tried. None is of proven value and some involve the risk of infecting staff; they include exchange transfusion, plasmaphoresis, haemodialysis, and extracorporeal circulation of the patient's blood through various animal livers, isolated or *in situ*, or through coated-charcoal columns. Corticosteroids, or gammaglobulin containing hepatitis B surface antibody in HBsAg positive cases, are of no value.

Chronic Parenchymal Disease

There are two main forms of chronic parenchymal liver disease: (1) chronic hepatitis, which comprises the two syndromes, persistent hepatitis and active chronic hepatitis, and (2) cirrhosis.

Aetiology. There are many causes of chronic hepatitis and cirrhosis. In Britain cirrhosis is usually associated with alcohol abuse, active chronic hepatitis and occasionally primary biliary cirrhosis. No cause can be found in 30 per cent of cases. Of less common causes, haemochromatosis accounts for about 5 per cent, all others being rare.

Alcohol. The mechanism whereby alcohol damages the liver is unknown; it is now, however, accepted as a direct liver toxin in man and in other primates. The production of cirrhosis requires a prolonged intake of alcohol of about 100 g or more daily for 5 to 15 years. A daily alcohol intake may be more likely to cause cirrhosis than episodic drinking.

Infection. Rarely, patients with severe type A or type B hepatitis may develop cirrhosis over a few months or years. In some patients with chronic hepatitis or cirrhosis, the proportion showing marked geographic variation (0–30 per cent), the HBsAg is found persistently in the blood and in such cases the hepatitis B virus is presumably the causative agent. Other patients with cirrhosis give a history of jaundice many years previously; the significance of this is, however, unknown. After an epidemic of type A hepatitis cirrhosis is very rare indeed; the hepatitis A virus may be less likely to cause chronic liver disease.

Metabolic Disorders. These include excess hepatic deposition of iron in haemochromatosis and of copper in Wilson's disease. Most metabolic conditions involving the liver occur in childhood, e.g. glycogen storage disease, fibrocystic disease and α_1-antitrypsin deficiency.

Drugs. Chronic hepatitis and cirrhosis have been reported in patients on long-term treatment with methotrexate or methyldopa.

Cholestasis. Prolonged cholestasis anywhere in the biliary tree may cause cirrhosis. In primary biliary cirrhosis, obstruction results from damage to interlobular bile ducts. Cirrhosis from large-duct obstruction may occur with biliary strictures or in sclerosing cholangitis. Neoplastic lesions do not cause cirrhosis as survival is short.

Congestion. Prolonged hepatic congestion may eventually result in cirrhosis. This is rare, as death usually occurs before cirrhosis develops. Congestion may be due to hepatic venous outflow obstruction as in the Budd-Chiari syndrome (p. 457) or, very rarely, chronic heart failure may cause 'cardiac' cirrhosis.

Immunological factors. Some patients with chronic liver disease of unknown cause have abnormal serum antibodies (p. 431). Though the autoantibodies themselves are not cytotoxic, their presence has suggested that liver damage may be produced by abnormal immune mechanisms. Currently, the possibility that sensitised lymphocytes may do this is being actively investigated; lymphocytes from patients with chronic liver disease have been shown to react to antigens in liver and bile and to be capable of damaging liver cells *in vitro*. The importance of these reactions in chronic liver disease, however, remains to be established. Immune reactions to the hepatitis B virus in chronic liver disease are mentioned above.

Malnutrition. This may occur secondarily in patients with cirrhosis, but it is unlikely that it is primarily responsible for cirrhosis. Permanent liver damage does not follow marasmus or kwashiorkor.

Cryptogenic cirrhosis. In this heterogeneous group, no cause can be found.

Pathology. CHRONIC HEPATITIS. Two types of chronic hepatitis are recognised histologically. Their names—persistent hepatitis and aggressive hepatitis—are easily confused with the clinical syndromes they underly—chronic persistent hepatitis and active chronic hepatitis; this should be avoided. In *persistent hepatitis* the essential feature is an infiltration of chronic inflammatory cells confined to the portal tracts which may be expanded or show short fibrous septa extending into the parenchyma. Changes in the hepatocytes are absent or slight; there may be small foci of liver cell necrosis with inflammatory cell infiltration (spotty necrosis) and sometimes the residual changes of viral hepatitis. Lobular architecture is normal and cirrhosis occurs only very rarely. In *chronic aggressive hepatitis*, the histological process underlying the clinical condition, active chronic hepatitis, both the portal tracts and the parenchyma are involved, lobular architecture is distorted and cirrhosis often develops. The portal tract infiltration of mononuclear cells extends irregularly into the surrounding parenchyma so that swollen liver cells become isolated in the inflammatory cell infiltrate. This process of hepatocyte destruction is called 'piecemeal necrosis' and it leads to septum formation linking portal tracts and central veins. The ensuing disruption of lobular architecture is accompanied by the development of regenerative nodules and thereby cirrhosis. Changes in the rest of the parenchyma are variable and resemble those of persistent hepatitis. These changes do not occur diffusely and may be more advanced in some areas than others, a point to be considered in interpreting sequential biopsies.

CIRRHOSIS. In cirrhosis widespread death of liver cells, resulting from many causes, is accompanied and followed by progressive fibrosis, regenerative (nodular) hyperplasia of surviving hepatocytes and distortion of liver architecture resulting in portal-systemic vascular shunts. The whole liver is involved, though not necessarily every lobule. Cirrhotic livers have an infinitely variable appearance limiting the usefulness of anatomical classifications. Currently, a simple classification into three types is used, namely micronodular, macronodular and mixed cirrhosis. *Micronodular cirrhosis* is characterised by regular connective tissue septa, regenerative nodules approximating in size to the original lobules (1 mm in diameter) and involvement of every lobule. This form, also called portal, septal, nutritional, monolobular, or Laënnec's cirrhosis, is characteristic but not pathognomonic of the parenchymal damage induced by alcohol. In *macronodular cirrhosis* the connective tissue septa vary in thickness and the nodules show marked differences in size, the larger ones containing histologically normal lobules. This form of cirrhosis is also called posthepatitic or postnecrotic cirrhosis. *Mixed cirrhosis* shows features of both micronodular and macronodular cirrhosis. None of these types of cirrhosis is static; micronodular cirrhosis may, for example, develop into a macronodular stage.

Chronic Hepatitis

It is important not to confuse gradually resolving acute hepatitis with chronic hepatitis. As there is no certain way to avoid this by clinical assessment or investigation, including biopsy, a diagnosis of chronic hepatitis should only be made firmly once liver disease has been present on clinical or other grounds for at least 6 months.

Persistent Hepatitis

Aetiology is discussed on page 447 and pathology on page 448.

Symptoms are mild and comprise fatigue, poor appetite, fatty food intolerance and upper abdominal discomfort, especially over the liver. The condition may be asymptomatic and revealed by biochemical tests done for other reasons. There may or may not be a history of acute hepatitis. Examination may show slight hepatomegaly, but is often normal. There are no features of chronic liver disease.

Serum bilirubin is normal or slightly raised, serum transferase is raised up to fivefold and alkaline phosphatase is generally normal. Serum albumin and globulin are normal. The HBsAg may be present but autoantibodies are not found. Liver biopsy shows persistent hepatitis.

Differentiation should be made from the posthepatitis syndrome (p. 441) and Gilbert's syndrome (p. 436), as well as from the pericholangitis associated with Crohn's disease and ulcerative colitis (p. 408). The prognosis is usually excellent, the patient should be reassured and no treatment is required. Rarely progression to active chronic hepatitis or cirrhosis may occur.

Active Chronic Hepatitis

(Lupoid Hepatitis, Plasma-cell Hepatitis, Juvenile Cirrhosis)

Aetiology is discussed on page 447 and pathology on page 448.

Clinical Features. This is a more severe disease than persistent hepatitis. It occurs predominantly but not exclusively in the second and third decades and more often in females. It shows a wide range of severity. The onset is usually insidious with fatigue, anorexia and jaundice. Other features include fever, arthralgia, epistaxis and ready bruising. Amenorrhoea is the rule. In about a quarter of cases the onset is acute, resembling viral hepatitis which, however, does not resolve normally. On examination, the general health appears good; jaundice is mild to moderate, or occasionally absent. Signs of chronic liver disease, especially spider telangiectasia and hepatosplenomegaly, are almost always present. Sometimes a 'Cushingoid' face with acne, hirsutism and pink cutaneous striae, especially on the thighs and abdomen, are present. Bruises may be seen.

Though liver disease usually dominates the clinical syndrome, many associated conditions occur in active chronic hepatitis emphasising its essentially systemic nature. These include migrating polyarthritis of large joints, a variety of rashes, most non-specific but including inflammatory papules and urticaria, lymphadenopathy, thyroid disorders such as Hashimoto's thyroiditis, thyrotoxicosis and myxoedema, Coombs'-positive haemolytic anaemia, pleurisy, transient pulmonary infiltration, ulcerative colitis and glomerulonephritis. Many patients have Sjögren's syndrome (p. 645).

Investigations. Liver function tests are markedly abnormal; serum transferase activity is much increased, albumin concentration is often reduced, globulin concentration very high and the prothrombin time prolonged. The serum bilirubin reflects the degree of jaundice but usually does not exceed 170 μmol/l (10 mg/100 ml). Autoantibodies are often found; antinuclear antibody in half the cases, smooth muscle antibody in two-thirds and antimitochondrial antibody in a quarter. The LE cell phenomenon is present in 10 to 20 per cent. The HBsAg may be found, but generally in males and less florid cases unassociated with many systemic features.

Diagnosis and Prognosis. Initially, differentiation from acute viral hepatitis may be impossible but the prolonged course and a biopsy at least 6 months after the onset will generally make the diagnosis clear. In all cases, Wilson's disease must be excluded (p.457). Where ulcerative colitis coexists, cholestatic features suggest pericholangitis rather than active chronic hepatitis. Difficulty in differentiation from persistent hepatitis usually occurs where the liver biopsy does not confirm the clinical diagnosis and in these cases a further biopsy is needed. The course is marked by exacerbations and remissions. Ultimately cirrhosis develops, about half the patients dying within 5 years of diagnosis, usually in the first 2 years. With the development of cirrhosis, ascites (p. 451), encephalopathy (p. 452), and portal hypertension (p. 451) occur. In patients with HBs antigenaemia, the progression of disease is slower so that survival is longer.

Treatment. Corticosteroids have been shown to be life-saving in this disease, especially in the early stages, reducing activity and improving hepatocellular function. Initially, prednisolone 40 mg/day is given orally and the dose reduced gradually as the patient and liver function tests improve. Treatment for at least 6 months is usually needed, when gradual withdrawal of prednisolone may be tried. Relapse is frequent and maintenance therapy (10–15 mg/day) may be required. Where severe corticosteroid side-effects occur, azathioprine 50 mg/day orally may be given and the dose of prednisolone reduced by half. Ascites, encephalopathy and portal hypertension are treated as described on page 454.

Cirrhosis of the Liver

Aetiology is discussed on page 447 and pathology on page 448.

Clinical Features. These vary greatly and may include any combination of the manifestations described below. None are specifically related to particular causes of cirrhosis, though florid spider telangiectasia, gynaecomastia and parotid enlargement are more common in alcohol-associated cirrhosis. Autopsy experience shows that cirrhosis may be entirely asymptomatic and in life it may be found incidentally or with minimal features such as isolated hepatomegaly.

Enlargement of the liver tends to be more common in the early stages of the disease, disappearing as hepatocyte destruction and fibrosis reduce liver size. The patient may complain of weakness, fatigue or weight loss. Non-specific digestive symptoms such as anorexia, nausea, vomiting and upper abdominal discomfort may occur as does gaseous abdominal distension. Otherwise, clinical features are due mainly to portal hypertension and/or hepatic insufficiency.

Portal Hypertension. This results from destruction and distortion of the hepatic vasculature leading to obstruction of blood flow. In addition, there may be transmission of arterial pressure to the portal venous system. Cirrhosis is the commonest but not the only cause of portal hypertension; obstruction of the portal vein, e.g. from thrombosis, may have the same effect (p. 457).

Splenomegaly. Some splenic enlargement in cirrhosis occurs as part of a general reticuloendothelial hyperplasia. Splenomegaly is, however, mainly caused by portal hypertension and in cirrhosis is its cardinal sign. The splenomegaly is seldom marked in adults, the spleen tip rarely reaching more than 5 cm below the costal margin. In children it may be much more marked. When the spleen is not enlarged clinically or radiographically, portal hypertension is unlikely.

Haematological Changes. Moderate leucopenia and thrombocytopenia frequently occur with splenomegaly and are attributed to hypersplenism (p. 625). Anaemia may occur and when hypochromic is usually due to blood loss from the gut. Macrocytes and target cells are common; though the marrow is usually normoblastic, megaloblastic anaemia sometimes occurs. Megaloblastic changes are usually due to nutritional folate deficiency; vitamin B_{12} deficiency is rare.

Collateral Circulation. This occurs where there are portal-systemic communications. These are in the distal oesophagus and proximal stomach, in the anus and distal rectum, in the falciform ligament and between the colonic, omental, splenic and retroperitoneal veins. Collateral vessels may be seen on the anterior abdominal wall and rarely they are very prominent around the umbilicus ('caput medusae'). The most important collateral vessels are in the oesophagus and stomach (oesophagogastric varices) as they may cause bleeding which may be severe and acute, or occult and chronic. Bleeding may occur from varices elsewhere in the gut but this is very rare. The presence of oesophagogastric varices establishes a diagnosis of portal hypertension. Special radiological procedures can demonstrate the patency of the splenic and portal veins, assess the extent of collateral circulation and allow the portal pressure to be measured (p. 433).

Ascites. In cirrhosis ascites is not due solely to portal hypertension. Several factors are responsible for general salt and water retention while portal hypertension and lymphatic obstruction in the cirrhotic liver predispose to the localisation of fluid in the abdomen. Liver failure leads to salt and water retention by decreasing renal blood flow which produces both a reduced glomerular filtration rate with excessive tubular resorption of water and sodium and an increased renal release of renin leading to secondary aldosteronism. Failure of the liver to metabolise aldosterone intensifies the secondary aldosteronism and failure to metabolise vasopressin reduces renal water clearance. Hypoalbuminaemia lowers the colloid osmotic pressure of the plasma, encourages the formation of oedema and may contribute to a poor renal blood flow.

Jaundice. This is mainly due to failure of bilirubin metabolism. Intrahepatic cholestasis may also be a contributing factor. In cirrhosis jaundice is generally mild or absent. Increasing jaundice implies progressing liver failure.

Circulatory Changes. In cirrhosis the circulation tends to be hyperdynamic with increased peripheral blood flow and reduced visceral blood flow especially to the kidneys. The cause for this is unknown. Increased peripheral blood flow is indicated by palmar erythema. Arteriolar changes result in cutaneous spider telangiectases; these lesions comprise a central arteriole, which may raise the skin surface, from which small vessels radiate. They are usually confined to the area above the nipples and occur especially on the face, necklace area, forearms and dorsum of the hands. At an early stage they may appear as white spots on cooling the skin. Reduced arterial oxygen saturation is frequent and central cyanosis may occur; this is probably due to the development of pulmonary venoarterial shunts and similar shunts may predispose to the development of clubbing of fingers.

Endocrine Abnormality. Gynaecomastia, sometimes unilateral, may occur. It can result from the liver disease but may be induced by spironolactone therapy. Loss of libido occurs in both sexes; there is impotence and testicular atrophy in men and breast atrophy and irregular menses or amenorrhoea in premenopausal women.

Haemorrhagic Tendency. This is found in advanced liver failure and is due largely to underproduction of coagulation factors (p. 424). Thrombocytopenia may also occur particularly when splenomegaly is present. It is seldom sufficient to cause spontaneous bleeding but may aggravate bleeding from other causes such as varices. Serum fibrinogen concentration is not reduced until the terminal stages, though in an occasional case fibrinolysis may be significant. Bruising, purpura, epistaxis, menorrhagia or gastrointestinal bleeding can all occur.

Skin Pigmentation. Generalised hyperpigmentation due to increased melanin deposition occurs in a minority of cases. When it occurs, haemochromatosis must be excluded.

Dupuytren's Contracture. Various studies have suggested that there is an increased incidence of Dupuytren's contracture in patients with cirrhosis but the statistical evidence for this is poor.

Fever. About a third of cirrhotic patients have a low-grade fever not due to infection.

Hepatic (Portal–systemic) Encephalopathy. The mental and neurological features described in fulminant hepatic failure (p. 443) occur in cirrhosis in a more chronic and intermittent fashion. This complication sometimes overshadows the liver disease and leads to a diagnosis of primary mental disorder. Rarely, irreversible central nervous system changes occur with paraplegia, parkinsonism, epileptic fits and dementia. In addition to liver failure, the collateral venous circulation in cirrhosis bypasses the liver and allows nitrogenous substances from the gut to reach the systemic circulation thereby increasing the tendency to encephalopathy. Where anastomoses are extensive, encephalopathy may even occur despite relatively good liver function; this is rare in cirrhosis alone, but may be seen following a surgical portal–systemic shunt. A number of factors precipitate hepatic encephalopathy in the cirrhotic patient, including sedative and hypnotic drugs, a high protein diet, infection, trauma including surgical operations, gastrointestinal bleeding, hypokalaemia and constipation.

Investigation. The serum bilirubin may be normal; increases are usually slight. Bilirubinuria may or may not be present, but excessive urobilinogenuria is usual. Serum transferase activity is usually slightly increased by up to three-fold and serum alkaline phosphatase is raised similarly. All these tests may be normal and they are of no prognostic value. The serum albumin is reduced and the prothrombin time remains prolonged in spite of parenteral vitamin K in those with poor liver function; these tests, especially sequential values, are of considerable value as deteriorating tests indicate a poor outlook. The serum globulin is raised. BSP retention is almost always increased, though falsely normal values may occur in hypoalbuminaemia. Autoantibodies or the HBsAg may be found.

Diagnosis. Alternative diagnoses to be considered depend on how the patient presents, for example with haematemesis (p. 370) or ascites (p. 451). In those with hepatomegaly, secondary carcinoma should be especially considered where enlargement is gross, irregular and hard and where the spleen is not palpable. The site of the primary tumour may be found. A primary liver tumour is also possible (p. 458). Cardiac failure, tricuspid disease and constrictive pericarditis should be sought especially where the liver is large, smooth and tender. Rarer causes of hepatomegaly include lymphoma, leukaemia, amyloidosis, sarcoidosis, abscess and hydatid cyst. In the tropics, kala azar, malaria or schistosomiasis may be present. Finally, a cause for cirrhosis must be sought, especially one which is treatable, such as haemochromatosis or Wilson's disease.

Prognosis. Although cirrhosis is a progressive disease, the rate of progression varies and the outlook is related to many factors. The prognosis is better where the cause of cirrhosis is corrected, as in alcohol abuse, haemochromatosis and Wilson's disease. Worsening liver function indicated by jaundice or ascites indicates a poor prognosis unless a treatable cause such as bleeding or infection is present. Encephalopathy not associated with an extensive collateral circulation is a poor prognostic sign and, as with ascites, a poor response to therapy is ominous. Acute bleeding from oesophageal varices is fatal in about one-third of cases. Marked hypoalbuminaemia (below 25 g/l), hyponatraemia (below 120 mmol/l) not due to diuretic therapy and a prolonged prothrombin time are bad prognostic signs. The course of cirrhosis is uncertain as unforeseen complications such as severe infection or hepatoma may lead to death.

Treatment is discussed on page 454.

Biliary Cirrhosis

Biliary cirrhosis is an uncommon condition resulting from prolonged obstruction anywhere between the small interlobular bile ducts and the ampulla of Vater.

Primary Biliary Cirrhosis

This disease affects predominantly women, usually in middle age. A chronic granulomatous inflammation of unknown cause destroys the interlobular bile ducts in the liver with the eventual development of cirrhosis. Pruritus is the commonest initial complaint and may precede jaundice by months or even years. When the patient is jaundiced pruritus is almost always present. Although there may be upper abdominal discomfort, the abdominal pain, fever and rigors of large bile-duct obstruction do not occur. In a few patients diarrhoea resulting from malabsorption of fat and pain and tingling in the hands and feet due to lipid infiltration of peripheral nerves may occur. Bone pain or fractures due to osteomalacia from malabsorption or osteoporosis may be prominent later in the disease.

Examination usually shows a well-nourished patient with or without scratch marks. Jaundice is only prominent late in the disease when the patient may become a bottle-green colour. Xanthomatous deposits occur in a minority especially around the eyes, in the hand creases and over the elbows, knees and buttocks. Hepatomegaly is virtually constant. Splenomegaly occurs later as portal hypertension develops. The disease generally lasts 5 to 10 years terminating in liver failure or alimentary bleeding.

The diagnosis is based on the clinical picture, on liver function tests showing cholestasis, especially a very high serum alkaline phosphatase activity greater than 250 units/l (30 KA units/100 ml), and on a positive antimitochondrial antibody test. It is confirmed by liver biopsy and the demonstration of normal large bile ducts on intravenous or retrograde cholangiography; occasionally laparotomy may be needed to determine the diagnosis.

In primary biliary cirrhosis no specific therapy is available. Azathioprine is of no value and corticosteroids are contraindicated as they exacerbate or precipitate bone disease. Palliative measures, e.g. for pruritus, are described on page 456.

Secondary Biliary Cirrhosis

This develops after very prolonged large duct biliary obstruction due to gallstones, bile duct strictures and, occasionally, sclerosing cholangitis (p. 465). It does not occur with neoplastic obstruction as survival is usually short. There is chronic cholestasis with episodes of ascending cholangitis or even liver abscess manifested by upper abdominal pain, tender hepatomegaly, fever, rigors, leucocytosis and sometimes a positive blood culture or septicaemic shock. Finger clubbing is common and xanthomas and bone pain may develop. Cirrhosis, ascites and portal hypertension are late features.

Treatment of Hepatic Cirrhosis

Although no treatment can reverse cirrhosis or even ensure that no further progression occurs, medical therapy can promote improved general health and alleviate symptoms. The main problems are to detect treatable causes, to correct malnutrition, to control fluid retention, encephalopathy and alimentary bleeding and to manage chronic cholestasis.

Aetiological Factors. Treatable conditions such as alcohol abuse, drug ingestion, haemochromatosis and Wilson's disease should always be sought. Relief of biliary obstruction will prevent biliary cirrhosis.

Nutrition. In the absence of encephalopathy or ascites, a high energy (3,000 kcal/day), protein-rich (80–100 g/day) diet should be advised. Where cholestasis is not a feature, fat intake need not be restricted. Alcohol must be forbidden. When a good diet is taken, vitamins and other supplements are not required.

Fluid Retention. Treatment of ascites and oedema may relieve symptoms but does not improve the prognosis and, if overvigorous, may lead to fatal complications. In mild cases, therefore, only salt restriction need be advised; by using salt in cooking while avoiding salt at table and especially salty foods such as soups, ham and bacon, daily salt intake may be reduced to about 2 g of sodium chloride daily (40 mmol of sodium). More severe ascites requires diuretics. Initially, a potassium sparing drug such as spironolactone (100–200 mg/day) or triamterene (100–200 mg/day) should be used. Additional diuresis may be obtained from a medium potency diuretic such as bendrofluazide (p. 162). Potassium supplements may or may not be necessary with this drug combination but hypokalaemia should be avoided as it may precipitate or worsen encephalopathy.

Patients with marked ascites should be admitted to hospital. They generally have more severe liver dysfunction and require more vigorous therapy to which they are apt to react adversely. Bed rest, restriction of water intake to 1 l/day and of salt to 22 mmol of sodium daily (1 g salt), and potassium supplements may induce diuresis. If this does not occur within 4 days spironolactone or triamterene should be added and potassium intake reduced. Only when this has failed should high potency diuretics such as frusemide (80–160 mg) be used. Treatment should aim to produce a weight loss not above 0·5 kg/day, and regular checks should be made of the blood urea and electrolyte concentrations. Occasionally patients do not respond to treatment; many are continuing to take salt and this should be checked. The temptation to remove fluid by paracentesis must be resisted as patients tolerate this very badly. In special centres a Rhodiascit machine to ultrafilter ascites and return its colloid to the patient can be used. Salt-poor albumin (25 g) intravenously over 3 hours with frusemide (40 mg i.v.) may initiate diuresis in resistant cases.

Hepatic Encephalopathy. Episodes of encephalopathy develop in many patients with cirrhosis and are usually readily reversed until the terminal stages occur. The principles of treatment are as in fulminant hepatic failure (p. 443). All dietary protein is stopped or reduced below 20 g/day, 1,500 kcal of glucose being given daily, orally or parenterally. The bowel flora is reduced with neomycin 2–4 g/day orally and laxatives are given to produce two stools daily. Lactulose (10–30 ml thrice daily) is often effective in those resistant to other laxatives; this non-absorbed disaccharide is split by colonic bacteria, and, in addition to increasing stool output, it reduces stool pH thereby limiting colonic ammonia resorption. As encephalopathy improves, dietary protein is increased by 20 g/day on alternate days to an intake of 40–60 g/day which is usually the limit in these cirrhotic patients. In those who respond partially to treatment, levodopa (0·5–2 g/day) may be tried.

Variceal Bleeding. Acute bleeding from oesophagogastric varices is frequently severe and requires blood transfusion. Every effort should be made to avoid hypotension which may reduce liver blood flow and produce significant liver damage. Vasopressin, 20 units in 100 ml of 5 per cent dextrose, should be given over 10 minutes to promote haemostasis by reducing portal venous pressure and blood flow to the variceal vessels. Abdominal colic, evacuation of the bowels and facial pallor from general arteriolar constriction indicate that vasopressin is active; absence of these suggests an inert vasopressin preparation. Cessation of bleeding is judged from nasogastric aspiration, pulse and blood pressure. This treatment can be repeated 2 hourly if bleeding recurs. When initial bleeding has been controlled its source should be determined by endoscopy as more than a third of patients with varices are bleeding from some other lesion, especially acute gastric erosions. Continued or recurrent bleeding from varices may then be controlled by a Sengstaken tube. This possesses two inflatable balloons which exert pressure in the lower oesophagus and gastic fundus. A useful modification, the Minnesota tube, allows secretions to be aspirated from the upper oesophagus when the balloons are inflated. If bleeding continues and liver failure has not occurred emergency surgery is necessary. Where oesophageal varices are bleeding, oesophageal transection or ligation of the varices may be done. Emergency portal–systemic shunt operations carry a high mortality and are reserved for those with good liver function.

In patients with chronic variceal bleeding and in those who have recovered from an acute bleed, the surgical creation of a portal–systemic shunt is the only way to stop further bleeding. The main shunts are the portacaval, the splenorenal and the mesocaval. Although they will reduce the likelihood of further bleeding, these operations have a relatively high mortality and a definite risk of postoperative hepatic encephalopathy, especially in older persons, which may be difficult to control. They do not increase life expectancy, predisposing rather to liver failure. Consequently, portal-systemic shunts should be considered only for those under 60 years of age with good liver function evidenced by good general health, no ascites or evidence of encephalopathy, serum bilirubin less than 35 μmol/l (2·0 mg/100 ml), and serum albumin over 35 g/l. There is no place for the prophylactic use of these operations in patients with varices who have not bled.

Chronic Cholestasis. Where this is associated with irremediable biliary obstruction, episodes of cholangitis require antibiotics. Such treatment should be reserved for exacerbations and not given continuously.

Pruritus, believed to be due to bile acids, is the main symptom demanding relief. This is best achieved with the anion-binding resin cholestyramine, which reduces the bile acids in the body by binding them in the intestine and increasing their excretion in the stool. A dose of 4–16 g/day orally is used. The powder is mixed in orange juice and the main dose (8 g) is taken with breakfast when maximal duodenal bile acid concentrations occur. Cholestyramine may bind other drugs in the gut (e.g. anticoagulants); the latter should therefore be taken one hour or more before the binding agent.

Anion-binding resins are not effective in complete biliary obstruction; then methyltestosterone (25 mg sublingually daily) or, for women, norethandrolone (10 mg orally thrice daily) are usually effective. These drugs, however, increase cholestasis at the canalicular membrane and jaundice invariably worsens. Anion-binding resins and the androgens usually relieve pruritus within a week.

Prolonged cholestasis is associated with steatorrhoea and malabsorption of fat-soluble vitamins and calcium. Steatorrhoea can be reduced by limiting fat intake to 40 g/day. Medium chain triglyceride supplements (Portagen) can be used to augment calorie intake. Monthly injections of vitamin K_1 (10 mg) and vitamin D (calciferol 300,000 units) and calcium supplements should also be given, the latter as effervescent calcium gluconate (2–4 g/day). This preparation, however, contains much sodium and, where there is fluid retention, calcium gluconate alone should be used.

Miscellaneous Diseases of the Liver

Haemochromatosis. This is an uncommon disease in which excessive iron absorption over years leads to a gross increase in total body iron from the normal level of 4 g to 20–60 g. Its aetiology has been the subject of much debate but the concensus favours haemochromatosis as inherited as an autosomal dominant with impaired penetrance. Clinical features generally occur in men aged over 45 years, menstruation and pregnancy providing protective mechanisms in women in whom the disease is 10 times less common.

Iron is deposited widely: the organs involved of greatest clinical significance are the liver, pancreas, endocrine glands and heart. In the liver, iron deposition occurs first in the peripheral hepatocytes extending later to all hepatocytes. The gradual development of fibrous septa leads to the formation of irregular nodules and finally regeneration results in macronodular cirrhosis.

Clinical features include the manifestations of hepatic cirrhosis, diabetes mellitus and heart failure. Leaden-grey skin pigmentation due to excess melanin and iron occurs especially in exposed parts, axillae, groins and genitalia, hence the term 'bronzed diabetes'. Impotence, loss of libido and testicular atrophy are also common.

The serum iron concentration is increased and the serum iron binding capacity is over 80 per cent saturated. The serum ferritin is also high (p. 432). The diagnosis is confirmed by liver biopsy.

Haemochromatosis must be distinguished from other forms of cirrhosis, especially that due to alcohol in which there may be excess liver iron. Differentiation must also be made from other causes of excess body iron discussed below.

Treatment is by weekly venesection of 500 ml (250 mg iron) until the serum iron is normal; this may take 2 years or more. Thereafter, venesection is done to keep the serum iron normal. Other therapy includes that for cirrhosis and diabetes mellitus.

Secondary Haemosiderosis. Many conditions are associated with widespread secondary siderosis. Though they may cause features similar to haemochromatosis, these are rare and the history suggests the true diagnosis. Primary conditions include chronic haemolytic disorders, sideroblastic anaemia (p. 601), multiple blood transfusion (generally over 150 *l*) and Bantu siderosis (p. 113). Marked hepatic siderosis may also occur in alcoholic cirrhosis.

Hepato-lenticular Degeneration (Wilson's Disease). This rare condition is described on page 732. It is important to note that any of its hepatic features, including cirrhosis, may occur without neurological abnormality. Kayser–Fleischer rings occur in virtually all patients with symptoms though their recognition may require slit-lamp examination. An episode of jaundice is often the first sign of disease; this may mimic acute viral hepatitis or be due to haemolysis consequent on red blood cell damage following sudden release of tissue copper. These episodes of jaundice may lead to fulminant hepatic failure. Later, the condition may proceed to active chronic hepatitis or a well-compensated cirrhosis. Slit-lamp examination of the cornea and measurement of the serum caeruloplasmin (p. 432) must be done in all young patients with recurrent acute hepatitis or chronic liver disease of unknown cause irrespective of associated neurological abnormality.

Non-cirrhotic Portal Hypertension. Any obstruction to the portal blood flow results in portal hypertension; cirrhosis is much the commonest but not the sole cause. Portal or splenic vein obstruction is followed by the development of collateral vessels by-passing the obstruction as well as portal hypertension. Umbilical infection in the neonatal period is believed to be an important cause but other conditions leading to thrombosis include polycythaemia rubra vera, malignant invasion from surrounding organs and pancreatitis. Portal tract lesions may also be responsible, including schistosomiasis, congenital hepatic fibrosis, myeloproliferative disease, exposure to arsenic or vinyl chloride and primary biliary cirrhosis. Other intraphepatic diseases causing portal hypertension include the Budd–Chiari syndrome.

Hepatic Venous Outflow Obstruction. *(Budd–Chiari Syndrome).* This is an uncommon condition in which venous obstruction occurs anywhere between the efferent centrilobular veins and the right atrium. Obstruction may be due to thrombosis, especially in polycythaemia rubra vera, invasion by tumours of the liver, kidney, or adrenal, or to congenital venous webs. The syndrome may develop in constrictive pericarditis or right ventricular failure. It also follows damage to the central hepatic veins in *veno-occlusive disease*, occurring especially in children in Jamaica due to ingestion of toxic alkaloids in 'bush tea' infused from plants. In up to three-quarters of patients no cause can be found for the obstruction.

The condition generally develops fairly rapidly with abdominal pain, tender hepatomegaly and ascites. Liver biopsy shows severe centrilobular congestion. Hepatic venous obstruction is demonstrated angiographically. Most patients die within a year but a few survive longer and develop cirrhosis.

Congenital hepatic fibrosis is a rare condition in which broad fibrous bands are found in the liver. Most patients have associated polycystic renal disease. Many die in early childhood of renal failure. Those who survive often develop gastro-intestinal bleeding due to portal hypertension, usually presenting between 5 and 30 years of age.

The Liver in Protozoal and Helminthic Infections. Protozoal infections associated with liver changes include malaria, trypanosomiasis, visceral leishmaniasis, toxoplasmosis and amoebiasis; the last is the most important as it causes liver abscesses which respond promptly to treatment (p. 844). In some cases of persistent malarial infection gross splenomegaly and portal hypertension develop (p. 839).

Schistosomiasis is the most significant helminthic infection as it may cause portal hypertension (p. 451). Echinococcosis, giving rise to hydatid liver cysts (p. 903), is the nest most important. Rarely the roundworm, *ascaris lumbricoides* (p. 906), may obstruct the common bile duct, and liver flukes (p. 900) may cause inflammation and adenocarcinoma of the bile ducts.

Cysts. Solitary cysts are rare, probably congenital, vary greatly in size and oc-cur more frequently in the right lobe. Polycystic disease is characterised by many cysts of variable size; half the patients have associated polycystic disease of the kidneys (p. 502). Cysts may be found elsewhere as in the pancreas and lungs. Some patients have cerebrovascular aneurysms. Hepatic cysts are usually found inciden-tally. Occasionally a large cyst may cause upper abdominal pain, nausea, vomiting and a palpable mass. Complications are rare and include obstructive jaundice, tor-sion, bleeding and rupture. Portal hypertension may occur in the polycystic form. Liver function tests are usually normal. Cysts show as rounded filling defects on liver scan.

Tumours of the Liver

Primary Neoplasms. *Hepatocellular carcinoma (hepatoma)* is the principal primary liver tumour. Its incidence shows great geographic variation. It occurs predominantly in males, and in 80 per cent of cases cirrhosis is present. Cirrhosis may be of any type, but hepatoma appears most commonly in haemochromatosis and alcoholic cirrhosis, dominantly male diseases, and rarely in primary biliary cirrhosis, which mainly affects women. Other aetiological factors include ingestion of aflatoxin-contaminated foods in tropical countries (p. 819) and exposure to toxins such as thorotrast, and arsenic. These last toxins usually produce angiosar-comas but they may also cause hepatomas. Oestrogens and androgens may cause adenomas or rarely hepatomas. The role of the HB virus is unknown.

Macroscopically, the tumour may be a single mass or there may be multiple tumour nodules. Microscopically, the tumour is made up of trabeculae of well-differentiated cells resembling hepatocytes. Bile secretion by tumour cells may be seen.

Deterioration in a patient with cirrhosis should always lead to suspicion of hepatoma, the clinical features of which include weakness, anorexia, weight-loss, fever, abdominal pain, abdominal mass and ascites. Hepatomas are vascular so that a bruit may be heard over the liver or intraabdominal bleeding may occur. Metabolic abnormalities are recognised increasingly and include polycythaemia, hyper-calcaemia, hypoglycaemia and porphyria cutanea tarda.

The detection of α-fetoprotein (p. 432) in the blood is virtually diagnostic. A liver scan almost always reveals a filling defect(s) and the diagnosis may be confirmed by liver biopsy. Positive α-fetoprotein tests occur in only-one third of patients in Western countries. Surgical removal requires a tumour confined to one lobe in the absence of cirrhosis and is rarely feasible; the possibility should always, however, be considered. No other therapy is of great value.

Other primary tumours are rare; they include haemangioendothelial sarcomas and adenomas. Cholangiocarcinoma is described elsewhere (p. 466).

Secondary Neoplasms are common and usually originate from carcinomas in the bronchus, breast, abdomen or pelvis. They may be single or multiple. Peritoneal dissemination frequently results in ascites.

Symptoms of the primary neoplasm are absent in about half the cases. Hepatomegaly may suggest cirrhosis, though splenomegaly is rare. There is usually rapid liver enlargement with fever, weight loss and jaundice. Liver function tests may be normal, a raised alkaline phosphatase activity being the commonest abnormality. Ascitic fluid has a high protein content, may be blood-stained and cytology may reveal malignant cells. Diagnosis can be made by needle biopsy in the area of a filling defect on liver scan or at laparoscopy.

THE GALL BLADDER AND BILE DUCTS
Anatomy and Physiology

The junction of interlobular bile ducts leads to the formation of the right and left hepatic ducts which exit from the liver in the porta hepatis. These join immediately to form the common hepatic duct which, with the common hepatic artery and portal vein, lies in the free edge of the lesser omentum. The common hepatic and cystic ducts join to form the common bile duct which varies in length (2–9 cm) depending on where the junction occurs. The common bile duct, passing towards the duodenum, is usually divided into supraduodenal, retroduodenal, intrapancreatic and intraduodenal portions; it is, however, more usefully separated into a thin-walled, wide-lumened proximal part up to 10 mm in diameter radiologically, and a thick-walled, narrow-lumened distal part 1–3 cm in length which may taper to a thread radiologically. The thick-walled part starts just outside the duodenal wall; it may be seen radiologically as a notch and is formed by the muscular choledochal sphincter (sphincter of Oddi). The common bile and pancreatic ducts fuse in the duodenal submucosa to enter the second part of the duodenum at the apex of the papilla of Vater. The gall bladder is a pear-shaped sac of about 50 ml capacity situated under the right hepatic lobe. Its fundus lies close to the tip of the right ninth costal cartilage, its body and neck passing posterosuperiorly into the cystic duct which runs in a series of S-bends to join the common hepatic duct. Congenital abnormalities of the biliary system are rare; a folded gall bladder fundus ('phrygian cap') may be seen radiologically and biliary atresia or a choledochal cyst may occur.

The liver secretes bile continuously, producing 1–2 litres daily at a pressure of 15–25 cm of water. As the resting pressure in the common bile duct is somewhat higher than that in the gall bladder, bile enters the latter where it is concentrated about 10-fold by water and electrolyte absorption. The intraluminal pressure in the common bile duct is probably maintained by the choledochal sphincter. Bile duct pressures above 30 cm of water inhibit bile secretion. Reflux of bile into the pancreatic duct often occurs normally. The gall bladder receives an autonomic nerve supply, mainly from the vagus; acetylcholine causes contraction of gall-bladder muscle and it is likely that vagal innervation controls gall-bladder tone while the sympathetic nerve supply has little or no effect. Gall bladder contraction is due mainly to cholecystokinin secreted by the duodenal mucosa in response to food (p. 347). The choledochal sphincter normally opens and closes rhythmically; cholecystokinin and glyceryl trinitrate cause it to relax, while secretin and the analgesic drugs morphine, pethidine and pentazocine cause contraction. Of the analgesic drugs, pentazocine causes least sphincteric contraction. Acetylcholine has variable effects. Peristalsis probably does not occur in the common bile duct.

Radiological Investigations

These are of particular value in biliary disease. An assessment can be made of the concentrating and contracting power of the gall bladder and of the patency of the biliary tree.

Abdominal X-ray. A plain film may show stones in the gall bladder or bile ducts, the soft tissue mass of an inflamed gall bladder, gas in the biliary tree due to a fistula into the intestine or pancreatic calcification. Only 10 per cent of gallstones are radio-opaque.

Cholecystography. This is the most useful single procedure in the diagnosis of gall bladder disease. An iodine-containing compound such as Telepaque is used which is absorbed from the gut, excreted into the bile by the liver and concentrated in the gall bladder so that it becomes radio-opaque; it is given (3 g orally) the night before the investigation. The normal gall bladder shows as a homogeneous ovoid or pear-shaped opacity which contracts in response to a fatty meal. Non-opaque gallstones may show as 'filling defects' within the opaque area; much less commonly a tumour may do the same. Failure of the gall bladder to opacify is a frequent finding in gall bladder disease (non-functioning gall bladder). However, failure to take or vomiting of the tablets, pyloric stenosis, diarrhoea, occasionally intestinal malabsorption, poor liver function or a serum bilirubin above 35 μmol/l (2 mg/100 ml) can produce the same result. In addition, for unknown reasons, a normal gall bladder may fail to opacify in up to 20 per cent of cases; for this reason the test should then be repeated, doses of Telepaque being given on each of the 2 days prior to the test. If the gall bladder still fails to opacify, it is virtually certain to be diseased.

Intravenous Cholangiography. Iodipamide methylglucamine (Biligrafin) given intravenously is excreted by the liver into bile. Provided liver function is good and the serum bilirubin not above 35 μmol/l it will allow the main biliary ducts and the gall bladder to be shown radiologically. This investigation may be used in those who have had a cholecystectomy. The extent of opacification of the biliary tree is much less than that achieved by cholecystography so that gallstones cannot be excluded confidently by this method. Furthermore, side effects due to Biligrafin are fairly frequent; these can be reduced by infusing the agent slowly over an hour rather than injecting it (infusion cholangiography).

Percutaneous Transhepatic Cholangiography. This is of value in patients with obstructive jaundice and may be done if the prothrombin time and platelet count are normal. Under local analgesia a needle or catheter is passed into the liver and if the biliary tract is entered it is filled with a contrast agent. Where there is large-duct obstruction, the dilated biliary tree is usually entered readily allowing demonstration of the site and often the nature of the obstruction. Less frequently the biliary tree is shown to be normal. Though modern methods using narrow-bore needles (Okuda needle) have increased the successful puncture of both normal and obstructed bile ducts, failure to enter the biliary tree cannot be taken to exclude fully a large duct obstruction. This procedure is usually carried out prior to surgery; though the use of narrow-bore needles has reduced the need for immediate surgery, facilities for operation should still always be available.

Endoscopic Retrograde Cholangiopancreatography. (ERCP, p. 351).

Operative and Postoperative Cholangiography. During operations on the biliary tract, the biliary tree should always be defined by injecting contrast material, either via the cystic duct or directly into the common bile duct. A similar procedure should be used postoperatively before withdrawing a draining tube (T tube) from the common bile duct.

Gallstones

Gallstone formation is the commonest disorder of the biliary tract. Indeed, gall bladder disease in its absence is a rarity.

Epidemiology and Pathology. The prevalence of gallstones is not known as in most instances they are asymptomatic; however, they are exceptionally common among certain American Indians and in Sweden, common in North America, Europe, Australia and among South African whites, but less frequent in India and the Far East, and rare in African blacks. Gallstones are generally twice as common in females as in males and their frequency rises with age. In prosperous countries the incidence of symptomatic gallstones seems to be increasing and occurring at an earlier age.

In the past, gallstones have been classified by their macroscopic appearance into metabolic, inflammatory and mixed types. Biochemical analysis, however, has shown this to be misleading. In countries where gallstones are common, cholesterol is the most usual and frequently the major component irrespective of appearance. It is found in over three-quarters of gallstones accounting for 10–98 per cent of their content. Some gallstones are composed almost wholly of calcium salts or bilirubin. The latter are commonest where there has been prolonged overproduction of bilirubin due to haemolysis; very little is known about the formation of calcium stones. Only the development of stones containing cholesterol will be considered further.

Aetiology. Current evidence suggests strongly that cholesterol gallstone formation is due mainly to physicochemical changes in bile predisposing to cholesterol precipitation. Cholesterol, which is insoluble in water, is held in solution in bile by its association with bile acids and phospholipid in the form of mixed micelles (p. 391). In gallstone disease, the liver produces bile containing reduced amounts of bile acid and phospholipid relative to cholesterol with which the bile therefore becomes saturated or even supersaturated. Such bile is termed lithogenic. These changes precede gallstone formation and seem to be due mainly to a reduction in the size of the bile acid pool associated with reduced bile acid secretion into the bile. In a few patients there is also an increased secretion of cholesterol into bile. Although the liver produces the abnormal bile, the gall bladder is important in gallstone formation as it provides sites of origin for cholesterol precipitation and a reservoir for gallstone growth. Infection and inflammation in the gall bladder may enhance the tendency to form stones.

Certain conditions predispose to gallstone formation. These include disease or loss of the terminal ileum and long-term cholestyramine therapy, all of which lead to loss of bile acids in the stool; in cirrhosis the secretion rate and pool of bile acids are low. Diets to lower serum cholesterol and long-term oral contraceptive therapy may also increase the frequency of gallstones.

Clinical Features. These are described below in relation to the various illnesses which may be caused by gallstones.

Treatment. Currently, the only satisfactory treatment is cholecystectomy with the removal of any stones elsewhere in the biliary tree. Chenodeoxycholic acid given orally has been shown to dissolve stones with a high cholesterol content. This therapy is, however, still under trial and is likely to be effective only for those with radiolucent (i.e. cholesterol) stones in a functioning gall bladder. A frequent problem results from the incidental finding of asymptomatic gallstones. Follow-up of persons with these shows a high incidence of subsequent symptoms, sometimes with the development of serious complications, especially in older patients. Whether or not cholecystectomy should be carried out remains controversial, but it should be considered only in those with no contraindication to surgery.

Acute Cholecystitis

Aetiology. Acute cholecystitis is almost always associated with obstruction of the gall bladder neck or cystic duct by a gallstone. Occasionally obstruction may be by mucus or rarely by a neoplasm. Initially, the inflammation is sterile being perhaps due to chemical irritation from an increasing concentration of the bile in the gall bladder. Later, enteric organisms, especially *Esch. coli* and *St. faecalis,* reach the gall bladder by unknown routes and secondary infection occurs. Culture of gall bladder contents within 24 hours of the onset of symptoms yields organisms in 30 per cent of cases, whereas after 72 hours organisms are obtained in about 80 per cent. Acute cholecystitis in the absence of stones is rare; it may develop in typhoid and paratyphoid fever or during bacteraemia.

Pathology. All degrees of inflammation from mild congestion to gross swelling and tenseness of the gall bladder with ulceration of its wall may occur. Occasionally, perforation takes place or the gall bladder may become distended with pus (empyema). Rarely, gas forms in the wall (emphysematous cholecystitis), a condition more frequent in males and in diabetes mellitus.

Clinical Features. The disease occurs at any age. Though more common in women, of the time-honoured factors—fair, fat, fertile, and 40 to 50—only the fat remains true. The disease is seen increasingly in persons aged under 40 years. The cardinal feature is upper abdominal pain mainly in the epigastrium and right hypochondrium. Though described as 'biliary colic', the pain is more fluctuant and with increasing severity radiates to the back and the right shoulder. There may be accompanying nausea and vomiting, fever is present and rigors occasionally occur. There may also be a history of previous similar pains. Examination shows right hypochondrial tenderness and rigidity worse on inspiration (Murphy's sign). Occasionally a gall bladder mass is palpable. Jaundice occurs in a minority and is usually slight; it suggests obstruction of the common duct.

Investigation. Plain X-ray of the abdomen may show gallstones. Cholecystography fails to show the gall bladder and intravenous cholangiography may show the common bile duct but not the gall bladder implying cystic duct obstruction. The serum amylase may be raised but is usually below 500 Somogyi units/100 ml. A moderate leucocytosis is common. Bilirubinuria may or may not be present.

Diagnosis. Differentiation has to be made from other causes of severe upper abdominal pain. These are mainly perforated peptic ulcer, acute pancreatitis, appendicitis (especially retrocaecal) and intestinal obstruction. Myocardial infarction should also always be considered. Investigations useful in this differentiation are the raised serum amylase (p. 386) in acute pancreatitis, chest and abdominal X-rays, and an electrocardiogram. Occasionally there may be confusion with renal colic, herpes zoster, epidemic myalgia, pleurisy and acute intermittent porphyria.

Course and Prognosis. Conservative therapy is followed by recovery in 80–90 per cent of cases though recurrences are common. Sometimes there is deterioration due to the development of empyema, perforation and peritonitis or ascending cholangitis. In these cases increasing abdominal pain and rigidity, high fever, tachycardia and hypotension occur.

Treatment. Initially, conservative therapy is usual. This consists of bed rest, relief of pain, maintenance of fluid balance and administration of antibiotics. Severe pain is relieved best by morphine 15–20 mg intramuscularly. Increased tone of the choledochal sphincter due to this drug may be minimised by atropine 0·6 mg intramuscularly. Less severe pain can be relieved by pethidine 100 mg or pentazocine 30 mg intramuscularly. Effective relief of pain may require repeated doses of analgesic every 2–3 hours. Provided persistent vomiting is not present oral fluids can be given. Nasogastric aspiration is required only when there is persistent vomiting, in which case fluid must be given by the intravenous route. An antibiotic, such as ampicillin 500 mg 6 hourly, is usually administered orally or parenterally in those who are more ill or vomiting; when given intravenously, it must not be put into dextrose solutions as these cause loss of antibiotic activity. During therapy, regular clinical examinations and records of temperature, pulse, blood pressure and fluid balance must be made to detect deterioration early. The development of complications, most common in the elderly, is the indication for surgery. However, over 90 per cent of patients recover; thereafter a cholecystogram is carried out. The finding of stones or a non-functioning gall bladder should lead to cholecystectomy within 2–3 months.

Early operation has been advocated for acute cholecystitis. Therapy is begun as above, cholecystography is carried out as soon as possible and operation done within a week of the onset of the illness. It is emphasised, therefore, that this is not an emergency operation. The results of such therapy are similar to those of conservative treatment. It does, however, require only the one hospital admission.

Chronic Cholecystitis

Clinical Features. Chronic cholecystitis is very common and almost always associated with gallstones. It usually manifests itself as recurrent episodes of biliary colic, unassociated with fever or leucocytosis. The pain lasts for several hours and may be followed by upper abdominal soreness for a number of days. An attack of biliary colic may develop into acute cholecystitis.

Sometimes a gallstone may pass into the common bile duct and cause obstructive jaundice. Upper abdominal pain is present in three-quarters of these patients and there is frequently a history of biliary colic. Biliary infection causes fever in one-third of cases; ascending cholangitis may then be severe, giving rise to liver abscesses or to septicaemia with shock. Obstruction is not usually complete so that the faeces remain pigmented and both bilirubin and excess urobilinogen are present in the urine. Occasionally, a gallstone may obstruct the common bile duct in the absence of abdominal pain or fever suggesting the presence of a pancreatic or biliary neoplasm. Alternatively, it may be associated with an attack of acute pancreatitis (p. 385). Rarely, a larger gallstone which has reached the intestinal tract, usually via a cholecystenteric fistula, may cause intestinal obstruction. This usually occurs in elderly patients. The clinical features are those of small intestinal obstruction with or without a history of biliary colic and the obstruction is usually in the terminal ileum. Abdominal X-ray shows small intestinal obstruction, perhaps the gall-stone and possibly gas in the biliary tree.

Some patients with gallstones complain of non-specific symptoms such as eructations, nausea, vomiting and upper abdominal discomfort mainly in the epigastrium or right hypochondrium. These may be precipitated by fatty foods. This symptom complex has been termed 'gall-bladder dyspepsia' and attributed to chronic cholecystitis. However, while such symptoms do occur in chronic cholecystitis and can be relieved by cholecystectomy, they also occur frequently in patients with other organic and functional bowel disease. Hence, when a patient complains only of these dyspeptic symptoms, other bowel diseases must be excluded carefully before they are attributed to the gall bladder.

Investigation. The results of liver function tests and of urine tests for bilirubin and urobilinogen will depend on the degree of obstruction to the common bile duct. Abdominal X-ray occasionally shows gallstones. Cholecystography will show either gallstones or a non-functioning gall bladder.

Diagnosis. In patients with recurrent biliary colic, pancreatitis is the main alternative diagnosis. Peptic ulcer should also be considered though the periodicity of the pain and its relation to meals is generally different. Reflux oesophagitis or gastric carcinoma may also need to be considered. Patients with biliary tract disease are usually in the older age range and other coincident alimentary disorders, especially hiatus hernia or diverticular disease, are often present. When a severe episode of pain occurs, other causes of an 'acute abdomen' should be considered. In the presence of obstructive jaundice the differential diagnosis lies between a stone in the common bile duct and pancreatic or biliary carcinoma (p. 466).

Treatment. Cholecystectomy and removal of gallstones from other parts of the biliary tree is the only satisfactory treatment. Biliary colic is treated as in acute cholecystitis.

Miscellaneous Diseases of the Gall Bladder and Biliary Tract

Non-calculous Cholecystitis. This is rare. It may occur in typhoid fever, in polyarteritis nodosa, as emphysematous cholecystitis due to *Cl. welchii* in diabetes mellitus and in those on corticosteroid therapy. It may follow trauma and may complicate septicaemia.

Cholesterolosis of the Gall Bladder. In this condition lipid deposits in the submucosa and epithelium appear as multiple yellow spots on the pink mucosa. The changes are restricted to the gall bladder, symptoms are due to associated gallstones and the condition is recognised only at operation.

Adenomyomatosis of the Gall Bladder. In adenomyomatosis there is hyperplasia of all elements in the gall bladder wall. This is usually localised to the fundus where it shows as a filling defect on cholecystography. It may also be generalised in which case cholecystography shows a distorted gall bladder possibly with intramural contrast medium in Rokitansky–Aschoff sinuses. Frequently there are associated gallstones. Although in most cases there are no symptoms, recurrent biliary colic sometimes occurs. In symptomatic cases treatment is by cholecystectomy though where there are no gallstones operation should not be done before excluding other diseases, especially peptic ulcer and pancreatitis. Cholecystectomy should be carried out if it is thought that the filling defect might be a neoplasm.

Postcholecystectomy Syndrome. Where cholecystectomy is carried out for gallstones, 70 per cent or more patients get complete relief of symptoms. When continuing or recurrent dyspepsia or biliary colic occurs, radiological examinations of the biliary tree for gallstones or unrecognised neoplasia should be carried out. Endoscopic retrograde cholangiopancreatography is specially valuable in these patients. In some patients neither this nor investigation for other diseases such as peptic ulcer or pancreatitis shows any abnormality. The patients are then often considered to suffer from a functional abnormality of the biliary tree—'biliary dyskinesia'. There is, however, no good evidence for such a condition and these patients should not be treated by procedures such as sphincterotomy or choledochoduodenostomy. Antacids, simple analgesics, sedatives, avoidance of foods clearly followed by symptoms and reassurance should be tried.

Sclerosing Cholangitis. In this condition there is fibrotic obliteration of the large bile duct system. It may be primary, associated with ulcerative colitis or retroperitoneal fibrosis, or secondary to cholelithiasis or surgery. There is gradually progressive cholestasis and abdominal pain punctuated by episodes of cholangitis. Secondary biliary cirrhosis (p. 454) may occur. Diagnosis is usually made by biopsy of the bile ducts at laparotomy.

Choledochal Cyst. This cystic dilation occurs in the common bile duct. It almost always presents by the age of 30 years with episodes of jaundice and abdominal pain. A mass is usually palpable in the right hypochondrium. Treatment is surgical, usually by drainage of the cyst or, rarely, excision.

Tumours of the Gall Bladder and Bile Ducts

Benign tumours of the gall bladder are uncommon and usually found incidentally at operation or autopsy. Papillomas, often really cholesterol polyps and sometimes associated with cholesterolosis of the gall bladder, and adenomas are the main types.

Carcinoma of the gall bladder is an uncommon tumour occurring more often in women and hardly ever under the age of 50 years. It usually is in the fundus or neck of the gall-bladder and some 90 per cent are adenocarcinomas. The remainder are anaplastic or, rarely, squamous tumours. Gallstones are usually also present and these are often held to be important in the aetiology of the tumour. Clinically, there is frequently a history of repeated attacks of biliary colic and cholecystitis followed by general deterioration in health, weight loss and constant right upper quadrant abdominal pain. The gall bladder or a mass is palpable in the right hypochondrium in half the patients. Jaundice is also present in half the patients and is occasionally an early feature in tumours of the gall bladder neck. Liver function tests most frequently show cholestasis. Gall bladder calcification (porcelain gall bladder), detectable on abdominal X-ray, is strongly associated with cancer. Cholecystography may show a filling defect in the gall bladder but frequently jaundice obviates the procedure or a non-functioning gall bladder is found. Endoscopic retrograde or percutaneous transhepatic cholangiography may be helpful but frequently the diagnosis is made only at laparotomy. In the majority of patients, the tumour is inoperable and survival is short.

Benign tumours of the bile ducts are extremely rare. Almost all are either papillomas or adenomas. They may cause biliary obstruction and generally are diagnosed only at operation.

Cholangiocarcinoma is an uncommon tumour arising anywhere in the biliary tree from the small intrahepatic bile ducts to the ampulla of Vater. It is not associated with cirrhosis. Virtually all the tumours are adenocarcinomas of varying degrees of differentiation and often with a marked connective tissue stroma.

Clinically, obstructive jaundice is the usual presenting feature though this may be delayed where the tumour involves only the right or left hepatic duct or an intrahepatic radical. Half the patients have upper abdominal pain and weight loss. Intrahepatic tumours are diagnosed as described for hepatoma (p. 458) with the exception that alphafetoprotein is hardly ever found. Transhepatic or retrograde cholangiography are the best methods for diagnosing large duct tumours preoperatively. Tumours at or above the junction of the hepatic ducts are often missed at operation despite operative cholangiography which may not show the intrahepatic ducts. Treatment is surgical; it is rarely possible to remove the tumour but palliative surgery to bypass it is worthwhile as growth is slow and survival may be prolonged for a few years.

Prospects in Liver Disease

Among the most important developments in recent years has been the discovery of the hepatitis B surface antigen as a marker of the hepatitis B virus. Further research has revealed other B virus antigens which will prove valuable not only in epidemiological studies but also in identifying virus infected patients likely to develop liver disease. In the foreseeable future, it is possible to look forward to the isolation of the virus itself and then to the development of effective vaccines. This would allow prevention of both acute and chronic liver diseases due to virus B. As a consequence of the progress in studies of virus B there are now efforts to identify the hepatitis A virus with encouraging but—so far—less dramatic results.

In chronic liver disease, prevention must be the long term objective. Much will depend on how society faces the problem of alcohol abuse. Where disturbance of immunity seems to be an aetiological factor, recent observations indicate that the T lymphocyte has a significant role and advances in this area may lead to more rational therapy.

The development of a liver support system for the management of patients with liver failure has, as yet, met with only limited success. Difficulties include perfecting of materials such as polymer-coated charcoal capable of adsorbing substances toxic to the liver. Further progress in this field is urgently required if we are to reduce the very high mortality in acute liver necrosis and also to facilitate liver transplantation. The latter is now seen to be technically feasible and there is steady progress in overcoming the immunity problems of organ transplantation and rejection.

Great advances have been made in understanding the pathogenesis of gallstones and perhaps these will lead to preventive measures in the future. Endoscopic retrograde cholangiography is an important adjunct in the diagnosis of biliary disease and as the expertise becomes more generally available the full impact of this new investigation should become apparent. This and other valuable diagnostic aids have been added to our repertoire and it will be necessary over the next few years to evaluate the many techniques in relation to effectiveness and expense.

N. D. C. FINLAYSON
J. P. A. MCMANUS
JOHN RICHMOND

Further reading:

Bouchier, I. A. D. (Ed.) (1973) Diseases of the biliary tract. *Clinics in Gastroenterology.* Vol. 2, No. 1. Philadelphia: Saunders.

Popper, H. & Schaffner, F. (Eds.) *Progress in Liver Diseases.* Vol. IV (1972) and Vol. V (1976). New York: Grune and Stratton.

Popper, H. (Ed.) (1975) Cirrhosis of the liver. *Clinics in Gastroenterology.* Vol. 4, No. 2. Philadelphia: Saunders.

Read, A. E. (Ed.) (1975) *Modern Trends in Gastroenterology.* No. 5. London: Butterworth.

Schiff, L. (Ed.) (1975) *Diseases of the Liver.* 4th edition. Philadelphia: Lippincott.—A very comprehensive reference book.

Sherlock, S. (1975) *Diseases of the Liver and Biliary System.* 5th edition. London: Blackwell.—The standard textbook for reference purposes.

Tygstrup, N. (Ed.) (1974) Viral hepatitis. *Clinics in Gastroenterology.* Vol. 3, No. 2. Philadelphia: Saunders.

10. Diseases of the Kidney and Urinary System

Structure and Mode of Action of the Kidneys

THE kidneys are each composed of approximately one million nephrons, the basic structure of one of which is illustrated in Figure 10.1.

The blood supply of the kidney is relatively large and amounts to about one-quarter of the cardiac output at rest, i.e. 1,300 ml per minute. The afferent arterioles which give rise to the glomerular capillaries arise from branches of the renal artery. Emerging from the glomeruli the capillaries unite to form the efferent arterioles which then supply blood to the proximal and distal convoluted tubules surrounding the glomeruli. The medulla is supplied by arterioles which arise from those glomeruli situated in the deeper regions of the cortex.

For a short distance the afferent arterioles and distal convoluted tubules are in contact, and at this point the tubular cells become tall and columnar in character, forming the macula densa. The wall of the arteriole is thickened by cells which contain large secretory granules. These structures together constitute the juxtaglomerular apparatus which is intimately concerned in the regulation of the volume of the extracellular fluids and blood pressure.

The hydrostatic pressure within the glomerular capillaries of about 45 mm Hg results in the filtration of fluid from the plasma into Bowman's capsule. This fluid is identical in its composition with plasma except that it normally contains no fat and very little protein. The filtrate thus formed then flows through the various parts of the tubule and is modified according to the needs of the body by tubular secretion and by the selective reabsorption of its constituents.

FUNCTIONS OF THE KIDNEYS

In health the volume and composition of the body fluids vary within narrow limits. The kidneys are largely responsible for maintaining this constancy and the excretion of the waste products of metabolism represents merely one aspect of this task. The various renal functions are conveniently considered under the following headings and some are shown diagrammatically in Figure 10.1.

1. **Regulation of the Water Content of the Body.** About two-thirds of the water filtered by the glomerulus is reabsorbed by the proximal tubules. The remaining water passes through the distal tubules and collecting ducts where its reabsorption is influenced chiefly by vasopressin, the antidiuretic hormone of the posterior pituitary. In the presence of vasopressin the collecting ducts become permeable to water which is then passively reabsorbed in response to the high concentration of sodium chloride and urea which exists in the medullary interstitium. The urine then becomes concentrated. In the absence of vasopressin the collecting ducts are impermeable to water. In these circumstances a dilute urine is formed by the tubular reabsorption of sodium without water. Disorders of the water-regulating mechanism which result in oliguria or polyuria are described on pages 472 and 473.

2. **Regulation of the Electrolyte Content of the Body.** The electrolyte content of the body is kept remarkably constant as a result of selective reabsorption by the renal tubules. A large part of the filtered sodium and probably all the potassium are actively reabsorbed in the proximal convoluted tubules. The

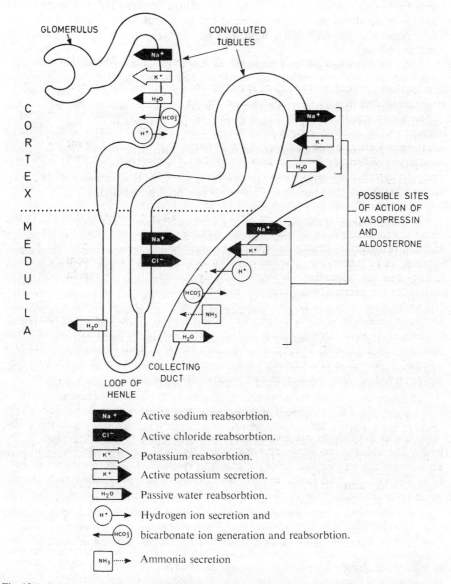

Fig. 10.1 Arrangements of some of the events concerned in urine formation. In the proximal tubule about two-thirds of the filtered sodium, potassium and water are reabsorbed. The greater part of the filtered bicarbonate is also reabsorbed here by a process which involves the secretion of hydrogen ions. The sodium and chloride reabsorbed in the ascending limb of the loop of Henle functions as a counter-current multiplier and is largely responsible for the hyperosmolality of the medullary interstitium. In the distal tubule and collecting duct potassium is secreted partly in response to the negative PD created by active sodium reabsorption. Hydrogen and ammonium ions are also secreted there and water is passively reabsorbed in the presence of vasopressin.

remainder of the sodium passes into the distal tubule and collecting ducts where its reabsorption appears to be under the influence of hormones of the adrenal cortex, especially aldosterone. With reduced secretion of these hormones, excessive quantities of sodium and chloride ions are lost in the urine, whereas with the administration of corticosteroids, sodium retention occurs. The reabsorption of sodium in the distal parts of the nephron creates a negative intraluminal potential with respect to the peritubular fluid; this encourages the secretion of potassium into the tubule.

The dual actions of the adrenocortical hormones and of the antidiuretic hormone on the renal tubules play an important role in determining the total volume of water and the electrolyte content of the body. The rate of secretion of vasopressin is determined mainly by changes in osmolality of the blood; aldosterone secretion is influenced *inter alia* by changes in the pulse pressure within the internal carotid and renal arteries; this influences the rate of secretion of renin by the juxtaglomerular apparatus. It has also been shown that proximal tubular reabsorption of water and salt is influenced by the volume of the blood and the extracellular fluid. How this control is mediated is unknown but the activity of a third so-called natriuretic hormone has been postulated.

3. **Maintenance of the Normal Acid-base Equilibrium of the Blood.** The ingestion and oxidation of a normal diet results in the formation of substances which yield hydrogen ions in aqueous solution. Carbonic acid is dealt with by its conversion to H_2O and CO_2, the latter being eliminated by the lungs. The other acids which include acetoacetic acid and the oxidative products of sulphur-containing proteins require the collaboration of an elaborate mechanism within the kidney for their disposal. These inorganic and organic acids are in the first instance partly neutralised by the blood and other buffer systems as described on pages 164 to 166. By itself this process leaves the blood abnormal in three respects, i.e. the hydrogen ion concentration remains increased above normal, the concentration of bicarbonate is reduced and the anions of the acids still require to be excreted. These abnormalities are corrected by mechanisms shown in Figure 10.2.

The degree to which these mechanisms operate is adjusted in accordance with the nature of the food ingested and the amount of endogenous acid production. In health, on a normal diet, 40–80 mmol of acid are excreted daily into the urine. When a diet consisting mainly of fruit and vegetables is taken alkaline sodium phosphate and bicarbonate are excreted in the urine and tubular secretion of hydrogen and ammonium ions is suppressed.

In disease states in which abnormally large amounts of organic acids are being formed, e.g. β-hydroxybutyric acid and acetoacetic acid in diabetic ketoacidosis, these processes are fully active and may be overwhelmed. Excess acid is retained in the blood and acidosis occurs. When renal tubular activity itself is severely affected by kidney disease these regulatory mechanisms fail and acidosis of renal origin develops.

4. **Retention of other Substances vital to Body Economy, e.g. Glucose, Amino Acids, Phosphate, Bicarbonate, Proteins.** Glucose is normally reabsorbed so completely by the proximal tubules that none can be detected in the urine by clinical tests. Renal glycosuria (p. 562) is a genetically determined benign defect of tubular reabsorption in which glucose appears in the urine in the presence of normal blood glucose levels. More rarely other *congenital or acquired abnormalities of tubular transport* result in abnormal loss in the urine of amino acids, phosphate,

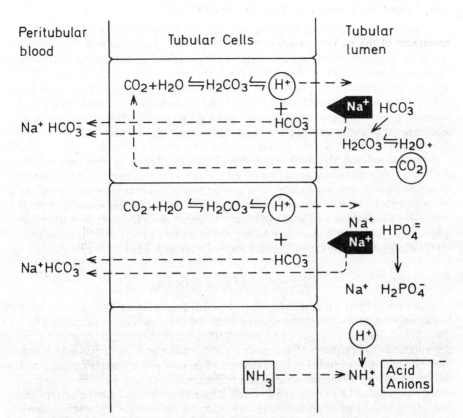

Fig. 10.2 (1) Carbonic acid is generated within the renal tubular cells from CO_2 and H_2O under the influence of carbonic anhydrase. The hydrogen ions of this acid are secreted into the tubular lumen in exchange for filtered sodium which is then reabsorbed into the blood.

The bicarbonate ions liberated from the carbonic acid made in the renal tubular cells are absorbed with the sodium into the blood; this restores the concentration of plasma bicarbonate to normal and also regenerates other buffers in the body which have been titrated by the invading acids.

(2) Some of the hydrogen ions are buffered in the urine by disodium hydrogen phosphate to form dihydrogen sodium phosphate and in the distal tubules by ammonia to form ammonium ions. The anions of the inorganic and organic acids are then excreted in the urine largely as ammonium salts.

sodium, potassium, calcium and water. These defects may occur singly or in combination. Examples of these disorders are cystinuria, familial hypophosphataemia, nephrogenic diabetes insipidus and the Fanconi syndrome, a disease chiefly of infancy and childhood.

In health the great bulk of the bicarbonate filtered by the glomeruli is removed from the urine by tubular reabsorption, and this becomes complete when the urine is acid. *Renal tubular acidosis* is a defect in the power either to reabsorb bicarbonate or to acidify the urine which then usually contains significant amounts of bicarbonate in the face of metabolic acidosis. Such defects may be acquired as a result of renal disease such as pyelonephritis; they also occur as a consequence of myelomatosis, hyperparathyroidism, Wilson's disease and the use of degraded tetracycline. Idiopathic renal tubular acidosis is a rare, inherited form. All types are apt to lead to osteomalacia, nephrocalcinosis and hypokalaemia.

In health only a small amount of protein (0·2 g/l) reaches the fluid in Bowman's capsule. The volume of glomerular filtrate, however, is so great that if this small amount were not reabsorbed, more than 3 g of protein rather than the normal 50 mg would be excreted in the urine in 24 hours.

5. **Excretion of Waste Metabolic Products, Toxic Substances and Drugs.** The end-products of metabolism, especially those of protein, include urea, uric acid, creatinine, phosphates and sulphates and are excreted in the urine.

6. **Hormonal and Metabolic Functions.** The juxtaglomerular apparatus within the kidneys is believed to secrete renin, which converts angiotensin I in the blood to angiotensin II. This substance increases the rate of aldosterone secretion by the adrenal cortex and also causes vasoconstriction. This may be the sequence of events by which renal ischaemia produces hypertension. The kidney is the main source of erythropoietin necessary for normal erythropoiesis and it is also responsible for the formation of 1,25 dihydroxycholecalciferol (p. 118).

Diagnosis of Renal Disease

In the majority of patients suffering from renal disease, symptoms and signs are not usually referred to the anatomical site of the kidneys. This is due to the fact that clinical features of renal disease most frequently arise from abnormalities in the chemical composition of the body or from hypertension. Their true origin therefore may be suspected only after the detection of urinary abnormalities, and the importance of a routine examination of the urine in clinical practice cannot be overemphasised. The examinations which may be of value include the determination of the volume of urine passed in 24 hours, the presence of abnormal urinary constituents and bacteriological examination. Under certain standardised conditions the determination of the specific gravity and pH of urine is of value. In addition it may be necessary to obtain further information by chemical analysis of the blood and urine, tests of glomerular and tubular function and radiological examination. The last includes plain X-ray of the abdomen, excretion urography (intravenous pyelography), cystoscopy, ureteric catheterisation with collection of urine samples from each kidney, retrograde pyelography, renal angiography, isotope renography and renal biopsy.

Urinary Volume

In health and in temperate climates the volume of urine excreted usually lies within the range of 800–2,500 ml per 24 hours. There is a limit to the power of the kidneys to concentrate urine and on a normal diet a minimum volume of 800 ml is required to excrete the solid urinary constituents which consist mainly of urea and electrolytes. Less solute has to be excreted when a diet rich in carbohydrate and fat and low in protein and salt is eaten, and as little as 250 ml of urine per 24 hours is sufficient in these circumstances.

Oliguria is the production of insufficient urine to enable solute to be excreted in adequate amounts and the *milieu intérieur* of the body to be preserved. If the concentrating power of the kidneys is seriously reduced or if the solute to be excreted in the urine is increased above the normal, as occurs, for example, in severe infections, a daily output of as much as 2–3 litres of urine may even be insufficient. Oliguria develops in conditions associated with a reduction in renal blood flow and rate of glomerular filtration, e.g. diseases giving rise to water and salt depletion, hypotension, cardiac failure, acute glomerulonephritis, and other parenchymal diseases of the kidneys. In these circumstances urine flow sometimes ceases completely and *anuria* develops. Anuria from this cause should be distinguished from urinary retention. In the latter case distension of the bladder will be found on examination of the abdomen, confirmed if necessary by catheterisation.

Polyuria denotes a persistent increase in urinary output. It must be distinguished from frequency of micturition, which may be defined as the frequent passage of small quantities of urine without an increase in the total volume.

There are two basic mechanisms which give rise to polyuria. It may be due either to the excretion of an abnormally large amount of solute so that elimination of an increased volume of water is required, or to a reduction in the ability of the kidney to concentrate urine so that an increased volume of water is needed to eliminate a given amount of solute. The latter defect may arise because of lack of circulating vasopressin or insensitivity of the concentrating mechanism within the kidney to its action. Polyuria occurs in the following clinical circumstances:

(*a*) Diabetes mellitus in which an osmotic diuresis occurs because of glycosuria due to hyperglycaemia.

(*b*) Renal disease with uraemia in which the elevated concentration of urea in the blood acts as the osmotic diuretic.

(*c*) Conditions in which there is decreased responsiveness of the collecting ducts to vasopressin, e.g. in some cases of chronic renal disease, during the recovery phase of acute renal failure, in hypercalcaemia such as may arise in hyperparathyroidism, in potassium depletion and in nephrogenic diabetes insipidus.

(*d*) The elimination of oedema, e.g. in recovery from heart failure or the nephrotic syndrome.

(*e*) Diabetes insipidus of neurohypophyseal origin in which there is diminished secretion of vasopressin.

(*f*) Inhibition of vasopressin secretion due to excessive drinking of fluid either from choice or from psychiatric causes, i.e. compulsive polydipsia.

Specific Gravity of Urine

The specific gravity of urine is defined as the ratio between the weight of a given volume of urine and the weight of an equal volume of distilled water. It is therefore a measure of the quantity of solids in solution and is an approximate measure of osmolality. For clinical purposes measurement of the specific gravity is made by a hydrometer (urinometer). In health, urea and sodium chloride are the main solutes contributing to the specific gravity of urine. In diabetes mellitus, on the other hand, the quantity of glucose in the urine may far outweigh the total of all the other solutes present; water containing 1 per cent glucose has a specific gravity of 1·004. Protein has almost the same effect in increasing the specific gravity as a similar quantity of urea. Urea, however, is present in a concentration of 20 g/*l* in normal urine, while protein, even in the most severe cases of the nephrotic syndrome, is seldom present in such large quantities. Thus 4 g protein per litre, which gives a strong reaction with Albustix, raises the specific gravity by only 0·001. The specific gravity of urine varies with the nature and quantity of food eaten as well as with the amount of water or other fluid taken.

The maximal capacity of the kidneys to concentrate urine may be determined after either depriving the patient of fluid or by the injection of vasopressin, but if a random or prebreakfast sample of urine is found to have a specific gravity of 1·020 or more there is clearly no need to carry out these tests. In health, fluid deprivation results in a rise in plasma osmolality which acts as a stimulus for production of antidiuretic hormone. The urine becomes progressively more concentrated as fluid deprivation is continued, and in experimental subjects increasing values for urine osmolality are found up to 3 days. This is far too long a period of time for clinical application but deprivation of fluid for at least 20 hours is necessary for consistently accurate results to be obtained in temperate climates. With this procedure urinary concentrations of above 800 mOsm/l, corresponding to specific gravity of from 1·022 to 1·040, are obtained in healthy individuals.

Reaction of the Urine and Acid Excretion

In health and on a normal diet, 40–80 mmol of acid are excreted daily in the urine. The greater part of this acid is excreted in buffered form, partly as dihydrogen phosphate, which constitutes the bulk of the titratable acidity of the urine, and partly as ammonium ions. A very small amount of free hydrogen ion is also excreted and it is this which is measured when the pH of the urine is determined. Little information is gained from the routine determination of urinary pH in random samples of urine. In certain circumstances the ability of the renal tubules to excrete hydrogen ions is depressed and the demonstration of this is of clinical significance. It is important to examine fresh specimens of urine since urea may decompose to form ammonia and give a false result if urine is left to stand. Infections of the urinary tract with organisms other than *Esch. coli* or tubercle bacilli also cause the urine to be alkaline owing to the breakdown of urea.

Failure to acidify urine following the oral administration of ammonium chloride is characteristic of distal renal tubular acidosis occurring either as an inherited or acquired defect, and may also occur in potassium deficiency and in some patients with hypercalciuria and nephrocalcinosis.

Measurement of Renal Clearance

The ability of the glomeruli to perform their function in health and disease may be estimated by the measurement of 'clearance'.

The term 'clearance' does not imply the complete removal of a substance from the plasma. It is an arbitrary, but quantitatively valid measurement which relates the amount of a substance present in the urine, produced over a unit of time, to its concentration in the plasma. It is measured from the following equation:

$$C = \frac{UV}{P}$$

in which C is the clearance, U is the concentration of the substance in the urine, P is the concentration of the substance in the plasma, V is the volume of urine in ml secreted per minute.

If a substance in the plasma passes freely through the glomerular filter, and is neither absorbed nor excreted by the tubules, the quantity excreted in the urine, UV, is identical with the quantity filtered by the glomeruli. The clearance of such a substance is therefore equal to the rate of glomerular filtration. Endogenous creatinine and the polysaccharide, inulin, appear to be excreted in this way and their clearances are used to estimate the rate of glomerular filtration, which for the average adult is about 120 ml per minute. Since urea is partly reabsorbed by the tubules its clearance is less than that of creatinine or inulin. The clearance of creatinine is determined by collecting urine over a 24-hour period and withdrawing one sample of blood during the day. It is advisable to check the accuracy of an abnormal result by repeating the test on one or more occasions.

Abnormal Constituents of Urine

1. **Protein.** The presence of protein in the urine, detectable by the use of Albustix or salicylsulphonic acid, is always of clinical significance. Proteinuria of this degree does not usually occur in disease of the lower urinary tract, though a small amount can be detected in severe urinary infection or obvious haematuria. Proteinuria almost invariably indicates the presence of parenchymal disease of the kidneys but its magnitude bears little relation to the degree of renal failure. In the absence of inflammation in the urinary tract, the protein is derived from plasma proteins which have penetrated the glomerular membrane in abnormally large amounts. Because of its smaller molecular size, albumin predominates over the globulins.

Small amounts of protein are usually found in the urine in severe chronic renal disease, in the course of febrile illness and in heart failure. Larger amounts of protein (e.g. 3 g/day or more) are found in the nephrotic syndrome. Bence Jones proteins (p. 37) may be present in myelomatosis and rarely in other diseases of the lymphoreticular organs.

Postural (Orthostatic) Proteinuria. In a number of apparently healthy children and adolescents, and less commonly in adults, protein is excreted in the urine in variable but usually small amounts without associated disease of the kidneys. The urine formed while these individuals are recumbent is free from protein so that examination of the first specimen voided immediately on rising in the morning is normal. On the other hand urine formed while the individual is in the erect position or following exercise is found to contain protein. Tests of renal function show no abnormality.

2. **Blood.** Blood is found in the urine in a wide variety of clinical conditions; haematuria commonly indicates serious disease of the urinary tract and the cause must always be sought without delay. The appearance of the urine varies with the amount of blood and is normal to the naked eye when traces only are present. When larger amounts of blood are present the urine may be smoky in appearance, bright red or reddish-brown. The brown discolouration is due to the formation of acid haematin from haemoglobin.

Red blood cells are found in varying numbers in the urine in acute glomerulonephritis, infective endocarditis, malignant hypertension, polyarteritis, systemic lupus erythematosus affecting the kidney, renal tuberculosis, congenital cystic disease, haemorrhagic diseases, renal infarction and trauma to the kidneys. Red cells occur in the urine also in inflammation and tumour of the kidney and of the urinary tract, in senile hyperplasia and carcinoma of the prostate, and in the presence of urinary calculi. They are absent, or very scanty, in minimal lesion and membranous glomerulonephritis and in most cases of the nephrotic syndrome due to other causes.

Many of these conditions can be diagnosed by the presence of characteristic symptoms and signs in addition to haematuria. When haematuria is the sole or presenting symptom the cause is most likely to be renal carcinoma, papilloma of the bladder, benign prostate hypertrophy or, in some localities, schistosomiasis (p. 894).

When blood appears only at the beginning of micturition, the rest of the urine voided being clear, the source of bleeding is distal to the bladder. When blood is uniformly mixed with the urine, it may have come from any part of the urinary tract other than the urethra. Renal colic accompanying haematuria indicates that the bleeding is renal or ureteric in origin.

To establish the presence of small quantities of blood in the urine it is essential to examine microscopically the centrifuged deposit of a fresh specimen. If the specimen is not fresh, the hypotonicity of a dilute urine or the hypertonicity of a concentrated urine may destroy or deform the red cells. Even if the urine is obviously red it is necessary to demonstrate the presence of red cells microscopically, in order to distinguish haematuria from other rarer causes of discolouration of the urine with which there may be confusion. These are:

(a) *Haemoglobinuria*, which accompanies various rare intravascular haemolytic crises. The urine gives the chemical and spectroscopic tests for haemoglobin, but no red cells are present.

(b) *Phenolphthalein* in an alkaline urine. Phenolphthalein is an ingredient of many proprietary purgatives, and self-medication with alkalis and purgatives is common. As urine tends to become alkaline on standing it may turn pink if phenolphthalein is present. The addition of acid dispels the colour.

(c) *Beetroot, senna, dyes* used to colour sweets and a few other substances taken by mouth may redden the urine.

(d) *Acute intermittent porphyria* in which large amounts of porphobilinogen are excreted in the urine. Fresh urine from such cases may appear normal, but on standing for some hours a dark red colour may develop. The presence of porphobilinogen may be suspected from the red colour produced by the addition of Ehrlich's aldehyde reagent. In contrast to that produced by urobilinogen, this colour is not extracted by chloroform.

3. **Pus Cells and Bacteria.** Pus cells may be found in the urine in inflammation of any part of the urinary tract. The urine should always be examined under the microscope and cultured when urinary tract infection is suspected. In obtaining the specimen for culture it is best to avoid catheterisation. A midstream specimen should be obtained from both male and female patients, and a culture should be made of this within 2 hours (p. 490).

4. **Urinary Casts.** Casts are cylindrical structures of microscopic size which are found in the urinary deposit. They are formed in the renal tubules by the coagulation of protein. Red blood corpuscles or epithelial cells may be impressed upon this matrix, producing blood and epithelial casts respectively; such casts are found in the early stages of acute glomerulonephritis and other diseases in which there is glomerular inflammation. Granular casts are formed by degeneration of the impressed cells. Epithelial and granular casts are indicative of inflammation and degeneration of the renal tubules. Hyaline casts are formed by coagulated protein without the addition of cellular elements and are found in chronic glomerulonephritis and occasionally in small numbers in normal urine, especially after vigorous exercise.

Although the number of cells and hyaline casts passed in the urine in the course of the day by the healthy adult is considerable, in practice microscopic examination of the centrifuged deposit reveals only an occasional cell or hyaline cast in each low power field.

5. **Bile and Urobilinogen.** These may also occur in the urine in abnormal amounts (p. 425).

Chemical Analysis of the Blood

With progressive impairment of renal function the composition of the body fluids becomes abnormal. These abnormalities may be detected by blood analyses. The products of metabolism which in health are excreted in the urine are retained in the blood, and the concentration of urea, creatinine and the anions such as phosphate and sulphate increases. Determination of the concentration of blood urea gives a useful indication of the degree of renal failure, but it should be remembered that this does not rise above the accepted normal maximum until renal function is reduced by at least 50 per cent. The diminishing capacity of the kidneys to secrete hydrogen ions results in their accumulation in the blood, and the severity of the consequent metabolic acidosis may be estimated by measurement of the concentration of bicarbonate. Estimation of plasma sodium, potassium, calcium and protein concentrations is of value in certain circumstances. A table of reference values for these and other biochemical factors, in SI and equivalent units, is given on page 949.

Glomerulonephritis

The term 'glomerulonephritis' is used to describe a bilateral disease of the kidneys which usually affects all the glomeruli. In practice, cases can usually be placed in one of three histologically defined categories which are described below under the headings of proliferative, minimal lesion and membranous glomerulonephritis. Renal biopsy now permits a degree of clinicopathological correlation hitherto unattainable. In the early stages of all three disorders the histological pictures are distinct. In cases of proliferative glomerulonephritis which fail to recover completely, and in the later stages of membranous glomerulonephritis which is a chronic disease, the histological features become less clearly distinguishable. The fact that hypertension may accompany some stage of these two diseases complicates the pathology still further by the changes due to arteriolosclerosis.

Proliferative Glomerulonephritis

This condition is characterised by a diffuse inflammatory reaction of the glomeruli of both kidneys. When the disease appears abruptly, the terms *acute glomerulonephritis* or *acute nephritis* are often applied.

Aetiology. The great majority of cases of proliferative glomerulonephritis are due to the deposition of circulating soluble antigen-antibody complexes on the endothelial side of the basement membrane of the glomerulus. The classical prototype of this type of disorder follows infection with haemolytic streptococci, especially of types 12, 1 or 49, and this may occur as acute tonsillitis, scarlet fever or upper respiratory infection. In developing countries streptococcal infection of wounds and skin infections are more often responsible but streptococcal infection anywhere may be the cause. Some viruses (e.g. varicella and E B) may also cause proliferative glomerulonephritis and a similar reaction can follow infection with organisms as different as staphylococci, pneumococci, *Myco. leprae*, *P. malariae* and schistosomiasis. It may also occur as a complication of infective endocarditis. In these latter conditions the glomerulonephritis appears as a complication of the underlying specific disorder.

Glomerular disease caused by immune complexes also occurs in systemic lupus erythematosus (antibody to DNA) and polyarteritis, in the course of some tumours and lymphomas which induce circulating antibodies and as a consequence of an immunological reaction to drugs. However, in many patients there is no clue to the nature of the responsible agent or disease.

Goodpasture's syndrome is a rare form of proliferative glomerulonephritis associated with haemoptysis; it develops as a consequence of the formation of IgG antibodies to glomerular basement membrane. Immunofluorescent studies show that these antibodies are deposited in a linear fashion along the basement membrane where they induce an inflammatory reaction.

Pathology. The earliest lesion is a diffuse reaction of the glomerular capillaries with variable swelling of the endothelial cells, proliferation of the mesangial cells and accumulation of polymorphonuclear leucocytes in the tuft and the glomerular space. There may be proliferation of the outer layer of Bowman's capsule to form epithelial crescents. In many cases these changes resolve with clinical recovery and the kidney returns to normal.

In persistent and progressive cases the epithelial crescents, which arise as a result of the presence of red blood cells, fibrin and inflammatory exudate in Bowman's space, increase in size. Progressive fibrosis of crescents and glomeruli occurs and the glomerular capillaries gradually become obstructed, resulting in secondary degeneration in the tubules. Ultimately many nephrons may be replaced by fibrous tissue, leading to small contracted kidneys. It appears likely that the antigen-antibody complexes activate both the coagulation and the complement system. The degree of intravascular glomerular thrombosis partly determines the rapidity of the deterioration and possibly also whether the condition resolves. This component of the disorder may be assessed by estimation of the breakdown products of fibrinogen and fibrin (FDP) in the urine. Another factor influencing the outcome is the way in which the mesangial cells fulfil their phagocyte role. In some cases proliferation of the mesangial cells is so marked that they project into the glomerular capillaries and seriously interfere with their function. This variant is called *mesangiocapillary glomerulonephritis*. The activation of complement in streptococcal glomerulonephritis is reflected in a transient fall in the component of complement C3 (p. 28) during the illness. In mesangiocapillary glomerulonephritis there is a persistent reduction of serum complement which probably antedates the disease. This abnormality, which is possibly genetically determined, may increase the susceptibility of the host to circulating immune complex disease.

The appearance of generalised oedema, which especially affects the face, gave rise to a theory that there is generalised capillary damage; it is now believed that the oedema is caused by fluid retention consequent on reduced filtration due to glomerular damage and to a relative increase in the reabsorption of water and salt by the tubules. The facial oedema is marked possibly because the skin here is more loosely attached to the subcutaneous tissues than elsewhere and the patient can lie flat in the absence of heart failure.

Clinical Features. The condition occurs most commonly in childhood and adolescence but may develop at any age. When it follows streptococcal infection a latent period is usual, the features of glomerulonephritis developing 1 to 3 weeks after the infection has subsided. The infection itself may be slight and may even pass unnoticed, and there is no relationship between its severity and the probability of the development of the disease. In children the onset is usually abrupt, the most constant features being puffiness of the face, low urinary output and blood-stained urine. The puffy face gives an appearance which is almost pathognomonic. Oedema may be detected around the ankles if the patient is ambulant. Breathlessness due to pulmonary oedema may be present and in severe cases pleural effusions develop. Occasionally there is discomfort in the renal angles and epistaxis may occur. In acute cases there may be malaise, fever, anorexia, vomiting and headache.

In adults, a history of acute streptococcal or other infection is less commonly obtained and the onset is usually insidious with progressive tiredness and slowly developing oedema of the lower limbs. Virtually asymptomatic cases may be discovered after routine examination of the urine.

In most cases there is a moderate rise in diastolic blood pressure. In a few hypertensive encephalopathy occurs (p. 222).

Urine. The daily output is usually reduced in volume due to a fall in the rate of glomerular filtration and increased tubular reabsorption of water and salt. Anuria may occur in very severe cases. The urine may appear red or smoky owing to the presence of blood and is usually concentrated. Proteinuria is of moderate degree, seldom exceeding 4 g per day, but the amount present is out of proportion to the haematuria. Microscopic examination of the urinary deposit reveals erythrocytes, some leucocytes, and red blood cell, epithelial and granular casts.

Renal function tests. In the early stages concentrating power is usually unimpaired, and the specific gravity of the urine is high. The rate of glomerular filtration is reduced and the concentration of urea in the blood is raised. A moderate degree of acidosis is usual. When recovery occurs the filtration rate rises and the blood urea concentration falls to normal.

Course and Prognosis. Complete recovery occurs in about 90 per cent of children who suffer from the disease. The prognosis is worse in adults and after middle age when recovery occurs in only about 50 per cent of cases. In most instances the acute manifestations lessen in the course of 3 to 4 days, the temperature, pulse rate and blood pressure falling to normal. Diuresis occurs, and the oedema, haematuria and number of casts in the urine diminish. Small amounts of blood may be present in the urine for 10 to 14 days, while proteinuria may persist for several weeks or months.

In about 10 per cent of cases hypertension and haematuria subside and the patient apparently regains normal health. Proteinuria however persists, and after many years chronic glomerulonephritis, hypertension and renal failure develop.

In a small number of cases the symptoms and signs persist for months or years. In some the proteinuria becomes massive and gross generalised oedema develops. Some call this stage subacute glomerulonephritis. Uraemia and acidosis slowly increase and the patient may die of renal failure while oedema persists.

Rarely, in rapidly progressive glomerulonephritis, marked hypertension, extreme oliguria, recurrent convulsions and death may occur within a few days from acute cardiac failure and pulmonary oedema or in 2 or 3 weeks from uraemia. Treatment by dialysis has improved the mortality in this group but it still remains high.

Differential diagnosis. Poststreptococcal nephritis may be diagnosed if group A haemolytic streptococci can be isolated or if there is evidence of streptococcal infection as shown by a rising titre of ASO (antistreptolysin) antibody. Unfortunately this reaction is negative in a significant number of cases. In the absence of other infective causes, acute glomerulonephritis should be distinguished from:

Angio-oedema, in which sudden swelling of the eyelids is a frequent feature. This condition is usually associated with swelling of the lips or tongue; urinary abnormalities are absent. In addition, the patient may be known to be an allergic subject, similar attacks may have occurred previously, and eosinophilia is often present.

Henoch-Schönlein purpura (p. 629) in which focal or diffuse glomerulonephritis is associated with purpura and swollen joints and sometimes abdominal pain and melaena.

Polyarteritis and systemic lupus erythematosus in which red blood cell casts may also be found in the urine. Other organs are usually involved in the pathological process, and the diagnosis of these two diseases is suspected on this basis. Polyarteritis and systemic lupus erythematosus are occasionally confined to the kidney, when renal biopsy is necessary to establish the diagnosis.

Acute pyelonephritis, in which oedema is absent while pain and tenderness in the lumbar region and frequency of micturition may occur. The urine contains microorganisms, more pus than red blood cells and red cell casts are absent.

Haematuria due to tuberculosis or tumours of the kidney or urinary tract in which oedema does not occur and there are no cellular casts in the urine.

Infective endocarditis, in which microscopic haematuria is a valuable diagnostic sign, and uraemia may develop.

Acute recurrent focal nephritis, a condition of unknown but probably multiple aetiology in which recurrent episodes of haematuria occur over a period of months or years. There are no other symptoms or signs of acute proliferative glomerulonephritis. The diagnosis is made by renal biopsy in which mesangial proliferation is found affecting only some glomeruli. Repeated episodes may lead to progressive glomerular destruction with renal failure and hypertension.

Treatment. The three principal needs in the treatment of acute proliferative glomerulonephritis are rest and warmth, dietary regulation, and the elimination of infection. The patient should be kept warm in bed and protected from cold and draughts; ideally rest in bed should be maintained until haematuria, hypertension, oedema and proteinuria have disappeared.

DIETARY REGULATION. There is no evidence that modifications of the diet make any significant difference to the healing process in nephritis, but protein restriction controls the degree of uraemia. Complete restriction of protein with an adequate energy intake from carbohydrate and fat ensure minimum protein breakdown. For most cases, however, reduction of the protein intake to 40 g/day appears to be satisfactory.

In addition to protein restriction, treatment should be directed to maintaining fluid and electrolyte balance. In cases of *mild to moderate* severity:

1. *Fluid* should be restricted while oedema is present to $\frac{1}{2}$ litre per day plus the volume of the previous day's output. If there is evidence of pulmonary oedema, fluid should be withheld entirely.

2. *Food* should be given in such quantities as the patient desires, but consisting mainly of carbohydrate and fat, e.g. bread, biscuits, cereals, jam, syrup, sugar and vegetables. Not more than half a pint of milk per day may also be taken. Sufficient

protein is present in such foods to reduce the breakdown of body protein for essential needs to a low level.

3. *Salt* should not be used in cooking nor added to food. If the oedema is severe a low salt diet should be given.

In the occasional rare case of *severe* nephritis with anuria or extreme oliguria which shows no improvement within 3 or 4 days on the measures mentioned above, the regime described on page 497 should be adopted.

When hypertension and haematuria have subsided and diuresis has occurred, a light diet with a moderate restriction of protein (an egg at one meal and a small helping of fish, or meat at another meal) is given for a few days before the resumption of a normal diet.

ELIMINATION OF INFECTION. Streptococcal infection should be treated with penicillin. Removal of infected tonsils or other septic foci should be delayed until convalescence is advanced, as operation may be followed by an exacerbation, especially if carried out during the acute stage. However, in a few cases with persistence or repeated recurrence of symptoms and signs, these features may disappear only after the removal of a focus of chronic infection, e.g. apical teeth abscesses or mastoiditis. In the event of operative treatment being needed, benzylpenicillin should be given on the day of operation and for 3 days after it. When the condition is associated with other infections appropriate antimicrobial treatment should be given.

OTHER MEASURES. Hypertension does not require treatment in the majority of cases; the treatment of hypertensive encephalopathy is described on page 225. Attempts to influence the course of the disease by the use of corticosteroids or immunosuppressive drugs have not been successful.

Minimal Lesion Glomerulonephritis and Membranous Glomerulonephritis

Minimal lesion and membranous glomerulonephritis are conditions associated with a marked increase in the permeability of the glomerular basement membrane. This leads to proteinuria which is often so severe that hypoproteinaemia and oedema develop. The two conditions are described together because, although they tend to affect different age groups, they present with identical clinical features.

Aetiology and Pathology. The aetiology of both types of glomerulonephritis is unknown. Unlike proliferative glomerulonephritis neither disease is preceded by any recognisable infection.

In membranous glomerulonephritis the histological appearances consist of a diffuse hyaline thickening of the glomerular capillary walls. As the disease progresses the thickening becomes more severe and the glomerular tufts are converted into structureless hyaline tissue. Immunofluorescent studies show that while immunoglobulins are deposited in the basement membrane, there is little or no mesangial cell proliferation characteristic of proliferative glomerulonephritis. Some take the view that membranous glomerulonephritis is the result of antigen-antibody complexes sufficiently small to pass through most of the thickness of the glomerular basement membrane and become deposited on its external subepithelial aspect. While this could explain the lack of mesangial cell proliferation, the possibility of glomerular injury from other mechanisms cannot be excluded and the nature of the antigen or antigens is unknown in the vast majority of cases. It has now been shown that antibodies to type B hepatitis are occasionally associated with membranous glomerulonephritis.

In minimal lesion glomerulonephritis, the glomeruli show no lesion when examined by light microscopy. However, abnormalities of glomerular structure involving especially the epithelial cells are revealed by the electron microscope. The evidence suggests that this condition does not progress to glomerular destruction as is usually the case with membranous glomerulonephritis, and there is no evidence that the condition is due to the deposition of antigen-antibody complexes. Minimal lesion glomerulonephritis may occasionally follow exposure to pollen and this suggests a Type I allergic response; however there is no immunofluorescent or other evidence to implicate IgE in the disease process.

Clinical Features. Minimal lesion glomerulonephritis occurs predominantly in children and young adults while membranous glomerulonephritis mainly affects those over 30 years of age. Both diseases are insidious in onset. If the proteinuria is slight they may persist without symptoms and remain undetected for months or years. When proteinuria increases in severity, oedema occurs and it is in this way that attention may be drawn to their existence. The patient may also notice the urine becomes frothy. The oedema is generalised, involving first the subcutaneous tissue and later the serous sacs and lungs. The face presents a pale and puffy appearance. The general health may remain good for some considerable time but eventually becomes progressively impaired, with increased liability to infection of the oedematous tissues or the serous cavities.

The urine contains protein in moderate amounts though as much as 30 g may be excreted per day in occasional patients. Granular and hyaline casts are seen on microscopic examination, red cells being scanty or absent.

At first chemical examination of the blood shows little or no increase in urea. Plasma cholesterol is raised commonly to 5–8 mmol/l and the plasma and ascitic fluid may look milky due to an increase in fat and β-lipoproteins. Total plasma proteins are greatly reduced, e.g. to 3–4 g per 100 ml. There are quantitative changes in the various globulin fractions, but the chief reduction affects albumin. Proteins of larger molecular weight, especially α_2-globulin, are retained in the blood and hence are increased relative to the other plasma proteins. The resulting fall of colloid osmotic pressure of the plasma is mainly responsible for the massive oedema which is the prominent clinical feature. The ensuing oligaemia stimulates the secretion of aldosterone which promotes further electrolyte and water retention and sometimes potassium loss.

In the early stage of the diseases renal function tests reveal no impairment of glomerular filtration rate or of the ability to concentrate urine.

Course and Prognosis. In the majority of cases the oedema persists for months or years, with occasional spontaneous but temporary remissions. Prior to the use of effective diuretics, antibiotics and corticosteroids, recovery rarely occurred. The majority of patients died either from intercurrent infection in the oedematous phase or from renal failure. Protein malnutrition with striae in the skin and osteoporosis may occur. There is now ample evidence that in patients with minimal lesion glomerulonephritis, corticosteroids and immunosuppressive treatment causes the proteinuria to subside and the condition to resolve. In membranous glomerulonephritis, however, the prognosis is less favourable. Arterial hypertension and hypertensive retinopathy develop and progressive renal destruction ultimately reduces the rate of glomerular filtration in the majority of cases.

Proteinuria diminishes, and consequently the plasma proteins rise and oedema becomes less. There is gradual impairment of renal function as the disease progresses to chronic glomerulonephritis with uraemia (p. 484). In a minority of cases, however, slow resolution of the glomerular lesion occurs and patients may recover completely.

Differential Diagnosis of the Nephrotic Syndrome. The term 'nephrotic syndrome' is used to describe the clinical state of hypoproteinaemic oedema associated with marked proteinuria irrespective of its aetiology. Minimal lesion glomerulonephritis is the most common cause of the nephrotic syndrome in children and is responsible for about 20 per cent of cases in the adult. Membranous glomerulonephritis is more common in adults and both must therefore be distinguished from other renal disorders which give rise to a similar clinical picture. Sometimes the aetiology of the nephrotic syndrome is obvious from the presence of other clinical features of the causative disease. In many patients it is necessary to carry out a renal biopsy in order to make the diagnosis. .

Proliferative glomerulonephritis is occasionally associated with marked proteinuria and massive oedema. In many patients the clinical history and the course of the disease are sufficient to make this diagnosis clear, but in others the true nature of the syndrome is detected only after renal biopsy.

Diabetic nephropathy is discussed on page 579.

Amyloid disease is usually secondary to rheumatoid arthritis, myelomatosis, tuberculosis or chronic suppuration. It gives rise to proteinuria as a result of the deposition of amyloid material in the glomerular capillaries. Renal biopsy is usually necessary to provide histological evidence of amyloid infiltration. Primary amyloidosis is rare and affects other tissues, e.g. tongue, myocardium or peripheral nerves.

Drugs, e.g. mercury, troxidone, penicillamine and gold may cause the nephrotic syndrome.

Renal vein thrombosis is a rare cause of the nephrotic syndrome. It should be suspected when proteinuria occurs in a patient with evidence of deep venous thrombosis in the lower limbs or if an illness is complicated by pain in the loins and the subsequent development of the nephrotic syndrome.

Occasionally the nephrotic syndrome develops as the presenting feature in the course of *systemic lupus erythematosus* and *polyarteritis* or it arises in association with *tumours* when it may be due to circulating autoantibodies being deposited in the glomerulus.

P. malariae infection is an important cause of the syndrome in children in parts of Africa (pp. 839 and 935).

The nephrotic syndrome must also be distinguished from:

Cardiac failure with severe oedema, in which dyspnoea is present, the venous pressure is increased, signs of underlying cardiac disease are present, oedema is usually absent from the face, and proteinuria is less severe.

Hypoproteinaemic oedema, due to causes other than loss of protein in the urine, namely impairment of intake, digestion, absorption or synthesis of protein and in protein-losing enteropathy.

Treatment is directed at relief of oedema and control of proteinuria.

RELIEF OF OEDEMA. 1. Protein intake. So long as the blood urea is not elevated, a liberal intake of protein is desirable in an attempt to make good the urinary loss of protein. At least 90–100 g protein per day should be given. This may be supplemented with Casilan or Lonolac which are salt-free protein concentrates.

2. Salt intake should be restricted by prohibiting extra table salt, avoiding salty foods and reducing the amount used in cooking. Although drastic salt restriction occasionally produces dramatic results, 'salt-free' diets are so unappetising that patients will not tolerate them for more than a few weeks.

3. Diuretics are of great value in controlling the oedema e.g. frusemide (p. 161). Because of the associated oligaemia these diuretics occasionally induce renal failure by causing further salt loss. In this event, or if the oedema is resistant, relief is obtained by giving plasma, salt-free albumin or dextran intravenously.

4. Spironolactone is indicated in patients who show marked features of secondary aldosteronism, e.g. hypokalaemia.

CONTROL OF PROTEINURIA. *Corticosteroids* provide the main chance of cure in the treatment of minimal lesion glomerulonephritis. In the majority of cases this treatment abolishes proteinuria. Prednisolone should be given in doses of 1 mg/kg/day for about 3 weeks and then reduced to about one-third of this dose and continued for 2–3 months.

Immunosuppressive Therapy. In a minority of patients with minimal lesion glomerulonephritis the condition relapses after treatment when prednisolone is stopped. Such individuals are then best treated with cyclophosphamide in doses of 3 mg/kg body weight for 8 weeks. A weekly check of the white blood cell count should be made and the dose reduced if leucopenia develops. Temporary alopecia and chemical cystitis are the adverse effects.

Corticosteroids, cyclophosphamide and other immunosuppressive drugs are ineffective in membranous glomerulonephritis.

Chronic Glomerulonephritis

Aetiology. Chronic glomerulonephritis develops when proliferative glomerulonephritis becomes progressive and in most cases of membranous glomerulonephritis. Frequently, however, no history of either disease is obtained and in these, post-mortem studies of the kidney suggest that the pathological change has been developing insidiously over many years. Both conditions lead to chronic renal failure (p. 494).

Pathology. The kidneys are small; the capsules strip with difficulty, leaving a granular surface; the peripelvic fat is increased and there is great reduction in renal cortical tissue. The normal distinction between cortex and medulla is obscured.

On microscopical examination there is fibrosis or hyalinisation of most of the glomeruli with fibrous replacement of many tubules. Remaining nephrons may show hypertrophy and arteriolosclerosis is usually present.

Pathogenesis. The clinical features of chronic glomerulonephritis are attributable to the effects of chronic renal failure combined usually with arterial hypertension. As renal failure develops, the composition of the body fluid becomes abnormal, particularly with regard to its water and salt content, its acid-base equilibrium, and the concentration of nitrogenous compounds which are normally excreted by the kidney. These alterations ultimately combine to produce the clinical picture of severe uraemia which is the terminal stage of renal failure.

Clinical Features. A history of acute glomerulonephritis or of the nephrotic syndrome is obtained in some cases. The earlier stages of the disease may be unattended by symptoms but may come to light only by discovery of proteinuria or hypertension during the course of a routine examination. Later, because of the widespread consequences of renal failure, the symptoms and signs are referable to almost every system and patients suffering from the disease present with complaints which at first sight may not suggest their renal origin. The patients may seek medical advice because of polyuria, thirst, loss of energy, weakness, nausea, vomiting, or diarrhoea. Polyuria develops both because of diminished power for tubular reabsorption of water and because the elevated blood urea produces an osmotic diuresis. Anaemia is the main cause of the loss of energy and it is usually normocytic. The high blood pressure may have been detected in the course of a general examination or the patient may have sought advice for headache, loss of vision or breathlessness or because of the occurrence of cerebrovascular insufficiency.

As the disease progresses, renal function deteriorates and uraemia increases. The blood concentration of urea and other nitrogenous compounds steadily rises. The patient looks more ill and the complexion is sallow, often accompanied by a yellow-brown discolouration attributed to the retention of urinary pigment. With the exception of those who develop cardiac failure from hypertension and those in whom the chronic stage of membranous glomerulonephritis has followed rapidly upon the initial oedematous stage, the patients are not only free from oedema but usually exhibit signs of water and salt depletion. The skin and tongue are dry and the blood pressure may fall from its previous high level. Acidosis contributes to the dyspnoea and the respirations are deep (Kussmaul's respiration). Hiccough, muscular twitchings, fits, drowsiness and coma may occur. A tendency to bleed may develop in the terminal phase, as evidenced by epistaxis, bleeding gums, bruises, purpura, haematemesis and melaena. Hypertensive retinopathy of any degree may be present and visual impairment may result from numerous hard exudates arranged in star shape around the macula. Some patients complain of vague muscle or bone pain and in a few cases this becomes severe. Peripheral neuropathy due to uraemia also occurs.

Radiological examination occasionally reveals the appearances of osteomalacia, osteitis fibrosa (p. 531) and areas of osteosclerosis. Osteomalacia is due to the development of resistance to the action of vitamin D which probably owes its origin to failure by the kidney to convert vitamin D taken in the diet to the active metabolite (p. 118). In young individuals this interferes with normal growth and the condition has been called renal rickets. Osteitis fibrosa arises as a result of secondary hyperparathyroidism, the parathyroid glands being stimulated by the low concentration of plasma calcium. The cause of osteosclerosis is unknown.

Laboratory Data. During the early stages of the disease, and before nitrogen retention in the blood is detectable, the urine is found to contain protein, usually in small amounts; red blood cells and granular and hyaline casts are present in small numbers. Glomerular filtration may be reduced to less than 10 per cent of normal and there is a gradual rise in the concentration of plasma urea, creatinine and phosphate. The ability of the kidneys to form concentrated or dilute urine is impaired. Ultimately this power is lost completely and the urine is of a fixed specific gravity (1·010). The plasma concentration of bicarbonate diminishes as acidosis occurs. The plasma concentration of calcium is frequently reduced possibly due to defective vitamin D metabolism (p. 118). Potassium occasionally accumulates in the blood and is one of the factors causing death by its effect on the heart.

Course and Prognosis. The disease progresses steadily over months or years to a fatal termination. The course may be punctuated by exacerbations of acute glomerulonephritis which hasten the progress of the disease. When nitrogen retention and acidosis are severe, the outlook is grave and most patients die in a few months or a year. Papilloedema is a bad prognostic sign and unless treatment with antihypertensive drugs is begun before uraemia becomes severe, most patients who show it die within a few months. The cause of death is generally uraemia frequently complicated by infection to which such patients are susceptible; in other cases the patient dies from a cerebral haemorrhage, cardiac failure or myocardial infarction. A terminal non-bacterial pericarditis is common. Haemorrhage from any site or enterocolitis are also ominous features.

Differential Diagnosis. The distinction between chronic glomerulonephritis and other causes of chronic renal failure with hypertension is difficult and may be impossible. A similar clinical picture may arise in the following diseases.

1. Other conditions which primarily affect the glomeruli with their eventual destruction include polyarteritis, systemic lupus erythematosus, amyloid disease and diabetes mellitus. Patients suffering from these conditions may die ultimately of renal failure and uraemia.

2. Essential hypertension may occasionally lead to nephrosclerosis and uraemia. This should be suspected if there is a clear family history of high blood pressure; also in the malignant phase of hypertension from any cause evidence of renal disease is invariably present and renal failure is rapidly progressive.

3. Congenital polycystic disease of the kidneys may be diagnosed by the family history, by palpation of the enlarged, firm and irregular kidneys and by intravenous or retrograde pyelography. Medullary sponge kidney is also occasionally responsible (p. 503).

4. Chronic pyelonephritis is more common in women, and hypertension may be absent. There may be a history of acute pyelonephritis and organisms can sometimes be cultured from the urine. However the diagnosis is often suggested by the radiological appearances seen after pyelography.

5. Analgesic nephropathy (p. 503) is suggested by a history of analgesic abuse.

6. Bilateral hydronephrosis may be confirmed by retrograde pyelography.

7. Congenital renal hypoplasia with bilateral small kidneys is occasionally the cause of death from uraemia in children.

Treatment. Although the natural history of the disease cannot be altered and there is progressive deterioration in renal function, the patient's health and feeling of well-being may be considerably improved with suitable treatment.

Diet. When there is nitrogen retention the onset of severe uraemia may be delayed by restricting protein intake to 40 g per day and by ensuring an adequate intake of carbohydrate (250 g) and fat (60 g), giving an energy value of 1,700 kcal. In the later stages when the blood urea concentration rises to 35 mmol/l (200 mg/100 ml) further protein restriction to 20 g/day is indicated. It is best to provide this as first class protein in the form of meat, milk and eggs and to avoid protein of lesser biological value in vegetables and cereals.

Fluid. Fluid restriction is contraindicated since, in view of the impaired concentrating power, a large volume of urine is needed to excrete end-products of metabolism. Except in the presence of cardiac failure a fluid intake sufficient to produce at least 2½ litres of urine per day should be advised.

Salt. In the absence of oedema, cardiac failure or arterial hypertension, salt restriction is contraindicated. In a few cases of chronic nephritis there is an excessive loss of salt in the urine due to a failure of tubular reabsorption, and this may be aggravated by an enforced high fluid intake. Water and salt depletion occur and this aggravates the uraemia. Clinical improvement results in such cases from the addition of 5–10 g salt per day. The limit to the additional salt is set by the occurrence of systemic or pulmonary oedema, or by an aggravation of the hypertension. Sodium bicarbonate should be substituted in part for sodium chloride when acidosis is severe and giving rise to symptoms.

When nausea, vomiting or coma make it impossible to control water and salt depletion and acidosis by oral administration, fluid and electrolytes should be given by intravenous infusion. The volume of fluid required depends upon the severity of the salt and water depletion and the degree of acidosis (p. 166). An average amount for a case of moderate severity is 5 litres given in 24 hours, one part of isotonic sodium bicarbonate, two parts of isotonic sodium chloride and two parts 5 per cent glucose. The infusion should be continued until the bicarbonate concentration of the blood has been increased, if possible to within the normal range and until the patient is adequately hydrated.

Infection. Obvious foci of infection, e.g. tonsils, infected sinuses or root abscesses should be removed in order to reduce the likelihood of an exacerbation of acute glomerulonephritis. Antibiotics, as with other medication, must be used with special care in the presence of chronic renal failure, notably benzylpenicillin, co-trimoxazole, streptomycin, gentamicin, kanamycin and cephaloridine. Tetracyclines should not be used because of their tendency to raise the blood urea.

Anaemia. This should be treated by slow blood transfusions though it is probably not desirable to increase the concentration of haemoglobin above 8·5 g, as a rapid rise in haematocrit causes a fall in renal plasma flow and a temporary aggravation of the uraemia; oral or parenteral iron therapy is ineffective unless there is evidence of a complicating iron deficiency.

Nausea, Hiccoughing or Vomiting. This may be relieved with chlorpromazine which should be given in reduced doses because of the danger of accumulation (25 mg intramuscularly).

Bone Pain. When the dominant radiological picture is that of osteomalacia, vitamin D should be given orally in doses of up to 5 mg calciferol daily for some weeks. The treatment should be controlled by chemical estimations of plasma calcium and alkaline phosphatase, for there is a significant risk of producing hypercalcaemia and calcification of the tissues.

Cardiovascular Complications. The presence of uraemia is no contraindication to the treatment of co-existing hypertension provided that care is taken to see that antihypertensive treatment does not cause a rise in the concentration of blood urea. The choice and use of drugs should be made according to the recommendations given on pages 223–225. Digoxin is normally excreted in the urine, and hence in renal failure the maintenance dose should not usually exceed 0·25 mg three times per week.

HAEMODIALYSIS AND RENAL TRANSPLANTATION. Within the last 10 years it has been possible by repeated intermittent haemodialysis to preserve the life of many patients with chronic renal failure who are devoid of all renal function. Repeated access to blood vessels is achieved by establishing an arteriovenous anastomosis usually in the arm. Facilities are limited but are likely to increase in the future; patients can be trained to carry out such treatment at home, where survival of up to 10 years is not uncommon.

The practicability of transplantation of a normal kidney from a healthy donor or a cadaver to patients with chronic irreversible renal failure is also under active investigation. Discreet enquiries should be made concerning the existence of an identical twin. If the healthy twin is willing to act as a donor the prospects of renal transplantation being successful are excellent. Most kidney transplantations are carried out using either kidneys from living but less closely related donors or from cadavers. It is customary to try to select donor kidneys on the basis of the pattern of HLA compatibility (p. 25), but there is little evidence that this is of importance in cadaver transplants. After 2 years the average survival rate is about 50 per cent, but the postoperative course is complicated by the need to give immunosuppressive drugs such as prednisolone, azathioprine or antilymphocytic serum.

Infections of the Kidney and Urinary Tract

Infection of the urinary tract is an extremely common clinical problem. The infection may involve the urethra, the bladder, the ureters and the kidneys themselves. In any individual case it is difficult on clinical grounds to be certain of the extent of the invasion of the various parts of the urinary tract. Formerly it was assumed that the kidneys and the upper urinary tract are involved in every case, even when the symptoms of the infection are those solely of cystitis or urethritis. However, the great majority of patients develop recurrent symptoms of lower urinary tract infection without apparently suffering deterioration of renal function in later life.

Acute Pyelonephritis

This is characterised by an acute inflammation of the parenchyma and pelvis of the kidney. The term 'pyelitis' is still used, but is inaccurate as the inflammation involves the renal tissue as well as the pelvis. The disease may be unilateral or bilateral.

Aetiology. Acute pyelonephritis is commonly associated with some obstruction in the urinary tract. In view of the importance of preventing chronic pyelonephritis, the existence of a predisposing lesion should be suspected in every case. In men this is commonly due to prostatic enlargement, in pregnant women to obstruction by the uterus and atonia of the ureters due to the action of progesterone, and in infants and children to congenital malformation of the urinary tract or severe ureterovesical reflux. Calculi, cervical prolapse, foreign bodies or tumours may also be responsible. Pyelonephritis may occur in infancy and in adult women, however, without evidence of an obstructive lesion. In most cases the infection ascends via the ureter but in some it is blood borne. About 75 per cent of the infections are due to *Esch. coli*, the remainder being mostly due to streptococci, staphylococci or the Proteus group of organisms.

The predominance of urinary infections in the female suggests that the anatomical relation of the short urethra to the rectum is a predisposing factor. Catheterisation of the bladder is particularly liable to introduce organisms into the urinary tract, and this procedure may be responsible for the later development of acute or chronic pyelonephritis in some patients. Catheterisation should be reduced to the minimum and when indicated should be carried out with strict aseptic precautions.

Pathology. The renal pelvis is acutely inflamed and there is often a coincident inflammation of the bladder. In those cases with macroscopic involvement of the renal parenchyma, groups of small abscesses may be seen on the surface of the kidney when the capsule has been stripped. On section, small cortical abscesses and linear streaks of pus in the medulla are often evident. On histological examination focal infiltration of the renal parenchyma by polymorphonuclear cells is evident.

Clinical Features. In many cases there is a sudden onset of pain in one or both loins, radiating to the iliac fossae and suprapubic area. There may be dysuria (difficult or painful micturition) and strangury (a painful desire to pass urine though the bladder is empty), with the frequent passage of small amounts of scalding, usually cloudy urine, due to an associated cystitis. The temperature rises rapidly to 38–40°C, with the general manifestations of fever. A rigor may occur, and there may be vomiting. Tenderness and muscular guarding may be present in the renal angle and the lumbar region. There is a leucocytosis. The urine in *Esch. coli* infections is nearly always acid; in other infections it may be acid or alkaline. On microscopic examination there are numerous pus cells and organisms, some red cells and epithelial cells. When the organisms are motile Gram-negative bacilli and the urine is acid, the infection may be assumed to be due to *Esch. coli.*

Pyelonephritis in infants and children, like infections of the throat and middle ear, often presents as a fever without any localising symptoms. The initial feature may be a convulsion. In the feverish child, particular attention should be paid to these sites and the urine should be examined for pus cells and organisms.

Pyelonephritis may occur with few or no symptoms referable to the urinary tract. This is particularly the case during pregnancy. Routine culture of a midstream specimen of urine has revealed the presence of asymptomatic bacteriuria in about 5 per cent of all pregnancies during the early months. If no antibiotics are given progression to acute pyelonephritis occurs in about 40 per cent of such cases, and this is rare in those in whom the urine was sterile at the original examination. Investigation by intravenous pyelography after the termination of pregnancy shows a high incidence of abnormalities of the urinary tract in those women with bacteriuria. Suppressive chemotherapy at the asymptomatic stage has been found to prevent the development of acute symptoms.

Course and Prognosis. With adequate treatment the disease subsides rapidly in the great majority of cases. Fever, pain, frequency and dysuria disappear in a day or two. The urine usually becomes sterile within a few days.

In some cases, although the acute symptoms subside, a low-grade infection may persist, and the disease may pass into the chronic stage. More rarely the disease may be severe and cause necrosis of the papillae (*acute necrotising papillitis*). Fragments of renal tissue are then excreted in the urine and can be identified histologically. This complication, which may lead to renal failure, is particularly liable to occur in diabetic patients and in those addicted to phenacetin (p. 503). In view of the frequency of acute pyelonephritis, the curable nature of the condition, and the fact that chronic pyelonephritis is a common cause of renal failure and hypertension, the importance of adequate treatment of the acute stage cannot be overstressed.

Differential Diagnosis. Acute pyelonephritis should be distinguished from:

Acute appendicitis, salpingitis, cholecystitis and *diverticular disease*, especially by the absence of pus and organisms in the urine.

Diaphragmatic pleurisy, with or without pneumonia. Pain is usually made worse by coughing or a deep breath. Tenderness with guarding similar to that occurring in pyelonephritis may be present, but there are no abnormalities in the urine and abnormal physical signs may be detected in the chest.

Perinephric abscess due to infection by *Staph. aureus*. The illness is severe and the characteristic clinical features are pain and tenderness in the renal region, high remittent fever and polymorphonuclear leucocytosis. Urinary symptoms are absent and there are usually no pus cells or organisms in the urine. Oedema may obliterate the normal hollow in the loin, and an abscess may eventually point in the loin or groin, or it may rupture into the peritoneal or pleural cavity. Careful enquiry frequently elicits the history of a recent boil.

Treatment. The patient should be confined to bed and the general measures for the treatment of fever applied. The precise treatment depends upon the infecting organism and its sensitivity, and a midstream specimen of urine should be sent to the laboratory before treatment is begun. This specimen should reach the laboratory within 2 hours of voiding or be refrigerated at 4°C for a period not exceeding 24 hours. Since infection is usually due to *Esch. coli* it has been customary for many years to start treatment with sulphadimidine in doses of 1 g three times a day after a loading dose of 2 g before the results of urine culture are available. On the other hand the sulphonamides are bacteriostatic drugs to which an increasing number of strains of *Esch. coli* are becoming resistant and they may induce serious adverse effects. Co-trimoxazole has been shown to be very effective in the acute attack but should not be given to pregnant women. Whatever drug is employed a second midstream specimen of urine should be sent to the laboratory from 4 to 6 weeks after the completion of the initial course of treatment to make sure that the infection has been eradicated. If this has not been accomplished further treatment with the appropriate antibiotic must be given, depending on the bacteriological findings. In the very severe case, and if septicaemia occurs, gentamicin or kanamycin are the drugs of choice. Ampicillin is of value in proteus infections and carbenicillin or gentamicin in infections with *Ps. aeruginosa*. Dosage of these antibiotics is given on pages 90 and 94.

In every case the possibility of calculus, an obstructive lesion of the urinary tract or renal tuberculosis must be considered and treated if found.

Chronic Pyelonephritis

Aetiology. The disease may follow an attack of acute pyelonephritis which has been treated inadequately but is more likely to have been caused also by infection above an unrelieved obstruction to the urinary tract, e.g. calculus, stricture or prostatic disease. Other cases may follow cystitis due to stasis as a result of a cystocele or interference with the innervation of the bladder, e.g. in paraplegia or multiple sclerosis. *Esch. coli* is the organism responsible for most cases. Other infecting agents are proteus, *Ps. aeruginosa*, staphylococci, etc. In conditions in which the outflow tract of the bladder is deranged, reflux of urine into the ureters may occur during micturition. It is not known if vesicoureteric reflux occurs in the absence of such a lesion nor to what extent it contributes to the development of pyelonephritis. Chronic pyelonephritis also occurs in conditions leading to nephrocalcinosis (p. 500).

Pathology. The changes may be unilateral or bilateral, and of any grade of severity. The fully developed case usually shows gross scarring of the kidneys, which may be much reduced in size with narrowing of the cortex and medulla. Microscopically there is patchy fibrosis with chronic inflammatory cell infiltration, tubular atrophy, periglomerular fibrosis and eventual disappearance of nephrons. The arteries and arterioles may show sclerosis and narrowing.

Clinical Features. In many cases no symptoms arise directly from the renal lesions, and the patient may consult the doctor because of lassitude, tiredness and vague ill-health or for symptoms of uraemia or arterial hypertension. Occasionally weakness and fainting may occur if the renal disorder is accompanied by excessive salt loss. The discovery of hypertension or proteinuria on routine examination may be the first indication of the presence of the disease. Symptoms arising from the urinary tract, however, may also be present and include frequency of micturition, dysuria and occasionally aching lumbar pain. The urine may contain pus cells, a small amount of protein and many epithelial cells, though in some cases it may be normal.

In all cases of chronic pyuria, investigations such as rectal or vaginal examination, cystoscopy and pyelography must be carried out to discover the nature of any underlying mechanical factor causing obstruction to the flow of urine and to determine the extent of the infection.

Course and Prognosis. The course is usually a long one and may be punctuated by acute exacerbations. The infection is difficult to eradicate, even when underlying mechanical obstructions are found and relieved. Pyonephrosis may occur, especially in the presence of renal calculi. It is characterised by persistent lumbar pain, intermittent pyrexia, often with rigors, emaciation, pyuria, and, if both kidneys are involved, uraemia. One or both kidneys may become palpable. Some cases progress to chronic uraemia, which may be alleviated for a year or two by treatment. In elderly people, in diabetic patients and in cases of tabes dorsalis or paraplegia, the infection may become fulminating and be the immediate cause of death.

Differential Diagnosis. Chronic pyelonephritis should be distinguished from renal tuberculosis by cystoscopy, pyelography and bacteriological examination of the urine. In the later stages, when hypertension and uraemia have developed, the condition may be difficult to distinguish from chronic glomerulonephritis and nephrosclerosis. The presence of pus and organisms in the urine and a past history of frequency and dysuria support the diagnosis of chronic pyelonephritis. The possibility of underlying analgesic nephropathy should always be considered. Evidence in favour of this includes a history of prolonged use of analgesics and a characteristic appearance on pyelography.

Treatment. Medical treatment of chronic pyelonephritis is similar to that described for the acute disease. The chronic infection is usually more difficult to eradicate. Attempts should be made to remove obstructive lesions or renal calculi by appropriate surgical procedures. An antibiotic to which the organism is sensitive should be given for 14 days (p. 490). If the infection is not eradicated suppressive treatment may be required for many months, the antibiotic used being indicated by the changing pattern and sensitivity of the organisms in the urine. Ampicillin, nitrofurantoin and nalidixic acid (p. 95) are valuable for this purpose. A moderate degree of uraemia may be present which progresses little for months or years. This is especially so when hypertension is absent or minimal; in such cases salt and water depletion is often present due to failure of tubular reabsorption, and this aggravates the uraemia. Considerable benefit may result from an additional intake of salt as described under chronic glomerulonephritis (p. 487). When the renal infection is unilateral or if pyonephrosis has developed, nephrectomy may be indicated; rarely, high blood pressure may be cured by the removal of the diseased kidney.

Cystitis, Urethritis and Prostatitis

Reference has already been made to the possibility that some infections of the urinary tract may be confined to the urethra or bladder. In these the features of systemic illness are slight and the symptoms are those of frequency and dysuria. Scalding pain is felt in the urethra during micturition. Suprapubic pain of cystitis is felt before, during and a few moments after voiding urine. Although the bladder is empty there may be an intense desire to pass more urine due to spasm of its inflamed wall. Tenderness is often present in the suprapubic region, and the urine may have an unpleasant odour and appear cloudy. Pus cells, red cells and organisms may be seen on microscopical examination of the urine. Sometimes the urine is grossly blood-stained. Cystitis is particularly common in women and young girls, and the infection is usually due to *Esch. coli.*

In some patients with symptoms suggestive of urethritis and cystitis, no bacteria can be cultured from the urine. The term *'urethral syndrome'* has been applied to this category of patients who are predominantly female. The cause of the symptoms is unknown although a variety of explanations, which include allergy to deodorants, etc., congestion of the urethra possibly related to sexual activity and infection of the urethral glands, have been put forward. Urethritis is associated with arthritis, conjunctivitis and sometimes diarrhoea in Reiter's disease (p. 639).

In acute prostatitis there may be considerable systemic disturbance. On digital examination of the rectum the prostatic gland is usually very tender.

Investigation. A possible predisposing cause for recurrent infections of the lower urinary tract should be sought though this is found in only a minority of cases. This may entail digital examination of the prostate, and gynaecological examination. Cystoscopy should be postponed until the acute condition has subsided. If there is reason to suppose that the kidneys are also involved, the examination should proceed with ureteric catherisation, the collection of samples of urine from each kidney, and retrograde pyelography.

Treatment. Therapy is similar to that of acute pyelonephritis (p. 490). In the majority of instances this is effective and there is no recurrence of the symptoms. In some patients, however, the clinical features of infection persist or recur. In patients with a normal urinary tract, particularly women with recurrent sexual intercourse-induced acute urinary infection, the great majority can be kept free of attacks by use of long-term low dose preventive antibacterial drugs, taken after voiding before going to bed. Such a regimen should be commenced after a curative course of treatment, as evidenced by bacteriological culture. Some women with recurrent infection can remain free of attacks by practising pre- and postcoital micturition, or by applying an antiseptic cream such as 0·5 per cent cetrimide to the periurethral area prior to sexual intercourse. It is perhaps preferable to attempt these simpler measures before embarking on a prophylactic course of treatment with an antibacterial agent.

The possible causes of failure to respond to treatment, or of relapse, are:

1. Infection with organisms including fungi or protozoa resistant to the chemotherapeutic agent employed.

2. Tuberculosis, with or without secondary infection.

3. Continued infection from above, e.g. pyelonephritis associated with calculi.

4. Obstruction below the base of the bladder by: (a) prostatic hyperplasia, carcinoma of the prostate, or urethral stricture in the male; (b) chronic urethritis or stricture in the female.

5. Atrophy of the urethra consequent upon oestrogen lack as in the postmenopause.

6. Involvement of the bladder by: (a) malignant tumour arising in the bladder or in adjacent organs; (b) vesical calculus; foreign bodies may have been inserted into the bladder; (c) inflammation from adjacent structures, e.g. diverticular disease.

7. The presence of urethral caruncle, cystocele, urethrocele or cervicitis in the female or a meatal fissure in the male. The latter may be noted as a tender induration on examination of the meatus.

8. Paraplegia, in which urinary infection is frequent, persistent and often the ultimate cause of death.

Renal Tuberculosis

Tuberculosis of the kidney is invariably secondary to tuberculosis elsewhere and occurs as a result of blood-borne infection. The initial lesion develops in the renal cortex and if untreated may ulcerate into the pelvis with consequent involvement of the bladder, epididymes, seminal vesicles and prostate. The disease tends to occur in young people and may manifest itself with recurrent haematuria and dysuria due to secondary involvement of the bladder. In addition the general features of tuberculosis, i.e. malaise, fever, lassitude and weight loss, may be present. Culture of the urine by ordinary methods may be sterile in spite of pyuria. The extent of the infection should be ascertained by cystoscopic examination, by pyelography, and by culture of the urine from both ureters. Chemotherapy should be given as for tuberculosis elsewhere (p. 292). Prednisone given concomitantly appears to prevent the development of stenosis of the ureter which is an important factor in causing deterioration of renal function. Partial or complete nephrectomy may be necessary in those in whom the disease has advanced to the stage of producing serious destruction of renal tissue with cavitation.

Renal Failure

The term *uraemia* has been used for more than a century to describe the clinical state which arises from renal failure. The retention of abnormal amounts of urea in the blood in renal disorders was amongst the early discoveries resulting from the application of biochemical methods to the elucidation of disease, and the symptoms of chronic renal failure were long attributed to it. The newer knowledge of renal physiology has shown that, as renal function becomes impaired, other complex biochemical changes occur and that these are probably more responsible for the clinical features of uraemia than the elevation of blood urea. These changes include disturbances in hydrogen ion concentration, abnormalities in water and electrolyte balance and the accumulation of many products of metabolism. In addition, renal failure is accompanied in the majority of cases by arterial hypertension, and this fact complicates still further the clinical picture.

Classification. Renal function may be impaired by disease affecting the renal parenchyma (*renal uraemia*), by extrarenal disorders such as acute circulatory failure (*prerenal uraemia*) or as a result of conditions in which there is obstruction to the outflow of urine (*postrenal uraemia*). The deterioration of renal function which ensues may be acute or chronic and of varying degrees of severity.

Acute Renal Failure may be due to a wide variety of conditions including acute proliferative glomerulonephritis, acute severe bilateral pyelonephritis, malignant hypertension, polyarteritis, renal involvement in systemic lupus erythematosus and eclampsia. In recent years, a condition in which disseminated intravascular coagulation occurs and in which the glomeruli may be predominantly affected has also been described as causing acute renal failure (p. 634).

Acute renal failure occurs also in patients in whom initially there is no primary renal disease but in whom acute circulatory failure leads to sudden reduction in renal blood flow; this reduces the capacity of the kidneys to perform their functions. Thus prerenal uraemia occurs in states associated with water and salt depletion, shock, haemorrhage, etc. (p. 495). With appropriate treatment, this type of uraemia is commonly reversible and the prognosis is generally good. In a proportion of cases of prerenal uraemia, renal ischaemia may be so severe and prolonged as to produce damage to the renal parenchyma. When this affects the tubules predominantly, the condition is called *acute tubular necrosis*. More rarely, but notably in cases of retroplacental haemorrhage occurring as a complication of pregnancy, the whole or a large part of the renal cortex is involved, the glomeruli as well as the tubules becoming necrotic. This is called *renal cortical necrosis*.

Chronic renal failure arises as a result of diseases which destroy renal tissue more slowly, i.e. chronic glomerulonephritis, chronic pyelonephritis, polycystic disease of the kidneys, hypertension, diabetic nephropathy, amyloid infiltration, tuberculosis and conditions causing hypercalcaemia.

For descriptive purposes, renal failure is conveniently subdivided into four categories based mainly upon the site of the lesion responsible:

1. Renal failure due to disease of the kidneys (renal uraemia).
2. Renal failure due to prerenal disease (prerenal uraemia).
3. Acute renal failure due to acute tubular necrosis.
4. Renal failure as a result of conditions in which there is obstruction of the renal tract resulting in impairment of renal function (postrenal uraemia).

I. Renal Failure due to Disease of the Kidney
(Renal Uraemia)

The clinical features and treatment of renal failure occurring as a result of glomerulonephritis are described on pages 485 and 487. The clinical features of renal failure occurring in the course of other chronic kidney diseases are essentially similar but are also those of the underlying disease.

II. Renal Failure due to Prerenal Disorder

(Prerenal Uraemia)

The performance of normal renal function is dependent upon the maintenance of an adequate renal circulation. The renal share of the cardiac output is normally about 25 per cent at rest. If the cardiac output falls the renal blood flow is disproportionately reduced. In this event, the glomerular filtration rate is reduced and oliguria results. While systemic hypotension often precedes prerenal uraemia, renal ischaemia may occur in its absence. Regional vasoconstriction is a means by which the blood pressure may be maintained in the face of oligaemia, and the success of this mechanism may deprive the kidneys of a large part of their blood supply. The urine is usually small in volume and the concentration of urea in the blood gradually rises. The more common causes of prerenal failure include:

1. *Loss of blood* from any cause including complications of pregnancy, trauma or gastrointestinal bleeding.

2. *Loss of plasma* as in burns and crushing injuries.

3. *Loss of fluid and salt.*
   (a) *from the gut* in severe vomiting, diarrhoea, acute intestinal obstruction, paralytic ileus and fistulous drainage.
   (b) *in the urine* in diabetic ketoacidosis and Addison's disease.
   (c) *from the skin* in excessive sweating (heat stroke).

4. *General anaesthetics* causing hypotension *and surgical operations* causing blood loss may reduce renal blood flow and precipitate renal failure in those whose blood volume is precariously balanced.

5. *Serious infection*, especially septicaemia from *Esch. coli*, peritonitis or severe pulmonary infection, may produce shock, and reduce renal blood flow.

6. *Acute cardiac failure* due to myocardial infarction or cardiac arrest.

7. Incompatible blood transfusion, haemolytic crises and acute liver disease are also sometimes responsible.

These conditions should be treated by appropriate fluids given intravenously and by specific measures as indicated in the treatment of diabetic ketoacidosis, Addison's disease, infection, etc. Prompt and effective replacement of blood, water and salt is essential. In many cases vigorous treatment in the early stages prevents the occurrence of significant degrees of renal failure. If oliguria or anuria persists in spite of the return of the blood pressure to normal, the functional integrity of the nephrons has become disrupted. The associated pathological changes which arise were originally called *acute tubular necrosis*. While this is a misleading term in that it does not accurately reflect the histological abnormalities, it is so widely used that it is employed here.

III. Acute Renal Failure due to Acute Tubular Necrosis

Acute renal failure with tubular necrosis is a disease affecting both kidneys, characterised by oliguria or anuria with urine of low specific gravity and rapidly developing uraemia. Much of the earlier information about acute renal failure was obtained from studies of the 'crush' syndrome which occurred during the air raids of the Second World War.

Aetiology. Acute tubular necrosis occurs as a complication of various conditions which are associated with renal ischaemia, and which are listed above as causes of prerenal uraemia. Certain drugs are also capable of producing acute renal failure, e.g. paracetamol, sulphonamides and cephaloridine. Poisoning by substances, such as sodium chlorate, which produce renal parenchymal necrosis, may also be responsible.

Pathogenesis. Severe shock and water and salt depletion are accompanied by widespread vasoconstriction. The blood supplied to the kidneys is reduced and afferent arteriolar vasoconstriction further curtails glomerular filtration. This sometimes occurs even when the systemic blood pressure is maintained. If the ischaemia is severe and of sufficiently long duration the basement membrane of the renal tubules is ruptured and focal necrosis of the cells occurs. Stasis of the circulation within the kidney is associated with some degree of intraglomerular coagulation. In addition, casts of haemoglobin or of plasma proteins sometimes form within the tubular lumen and interfere with the passage of fluid; interstitial oedema around the tubules may also raise the intrarenal pressure and constrict nephrons externally so contributing to the renal failure.

In cases following damage from agents, such as sulphonamides or sodium chlorate, direct damage to the renal tubular cells from toxic or allergic reactions is responsible.

Clinical Features and Course. The clinical features are those of the causal condition together with those of rapidly developing uraemia. Initially the urine volume is commonly but not invariably greatly reduced to between 200 and 500 ml/24 hours and this stage of the illness is called the *oliguric phase*. Any urine that is formed contains protein, casts and red and white blood cells. The specific gravity is usually about 1·010 early in the course of the disease, and this persists for several days or weeks. At first the patient may feel well, but after some days the features of uraemia appear. Initially these are anorexia, nausea and vomiting; apathy is followed by mental confusion and later muscular twitching, fits, drowsiness, coma, and bleeding episodes occur. At this stage the main dangers to life are (1) pulmonary oedema due to the injudicious administration of excessive amounts of fluid, (2) potassium intoxication due to the rise in the concentration of plasma potassium which is especially likely if there is haemolysis or massive soft tissue damage, (3) the occurrence of severe systemic infection to which such patients are susceptible, and (4) uraemia and metabolic acidosis.

The oliguric phase of the disease usually lasts for 1 to 3 weeks. If the patient does not succumb the daily volume of urine increases and rapidly may reach several litres. This is called the *diuretic phase* and coincides with healing of the renal tubules, reduction in intrarenal tension and resolution of intratubular casts and intraglomerular coagulation. During this phase there is uncontrolled water and sodium loss, and sometimes flaccid paralysis due to loss of potassium occurs in the absence of treatment. The concentration of blood urea ceases to rise and then gradually falls. Virtually complete recovery of renal function then takes place slowly over a period of 3 to 6 months.

Treatment

CAUSAL CONDITION. With a view to preventing or minimising the renal lesion, the underlying cause should be treated urgently. The blood volume should be quickly restored by appropriate transfusion and water and electrolyte deficits should be replenished. The adequacy of blood transfusion and fluid therapy is best monitored by the use of an in-dwelling atrial catheter (p. 193) and assessed by clinical response.

THE OLIGURIC PHASE. Treatment during the oliguric phase has undergone many changes which have reflected the understanding of the disease process. Formerly treatment was based upon the crude assumption that the kidneys could be forced to secrete urine by giving large amounts of fluids intravenously or by the use of osmotic diuretics such as sodium sulphate or by surgical renal decapsulation undertaken to relieve intrarenal tension. There seems little doubt that the former high mortality was largely due to these procedures which have now been abandoned.

Clinical and pathological studies have shown that the ischaemic renal lesions are usually reversible provided the patient can be kept alive during the oliguric phase. Treatment is therefore designed to minimise the need for renal function until healing occurs and this can often be achieved by simple dietary restrictions.

Water and Electrolyte Balance. This is maintained by replacing the obligatory losses of water through the skin and lungs, estimated to be about 600 ml water/day, and by giving no electrolytes since none are being lost from the body. In febrile patients an extra allowance of water is required to replace the fluid lost through visible perspiration and a further small supplement equal to the volume of urine passed each day should be added. Should abnormal losses of fluid occur, as in diarrhoea, additional fluid will be required in appropriate amounts.

Protein and Energy. Dietary protein is restricted to about 20 g/day and attempts are made to suppress endogenous protein catabolism to a minimum by giving as much energy as possible as fat and carbohydrate. For this purpose a diet restricted in its protein and electrolyte content may be supplemented by a liquid glucose preparation. In the event of vomiting, oral treatment should be avoided and carbohydrate should be given in the form of 10 per cent fructose through a large peripheral vein.

In many patients in whom the acute renal failure is mild in degree and relatively short in duration this treatment prevents the blood urea from rising more than 4 mmol/l (20 mg per 100 ml) per day, and the accumulation of potassium from protein catabolism is usually not sufficient to have serious consequences. If elevation of plasma potassium concentration should occur attempts should be made to reduce it by employing methods described on page 159; these include (1) the use of a sodium or calcium charged resin which removes potassium from the body, (2) giving 20 units of soluble insulin subcutaneously and an intravenous infusion of 50 g of glucose; and (3) controlling acidosis by intravenous administration of isotonic sodium bicarbonate.

Haemodialysis. In some patients, however, and especially in those suffering from severe infection or massive tissue damage, or in whom blood has become loculated in one of the tissue spaces, the rate of rise of blood urea and potassium is much more rapid and occurs in spite of the application of conservative methods; in these circumstances life may be threatened from acute renal failure within a few days. The patient should then be transferred to a centre equipped with the means for extracorporeal dialysis (artificial kidney). Daily haemodialyses may then be required over a period of several weeks before renal function returns. When this policy is adopted it is usually possible to be much more liberal regarding the intake of protein, fluid and energy. This is desirable from the point of view of encouraging repair of damaged or diseased tissues and is rendered possible by the daily correction of the composition of the blood and volume of body fluids achieved by the artificial kidney.

Peritoneal dialysis can sometimes be used as an alternative to haemodialysis. While this method has a place in the treatment of small children, it is a prolonged, uncomfortable, sometimes painful procedure and fraught with complications, notably peritonitis.

RECOVERY OR DIURETIC PHASE. When diuresis commences the concentration of blood urea tends to remain constant for a few days and then begins to fall. When this occurs, a light diet, containing not more than 40–60 g protein per day and ample fruit, should be provided. Sufficient fluid must be given to replace the increased and uncontrolled loss of water in the urine. The fluid intake must be increased by the volume of the previous day's urinary output. Salt supplements are usually needed during the diuretic phase to compensate for increased urinary loss. On average about 3 g of sodium chloride and 2 g of sodium bicarbonate are needed for each litre of urine passed. The fruit usually compensates for the potassium loss, though in many cases a supplement of potassium chloride by oral administration may also be required. As the blood urea concentration returns to normal values and renal function improves a normal diet may be taken.

Patients with severe acute renal failure are seriously ill and require skilled nursing, preferably in single rooms designed to prevent airborne or contact infection. Great care must be exercised in the use of drugs which are normally excreted by the kidneys.

Prognosis. The high mortality accompanying acute renal failure of ischaemic origin has been greatly reduced by the measures described above. Prognosis depends upon the speed and efficiency with which the therapeutic measures are put into operation, the prompt recognition and effective treatment of complicating infection, and the nature and the severity of the condition precipitating the syndrome. In cases of uncomplicated acute renal failure, such as those due to simple haemorrhage, the mortality should now be less than 10 per cent even when haemodialysis is required. In severe renal failure complicated by serious infection or multiple injuries it is about 50 per cent.

IV. Renal Failure due to Postrenal Causes

(*Postrenal Uraemia*)

Renal failure may result from obstruction at any point in the urinary tract due to the causes given below. In the presence of two functioning kidneys ureteric obstruction causes uraemia only when it is bilateral.

Diagnosis. The diagnosis may be suggested by a history of previous urinary symptoms such as pain in the loins, haematuria, renal colic, nocturia or difficulty in micturition. However, in many instances the onset is clinically silent and the cause of the obstruction discovered only after appropriate investigations. In contrast to acute renal failure associated with tubular necrosis, anuria is common and the complete absence of urine suggests the need for cytoscopy, ureteral catheterisation and retrograde pyelography.

Treatment. Surgical treatment is required for all cases of renal failure due to postrenal obstruction. Uraemia may be severe, yet relief of the obstruction followed by a high fluid intake results in recovery of adequate renal function in many patients, provided that this treatment has not been delayed too long.

Obstruction of the Urinary Tract

Obstruction to the flow of urine from the kidney through the pelvis, ureter, bladder and urethra is a common disorder; it causes stasis and a rise in pressure within the urinary tract which predisposes to infection, stone formation and renal failure. Obstruction may occur at any level but is most often found at the pelviureteric junction, in the ureter, at the neck of the bladder or in the urethra. Obstruction at the pelviureteric junction causes hydronephrosis; obstruction of the ureter results in hydroureter and later hydronephrosis; obstruction of the bladder neck or urethra distends the bladder, causes hypertrophy of its muscle seen on cystoscopic examination as trabeculation, and hydroureter and hydronephrosis. If obstruction is unrelieved, slow progressive destruction of renal tissue occurs; superimposed infection may cause cystitis, ureteritis or pyonephrosis in which renal damage may become more rapid.

Aetiology. Obstruction may be due to an organic lesion in the lumen or in or around the wall of the urinary tract, or it may arise because of a congenital defect in the muscles of the pelviureteric junction, ureter or bladder neck preventing the contraction wave and therefore the flow of urine. Organic causes include stone, blood clot, tumour, fibrosis following infection, or the precipitation of crystals due to sulphonamides. An aberrant renal artery, retroperitoneal fibrosis, accidental ligation at operation, carcinoma of the cervix, prostatic enlargement or phimosis may compress the lumen from outside.

Clinical Features. These vary with the cause and site of the lesion and in particular whether it is above or below the bladder. When the obstruction is supravesical, renal colic may occur, especially if the onset is sudden; more commonly the obstruction is gradual and an aching pain in the loins, sometimes aggravated by drinking, develops. Superimposed infection causes systemic manifestations with fever and dysuria. Haematuria is common.

When the obstruction is below the bladder, there is difficulty in micturition and the urinary stream is thin in calibre and poor in force. Complete urinary retention may occur with consequent distension of the bladder, which may be easily visible and palpable; either anuria or overflow incontinence ensues. In the latter event catheterisation reveals the presence of residual urine in the bladder after the patient has voided.

Treatment. In all cases the ultimate objective is to remove the source of obstruction; this is often possible, as in the case of a stone or prostatic hypertrophy. In the first instance it is necessary to relieve the obstruction in order to alleviate symptoms and preserve renal function. The action required varies with the nature of the underlying disease, but sometimes it may be dealt with initially and temporarily by draining the kidney, i.e. nephrostomy, the ureter, i.e. ureterostomy, or the bladder, i.e. suprapubic or urethral catheterisation. Antibiotics should be given if infection is severe but it is preferable to wait until the obstruction has been removed or relieved. When the hydronephrosis or pyonephrosis affects one kidney and this is severely damaged, nephrectomy is indicated. When obstruction affects both kidneys, appropriate treatment for renal failure should be given.

Renal and Vesical Calculi and Nephrocalcinosis

Aetiology. Urinary calculi have long presented fascinating aetiological problems which are still largely unsolved. Two or three centuries ago vesical calculus was so common in Britain that a respectable living could be made as a lithotomist, but the incidence is much lower at the present time for reasons that are not known. It is indeed surprising that renal and vesical calculi or nephrocalcinosis do not occur more frequently since some of the constituents of urine are present in a concentration in excess of their maximum solubility in water. It seems likely that urine contains certain substances, e.g. polypeptides, mucoproteins and citric acid, which, by forming complexes, keep otherwise insoluble salts in solution in the urine. Other authorities believe that the primary cause of urinary calculi is a pre-existing renal or vesical lesion which acts as a nidus on which urinary constituents precipitate.

The following conditions are frequently associated with stone formation:

(a) Climate or occupation which necessitates living or working under conditions where excessive loss of water from sweating occurs, thus causing constituents to be precipitated because of their high concentration in the diminished volume of urine excreted.

(b) Urinary infection, obstruction and stagnation.

(c) Conditions associated with hypercalciuria which increases the liability to the formation of stones consisting mainly of calcium phosphate and calcium oxalate. These include idiopathic hypercalciuria, excessive intake of milk or cheese, prolonged immobilisation, hyperparathyroidism, Cushing's syndrome, sarcoidosis, plasma cell myeloma and vitamin D intoxication.

(d) Certain rare inherited disorders, e.g. cystinuria and primary hyperoxaluria, which may lead to the production of cystine or oxalate stones respectively.

(e) Conditions causing increased excretion of uric acid, e.g. gout and leukaemia.

(f) The pH of the urine influences the extent to which some of these conditions lead to stone formation; thus an alkaline urine tends to increase the precipitation of calcium phosphate stones and so may be responsible for their occurrence in renal tubular acidosis from any cause. Likewise an acid urine reduces the solubility of uric acid and cystine.

Since the constituents of renal and vesical calculi are present in numerous articles of food it is not surprising that diet has been considered to be of aetiological importance. Many experimental investigations in animals have shown that by increasing the calcium content of the diet and reducing the intake of vitamin A, renal and vesical calculi can be produced regularly. Furthermore, the remarkable fall in the incidence of vesical calculi in children and young adults, which occurred in Britain in the nineteenth century, coincided with a marked improvement in the nutrition of the nation. Today, however, in prosperous countries the great majority of renal calculi occur in well nourished, healthy young men in whom the most careful investigations reveal no cause for stone formation.

Pathology. Urinary concretions vary greatly in size. There may be particles like sand anywhere in the urinary tract or large round stones in the bladder. Staghorn calculi fill the whole renal pelvis and branch into the calyces; they are usually associated with hydronephrosis and chronic pyelonephritis. Over 90 per cent of renal stones contain calcium but the nature of the salt varies with their origin. Deposits of calcium may also be present throughout the renal parenchyma, giving rise to nephrocalcinosis. This is especially liable to occur in cases of hyper-parathyroidism, renal tubular acidosis, vitamin D intoxication, and in healed renal tuberculosis.

Clinical Features. These vary according to the size, shape and position of the stone, and the presence and nature of the underlying condition. Renal calculi or nephrocalcinosis may be present for many years and yet themselves give rise to no symptoms. While nephrocalcinosis never gives rise to pain, the most common complaint arising from renal calculi is an intermittent dull pain in the loin or back, increased by movement or a sudden jolt. Some abnormal constituents of the urine, e.g. red cells, protein or pus cells, can be found at one time or another.

Renal Colic. When a stone is small enough to enter the ureter and large enough to obstruct it, an attack of renal colic develops. The patient is suddenly aware of pain in the loin, which soon radiates round the flank to the groin and often into the testis or labia in the sensory distribution of the first lumbar nerve. The pain steadily increases in intensity to reach a maximum in a few minutes. The patient is restless, and generally tries, unsuccessfully, to obtain relief by assuming various positions, both lying and sitting, and by pacing about the room. There is pallor, sweating, and often vomiting, and the patient may groan in agony. Frequency and haematuria may occur. Without treatment the intense pain usually subsides within two hours but may continue unabated for several hours or some days. In many cases the pain is constant during the attack, though slight fluctuations in severity may occur. Contrary to what is often believed, it is rare for attacks to consist of intermittent severe pains, coming and going every few minutes for some hours.

Diagnosis. When renal colic occurs the diagnosis is usually easily made as it can be established by the history and by the finding of red cells in the urine. All patients suspected of having renal calculus, including those with renal colic, should have a radiological examination of the urinary tract, including retrograde pyelography in some instances. If there is doubt about the cause of the abdominal pain, an intravenous pyelogram during the attack may be helpful. When the pain is due to a stone in the ureter, the radiograph shows a dense renal shadow with delay in the appearance of the dye in the renal pelvis. Appropriate investigations should be undertaken to discover the presence of any underlying condition which might be responsible for the development of renal calcification or lithiasis.

Prognosis. This varies greatly depending on the underlying cause and on whether the patient passes the stone in the urine or whether it continues to obstruct the ureter. In the latter case, if the stone is not removed surgically, hydronephrosis and pyelonephritis are likely to develop in time.

Treatment and Prevention. The immediate treatment of renal pain or renal colic is rest in bed, the application of warmth to the seat of pain, and the administration of analgesic drugs, e.g. pethidine (100 mg) or morphine (15–30 mg), and an-tispasmodic drugs, e.g. atropine sulphate (0·8 or 1·2 mg). These should be given intramuscularly and may be repeated within 2 hours. Attempts to dissolve calculi in the kidneys have not been successful. Stones in the renal pelvis and urinary bladder must be removed surgically. Stones in the ureter usually pass naturally if left alone and surgical removal is apt to be followed by stricture and its complications. When, however, pain persists or frequent bouts of pain become intolerable, the insertion of a ureteric catheter is often followed by the passage of the stone. Urgent surgical intervention is necessary in the event of anuria. It is also required if the stone has not moved for some months and hydronephrosis is developing or there is continuing infection in the urinary tract. A stone larger than 1 cm in diameter generally requires surgical removal.

Suitable medical or surgical measures should be instituted for the correction of any primary cause of renal lithiasis that may have been discovered.

Dietary restrictions prescribed with the object of preventing the formation of stones, are useful in the case of idiopathic hypercalciuria, with recurrent oxalate stones and in persons who have passed several uric acid stones. In idiopathic hypercalciuria a diet low in calcium, by reducing the intake of milk and cheese, is advisable. When dietary restriction is impracticable, bendrofluazide in a dose of 5 mg/day reduces urinary calcium excretion by about 30 per cent. The mechanism of this action is unknown but is probably renal. An alternative or supplementary treatment is the use of cellulose phosphate (5 g t.i.d.) which binds calcium in the diet and prevents absorption. In recurrent oxalate stones the elimination from the diet of articles which have a very high content of oxalate, such as rhubarb or spinach, may be worthy of trial.

The avoidance of liver, kidney, sweetbreads, fish roe, sardines and sprats, articles with a very high purine content, is advisable in persons who have passed several uric acid or urate stones, as may occur in gout or in patients with leukaemia. This may also be supplemented by the use of allopurinol (p. 650).

Since the distribution of phosphorus occurs so widely in foodstuffs, dietary restriction for the treatment of phosphate calculi is unlikely to be of any value. Phosphatic calculi are found only in alkaline urine, hence acidifying the urine by administering ammonium chloride daily may be effective. In contrast, cystine and urate stones may be prevented or sometimes dissolved by making the urine persistently alkaline, especially if combined with a high output of urine.

Lastly, the most important therapeutic and prophylactic measure for all forms of stones is the provision of an adequate fluid intake which assists in preventing deposition of crystalloids in the renal tissue. A daily output of urine of at least 3 l is advisable; hence the intake of fluid should be approximately 4 l daily. If the climate or the patient's occupation causes much sweating the fluid intake requires to be greatly increased.

Congenital Abnormalities of the Kidneys

Congenital anomalies of the urinary tract affect more than 10 per cent of infants and, unless they are immediately lethal, they are prone to lead to complications in later life. About 1 in 500 infants is born with only one kidney and, although usually compatible with a normal life, it is often associated with abnormalities in other organs.

Polycystic Disease. This genetically determined abnormality of renal structure may be associated with other congenital abnormalities, e.g. cystic liver (p. 458). There are two modes of inheritance. The commoner or adult type is inherited as an autosomal dominant trait. The infantile form is very rare and is inherited as an autosomal recessive; it is usually fatal within the first year of life.

The adult condition may be found during infancy, but symptoms often do not develop until adult life. Both kidneys are affected, are several times the normal size, and consist of masses of cysts, predominantly cortical, with a variable amount of renal parenchyma which often shows extensive fibrosis and arteriolosclerosis.

The clinical features include pain in the renal angles, haematuria, uraemia and usually a slowly developing arterial hypertension. Often one or both of the kidneys can be palpated and the surface may be nodular. In addition to polycystic disease, other diseases in which the kidneys may be palpable are hydro- or pyonephrosis, solitary cyst, renal carcinoma and other tumours. It should be remembered, however, that in some normal people all of the right kidney, and occasionally the lower pole of the left kidney may be felt on clinical examination. This is particularly true in slim women. On the other hand, pathologically enlarged kidneys are not always palpable. When a kidney can be felt, as in polycystic disease, it may be possible to appreciate departures from the normal size, smooth surface and firm consistency. Diagnosis can be confirmed by ultrasound or retrograde pyelography.

In course, prognosis and treatment, polycystic disease resembles chronic glomerulonephritis, and death occurs in middle age from uraemia, cerebrovascular accident or cardiac failure.

Medullary Cystic Disease. Medullary cysts are found in two widely different conditions. In *medullary sponge kidney* the cysts are confined to the collecting ducts in the medulla. Affected patients are usually middle aged and present with pain, haematuria or urinary tract infection. The diagnosis is made on radiographic examination and the prognosis is generally good.

In *uraemic medullary sponge kidney* small cortical cysts are also present and these lead to progressive destruction of the nephrons; this condition occurs in younger patients and there is often a family history. Sometimes affected kidneys are salt-losing; this aggravates the degree of renal failure but, even when treated appropriately, serious renal failure is usual.

Drug-induced Renal Disease

The susceptibility of the kidney to damage by drugs stems from its large blood supply relative to its weight and to the fact that it is the route of excretion for many water soluble compounds. Acute renal damage may arise in the course of treatment with a number of antimicrobial drugs which include sulphonamide, streptomycin and kanamycin. Sulphonamide compounds may precipitate in the renal tubules, calyces or ureter and cause obstruction to urine flow, and occasionally lesions similar to polyarteritis may develop. Streptomycin and kanamycin may induce proximal tubular damage with proteinuria. Tetracycline accentuates uraemia by its antianabolic effect on protein metabolism; tetracycline and amphotericin B, kept and used after the expiry date, can induce renal tubular acidosis and sometimes a Fanconi-like syndrome.

Analgesic Nephropathy. The occurrence of chronic renal damage as a consequence of long-continued ingestion of analgesics was first noted in Switzerland, and it is now recognised as an important potential cause of renal failure. Although phenacetin is the major culprit, the possibility that aspirin alone or in combination may also be responsible cannot be ruled out.

The majority of affected patients are women who suffer from anxiety or headaches or have personal or marital problems. They are commonly divorced, anxious, apprehensive and smoke or drink alcohol to excess. Other patients have taken analgesics over many years for rheumatoid arthritis or osteoarthrosis. Symptoms include polyuria and thirst, the features of recurrent urinary tract infection; renal colic caused by the passage of associated calculi, blood or fragments of necrotic renal papillae which can be recognised by microscopic examination of the urine also occur.

The pathological changes predominantly affect the corticomedullary junction with diffuse interstitial fibrosis and tubular atrophy. Ultimately there is loss of tubules in cortex and medulla and acute papillary necrosis may develop. The changes are probably the result of ischaemia due to interference with the blood flow through the postglomerular vessels of juxtamedullary glomeruli. A recognised complication is the development of transitional cell carcinoma of the renal pelves.

Treatment consists of withdrawing the offending drug and substituting another analgesic, e.g. paracetamol, if this therapy is essential. Provided the analgesic is withdrawn sufficiently early there is a reasonable prospect of some recovery of renal function; otherwise severe renal failure develops and becomes irreversible.

Tumours of Kidney and Urinary Tract

Renal Carcinoma

This is the most common tumour of the kidney. It was formerly called a hypernephroma on the mistaken view that it arose from adrenal rest tissue within the kidney. Haematuria is the most frequent presenting feature and blood clots may give rise to renal colic. Sometimes the tumour causes vague abdominal pain and it may also be responsible for long continued fever. Occasionally patients present first with symptoms arising from metastatic foci in the lungs, liver or bones. On rare occasions polycythaemia occurs, and this is believed to be due to excessive production of erythropoietin (p. 590). The diagnosis may be suspected from the history or the tumour may be palpable. Radiological investigation is usually essential, and aortography may distinguish the filling defect from that due to a simple cyst which is avascular. Early surgical treatment affords the only prospect of cure.

Nephroblastoma (Wilm's Tumour)

This is the second most common malignant tumour of the kidney and presents in the first decade, and often the first year of life. The tumour is radiosensitive and the best hope of cure is early diagnosis and surgical removal followed by radiotherapy.

Tumours of Renal Pelvis, Ureter, Bladder and Prostate Gland

Tumours of the renal pelvis, ureter and bladder are histologically similar and are almost always transitional cell carcinomas. They tend to spread locally by direct invasion but also by implantation to other parts of the urinary tract. While some are benign, e.g. papillomata, all urinary tract tumours are liable to recur even after apparently adequate treatment. The bladder is by far the most common site and epidemiological studies have shown that it is particularly likely to develop in patients who work in industries where exposure to analine is likely such as dyeing and printing. Haematuria as a sole presenting symptom is almost universal. Features due to obstruction to the urinary tract also occur and symptoms of urinary tract infection may be superimposed. Diagnosis is made by cystoscopy, biopsy and radiography. Bladder tumours are treated by diathermy or radiotherapy. Cystectomy with transplantation of the ureters to colon or skin may be necessary.

Prostatic carcinoma usually presents with symptoms of urethral obstruction similar to those of benign prostatic hypertrophy. On digital examination of the rectum the prostate is felt to be very hard and the median furrow may be obliterated. Spread through the capsule and metastases in bone occur and are often associated with a rise in the serum acid phosphatase. Both the primary growth and metastases can be controlled with oestrogens, e.g. dienoestrol. Gynaecomastia is a troublesome side-effect. In some cases orchidectomy may also be necessary.

Benign enlargement of the prostate gland is of unknown cause but it may be associated with a fall in androgen secretion. It is most commonly found in men over 60 years. Histologically the inner zone of the gland undergoes hyperplasia and hypertrophy and there is an increase in the fibromuscular stroma. The enlarged prostate obstructs the outflow of urine from the bladder by compressing, displacing, distorting and elongating the prostatic urethra with the effects on bladder and renal function referred to on page 499.

The clinical features are those of progressive obstruction to urinary flow. Acute urinary retention may arise if the gland suddenly increases in size because of superimposed infection or congestion, or when cardiac failure develops in the elderly. Then the patient has a sudden desire to micturate but is unable to do so, the bladder becomes tense and is tender. More chronic retention may pass unnoticed for some time but there is a gradual increase in the volume of urine which remains in the bladder after micturition. Haematuria and bleeding from the urethra may also occur and may be the presenting symptom. On rectal examination the prostate may feel large, elastic and is uniform in consistency; however, when the median lobe alone is affected, the prostate feels normal and the condition can be recognised only by cystoscopy.

Prostatectomy is the only effective treatment and the important decision is when to operate. Acute retention should be relieved by catheterisation and drainage; sometimes this reduces congestion and the ability to pass urine spontaneously can be regained. If this does not occur, operation should be carried out in a few days.

Testicular Tumours

Tumours of the testes are uncommon but are usually malignant, sometimes spreading to the lungs at an early stage. A seminoma presents as a painless and often rapid uniform enlargement of the testes while a teratoma causes nodular enlargement. Some teratomas produce gonadotrophic hormones and cause gynaecomastia. Treatment is by orchidectomy and radiotherapy. Teratomas are more radio-resistant and the prognosis is poorer.

Prospects in Nephrology

The last 25 years have seen major advances in understanding the nature of renal disease and in its therapeutic control. Since 1950, renal transplantation and haemodialysis for acute and chronic renal failure have passed through a tentative and experimental phase and become established clinical procedures. Studies of renal biopsies by light, electron and immunofluorescence microscopy have transformed concepts of glomerular disease; knowledge of immunological mechanisms and their associated effects on complement, the mediators of inflammation and coagulation, are beginning to clarify the origin of glomerular damage, and awareness that the kidney acts as an endocrine organ has increased understanding of some forms of hypertension, of vitamin D resistance and renal osteodystrophy and of renal anaemia.

Progress in the foreseeable future is likely to consist of a steady consolidation of these foundations rather than any dramatic discovery that might otherwise transform the picture. Knowledge of renal structure will be further advanced by the use of scanning electron microscopy and the application of immunofluorescent techniques to electron microscopic preparations. Improved methods of detecting and measuring antigen-antibody complexes and the identification of further unknown specific antigens, including viruses, will add to the list of agents known to be responsible for glomerulonephritis. At present immunosuppressive therapy is disappointing in controlling both the naturally occurring immunological renal disorders and in the immunologically based rejection of transplanted kidneys. The non-specific nature of the action of immunosuppressive drugs gives rise to serious problems of toxicity and of opportunist infection. The ultimate goal in renal transplantation is the induction of specific tolerance by which ideally the immune response against the transplantation antigens of a grafted kidney only is suppressed and all other immunological responses remain normal. Experimental work in rats gives rise to optimism that this might be ultimately achieved.

Estimates of plasma 1–OH and 1–25 OH cholecalciferol and of parathyroid hormone and calcitonin will increase the capacity to prevent renal osteodystrophy, but the isolation, precise measurement and therapeutic availability of erythropoetin appear to be more distant.

The prevention of chronic pyelonephritis and renal failure by the eradication of urinary tract infection at an early stage appear to be a goal which recedes with the passage of time. Even if it is accepted that a significant proportion of chronic pyelonephritis arises from recurrent infections in infancy, the cost and difficulties of screening large numbers of children sufficiently often to detect them present formidable obstacles.

Finally, steady miniaturisation of artificial kidneys using improved synthetic membranes and adsorbents with the ultimate aim of producing a portable, round-the-clock working artificial kidney is likely to continue.

J. S. ROBSON

Further reading:

Black, D. A. K. (1973) *Renal Disease*. 4th edition. Oxford: Blackwell.
Macleod, J. (1976) *Clinical Examination*. 4th edition. Edinburgh: Churchill Livingstone.—For further information about examination of the kidneys and the urine.
Passmore, R. & Robson, J. S. (1976) *Companion to Medical Studies*. Vol. 1, p. 35.1. Oxford: Blackwell.
Passmore, R. & Robson, J. S. (1973) *Companion to Medical Studies*. Vol. 2, p. 11.1. Oxford: Blackwell.
Passmore, R. & Robson, J. S. (1974) *Companion to Medical Studies*. Vol. 3, p. 22.1. Oxford: Blackwell.
de Wardener, H. E. (1973) *The Kidney*. 4th edition. Edinburgh: Churchill Livingstone.

11. Endocrine and Metabolic Diseases

THE advances that have been achieved in the technology of hormone assay have resulted in a better understanding of clinical endocrinology in physiological terms. The isolation and synthesis of hormones or biologically active analogues have made many endocrine diseases eminently amenable to treatment. Formerly many hormone assays were confined to research laboratories but with improved techniques and understanding of their clinical application an increasing range of assays is becoming available to the clinician. Among the methods in use are radioimmunoassay, competitive protein binding and fluorimetry. In addition, cytochemical techniques provide a new degree of sensitivity in the measurement of certain pituitary hormones. In order to take full advantage of such improvements in laboratory aspects of endocrinology the clinician, while clearly having to maintain his clinical acumen, must also be familiar with the investigative aspects of the subject. This is discussed in some detail in this chapter.

The application of the science of immunology to endocrinology has been responsible for many of the advances, notably radioimmunoassay of all the hormones produced by the anterior pituitary gland and of many of the hormones produced by its target glands, thyroid, adrenal, testis and ovary. The study of immunology has thrown much light on the possible pathogenesis of many endocrine diseases in terms of autoimmunity, including certain of the thyroid diseases, a form of adrenal insufficiency and of parathyroid insufficiency, certain types of gonadal failure and possibly insulin-dependent diabetes mellitus.

Among the advances in clinical endocrinology has been the recognition of a form of thyrotoxicosis which is due to the excessive secretion of triiodothyronine alone. Understanding of the role of the hypothalamus in disease followed the identification and synthesis of hypothalamic releasing and inhibitory hormones which affect the pituitary gland. Pharmacological control of excessive prolactin secretion and reduction of growth hormone secretion in acromegaly has become possible with the introduction of bromocriptine, a dopamine agonist. It is also now known that certain non-endocrine tumours synthesise and secrete trophic hormones such as ACTH or biologically active analogues.

While the metabolic aspects of the commonest of the endocrine diseases, diabetes mellitus and thyrotoxicosis, can be readily controlled, some of the complications of these conditions remain poorly understood, particularly angiopathy in diabetes mellitus and exophthalmos in thyrotoxicosis.

Endocrinology also permeates many other clinical disciplines, not only because disordered function of the endocrine glands may affect every organ in the body, but because corticosteroids are extensively used for the control of inflammation and adverse immune reactions in a variety of serious disorders. When used in pharmacological doses for these purposes there may be both beneficial and adverse effects because the anti-inflammatory action of the corticosteroids cannot be separated from their hormonal activity.

Among the benefits which will accrue if clinicians make full use of new knowledge in endocrinology is that disease will be more readily detected in its early stages and unnecessary morbidity avoided.

THE HYPOTHALAMUS AND THE PITUITARY GLAND

Anatomy and Physiology. The pituitary gland is enclosed in the sella turcica, bridged over by the diaphragma sellae, with the sphenoidal air sinuses below, and the optic chiasma in the subarachnoid space above. The gland is composed of two lobes, anterior and posterior, and is connected to the hypothalamus by the infundibular stalk carrying the portal vessels from the median eminence of the hypothalamus to the anterior lobe of the pituitary gland and nerve fibres to the posterior lobe.

The anterior lobe consists of three main histological types of cell, chromophobe, eosinophil and basophil. It affects growth, thyroid activity, sexual function, lactation and water, carbohydrate, protein and fat metabolism by regulating the secretions of the other endocrine glands.

The posterior lobe (pars nervosa or neurohypophysis) contains neuroglial fibres which emanate from the supraoptic and paraventricular nuclei of the hypothalamus.

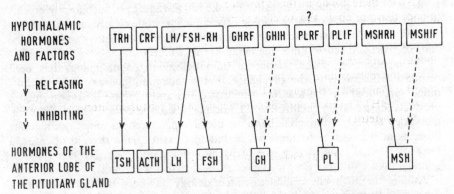

Fig. 11.1 The principal direct relationships between the hypothalamus and the anterior lobe of the pituitary gland. Hypothalamic releasing (R) and inhibiting (I) activities are described as hormones (H) when they have been chemically identified and synthesised, and as factors (F) while their recognition still depends upon biological activity only, as determined in animal studies.

HORMONES OF THE ANTERIOR LOBE. Secretion of each of the seven hormones formed by the anterior lobe of the pituitary gland is influenced by a stimulus provided by the hypothalamus, either in the form of a releasing hormone or factor, or by an inhibitor which suppresses secretion (Fig. 11.1).

The secretion of the hypothalamic factors in turn is dependent upon a wide variety of stimuli of nervous, metabolic, physical or hormonal origin, in particular from the appropriate target organs of the pituitary hormones, the thyroid gland, the adrenal cortex and the gonads. The secretion of corticotrophin, and presumably of the hypothalamic corticotrophin releasing factor (CRF), is partly time-dependent, being most active in the morning, and least in the evening, except when this physiological diurnal (circadian; nyctohemeral) rhythm is overridden by other stimuli, particularly emotional or physical stresses.

The thyrotrophin releasing hormone (TRH) formed in the hypothalamus, like the other hypothalamic releasing or inhibiting factors, passes through the portal system of vessels connecting the hypothalamus to the pituitary gland, where it promotes the secretion of the thyroid stimulating hormone (TSH). The luteinising hormone and follicle stimulating hormone releasing hormone (LH/FSH-RH) acts on the pituitary to release both LH and FSH, and is now known simply as LHRH. In the male LH is known as interstitial cell stimulating hormone (ICSH). Growth hormone (GH) however is controlled by a dual system, namely growth hormone releasing factor (GHRF) and an inhibitory hormone (GHRIH). The latter is known also as somatostatin and has many other functions, including reduction in plasma gastrin, glucagon, insulin and in platelet stickiness. It is probably also produced in sites other than the hypothalamus. Prolactin is under the control of an inhibitory factor (PLIF) and may also be influenced by a releasing factor (PLRF), but this is less certain; likewise the section of the melanocyte stimulating hormones (α and β MSH) may be under dual control. It is noteworthy that the pituitary hormones with target glands (TSH, ACTH, FSH and LH) appear to be controlled by hypothalamic releasing hormones alone. By contrast, the pituitary hormones without target glands (GH, PL and MSH) may have a dual control mechanism from the hypothalamus, namely a releasing factor, opposed by a specific inhibitory factor. The hypothalamic hormones, TRH for example, may not be as specific in their action as their names imply.

To date there are no methods for measuring plasma levels of hypothalamic hormones that are applicable to clinical practice.

HORMONES OF THE POSTERIOR LOBE. The neurohypophysis secretes two hormones, vasopressin and oxytocin. The principal action of vasopressin is to increase the reabsorption of water by the renal tubules, so that the osmolality of the blood is maintained. Because of this action it is also known as the antidiuretic hormone (ADH). Oxytocin induces contraction of the parturient uterus and is widely used in obstetrics for this purpose.

Diagnosis of Disordered Pituitary Function

All the protein and peptide hormones of the pituitary gland can now be measured in body fluids by radioimmunoassay. In addition, three hypothalamic hormones, namely TRH, LH/FSH-RH and GHRIH, have been synthesised and can be used clinically to stimulate or inhibit the release of the appropriate pituitary hormones. Furthermore, the methods of assay for the hormones produced by the target glands of the pituitary are more reliable and more readily available than previously. Thus it is now possible to assess very fully and specifically the functional activity and the secretory capacity of the pituitary gland and its target organs. Several pituitary hormones, namely TSH, ACTH, GH, and gonadotrophins are available in suitable forms for the investigation and treatment of endocrine disorders, and are particularly valuable in distinguishing between primary insufficiency of the adrenal cortex, the thyroid gland and the gonads, and secondary failure due to reduced or absent secretion of one or more pituitary trophic hormones.

The methods used in applying assay procedures to the diagnosis of pituitary disease must always be discussed in advance with the laboratory staff responsible for the hormone assays, so that the overall procedure is standardised. For example, in assessing increased production of growth hormone in acromegaly (p. 511), a standard glucose tolerance test is performed with radioimmunoassay of growth hormone at half-hourly intervals along with measurements of blood glucose. Under physiological conditions growth hormone secretion is promptly suppressed by a rise in the blood glucose level, while there is no significant suppression in patients with pituitary tumours secreting growth hormone.

In assessing impaired secretion of growth hormone, insulin hypoglycaemia may be used (p. 544); this has the added advantage of stimulating the pituitary to secrete ACTH, which may be measured directly or can be monitored by estimating plasma 11-OH corticosteroids and also prolactin. In children more convenient screening tests are the rebound increase of plasma growth hormone at $2\frac{1}{2}$ to 3 hours after oral glucose or the response of GH secretion to exercise, to oral arginine or to beef extracts such as Bovril.

In the case of the thyroid gland, TRH can be given intravenously and the pituitary response assessed by measuring the serum TSH concentration after 20 minutes. LH/FSH-RH can be given intravenously at the same time and the plasma LH and FSH measured also. The precise timing of the samples to be taken, the number of samples, usually several, the separation of plasma or serum from the red cells, and the conditions of storage are critical factors in making a reliable assessment of the function of the pituitary gland.

Tumours of the Pituitary Gland

Pathology. About 80 per cent of pituitary tumours are non-secretory, chromophobe adenomas, and are associated with hypopituitarism. Eosinophil adenomas, associated with excess secretion of growth hormone, present clinically as acromegaly (p. 511), or rarely, in the adolescent, as giantism (p. 511). Basophil adenomas secrete corticotrophin and MSH, and may present as Cushing's disease (p. 536). These basophil tumours are usually too small to produce local pressure effects, except in cases of long standing, or after bilateral adrenalectomy undertaken several years earlier (Nelson's syndrome, p. 538). Mixed or transitional cell tumours resembling chromophobe adenomas may be capable of secreting GH and ACTH.

Craniopharyngiomas are tumours or cysts developing in cell rests of Rathke's pouch, and may be located within the sella turcica, or commonly in the suprasellar space, where they frequently calcify. In either situation their clinical presentation is likely to be due to pressure on one or both lobes of the pituitary gland, on the stalk, on the hypothalamus, or on the visual pathways. Primary carcinoma of the pituitary gland is particularly rare, but a metastatic tumour from a primary in the breast, lung, kidney or elsewhere may occur in the hypothalamus. Other tumours, for example pinealoma, ependymoma or meningioma, may occasionally be associated with some disturbance of pituitary function. Granulomatous lesions of the pituitary or hypothalamus such as sarcoidosis or syphilis may mimic pituitary tumours.

Clinical Features. The clinical features of pituitary tumours vary, depending on the type of lesion in the pituitary gland, whether both lobes are involved or only one and whether there is any hypothalamic involvement. Destruction of the gland in part or in its entirety will be followed by hypopituitarism (p. 513). Enlarging tumours of the gland may present with signs attributable to increased output of hormones (p. 511) or, more commonly, to failure of secretion. Some tumours secreting hormones compress the remaining pituitary tissue, so that there may be failure of some functions of the gland in the presence of an excess of others. Failure of function may be progressive and sequential; secretion of gonadotrophins usually declines first, followed by GH, ACTH and finally TSH.

Clinical features also depend upon the site and size of the tumour. Headache is the most constant but least specific symptom. Involvement of an optic nerve, the optic chiasma, or an optic tract may lead to impaired visual fields. The patient occasionally notices a visual field defect, but, more commonly, examination of the visual fields by confrontation or by perimetry will be required to identify the likely point of interference within the visual pathway (Fig. 14.4, p. 671), bitemporal visual field defect being the characteristic finding. Optic atrophy may be apparent on ophthalmoscopy. Diplopia and strabismus may follow pressure on the third, fourth or sixth cranial nerves. Some tumours expand sufficiently to interfere with vasopressin secretion and so cause diabetes insipidus. Tumours which expand upwards to impinge on the hypothalamus may be associated with disturbances of sleep and of appetite. Obesity arising in this way is part of the rare Frohlich's syndrome.

Enlargement of the sella turcica and erosion of the clinoid processes may be detected on radiological examination, or suprasellar calcification may be seen in a craniopharyngioma. A 'double floor' may be apparent on tomography of the sella if the tumour is expanding downwards. Air encephalography may be particularly helpful in delineating tumours which have spread beyond the sella turcica and computerised axial tomography (p. 692) is also available.

Treatment of Pituitary Tumours. Two main considerations determine whether surgical treatment is required. If there is evidence of pressure on the visual pathways, for example a visual field defect, surgical treatment is appropriate. Secondly, if hyperfunction, as judged by suitable assays, is sufficiently severe to affect the patient's welfare and prognosis, then treatment aimed at destroying the tumour or its capacity to secrete should be considered. Hypophysectomy may be performed from below by a trans-sphenoidal approach or, if there is suprasellar extension, through a transfrontal craniotomy.

Adequate suppression of secretory capacity may be achieved without open operation using either radiotherapy applied externally, or internally by placing a source of radiation, for example ^{90}Yttrium in pellet form, within the pituitary gland. This latter technique is now viewed with less favour than previously on account of the complications it may cause. Replacement therapy (p. 514) is likely to be required during and after treatment in this way.

Syndromes due to Anterior Pituitary Hypersecretion

Giantism and Acromegaly. Hypersecretion of growth hormone by eosinophil cells may develop very rarely before the epiphyses have united, to produce giantism. Much more frequently it occurs in adult life, after union of the epiphyses, and the condition is described as acromegaly (large extremities). If hypersecretion begins in adolescence and persists into adult life, giantism and acromegaly may be associated.

Acromegaly is characterised by an increase in the size of the bones and soft tissues of the hands, feet, supraorbital ridges, sinuses and the lower jaw. The skin becomes thick and coarse; the subcutaneous tissues increase in depth, while enlargement of the tongue, lips, nose and ears may be conspicuous. The viscera, for example the heart, thyroid and liver, enlarge. Sweating is common. Carbohydrate tolerance is reduced in about 30 per cent of cases to the extent that diabetes mellitus develops. As the disease progresses, the patient often develops a kyphosis and muscular weakness. Hypertension is a common complication. The disease tends to progress slowly over several years, but patients are frequently seen with certain features of acromegaly in whom the progress of the condition has apparently been arrested, or a phase of hyperpituitarism may pass into hypo-pituitarism. Sensitive radioimmunological methods of assaying growth hormone in blood (p. 509) now make it possible to assess with precision the activity of these tumours as well as the results of treatment. Bromocriptine (p. 512) is being used to reduce GH levels until hypophysectomy or irradiation has achieved this result, and may also be given in combination with these procedures.

Cushing's Disease. Hypersecretion by basophil cells or sometimes by chromophobe cells leads to Cushing's disease (p. 539).

Syndromes due to Anterior Pituitary Hyposecretion

Pituitary Dwarfism and Infantilism

In children hyposecretion causes dwarfism and pituitary infantilism. The term 'dwarfism' means that growth is retarded; 'infantilism' implies that sexual develop-ment is subnormal for the individual's age, though it is also used to indicate reten-tion of infantile as opposed to adult proportions of the head, limbs and trunk.

While pituitary tumours are an uncommon cause of dwarfism, delayed growth and development is characteristic of most pituitary tumours in children. In addi-tion to requiring full assessment by assays of pituitary hormones, for example TSH, GH, ACTH and gonadotrophins, or if the techniques are not available, by the assay of target organ hormones, it is essential that accurate records be kept of the child's height, weight and bone age. Radiographs of the left hand and wrist taken at intervals of 1 year can be compared with the standard atlas prepared by Greulich and Pyle, so that the progress of bone development is assessed. Adequate supplies of growth hormone are available in Britain from the Medical Research Council for the treatment of children in whom growth hormone secre-tion has been shown to be absent following appropriate stimulation. Intramuscular injections are given twice weekly for several years according to the response. Height and weight should be recorded on a Tanner and Whitehouse chart which can be purchased from Creaseys Ltd., Bull Plain, Hertford, England.

DIFFERENTIAL DIAGNOSIS OF DWARFISM

Growth may be delayed or impaired for many reasons. Tallness and shortness of stature have genetic components. One form of dwarfism is Turner's syndrome (p. 12). Premature birth may be associated with persistent stunting of growth; this also occurs in anoxic forms of congenital heart disease, in chronic liver disease, in many chronic infections, and in persistent undernutrition for any reason. Pituitary dwarfism must also be distinguished from:

(a) *Infantilism due to coeliac disease* (p. 394). This disability is as-sociated with steatorrhoea and defective absorption, especially of fat, minerals and vitamins. Dwarfs of this type are usually larger than the pituitary type; they may be further distinguished by a prominent abdomen due to intestinal distension, and by a history of the passage of pale, bulky, offensive stools. Fibrocystic disease of the pancreas (p. 388) may simulate malabsorption due to gluten induced enteropathy.

(b) *Rickets* (p. 119). A defective diet or malabsorption may be responsible; kyphosis, pigeon-chest deformity and bowing of the legs are common sequelae.

(c) *Achondroplasia.* This hereditary disorder of endochondral ossification is characterised by failure of the long bones of the arms and legs to grow properly, while the trunk and head develop normally. Dwarfs of this type are sexually and intellectually normal and frequently used to appear in circuses.

(*d*) *Renal dwarfism*. Renal failure arising in early childhood may be caused by neuromuscular incoordination at the outlet of the bladder, which produces back-pressure and hydronephrosis, or it may be due to congenital cystic disease, congenital hypoplasia of the kidneys or, most commonly, chronic nephritis. Many of the characteristic features of renal failure may be found, for example hypertension, a raised blood urea and changes in the fundus of the eye. In some cases hereditary defects of renal tubular function may be responsible (p. 470).

(*e*) *Cretinism and juvenile hypothyroidism*. If these conditions are not recognised and treated promptly, stunting of growth will occur (p. 526).

Hypopituitarism

Aetiology. At one time destruction of the anterior lobe of the hypophysis was commonly due to infarction and this was often a sequel to post-partum haemorrhage (*Sheehan's syndrome*). Improvements in obstetrical care have greatly reduced the incidence of this accident and the disorder is now most commonly due to a chromophobe adenoma. Other causes include nonsecretory tumours, a fractured skull, infection, granulomas (syphilis, sarcoidosis) and the presence of simple cysts. In some, an 'empty sella' may be due to a previous granuloma. Idiopathic cases are probably the result of failure of the hypothalamus to secrete the appropriate releasing hormones or may be due to an autoimmune hypophysitis. Surgical treatment of tumours of the gland is often followed by a degree of hypopituitarism calling for replacement therapy, and complete hypophysectomy is sometimes performed in the treatment of malignant disease, for example carcinoma of the breast.

Clinical Features. In Sheehan's syndrome, a history is usually obtained that several years before the onset of the presenting illness, the patient had a difficult confinement with haemorrhage and a need for blood transfusion. Lactation failed or was never established, amenorrhoea persisted indefinitely and other changes attributable to the absence of the trophic hormones gradually made their appearance. Some of the features of hypothyroidism (p. 526) may be present, but myxoedema is seldom prominent. Absent or scanty axillary and pubic hair are characteristic findings. Symptoms of adrenal insufficiency (p. 541) may be noted, but the changes in serum electrolytes found in severe adrenal insufficiency do not occur in hypopituitarism and the blood pressure is usually not so low. This is probably because aldosterone continues to be secreted by the glomerulosa layer of the adrenal cortex, since this function is largely independent of corticotrophin. Cortisol production, however, falls to a minimum because the essential corticotrophic stimulus from the pituitary gland is absent or inadequate. In contrast to the pigmentation of the skin in Addison's disease (p. 541) a striking degree of pallor is often one of the signs suggesting hypopituitarism. Although a mild degree of normochromic anaemia is usually present, this is insufficient to explain the pallor of the skin. Capillary vasoconstriction and the absence of melanin together account for this conspicuous sign.

COMA IN HYPOPITUITARISM. Patients with hypopituitarism are peculiarly liable to go into coma if inadequately treated. While the onset of coma may occur for no apparent reason, it usually follows some mild infection or injury, in the same way that an Addisonian crisis may follow some relatively trivial stress (p. 541). The coma may be due to one or more of the effects of hypopituitarism. These include increased sensitivity to insulin and spontaneous or reactive hypoglycaemia. Water intoxication is another important factor, due to a disturbance of water metabolism in patients with adrenal insufficiency (p. 543). Hypothyroidism (p. 525) is also an important component in the causation of coma; hypothermia with a rectal temperature as low as 32°C or less may develop. Failure of ventilation with anoxia and respiratory acidosis should also be considered in treating what is frequently a lethal complication of hypopituitarism.

Diagnosis. Hypopituitarism is sometimes confused with anorexia nervosa (p. 777). The distinguishing features lie in the history and the presence of pubic, axillary and lanugo hair in anorexia nervosa. In addition, anorexia nervosa is characterised by an absent appetite and gross wasting, whereas in hypopituitarism neither is striking unless some other cause is present. Assays of pituitary trophic hormones or of the products of the target glands will help to distinguish these two disorders and others which might be confused with hypopituitarism. In anorexia nervosa the endocrine failure is restricted to the gonadotrophins and ovarian hormones. The excellent response of patients with hypopituitarism to treatment with corticosteroids will also help to distinguish between the two conditions.

Treatment. The aim should be to provide adequate substitution therapy, according to the deficiencies demonstrated, so that the patient can lead a normal life. Cortisol should be given by mouth in doses of 20 mg in the morning and 10 mg in the evening or according to the cortisol blood profile levels. Thyroid hormone will usually be required and should be given orally as thyroxine 0·1–0·2 mg daily. It is dangerous to give thyroid hormone to these patients until they have been protected by cortisol against the possibility of an Addisonian type of crisis. Excessive doses of corticosteroids may lead to hypertension. Oedema occasionally is troublesome, and may be corrected by substituting a corticosteroid without electrolyte effects, for example prednisolone, in a dose of 5 mg in the morning and 2·5 mg in the evening. In some circumstances it may be helpful to add an oestrogen, such as ethinyl oestradiol 50 µg daily, and for adolescent or adult men an androgen may be required (p. 522). Fertility may be restored in young patients with appropriate gonadotrophin therapy.

Diabetes Insipidus

This uncommon disease is characterised by the persistent excretion of excessive quantities of urine of low specific gravity, and by constant thirst.

Aetiology. The disease develops after damage to the neurohypophyseal mechanism for the production of vasopressin. It may occur with tumours of the pituitary, with a craniopharyngioma, or after operations in this region, and as a sequel to encephalitis, basal meningitis, syphilis, and fractures at the base of the skull. Metastatic disease involving the neurohypophysis may occasionally be responsible. In panhypopituitarism, the symptoms of diabetes insipidus may not be apparent until corticosteroid therapy has been provided. An adequate level of corticosteroids is required for the condition to be expressed. A rare genetic form exists due to unresponsiveness of the renal tubules to vasopressin (nephrogenic diabetes insipidus), but in some cases no cause can be identified.

Symptoms. The most marked symptoms are polyuria and polydipsia. The patient may pass 5–20 or more litres of urine in 24 hours. The urine is clear and of low specific gravity and osmolality, i.e. less than the plasma osmolality, ≈ 300 m Osm/kg, even when fluid intake has been withheld.

Diagnosis. A positive diagnosis of diabetes insipidus depends on demonstrating that a rise of plasma osmolality induced either by withholding fluids or infusing hypertonic saline is not accompanied by a rise in the osmolality or specific gravity of the urine, but that when vasopressin is given, such a rise does occur. This final test is necessary in order to show that the kidney is capable of concentrating the urine which it cannot do in familial nephrogenic diabetes insipidus.

It may be difficult to differentiate the polyuria of diabetes insipidus from that found in *hysterical polydipsia*. In such cases, if fluids are withheld for 24 hours, the urine is found to concentrate to a normal specific gravity. Accurate weighing of the patient will show whether she has been drinking surreptitiously meanwhile and should be undertaken at regular intervals during such a test in order to avoid the risks inherent in excessive dehydration. If the patient's weight falls by more than 3 per cent the test should be terminated.

Other causes of polyuria are discussed on page 473.

Treatment. The minimum amount of vasopressin required to keep the patient in water balance must be determined by controlling the fluid output and then reducing the dose of hormone without permitting polyuria or excessive thirst to recur.

A synthetic analogue of vasopressin, desmopressin (DDAVP), has now been introduced; this can be given intranasally, and the action is sufficiently prolonged for administration once or twice daily to elicit a response as effectively as vasopressin when given by injection. It is now the preferred form of treatment.

Chlorothiazide, clofibrate and carbamazepine have been used with some success to suppress the thirst and hence to improve the polydipsia and polyuria of diabetes insipidus. Their modes of action are not understood.

THE THYROID GLAND

Anatomy and Physiology. The thyroid gland consists of an isthmus and two lateral lobes, and lies in front of and on either side of the upper part of the trachea and the laminae of the thyroid cartilage. Posteriorly it is closely related to the recurrent laryngeal nerves which lie between the trachea and the oesophagus; the gland is separated from these nerves by its fibrous sheath. The thyroid gland is provided with a rich blood supply through the superior and inferior thyroid arteries. The parathyroid glands are usually to be found lying on the posterior aspect of the thyroid in its substance or in the sheath of the gland and in relation to the upper cornu of the thymus.

Thyroxine (T_4) and triiodothyronine (T_3), the hormones secreted by the gland, are bipeptides containing respectively 4 and 3 atoms of iodine in each molecule. Both are normally stored in the colloid vesicles as thyroglobulin. Because it is less strongly bound to serum proteins, T_3 acts more rapidly than T_4. It is also effective in smaller doses than T_4. Thus the effects of T_3 may be apparent in a number of hours while an equivalent dose of T_4 may take several days to be effective. Both hormones act directly on most of the tissues of the body to increase cellular metabolism.

Thyroid function is controlled by thyroid stimulating hormone (TSH) secreted by the anterior pituitary gland which in turn is controlled by thyrotrophin releasing hormone (TRH) secreted by the hypothalamus. TRH is a tripeptide which has been synthesised and is available for clinical use. There is also a negative feed-back mechanism whereby the thyroid hormones act principally on the anterior pituitary to suppress the secretion of TSH. TSH stimulates the release of thyroid hormones from the colloid into the circulation and also stimulates the synthesis of these hormones.

Calcitonin, secreted by the parafollicular C(calcitonin)-cells of the thyroid gland, is discussed on page 530.

Hyperthyroidism

The clinical condition consequent upon overproduction of T_3 or of both T_3 and T_4 is referred to as hyperthyroidism or thyrotoxicosis. In a small minority of patients the excess production of thyroid hormone is confined to T_3, but it is likely that a greater number of cases have an initial phase of excess T_3 production followed by an overproduction of both T_3 and T_4, and it is usually at the latter stage that the diagnosis is made.

Aetiology and Pathology. The serum TSH levels in patients with thyrotoxicosis are either reduced or undetectable using current radioimmunoassay techniques. Cases of thyrotoxicosis due to excess TSH production by pituitary tumours are exceptionally rare.

In many patients with hyperthyroidism the IgG autoantibody, human specific thyroid stimulator (p. 44), can be detected in the serum by radioimmuno-TSH-receptor assay and it is possible that this antibody may be the cause of hyperthyroidism in most instances. Other evidence of autoimmune activity directed against the thyroid gland in hyperthyroidism is the presence of lymphocytic infiltration in the gland which may be negligible, focal or extensive.

In a small percentage of patients, thyrotoxicosis is due to the presence of a hyperactive solitary nodule with suppression of the remainder of the gland through the normally functioning feed-back mechanism. In the majority of patients with hyperthyroidism the thyroid gland is either diffusely hyperactive (*Graves' disease*) or the gland consists of multiple active nodules interspersed with inactive areas. This latter state is probably the outcome of alternate stimulation and degeneration or results from the development of thyrotoxicosis upon a multinodular goitre. Toxic nodular goitres tend to occur in older patients and diffuse goitres in younger subjects. Histologically, in Graves' disease, the increased activity of the gland is manifest by reduction in the size of the thyroid vesicles which are relatively empty of colloid; the epithelium is tall and columnar in contrast to the flat cuboidal epithelium of the normal gland. The vasculature is markedly increased.

Clinical Features. Thyrotoxicosis is found much more frequently in women than in men (8:1), usually in the third to sixth decades, but it may occur at any age.

There may or may not be clinically detectable enlargement of the thyroid gland (goitre). The increased blood supply to the thyroid may be manifest by a bruit, which should not be confused with a murmur transmitted from the aortic area into the neck or arising in the carotid artery, or in the jugular veins as a venous hum. If the increased blood supply is sufficiently pronounced there may be a thrill and the thyrotoxic gland may even be pulsatile.

Most of the clinical features of thyrotoxicosis may be explained in terms of excess production of T_3 or of $T_3 + T_4$. The increased metabolism accounts for the loss of weight in spite of the increased appetite that is so often a striking feature in the clinical history. Occasionally, however, the patient overcompensates in terms of food intake and may gain weight.

Thyroid hormones potentiate the action of the sympathetic nervous system and of adrenaline and noradrenaline. The increased cardiac output required to meet the metabolic demands, together with the effect of T_3 and T_4 on the sympathetic nervous system, tends to produce a tachycardia or, particularly in elderly patients, arrhythmias such as atrial fibrillation or ectopic beats. The patient may complain of palpitations with or without the symptoms of cardiac failure. Sinus tachycardia, persisting during sleep, is one of the earliest and most constant signs. The pulse pressure is increased and capillary pulsation may be detectable. In the presence of coincident systolic hypertension a collapsing pulse may be noted. In the older patient cardiovascular manifestations may be the only clinical evidence of hyperthyroidism and it should be remembered that thyrotoxicosis is one of the three commonest causes of atrial fibrillation.

There are other consequences of the effect of excess thyroid hormones on the sympathetic nervous system. Patients commonly complain of increased frequency of bowel motions, usually with formed stools and there may be an element of malabsorption. A lag curve in a glucose tolerance test may be demonstrable partly as a result of intestinal hurry. A fine tremor of the fingers and retraction of the upper eyelids may occur, while the hands are often hot and sweaty because of the increased metabolic rate and the need to lose excess heat. Intolerance of warm temperatures is characteristic. Thyrotoxic patients, although they are hyperdynamic, have a low efficiency in terms of what they achieve. They suffer from an inability to relax both mentally and physically; anxiety is a frequent feature.

Less common clinical features that cannot be so readily explained in terms of disturbed physiology include exophthalmos (p. 524), pretibial myxoedema and finger clubbing, reduced fertility and menstrual irregularities. In addition there may be weakness and wasting of the proximal muscles in the arms and legs (thyrotoxic myopathy), which recovers when normal thyroid function is restored.

Thyrotoxic crises are now uncommon, as cases of hyperthyroidism are recognised and treated earlier and more effectively. They may be seen shortly after thyroidectomy in patients who have not been adequately prepared for operation or in patients who have been operated on for some other disability without hyperthyroidism having been recognised. Alternatively, some severe infection, for example pneumonia, may so aggravate a thyrotoxic state that a crisis is precipitated. The patient in crisis suffers from severe mental and physical exhaustion with delirium, delusions or mania, dehydration, ketosis, tachycardia, cardiac failure and inability to control body temperature, with hyperthermia.

Progress. In some cases thyrotoxicosis undergoes spontaneous remission within a period of months or years, while in other cases it follows a course of intermittent and unpredictable remission and relapse. Before modern therapy became available it was commonly fatal, but spontaneous and permanent remissions also occurred.

Hyperthyroidism in the newborn and in children. Thyrotoxicosis may occur rarely in the newborn when it is thought to be due to the transplacental transmission of thyroid stimulating antibody. This form of hyperthyroidism is self-limiting. If thyrotoxicosis occurs before puberty there is an increase in the growth rate so that affected children are unusually tall for their age.

Diagnosis. The investigative facilities are now so precise that it should not be necessary to treat patients in the absence of a high degree of certainty concerning the diagnosis. Anxiety neurosis presents the commonest problem in differential diagnosis.

Protein-bound iodine (PBI). This used to be the most widely used test of thyroid function. It is however affected by many drugs including those which contain iodine so that high values are found in euthyroid patients prescribed expectorants containing iodine or tablets or capsules in which tetraiodofluorescein is the colouring agent. In addition certain radiographic studies, e.g. cholecystography, pyelography and myelography, utilise contrast media which contain iodine. Another disadvantage is that increased concentration of thyroid hormone-binding proteins, of which thyroxine-binding globulin is the most important, occurs in pregnancy and in patients on oestrogen therapy including most varieties of oral contraceptives. This results in an elevation of the PBI without a change in concentration of free thyroid hormones which are metabolically active. The PBI is therefore of limited value in the diagnosis of thyrotoxicosis.

Total serum thyroxine. The total serum thyroxine measured by competitive protein binding or radioimmunoassay is not influenced by exogenous iodine, but is altered in a similar manner to the PBI by factors which affect the concentration of thyroid hormone-binding proteins. It is a more useful test than the PBI.

T_3 resin uptake and free thyroxine index. The T_3 resin uptake test is an indirect measure of circulating thyroid hormone levels. It measures the degree of saturation of the binding sites on the thyroid hormone-binding proteins. High values are found in thyrotoxicosis but low values are recorded in euthyroid patients either pregnant or on oestrogen medication. The role of such a test is in the calculation of the *free thyroxine index* derived from the product of either the PBI or the total serum thyroxine and the T_3 resin uptake. In euthyroid patients with abnormalities of the thyroid hormone-binding proteins and in whom the PBI or the total serum thyroxine is elevated, the T_3 resin uptake will be depressed and the free thyroxine index is more likely to lie in the normal range. The need for a free thyroxine index has been largely superseded by the simplicity of the effective thyroxine ratio.

The effective thyroxine ratio (ETR). This integrates into a single procedure the measurement of total serum thyroxine and the binding capacity of thyroid hormone-binding proteins. At the present time the ETR provides the most reliable single test of thyroid function available which can be readily carried out on a sample of serum and requires only simple radio-isotope equipment. It is not affected by oral contraceptives, pregnancy, excess iodine, or as far as is known at present, by any other drug.

The measurement of the in vivo uptake of radioactive iodine or technetium by the thyroid gland. The overactive gland synthesising excess T_4 has an increased uptake of iodine which can be simply shown by measuring the proportion of an oral tracer dose of ^{131}I (half-life 8 days) or ^{132}I (half-life 2·3 hours) taken up by the thyroid gland in a given time (e.g. 4 hours) by using an appropriate 'counter' over the neck. Alternatively, an isotope of technetium (Tc99m: half-life 6 hours) may be used intravenously with the thyroid uptake measured at 20 minutes, giving an even smaller dose of radiation to the gland which can be regarded as insignificant. The major fallacies in such studies are caused by iodine deficiency (which can give an increased uptake measurement without the presence of thyrotoxicosis) and iodine excess (which can give a low uptake measurement in spite of the presence of thyrotoxicosis).

Either ^{131}I or Tc99m may be used to obtain a scan of the gland, indicating the amount and the distribution of functioning tissue. Scans are also useful in thyrotoxic patients for detecting a solitary 'hot' nodule or a retrosternal extension of the gland.

T_3 *suppression test.* In patients giving equivocal results it can be determined whether or not the gland is under the control of the anterior pituitary by repeating the thyroid gland iodine uptake measurement after the patient has taken 120 μg T_3/day in divided doses for 7 days. Failure of suppression is characteristic of thyrotoxicosis. The test should be avoided if there is any risk of cardiac failure being induced and in pregnancy. In terms of radiation the risk in pregnancy of using ^{132}I or Tc 99m is negligible.

Serum TSH levels in response to TRH stimulation. In thyrotoxicosis the secretion of TSH by the anterior pituitary is suppressed so that serum levels of TSH are either reduced or absent. Moreover, the TSH response of the pituitary 20 minutes after the injection of TRH is absent (Fig. 11.2). This is one of the most useful tests of thyroid function and has largely replaced the T_3 suppression test.

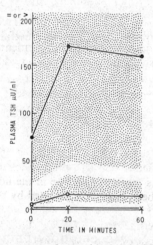

Fig. 11.2 The mean plasma TSH response and range (shaded area) following 200 μg TRH i.v. in 49 patients with primary hypothyroidism (●——●), 74 normal subjects (O——O) and 63 patients with thyrotoxicosis (×——×). (From Irvine *et al.* (1974), by permission of the Editors of *Companion to Medical Studies.* Vol. 3. Oxford: Blackwell.)

T_3 *Thyrotoxicosis.* When thyrotoxicosis is due to excessive production of T_3 alone, the PBI, ETR, total serum T_4, and thyroid uptake of radio-isotopes may give normal results. The measurement of the plasma concentration of total serum T_3 together with the TRH test are therefore the two most useful diagnostic aids in relation to thyrotoxicosis.

Treatment. Three effective methods of treating thyrotoxicosis are available:

1. Antithyroid drugs, such as carbimazole, initially supplemented as necessary by beta-adrenergic blocking agents, for example propranolol.

2. Surgery, after a euthyroid state has been achieved with antithyroid drugs or under propranolol cover.

3. Radioactive iodine, with or without the use of propranolol or antithyroid drugs.

ANTITHYROID DRUGS. The site of action of the different antithyroid drugs is indicated in Figure 11.3. Most commonly used are those that act by blocking the organic binding of iodine to tyrosine, carbimazole in Europe and methimazole in North America. Other drugs which act in this way are propyl and methyl thiouracil, which may occasionally be useful in the event of hypersensitivity to the drug of first choice.

Carbimazole is given initially in full suppressive doses of 15–20 mg at 8-hourly intervals for 3 to 4 weeks according to the severity of the condition and the size of the goitre. Thereafter the dose can generally be reduced, and, as the patient's clinical state responds, the aim should be to give as little of the antithyroid drug as necessary to achieve a euthyroid state, which may vary between 5–30 mg per day. Overtreatment with antithyroid drugs will result in TSH production by the anterior pituitary with a risk of increase in size of the thyroid. In patients in whom the natural history of the underlying process is one of exacerbation and remission, stable control may only by achieved with drugs when an excess dose of carbimazole (but not greater than 45–60 mg/day) is combined with continuous thyroxine administration in a dose of 0·15 mg/day.

Carbimazole or methimazole may be selected as the definitive therapy or, as discussed below, may be used to prepare the patient for surgery. If antithyroid drugs are being used as definitive therapy they should be continued for a period of

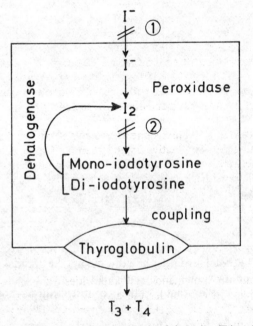

Fig. 11.3 Diagrammatic representation of the synthesis of thyroxine (T_4) and of triiodothyronine (T_3), illustrating the main sites of block induced by (1) potassium perchlorate and (2) by carbimazole, methimazole and the thiouracil group of drugs. The possible sites for enzyme deficiency in thyroid dyshormonogenesis (p. 528) are also shown.

at least 1 year and restricted to children or young adults (especially girls) who do not have marked enlargement of the gland. It is considered that by selecting cases in this way rather less than 50 per cent of thyrotoxic patients will go into lasting remission and will not require further therapy. Attempts to estimate the probability of achieving lasting remission by doing T_3 suppression tests while the patient continues on antithyroid drugs have given uncertain results.

Carbimazole, methimazole and the thiouracil group of drugs as well as potassium perchlorate, are liable to produce toxic effects, of which the commonest is skin rash and the most serious are the blood dyscrasias, agranulocytosis being most frequent. Routine white cell counts are of little value in its early detection as it occurs with dramatic suddenness, usually, but not necessarily, in the first few weeks of treatment. Patients taking these drugs must be told to report a sore throat and to stop the drug immediately until it is clear whether agranulocytosis has occurred or not. By stopping the drug promptly and by using antibiotics prophylactically serious consequences will be avoided and the leucocyte count will return to normal within 1 to 2 weeks. Potassium perchlorate induces blood dyscrasias more commonly than other antithyroid drugs, including red cell aplasia which is usually lethal. For this reason, potassium perchlorate should be used only as a temporary expedient if hypersensitivity to other drugs has occurred and if radioactive iodine therapy or surgery under propranolol cover are not acceptable alternatives. It should never be used in a dose greater than 1 g/day.

There is no place for the use of potassium iodide as an antithyroid drug except in the final preparation for surgery of a patient already made euthyroid with other antithyroid drugs, or in the management of a thyrotoxic crisis.

BETA-ADRENERGIC BLOCKING DRUGS. These are very useful as they can produce much symptomatic improvement by countering the increased action of the sympathetic nervous system. Thus palpitations, finger tremor, anxiety, lid retraction and increased bowel activity may be alleviated with propranolol, 40 mg 8 hourly, or greater doses if required. It can therefore be useful during the interval of several weeks which is required for antithyroid drugs or radioactive iodine to be fully effective. Contraindications to propranolol include bronchial asthma; these and the side effects of the drug are discussed on page 224.

SURGICAL TREATMENT. This is the treatment of choice if the patient is considered too young for radioactive iodine therapy (i.e. during the reproductive years), if the antithyroid drug therapy has failed to produce a lasting remission, or there have been sensitivity reactions to antithyroid drugs. Thus a thyrotoxic patient younger than 40 years with a large goitre should be treated by surgery rather than by a prolonged course of antithyroid drugs in the somewhat vain hope that the condition will remit in the interval and not recur when antithyroid drugs are withdrawn.

For a girl a thin thyroidectomy scar may be more acceptable cosmetically than a goitre. Men are thought to relapse more frequently after prolonged antithyroid drug therapy than are women and some authorities would advocate surgery as the treatment of choice in men under the age of 40, irrespective of the size of the goitre. The patient may state a preference once the possibilities have been explained.

The patient may be prepared for subtotal thyroidectomy either by propranolol alone or by carbimazole until euthyroid, followed by 14 days of potassium iodide in a dose of 60 mg twice daily. Potassium iodide should not be used as a means of achieving a euthyroid state except in thyrotoxic crisis. It reduces the vascularity of the gland making it appreciably firmer and operation easier for the surgeon. The effects of potassium iodide are transitory so that it is important to reserve the drug for use in the circumstances described.

If propranolol is used alone as preoperative preparation it is essential that tachycardia is controlled (by increasing the dose above 40 mg 4 times per day if necessary), that the dose on the morning of operation is not omitted and that propranolol is continued for 7 days after operation. The advantages of propranolol preparation are greater flexibility in the timing of surgery, less blood loss and quicker permanent control of the thyrotoxicosis.

Some 80 per cent of thyrotoxic patients treated by subtotal thyroidectomy should have no complications at least within 3 to 5 years thereafter. In some 15 per cent there will be either recurrence of the thyrotoxicosis or post-operative hypothyroidism requiring continuous thyroxine replacement therapy. The relative proportion of each depends on the amount of thyroid tissue left at operation. Thyrotoxic patients with high titres of thyroid complement fixing antibody in the serum before operation tend to have an appreciable degree of lymphocytic infiltration in the gland and tend to develop hypothyroidism post-operatively. While the majority of patients who become hypothyroid after surgery do so within the first 6 months or a year, there is a low but steady further incidence with each year after surgery making annual review of the patient desirable.

Damage to the recurrent laryngeal nerves occurs in a small percentage of patients and will produce temporary hoarseness with subsequent appreciable recovery as the other vocal cord compensates. Any malfunction of a vocal cord found during routine examination prior to operation would be a contraindication to thyroid surgery, as the risk of malfunction of both cords would not be justifiable.

The parathyroid glands may be rendered temporarily ischaemic by interruption of their blood supply or they may be inadvertently removed, producing transient or permanent hypoparathyroidism respectively. The late onset of hypoparathyroidism is a complication of partial thyroidectomy which should be looked for in the follow up of surgical patients, as cataract and mental disturbance may develop insidiously in the presence of persistent mild hypocalcaemia. On account of the high incidence of recurrent laryngeal nerve damage and of hypoparathyroidism following second operations, thyrotoxic patients who relapse after surgery should be treated with radioactive iodine.

RADIOACTIVE IODINE. Radioactive iodine is the treatment of choice for thyrotoxic patients over the age of 40 years and also for younger patients who for some other reason appear to have a short life expectancy. It has no established complications other than the incidence of hypothyroidism in the years following therapy (Fig. 11.4). The incidence of thyroid cancer or leukaemia following ^{131}I therapy has been shown not to be increased. Although an effect on the spontaneous mutation of the gametes in the ovary or testis has not been proved it is difficult to disprove and therefore the administration of radioactive iodine to persons of reproductive age who have not been sterilised should be discouraged unless there is no suitable alternative.

The assessment of the appropriate therapeutic dose of [131]I (half-life 8 days) presents some difficulties for the following reasons. The amount of functional thyroid tissue is not easy to assess with accuracy, the amount of radiation to the gland following a given dose can only be assessed by time-consuming dynamic studies, and even if a predicted amount of radiation per gram of thyroid tissue could be given, there remains the variation in radiosensitivity among thyroid glands of different patients. For these reasons the empirical assessment of dosage using clinical criteria gives results as good as those dependent on sophisticated physical methods, provided that an avid uptake of the isotope by the gland has been established.

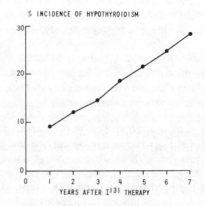

Fig. 11.4   The cumulative incidence of hypothyroidism after ^{131}I therapy for thyrotoxicosis.

Using a dose as small as 3 mCi ^{131}I with a diffuse uptake of the isotope as shown on a scan in a small thyroid or as high as 15–30 mCi for a large multinodular gland, the patient's thyrotoxicosis will be controlled in some 70 per cent of cases following a single oral administration. It may take 2 months or longer for the dose to be effective. If the thyrotoxicosis is severe, more rapid relief may be obtained by the addition of propranolol. Carbimazole should preferably not be given prior to the administration of ^{131}I as there is some evidence that it reduces the effective radiation dose by virtue of the enzyme block which it induces. When given after ^{131}I carbimazole masks the effectiveness of the ^{131}I and makes the assessment of the need for a further dose of ^{131}I more difficult. The use of carbimazole in conjunction with ^{131}I should therefore be reserved for patients with cardiac failure or asthma, in whom propranolol is contraindicated. After 2 months a further dose of ^{131}I should be given in the 30 per cent who have not responded adequately to the first dose, using a 50 to 100 per cent higher dose in order to avoid the undesirable occurrence in a few patients of the need for repeated doses of the isotope. Large doses of ^{131}I should be given to thyrotoxic patients in cardiac failure or atrial fibrillation to ensure prompt control of thyroid function with a single dose, even though this will produce a high incidence of hypothyroidism. The patient's thyroid state can then be stabilised by replacement doses of thyroxine.

The continuing incidence of new cases of hypothyroidism for many years following radioactive iodine therapy makes annual review essential until such time as the patient has become hypothyroid and is on a suitable life-long replacement dose of thyroxine. Some patients may maintain a euthyroid state after ^{131}I therapy for thyrotoxicosis by secreting adequate amounts of T_3 although their T_4 secretion may be subnormal.

THYROTOXIC CRISIS. The treatment of thyrotoxic crisis consists of intravenous fluid and glucose replacement; parental hydrocortisone on account of possible adrenocortical exhaustion; sedation and suppression of hyperpyrexia with chlorpromazine; digoxin for cardiac failure; propranolol if cardiac failure is not pronounced; intravenous potassium iodide 60 mg twice daily as the most rapidly acting antithyroid drug; and control of body temperature by tepid sponging. Antithyroid drugs such as carbimazole are administered as soon as the patient is capable of taking medicaments orally. Precipitating causes must be dealt with, e.g. acute infection. Thyrotoxic crisis carries a high mortality; prevention and early recognition are essential if deaths are to be avoided.

HYPERTHYROIDISM IN CHILDREN. Children, including young teenagers, have a high relapse rate following subtotal thyroidectomy, and radioactive iodine therapy is contraindicated. They should therefore be treated with carbimazole or methimazole for as many years as is necessary.

HYPERTHYROIDISM IN PREGNANCY. This may be treated with antithyroid drugs or by surgery provided the operation can be carried out in the middle trimester after appropriate preparation with antithyroid drugs and preoperative potassium iodide. If antithyroid drugs are used throughout it is important to give the smallest dose that will control the thyrotoxicosis and to use an indicator of thyroid function such as the ETR that is not altered by pregnancy. Towards term, the dose of antithyroid drugs should be further reduced in the hope of withdrawing them for the last 3 weeks of pregnancy. In this way the uncommon complication of the fetus being born with a goitre may be avoided. If antithyroid drugs are to be continued after pregnancy the baby must not be breast fed. Radioactive iodine treatment should never be used for therapy in pregnancy.

Exophthalmos

The pathogenesis of exophthalmos is unknown. An exophthalmos producing substance is thought to emanate from the pituitary but its existence and nature are uncertain. Defined as the protrusion of one or both eyeballs, exophthalmos may be detected clinically in the majority of cases by observing the white sclera both above and below the iris. In other cases periorbital oedema which is frequently also present may obscure this sign. The degree of protrusion and especially any progression or regression of exophthalmos should be recorded by use of an exophthalmometer.

Exposure of the cornea as a consequence of the eyelids failing to close properly will result in keratitis producing a feeling of grit in the eye and excessive watering. The conjunctiva may become injected and oedematous (chemosis).

Weakness of the extraocular muscles may give rise to an ophthalmoplegia with double vision, which is often first detected when the patient is asked to look upwards and outwards.

In a small minority of cases the exophthalmos takes a relentlessly progressive course so that the increased intra-orbital pressure causes a severe aching in the eyes and reduction in visual acuity. This constitutes an emergency situation in which relief of pressure within the orbit must be achieved if permanent deterioration in vision is to be avoided. Decompression of the orbital cavity by surgical means may be required, but large doses of oral corticosteroids may be used as an interim measure if surgery is not immediately possible. Fortunately, in most cases of exophthalmos the condition is less severe and after a phase of progression enters into a prolonged phase of gradual improvement although the eyes seldom return to the normal state. A lateral tarsorrhaphy, stitching together the outer margins of the eyelids, may be all that is required, thereby improving their appearance and preventing exposure keratitis. In even milder cases, chloromycetin eye drops or ointment applied at night and the wearing of slightly tinted spectacles with protective side pieces to the frames will prevent the irritation of glare, dust and wind.

In relation to the treatment of thyrotoxicosis it is particularly important that hypothyroidism is avoided as this does seem to aggravate any associated exophthalmos.

In some patients exophthalmos may precede the development of frank thyrotoxicosis and present a problem in differential diagnosis, especially if the exophthalmos is unilateral when orbital or retro-orbital tumours and infections may require consideration. Support for an endocrine aetiology may be obtained by demonstrating an abnormal TRH or T_3 suppression test or thyroid or gastric antibodies in the serum, or by eliciting a family history of thyroid disease.

Hypothyroidism

Hypothyroidism may be due to causes within the thyroid gland itself (primary) or, less commonly, to failure of TSH production following pituitary or hypothalamic disease (secondary). Hypothyroidism, especially when it is due to primary thyroid failure, is often, but not necessarily, associated with myxoedema, a thickening of the skin by deposition of a mucinous material giving the patient a characteristic appearance.

Incidence and Aetiology. Hypothyroidism commonly occurs as a sequel to ^{131}I therapy for thyrotoxicosis. Primary spontaneous hypothyroidism is much less common than thyrotoxicosis and principally affects middle-aged females, although it can occur in either sex at any age.

Spontaneous primary hypothyroidism may be associated with a goitre or with thyroid atrophy. The commonest cause of spontaneous goitrous hypothyroidism in an adult female is Hashimoto's thyroiditis. It is believed that thyrotoxicosis, Hashimoto's thyroiditis and primary atrophic hypothyroidism belong to a continuous spectrum of disease. This is characterised by: (1) a common familial trait towards organ-specific autoimmune disease in general; (2) the frequent occurrence in the serum of thyroid and gastric parietal cell antibodies, and (3) evidence of delayed cellular hypersensitivity to thyroid components as well as to such non-tissue specific antigens as mitochondria.

Less commonly hypothyroidism may be associated with other types of goitre; for example an enzyme deficiency in the synthesis of thyroid hormones (dyshormonogenesis, Fig. 11.3). This form is more likely to present in children or in young adults. When hypothyroidism is secondary to pituitary insufficiency, myxoedema is unusual.

Clinical Features of Primary Hypothyroidism. *Adults.* In contrast to thyrotoxicosis the symptoms are the result of decreased metabolism, with slowing of mental and physical activity. The onset is gradual and often mistaken for ageing alone. Often the patient is the last to complain and has to be persuaded by relatives or friends to seek medical help. Frequently, the general practitioner will recognise the condition on meeting the patient for some other reason, especially after a long interval. On questioning, the patient may admit to sensitivity to cold, dryness of the skin, coarse and dry hair, constipation, gain in weight, tiredness, vague generalised pains, deafness, forgetfulness and disordered menstrual function. The patient may also complain of tingling in the fingers since the deposition of mucopolysaccharide may produce a carpal tunnel syndrome (p. 748), although it is to be remembered that patients with primary spontaneous hypothyroidism are also predisposed to Addisonian pernicious anaemia which may give rise to similar symptoms from polyneuropathy. Anaemia may also be a direct result of thyroxine deficiency (p. 605).

In an advanced case the face appears swollen with puffy eyelids, thick lips and an enlarged tongue. The skin is pale as a consequence of thickening with myxoedema. Sweating is conspicuously absent and the skin is dry and readily flakes on rubbing. The hair tends to be more sparse than normal and lustreless. Speech is slow, monotonous and husky or, in advanced instances, deep and croaky. In a milder case her friends may be repeatedly asking if she has a 'cold'.

Characteristically the pulse rate is slow, but if the condition has progressed to cardiac failure, tachycardia may be found. Commonly there is evidence of coronary artery insufficiency with angina pectoris or ECG evidence of myocardial ischaemia. On radiological examination the heart is frequently seen to be enlarged; in some cases there may be a pericardial effusion which is usually reversible with treatment. The blood pressure in uncomplicated hypothyroidism is usually normal. However, since degenerative vascular disease is common in hypothyroidism, the patient may have systolic hypertension. Marked slowing of the recovery phase of the ankle jerk due to delayed relaxation of the calf muscles is a useful clinical sign. Patients with severe hypothyroidism may show frank psychosis with hallucinations and delusions ('myxoedema madness') or pass into a state of coma. In a severe case, failure to control body temperature is one of the most lethal complications; mortality rises markedly as the body temperature (measured by a low reading rectal thermometer) falls below 32°C.

While it is easy to detect the advanced case, a high index of suspicion is required to avoid missing the early case and so prevent unnecessary morbidity.

Children. In children hypothyroidism presents as a deterioration in performance at school, lack of interest in games and an arrest or slowing of growth. These features will precede the development of clinically obvious myxoedema. As in adults there may or may not be a goitre.

Infants. Failure of thyroid development is responsible for the condition of *cretinism.* It is important to diagnose the state and initiate thyroxine replacement therapy as early as possible. The development of the brain is dependent on the thyroid hormones so that delay in starting treatment will inevitably lead to permanent mental impairment which will be the more severe the longer the delay. The diagnostic features are failure to achieve the normal milestones of development, constipation, poor feeding and a characteristic cry. Only in advanced cases will the child develop the obvious features of cretinism, which include a pot belly with umbilical hernia, coarse facial features with a broad flat nose, thick lips and a large tongue protruding from the mouth.

The defects leading to failure of thyroid development are genetic and are inherited as Mendelian recessives: in the heterozygous state the child may be goitrous only, but in the homozygous state both goitrous and a cretin.

Investigation of Hypothyroidism. *Serum PBI and Total Serum T_4.* The measurement of the PBI has been largely replaced by serum T_4, which ideally should be combined with a plasma TSH measurement. If abnormalities of thyroxine binding proteins are suspected, a form of free thyroxine index should be used.

Plasma TSH and TRH. All patients with primary hypothyroidism have an elevated plasma TSH level but not all patients with an elevated plasma TSH necessarily have a significant degree of hypothyroidism. While a normal or low TSH level may be associated with secondary hypothyroidism due to pituitary or hypothalamic disease, a normal serum TSH level would exclude primary hypothyroidism. No purpose is achieved by doing TRH tests in primary hypothyroidism but a TRH test may be helpful in deciding whether secondary hypothyroidism is due to pituitary or hypothalamic disease.

Radioactive Iodine Studies. A single measurement of uptake by the gland is of very little value in the diagnosis of hypothyroidism, but the response in the uptake to adequate stimulation by parenteral TSH (10 i.u. bovine TSH on each of 3 consecutive days) is a good index of the capacity of the gland to function. Patients with primary hypothyroidism fail to respond. Radioimmunoassay of plasma TSH has largely superseded the need for TSH stimulation tests, but the latter is still useful in determining whether thyroxine medication empirically started in the past for suspected primary hypothyroidism is actually required.

Radiological Studies. X-ray of the epiphyses in children or of ossification centres in the wrist or heel, in infants, will indicate whether the bone age is delayed relative to the chronological age. Hypothyroidism in young people is invariably associated with impaired bone development; fragmentation of the epiphysis at the head of the femur is a striking radiological sign.

Treatment. In uncomplicated adult cases treatment with thyroxine should start with 0·05 mg/day increasing to 0·1 mg/day after 3 weeks provided cardiac failure or angina have not arisen. After a further 3–6 weeks the dose may be increased to 0·15–0·2 mg/day. This is now considered to be the normal full replacement dose, but a few patients may require up to 0·3 mg thyroxine/day. Patients must understand that their well-being depends on continued treatment and that they must not stop thyroxine when they feel better. There is no advantage in divided doses or taking tablets that consist of a mixture of T_3 and T_4.

In a patient known to have ischaemic heart disease it will usually be desirable to keep the dose of thyroxine between 0·05 and 0·1 mg/day and to use a beta-adrenergic blocking agent such as propranolol. In patients with secondary hypothyroidism it is essential to treat any adrenocortical insufficiency before starting thyroxine.

Myxoedema Coma with Hypothermia. Small doses (10 μg) of triiodothyronine (liothyronine) may be given intravenously 8 hourly together with hydrocortisone and glucose and very slow restoration of the body temperature to a level of 32°C; conservation rather than active heating should be the principle of restoration above 32°C.

Goitre

This term is applied to any enlargement of the thyroid gland and on clinical examination its size, shape, consistency, symmetry, irregularity of surface, mobility or fixation relative to adjacent tissues, and the presence or absence of a bruit should be established. The level of thyroid activity should be determined in the manner already described. Goitre associated with thyrotoxicosis will not be discussed further. The common diagnosis of simple goitre is arrived at by the exclusion of other causes, such as Hashimoto's thyroiditis, subacute thyroiditis, dyshormonogenesis, or carcinoma of the thyroid gland.

Hashimoto's Thyroiditis

Hashimoto's thyroiditis is characteristically a firm diffuse enlargement of the thyroid gland with or without hypothyroidism. It may give rise to an aching discomfort in the neck and to mild, but never severe, obstructive symptoms. It occurs most commonly in middle-aged women. Almost all cases have antibodies in the serum to thyroglobulin or to the microsomal fraction of thyroid cytoplasm (p. 41), frequently in high titre. The ESR is often elevated. Histologically the gland consists of rather small thyroid vesicles with columnar epithelium showing eosinophilic granularity, infiltration by lymphocytes and plasma cells, sometimes with germinal centre formation and an increase in the fibrous tissue stroma. Some of these histological features may be more marked in some glands than in others or in different parts of the same gland.

In most instances there will be a satisfactory regression in the size of the goitre in response to thyroxine 0·2 mg/day, which can be hastened by giving 20 mg prednisolone 8-hourly for 10 days only. Patients with Hashimoto's thyroiditis should remain on life-long thyroxine therapy irrespective of whether or not they were initially hypothyroid. In cases of diagnostic doubt a needle biopsy of the gland under local anaesthesia may be helpful. Partial thyroidectomy in such patients rapidly produces hypothyroidism if it did not already exist and is usually unnecessary.

Subacute (de Quervain's) Thyroiditis

This is a painful condition generally associated with some thyroid enlargement. It is thought to be due to a virus infection of the thyroid (e.g. Coxsackie B) and viral antibody studies are sometimes helpful diagnostically. Thyroid function is suppressed as indicated by a very low uptake of radioactive iodine or technetium by the gland and histologically the characteristic feature is the presence of giant cells. The ESR may be markedly elevated and thyroid antibody tests are generally negative. The condition tends to regress spontaneously but may be persistent.

Thyroxine 0·2–0·3 mg/day should be given to suppress TSH secretion and, in some cases, it may be necessary to give a course of oral corticosteroids or parenteral ACTH. Surgery is seldom required even in the protracted case.

Dyshormonogenesis

The patient who has a partial enzyme defect related to one of the steps in the synthesis of thyroid hormones (Fig. 11.3) is likely to develop a goitre in response to continued TSH secretion in the attempt to overcome the enzyme block; the increased vascularity may produce a bruit. While all these defects are rare, the commonest and the easiest to detect is a genetically determined defect in the binding of iodine to tyrosine which, when associated with nerve deafness, is known as *Pendred's syndrome*. Such an enzyme defect may be detected by a test with potassium perchlorate following an oral tracer dose of ^{131}I or ^{132}I; potassium perchlorate discharges out of the gland any iodine which is not organically bound.

Tumours of the Thyroid Gland

Carcinoma. This is uncommon, forming about 1 per cent of all cases of cancer in Britain. It may be anaplastic or differentiated, and follicular or papillary or a mixture of the two. Advanced cancers are obvious by their hardness, irregularity, adhesion to surrounding tissues and associated lymphadenopathy. Early carcinoma of the thyroid gland presents as a single nodule which almost invariably has poorer function than the surrounding normal thyroid tissue. If the nodule is sufficiently large it will be detectable as a 'cold' area on thyroid scanning. It is not possible to distinguish clinically between a single nodule that is malignant and one that is benign; all single (solitary) nodules should therefore be removed for histological examination. The proportion of solitary nodules in which malignancy is demonstrated is variously estimated at 1–10 per cent according to the histological criteria adopted.

Well differentiated thyroid tumours should be treated by total thyroidectomy followed by life-long oral thyroxine 0·2–0·3 mg/day according to the patient's age. Occasionally metastases from a well differentiated tumour may take up sufficient radioactive iodine, after all normally functioning thyroid tissue has been ablated by surgery and ^{131}I, to allow effective treatment with a further large dose of ^{131}I. Anaplastic tumours may show a good initial response to external radiotherapy, but invariably recur.

Medullary carcinoma of the thyroid arises from the parafollicular C-cells; although rare, it is of particular interest as it is associated with high levels of plasma calcitonin (p. 530), prostaglandins or 5-hydroxytryptamine, causing symptoms such as flushing, borborygmi and diarrhoea. Patients with this form of thyroid cancer may have neuromas on the tongue, lips or eyelids, Marfanoid skeletal proportions (p. 241), and, occasionally, phaeochromocytomas.

Benign Tumours. Solitary lesions in the thyroid may consist of adenomas or cysts; calcification in these cysts is common. Haemorrhage occasionally occurs into adenomas and on these grounds as well as others their removal is justified.

Simple Goitre

Simple goitre may occur sporadically, but in certain parts of the world it is found more frequently and is then referred to as endemic goitre.

Aetiology. This is not fully understood, but it is generally believed to be closely related to iodine deficiency, either (*a*) because of iodine deficiency in the diet or (*b*) because of factors in the diet or water such as excess calcium that may interfere with iodine absorption or (*c*) because of goitrogens in the diet that prevent concentration of iodine by the thyroid. Fish is a main source of iodine and thus simple goitre due to iodine deficiency is endemic in the mountains of New Guinea, in the Alps and in the Himalayas.

Apart from the antithyroid drugs, a number of other drugs are known to interfere with the synthesis of thyroid hormones; thus prolonged treatment with sulphonamides or PAS may produce a goitre. Iodides taken persistently in large doses in the form of cough mixtures or 'asthma cures' may likewise cause a goitre. In each of these examples the secretion or release of thyroid hormones is suppressed and presumably the goitre results from continuing increased secretion of TSH. An intermittent shortage in supply of iodine to the gland over prolonged periods is thought to result in the multinodular character of long-standing goitres, or alternatively they may result from a patchy defect of colloid storage throughout the gland.

Clinical Features. A small soft diffuse simple goitre may occur at puberty or during pregnancy and may regress spontaneously thereafter, but in other cases it persists. If already present, it may enlarge further at these times. A simple goitre of long standing may achieve considerable size, become grossly nodular and give rise to obstructive symptoms, particularly if there is a retrosternal extension. Compression or deviation of the trachea may be noted clinically or radiologically and obstruction in the thoracic inlet may lead to venous engorgement of the head and neck. Bruits and thrills do not occur in simple goitres.

Treatment and Prevention. The treatment of sporadic simple diffuse goitre at puberty should be with thyroxine for 1 to 2 years and not potassium iodide. An adequate dietary intake of iodine should be ensured. Multinodular simple goitres are unlikely to respond to thyroxine and may require partial thyroidectomy for cosmetic reasons, or if obstructive symptoms are present or likely to occur. Postoperative life-long treatment with thyroxine may prevent a recurrence, although hypothyroidism after partial thyroidectomy for simple goitre is uncommon.

An adequate intake of iodine, particularly in the early years of life, is the only really satisfactory way of preventing sporadic simple goitre (p. 529). The incidence of endemic goitre can be greatly reduced by correcting iodine deficiency, for example, by an injection of iodised oil in the case of the New Guinea population or by legislation that ensures that table salt contains traces of iodine.

Calcitonin

The parafollicular cells (C-cells) of the thyroid gland secrete a polypeptide hormone, calcitonin, apparently unrelated to the other functions of this gland. When administered by injection, the hormone lowers the serum calcium concentration. Its main effect on bone is to inhibit resorption, so that in these two important respects it could be regarded as a physiological antagonist of parathyroid hormone. It is secreted in very large quantities by medullary carcinomas of the thyroid gland, without however producing significant hypocalcaemia, and after complete removal of the source of the hormone, namely the thyroid gland, hypercalcaemia is not a feature.

Therapeutically, the hormone has been used to reduce hypercalcaemia, but corticosteroids may be more effective in doing so in sarcoidosis, vitamin D intoxication and in metastatic malignant disease in bone. In Paget's disease of bone calcitonin has proved valuable in providing relief from pain in the minority of cases where pain is a dominant feature. Intramuscular injections of $50\,\mu g$ of salmon calcitonin thrice weekly for 6 weeks may be followed by relief of pain for many months, after which the course of treatment can be repeated if necessary.

THE PARATHYROID GLANDS

Anatomy and Physiology. These glands, usually four in number, each measure about 5 mm in diameter. Their relation to the thyroid gland is described on page 515. The parathyroid glands control the concentration of calcium and inorganic phosphorus in the blood plasma, both by enhancing the removal of mineral from the skeleton, and by promoting the excretion of phosphorus by the kidney.

Calcium occurs in plasma in two forms, 'diffusible' and 'non-diffusible'. The diffusible calcium consists of ionised calcium, and a small amount of non-ionised calcium salts of organic acids. From the point of view of neuromuscular function and the occurrence of tetany, as well as the secretion of parathyroid hormone, it is the ionised plasma calcium concentration which is important. The non-diffusible fraction is that portion which is bound to the plasma albumin; if this is very low, the total plasma calcium might be 2·0 mmol/l (8 mg/100 ml) or less and yet the ionised calcium could be normal. When the plasma protein concentration is high, the plasma calcium might be 3·0 mmol/l or even more, but this would not necessarily constitute evidence of hyperparathyroidism.

In addition to parathyroid hormone, calcitonin and vitamin D metabolites also affect the metabolism of calcium and phosphorus, so that these factors must be considered in disorders of these elements. Assays of parathyroid hormone are becoming more widely available; controversy continues regarding the reliability and relevance of calcitonin assays, except in the diagnosis of medullary carcinoma of the thyroid gland.

Hyperparathyroidism

This term is used to describe the consequences of excessive secretion of parathyroid hormone, due either to primary disease in the parathyroid glands, or secondary usually to renal disease. *Primary hyperparathyroidism* is uncommon and is usually due to a single parathyroid adenoma. Very occasionally it may be caused by simple hyperplasia or multiple adenomas: a functioning parathyroid carcinoma can also occur.

Secondary hyperparathyroidism with hypertrophy of the glands is found in chronic renal failure. The chemical pathology involved is complex because of the primary metabolic changes of renal origin, modified in turn by the increased parathyroid activity. It also occurs as a sequel to osteomalacia.

The term *tertiary hyperparathyroidism* is used to describe cases of the secondary variety of long standing in which a continuing stimulus is responsible for parathyroid hyperplasia being replaced by autonomous function in one or more parathyroid adenomas.

When hyperparathyroidism involves the bones to such an extent that cyst formation occurs, the condition is sometimes known as *osteitis fibrosa* or *von Recklinghausen's disease of bone*. Radiological evidence of involvement of the bones is seen only in a minority of cases.

Clinical Features. Some of the clinical findings in primary hyperparathyroidism are more readily understood if the action of the parathyroid hormone is recalled. In the first place the excretion of phosphorus in the urine is increased, and often that of calcium also; both phosphorus and calcium are mobilised from bone. The most significant chemical finding is an increase in the plasma concentration of calcium, occasionally to as much as 5·0 mmol/l. The plasma concentration of inorganic phosphorus may fall below 0·7 mmol/l. The plasma alkaline phosphatase, an index of osteoblastic activity, may be raised above the normal range of concentration of 22–87 i.u./l depending on the degree of involvement of bone.

Renal calculi frequently form in association with the increased excretion of calcium in the urine. While many patients with hyperparathyroidism develop symptoms due to renal calculi, relatively few presenting with renal calculi owe their disorder to increased parathyroid activity. In other cases of hyperparathyroidism, deposits of calcium form in and around the renal tubular epithelium (nephrocalcinosis), so that in severe cases scattered radiological opacities may be visible within the renal outline. Tubular reabsorption of water may be impaired as a consequence of deposition of calcium in the renal medulla, secondary infection, or the direct effects of parathyroid hormone. Polyuria and thirst may be sufficiently severe to suggest diabetes insipidus. In cases of long standing, and in those with associated pyelonephritis, the renal disease may progress to uraemia in spite of the relief of the hyperparathyroidism.

Patients with hypercalcaemia frequently complain of weakness, loss of appetite, drowsiness, nausea and vomiting. Some of these patients also have a peptic ulcer, and the symptoms from this source may obscure those of hyperparathyroidism. Acute pancreatitis is sometimes a presenting feature in hyperparathyroidism. In patients with bone disease, backache is a common complaint.

A parathyroid adenoma may occasionally coexist with secreting adenomas or hyperplasia in the pituitary, pancreas or adrenals. This association is known as *multiple endocrine adenomatosis* and may account for unusual symptoms.

Physical examination is usually unhelpful. Occasionally a parathyroid adenoma is sufficiently large and suitably placed to be palpable or even visible as a swelling in the region of the thyroid gland. Measurement of calcium excretion in the urine is a useful investigation in this disease. Provided the intake does not exceed 12·5 mmol daily, amounts of calcium in the urine persistently in excess of 7·5 mmol daily should be regarded as abnormal.

In some, only radiological evidence of demineralisation may be found, or subperiosteal erosions may be noted in the phalanges. The 'pepperpot' appearance seen in lateral radiographs of the skull is virtually diagnostic of hyperparathyroidism. Occasionally characteristic cysts composed of fibrous tissue, osteoblasts and osteoclasts may be seen, but preoccupation with the search for bone cysts may mean that the other less arresting changes are overlooked.

Diagnosis. Much the most important single diagnostic feature of hyperparathyroidism is a raised plasma calcium concentration, and it may be necessary to carry out a series of estimations at intervals in doubtful cases, since the hypercalcaemia may be episodic. It is important that a tourniquet should not be used in obtaining blood samples, since this may be responsible for raising the plasma calcium concentration appreciably. Plasma calcium levels should be adjusted if necessary for variations in plasma albumin concentration. Taking 46 g/l as normal, 0·022 mmol/l of calcium should be subtracted from the total plasma calcium value for each 1·0 g/l by which the plasma albumin concentration exceeds 46 g/l and vice versa for lower readings.

Other causes of hypercalcaemia include metastatic malignant disease in bone, particularly from carcinoma of the breast, sarcoidosis, myelomatosis and overdosage with vitamin D. The plasma inorganic phosphate concentration is usually lowered in hyperparathyroidism, but more diagnostic support may be obtained by measuring the renal threshold for inorganic phosphate.

Radioimmunoassays of parathyroid hormone are proving valuable in diagnosis and in localising small tumours by identifying high concentrations of hormone in specific veins in the root of the neck or mediastinum. However, a negative assay does not exclude the presence of a tumour.

Treatment. Removal of a solitary adenoma is usually sufficient to produce clinical cure, provided advanced renal disease is not already present. Patients with multiple adenomas or generalised hyperplasia of all the parathyroids may be difficult to manage, especially when the glands lie in unusual situations such as the superior mediastinum, but surgical treatment offers the only prospect of cure.

Hypoparathyroidism

This unusual condition may arise from a variety of causes, but with each the common clinical feature is tetany. Biochemically, a depressed concentration of calcium and a raised concentration of phosphate in plasma are characteristic.

POSTOPERATIVE HYPOPARATHYROIDISM. A transitory form of the disorder is common after a partial thyroidectomy, presumably due to interference with the blood supply of the parathyroid glands. After a complete thyroidectomy, undertaken for example for a thyroid carcinoma, permanent hypoparathyroidism may occur. Following removal of a parathyroid adenoma or carcinoma, hypoparathyroidism is likely to occur, depending partly on the extent to which biopsies of parathyroid tissue have been undertaken. The degree and duration of postoperative hypocalcaemia is largely determined by the severity of the accompanying bone disease.

INFANTILE HYPOPARATHYROIDISM. This may be transient and associated with maternal hyperparathyroidism or calcium deficiency, or it may be associated with thymic aplasia (Di George syndrome, p. 35).

IDIOPATHIC HYPOPARATHYROIDISM. This form may develop at any age, and is sometimes associated with autoimmune adrenocortical disease, thyroid disease or premature ovarian failure; antibodies to parathyroid, adrenal and thyroid tissue have been demonstrated in some of these patients, so that autoimmunity is a probable cause. In these patients, in addition to tetany there may be other characteristic features including psychoses, cataracts, papilloedema, calcification in the basal ganglia, and moniliasis, particularly of the finger nails. Familial cases have been described.

PSEUDOHYPOPARATHYROIDISM. This is the term applied to a congenital variety, which may be familial. It presents with the biochemical features of hypoparathyroidism, and in addition aberrant calcification or even ossification, cataracts, mental retardation and skeletal abnormalities, for example short metacarpals. These patients are resistant to the action of administered parathyroid hormone; their own parathyroid glands appear to be normal histologically, plasma parathyroid hormone levels are raised, and high concentrations of calcitonin have been found in their circulation and in their thyroid glands.

Treatment. Commercial preparations of parathyroid hormone available for the treatment of parathyroid insufficiency are unsatisfactory because they have to be given by frequent injections, and soon become ineffective because of antibody formation. In the acute phase, calcium is given intravenously as for tetany; substitution therapy for persistent hypoparathyroidism is provided by calciferol, or an analogue of vitamin D, dihydrotachysterol (p. 535).

Tetany

Aetiology. There is an increased excitability of peripheral nerves due either to a low plasma calcium concentration or to alkalosis in which the proportion of the plasma calcium in the ionised form is decreased, although the total calcium concentration remains unaltered. Magnesium depletion should also be considered as a possible contributing factor, particularly in the malabsorption syndrome.

CAUSES OF DEPLETION OF PLASMA CALCIUM. (1) *Inadequate intake or absorption of calcium*. This occurs in rickets, osteomalacia and the malabsorption syndrome. (2) *Hypoparathyroidism*. (3) *Chronic renal failure* where, although the plasma calcium is often low, coincident acidosis usually prevents tetany.

CAUSES OF ALKALOSIS. (1) *Repeated vomiting* of acid gastric juice, as in gastric outlet obstruction from peptic ulceration. (2) *Excessive quantities of absorbable alkalis* given by mouth especially when associated with repeated vomiting. (3) *Hyperventilation*, most commonly due to hysteria, lowers the arterial Pco_2. (4) *Primary aldosteronism* (p. 539).

Clinical Features. In *children* a characteristic triad of carpopedal spasm, laryngismus stridulus and convulsions may occur, though one or more of these may be found independently of the others. The hands in carpal spasm adopt a characteristic position. The metacarpophalangeal joints are flexed and the interphalangeal joints of the fingers and thumb are extended (*main d'accoucheur*). Pedal spasm is much less frequent. Laryngismus stridulus is caused by spasm of the glottis.

In *adults* convulsions and laryngismus stridulus are rarely encountered. Carpopedal spasm is the usual finding, the patient complaining of painful cramps in the limbs and tingling in the hands and feet.

Latent tetany may be present when signs of overt tetany (e.g. spontaneous carpopedal spasm) are lacking. It is recognised by eliciting the following signs:

1. *Trousseau's Sign*. Inflation of the sphygmomanometer cuff on the upper arm to more than the systolic blood pressure is followed by characteristic spasm in the forearm muscles within 4 minutes.

2. *Chvostek's Sign*. A tap over the facial nerve in the parotid gland stimulates the hyperexcitable nerve, and the facial muscles contract. However, a response may frequently be elicited in normal persons.

Treatment
Control of Tetany. Injection of 20 ml of a 10 per cent solution of calcium gluconate slowly into a vein will raise the plasma calcium concentration immediately. An intramuscular injection of 10 ml may also be given to obtain a more prolonged effect. In severe cases of alkalotic tetany intravenous calcium gluconate often relieves the spasm, while more radical treatment of the alkalosis, which will vary with the cause, is being applied. If tetany is not relieved by giving calcium the administration of magnesium may be required.

Correction of Alkalosis. 1. In persistent vomiting, intravenous isotonic saline is the most effective treatment.

2. When alkalis have been given to excess their withdrawal may suffice to stop the tetany, but if not, ammonium chloride 2 g should be given 4-hourly until relief has been obtained.

3. The inhalation of 5 per cent carbon dioxide in oxygen may be prescribed for the correction of the alkalosis of hyperventilation, or more simply, the patient should be made to rebreathe her own expired air from a suitable bag. If the patient

is then asked to overbreathe until tingling is again felt in the fingers (usually within 5 minutes), she is so impressed by the demonstration of the origin of her symptoms that this sequence of events does not recur. The hysterical patient should also be treated by appropriate psychotherapy (p. 778).

Treatment of the underlying condition. When tetany follows removal of a parathyroid gland and if there is any residual parathyroid tissue, this usually undergoes compensatory hypertrophy. In the interval intravenous calcium gluconate may be required to control the tetany. If all the parathyroid tissue has been removed, prolonged replacement therapy with calciferol is commonly used to maintain a normal plasma calcium concentration. One tablet (1·25 mg) daily is usually adequate, but less, or more, may be required. The maintenance dose is determined by careful monitoring of the plasma calcium at intervals, as persistent hypercalcaemia which might follow prolonged high doses of vitamin D would lead to widespread metastatic calcification and rapidly progressive renal failure.

Dihydrotachysterol, an analogue of vitamin D, is also a useful substitute in parathyroid insufficiency, but it is more expensive than calciferol.

In chronic renal failure (p. 486) temporary benefit is usually the most that can be expected unless haemodialysis or transplantation is being employed; symptoms should be treated with parenteral calcium as they arise.

Treatment may also be required for rickets (p. 120), osteomalacia (p. 123) or malabsorption (p. 394).

THE ADRENAL GLANDS

Anatomy and Physiology. The adrenal glands lie in relation to the upper poles of the kidneys. Each consists of an inner medulla which secretes adrenaline and noradrenaline and an outer cortex formed of three layers. These, from without inwards, are the zona glomerulosa, fasciculata and reticularis. Although over 40 steroid compounds have been extracted from the adrenal cortex, the principal hormones secreted are cortisol, corticosterone, aldosterone, androstenedione, androsterone and dehydroepiandrosterone. These hormones are grouped according to their main metabolic activity, i.e. glucocorticoids, mineralocorticoids or androgens.

Adrenocorticotrophic hormone (ACTH) is the only substance so far recognised that will alter the rate of biosynthesis and secretion of the glucocorticoid cortisol from the zona fasciculata and reticularis. ACTH also increases the secretion of the adrenal androgens such as androstenedione. Aldosterone (mineralocorticoid) secretion by the zona glomerulosa is primarily controlled by the renin-angiotensin mechanism (p. 472) and is not markedly affected by physiological alterations in ACTH levels.

Three major mechanisms appear to control ACTH release and thus cortisol secretion, namely, negative feedback, diurnal (nyctohemeral) rhythm and stress.

The negative feedback mechanism is thought to operate via the hypothalamus rather than directly on the pituitary but there is still uncertainty about this. The corticotrophin releasing factor (CRF) from the hypothalamus has not yet been isolated in man and cannot be measured in serum. Reduction in the level of plasma cortisol leads to an increased secretion of ACTH from the basophil cells of the anterior pituitary, probably effected by increased release of CRF from the hypothalamus. Conversely, a rise in plasma cortisol produces a rapid suppression of the secretion of ACTH. Cortisol secretion is thus presumably determined at the hypothalamic level, controlled by an inherent diurnal rhythmicity of CRF secretion and consequently of ACTH release. The normal range of plasma cortisol levels in an unstressed subject would be 220–720 nmol/l (8–26 μg/100 ml) at 0800 to 1000 h and less than 275 nmol/l (10 μg/100 ml) at 2200 to 2400 h.

Stress can override the negative feedback mechanism and the diurnal rhythm. Trauma, pain, apprehension, nausea, fever and hypoglycaemia have all been shown to be effective forms of stress in this regard.

It is from an understanding of the normal physiological mechanisms involved in adrenocortical hormone secretion that procedures have been developed to test various components of the hypothalamo-pituitary-adrenal axis and so determine the site of the lesion in cases of adrenocortical over- or underactivity.

The glucocorticoids have effects which are antagonistic to insulin, tending to raise the blood sugar by converting amino acids derived from protein breakdown into glucose (gluconeogenesis). Glucocorticoids such as cortisol have other important actions including the suppression of inflammatory reactions which may occur in response to injury, infection or immunological mechanisms. Glucocorticoids are also lipogenic and have some mineralocorticoid effects especially when used in pharmacological doses.

Aldosterone is the naturally occurring mineralocorticoid. It produces retention of sodium and increased excretion of potassium and if given in pharmacological doses over a prolonged period also causes hypertension. Weight for weight aldosterone has far greater mineralocorticoid activity than the glucocorticoids.

In addition to androgens, the adrenal cortex also synthesises oestrogen and progesterone in small quantities in both sexes. The nitrogen-retaining (anabolic) activity of the androgenic hormones is antagonistic to the catabolic effect of the glucocorticoids.

Hyperfunction of the Adrenal Gland

Cushing's Syndrome. This can be defined as the symptoms and signs associated with prolonged exposure to inappropriately elevated plasma corticosteroid levels. The patients may be divided into two main groups depending on whether or not the condition derives from exposure to excessive ACTH.

ACTH dependent causes of Cushing's syndrome:

1. Iatrogenic—administration of excessive quantities of ACTH or its synthetic analogues (p. 548).
2. Pituitary-dependent bilateral adrenocortical hyperplasia, conventionally called *Cushing's disease*.
3. The ectopic ACTH syndrome—secretion of ACTH by malignant or benign tumours of non-endocrine origin.

Non-ACTH dependent causes of Cushing's syndrome:

1. Iatrogenic—administration of supraphysiological doses of corticosteroids.
2. Adenomas or carcinomas of the adrenal cortex.

Cushing's syndrome associated with pituitary-dependent adrenocortical hyperplasia and adrenal tumours is four times more common in women than in men. This contrasts with the male predominance found in Cushing's syndrome secondary to the ectopic production of ACTH by non-endocrine tumours, commonly carcinoma of the bronchus. In the non-ectopic group the peak age incidence is between 35 and 50 years whereas it is later in the others.

Clinical Features of Cushing's Disease. These can be interpreted largely in terms of the action of the glucocorticoids described above. Thus the gluconeogenic effect is seen as an elevation of the blood glucose level and glycosuria if the renal threshold is exceeded. A proportion of patients develop diabetes with characteristically abnormal glucose tolerance curves. The effect on the blood sugar is however not invariable because of other mechanisms that counteract any disturbance in carbohydrate metabolism, such as insulin secretion. The breakdown of protein to form glucose is reflected in the reduction of muscle, skeletal and connective tissue, leading to weakness, proximal myopathy, osteoporosis, easy bruising and purple striae of the skin over the abdomen, buttocks and thighs. Osteoporosis may be sufficiently severe to produce backache with or without radiological changes in the vertebral bodies progressing to collapse and kyphosis with shortening of the vertebral column and loss of height.

The most striking features of Cushing's disease are the moon face, central obesity, buffalo hump (accumulation of fat at the lower part of the back of the neck), plethora and hypertension that are associated with the redistribution of body fat, and sodium and fluid retention produced by the weak but unopposed mineralocorticoid action of glucocorticoids. The loss of potassium may also contribute to muscular weakness. The overproduction of adrenal androgens may lead to the development of hirsutism and acne in some patients with perhaps temporal recession of scalp in females. Amenorrhoea or other disorders of menstrual function are common. Mental symptoms, in particular depression, may be prominent.

The pituitary gland in Cushing's disease is seldom grossly enlarged either in the presence of hyperplasia or of an adenoma of the basophil or chromophobe cells. Although some enlargement may be detectable on X-ray of the pituitary fossa, often no radiological abnormality can be seen. Expansion of the pituitary fossa

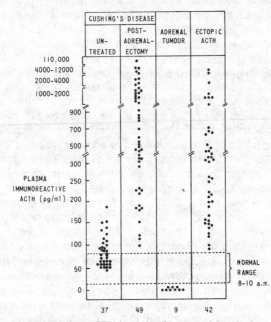

Fig. 11.5 Plasma immunoreactive ACTH levels in 137 cases of Cushing's syndrome. (From Besser and Edwards (1972), *Clinics in Endocrinology*, Vol. 1, No. 2, p. 451.)

and pressure on the optic chiasma may occur due to an adenoma following treatment by bilateral adrenalectomy and replacement doses of steroids. In such cases the very high levels of ACTH in the serum (Fig. 11.5) together with the secretion of melanocyte stimulating hormone (MSH) cause marked brown pigmentation of the skin (*Nelson's syndrome*).

In the case of an adrenocortical tumour affecting the zona fasciculata/ reticularis, the clinical features will depend on the type of steroid that the tumour is synthesising. If the tumour is making glucocorticoids almost exclusively the clinical features will be indistinguishable from Cushing's disease, whereas if the tumour is making androgens predominantly the female patient will be virilised, with pronounced hirsutism, deepening of the voice, recession of the hair on the forehead, acne and clitoral enlargement, possibly with increased libido. In males an adrenal tumour may induce feminisation if the tumour is mainly making oestrogens. Although many adrenocortical adenomas are benign, functional carcinomas do occur with metastases to other organs.

When Cushing's syndrome is due to the production of ectopic ACTH the striking features are the rapid development of brown pigmentation due to the very high plasma levels of ACTH or MSH or biologically active analogues. Frequently such patients show a marked alkalosis and potassium depletion. Characteristically they do not appear Cushingoid (moon face and central obesity) presumably because the underlying malignant process and the short survival time prevent this. The prognosis for such patients is generally measured in weeks or months.

Differential Diagnosis. The main differential diagnosis of Cushing's disease or syndrome is simple obesity and simple hirsutism, especially when either is associated with mild hypertension and menstrual irregularity or when both coexist. Functional ovarian tumours may give a similar clinical picture. It can sometimes be difficult to decide when to investigate and when to exclude the possibility of Cushing's disease or syndrome on clinical grounds alone. Overactivity of the adrenal cortex is comparatively rare while simple obesity, hirsutism, menstrual irregularities and hypertension are common.

Investigation of Suspected Overactivity of the Zona Fasciculata/Reticularis. Disordered function of the zona fasciculata/reticularis is almost invariably reflected in an alteration of the normal diurnal rhythm of cortisol secretion with high levels of plasma cortisol in the evening; the simple measurement of plasma fluorogenic corticosteroids by Mattingly's method can be taken as a close approximation to the level of plasma cortisol. The demonstration of such an abnormality does not establish the diagnosis since stress, obesity or hypertension may produce similar findings. In subjects with normal adrenocortical function the secretion of cortisol should be readily suppressible with biologically active analogues of cortisol such as dexamethasone. These substances do not contribute to the measurement of fluorogenic corticosteroids which therefore continue to reflect the endogenous level of cortisol in the plasma. Normal subjects and patients suffering from simple obesity or from hypertension due to causes other than Cushing's syndrome will show suppression of cortisol secretion following 0·5 mg oral dexamethasone 6-hourly for 48 hours. The majority of patients with Cushing's disease will show significant suppression following 2·0 mg dexamethasone 6-hourly for 48 hours, while most patients with adrenal tumours and the ectopic ACTH syndrome will fail to do so at this dosage. A further test of glucocorticoid production is the cortisol secretion rate (normal range 250–850 μmol/

24 hours); this involves the administration of ^{14}C-labelled cortisol and the measurement of one of its metabolites in a 24-hour collection of urine.

An assessment of adrenal androgen secretion may be made by measuring the 17-oxosteroid excretion in 24-hour urine samples and in the rare feminising adrenal tumour in males the oestrogen output may also be estimated in urine.

Once a diagnosis of excess activity of the zona fasciculata/reticularis has been made, some indication of the cause may be obtained by radioimmunoassay of the plasma ACTH concentration. As shown in Figure 11.5, moderately elevated levels are seen in Cushing's disease, low or undetectable levels occur in adrenal adenoma and strikingly high levels are found in the ectopic ACTH syndrome. Further information may be obtained by adrenal arteriography or scan. In the ectopic ACTH syndrome the tumour producing the ACTH is frequently highly malignant and is usually only too obvious.

About 70 per cent of cases with overactivity of the zona fasciculata/reticularis are due to Cushing's disease, (i.e. pituitary dependent bilateral adrenal hyperplasia), 20 per cent to an adrenal adenoma or carcinoma and 10 per cent to the ectopic ACTH syndrome.

Treatment of Overactivity of the Zona Fasciculata/Reticularis. This clearly depends on establishing the cause. The adrenal which is the site of an adenoma or carcinoma should be removed surgically. In the case of the ectopic ACTH syndrome the primary tumour should be removed but unfortunately this is rarely possible. Transitory improvement may be achieved by using metyrapone (p. 545) or aminoglutethimide to block cortisol synthesis together with appropriate electrolyte replacement with particular reference to potassium.

In relation to the more common Cushing's disease opinions vary as to the best treatment. The most usual is bilateral adrenalectomy preceded by the control of adrenocortical function with metyrapone and followed by replacement steroid therapy (p. 546). Nelson's syndrome (p. 538) may be a later postoperative complication; this can be prevented either by giving external irradiation to the pituitary at the time of bilateral adrenalectomy or should there be evidence of rising plasma ACTH levels in excess of 1,000 pg/ml after the operation. Those who endeavour to treat the condition more rationally by implantation of radioactive yttrium into the pituitary achieve somewhat variable results. Proton beam irradiation to the pituitary gland is another possible form of treatment but has not yet been fully assessed.

Aldosteronism (Overactivity of the Zona Glomerulosa)

This necessarily means hypersecretion of aldosterone and it may be primary in origin or secondary to some other pathology.

In *primary aldosteronism*, usually associated with an adenoma and known as *Conn's syndrome*, the most consistent symptom is weakness, often episodic, and attributable to potassium deficiency. Polyuria and polydipsia, also due to the effects of potassium depletion and impaired renal tubular reabsorption of water, commonly occur. Tetany may be an occasional presenting symptom precipitated by the metabolic alkalosis associated with potassium depletion. The blood pressure is usually raised and the condition may be mistaken for essential hypertension, or for myasthenia gravis because of the weakness. Oedema is most unusual. Primary aldosteronism should be treated by removal of the affected gland or, if this is not possible, spironolactone should be given.

Secondary aldosteronism occurs in cirrhosis of the liver with ascites, in the nephrotic syndrome and less consistently in severe cardiac failure. Potassium depletion may not be detected in the plasma, hypertension is less likely to occur and oedema is usual. The use of spironolactone in the management of these conditions is dicussed on page 162. Secondary aldosteronism may also occur in patients with unilateral renal ischaemia due to renal artery stenosis, a form which can occasionally be cured by surgical correction of the arterial defect.

Plasma renin (p. 220) and plasma and urinary aldosterone assays are important in identifying these disabilities.

Insufficiency of the Adrenal Cortex

Inadequate secretion of the adrenocortical hormones may be primary from acquired disease of the adrenals (Addison's disease) or because of congenital deficiency of the enzymes required for the synthesis of adrenocortical hormones (congenital adrenal hyperplasia). It may be secondary to failure of ACTH secretion due to pituitary or hypothalamic disorders (Fig. 11.6).

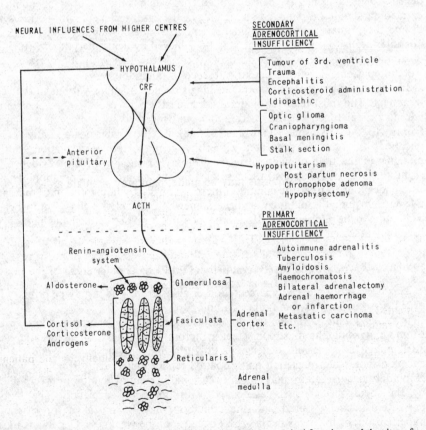

Fig. 11.6 Diagrammatic representation of the control of adrenocortical function and the sites of action of the various causes of disordered function. (Irvine & Barnes (1972) *Clinics in Endocrinology*, Vol. 1, No. 2.)

Addison's Disease

Autoimmune adrenal failure (78 per cent) and tuberculous destruction of the adrenal (21 per cent) are the commonest causes of Addison's disease in the developed countries, while other causes such as those listed in Figure 11.6 are rare. When acute adrenal failure occurs during the course of an infection with septicaemia (usually meningococcal) it has the eponym Waterhouse-Friderichsen syndrome.

Autoimmune adrenal failure (previously referred to as 'idiopathic' or 'simple' atrophy) affects females twice as frequently as males and may occur at any age. It is characterised by adrenocortical antibodies in the serum, by cell mediated hypersensitivity to adrenocortical antigens and by a high incidence of other organ-specific autoimmune diseases such as thyrotoxicosis, Hashimoto's thyroiditis, primary atrophic hypothyroidism, pernicious anaemia, premature ovarian failure, idiopathic hypoparathyroidism and also insulin dependent diabetes. Histologically both adrenals show atrophy of the cortical cells in all three zones with lymphocytic infiltration and increase in fibrous tissue. The medulla is not significantly affected. The adrenals are usually smaller than normal and appear atrophic.

In tuberculous destruction of the adrenal there is caseation with giant cells and calcification which may be detected radiologically in long-standing cases.

Clinical Features. The onset of adrenal insufficiency may be acute or chronic, or more commonly acute following upon chronic. The main clinical features of chronic primary adrenal insufficiency are weakness, weight loss, hyperpigmentation or vitiligo, hypotension and gastrointestinal disorders. The invariable symptoms of tiredness and malaise, both physical and mental, gradually increase. Loss of weight does not occur until the adrenal failure is well advanced and then it is invariable. Anorexia, nausea and constipation alternating with diarrhoea occur with increased frequency as the disease progresses. Eventually in *adrenal crisis* the gastrointestinal complaints may be the outstanding feature and an erroneous diagnosis of severe gastroenteritis may be made; pain may simulate an acute obdomen. A wrong diagnosis may cost the patient his life.

Pigmentation of the skin is often the clinical sign that first raises the suspicion of primary hypoadrenalism. A history of its recent onset is more significant than pigmentation of long standing. This feature is due to increased melanin and is most obvious in regions normally pigmented and exposed to light or pressure, e.g. face, neck, back of hands, knuckles, elbows and knees, or in areas of the body subject to friction and in skin creases, particularly in the palms. The mucous membranes of the mouth, the conjunctivae and the vagina may also become pigmented. Scars that have been present before the onset of primary adrenal failure remain unpigmented in contrast to those that are acquired after the onset of adrenal failure. Pigmentation may precede the other features of hypoadrenalism by many years. It often manifests itself initially by the patient acquiring a much better suntan than usual and the tan taking longer to disappear. The progressive pigmentation is believed to be due to increased secretion of MSH by the pituitary which occurs simultaneously with augmented ACTH release and possibly in part to ACTH itself. Vitiligo, patchy areas of depigmentation of the skin surrounded by increased pigmentation, occurs in 10 to 20 per cent of patients with Addison's disease, particularly in dark-skinned races.

The patient may give a history of very slow recovery from an illness or operation, having escaped an acute crisis at such a time. Likewise, there may be a history of extreme sensitivity to drugs such as morphine or pethidine.

Hypotension is almost invariable whether the patient is erect or supine. It is uncommon for a patient with primary adrenocortical failure to have a systolic blood pressure greater than 110 mm Hg before appropriate replacement therapy is started. Normal reflex maintenance of the blood pressure is impaired and dizziness and syncopal attacks may result from postural hypotension.

Reactive hypoglycaemia after a carbohydrate meal may occur, cortisol being one of the physiological antagonists of insulin. Hypoglycaemia is usually manifest by tiredness and lethargy, the patient having more than usual difficulty in getting up in the morning.

Loss of body hair, especially in the female, is occasionally found but is generally not so marked as in hypopituitarism. Menstrual disorders, usually amenorrhoea, are common during the onset of the disease before treatment is instituted. A significant proportion of patients with autoimmune Addison's disease suffer from premature failure of ovarian function on account of an immunological reaction against antigens that are shared between the adrenal cortex and the steroid producing cells of the ovary.

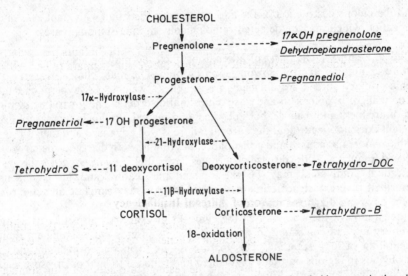

Fig. 11.7 The enzymatic steps involved in the synthesis of cortisol and aldosterone in the adrenal cortex and the urinary metabolites (underlined in italics) that are likely to be increased should there be an enzyme block (e.g. in congenital adrenal hyperplasia) at the next enzymatic step. The fall in the secretion of cortisol will activate the anterior pituitary to secrete ACTH with increased stimulation of the enzymatic steps preceding the block.

Secondary Adrenal Insufficiency

The secretion of ACTH and TSH is more resistant to pituitary damage than is the secretion of the gonadotrophins or growth hormone, so that patients with adrenal insufficiency secondary to organic pituitary disease generally show clinical features of impaired gonadotrophin secretion or of growth hormone secretion if the patient is of appropriate age for such features to be manifest. Thus a patient with secondary adrenal insufficiency will differ from one with Addison's disease by showing pallor instead of increased pigmentation of the skin. The skin is usually fine provided hypothyroidism is not pronounced, and there is marked loss of axillary and pubic hair. Because the secretion of aldosterone is largely independent of the pituitary, the blood pressure is better maintained than in primary adrenal insufficiency and the threat to life is less marked. Otherwise the symptoms are similar to those of primary adrenal insufficiency. In the absence of ACTH secretion the zona fasciculata/reticularis undergoes disuse atrophy.

Adrenal insufficiency induced by the prolonged use of therapeutic doses of corticosteroids is discussed on page 549.

Congenital Adrenal Hyperplasia with Insufficiency

The synthesis of aldosterone and of the glucocorticoids involves a series of enzymatic steps involving hydroxylases. Congenital adrenal hyperplasia with insufficiency may present at birth, in infancy, or in childhood, depending on the precise type and severity of the hydroxylase deficiency. In the attempt to overcome the enzyme block, negative feedback control results in increased secretion of ACTH with overproduction of the compounds synthesised before the enzyme block is encountered. This usually means the production of large quantities of androgenic steroids. The metabolic consequences of deficiency of enzymes at the different stages of synthesis of cortisol and aldosterone are illustrated in Figure 11.7. Thus at birth, female infants may show signs of virilisation with clitoral hypertrophy and variable degrees of fusion of the labia. Male infants particularly may die in adrenocortical insufficiency, because the genital stigmata to be seen in female infants are not present to provide an appropriate warning of adrenal disease. If the enzyme defect is less severe the patient may survive infancy and present in childhood with evidence of precocious puberty. Growth may be abnormally advanced at first but is restricted later by early fusion of the epiphyses. Thus patients with mild examples of the enzyme defects usually come under supervision when excessive tallness, premature appearance of secondary sexual characteristics or libidinous tendencies arouse parental anxieties.

Investigation of Adrenal Insufficiency

The symptoms and signs of adrenal insufficiency are so non-specific that confirmation of the diagnosis must be sought whenever suspicion arises. Tests of adrenocortical function are based on: (1) The metabolic effects of corticosteroids. (2) The measurement of cortisol levels in the resting state and following stimulation. (3) Measurement of ACTH levels in the plasma.

1. **Metabolic Effects.** Patients with Addison's disease, in contrast to those with secondary adrenal insufficiency, may show alteration in their serum electrolytes with depressed sodium and elevated potassium levels; this is by no means invariable even in advanced cases and must not be depended upon for diagnosis. Some degree of hypoglycaemia may occur but this also is of little diagnostic value. In past years the inability of patients with adrenal insufficiency to excrete a water load rapidly was used as a diagnostic test.

2. **Cortisol Levels.** Provided the patient is not in crisis or approaching crisis, time may be taken to determine the presence of absence or a diurnal rhythm in plasma cortisol levels by taking blood at 0900 hours and 2300 hours for 2 or 3

consecutive days for determination of fluorogenic corticosteroid levels before treatment is started. Low levels and the absence of a diurnal rhythm could be due to a lesion at any point in the hypothalamic-pituitary-adrenal axis. Normal levels and a normal rhythm would suggest that the whole axis is normal, but the possibility exists that, while overall function is maintained, there has been a significant reduction in reserve function which could be of paramount importance in times of stress. For this reason, if either primary or secondary adrenal insufficiency is suspected clinically, the diurnal rhythm studies should be supplemented by stimulation tests.

ACTH Test. The stimulation tests should be done in a logical sequence, starting with the administration of ACTH or a potent analogue. The preparation of choice is tetracosactrin depot, which consists of the biologically active first 24 amino acids of human ACTH adsorbed to zinc phosphate to give a preparation with a duration of action of at least 24 hours when given in an intramuscular dose of 1·0 mg. Special care is required with this drug: occasional patients have collapsed within 1 hour of administration, even after many previous injections, and it is advised that they should remain under direct observation for at least such an interval.

The plasma fluorogenic corticosteroid level may be measured at 30 minutes, 60 minutes and 5 hours after the injection. For a normal result the initial basal level should be greater than 140 nmol/l, the increment after 30 minutes should be more than 200 nmol/l and the level eventually exceed 690 nmol/l. If all three of these criteria are met it is unnecessary to proceed further but if this initial response is impaired the procedure should be repeated on the following 2 days.

In secondary adrenal insufficiency there is a characteristic stepwise increase in plasma cortisol levels on each day of tetracosactrin depot administration, while in primary adrenal insufficiency (Addison's disease) there is little or no response. For practical purposes the criteria for primary adrenal insufficiency would be failure of the plasma fluorogenic corticosteroid levels to rise above 700 n mol/l by 5–12 hours after the third intramuscular injection of 1·0 mg tetracosactrin depot given on three consecutive mornings.

Since highly biologically active analogues of cortisol, such as betamethasone or prednisolone, do not cause fluorescence in the Mattingly procedure, ACTH stimulation tests can be effectively carried out even though the patient may have recently started replacement therapy using these analogues.

Insulin Induced Hypoglycaemia. In a patient in whom secondary adrenocortical insufficiency is suspected, the next procedure should be insulin induced hypoglycaemia. Unless radioimmunoassay of ACTH levels is readily available, insulin induced hypoglycaemia should be undertaken only after it has been shown that the patient's adrenal cortex is fully responsive to ACTH stimulation, because the patient's own adrenals will be used to assay the ACTH secreted from the pituitary in response to the hypoglycaemia. Insulin induced hypoglycaemia is a safe procedure provided certain precautions are taken. A history of epilepsy is a contradindication. Patients with hypopituitarism are very sensitive to small doses of insulin and the dose should not exceed 0·1 unit soluble insulin/kg body weight. This is given in the form of a single intravenous injection, an in-dwelling cannula with a slow infusion of saline having previously been established. The patient must be observed throughout the test with the physician at hand checking the condition of the patient repeatedly. A good index of adequate hypoglycaemia is the presence of sweating. Should hypoglycaemia become profound and the clinical features indicate that the test should be abandoned, the situation can be readily corrected by giving glucose via the intravenous cannula and hydrocortisone if necessary. In addition to the clinical criteria of sweating, the blood sugar should fall to less than 2·2 mmol/l or to less than 50 per cent of the basal level at 30 minutes, whichever is the lower. Blood glucose and plasma fluorogenic corticosteroid levels should be estimated half-hourly for 120 min. Normal peak values of the latter show a mean of 785 nmol/l with a range of 560–1060 nmol/l, the increment being a mean of 400 with a range of 200–670 nmol/l.

Useful information on growth hormone secretion and prolactin can be obtained from the same samples. The corticosteroid response to insulin induced hypoglycaemia is probably the most sensitive of the tests currently available for assessing hypothalamic-pituitary-adrenal function.

As shown in Figure 11.8, insulin induced hypoglycaemia measures the function of the entire hypothalamic-pituitary-adrenal axis. If a patient has a normal diurnal rhythm of plasma cortisol, a normal response to ACTH stimulation and a normal plasma cortisol response to insulin hypoglycaemia, there is no abnormality of the hypothalamic-pituitary-adrenal axis. If adequate insulin hypoglycaemia does not give a normal rise in plasma cortisol, it is sometimes possible to localise the lesion further by proceeding to a metyrapone test.

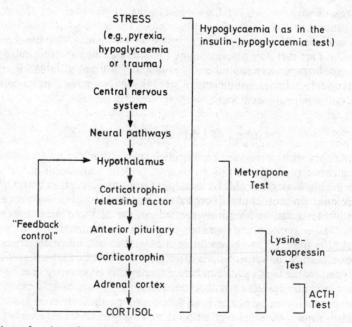

Fig. 11.8 Sites of action of test procedures used in assessing hypothalamic-pituitary-adrenal function.

Metyrapone Test. Metyrapone inhibits the enzyme 11-beta-hydroxylase that is involved in the final step in the synthesis of cortisol (Fig. 11.7). Its oral administration in a dose of 750 mg 4-hourly for 24 hours therefore produces a fall in the secretion of cortisol which activates the hypothalamic-pituitary axis via the feedback mechanism so that the secretion of ACTH is increased. Consequently, there is a build-up of the immediate precursor of cortisol, 11-deoxycortisol, which is released into the circulation. After being metabolised in the liver to its tetra-hydro-derivative, it is excreted in the urine in the 17-oxogenic steroid fraction. In carrying out a metyrapone test the plasma fluorogenic steroids and the 24-hour urinary 17-oxogenic steroids should be measured during the preceding 48 hours, the 24 hours during the administration of metyrapone, and the following 24 hours. If the hypothalamic-pituitary axis is normal there should be a fall in the plasma fluorogenic steroids and a rise in the urinary excretion of 17-oxogenic steroids. The latter will not occur with lesions in the hypothalamus or pituitary that affect CRF or ACTH secretion. Unlike ACTH stimulation tests, the metyrapone test cannot be done if the patient is taking exogenous corticosteroids in any form. The normal response in the urinary 17-oxogenic steroid is a mean maximum level of 100 μmol/day with a range of 63–127 μmol/day. The mean increment in normal subjects is 66 with a range of 30–107 μmol/day. The metyrapone test should be avoided in pregnancy and not attempted in suspected primary adrenal failure.

Abnormal findings in the metyrapone test sometimes occur in subjects in whom the hypothalamic-pituitary-adrenal axis is normal by all other criteria; this is thought to be due to failure to achieve a sufficient block of hydroxylation in the adrenal, either because of inadequate absorption of metyrapone or because of its very short half-life in plasma.

3. **Measurement of ACTH Levels in Plasma.** In the presence of low levels of plasma fluorogenic steroids, if the plasma ACTH level is high, one would have strong evidence of primary adrenocortical insufficiency. The measurement of plasma ACTH levels greatly facilitates the study of hypopituitarism as it is no longer necessary to use the patient's potentially normal adrenals in an *in vivo* bioassay. Such direct measurements of ACTH are also particularly helpful in relation to insulin hypoglycaemia and metyrapone tests.

Treatment of Adrenocortical Insufficiency

All patients with adrenocortical insufficiency will require replacement therapy with a glucocorticoid, while the majority of patients with Addison's disease will also need a mineralocorticoid. In congenital adrenal hyperplasia, full replacement doses of glucocorticoid will suppress ACTH secretion and prevent excessive formation of metabolites with consequent regression of the clinical features. If the nature of the enzymic block demands it, a mineralocorticoid should be added.

Cortisol is the drug of choice for routine glucocorticoid replacement therapy. Cortisone acetate, although widely used, has the disadvantage that it has to be metabolised by the liver to cortisol before having any physiological action. Abnormal liver function results in reduced conversion of cortisone acetate to cortisol and the possibility of impaired liver function is particularly relevant in cases of secondary adrenal insufficiency who are taking oral androgen therapy for concomitant hypogonadism. Other synthetic glucocorticoids, e.g. prednisone, prednisolone, dexamethasone and betamethasone are useful in keeping a patient in good health while adrenal function tests are being done, but have the disadvantage in terms of continual replacement therapy in that they do not react in the fluorogenic corticosteroid assay so their dosage cannot be monitored. Cortisol, cortisone acetate and the synthetic glucocorticoids have a biological action of some 6 to 8 hours.

For maintenance treatment it is best to give the glucocorticoid medication in a regime which mimics the normal diurnal variation of cortisol output. For most patients this would be 20 mg cortisol at breakfast time and 10 mg at about 1800 hours. The equivalent doses of cortisone acetate would be 25 mg and 12·5 mg respectively. While it is not possible to be dogmatic about how much glucocorticoid any individual may require as absorption and metabolism may vary, the regime described will meet the needs of most patients. To assess the requirements of those whose response appears to be unsatisfactory a *corticosteroid profile* should be carried out. Plasma fluorogenic corticosteroids should be estimated before and half an hour, 1 hour and then at 2-hourly intervals after an oral dose of 20 mg of cortisol, or whatever dose seems to be clinically indicated. The plasma level usually reaches a peak after 30–60 minutes and the amount of cortisol should be adjusted to give a peak of 700–830 nmol/*l* and a level of about 165 nmol/*l* before the evening dose.

Fludrocortisone is the most useful mineralocorticoid for maintenance therapy, and the dose should be adjusted according to the serum electrolytes, the state of hydration of the patient and the blood pressure. Most patients require 0·05–0·15 mg in a single morning dose. The signs of overdosage of mineralocorticoid are those of sodium retention, i.e. hypertension, oedema, headaches and arthralgia, and also potassium depletion, hypokalaemic alkalosis and muscular weakness. The occasional patient is unable to tolerate fludrocortisone and in these cases subcutaneous or intramuscular injection of deoxycortone acetate (DOCA) in oil may be given in a dose of 2·5 mg daily or on alternate days. A long-acting preparation may be given in a single dose of 50 mg every 3 to 4 weeks, e.g. desoxycortone trimethyl acetate (DCTMA); 2·5 mg DOCA, 0·1 mg fludrocortisone daily, and 75 mg DCTMA monthly are equivalent in terms of sodium retention.

The regime to be followed in secondary adrenocortical insufficiency is the same as in Addison's disease except that a mineralocorticoid is not required as aldosterone production is little affected. Any associated condition due to lack of other trophic hormones will require therapy along the usual lines.

During periods of stress, e.g. trauma, infection or operations, it is necessary for the dose of glucocorticoid to be increased to mimic what would happen in an individual with normal function of the hypothalamic-pituitary-adrenal axis. Thus if a patient develops a severe cold or influenza he should increase the dose of oral steroids to twice their normal maintenance level for 2 to 3 days. Should gastroenteritis with or without vomiting occur the oral glucocorticoid should be changed to intramuscular hydrocortisone at an increased dose level. Consequently, it is essential that patients with impaired adrenal function, either primary or secondary, should have available ampoules of hydrocortisone hemisuccinate for injection which are not outdated and which they know how to use.

Every patient on oral steroids of whatever form should have a steroid card or preferably a bracelet giving details of the condition from which he is suffering, dose of steroids that he is taking and the address of his physician. The opportunity should be taken when the patient is initially seen and during the hospitalisation period to indoctrinate him in the importance of carrying this means of identification everywhere, and to increase the dose of corticosteroids if he develops an infection or incurs an injury. Should the patient be involved in an accident and be taken unconscious to a casualty department the outcome may be avoidably disastrous if the information that the patient is taking steroids is not available.

Any operation, even the most minor such as a dental extraction, is a potential hazard to a patient with adrenocortical insufficiency. On no account should such a patient be given morphine or pethidine. For dental extraction the patient should be admitted to hospital for the day. It is usually only necessary to give twice the normal dose of glucocorticoid on the day of the extraction and possibly the morning following and to resume normal replacement dosage thereafter provided there are no complications. Larger doses of steroids and more careful monitoring both pre- and post-operatively are required for more major surgery.

ACUTE ADRENAL CRISIS. This is a medical emergency. If promptly treated with intravenous hydrocortisone hemisuccinate (or hydrocortisone sodium succinate) and intravenous fluids there is in most cases a dramatic improvement in a previously moribund patient over 12 to 24 hours. Occasional cases will need more protracted treatment depending upon how quickly the precipitating cause, e.g. infection, is brought under control. In incipient crises, intravenous fluids may not be necessary, but in frank crises with peripheral circulatory failure the patient may succumb in spite of massive doses of intravenous hydrocortisone. Hypertensive agents are not helpful in this situation. The intravenous fluids should consist of 5 per cent dextrose to correct hypoglycaemia and isotonic saline to correct sodium loss. Hydrocortisone hemisuccinate is best given parenterally over the first 24–48 hours until gastrointestinal symptoms settle completely and one can be sure that oral medication will be effective. The initial dose should be 100 mg intravenously 6 hourly for the first 24 hours and then 50 mg 6 hourly for the next 24 hours. If progress is satisfactory, oral cortisol can be given thereafter in a dose of 20 mg 8 hourly. The dose of oral cortisol can then be further reduced in a stepwise fashion by 10 mg daily until normal maintenance levels are reached. Below 40 mg of oral cortisol per day a mineralocorticoid is best added to the therapeutic regime, initially in a single morning dose of 0·1 mg fludrocortisone.

Prognosis in Adrenal Insufficiency

With modern therapy the life expectancy of patients with adrenal insufficiency should be normal, within the limits imposed by any associated disease such as pituitary tumour, or other clinical disorder such as diabetes mellitus which may co-exist with autoimmune adrenal insufficiency. Otherwise the main risk to life is the avoidable occurrence of acute adrenal crisis and delay in its prompt management.

Corticosteroids and ACTH in the Treatment of Disease

Extensive use has been made of the anti-inflammatory actions of corticosteroids and of their synthetic analogues since cortisone became available in 1948. Alternatively, ACTH may be administered parenterally to augment the endogenous production of cortisol. Some of the steroid analogues are listed in Table 11.1 with the dosage which is therapeutically equivalent to 20 mg cortisol. Of these prednisolone is the most commonly used for purposes other than replacement therapy. It is widely prescribed in the treatment of connective tissue diseases, of autoimmune disorders and conditions involving other forms of immune reaction. Corticosteroids may be used to suppress inflammation, for example in conjunction with chemotherapy in acute tuberculosis (p. 292). The distinction between inflammation and immune reaction may be difficult to make. The use of corticosteroids in pharmacological doses is discussed under the heading of the various diseases for which they may be employed.

Table 11.1 Relative potencies of corticosteroids and their synthetic analogues

Compound	Size of oral tablet (mg)	Approximate Relative Potency		Equivalent dosage (for anti-inflam-matory effect) (mg)
		Anti-inflammatory (glucocorticoid) effect	Sodium-retaining (mineralo-corticoid) effect	
Cortisone	25	1	1	25
Cortisol	20	1·2	1	20
Prednisolone/ prednisone	5	5	0·8	5
Betamethasone	0·5	40	negligible	0·5
Dexamethasone	0·5	37	minimal	0·5
Fludrocortisone	0·1	0·05	200	—
Aldosterone*	—	none	500	—

* Not used in clinical practice.

The Dangers of Corticosteroid Therapy

The use of corticosteroids in doses exceeding those required for replacement therapy carries certain risks which must be balanced against the possible therapeutic advantages. These risks can be subdivided into two types: (1) the undesirable metabolic consequences that cannot be separated from the anti-inflammatory effect of the steroid and (2) the suppression of the hypothalamic-pituitary-adrenal (HPA) axis that may follow the use of pharmacological doses of steroids over a prolonged period.

1. *The metabolic consequences* are those that are encountered in Cushing's syndrome and are naturally more pronounced the higher the dose and the longer the treatment. Thus, although certain corticosteroid analogues may have slightly less mineralocorticoid activity than cortisol, fluid retention, moon face, central obesity, striae, etc., may all be induced. The glucocorticoid action not infrequently precipitates diabetes mellitus and the catabolic effect is responsible for os-teoporosis as an insidious but frequent complication of long term steroid therapy. Corticosteroids may modify the normal response to a major illness so that pain, tenderness, fever or a raised ESR may be abolished, while the response to inflam-mation and therefore the defences against infection may be poor and healing im-paired. In this way treatment with these drugs may be responsible for masking the more typical and sometimes dangerous consequences of a variety of illnesses. For example, oral corticosteroids may induce peptic ulceration with perforation without pain and the physical signs indicative of inflammation in the peritoneal cavity may not be present. As in Cushing's syndrome, mental symptoms may be troublesome, ranging from euphoria to depression which may be so severe as to lead to suicide.

2. *The suppression of the HPA axis* following prolonged corticosteroid therapy in doses greater than 7·5 mg prednisolone per day or its equivalent may be long standing, especially with regard to the hypothalamic-pituitary portion of the axis. This may make it difficult to withdraw steroid, the patient being as vulnerable as someone with secondary adrenocortical insufficiency due to organic pituitary dis-ease. Stimulation of the adrenal cortex in such cases is usually possible with adequate ACTH dosage, but there is no known way of producing a comparably strong and prolonged stimulus to the hypothalamic-pituitary axis without risking

adrenocortical failure. When trying to wean a patient off corticosteroid therapy, one should first ensure that the adrenal cortex is functional by giving tetracosactrin depot 1·0 mg i.m. on 3 consecutive mornings and measuring the plasma cortisol response at 30 minutes, 1 hour and 5 hours (p. 544). Then, after gradually reducing the dosage of oral steroid, a maintenance dose of 20 mg cortisol should be given at 0800–0900 hours and no cortisol in the evenings; the hypothalamo-pituitary axis will then have no exogenous steroid to suppress the secretion of CRF or ACTH in the early hours of the morning. In this way a normal diurnal rhythm may be restored and the HPA axis should thereafter respond normally to stress. This may take many months to achieve, while in other cases, normal function may be restored shortly after steroid therapy has been withdrawn.

Because it can be such a difficult task to withdraw corticosteroid therapy when it has been used in pharmacological dosage for a prolonged period, attempts have been made to use synthetic ACTH preparations such as tetracosactrin depot in place of oral corticosteroids. When used in appropriate dose, there is evidence that therapeutically useful elevation in the plasma cortisol levels may be achieved without risk of suppression of the HPA axis. ACTH therapy is therefore probably better than oral corticosteroid treatment for chronic relapsing conditions when it is hoped that the steroids can be withdrawn during periods of remission. In children ACTH therapy has the distinct advantage over treatment with oral steroids in that it causes less inhibition of growth. Porcine ACTH gel should no longer be used on account of the hypersensitivity reactions that it may cause.

The incidence of mooning of the face and obesity is similar with oral corticosteroids and ACTH. Peptic ulceration and bruising are commoner with corticosteroids, and hypertension, pigmentation and acne with ACTH. In view of the serious risks involved very careful consideration must be given before either is employed and the practitioner must be convinced that the therapeutic benefits outweigh the disadvantages.

Phaeochromocytoma

Phaeochromocytomas are tumours of chromaffin tissue which secrete catecholamines, predominantly noradrenaline but also adrenaline. The tumours, most of which are benign, may occur at any site along the sympathetic chain, but 90 per cent are found in the adrenal glands. Rarely the lesions may be multiple. Phaeochromocytoma is an uncommon tumour but of considerable interest because of its pharmacological effects. The clinical presentation depends upon the relative amounts of noradrenaline and adrenaline secreted. The most common sign is hypertension which may be paroxysmal or sustained and associated with episodes of extreme skin pallor, sweating, palpitations, headache, epigastric pain and chest discomfort. Apprehension is common during a paroxysm.

The diagnosis of phaeochromocytoma depends on the demonstation of increased levels of catecholamines or their metabolites in the urine, e.g. metanephrine and normetanephrine or HMMA (4 hydroxy-3-methoxy mandelic acid, known also as VMA). The location of the tumour is best shown by adrenal venography.

The treatment of phaeochromocytoma is by excision of the tumour if it can be identified or, failing this, alpha and beta receptor blockade may be used. In order to avoid hypertension and arrhythmias during induction of anaesthesia and handling of the tumour at operation, the preoperative preparation of the patient with α- and β-adrenergic blocking agents (phenoxybenzamine and propranolol) is essential.

Emergencies associated with hypertensive crises should be dealt with by the intravenous administration of phentolamine in doses of 5 mg.

Sexual Disorders in the Male

Disabilities of this type may present in many forms. Some are due to faults arising in the mechanism of sex determination as early as conception, others to errors later in sexual differentiation of the embryo and fetus, and after birth, in sexual development. Abnormalities of the sex chromosomes may be associated with failure of sexual development so that the individual may show some of the characteristics of both sexes, a state known as intersex. The term hermaphroditism is reserved for patients in whom male and female gonadal tissue is found to coexist; it occurs much less commonly than the intersexes.

The anatomical characteristics of the male are influenced by essential hormonal factors, particularly androgen secretion. The personality and behaviour of the male are further attributes which must be considered in assessing the individual patient's needs. A few only of the more common sexual disorders occurring in the male will be discussed here.

Hypogonadism

This term is used to include failure of one or both of the main functions of the testis, namely the production of spermatozoa and the secretion of androgens. The defect may involve only impaired spermatogenesis in the seminiferous tubules of the testis, or the interstitial (Leydig) cells of the testis may also be affected so that the secretion of testosterone by these cells is reduced or abolished. If the function of the interstitial cells is defective, then tubular dysfunction is inevitable.

Aetiology. Hypogonadism may be part of the syndrome of hypopituitarism. Hypogonadotrophic hypogonadism with an apparently normal pituitary gland appears to be due to failure of the hypothalamus to secrete the appropriate gonadotrophin releasing hormones. In addition there are cases in which the anterior pituitary is intact but the testes have been destroyed or damaged (primary testicular failure). Trauma, tuberculosis, gonococcal infections, syphilis, malignant disease, orchitis as in mumps, and surgical castration are recognised causes of primary testicular failure. Maldescent or failure of descent will also lead to failure of the tubular epithelium to develop. Haemochromatosis, cirrhosis of the liver and oestrogen administration may all be associated with testicular insufficiency. The disorder may also be due to abnormalities of the sex chromosomes (p. 10). Many cases remain, however, for which an aetiological diagnosis is still not possible, and these form the majority of patients who present with infertility as their only complaint (idiopathic oligospermia). The normal sperm count is about $6 \times 10^7/ml$.

Clinical Features. The nature of the sequelae from failure of function of the interstitial cells depends upon the age of the patient at the time of the onset of the disease. When this occurs *before puberty* the external genitalia and the secondary sex characteristics fail to develop. In these circumstances the epiphyses of the long bones do not close at the usual age and in consequence the patient may grow to an excessive height. The typical pre-pubertal eunuch develops into a tall man with a hairless face, a high-pitched voice, small genitalia and an immature personality.

Anosmia is not infrequently associated with hypogonadotrophic hypogonadism.

When the onset of the disease is *postpubertal* the changes are less striking. Growth is not affected and there is regression rather than disappearance of the secondary sex characteristics. The external genitalia undergo partial atrophy. Fatigue, loss of initiative and libido are common complaints. In some patients, particularly when the deprivation is sudden as after surgical castration, there may be 'menopausal symptoms' such as hot flushes and profuse sweating, unless full replacement therapy is provided.

Treatment. Hypogonadism due to deficiency of androgens may be corrected by replacement therapy with testosterone. The most satisfactory and economical form of therapy is the implantation of 600 mg of testosterone, in the form of 100 mg pellets, into the subcutaneous tissue of the anterior abdominal wall. Such an implant is gradually absorbed over a period of about 6 months, after which it may be renewed. Alternatively fluoxymesterone, a synthetic analogue of testosterone, can be given sublingually in doses of 10–20 mg daily.

In some cases of deficiency of the germinal epithelium, especially when this is due to lack of FSH, increased spermatogenesis may be achieved by treatment with human chorionic gonadotrophin and Pergonal, a proprietary preparation of human postmenopausal urine with both FSH and LH activity.

Cryptorchidism

Cryptorchidism (undescended testis) may be the presenting feature of hypogonadotrophic hypogonadism or may be due to an anomaly of the pathway of descent which occasionally may be surgically remediable. Highly retractile testes, particularly in an obese boy, may be mistaken for cryptorchidism. Carcinoma is more common in undescended than normal testes. If the glands remain in the inguinal canal they are more liable to trauma than if situated in the scrotum. The seminiferous tubules will fail to develop in an undescended gland, and if the condition is bilateral, sterility will follow. Even in testes which remain undescended into adult life the interstitial cells function normally, so that the secondary sex characters develop in the usual way.

A course of chorionic gonadotrophin, 4,000 i.u. thrice weekly for a month, should be given at about 6 years of age. If this is unsuccessful the testis or testes should be placed in the scrotum surgically.

Impotence

Impotence, that is inability of the male to have sexual intercourse, is due to psychological causes in the majority of cases, and in these circumstances is not due to abnormality of the testes. Rarely it may be an important early symptom in organic disease such as diabetes mellitus, multiple sclerosis and tabes dorsalis. In hypogonadism due to anterior pituitary deficiency, a complaint of impotence is unusual; such patients usually have little interest in sexual function, and are unlikely to make this complaint spontaneously until they have received treatment for adrenal and thyroid insufficiency. They may then become aware of their impotence and require treatment with an androgen, e.g. testosterone. Gonadotrophins may be used to restore fertility if desired. Some cases of impotence are known to be associated with hyperprolactinaemia. Some patients of this type have been treated successfully with bromocriptine (p. 512).

Infertility in the Male

Sterility in the husband is believed to be responsible for the infertility of approximately one-half of all childless marriages. The cause is usually defective development of the germinal epithelium in the seminiferous tubules, with oligospermia or azoospermia, but may follow hypogonadism due to any of the causes described earlier.

Chromosomal abnormalities may be recognised by examination of a buccal smear for Barr bodies, but usually confirmation requires a full karyotype analysis (p. 7). Seminal analysis is a simple procedure and a low sperm count, or the presence of abnormal and immotile forms may be detected in this way. Testicular biopsy frequently provides valuable information on the development of the spermatic tubules and on the maturation of the germinal epithelium. This investigation should be undertaken before declaring a hopeless prognosis since the use of clomiphene for a period of 6 months or longer as a means of promoting gonadotrophin secretion, may occasionally stimulate spermatogenesis.

Treatment of a varicocele has sometimes corrected infertility. Obstruction of the vas deferens may also be amenable to surgery.

Sexual Disorders in the Female

Many conditions regarded as primarily gynaecological in nature may have much wider implications. Primary amenorrhoea, for example, may provide an important indication of systemic disorder or it may be due to a chromosomal anomaly such as Turner's syndrome. Hermaphroditism may present with amenorrhoea. Congenital adrenal hyperplasia, if unrecognised and untreated in childhood, pituitary tumours and developmental disorders in the genital tract may all require full gynaecological and endocrine assessment for precise diagnosis. Secondary amenorrhoea must also be regarded as a symptom requiring further investigation, but it is so common a feature of a wide range of conditions that by itself it has little specific diagnostic value.

Disorders of the Menopause

The term menopause is used to describe the cessation of the menstrual cycle, which occurs in most women between the ages of 45 and 50, abruptly or gradually, and as a direct result of the failure of the ovaries to produce oestrogens and progesterone. As a consequence the pituitary gland becomes more active and produces FSH and LH in greater quantity. Assays for these hormones may be of value in distinguishing amenorrhoea due primarily to failure of the ovaries from amenorrhoea due to failure of the pituitary to secrete gonadotrophins.

Clinical Features. The ease with which a woman adapts herself to the change of circumstances associated with the menopause varies widely. In some the loss of reproductive capacity is associated with depression and other psychological symptoms; in others adjustment is readily achieved and may be unattended by any emotional reaction. In the group of patients who are troubled by symptoms, anxiety, emotional instability, irritability, insomnia, and particularly hot flushes and cold sweats are common complaints. Depression is frequent and occasionally may be severe with suicidal tendencies. Obesity may first appear, or, if previously present, may increase at this time. Hirsutism, especially the appearance of dark hair on the upper lip and chin, is not uncommon. Osteoarthrosis may be responsible for considerable disability, particularly in the obese. Osteoporosis commonly presents for the first time in the early years after the menopause (p. 124).

Pruritus vulvae is a common complication which is frequently associated with changes in the mucous membranes of the genital tract. Leukoplakia vulvae may develop, and if untreated may progress to carcinoma. Senile vaginitis, which not infrequently occurs, may cause considerable distress from irritation, dysuria and vaginal discharge, especially if complicated by secondary infection.

Treatment. The essential treatment is explanation of the nature of the condition, coupled with specific treatment for the complications. Tranquillisers may occasionally be helpful. Features attributable to oestrogen deficiency call for replacement therapy with a synthetic oestrogen such as ethinyl oestradiol. The daily dose required to suppress menopausal symptoms in different individuals varies from 10 to 50 μg daily, but 20 μg daily is often adequate; this should be given in courses lasting for 21 days, repeated if necessary after an interval of 7 days. The patient must be warned that treatment in this way can be expected to be followed by vaginal bleeding as in a normal menstrual period.

Other appropriate measures, such as treatment of obesity and osteoarthrosis, may also be required. Excessive growth of hair on the face may be removed by shaving or depilatory cream, or may be made less conspicuous by bleaching with hydrogen peroxide. Depression complicating the menopause responds well to psychiatric treatment.

W. J. IRVINE
J. A. STRONG

DIABETES MELLITUS

Diabetes mellitus is a clinical syndrome characterised by hyperglycaemia, due to deficiency or diminished effectiveness of insulin. The disease is chronic and affects the metabolism of carbohydrate, protein, fat, water and electrolytes, sometimes with grave consequences. The metabolic derangement is frequently associated with permanent and irreversible functional and structural changes in the cells of the body, those of the vascular system being particularly susceptible. The changes lead in turn to the development of well-defined clinical entities, the so-called 'complications' of diabetes, which most characteristically affect the eye, the kidney and the nervous system.

Diabetes mellitus is the most common of the endocrine disorders. The prevalence in Britain is over 1 per cent, although about half of those remain undetected.

Aetiology. On the basis of aetiology two main types of diabetes are recognised, namely primary (idiopathic) diabetes and secondary diabetes.

PRIMARY (IDIOPATHIC) DIABETES. The great majority of cases seen belong to this group, which consists of two main clinical types: juvenile-onset or *insulin-dependent diabetes* and maturity-onset or *insulin-independent diabetes* (p. 559). Although the precise aetiology is still uncertain, several contributing factors are known to be involved and in both types heredity and environment interact to determine which of those with a genetic predisposition actually develop the clinical syndrome and the timing of its onset. However, both the pattern of inheritance and the environmental factors differ in younger and older-onset diabetics.

Age. The disease may appear at any time, but 80 per cent of cases occur after the age of 50 years and the highest incidence of new patients is in the 60–70 age group. Diabetes is, therefore, principally a disease of the middle-aged and elderly.

Sex. There are rather more young male diabetics than female; in middle age women are more often affected. Repeated pregnancy may add to the likelihood of developing diabetes in middle age, particularly in obese women.

Heredity. In both types of diabetes a familial tendency exists and twins are more often both diabetic when they are identical than when they are non-identical. Genetic factors are probably more important in those who develop diabetes after the age of 40 and evidence of dominant inheritance has been obtained in this type of diabetes. In younger subjects susceptibility to diabetes is associated with particular HLA phenotypes. The risk of developing diabetes is 2 to 3 times greater in those who are HLA-B8 or BW15, and affected diabetic siblings tend to have at least one and, in many cases, both HLA haplotypes in common. Both these findings are consistent with the presence of a diabetogenic gene or genes at a locus closely linked to the HLA chromosomal loci. Since genes closely linked in this way probably influence immune responses, a possible mode of action for the HLA-linked gene may be to permit a rapid immunological destructive process of the pancreas to occur, perhaps in response to a virus infection.

Autoimmunity. Considerable evidence now exists in support of the hypothesis that insulin-dependent diabetes is an autoimmune disorder irrespective of the age of onset of the disease. Diabetes coexists with other autoimmune disease such as pernicious anaemia, hyperthyroidism, Hashimoto's thyroiditis, primary hypothyroidism and Addison's disease more often than can be accounted for by chance. Thyroid, gastric, cytoplasmic, intrinsic factor and adrenal antibodies are all many times more common in diabetic than in non-diabetic populations. More direct evidence is provided by: (1) the lymphocytic and plasma cell infiltration found in the pancreas of young diabetic patients dying within 6 months of developing the disorder; (2) the demonstration of T lymphocytes sensitised against antigens derived from the pancreas in 20–30 per cent of young insulin-dependent patients; and (3) the fact that antibodies reacting with human pancreatic islet cells have been found by immunofluorescence in the serum of over 50 per cent of insulin-dependent diabetic patients soon after diagnosis, irrespective of age. In contrast, islet-cell antibodies are not found more commonly in the serum of diabetics requiring only dietary restriction than in control subjects. A number of diabetics requiring oral hypoglycaemic agents have islet-cell antibodies in the serum; such patients have an increased risk of becoming insulin-dependent eventually.

Infection. There is some evidence that viral infection may be involved in the aetiology of juvenile insulin-dependent diabetes. It is known that certain viruses can induce diabetes experimentally in some laboratory animals and a high incidence of diabetes has been known to occur after outbreaks of mumps. A seasonal variation in the incidence of diabetes in children has been demonstrated, with peaks occurring in October and June, and antibodies to Coxsackie B4 virus have been found significantly more often in the plasma of recently diagnosed young diabetics than in controls. Older diabetics do not show this excess of Coxsackie B4 infection, but infection of any kind may be important in unmasking latent diabetes in the middle-aged and elderly. Staphylococcal infections, in particular, are frequently associated with the development of clinical diabetes.

Obesity. The association of obesity and diabetes has long been recognised but it is still uncertain whether obesity is the result or the cause of diabetes. The majority of middle-aged diabetic patients are obese, but only a minority of obese people develop clinical diabetes. Most of the evidence supports the view that obesity is diabetogenic in those genetically predisposed to the disorder and that the rising incidence of diabetes in older people is related to the increasing prevalence of obesity in the population as a whole.

Diet. Overeating, especially when combined with underactivity, is associated with a rise in the incidence of diabetes in the middle-aged and elderly. Studies of the incidence in war and peace and in immigrants whose material standards of living suddenly rise provide evidence of this. Studies of diabetic sibships also demonstrate that diabetic patients eat significantly more than their non-diabetic siblings.

SECONDARY DIABETES. A minority of cases of diabetes occur as a result of a recognisable pathological process or secondary to the treatment of some other condition.

1. In *pancreatic diabetes* diseases such as pancreatitis, haemochromatosis and carcinoma cause destruction of the pancreas and lead to impaired secretion and release of insulin. Diabetes will also follow pancreatectomy.

2. In another group of cases, diabetes occurs because there are abnormal concentrations of hormones in the circulation which are *insulin antagonists*.

(a) Administration of *growth hormone* can produce permanent diabetes in experimental animals and about 30 per cent of patients with acromegaly are diabetic.

(b) *Adrenocortical hormones*, such as cortisol, raise the concentration of glucose in the blood by increasing protein breakdown and by inhibiting utilisation of glucose by the peripheral tissues. Thus, many patients with Cushing's syndrome show impaired carbohydrate tolerance; diabetes may be precipitated by ACTH or corticosteroid therapy and the stress of physical injury may operate in this way. Conversely increased sensitivity to insulin is an important feature of Addison's disease and of hypopituitarism, and this can be corrected by the administration of corticosteroids.

(c) *Adrenaline* raises the blood glucose concentration by increasing the breakdown of liver glycogen and by suppressing the secretion of insulin. Patients with phaeochromocytoma frequently show a diabetic blood glucose curve on glucose tolerance testing and the incidence of these uncommon tumours is relatively high among diabetic patients.

(d) *Thyroid hormone* in excess will aggravate the diabetic state and some patients with hyperthyroidism show impaired glucose tolerance.

(e) *Gestational diabetes* refers to the hyperglycaemia which can occur temporarily during pregnancy in individuals who have an inherited liability to develop the disorder. During normal pregnancy there is an increased production of hormonal antagonists to insulin, which in turn demands an increased rate of secretion and release of insulin. A failing pancreas may be unable to meet this demand.

3. *Iatrogenic diabetes*, in those genetically susceptible, may be precipitated by

various forms of therapy, notably corticosteroids and thiazide diuretics.

4. *Liver disease*, particularly cirrhosis and hepatitis, may be associated with impaired glucose tolerance.

Chemical Pathology. Although it has already been emphasised that diabetes is a clinical syndrome combining several different pathological processes in a common clinical picture, it can be asserted that in every case the hyperglycaemia results from the fact that the insulin secreted by the pancreas is either insufficient in amount or ineffective in action for one or more reasons. In any event increased gluconeogenesis and lipolysis will follow as compensatory reactions under the influence of such hormones as growth hormone and adrenocortical hormones, in what is basically a situation of glucose lack. Thus the hyperglycaemia characteristic of diabetes arises from two main sources, namely a reduced rate of removal of glucose from the blood by the peripheral tissues and an increased rate of release of glucose from the liver into the circulation. Although significant amounts of insulin can be detected in the plasma of some cases of primary diabetes, the majority of cases presenting spontaneously with classical symptoms of diabetes are characterised, prior to treatment, by a marked absolute deficiency of plasma insulin when compared with normal subjects. Moreover the level of plasma insulin correlates well with the clinical picture and the type of treatment subsequently required. It seems most likely that the abnormalities in carbohydrate tolerance and lipid metabolism result directly from the lack of insulin. However, the sequence of events which culminates in the development of this insulin-deficient state is still uncertain, as already discussed on page 555.

CONSEQUENCES OF HYPERGLYCAEMIA AND GLYCOSURIA. When the glucose concentration in the blood exceeds the capacity of the renal tubules to reabsorb it from the glomerular filtrate, *glycosuria* occurs. In most people the level of blood glucose at which this happens is approximately 10 mmol/l(180 mg/100 ml). Glucose increases the osmolality of the glomerular filtrate and thus prevents the reabsorption of water as the filtrate passes down the renal tubular system. In this way the volume of urine is markedly increased in diabetes and *polyuria* and *nocturia* occur. This in turn leads to loss of water and minerals which results in *thirst* and *polydipsia*.

In acute cases, or in more slowly progressive cases where the condition remains undetected for a long period of time, and particularly if the fluid intake has been low because of mental confusion or for other reasons, severe depletion of water and electrolytes may occur. As the concentration of glucose in the blood rises the extracellular fluid becomes hypertonic, and water leaves the cells. In the early stages, before the volume of the extracellular fluid is grossly reduced the patient will show relatively few clinical signs, but if the loss of water and electrolytes continues, depletion of extracellular fluid will occur, with the development of the clinical features of severe dehydration.

CONSEQUENCES OF POOR GLUCOSE UTILISATION. Impaired utilisation of carbohydrate results in a sense of *fatigue*, and causes two main compensatory mechanisms to operate in an attempt to provide alternative metabolic substrate. Both of these lead to loss of body tissue, that is *wasting*, which may occur in spite of a normal or even an increased intake of food, and which is additional to any loss of weight resulting from loss of body fluid. The compensatory mechanisms are:—

1. *Increased Glycogenolysis and Gluconeogenesis*. Glycogen and protein are present in cells associated with water and intracellular electrolytes. As glycogen and protein are catabolised, glucose, nitrogen, water and electroytes, particularly potassium, are released into the extracellular space. An increased urinary excretion of potassium,

magnesium and phosphorus therefore occurs.

2. *Increased Lipolysis*. This is seen as a raised fasting plasma concentration of non-esterified fatty acid (NEFA), and a diminished fall in plasma NEFA in response to a carbohydrate load. The extent to which increased lipolysis occurs is proportional to the degree of insulin deficiency. If the latter is marked, the normal response to feeding, namely suppression of lipolysis, may be completely lost and the plasma concentration of NEFA may remain consistently elevated to three or four times the normal level.

Fatty acids are taken up by the liver and degraded through eight steps within the mitochondria of the liver cells. Each stage yields one molecule of acetyl coenzyme A. Normally most of these molecules enter the citric acid cycle by condensing with oxaloacetic acid, but in severe diabetes more is formed than can enter the citric acid cycle. Instead acetyl coenzyme A is converted to acetoacetic acid. Most of this is then reduced to beta-hydroxybutyric acid, while some is decarboxylated to acetone. These *ketone bodies*, when formed in small amounts, are usually oxidised and utilised as metabolic fuel. However the rate of utilisation of ketone bodies is limited. When the rate of production by the liver exceeds that of removal by the peripheral tissues, then the blood level rises. Ketone bodies raise the osmolality of the plasma and so also lead to the withdrawal of water from the cell. They are strong acids which dissociate readily and release hydrogen ions into the body fluids. The fall in pH is reduced by the buffers of the blood, the most important being bicarbonate. The dissociation of carbonic acid is reduced, and the ratio of bicarbonate ions to carbonic acid falls, and measurement of plasma bicarbonate will show a lower value than normal. This state is called *ketoacidosis*. The rise in hydrogen ion concentration and increase in Pco_2 in the arterial blood stimulate pulmonary ventilation so that clinically *hyperpnoea* or 'air hunger' is observed.

The extent to which the clinical features of dehydration and ketoacidosis are seen in the individual case will depend on such factors as the speed at which the condition develops and the extent to which the patient himself increases his intake of fluid, as well as on the degree of insulin deficiency present.

Pathology. Histological examination of the pancreas at necropsy shows abnormalities in the islets of Langerhans in most cases of clinical diabetes. However it should be noted that these abnormalities are mostly of a quantitative nature; nearly all the types of lesion in the islets in diabetes can also occur in non-diabetics, although the lesions are much less common in the latter.

In the younger age group, that is those under the age of 40, the majority of whom require treatment with insulin, marked changes can be seen in the islet tissue of the pancreas which, regardless of the primary cause of diabetes, is sufficient in itself to account for the disease. The abnormality consists essentially of the degeneration of the islet tissue, from which the beta cells have largely disappeared, leaving behind a variable number of alpha cells and a majority of small undifferentiated cells. The remaining beta cells show evidence of excessive activity; the nuclei are commonly enlarged with degranulation of the cytoplasm. These appearances of the pancreas are consistent with the fact that most young diabetics have extremely low plasma insulin levels when first seen.

In the midde-aged and elderly, the majority of whom do not require treatment with insulin, the moderate reduction in the total mass of islet tissue which is commonly seen does not appear to be sufficient in itself to account for the degree of impaired carbohydrate tolerance shown by many of these patients. On the other hand, the observation that in many cases the beta cells, despite prolonged hyperglycaemia and their reduced number, fail to develop cytological signs of hyperactivity, suggests that in these diabetics the beta cells may be relatively insensitive to the stimulus of an elevated blood glucose. Failure to respond to hyperglycaemia could result from vascular lesions or from alterations in the islet stroma, interfering with the exchange between the blood and the islet cells. Fibrosis, hyalinisation, and fibrin deposits in the pericapillary space and changes in the islet epithelial basement membrane are often present in older diabetics.

Long-standing diabetes is commonly associated with a general disorder of small blood vessels which is seen as an abnormal thickening of the basement membrane of the capillaries throughout the body. It is uncertain whether this occurs in the prediabetic period, but its development thereafter seems to be mainly related to the duration of clinical diabetes. Thickening of the basement membrane *per se* is not pathognomonic of diabetes. It occurs for example as part of the normal ageing process; however the increased permeability of the thickened basement membrane in diabetes is a unique pathological feature. The widespread involvement of small blood vessels appears to be the common denominator of the complications associated with long-term diabetes. The main clinical and pathological impact of this micro-angiopathy is to be found in the retina, the kidney and the nervous system.

Clinical Features. Two main types of diabetes have long been recognised, and it is now clear that the level of plasma insulin correlates well with the clinical picture and the type of treatment subsequently required.

1. The juvenile-onset type usually develops during the first 40 years of life in patients of normal or less than normal weight. The majority develop severe symptoms of diabetes acutely, over a period of several weeks or months and if treatment with insulin is withheld they rapidly develop fatal ketoacidosis. Since administration of insulin is required for their survival, an alternative and preferable name for this group of patients is *insulin-dependent*.

2. The adult or maturity-onset type usually appears in middle aged or elderly patients who are often obese and in whom hyperglycaemia can usually be controlled by dietary means alone or, if not, by an oral hypoglycaemic compound. For this reason it is sometimes described as the *insulin-independent type*. Insulin is detectable in the plasma of nearly all patients in this category, and they are therefore less prone to develop ketosis. In this sense the disease is less severe than in the juvenile-onset type; however, the complications associated with long-term diabetes occur in both types. Many patients with maturity-onset diabetes have a long history of mild symptoms which may come and go, and which may frequently be ignored or misdiagnosed for years before the true diagnosis is made.

Apart from patients with established clinical diabetes, two other categories are recognised.

Potential diabetics are persons with a normal glucose tolerance test who nevertheless have an increased liability to develop diabetes for genetic reasons, e.g. the children of two diabetic parents; the children of parents where one is diabetic and the other has a first degree relative who is diabetic; the non-diabetic members of pairs of identical twins where one is known to be diabetic.

Latent diabetics are persons in whom the glucose tolerance test is normal, but who are known to have given an abnormal result under conditions imposing a burden on the pancreatic beta cells, e.g. during pregnancy, infection or other severe stress, mental or physical, during treatment with cortisone or other diabetogenic drugs, or when overweight.

PRESENTATION. Diabetes may be discovered in one of several ways:

1. Many patients are first noted to have glycosuria in the course of some routine examination. They may have had few or no symptoms, and no abnormal physical signs may be found.

2. Some patients present complaining of some or all of the classical symptoms of diabetes including thirst, polydipsia, polyuria, nocturia, tiredness, loss of weight, white marks on clothing, pruritus vulvae or balanitis, a change in refraction usually in the direction of myopia, paraesthesiae or pain in the limbs and impotence.

3. Diabetes may first present as a fulminating ketoacidosis associated with an acute infection or even without evidence of a precipitating cause, and in such cases epigastric pain and vomiting may be the presenting complaints. This is more likely to occur in the juvenile-onset type and such cases are acute medical emergencies.

4. Finally, patients may present with symptoms due to the complications of diabetes.

The severity of many of the classical symptoms of clinical diabetes are directly related to the severity of glycosuria. If relatively mild hyperglycaemia has developed slowly over many years the renal threshold for glucose will rise, glycosuria may be slight, and the symptoms of diabetes correspondingly trivial.

Physical Signs depend very much on the mode of presentation. Cases without complications will usually show no abnormal physical signs attributable to diabetes. In some cases vulvitis or balanitis may be found, since the external genitalia are especially prone to infection by fungi (Candida) which flourish on the skin and mucous membranes contaminated by glucose. In the fulminating case the most striking features are those of dehydration. The intraocular pressure may be obviously reduced. A rapid pulse and a low blood pressure may then be anticipated. Breathing may be deep and sighing in the acidotic patient; the breath is usually fetid and the sickly sweet smell of acetone may be noticeable. Mental apathy and confusion may be present or there may be stupor or even coma.

Evidence of complications of diabetes may be noted. Ophthalmoscopy may show the typical appearance of diabetic retinopathy (p. 579). The most constant early signs of diabetic neuropathy are depression or loss of the ankle jerks, and impaired vibration sense in the legs (p. 582).

The presence of diabetic nephropathy may be indicated by proteinuria in addition to glycosuria; rarely the other features of the nephrotic syndrome may be apparent.

Potential and latent diabetics may complain of no symptoms and there may be no abnormality detectable on examination. However certain features are recognised as being characteristic of potential diabetes without necessarily implying that individuals who show these features will progress inevitably to clinical diabetes. For example it has been demonstrated that genetically constituted potential diabetics are predisposed to coronary arterial and peripheral vascular disease. They may show abnormal lipid patterns in response to oral contraceptives. They have a high incidence of still-born babies, abnormally large and heavy babies and babies with congenital defects. They may be much overweight at a time when there is no detectable abnormality in terms of carbohydrate intolerance.

Diagnosis. By definition hyperglycaemia remains the *sine qua non* of the clinical diagnosis of diabetes mellitus. In the individual case when the classical symptoms are present, the diagnosis is often beyond reasonable doubt by the time the history taking and physical examination are complete, and it may then be confirmed by the finding of marked glycosuria, with or without ketonuria, and a random blood sugar greater than 13·9 mmol/*l* (250 mg/100 ml). However in many cases, particularly those with diabetes of later onset who have few if any symptoms, and where glycosuria is frequently discovered by chance, the diagnosis is less obvious and a glucose tolerance test will be required.

URINE TESTING. *Glycosuria*. For individual screening purposes sensitive and glucose-specific dip-stick methods are available. Clinistix consists of a paper stick impregnated with an enzyme preparation which turns purple when dipped in urine containing glucose. No other urinary constituent gives this reaction: it therefore provides a rapid and specific qualitative test for glucose. A positive response indicates that the urinary glucose concentration exceeds 0·55–1·11 mmol/*l* (10–20 mg/100 ml), but does not measure the amount accurately. Semiquantitative measurement of urinary reducing activity can be obtained using copper reduction methods, most conveniently with the Clinitest tablet.

When Clinitest tablets only are used to detect reducing substances in the urine, it may be necessary to establish the identity of the urinary reducing agent. Glucose can easily be identified with Clinistix. Other reducing substances, however, occasionally occur in urine, including lactose, which may be found in the later stages of pregnancy or during lactation. Pentosuria, fructosuria and galactosuria may all occur as manifestations of rare genetic disorders and special methods are required for the identification of these reducing substances when they occur in urine.

It is common practice to examine overnight specimens of urine for glucose. By using such a procedure the milder cases of diabetes will be overlooked. If a sample collected during the 2 hours following a meal is examined, then more of the milder cases will be recognised. There is at present no comparably simple procedure which in the individual case is of so much value in indicating the presence of grosser degrees of hyperglycaemia as testing the urine for sugar. The most serious disadvantage in the use of the urine test diagnostically arises from individual variations in renal threshold, so that on the one hand some undoubtedly diabetic people have a negative urine test for glucose due to a raised renal threshold, and on the other those with a low renal threshold give a false positive test. In order to distinguish cases of this type from patients with mild diabetes, suitable tests of carbohydrate tolerance are required.

Detection of Ketone Bodies in Urine. The amounts of ketone bodies normally excreted by healthy persons are not detected but clinically important amounts can be recognised by the nitroprusside reaction which is conveniently carried out using Acetest tablets or Ketostix test papers. Ketonuria may be found in normal people who have been fasting for long periods, who have been vomiting repeatedly or who have been eating a diet very high in fats and low in carbohydrate. Ketonuria is therefore not pathognomonic of diabetes, but if both ketonuria and glycosuria are found, the diagnosis of diabetes is practically certain.

RANDOM BLOOD SUGAR. In many cases the clinical diagnosis of diabetes can be made with the help of a single blood sugar estimation, which may be used as the final confirmatory test when the symptoms strongly suggest the diagnosis. In these circumstances a random blood sugar exceeding 13·9 mmol/*l* (250 mg/100 ml) is almost certain to indicate diabetes. However, a random blood sugar below this level does not exclude diabetes, and in this case some degree of standardisation of the conditions under which the blood sugar is measured is necessary. In practice, the oral glucose tolerance test is the cornerstone of the diagnosis of diabetes unless a grossly elevated single blood sugar measurement, with or without clinical symptomatology, has already made this clear.

THE ORAL GLUCOSE TOLERANCE TEST (Fig. 11.9). The patient, who should have been on an unrestricted carbohydrate intake of at least 250 g for 3 days or more, fasts overnight. Out-patients should rest for at least half an hour before starting the test, and should remain seated and refrain from smoking during the test. A sample of blood is taken to measure the fasting blood glucose level and 50 g glucose dissolved in about 200 ml of water is then given by mouth. Thereafter samples of blood are collected at half-hourly intervals for 2 hours, and their glucose content is estimated.

The WHO Committee on Diabetes (1965) recommended that the following levels of glucose, either fasting or 2 hours after the glucose load, should be accepted as normal or diabetic respectively.

	Glucose concentration mmol/l (mg/100 ml)	
Sample	Normal	Diabetic
Venous blood	<6·1 (110)	>7·2 (130)
Capillary blood	<6·6 (120)	>7·7 (140)
Plasma	<7·5 (135)	>8·6 (155)

Intermediate readings call for scrutiny of the curve as a whole and further evaluation of the patient, including the history obtained. It may be necessary to keep the patient under observation and to repeat the test at a later date.

The particular method of estimating the blood sugar and the precise technique used for carrying out the glucose tolerance test should be taken into account. In elderly persons and in patients after myocardial infarction or with malignant disease, blood glucose concentrations may be somewhat higher than those quoted above, without the patient necessarily having diabetes.

Differential Diagnosis of Glycosuria. *Renal Glycosuria.* Apart from diabetes, the commonest cause of glycosuria is renal glycosuria. If glucose regularly and consistently appears in the urine when the blood level is less than 10·0 mmol/l the individual is said to have a low renal threshold for glucose, or renal glycosuria. This is a benign condition which may run in families and which commonly occurs temporarily in pregnancy, due probably in this case to an increase in the glomerular filtration rate. Renal glycosuria is unrelated to diabetes, and is not accompanied by the symptoms of glycosuria in diabetes, i.e. thirst and polyuria, although pruritus vulvae and even ketonuria may occur.

Renal glycosuria is a much more frequent cause of glycosuria than diabetes in young persons, particularly in the age group 20 to 30 years, when they are commonly examined prior to entering the armed services, professions and industry. In the older age groups the reverse holds, and hyperglycaemia in excess of 11·1 mmol/l can occur without any glycosuria. For this reason if urine tests for glucose are used as a method of screening for diabetes, some cases will be missed, so that a glucose tolerance test or at least a single blood glucose estimation 2 hours after an oral dose of 50 g of glucose should be used whenever possible.

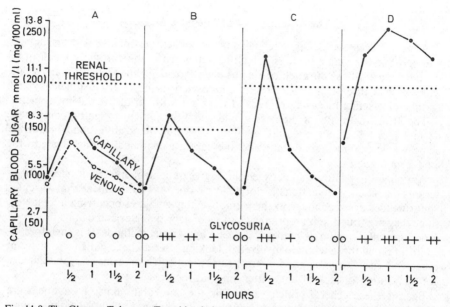

Fig. 11.9 The Glucose Tolerance Test: blood glucose curves after 50 g glucose by mouth, showing (A) normal curve, (B) renal glycosuria, (C) alimentary (lag storage) glycosuria and (D) diabetes mellitus of moderate severity.

It may be important to determine the renal threshold for glucose, and this can be done reliably only by testing samples of urine for glucose taken at intervals of half an hour in the course of a glucose tolerance test and relating the results to the blood glucose concentration. This information may be specially important in the occasional diabetic with a low renal glucose threshold who, if attempts are made to control his diabetes on urine tests alone, is likely to be kept in a persistent state of hypoglycaemia.

Alimentary (Lag Storage) Glycosuria. In some individuals an unusually rapid but transitory rise of blood glucose follows a meal and the concentration exceeds the normal renal threshold; during this time glucose will be present in the urine. This response to a meal or to a dose of glucose is traditionally known as 'lag storage', although alimentary glycosuria is a better term; it is not uncommon as a cause of symptomless glycosuria. It may occur in otherwise normal people or after a partial gastrectomy, when it is due to rapid absorption, or in patients with hyperthyroidism or hepatic disease. This type of blood glucose curve is usually regarded as benign and unrelated to diabetes; although the peak blood glucose is abnormally elevated, the value 2 hours after oral glucose is normal (Fig. 11.9).

Other Metabolic Disorders. Impaired carbohydrate tolerance with associated glycosuria may occur with any of the forms of secondary diabetes (p. 556).

Raised Intracranial Pressure. A cerebral tumour, haemorrhage or injury may be associated with glycosuria.

Starvation. Carbohydrate deprivation can lead to the development of a diabetic type of blood glucose curve with associated glycosuria in normal people. It would seem, however, that the daily carbohydrate intake has to be less than about 50 g before it has a notable effect. This effect of a low carbohydrate intake may be of importance clinically in relation to the diagnosis of diabetes in a person on a reducing diet or if acutely ill with a low daily intake of food.

The Management of Diabetes Mellitus

Aims of Treatment. Diabetic patients no longer die in ketoacidosis in any number, but the major problem which has emerged is the chronic invalidism of many of those whose duration of life has been extended. They live for many years with vascular disease such as cerebral atherosclerosis, coronary insufficiency and peripheral vascular disease, with renal disease and with serious visual impairment.

The ideal treatment for diabetes would allow the patient to lead a completely normal life, to remain not only symptom-free but in positive good health, to achieve a normal metabolic state, and to escape the complications associated with long-term diabetes.

Although the relationship between the degree of control and the development of serious diabetic complications is not a simple one, it would appear that vascular abnormalities are secondary to the metabolic abnormalities occurring in diabetes, since they are found in both primary and secondary diabetes and can be produced experimentally in animals rendered diabetic by various methods. It is therefore incumbent on all those who are involved in looking after diabetic patients to strive in every way to achieve as good control as is practicable in terms of blood glucose concentration, for lack of any better index at the present time.

Bearing these general principles in mind the immediate aims of treatment are therefore, first, the abolition of symptoms of diabetes while avoiding hypo-glycaemia, second, the correction of hyperglycaemia and glycosuria and, third, the attainment and maintenance of an appropriate body weight.

The patient should realise as early as possible that it is upon him that success or failure will depend. The doctor can only advise. As adherence to a diabetic regimen demands from the patient self-discipline and a sense of purpose, every effort should be made to ensure that he understands the object of each aspect of his management. Accordingly, time must be spent on the education of the patient, and the doctor must be responsible for ensuring that his diabetic patients are educated to the limit of their abilities and that as far as possible they have adjusted adequately to their condition and have sufficient knowledge to undertake the day-to-day management of their diabetes competently.

As soon as the diagnosis is certain the patient should be told that he has diabetes, he should be reassured, and instruction and treatment begun forthwith. The average patient suffers from an acute anxiety reaction on being told that he has diabetes. If he understands what is wrong with him, why he has certain symptoms, and what he must do to correct the abnormalities present, it will be found that he is much less afraid and much more co-operative in carrying out the regime prescribed.

Types of Treatment. There are three methods of treatment and each involves an obligation for the patient to adhere to a dietary regimen for the remainder of his life, namely diet alone, diet and oral hypoglycaemic drugs and diet and insulin.

Approximately 50 per cent of new cases of diabetes can be controlled adequately by diet alone, about 20 per cent require insulin and another 30 per cent will need an oral hypoglycaemic drug. The principles governing the choice of therapeutic regimen when a diabetic patient is seen for the first time are discussed on page 571. A patient may pass from one group to another temporarily or permanently.

Diet. GENERAL PRINCIPLES. The treatment of all diabetic patients, especially those who require insulin, involves some dietary restrictions if control is to be satisfactory. By regulating the amount and the times of food intake, particularly the carbohydrate intake, and by dove-tailing the dose of insulin, or of oral hypoglycaemic agent, an attempt is made to achieve a flat profile of glycaemia throughout the day and night. It is obvious that if the intake of food varies from day to day it is impossible to work out a steady insulin or other regime to cover it. It is extremely important that patients should understand that this is the main reason for dietary restriction. Many have the mistaken idea that the main purpose of dietary measures in their treatment is the avoidance of certain 'bad' foods.

If one is to achieve a fixed daily intake and avoid the monotony of a static diet sheet, some kind of exchange system is necessary, and this is the basis for the construction of nearly all diets in use today. Many doctors are intimidated by the number and variety of diet sheets published and feel that, since they are not trained dietitians, they cannot treat diabetes. A dietitian is certainly most helpful but is not indispensable; the basic principles of an exchange system of dietary treatment are simple, although the education of a patient in their use is time-consuming.

The first step in preparing any dietary regimen is to map out a time-table of the patient's day including a description of his usual meals. This is an essential step and one which is too often omitted. The total daily requirement of calories must next be decided. The diet must be nutritionally adequate for the patient's needs, and it must, therefore, be estimated for each individual patient after considering such factors as age, sex, actual weight in relation to desirable weight (Table 18.2 p. 948), activity, occupation, and financial resources. An approximate range for the various groups might be (1) an obese, middle-aged or elderly patient with mild diabetes, 1,000–1,600 kcal daily, (2) an elderly diabetic but not overweight, 1,400–1,800 kcal daily, (3) a young, active diabetic, 1,800–3,000 kcal daily. The importance of maintaining the body weight at or slightly below the ideal for the patient's height cannot be overemphasised. Thus the calorie range of group 2 may have to be extended if it is not sufficient to maintain weight, and young patients in group 3 who are overweight may have to reduce their daily intake to below 1,800 kcal, perhaps temporarily.

Next the proportion of calories derived from carbohydrate, protein and fat must be allocated. The approximate ratio in British diets is, protein 12 per cent, fat 42 per cent and carbohydrate 46 per cent. Although all sucrose should be eliminated from the diet the percentage of calories derived from carbohydrate should usually remain about the same, those from protein increased if this is practicable, and those from fat reduced. In most diabetic diets, therefore, the percentage of calories derived from carbohydrate should be 45–48 per cent, from protein 15–18 per cent and less than 40 per cent from fat.

The daily intake of *carbohydrate* to be prescribed ranges from the minimum sufficient to prevent ketonuria, that is, 100 g daily, to a maximum of 240–260 g. The upper limit is imposed by the fact that it is difficult to achieve satisfactory blood glucose levels throughout 24 hours with a daily carbohydrate intake greater than this. If the daily intake of carbohydrate is 240 g, approximately 50 g of carbohydrate will usually be provided by each of the three main meals, 20 g by each of three snacks and 30 g by one pint of milk (540 ml) taken in the course of the day. Experience has shown that it is very difficult to prevent an excessive rise in the blood glucose concentration after each meal with amounts larger than this even when all the carbohydrate consumed is in the form of starch. A simple method of calculating the carbohydrate content of the diet is to allocate a figure equivalent to one-tenth of the total calories plus approximately 30 g to carbohydrate, that is, if a diet of 1,800 kcal is prescribed it should contain about 210 g of carbohydrate, providing 840 kcal or 46 per cent of the total. All the carbohydrate eaten should be in the form of starch. Readily absorbed carbohydrates, such as glucose and sucrose, should generally be avoided because they produce sudden rises in the blood glucose level.

The consumption of *protein* is largely determined by social and economic considerations and will frequently be lower than would be considered desirable. If this is the case, every effort should be made to increase the protein intake and to try to ensure that some protein is eaten at each main meal. An adequate consumption of protein is necessary in children and adolescents to ensure satisfactory growth, and since amino acids stimulate the beta cells of the pancreas to secrete insulin, in both normal subjects and in those with insulin-independent diabetes, a smaller rise in blood glucose concentration occurs when carbohydrate is consumed along with protein. In both categories of diabetic patients consumption of protein will also promote satiety and so help them to keep more strictly to their carbohydrate allowance. A minimum amount of protein should therefore be specified in all diabetic diets, but in the case of those who are not obese it should be emphasised that more than the amount specified may be taken if desired. The daily consumption of protein will usually lie in the range of 60–110 g.

The *fat* intake should be adjusted to bring the total calories to the level desired, and will usually amount to 50–150 g daily. Because diabetic patients have an increased risk of death from ischaemic heart disease, and because ischaemic heart disease may be related to the amount of saturated fat in the diet, the total amount of fat should be restricted even in those who are not obese. Plasma lipids, particularly cholesterol, should be checked regularly and if significantly elevated the diabetic diet may be appropriately modified (p. 589).

When the patient's requirements have been assessed the figures must be translated into practical and comprehensible instructions for the patient, using one of the types of diet prescription sheets described below.

Each patient should be given a cyclostyled or printed copy of the list of exchanges (p. 922) with instructions regarding the meals at which they may be taken. The diet sheet and exchanges must be discussed with the patient repeatedly and with a relative if necessary until the system is fully understood.

TYPES OF DIET. Basically there are two types of diet: (1) measured, in which the amount of food to be eaten at each time of the day is specified, and (2) unmeasured, in which the patient is supplied with a list of foods grouped in three categories: foods with a high sucrose content which are to be avoided altogether; foods containing carbohydrate in the form of starch which are to be eaten in moderation only; and non-carbohydrate foods which may be eaten as desired. An example is shown on page 946.

Measured Diets. In these diets the portions of food may be measured either by weighing with scales or more simply by using household measures. Measured diets are required for two groups of patients, (a) those who require insulin or an oral hypoglycaemic agent, and (b) those who are overweight and require a strict reducing regimen.

Patients in group (a) should if at all possible weigh out the portions of food initially. They should be provided with a simple balance (available on NHS prescription) for this purpose. After a few weeks most patients are capable of assessing the weight of portions with sufficient accuracy by eye, and regular weighing becomes less necessary. However it is often valuable to check visual assessments by weighing from time to time. A method of constructing a sample diet of 1,800 kcal suitable for patients in group (*a*) is described on pages 941 to 945. The exchanges for carbohydrate, protein and fat on which it is based are set out on pages 942 to 944. It is important to realise that the exchanges or portions employed as units are arbitrary and are decided mainly in the light of the food habits of the population as a whole. The British Diabetic and Dietetic Associations have recommended that the carbohydrate unit should contain 10 g carbohydrate. In Britain the staple carbohydrate food is bread, and the basic carbohydrate exchange for the purposes of calculation is therefore taken to be $\frac{2}{3}$ oz bread which contains 10 g carbohydrate, along with 2 g protein and $\frac{2}{3}$ g fat. This is the reason why a carbohydrate exchange (p. 941) contains some protein and fat in addition to carbohydrate. Note also that a protein exchange contains some fat.

Diabetics who are obese should be urged to accept a reducing regime (p. 147). The method of achieving reduction in weight is the same for obese diabetic patients as for those with simple obesity. Diet No. 1 (p. 939) will meet the needs of many. The portions in this diet can be weighed out with scales but more usually are dispensed using household measures as described in this diet. It should be explained that such a strict diet is to be followed temporarily only until the standard weight is reached; thereafter the diet may be increased, and if the patient is sufficiently intelligent, advice can then be given on how to avoid monotony by using the list of exchanges for diabetic diets provided on pages 942 to 945.

Unmeasured Diets. If insulin or oral hypoglycaemic agents are not required and marked obesity is not present, it may not be necessary for the patient to follow such an accurate diet. Sometimes it may be impracticable to do so because of the patient's mental, visual or other physical incapacity or unwillingness to co-operate. Many patients develop the disease when they are already middle-aged or elderly and have a mild type of diabetes often associated with moderate obesity. For such patients an unmeasured diet of the type described on page 946 may be adequate.

Alcohol. There is no medical objection to taking alcoholic drinks in moderation provided the patient realises that he must take account of their calorie value and sometimes of their carbohydrate content. Beer for example may contain 10–30 g of carbohydrate per half litre (1 pint approx.) and with the alcohol this will provide 150–400 kcal, depending on the strength of the beer. Sweet wines and cider all have a high carbohydrate content, and spirits such as whisky and gin, while free of carbohydrates, contain about 70 kcal per 30 ml.

Sweetening Agents. Advice may also be asked about sweetening agents and so-called diabetic foods and drinks. Saccharin has been employed as a sweetening agent for many years. It has no calorie value. Sorbitol, a glucose derivative, and fructose are also added to 'diabetic' foods and drinks for sweetening purposes. In moderate quantities neither will interfere with the action or requirements of insulin. If a patient is having difficulty in reducing weight or in maintaining a normal weight, then the use of substitutes for sugar should be discouraged, since they may perpetuate the patient's desire to eat sweet foods and thus make it more difficult for him to tolerate dietary restrictions. Diabetic chocolate has a high fat content and this must be taken into account.

Oral Hypoglycaemic Drugs. A number of compounds are effective in reducing hyperglycaemia in patients who would otherwise require insulin. The sulphonylureas, tolbutamide and chlorpropamide, and to a lesser extent the biguanides, metformin and phenformin, have a place in the management of about 30 per cent of diabetic patients. Although their mechanism of action is different, the action of both groups depends upon a supply of endogenous insulin, and it is therefore futile and dangerous to attempt to control juvenile-onset diabetes with these compounds.

SULPHONYLUREAS. *Tolbutamide* is the mildest, and probably also the safest, of the sulphonylureas. Since its effective action does not exceed 6 to 8 hours it should be administered two to three times a day. The dose varies between 1 and 2 g daily. It is very well tolerated and toxic reactions such as skin rashes occur only rarely. Unfortunately, the relapse rate is relatively high.

Chlorpropamide has a biological half-life of about 36 hours, and an effective concentration can be maintained in the blood by a single dose at breakfast. The usual maintenance dose is between 100 and 375 mg daily; larger doses should not be used on a long-term basis, since above this level there is an increased risk of toxic effects, such as jaundice, drug rashes, and blood dyscrasia. Two other effects of clinical importance should be noted. If alcohol is taken following chlor-propamide an unpleasant flushing of the face occurs in some patients. Chlor-propamide may lead to severe hypoglycaemia, which can be very refractory to treatment. Great care must be taken to avoid this, particularly in elderly patients, and once glycosuria has been abolished and symptoms relieved, the daily dose of chlorpropamide must be reduced to the minimum required to maintain control. In fact many patients who require 375–500 mg daily initially can be maintained on a long-term basis on 100 mg or less per day.

Newer Sulphonylureas. Acetohexamide, tolazamide, glibenclamide, glipizide and glymidine usually offer little advantage over these two older compounds but may be useful in individual cases.

Sulphonylureas are valuable in the treatment of patients with maturity-onset diabetes who fail to respond to simple dietary restriction and who are not overweight. Sulphonylureas should not be given to obese patients since their use may be associated with a considerable increase in weight and with a consequent reduction in life expectancy.

BIGUANIDES. The biguanides are less widely used in Britain than the sul-phonylureas, because of the higher incidence of side-effects, particularly gas-trointestinal symptoms and because there have been a significant number of deaths from lactic acidosis in patients taking these drugs. However, the biguanides are valuable in two clinical situations. Firstly, since their administration is not associated with an increase in weight, they are to be preferred when it is essential to treat a patient with maturity-onset diabetes who is overweight but in whom hyperglycaemia persists despite efforts to adhere to a diet and reduce weight. Secondly, as the hypoglycaemic effect of the biguanides appears to be synergistic with that of the sulphonylureas, there is a place for combining the two when the sulphonylureas alone have proved inadequate (primary failure), and when, as happens with 5 to 10 per cent of patients, initial success is followed after several months or even 1 to 2 years by loss of control (secondary failure).

Metformin is less likely to cause gastrointestinal side-effects and lactic acidosis than *phenformin*, and is given with food in two or three daily doses of 0·5–1·0 g each. Its use is contraindicated in patients with chronic renal or hepatic disease and in those who take alcohol in excess, as the risk of lactic acidosis occurring is significantly increased in such patients. Its administration should be discontinued, at least temporarily, if any other serious medical condition develops, and treatment with insulin substituted.

CLINICAL USE OF SULPHONYLUREAS AND BIGUANIDES. Patients may be started on an oral hypoglycaemic drug as soon as it is clear that dietary measures alone are inadequate. It is usually possible to reach a decision on the success or failure of these drugs within a week, though occasionally a full response may not be apparent for considerably longer. Diabetics treated successfully in this way for prolonged periods may ultimately need an alteration of dose or a change of regime temporarily or permanently; in particular they may require insulin to meet the needs created by a severe infection, an operation or other stress.

A report from America suggests that those taking an oral hypoglycaemic drug are at increased risk of dying from ischaemic heart disease. This may be due to a high incidence of ventricular fibrillation in diabetic patients on oral therapy who sustain a myocardial infarct. Although the case against these drugs is not yet proven, strenuous efforts should be made to control as many patients as possible by diet alone for this and other reasons (p. 568). Furthermore those taking oral hypoglycaemic drugs who develop a myocardial infarct should have these replaced by insulin during the acute illness and have a longer period of close supervision than non-diabetics, preferably in a coronary care unit.

Insulin. With one or more of the preparations of insulin available it is usually possible to keep the blood glucose within reasonable, although not physiological, limits throughout the day and night without undue risk of hypoglycaemia.

Two main therapeutic forms of insulin are available, namely (1) rapid-onset, short-acting and (2) delayed-onset, long-acting or 'depot' preparations. There are various varieties of each type as shown in Table 11.2 (p. 570). The older beef insulins contain varying amounts of glucagon, pro-insulin, altered insulin and other peptides, and these, rather than insulin itself, are largely responsible for the insulin-binding antibodies found in the plasma of all patients treated with conventional insulins. Highly purified, 'monocomponent' or 'single peak' porcine insulins are available which are virtually non-antigenic (e.g. Actrapid MC and Leo Neutral insulin). These new insulins are more expensive and their use is largely reserved for patients with either abnormal resistance or allergy to the older preparations, e.g. fat atrophy at injection sites. However, the purer preparations will probably supersede the older preparations. Care must be taken to avoid hypoglycaemia when transferring patients from the older to the newer preparations, and the higher the dose of conventional insulin, the stricter the supervision required. All the therapeutic preparations of insulin are made in concentrations of 40 and 80 units per ml, and soluble insulin is also available in a concentration of 20 units per ml and 320 units per ml.

SOLUBLE INSULINS. These are clear solutions in contrast to the depot insulins which are cloudy. When injected subcutaneously, soluble insulin is rapidly effective (Table 11.2) but the action is relatively short-lived. A patient stabilised on soluble insulin alone would therefore need at least two injections in the day.

Soluble insulin is essential in the following circumstances:

(a) For new cases with severe dehydration or ketoacidosis.

(b) For emergencies associated with ketosis, such as acute infection, gastroenteritis and some surgical operations.

(c) For the treatment of nearly all young patients.

Table 11.2

Preparation of insulin	Antigenicity	Hypoglycaemic effect	Approximate duration of effect in hours		
			Start	Maximum	Termination
Soluble	++	Rapid onset and short duration			
Actrapid MC	0		½	4–6	6–10
Insulin Leo Neutral	0				
Globin	+++	Intermediate			
IZS Amorphous (semilente)	+				10–14
Semitard MC	0		2–3	6–10	
Isophane (NPH)	+++				12–22
Insulin Leo Retard	0				
PZI	+++	Slow onset and long duration			
IZS Crystalline (ultralente)	+		4–6	8–14	20–30
Monotard MC	0				

DEPOT INSULINS. In a relatively small number of cases an adequate degree of control can be established by a single morning injection of depot insulin. Such patients are usually elderly with relatively mild diabetes. Most insulin-requiring diabetics however do best on a depot insulin with one or two supporting doses of soluble insulin. The choice of depot insulin in an individual case is determined by consideration of the patient's way of life, including his meal pattern, type of occupation, hours of work and recreation, in relation to the time of action of the various depot insulins. More insulin will be required to cover main meals and periods of inactivity, and vice versa.

Protamine Zinc Insulin (PZI). The addition of zinc and protamine to soluble insulin delays its release from the site of injection, so that PZI exerts its maximum effect on the blood glucose later, and the duration of action is longer, than soluble insulin (Table 11.2). Despite its prolonged action PZI does not always keep the blood glucose within acceptable limits throughout the 24 hours. Glycosuria is most likely to occur before the morning injection has taken full effect, and a dose of soluble insulin is generally required in the morning and sometimes in the evening, especially in young patients. Merely to increase the morning dose of PZI may result in severe hypoglycaemia later in the day or night. Indeed it is a good rule that the dose of PZI should not exceed 40 units at a single injection. When giving soluble insulin and PZI together, the two should not be mixed in the syringe, but may be given through the same skin puncture. If the two are mixed the protamine in the PZI will convert some of the soluble insulin into PZI.

Insulin Zinc Suspensions (IZS). The rate of release of these insulins from the tissues is related to the size of the insulin particles which are suspended in acetate buffer. Three preparations are available:

(*a*) IZS amorphous (*semilente*) insulin has a duration of action which is intermediate between that of soluble and protamine zinc insulin.

(*b*) IZS crystalline (*ultralente*) insulin is slower in action than IZS (amorphous) insulin (Table 11.2).

(*c*) IZS (*lente*) insulin is a mixture of three parts of amorphous with seven parts of crystalline material. It is dispensed when IZS is prescribed unless the prescription specifically orders semilente (amorphous) or ultralente (crystalline).

There are two highly purified IZS preparations: Semitard MC, its time of action corresponding to semilente; and Monotard MC, corresponding to lente.

Globin Insulin. This is another depot insulin, intermediate in duration of action between soluble and protamine zinc insulin.

Isophane (NPH) Insulin. This is similar in action to globin insulin, though its effect is slightly more prolonged. Since isophane insulin contains an excess of soluble insulin it can be mixed in the same syringe as soluble insulin. This is convenient particularly if an automatic injector (for example a 'Hypogard' or a 'Palmer Injector') is used. Many younger patients are best treated with isophane and soluble insulin taken twice daily.

A highly purified depot insulin, corresponding to isophane insulin, is also available (Leo Retard).

In practice one must be prepared to try combinations of the various insulin preparations, and to vary the time at which they are administered in the light of the results of urine tests and blood glucose estimations at different times of the day until smooth control is achieved over the 24-hour period. It is impossible to forecast the response of a patient to insulin, and the daily dose required to establish control varies from 10 to 100 units or more.

A practical point worth mentioning, since it may give rise to distress if not anticipated, is that blurring of vision (which may occur in a severe diabetic before treatment) may become noticeably worse after starting treatment with insulin. It is due to transitory osmotic abnormalities in the eye, especially the lens, and may persist for as long as several weeks after initiating treatment.

Choice of Therapeutic Regime. It must be emphasised that the regime eventually adopted in each case of diabetes is chosen by a process of trial, and that changes may be needed as more is learned about the patient and the kind of diabetes which he has.

The chief indications for the main types of therapeutic regimen are:

1. Practically all young patients who develop diabetes before the age of 40 require treatment with insulin. The majority will be best controlled by taking soluble insulin in the morning along with one of the depot insulins, most usually protamine zinc insulin or isophane insulin. In addition a second dose of soluble insulin, or of soluble and depot insulin (most commonly isophane insulin), may be required before the evening meal.

2. The majority of patients developing the disease over the age of 40 can and should be controlled by diet alone. This applies particularly to obese patients, but others who are not overweight may also do well on dietary therapy alone.

3. Those over the age of 40 who fail to achieve satisfactory control by dietary measures alone will usually respond well to a sulphonylurea if they are not obese, or to a biguanide if they are obese. If adequate control is not achieved by one drug, a combination of sulphonylurea and biguanide may be tried. If this fails insulin will be required.

4. Elderly patients who require insulin will often do well with a relatively small dose (20 units) of a depot insulin alone, such as PZI, IZS (lente) or isophane insulin. A few, particularly those who would otherwise require more than 40 units of PZI a day to be adequately controlled, should be given soluble insulin in addition.

It must be stressed again that obese patients should be treated by dietary restriction and weight reduction rather than by the administration of insulin or other hypoglycaemic agent. The advent of the 'insulin era' has obscured the remarkable improvement in glucose tolerance which usually results from reduction in weight. Insulin and the sulphonylureas increase the appetite, and thus may increase weight and intensify the total disability.

Initiation of Treatment. It is rarely necessary to admit diabetic patients to hospital for initial stabilisation. Indeed it is desirable that the patient learns to manage all aspects of his disorder as quickly as possible, and this can best be done as an outpatient while leading a relatively normal existence at home and at work. However, patients being stabilised on insulin have to be seen daily at first and if this is not otherwise possible, admission to hospital will be necessary. Hospital admission will also be necessary for patients with severe ketoacidosis.

As soon as the diagnosis is made a careful search is necessary to detect early evidence of the complications to which the diabetic is prone (pp. 578–583). These include coronary artery disease and hypertension, obliterative arterial disease, peripheral neuropathy, cataract, retinopathy, nephropathy, pulmonary tuberculosis and other infections, particularly of the skin and urinary tract.

PATIENT'S EDUCATION. 1. Every patient who is capable of learning must be taught how to test his urine with a Clinitest set (and sometimes with Acetest tablets also), to keep a record of the results and to understand their significance.

2. All patients requiring insulin must learn to measure their dose of insulin accurately with an insulin syringe (B.S. 1619), to give their own injections and to adjust the dose themselves on the basis of urine tests and other factors such as illness, unusual exercise and insulin reactions. They should be made to experience an insulin reaction (p. 573) at an early stage, so that they know what this involves, can recognise the early signs and take appropriate action.

3. All patients must have a working knowledge of diabetes, i.e. they must be able to recognise the symptoms associated with marked glycosuria and to understand their significance. They must be told that many drugs have undesirable effects on the diabetic state, as may also such other factors as illness of any kind or emotional upset. They should be advised to come to the doctor or the clinic at once, without prior appointment, as soon as they are aware of any deterioration in health or urine tests which does not respond rapidly to the simple measures that they take themselves.

4. All patients must know how to take care of their feet, and learn to treat any infected lesion with respect.

Education of the patient is time-consuming and repeated practical demonstrations may also be required. It may be supplemented by reading appropriate booklets. However, it is only in this way that diabetic patients can safely undertake all normal activities while maintaining good control of their disease. If the patient is a child, or is blind, mentally defective or otherwise incapable, instructions in these matters must be given to a parent, or other attendant.

It is a wise precaution for diabetic patients who are taking insulin or oral hypoglycaemic drugs to carry a card with them at all times stating their name and address, the fact that they are diabetic, the nature and dose of any insulin or other drugs they may be taking, and, in addition, giving the name, address and telephone number of their family doctor and any special diabetic clinic they may be attending. Suitable cards are provided by the British Diabetic Association for the use of members.

SUPERVISION OF PATIENT. Diabetics should be seen at regular intervals for the remainder of their lives. The object is to check the degree of control and if necessary to make appropriate alterations in treatment and to watch for any complications. Records should be kept so that the doctor is immediately on the alert if changes in health occur. The frequency of visits is determined by the severity of the disability, the reliability of the patient and his ability to manage his own condition.

For the general practitioner with diabetic patients scattered widely in his practice, this supervision may be difficult. For this reason and because of the need to develop and apply new and better techniques for the control of diabetes, many hospitals arrange diabetic clinics.

ASSESSMENT OF CONTROL. At the patient's regular visit to the diabetic clinic or to his general practitioner, the degree of control should be assessed by considering the patient's weight in relation to his standard weight; the results of urine tests; the blood glucose estimation; the presence or absence of symptoms of either hyper- or hypoglycaemia.

Urine Testing. Proper assessment of control is impossible unless in the course of his normal activity the patient tests samples of urine regularly. By selecting suitable times for the tests and tabulating the results, it is easy for the doctor or the experienced patient to decide whether the dose of insulin or hypoglycaemic drug should be increased or reduced, or whether the carbohydrate content of the diet or the time when it is taken should be altered.

Diabetics taking insulin should test samples of urine obtained before breakfast, before the mid-day and evening meals, and at bedtime (prior to a bedtime snack if this is taken). The patient must empty his bladder and discard this urine about 30 minutes before passing a specimen for testing. Otherwise the premeal specimen will include urine secreted into the bladder after the previous meal and will give the impression that the blood glucose concentration before meals is higher than it really is. Patients treated by diet alone or with oral hypoglycaemic agents should test the first morning specimen and a sample passed about 2 hours after the main meals of the day. The majority of all the above specimens should be either free of or contain $\frac{1}{4}$ per cent of glucose or less.

While the patient is being stabilised, tests will have to be carried out three or four times daily; when control is established the frequency can be greatly reduced. Three or four tests on a single day once or twice weekly are much more informative about the state of control than a single test carried out daily. A full series of tests should be undertaken therefore on one or more selected days each week.

Blood glucose Estimations. At the patient's regular visits to the diabetic clinic, it is advisable to measure the blood sugar level as an additional index of the degree of control. In assessing the result it is important to consider the interval between taking the sample and the last meal and also previous physical activity. A series of estimations made over several months, or even years, provides a useful record of the patient's ability to control his disease. This is particularly important during pregnancy when the renal threshold may fall temporarily.

Insulin Reactions and Hypoglycaemia. If soluble insulin is administered to a normal person the blood glucose falls, producing symptoms that may begin to appear when the concentration is about 2·7 mmol/l (50 mg/100 ml) and are fully developed at about 2·2 mmol/l. In diabetics who are constantly hyperglycaemic, the same symptoms may develop at much higher levels, e.g. 6·6 mmol/l or more.

In order of frequency the symptoms include a feeling of being weak and empty, hunger, sweating, palpitation, tremor, faintness, dizziness, headache, diplopia and mental confusion. Abnormal behaviour, leading occasionally to arrest by the police on a charge of being drunk and disorderly may also occur. Alternatively, and particularly in children, there may be lassitude and somnolence, muscular twitchings, deepening coma and convulsions.

Hypoglycaemia induces secretion of adrenaline, and this in turn causes tachycardia and tremor. Adrenaline, by mobilising liver glycogen, combats the hypoglycaemia. This homeostatic reaction on the part of the body partly explains why patients rarely die of hypoglycaemic coma from too much soluble insulin. By contrast, coma is dangerous when it arises from a large dose of depot insulin or from an overdose of a sulphonylurea, particularly chlorpropamide. The latter condition although relatively uncommon is resistant to treatment, since the drug reduces the hepatic release of glucose, and because the half-life of the drug is so long. The brain is dependent on the blood glucose for the energy necessary for its activity. For this reason, hypoglycaemia should be prevented from recurring by prompt reduction of the dose of insulin or of sulphonylurea.

Hypoglycaemia due to overdosage with soluble insulin comes on rapidly, at the time when the insulin is having its maximum effect (Table 11.2, p. 570), and usually passes off soon. Reactions from excessive IZS (lente) given before breakfast usually occur in the later afternoon and those from PZI at night or early next morning. These reactions begin gradually with little adrenaline response and become persistent and profound unless vigorously treated. The predominant symptoms are very variable and include headache, malaise, night sweats, nausea leading sometimes to troublesome vomiting, mental confusion and drowsiness, especially in the morning. Coma may follow.

TREATMENT OF HYPOGLYCAEMIC REACTIONS. Since hypoglycaemia can easily be corrected if recognised early, it is useful for diabetic patients to experience the condition under supervision. In this way they learn to recognise the early symptoms. They must be made to realise that the most frequent causes of the condition are unpunctual meals and unaccustomed exercise, and seek to avoid both or to make adjustments to meet these circumstances. They should always carry some tablets of glucose or a few lumps of sugar for use in an emergency. Unless an attack of hypoglycaemia is adequately accounted for, the patient should reduce the next and subsequent doses of insulin by 20 per cent, and seek medical advice.

If the patient is so stuporous that he cannot swallow, he should be given an intravenous injection of 25 g of glucose (50 ml of a 50 per cent solution). This may have to be repeated. If this is not available, a subcutaneous injection of 0·5 ml of 1 in 1,000 solution of adrenaline may be tried, but it is relatively ineffective. Alternatively, the insulin-dependent patient may be given a subcutaneous or intramuscular injection of 1 mg of glucagon, repeated if necessary after 10 minutes. This raises the blood glucose by mobilising liver glycogen, and has the advantage of convenience in that it can be given by anybody capable of learning to use a syringe, but it may not be effective in severe and prolonged hypoglycaemia due to depot insulins. In addition to increasing hepatic glycogenolysis, glucagon stimulates the secretion of insulin and it should not be used to treat hypoglycaemia induced by an oral hypoglycaemic agent, since this may simply aggravate the disability by provoking further insulin secretion.

As soon as the patient is able to swallow, he should be given 30 g of sugar by mouth. Full recovery may not occur immediately. Further, when hypoglycaemia

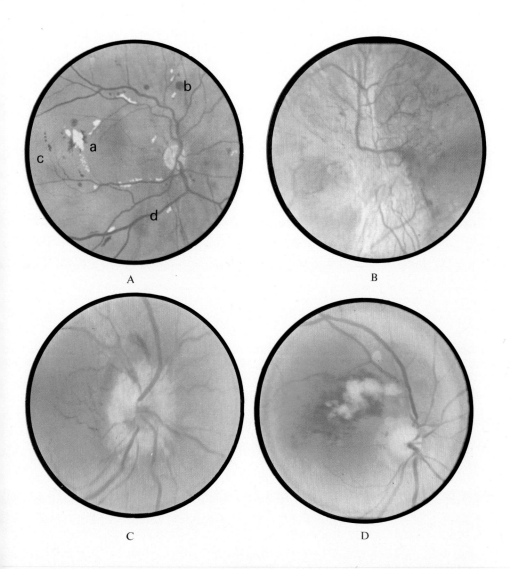

PLATE II

A, Diabetic retinopathy; (*a*) Exudates; (*b*) Dot haemorrhages; (*c*) Microaneurysms; (*d*) Congested veins. B, Advanced proliferative diabetic retinopathy. Heavily vascularised sheets of fibrous tissue are forming in the vitreous, mainly derived from the optic disc. C, Papilloedema. Note swelling of the disc and haemorrhages on or very near the disc. D, Thrombosis of the lower temporal branch of the central retinal artery. Note haemorrhages and exudates. There is also pathological cupping of the disc due to raised intra-ocular pressure which probably predisposes to retinal thrombosis.

(*By permission of Professor C. I. Phillips, Department of Ophthalmology, University of Edinburgh*)

has occurred in a diabetic using a depot preparation of insulin or a sulphonylurea, particularly chlorpropamide, the possibility of relapse within a day or more should be anticipated.

Repeated episodes of hypoglycaemia may lead to permanent intellectual deterioration; accordingly, adjustments to prevent recurrences are essential.

The Complications of Diabetes Mellitus

Diabetic Ketoacidosis

Prior to the discovery of insulin more than 50 per cent of diabetic patients ultimately died of ketoacidosis. Today this complication is preventable and accounts for less than 2 per cent of diabetic deaths. However, both the incidence and the mortality rate are still regrettably high. Failure of the patient to understand his disease, and failure to appreciate the significance of symptoms of poor control are the most common causes. Thus its prevention is largely a problem of education of patients and at times of their physicians. A clear understanding of the biochemical disorders involved (p. 557) is essential for its efficient treatment which should aim at having the patient out of danger within 24 hours.

Water and Mineral Depletion. The deficit of total body water in a severe case may be about 6 litres. About half of this is derived from the intracellular compartment and occurs comparatively early in the development of acidosis with relatively few clinical features; the remainder represents loss of extracellular fluid sustained largely in the later stages. It is at this time that marked contraction of the size of the extracellular space occurs, with haemoconcentration, a decrease in plasma volume, and finally a fall in blood pressure with associated renal ischaemia and oliguria.

The concentration of sodium and potassium in the serum gives very little indication of total body losses, and may even be raised due to disproportionate losses of water. Sodium loss, mainly from the extracellular space, may amount to as much as 500 mmol. Potassium loss from the cell may be 400 mmol or more. The concentration of potassium in the plasma in these circumstances is dependent on the balance between catabolism of protein and glycogen and haemoconcentration on the one hand, and urinary excretion on the other. Since the former generally exceeds the latter a high level of plasma potassium is likely to be present initially, in spite of a total body deficit. However, within a few hours of beginning treatment with insulin, there is likely to be a precipitous fall in the plasma concentration of potassium. At least three mechanisms are responsible for this: dilution of extracellular potassium by the administration of potassium-free fluids, the movement of potassium into the cells as the result of insulin therapy, and the continuing renal loss of potassium.

Ketoacidosis. The mechanism of the development of this state has been described (p. 558). Apart from the clinical findings, its severity can be rapidly assessed by measuring the plasma bicarbonate, less than 12 mmol/l indicating severe acidosis. The hydrogen ion concentration in the blood is an even more valuable guide but it may not be as readily available. There are no simple and accurate quantitative methods for the determination of plasma ketones.

Clinical Features. Any form of stress, particularly an acute infection, can precipitate severe ketoacidosis in even the mildest diabetic. The most common cause is neglect of treatment due to carelessness, misunderstanding or illness, and failure to adjust the therapeutic regimen in the event of an acute infection.

The *symptoms* of diabetic ketoacidosis invariably include intense thirst and polyuria. Constipation, muscle cramps and altered vision are common. Sometimes, especially in children, there is abdominal pain, with or without vomiting. Hence diabetic ketoacidosis is important in the differential diagnosis of the acute abdomen. Weakness and drowsiness are commonly present, but it should be remembered that the state of consciousness is very variable and a patient with dangerous ketosis requiring urgent treatment may walk into hospital. For this reason the term diabetic ketoacidosis is to be preferred to the traditional 'diabetic coma', which suggests that there is no urgency until unconsciousness occurs. In fact it is imperative that energetic treatment is started at the earliest possible stage.

The *signs* include a dry tongue and soft eyeballs due to dehydration: 'air hunger' indicated by long, deep, sighing respirations; a rapid, weak pulse, and low blood pressure; sometimes abdominal rigidity and tenderness; the smell of acetone in the breath; ultimately coma supervenes.

Laboratory tests show (1) ketonuria and severe glycosuria; (2) blood glucose usually between 22·2 and 44·4 mmol/l (400 and 800 mg/100 ml), but it may be much higher and in some cases lower; (3) low plasma bicarbonate and blood pH; (4) normal or raised serum sodium and potassium; (5) leucocytosis.

It should be noted that the degree of hyperglycaemia and ketoacidosis do not always necessarily correlate well. Even at a level of blood glucose as low as 19·4 mmol/l (350 mg/100 ml), life-threatening acidosis may be present; on the other hand diabetic coma can occur, usually in elderly patients, with extreme hyperglycaemia and dehydration but no ketoacidosis, *hyperosmolar diabetic coma*.

Treatment. This condition should be treated with the utmost urgency in hospital. Intravenous therapy is required since even when the patient is able to swallow, fluids given by mouth may be poorly absorbed. Establishing an intravenous infusion can be technically difficult because of collapsed veins, but cutting down and tying in a cannula should be avoided if at all possible, because the veins may be needed again. Treatment must be checked against the blood concentration of glucose, potassium and bicarbonate estimated at intervals at first of not longer than 2 hours. Only in this way can the metabolic disorder be corrected accurately and rapidly. The aim should be to overcome with all speed:

1. Ketosis, by means of insulin to permit glucose utilisation.
2. Peripheral circulatory failure, acidosis, and water and electrolyte depletion, by means of appropriate intravenous fluids.
3. Infection, if present, by means of antibiotics.

Only rapidly acting insulins should be used, i.e. soluble or Actrapid. Ketosis and dehydration render the comatose patient relatively resistant to insulin. The conventional treatment of diabetic ketoacidosis has, therefore, involved the use of large doses of soluble insulin, 100 units normally being given immediately the diagnosis is made, half intravenously and half intramuscularly. The total amount of insulin used subsequently varies widely and is assessed in the light of changes in the blood glucose level every 2–4 hours; severe cases are usually given at least 500 units in the first 24 hours and often considerably more. As long as there is evidence of peripheral circulatory failure some of the insulin should be given intravenously.

It has now been suggested that such large doses of insulin are unnecessary and that low-dose regimens are just as effective, are less complicated and may be safer. Twenty units of soluble insulin may be given intramuscularly immediately and then five units (i.m.) hourly thereafter. The blood glucose concentration should fall by 3–6 mmol/l/hour. If the patient is severely hypotensive and/or there is no fall in the blood glucose concentration by 2 hours after the first dose, then 2–6 units insulin/hour can be given with a continuous infusion pump. When the blood glucose concentration has fallen to 13·9 mmol/l (250 mg/100 ml) insulin may then be given by subcutaneous injection as required.

The deficit of extracellular fluid, which is likely to be about 3 litres, should be made good by infusion of saline isotonic with plasma (0·9% NaCl). In cases which are also severely acidotic (bicarbonate <12 mmol/l), ½ litre of the isotonic saline may be replaced by isotonic sodium bicarbonate (1·4%) or, if this is not available, by isotonic sodium lactate solution (M/6). The intracellular deficit of water, usually about 2–3 litres, must be replaced by giving 5 per cent glucose and not by more saline. It is best given when the blood glucose is approaching normal. It is important to continue the intravenous glucose together with appropriate doses of soluble insulin subcutaneously until the ketonuria has disappeared and the water deficit has been made good.

If the patient is admitted in profound circulatory failure, or the blood pressure remains low after the administration of saline and bicarbonate, it may be necessary to give blood or plasma.

Every patient in diabetic ketoacidosis is potassium depleted and many will require intravenous potassium (p. 158) to prevent the development of dangerously low levels of potassium during the course of treatment. As the serum potassium is often high at the time of diagnosis it is important not to start potassium therapy until the level in the serum has fallen to normal, the peripheral circulation has been restored, and the urinary output is adequate. Approximately 80 mmol of potassium may safely be given by vein in the first 16 hours but much more than this may be required. It is important to realise that sufficient potassium must be given to maintain a normal serum concentration, and this can be confirmed only by frequent estimations. It is customary to add 1·5 g potassium chloride (20 mmol potassium) to each 500 ml of glucose and water given intravenously. Once oral feeding has started potassium chloride (p. 158) should be given 4-hourly for 2 to 3 days to restore the total body deficit.

In a stuporous or comatose patient, gastric aspiration should be undertaken to avoid the risk of inhaling vomitus.

Infections must be carefully sought and vigorously treated since it may not be possible to abolish ketosis until they are controlled. Once ketosis has been overcome, and the water and salt deficit made good (usually in about 24 hours), feeding by mouth can be started with frequent small fluid feeds each containing about 25 g of carbohydrate. Three examples of such feeds are:

1. 100 ml (3½ oz) fruit juice plus 15 g (½ oz) of cane sugar or glucose.
2. 200 ml (7 oz) milk plus 180 g (6 oz) of porridge.
3. 200 ml (7 oz) milk plus 10 g (⅓ oz) cereal plus 7 g (¼ oz) sugar.

Enough insulin should be given to prevent any further ketonuria or glycosuria. Control can be lost very quickly; frequent blood sugar estimations are needed and soluble insulin should be given before each oral feed, even if the urine is free of sugar and only very small doses of insulin are required.

Differential Diagnosis of Coma in a Diabetic. Confusion between coma due to hypoglycaemia and that associated with ketosis should seldom arise; the distinction is clear (Table 11·3). Diabetic coma may occasionally pass undetected into hypoglycaemic coma through too enthusiastic treatment; likewise, vomiting induced by hypoglycaemia from a depot insulin may continue until diabetic coma develops.

Table 11.3 Differential diagnosis of coma in a diabetic

	Hypoglycaemic Coma	Coma with Ketosis
History:	no food; too much insulin; unaccustomed exercise	too little or no insulin; an infection; digestive disturbance
Onset:	in good previous health related to last insulin injection	ill-health for several days
Symptoms:	of hypoglycaemia; occasional vomiting from depot insulins	of glycosuria and dehydration; abdominal pain and vomiting
Signs:	moist skin and tongue full pulse normal or raised BP shallow or normal breathing brisk reflexes plantars usually extensor	dry skin and tongue weak pulse low blood pressure air hunger diminished reflexes plantars usually flexor
Urine:	no ketonuria no glycosuria, if bladder recently emptied	ketonuria glycosuria
Blood:	hypoglycaemia normal plasma bicarbonate	hyperglycaemia reduced plasma bicarbonate

Vascular Disorders

Vascular disease, arterial, arteriolar and capillary, is the largest and most intractable problem in clinical diabetes. Arterial disease is easily the commonest cause of death in diabetics over the age of 50, and the mortality rate is far higher than expected, while nephropathy accounts for more than half the deaths under 50. Moreover, diabetes is the most important systemic disease causing blindness. Strict control probably offers the best chance of delaying the onset and progress of the vascular complications of diabetes.

Atherosclerosis occurs commonly and extensively in diabetics. The pathological changes in diabetics are not specific in a qualitative sense but they occur earlier and are more widespread than in non-diabetics. Thus diabetics are more prone at an earlier age than other people to intermittent claudication, gangrene of the toes and feet and myocardial infarction. The peripheral pulses in the legs are often diminished or impalpable, and particularly in elderly patients, ischaemic changes in the feet are frequently apparent. Defective circulation in the legs resulting in poorly nourished tissues predisposes to the dangerous complication of gangrene. If a painless peripheral neuropathy is present, this may also be of aetiological importance, since the patient will tend to ignore or neglect injuries and other damage to the tissues. Diabetic gangrene usually starts in one foot, following a trivial injury—the cutting of a corn, or a burn from a hot water bottle. Toxic absorption from necrotic tissue and secondary infection may kill the patient unless the limb is amputated. Amputation of a toe, a foot, or even a whole leg is sometimes necessary to save life.

A great deal can be done to prevent this serious complication by instructing diabetics with a poor circulation to wear properly fitting shoes, to use bed-socks rather than hot water bottles, never to cut their own corns and to 'keep their feet as clean as their face'. The services of a skilled chiropodist are invaluable.

Diabetic Nephropathy

Diabetic Glomerulosclerosis. A specific type of renal lesion may occur as a result of the changes in the basement membrane of the glomerular capillaries; there are two types, diffuse and nodular. The former is the more common and consists of a generalised thickening of glomerular capillary walls. The nodular type is a development of this, and in these cases rounded masses of acellular, hyaline material are superimposed upon the diffuse lesion in the glomeruli. These nodules are sometimes called Kimmelstiel–Wilson bodies. Diabetic glomerulo-sclerosis can be seen by light microscopy in about 70 per cent of diabetic patients at autopsy. In the early stages of diabetes there may be little or no clinical evidence of renal involvement, and even with well-established diabetic glomerulosclerosis the patient may exhibit only slight to moderate proteinuria. In some cases, however, the patient develops marked proteinuria and the nephrotic syndrome with increasing renal failure and uraemia.

There is no way of preventing or modifying the progression of nephropathy once this is clinically apparent as proteinuria. In the later stages the management is the same as in other forms of chronic renal disease. Regular haemodialysis is technically possible although access to the circulation or maintenance of a shunt may be affected by diseased peripheral vessels. Results are less good than in non-diabetics and may not justify the burden placed on the patient. Renal transplantation is more hopeful and in some centres results are almost as good as in non-diabetics.

Diabetic Retinopathy

Retinopathy is the commonest long-term complication of diabetes. In most cases it produces no symptoms but it can cause blindness and in Britain diabetic retinopathy is now the single most common cause of blindness in those aged 30 to 64 years.

Clinical Features. These are shown in Plate II and occur in varying combinations in different patients. Abnormalities of the capillary bed are the earliest lesions. They include capillary dilation and closure which are not clinically visible. In most cases *microaneurysms* are the earliest clinical abnormality detected in diabetic retinopathy. They appear as minute, discrete, circular, dark-red spots near to, but apparently separate from, the retinal vessels. They look like tiny haemorrhages but photography of injected preparations of retina show that they are in fact minute aneurysms arising mainly from the venous end of capillaries near areas of capillary closure. *Venous abnormalities* are among the commonest manifestations of diabetic retinopathy. Dilation, irregularity and increased tortuosity of the retinal veins are all seen. *Haemorrhages,* most characteristically occurring in the deeper layers of the retina and hence round and regular in shape, are also a relatively early feature of diabetic retinopathy. The smaller ones may be difficult to differentiate from microaneurysms and the two are often grouped together as 'dots and blots'. *Soft exudates,* similar to those seen in hypertension, occur and represent areas of infarction. *Hard exudates* are more common and are specific to diabetic retinopathy. They are yellow, with irregular, sharply defined edges, varying in size from tiny specks to large confluent often circular patches. They probably result from leakage of serum from abnormal retinal capillaries and lie over areas of neuronal degeneration. *New vessels* may arise from mature vessels on the optic disc or the retina. The earliest appearance is that of fine tufts of delicate vessels forming arcades on the surface of the retina. As they grow they may extend forwards towards the vitreous. They are fragile, readily leak and at first have no visible connective tissue covering. They are liable to rupture causing haemorrhage which may be intraretinal, preretinal (subhyaloid) or into the vitreous. Irritative serous products leaking from these new vessel systems stimulate a connective tissue reaction: *retinitis proliferans*. This first appears as a white cloudy haze among the network of new vessels. As it extends the new vessels are obliterated and the surrounding retina is covered by a dense white sheet. At this stage bleeding is less common but retinal detachment can occur due to contraction of adhesions between the vitreous and the retina.

CLASSIFICATION. Patients with only microaneurysms, retinal haemorrhages and exudates are classified as having *simple or background retinopathy*, while those with preretinal haemorrhage, new vessel formation, or fibrous proliferation are classified as having *proliferative or malignant retinopathy*. As with nephropathy duration of diabetes is the most important factor influencing the occurrence of retinopathy and some abnormality, even if only a single microaneurysm, can be seen in the fundi of at least 60 per cent of diabetics who have had the condition for 30 years. The course is very variable. In general prognosis for vision is good for patients with simple retinopathy and bad for those with proliferative retinopathy, of whom half are blind within 5 years.

INTERFERENCE WITH VISION. Microaneurysms, abnormalities of the veins, blot haemorrhages and exudates will not interfere seriously with vision unless they are associated with macular oedema or directly involve the macula. Unfortunately all these lesions occur most commonly in the perimacular area. New vessels may be completely symptomless until sudden visual loss occurs from a haemorrhage into the vitreous. Although these frequently clear, the risk of recurrence is high and the more frequent the haemorrhage the slower and less complete the recovery. New vessel formation is potentially reversible and therefore treatable. Fibrous tissue may obscure the retina and seriously damage sight, and retinal-vitreal adhesions may pull the retina forward and produce retinal detachment causing blindness. Retinitis proliferans is the irreversible end-stage of diabetic retinopathy which cannot be influenced by any form of treatment at present available. Early diagnosis and treatment of new vessel formation is therefore of vital importance.

Prevention. This is difficult. As the development of microangiopathy seems to be secondary to the metabolic abnormality and there is evidence to suggest that good control of the diabetes reduces the chance of the development and may delay the progression of severe diabetic retinopathy, every effort should be made to maintain a normal metabolic state in all diabetic patients. It is a common error to suppose that diabetes which is 'mild', i.e. controlled by diet alone, carries little risk of complications.

Treatment. There is no specific treatment for simple retinopathy without maculopathy which is usually not associated with significant impairment of vision.

The administration of clofibrate will clear hard exudates from the retina but will not affect the underlying neuronal degeneration. It may be of value in preventing further exudation. The diabetes and any hypertension must be well controlled.

In simple retinopathy visual loss results from macular exudates, haemorrhage or oedema. Photocoagulation by either the white light of the xenon arc or by the green light of the argon laser can be used to destroy abnormally leaking vessels in the perimacular area and thus reduce oedema. Coagulation of the centre of rings of hard exudates may hasten absorption of the exudates. The smaller spot size and shorter duration of the argon laser enables lesions nearer the macula to be treated.

The primary aim in treating proliferative retinopathy is to destroy new vessels by photocoagulation before vitreous haemorrhage, macular damage or retinal detachment occur. The white light of the xenon arc is absorbed and converted to heat energy by the pigment epithelium and is effective in destroying intraretinal new vessels and those lying flat on the surface of the retina; it is ineffective where new vessels grow forwards from the surface of the retina or lie on the disc. These can, however, sometimes be destroyed by the green light of the argon laser, as this light is absorbed at the level of the pigment epithelium and by haemoglobin. If photocoagulation fails, pituitary ablation can be considered in a few, carefully selected patients. However, the morbidity and mortality associated with this procedure is particularly high in diabetics.

Light coagulation of new vessels on the retina can be done under local anaesthesia, and in skilled, experienced hands is a simple procedure which carries little risk and can be very effective. Because diabetic retinopathy is now a treatable condition if diagnosed early, when it is commonly symptomless, diabetic patients must have their eyes examined regularly, every 6 to 12 months, by a competent observer. To obtain adequate visualisation of the retina the pupils must be dilated with a mydriatic. Once there is evidence of progression of simple retinopathy, and particularly whenever new vessels are seen, the patient must be referred to an ophthalmologist for further supervision and treatment.

Cataract

Very rarely a specific type of opacity of the lens (cataract) occurs in diabetic children whose disease has not been adequately controlled. Cataract also occurs in elderly diabetics, but is said to be no more common than in other elderly people.

Infections

Lowered resistance to infection is associated with poor control of diabetes.

Carbuncle. The development of a carbuncle may unmask latent diabetes; it may even precipitate ketosis and coma. The diabetic state brought on by a carbuncle is not invariably permanent; glucose tolerance may return to normal (at least temporarily) when the infection subsides. Cleanliness is a special virtue in the prevention of skin infection in diabetes. Once infection has occurred a suitable antibiotic must be used.

Pulmonary Tuberculosis. If a diabetic under treatment shows unexplained loss of weight, increase in insulin requirements or symptoms of pulmonary disease, clinical and radiological examination of the lungs should be undertaken. Pulmonary tuberculosis can be arrested in its early stages by prompt recognition and specific treatment, and every newly diagnosed diabetic should have a radiological examination of his chest.

Urinary Tract Infections. The presence of glucose in the urine provides a favourable medium for the growth of bacteria. Persistent infections of the urinary tract frequently occur, and for this reason catheterisation in particular should be avoided. Treatment consists of controlling the glycosuria and the use of chemotherapy or an antibiotic as for any other urinary tract infection.

Vulvitis. Pruritus vulvae is very commonly associated with moniliasis in the diabetic woman. *Candida albicans* is nearly always present. In the majority, the treatment is abolition of glycosuria which brings rapid relief. In a few cases local treatment with nystatin cream and pessaries may be required.

Diabetic Neuropathy

Peripheral neuropathy is a frequent complication of diabetes at any stage, which in the majority of cases may be unnoticed by the patient, but in some may give rise to troublesome symptoms. Motor, sensory or autonomic nerves may be involved in varying combinations to give the following clinical pictures.

Chronic peripheral neuropathy is the most common form of this disability. It occurs only rarely in diabetics under 20 years of age, but is frequent in elderly diabetics with long-standing disease. Since it also occurs in elderly people who do not have diabetes, degenerative disease of the vasa nervorum is thought to contribute to its development. While there may be some weakness and wasting of the muscles of the lower limbs, in most cases the sensory component predominates and symptoms are slight or absent; in others there may be pain, muscle tenderness and paraesthesiae in the limbs. The pain is characteristically confined to a leg or foot, its distribution is commonly in the anterior femoral region and it tends to be worse in bed at night.

The findings are confined to the lower limbs. Absent or diminished tendon reflexes are characteristic, the ankle jerks being mainly affected. Diminution or loss of vibration sense at the ankle or knee is also common. In advanced cases loss of other forms of sensation may be detected. Trophic changes may appear on the feet and ankles in severe chronic neuropathy; ulceration may develop secondarily to trivial trauma and disorganisation of joints may occur, resembling the Charcot joints seen in tabes dorsalis.

This type of neuropathy bears little relation to the quality of control and is unresponsive to treatment.

Involvement of the autonomic nervous system may cause diarrhoea, overflow incontinence of urine, impotence, postural hypotension and disturbances of sweating and skin temperature regulation. Involvement of the autonomic nervous system may result in an impaired sympathetic response to hypoglycaemia so that the patient no longer experiences the classical warning symptoms.

Like chronic peripheral neuropathy, autonomic neuropathy seems to bear little relation to the degree of control and to be unresponsive to treatment.

Acute peripheral neuropathy is distinguished by its association with poor control, and by its improvement with adequate control of the diabetes. Pain and paraesthesiae are usually more severe than in the chronic type.

Diabetic amyotrophy is a predominantly motor form of acute diabetic neuropathy. It consists of bilateral, often asymmetrical wasting and weakness, particularly of the quadriceps, with concomitant pain. With good control of diabetes, recovery is the rule after months or even years.

Mononeuropathy. Isolated nerve palsies occur in diabetics and are usually associated with poor diabetic control. Cranial nerve palsies are not uncommon;

foot drop is relatively frequent, may develop suddenly and can be the presenting symptom of diabetes. There is a high incidence of the carpal tunnel syndrome.

Special Problems in the Management of Diabetes

Diabetes in Children. Fortunately diabetes is not common in childhood, but when it occurs it is relatively severe and always requires treatment with insulin. The therapeutic problem of matching the dose of insulin to the food intake raises practical difficulties but the principles of treating children with diabetes are the same as for adults who have insulin-dependent diabetes. It is important to achieve as good a control of the diabetes as possible and diabetic children and their parents need to be educated in the management of their disorder to the limit of their ability.

Food. The nutritional needs of diabetic children are essentially no different from those of other children. Since they should be growing, their caloric requirements are large in proportion to their size, by comparison with adult standards. Difficulties may be experienced in finding the best means of providing the requisite calories. In children, likes and dislikes for particular foods are often fickle and unpredictable. It is important to make sure that the child does not become too fat; hypoglycaemia due to too much insulin can lead to excessive appetite and hence to obesity. A dietitian can do much to help the child and his parents. A diabetic child must not have sugar or sweets, but the essential composition of his diet need differ little from that of his friends. It is important that everything possible should be done to avoid distinguishing him from his contemporaries. Once properly trained, he may go with them to a summer holiday camp if he so desires, provided that the camp organiser understands his disease. The British Diabetic Association runs special camps for diabetic children.

Insulin. Day-to-day requirements for insulin are often very variable. Children must not be expected to lead the steady life of a business man or housewife; their emotions and activities fluctuate unexpectedly—sometimes wildly active and sometimes sulking. This may have an important effect on their daily needs for insulin; excessive activity may result in hypoglycaemia, whilst lethargy may lead to hyperglycaemia. The latter may also be caused by any one of the numerous infectious diseases to which all children are prone. A combination of one of the depot insulins and soluble insulin before breakfast and usually a second dose of soluble insulin and if necessary a depot preparation before supper is a suitable arrangement for most diabetic children, providing the necessary flexibility. Children and parents need to have sufficient knowledge to make daily alterations in the dose of insulin on the basis of the results of preprandial urine tests and other relevant factors such as exercise and illness.

Diabetes in Pregnancy. One of the important consequences of the discovery and use of insulin is that diabetic women can now have children, whereas in the preinsulin era they were almost always amenorrhoeic and infertile. If a diabetic woman wishes to have a child there is no reason why she should avoid pregnancy, provided that she suffers from none of the more serious complications of diabetes and provided she remains constantly under expert medical care.

Nevertheless pregnancy in a diabetic woman carries certain definite risks; in the later stages of pregnancy she may develop an excessive accumulation of amniotic fluid; in addition the fetus is sometimes unusually large leading to difficulty in labour. Moreover the chances that a diabetic mother may lose her baby either from a stillbirth or in the early neonatal period are greater than those of a non-diabetic mother, even with the most careful supervision.

The proper treatment of a pregnant diabetic patient requires the close and co-ordinated supervision of a team consisting of physician, obstetrician, anaesthetist, nurse and dietitian. The sooner the pregnancy is diagnosed the better. Some non-pregnant diabetic women often miss one or more menstrual periods, especially if their disease is poorly controlled. For this reason a laboratory test for pregnancy is often helpful. There are grounds for suggesting that oral hypoglycaemic agents might be teratogenic, and any diabetic patient who is taking these drugs and becomes pregnant should change to a preparation of insulin as soon as the pregnancy is diagnosed.

It is desirable that the expectant mother should spend a week as an ambulant in-patient in hospital towards the end of the third month of pregnancy. This will enable the patient and the team to get to know each other. Every effort must be made at this time to see that her diabetes is under the best possible control; further education of the patient may be needed in the proper management of her diet and insulin while at home. The diet, at first at least, need differ in no important respect from the diabetic diet (Diet No. 2, p. 945) to which she has been accustomed, but may need adjustment later, particularly with additional milk. Practical problems may be created for the physician and dietitian by bouts of vomiting that common-ly occur in the early stages of any pregnancy, and by the peculiar food fads which many pregnant women develop.

After the diagnosis of pregnancy has been made the patient should be seen at first at fortnightly and later at weekly intervals. Continued full control of the diabetes may be complicated by other factors. First, the renal threshold for glucose often falls as pregnancy advances. This is a normal phenomenon, but in the diabetic it means that the tests for glycosuria which she carries out at home may cease to be a reliable index of diabetic control. Further, in the later stages of pregnancy, lactosuria may occasionally occur and may lead to confusion. If excessive amounts of glucose are lost in the urine because of the lowered renal threshold, it may be necessary to give additional carbohydrate feeds between meals and sometimes at night, covered by suitable amounts of soluble insulin to avoid ketosis. Then, too, the requirements for insulin usually increase as pregnan-cy advances. Frequent estimations of blood glucose are needed to ensure that an increase in insulin dosage, based on misleading urine tests, is not producing hypoglycaemia; or alternatively, that hyperglycaemia is not insidiously building up through failure to give enough insulin to meet an increase in insulin requirements.

Pregnancy in a diabetic woman should seldom if ever be allowed to proceed to term. The chances of survival for the infant are greatly enhanced if it is delivered between the thirty-sixth and thirty-eighth weeks by induction of labour or if necessary by Caesarean section. Following delivery the insulin requirements of the mother fall considerably. Frequent blood glucose estimations and co-operation between the physician and dietitian are needed to ensure an uneventful return to the former diet and insulin dosage.

A final word of warning is necessary. It has already been indicated that sugar in the urine is not unusual during normal pregnancy, either because of a fall in the renal threshold for glucose or through lactose appearing in the urine. The finding, however, of reducing substances in the urine of a pregnant woman should never be lightly dismissed as a normal phenomenon. Full clinical investigation to exclude diabetes is essential; otherwise a preventable catastrophe may follow.

Diabetes and Surgery. Any surgical operation, however minor, and the accompanying anaesthetic cause a metabolic stress which the diabetic is less well able to meet than the normal person. The stress is temporary and will not be aggravated by a mild hyperglycaemia, but an accompanying acidosis will prejudice normal recovery. The position is worse if there is tissue wasting with much breakdown of fat and protein and the excretion of large amounts of potassium, phosphate and other intracellular electrolytes.

Two points must be kept in mind: the need to provide an adequate supply of energy for the tissues, and the need to be constantly on the alert for acidosis.

In practice there are two separate problems. The first is the management of a stabilised diabetic who has to undergo an operation at a time which can be chosen by the surgeon and physician. The second is that of a diabetic whose disease may not be well controlled and who suddenly has to be operated upon because of trauma, acute sepsis or a major abdominal or other catastrophe, or one who is first discovered to be diabetic immediately before operation.

1. *Elective Surgery in a Stabilised Diabetic.* All diabetics must be admitted to hospital about three days before an operation, even a minor one. During this period the control of the diabetes can be checked thoroughly. Provided a diabetic goes to the theatre in good condition, there is unlikely to be any significant change in the blood glucose, plasma bicarbonate or ketone levels during the time he is undergoing surgery. In fact, hypoglycaemia is more likely to occur than acidosis. For this reason it is generally advisable to give no insulin immediately before operation. During the day preceding the operation the patient's usual diet and doses of insulin should be given though doses of depot insulin of more than 20 units should be reduced by half and a supplementary dose of soluble insulin given later that day instead. It will usually be possible to arrange for the operation to take place in the morning. The patient should receive no breakfast and nothing by mouth before operation. Before being transferred to the theatre the fasting blood glucose level should be determined. If this lies between 6·6 and 11·1 mmol/*l* (120 and 200 mg/100 ml) then no glucose or insulin need be given. If the level is below 6·6 then about 25–40 g of glucose should be given intravenously, preferably in hypertonic solution, in order to prevent possible hypoglycaemia during the operation. No insulin is necessary. If the fasting blood sugar is over 11·1, which is infrequent, then some insulin will be required. About one-third of his usual total daily dose is indicated, in the form of soluble insulin, but its administration can usually be postponed until after operation.

Recovery from the anaesthetic must be carefully supervised. The sooner the patient returns to his usual diet the better. This interval may be a few hours or several days, depending on the nature and severity of the operation. Within a few hours of recovery from the anaesthetic many patients are able to take a fluid or semifluid feed containing 25 g of carbohydrate (p. 577) at 3- to 4-hourly intervals, covered by suitable doses of soluble insulin. Some insulin-dependent diabetics after a major operation may need to have most of their energy requirements supplied as glucose, either intravenously or by mouth. If all has gone well, a single determination of the fasting blood glucose each morning will suffice. If recovery is stormy, measurements may be necessary at 4-hourly intervals or even more frequently. Determination of the plasma bicarbonate and electrolytes in the blood will also be helpful. The insulin dosage will depend on these findings, and until stability has been regained only soluble insulin should be used.

Each specimen of urine must be tested for sugar and ketone bodies. If ketosis develops it is essential to take immediate steps to increase the metabolism of glucose by adjusting the dose of insulin.

2. *Diabetes and Surgical Emergencies.* Circumstances vary so much that it is impossible to consider them except in the most general way. The essentials are to maintain the oxidation of glucose by the tissues at a sufficient rate and to combat acidosis and electrolyte disturbances when they occur. This can be done effectively only if the state of the diabetic control is assessed continuously and accurately. A laboratory service that can provide rapid results is thus essential. As long as the surgical condition remains untreated and the 'metabolic stress' continues, the diabetic condition is likely to get worse. Once the patient's surgical condition is under control he may be expected to respond promptly to the appropriate therapy for his diabetes.

Prognosis of Diabetes

The prognosis in diabetes has improved steadily since the introduction of insulin; but even with its use the average expectation of life is still rather less than that of a non-diabetic. It may be difficult to estimate the prognosis of an individual patient because so many variable factors have to be considered. Thus the child of parents poor in means and education, who is first seen in coma, obviously has a very different future compared with the middle-aged lady in easy circumstances who complains of nothing but a little thirst and pruritus, and can afford the time and the means to follow precisely the diet prescribed for her. The incidence of the complications of diabetes is mainly related to the duration of the disease but probably also to the precision with which it has been controlled.

Prevention of Diabetes

Diabetes is a disease of the prosperous, and in wealthy countries it is one of the major health problems. The hardships of the Second World War were associated with a marked decline in the incidence of diabetes in European countries; rationing of both food and petrol was probably responsible. The importance to health of sufficient exercise and of avoiding dietary excess has been stated repeatedly. Diabetes, like obesity and atherosclerosis, is likely to arise in predisposed persons who eat too much and exercise too little. Excess of dietary carbohydrate may strain the limited capacity of the pancreas to produce insulin, especially if it is in the form of sugar or other refined carbohydrate; excess of dietary fat may accelerate the complications of diabetes; atherosclerosis is a common cause of death in diabetics. In any event the public should be warned primarily against an overall excess of calories.

Screening. It is much easier to control the disease and to maintain the health of the patient in a state which allows him to lead a normal life, if the diagnosis is made early in the course of the disease. In many patients, the biochemical changes can be detected before the symptoms are sufficiently severe to make them seek medical advice. Any screening technique is expensive and should be used only if it is likely that a significant number of new diabetics will be recognised. High-risk groups, for example the first degree relatives of known diabetics, the obese and the mothers of babies weighing more than 10 lb at birth, will give a particularly high yield. The prevalence of diabetes in different communities varies from 0·5 to 5 per cent. These figures vary widely according to the social and economic state of the people and the educational and medical services available.

Urine testing has been widely used as a screening procedure. As up to 3 per cent of people may have renal glycosuria and so will have to be recalled for blood tests, and as a number of undoubted diabetics will be missed owing to their raised renal threshold for glucose, this is an unsatisfactory procedure. Whenever practicable, estimation of the blood glucose 2 hours after 50 g glucose orally is recommended as the screening procedure. Auto-analysers enable large numbers of samples to be tested daily.

Quite apart from screening high-risk groups it is not difficult to make out a case for a routine test of the urine for glucose in every full clinical examination; and all those with glycosuria (albeit of minor degree) should be considered diabetic until proved otherwise.

Genetic Counselling. Diabetic patients will often consult their doctor about the advisability of having children and sometimes it is his duty to warn them of the dangers. They can be told that the risks of pregnancy and delivery are little greater for a diabetic mother than for a normal woman, provided she submits to the strict discipline required. The chances that she will produce a healthy baby are also good, but not quite so good as for a normal mother. The chances that her child will subsequently develop diabetes are higher than normal. If both parents have diabetes, the probability is that about 25 per cent of their children will develop the disease at some stage in life. The risk is about half this if only one parent is affected. Many diabetics have healthy children, and how strongly a doctor should word these necessary warnings is a matter for judgement in each case. The family history, the severity of the disease in the parents and their educational and economic background, must all be considered.

Conclusion. The management of a patient with diabetes mellitus offers a special opportunity for good medical practice, there being few other chronic diseases in which efficient management makes so much difference to the patient's life. The problems presented by the aetiology of diabetes and its long-term complications continue to offer some of the most demanding and fascinating challenges in medical research today.

Other Metabolic Disorders

Metabolism is as fundamental as life itself; in medicine the term is usually restricted to disorders which can best be described in biochemical terms.

Many metabolic disorders are acquired. Others are congenital. The genetic aetiology of numerous inborn errors of metabolism has been identified with abnormalities of the structure or function of DNA and the pattern of their inheritance mapped by the study of a particular biochemical disorder. Metabolic disorders therefore may be classified in many ways, for example by the mode of inheritance or by the chemical factors involved. The specific enzyme deficiency responsible for the disorder, or the body system principally affected may be named. Disorders of carbohydrate, protein or amino acid, lipid or mineral metabolism may be predominant features, and a few examples of these are given below.

The vast majority of inborn errors of metabolism are rare and it would be inappropriate to describe them here. The reader will find much further information in specialised textbooks (p. 589).

Carbohydrate. Diabetes mellitus is by far the most frequent and important metabolic disorder of carbohydrate. Rare genetic errors lead to abnormalities in the metabolism of galactose (galactosaemia), fructose (fructosuria), and glycogen (glycogen storage diseases, such as von Gierke's disease).

Amino acids. Inborn errors account for many relatively rare diseases such as cystinuria (p. 471) and the Fanconi syndrome (p. 471). Phenylketonuria is also rare but leads to mental retardation if not detected in the neonatal period and treated with a special diet.

Purines. Gout (p. 649) is a classical example of a metabolic disorder but in practice is best considered along with other causes of arthritis.

Lipids. Serum lipids are complex mixtures among which cholesterol and triglyceride are the most useful indices for the detection and monitoring of hyperlipidaemia. Lipids circulate as lipoproteins, while free fatty acids are bound to albumin (p. 424). Analysis of fasting serum lipids and particularly of lipoproteins provides a useful classification of the hyperlipidaemias as devised by WHO, and based particularly on the work of Fredrickson (p. 589). In this classification there are five major types (I–V) of hyperlipidaemia due to either genetic defects in lipid metabolism or environmental factors such as diet, alcohol and drugs, including oestrogens and corticosteroids.

Primary Hyperlipidaemias

Patients with primary hyperlipidaemia can for most clinical purposes be classified into three groups. Two of these are metabolically heterogeneous but treatment can usually be allocated on a group basis.

Group I consists of Fredrickson's Type IIa. Serum is clear, cholesterol concentration raised, triglyceride levels normal, and β-lipoproteins increased. Most patients have mild to moderate hypercholesterolaemia (7–10 mmol/l) and physical signs are usually absent although early arcus senilis or xanthelasma may be present. The disorder is relatively common in Britain and is a risk factor for ischaemic heart disease. It is usually weakly inherited and environmental factors, such as the dietary intake of saturated fat and cholesterol, are probably important in its aetiology.

About 5 per cent of patients with hypercholesterolaemia have a more sharply defined disorder transmitted as an autosomal dominant and present from birth. Serum cholesterol levels range from 8–16 mmol/l in heterozygotes and from 16–32 mmol/l in the rare homozygotes. In this disorder clinical stigmata of hyperlipidaemia are frequent. Tendon xanthomas are common on the dorsum of the hand and in the Achilles tendons. Arcus senilis and xanthelasma on the eyelids are often prominent and 50 per cent have ischaemic heart disease by the time they are 50 years old.

Group II comprises Fredrickson's Type IIb, III, IV and V. The serum is cloudy, triglyceride and pre-β-lipoproteins increased, and cholesterol may be normal or, if increased, the rise is usually less pronounced than that of triglyceride. Specific physical signs are uncommon although xanthomas can occur. Obesity, impaired carbohydrate tolerance and hyperuricaemia often coexist. There is a strong association with ischaemic heart disease and this group is also relatively common in Britain.

Group III is represented by Fredrickson's Type I. This is a rare disorder consisting of chylomicronaemia resulting from deficiency of extrahepatic lipoprotein lipase.

Secondary Hyperlipidaemia

This occurs in association with diabetes mellitus, in hypothyroidism, the nephrotic syndrome, biliary obstruction and in pancreatitis.

Treatment of Hyperlipidaemia. Control of primary hyperlipidaemia always requires dietary measures. Obesity must be corrected in every case.

Groups I and II should have a fat-modified diet in which the intake of cholesterol is restricted and the total fat intake is reduced to provide about 36 per cent of the total calories. The intake of saturated fat is reduced, while the intake of polyunsaturated fat is increased to provide a polyunsaturated:saturated fat ratio of more than 1 : 1. A list of foods to be avoided is given on page 942.

If dietary measures alone are insufficient to control the hyperlipidaemia, Group I patients with multifactorial hypercholesterolaemia often respond well to clofibrate, while those with a single dominant gene should first be given cholestyramine. An incomplete response in these patients may be improved by the addition of clofibrate or nicotinic acid. Patients in Group II usually respond to clofibrate or nicotinic acid.

Group III patients improve dramatically with restriction of fat intake to about 25 g daily.

Secondary hyperlipidaemia usually responds to treatment of the underlying condition when this is possible.

JOYCE D. BAIRD
J. A. STRONG

Further reading about endocrinology:

Passmore, R. & Robson, J. S. (1974) *Companion to Medical Studies.* Vol. 3. Oxford: Blackwell.
Williams, R. H. (1974) *Textbook of Endocrinology.* 5th edition. London: Saunders.
Irvine, W. J. (Ed.) (1975) *Autoimmunity in Endocrine Disease.* Clinics in Endocrinology. Vol. 4 No. 2. London: Saunders.
Williams, D. I. & Chisholm, G. D. (Eds.) (1976) *Scientific Foundations of Urology.* London: Heinemann. This includes an account of male sexual and endocrine disorders and their investigation.

Further reading about diabetes mellitus:

Oakley, W. G., Pyke, D. A. & Taylor, K. W. (1968) *Clinical Diabetes and its Biochemical Basis.* Oxford: Blackwell.
Oakley, W. G., Pyke, D. A. & Taylor, K. W. (1975) *Diabetes and its Management.* Oxford: Blackwell.
Keen, H. & Jarrett, R. J. (1975) *Complications of Diabetes.* London: Arnold.

Further reading about metabolic disorders:

Bondy, P. K. & Rosenberg, L. E. (1974) *Duncan's Diseases of Metabolism.* 7th edition. London: Saunders.
Stanbury, J. B., Wyngaarden, J. B. & Fredrickson, D. S. (1972) *The Metabolic Basis of Inherited Disease.* 3rd edition. New York: McGraw-Hill.
Lewis, B. (1970) Hyperlipidaemia. *Medicine,* 668–673.
Beaumont, J. L., Carlson, L. A., Cooper, G. R., Fejfar, Z., Fredrickson, D. S. & Stasser, T. (1970) *Classification of Hyperlipidaemias and Hyperlipoproteinemias.* Bulletin World Health Organisation, **43**, 891. This is a definitive classification agreed by a W.H.O. specialist committee.

12. Diseases of the Blood and Blood-forming Organs

Blood Formation

Up to the fifth month of fetal life blood cells are formed both in the liver and spleen. Thereafter normal formation of the red cells, the granular series of white cells and the platelets takes place increasingly in the medullary cavities of bones and from birth onwards is restricted to these sites. During childhood there is a progressive diminution in the amount of red haemopoietic marrow so that in the young adult it is restricted to the heads of the femora and humeri, to flat bones such as the sternum, ribs and ilia and to the vertebrae. The red marrow may extend into the shafts of the long bones when there is an increased demand for blood formation.

All the cells of the blood are derived from mesenchymal stem cells which belong to the reticuloendothelial system (Table 12.1). These are present in the bone marrow; in other sites such as the lymph nodes and spleen they give rise to the non-granular white cells.

The Red Blood Cells (Erythrocytes)

The earliest red cell precursor in the marrow is the proerythroblast, a large cell with a nucleolated nucleus and deeply basophilic cytoplasm. Maturation proceeds through the various stages of normoblasts in which there is progressive condensation of the nuclear chromatin and the development of haemoglobin in the cytoplasm. Disappearance of the nucleus completes the formation of the young erythrocyte which is larger than the mature form, shows a faintly bluish colour with Romanowsky stains and still contains fine reticular material, residual RNA from the nucleus, which can be shown by supravital staining with cresyl blue (reticulocyte). The mature erythrocyte stains as an eosinophilic, circular, biconcave disc with a diameter of 7·2 microns. Its shape is adapted to its function in gas transfer and the cell membrane is an elastic and dynamic structure through which water and potassium and sodium ions are passed by active processes, the energy for which is derived from glucose. The red cell membrane carries the blood group characters on its surface. After the first few days of life there are in health no nucleated red cells and less than 1 per cent of reticulocytes in the peripheral blood. The presence of normoblasts indicates excessive or abnormal blood formation or irritation of the bone marrow. An excessive number of reticulocytes reflects increased erythropoiesis. The megaloblast, an abnormal red cell precursor, is considered on page 601.

The number of erythrocytes remains remarkably constant in a healthy individual. There is evidence to suggest that the natural controlling stimulus of erythropoiesis is a hormone-like factor called erythropoietin which is produced mainly in the kidney. It is known that anoxaemia stimulates red cell formation and that those who live at high altitudes have an increased rate of production. In addition vitamin B_{12}, folate, protein, iron, vitamin C, thyroxine and possibly some

Table 12.1   Origin and development of blood cells

STEM CELL

Erythrocyte Series	Granulocyte Series	Lymphocyte Series	Monocyte Series	Thrombocyte Series
Proerythroblast	Myeloblast	Lymphoblast	Monoblast	Megakaryoblast
Early normoblast	Promyelocyte			Megakaryocyte
Intermediate normoblast	Neutrophil, eosinophil, basophil myelocyte			
Late normoblast				
Reticulocyte	Neutrophil, eosinophil, and basophil polymorph	Lymphocyte	Monocyte	Platelet
Erythrocyte				

Present in normal peripheral blood

trace elements such as copper and manganese are necessary for the continuation of normal erythropoiesis.

Haemoglobin. The role of the erythrocytes depends on their content of haemoglobin which is formed in the bone marrow in the maturing red cells. It is the oxygen transport mechanism of the blood and is also important in the buffering of carbonic acid (p. 165). Haemoglobin is a complex molecule being a conjugate of a protein (globin) with a red pigment (haem), the latter being a combination of a porphyrin with ferrous iron. In normal adult haemoglobin (haemoglobin A) the molecule of globin consists of four paired polypeptide chains, two alpha chains of 141 amino acids and two beta chains of 146 amino acids. Many variants of haemoglobin can occur according to the make-up of the chains, but only three forms are present physiologically. Haemoglobin F is present in the fetus and disappears during the few months after birth. It is replaced by haemoglobin A together with a small percentage of haemoglobin A_2. Other variations of the haemoglobin molecule are associated with the clinical states known as the haemoglobinopathies (p. 822).

Vitamin B_{12} and Folate. These members of the vitamin B complex are important factors in nucleic acid synthesis. In the developing red cell they are required for the maturation of the nuclei of primitive erythroblasts to form normoblasts. If the bone marrow receives an inadequate supply of either vitamin, erythropoiesis changes to an abnormal type characterised by the formation of megaloblasts and there is a diminished output of red cells.

VITAMIN B_{12}. This is the name given to various cobalamins that play a vital role in DNA synthesis (p. 1). The active form in the body is probably 5'-deoxyadenosylcobalamin. In man the assimilation of vitamin B_{12} from the lower ileum is facilitated by the gastric intrinsic factor. Two forms of the vitamin are used in treatment. The first used is cyanocobalamin, but hydroxocobalamin is to be preferred as it is less rapidly excreted in the urine and is therefore more effective.

FOLATE. This vitamin occurs in varying concentrations in many foodstuffs (p. 138). Either in the small intestinal lumen or mucosal cells it is broken down to simpler forms by folate conjugase. At some stage after absorption the enzyme dihydrofolate reductase produces reduced forms. Folate is essential for many metabolic processes in the body leading ultimately to DNA formation in cells. The therapeutic agent mainly employed, and given the name folic acid, is pteroylglutamic acid. When a drug such as methotrexate (p. 619) inhibits dihydrofolate reductase, it is possible to employ folinic acid to overcome the metabolic block.

Iron. This is essential for the synthesis of haemoglobin and is present also in myoglobin and certain enzymes such as cytochrome. Present in various foods (p. 113), it is absorbed from the upper small intestine in the ferrous form, and reducing agents such as vitamin C and some amino acids facilitate its absorption in an acid medium. The amount absorbed is largely determined by the activity of erythropoiesis and the level of the iron stores in the body. There is still speculation about the exact mechanism of iron absorption from the intestine. The cells of the small intestinal mucosa are believed to contain a protein named apoferritin which combines with some of the iron to form ferritin. If excessive amounts of iron enter the cell, they are lost to the body because the effete mucosal cell is shed into the gut lumen with its ferritin content. Meantime the iron that is needed has been attached to the iron-binding globulin of the plasma, transferrin, which is not normally fully saturated. The body conserves its iron content so that almost all of that liberated by the breakdown of effete red cells is utilised for fresh haemoglobin synthesis. Hence only about 1 mg daily is lost from the skin and alimentary and urinary tracts. In men this small iron loss is easily replaced by the iron in the food, but balance is more difficult to maintain in women who need to absorb about a further 1 mg daily to cover menstrual blood loss and whose requirements are even greater during pregnancy and lactation.

The iron content of the body gradually increases from 0·5 g at birth to about 5 g in the average adult. Of this some 60 per cent is in the erythrocytes and a reserve is held in the liver, spleen and bone marrow for the replacement of about 25 per cent of the circulating haemoglobin following haemorrhage. This reserve is stored in the body in two forms, ferritin and haemosiderin.

The White Blood Cells (Leucocytes)

(a) *The Granular Series.* These are so called because of the granules shown by Romanowsky stains in the cytoplasm of the more mature forms. They are derived from the stem cells in the active bone marrow (Table 12.1) where their earliest recognisable precursors are myeloblasts which have large nuclei containing nucleoli and no cytoplasmic granules. The latter mature to the myelocytes which are smaller cells with coarser nuclei and no nucleoli. About 30 per cent of white cells in the bone marrow are myelocytes. Condensation of the nuclear chromatin proceeds to the formation of metamyelocytes, with kidney-shaped nuclei and finally to the young granulocytes or polymorphonuclear leucocytes which have lobulated nuclei. The older the granulocyte, the more lobes there are in the nucleus. The cells are classified as neutrophil, eosinophil or basophil according to the staining reactions of their granules. The mature neutrophil cells have a high enzyme content and are actively phagocytic to infective organisms which they digest. The products of autodigestion from cells killed by organisms (pus cells) are potent stimulants of fresh neutrophil formation by the marrow. The eosinophils are also phagocytic and their granules contain histamine. They are concerned in processes involving foreign proteins such as hypersensitivity reactions. The basophil granulocytes are non-phagocytic and have granules containing heparin and histamine.

Mature neutrophil granulocytes account for about 70 per cent of the total leucocytes in the peripheral blood of a healthy adult though a huge reserve of them is held in the marrow and they are present in large numbers in various organs and tissues. Physiological factors which increase their number in the peripheral blood include exercise, emotional stress and pregnancy. Immature granulocytes, represented by metamyelocytes, are found when the production of leucocytes is being stimulated by severe pyogenic infections but in adults the occurrence in the blood of myeloblasts reflects a serious disturbance of marrow function such as leukaemia.

(b) *Lymphocytes*. These are mainly derived from stem cells in lymphoid tissue throughout the body though some are found in the bone marrow. The immature form, the lymphoblast, is a large cell with a nucleolated nucleus and so closely resembles the myeloblast that special staining methods are required to differentiate them. From lymphoblasts are derived the large and small lymphocytes both of which are found in the peripheral blood and widely distributed throughout body tissues. It seems that some small lymphocytes are resting cells and are capable of transformation to large lymphocytes in lymphoid follicles. The thymus plays an important role in the production of long-lived lymphocytes which are concerned in the phenomenon of immunocompetence (p. 26). Lymphocytes are mainly concerned with the formation and transport of antibodies (p. 27).

(c) *Monocytes*. These are formed from stem cells in the spleen and lymphoid tissue and to a lesser extent in the bone marrow. Immature cells, monoblasts, are large nucleolated forms, very similar to myeloblasts and lymphoblasts, and they mature into adult forms with a lobulated nucleus and a cloudy blue cytoplasm containing a few minute red granules. The monocytes are actively motile and phagocytic.

The Platelets (Thrombocytes)

These are derived in the bone marrow from megakaryocytes, which are very large cells containing multilobulated nuclei and granular cytoplasm from which the platelets are formed. Platelets are small (2–4 microns) hyaline non-nucleated bodies with blue or purple granules.

Range of Normal Haematological Values

In the newborn the red cell count is approximately $6 \cdot 0 \times 10^{12}/l$ ($6 \times 10^6/\text{mm}^3$) and the haemoglobin level about $18 \cdot 0 \, \text{g/dl}$ ($18 \cdot 0 \, \text{g/100 ml}$). Occasional normoblasts and up to 6 to 7 per cent of reticulocytes may be found during the first 2 to 3 days of life. By 3 months the red cell count and haemoglobin concentration have fallen to around $4 \cdot 0 \times 10^{12}/l$ and $11 \cdot 0$ g/dl. Thereafter as erythrocyte production increases the figures rise gradually to the adult range by about the age of 11 years, i.e. red cell count of approximately $4 \cdot 5 \times 10^{12}/l$ and haemoglobin of about $14 \cdot 4$ g/dl.

The total white cell count in the peripheral blood at birth is of the order of $15 \cdot 0 - 25 \cdot 0 \times 10^9/l$ ($15 \cdot 0 - 25 \cdot 0 \times 10^3/\text{mm}^3$), accounted for largely by neutrophil granulocytes. Their numbers fall rapidly in the first 2 days of life and thereafter until about the age of 4 years lymphocytes comprise the majority of the total white cell count of $4 \cdot 0 - 10 \cdot 0 \times 10^9/l$. In adults the differential white cell count is constituted as follows:

Neutrophil Granulocytes—60–70 per cent ($2 \cdot 5 - 7 \cdot 0 \times 10^9/l$).
Basophil Granulocytes—0–1 per cent ($0 - 1 \cdot 0 \times 10^8/l$).
Eosinophil Granulocytes—1–4 per cent ($4 \cdot 0 \times 10^7/l - 4 \cdot 0 \times 10^8/l$).
Lymphocytes—23–35 per cent ($1 \cdot 0 - 3 \cdot 5 \times 10^9/l$).
Monocytes—4–8 per cent ($1 \cdot 6 - 8 \cdot 0 \times 10^8/l$).

The erythrocyte sedimentation rate (ESR) is less than 15 mm in 1 hour (Westergren). In the healthy elderly it may be as high as 30 mm in 1 hour.

Other normal haematological values for adults are given on page 950.

Blood Destruction

Destruction of all formed elements of the blood occurs in cells of the reticuloendothelial system. The survival time of the mature erythrocytes in the peripheral blood is approximately 110 to 120 days. This is the time as estimated by cross-transfusion experiments and represents the mean life-span. A more practical technique is one in which red cells incorporating ^{15}Cr are transfused and the time taken for half of the radioactivity to disappear is estimated. By this method the half-life of the red cells is 25 to 35 days because of the elution of chromium from the cells. As the cell ages and its enzyme activity declines, its membrane becomes defective so that the cell is removed from the blood and broken down in the reticuloendothelial system. The degradation of haemoglobin yields iron from haem and this is mostly reutilised by the marrow for fresh haemoglobin synthesis. The iron-free residual pigment, biliverdin, is converted to bilirubin and carried by the plasma to the liver for excretion.

The life-span of the platelets has also been measured and found to be 9 to 11 days but much less is known about the survival time of the leucocytes. The granulocytes probably last 3 to 4 days but the life-span of the monocytes and lymphocytes is less certain. It appears that some small lymphocytes may re-enter the circulation at intervals for years (p. 28).

Terms relating to Blood Disorders

(a) *Anaemia.* This is said to be present when the concentration of haemoglobin in the blood falls below the normal level for the age and sex of the individual.

(b) *Microcytosis.* The average diameter of the red cells is reduced. This is commonly found in iron deficiency anaemia.

(c) *Macrocytosis.* The average diameter of the red cells is greater than normal. This is seen, for instance, in pernicious anaemia.

(d) *Hypochromia.* This exists when the red cells contain less than the normal amount of haemoglobin. They stain less deeply and show central pallor and the mean corpuscular haemoglobin concentration (MCHC) is lower than normal. Hypochromia is commonly associated with microcytosis and is the characteristic feature of iron deficiency anaemia.

(e) *Anisocytosis.* This is the name given to inequality in the size of the red cells. It is found in many forms of anaemia but is most prominent in pernicious anaemia. It is an indication of abnormal activity of the bone marrow.

(f) *Poikilocytosis.* This name is applied to marked irregularity in the shape of the red cells. It is never present without anisocytosis and usually reflects dyserythropoiesis.

(g) *Elliptocytosis.* This means the red cells have an elliptical shape. It is an abnormality of the erythrocytes inherited as a Mendelian dominant and minor degrees of it are quite common and of no pathological significance. In its more severe forms it may be associated with a haemolytic process.

(h) *Polychromasia and Reticulocytosis.* Young red cells when stained by the Romanowsky method have a faint bluish colour. A blood film in which such cells are present along with those of normal pink colour is said to show polychromasia. When stained supravitally by cresyl blue the young cells, which are slightly larger than adult erythrocytes, show up as reticulocytes. Polychromasia and reticulocytosis indicate active production of new red cells by the bone marrow.

(i) *Punctate Basophilia.* Pathologically damaged young red cells may show several deep blue dots in the cytoplasm when stained by Romanowsky stains. Punctate basophilia may be found in any severe anaemia, but the presence of many cells affected in this way is most commonly seen in chronic lead poisoning, where it may occur when anaemia is slight.

(j) *Nucleated Red Cells.* These are usually normoblasts, and are occasionally found when erythropoiesis is very vigorous or more often where there is irritation of the bone marrow, as in leukaemia.

(k) *Leucocytosis.* This means an increase in the total number of white blood cells to over $10 \cdot 0 \times 10^9/l$ ($10 \cdot 0 \times 10^3/mm^3$). This may take the form of a polymorphonuclear leucocytosis in which the increase is due to the outpouring of many young neutrophil granulocytes, as occurs in the presence of pyogenic infections such as tonsillitis or pneumonia. Alternatively it may take the form of a lymphocytosis, as is frequently found, for example, in whooping-cough. Infants commonly respond to infections by producing a lymphocytosis.

(l) *Leucopenia.* This means a decrease in the total number of white cells below $4 \cdot 0 \times 10^9/l$ and usually involves a reduction only of the granulocytes (granulopenia). Leucopenia is found in tuberculosis, enteric fever, many acute viral infections, undulant fever, etc. Occasionally a leucopenia is found in overwhelming infections and is then a bad prognostic sign.

(m) *Eosinophilia.* This is the term used when the number of eosinophil granulocytes exceeds $4 \cdot 0 \times 10^8/l$. Eosinophilia is found most commonly in infection with worms, in allergic diseases such as asthma, hay fever, urticaria, pulmonary eosinophilias (p. 305), lymphadenoma (p. 622), and in certain skin diseases.

(n) *Monocytosis* (over $8 \cdot 0 \times 10^8/l$). This is found in, for example, infectious mononucleosis, advancing tuberculosis and malaria.

(o) *Thrombocytopenia* means a diminution in the number of blood platelets (normal figure $150–400 \times 10^9/l$). Bleeding tends to occur when the platelet count falls to below $40 \times 10^9/l$, but there is no exact relationship between the platelet level and a bleeding tendency.

(*p*) *Leucoerythroblastic Anaemia*. This name describes the blood picture in which myelocytes and normoblasts are simultaneously present in the peripheral blood of an anaemic patient. It reflects bone marrow irritation, e.g. in malignant disease or myelofibrosis.

(*q*) *Extramedullary Haematopoiesis*. This term is applied when in an adult patient the bone marrow is replaced by fibrous tissue (*myelofibrosis*) and the production of blood cells takes place in the spleen and liver as in fetal life. This can result in progressive enlargement of the spleen and liver and is accompanied by a leucoerythroblastic anaemia. Extramedullary haematopoiesis occurs not uncommonly in the first year of life when the available bone marrow space is insufficient to allow for an increased demand for blood formation.

DISORDERS OF THE RED BLOOD CELLS

The Anaemias

A simple clinical approach to the diagnosis of a patient with anaemia is to keep in mind that the condition results from one of the three following causes, though more than one may be present:

1. Diminished production of normal red cells by the bone marrow. This implies failure or suppression of the normal mechanisms promoting erythropoiesis or deficiency of factors required for the maturation of the red cell.

2. Excessive destruction of red cells.

3. Loss of blood, which may be acute or chronic.

In a more detailed classification of the anaemias it must be remembered that those resulting from iron deficiency constitute by far the largest group and it is thus logical to deal with them first. Hundreds of such patients are encountered for every case of megaloblastic anaemia, haemolytic anaemia or pancytopenia. Blood loss results in loss of iron from the body with a consequent deficiency of haemoglobin synthesis. It is also necessary to group together a number of anaemias of uncertain origin in which the specific cause is not known and in which more than one causal factor may be present. The special problems presented by anaemia in the tropics are discussed on page 819.

Classification of the Anaemias

I. Anaemias due to Diminished Production of Normal Red Cells

A. DEFICIENCY OF IRON

Chronic nutritional hypochromic anaemia.
Posthaemorrhagic anaemia resulting in a relative deficiency of iron.
Hypochromic anaemia due to malabsorption of iron.
Sideroblastic anaemia, a failure of iron utilisation rather than deficiency.

B. DEFICIENCY OF VITAMIN B$_{12}$ OR FOLATE—THE MEGALOBLASTIC ANAEMIAS

Addisonian pernicious anaemia.
Nutritional megaloblastic anaemia.
Megaloblastic anaemia due to disease of the gastrointestinal tract (p. 392).
Megaloblastic anaemia in pregnancy.
Megaloblastic anaemia in infancy.

Megaloblastic anaemia complicating haemolytic anaemia or leukaemia.
Megaloblastic anaemia due to various drugs.

C. DEFICIENCY OF VITAMIN C. The anaemia of scurvy.

D. DEFICIENCY OF THYROXINE. The anaemia of myxoedema.

E. PANCYTOPENIA. (Aplastic anaemia).

II. Anaemias due to Excessive Blood Destruction (Haemolytic Anaemias)

A. Due to hereditary abnormalities of the erythrocyte. (*a*) Hereditary spherocytosis. (*b*) Glucose-6-phosphate dehydrogenase deficiency. (*c*) Haemoglobinopathies, e.g. sickle-cell anaemia and thalassaemia.

B. Due to infective or toxic factors.

C. Due to erythrocyte antibodies. (*a*) Haemolytic disease of the newborn. (*b*) Autoimmune (acquired) haemolytic anaemia. (*c*) Symptomatic haemolytic anaemia. (*d*) Paroxysmal haemoglobinuria.

III. Anaemias of Uncertain Origin

This group includes the anaemias associated with chronic infection, uraemia, rheumatoid arthritis, liver disease and widespread malignant disease.

Clinical Features of Anaemia

Anaemic patients have clinical features which are the direct consequence of the diminished oxygen-carrying power of the blood on the tissues and organs of the body. Their occurrence and severity depend on the degree of anaemia, and especially on the rapidity of its development, but are independent of its type. The clinical features of anaemia are:

Fatigue and lassitude.

Breathlessness on exertion.

Dizziness, dimness of vision, headache, insomnia.

Pallor of the skin and, much more significant, of mucous membranes.

Palpitation, tachycardia, cardiac dilatation, systolic murmurs.

Anorexia and dyspepsia.

Tingling and 'pins and needles' in the fingers and toes (paraesthesiae). This occurs particularly in pernicious anaemia.

In severe cases there may be oedema of the ankles and basal crepitations.

Angina pectoris (due to myocardial anoxaemia), especially in older patients with coronary artery disease.

I. Anaemias due to Diminished Production of Normal Red Cells

A. Anaemia due to Deficiency of Iron

Chronic Nutritional Hypochromic Anaemia

Aetiology. This is the most common type of anaemia not only in Britain but in every country of the world. It occurs mainly in women of the child-bearing age because of the enhanced demands for iron resulting from blood loss from menstruation, and the increased nutritional requirements of pregnancy and lactation.

Clinical Features. The symptoms are of gradual onset. In addition to the general features of anaemia described on page 597 there are other features of nutritional deficiency, particularly glossitis, angular stomatitis, koilonychia and atrophy of the mucosa of the pharynx and stomach, sometimes giving rise to dysphagia. Koilonychia is the name given to certain changes in the nails first evidenced by brittleness and dryness. Later there is flattening and thinning and finally concavity (spoon-shaped nails). In a small proportion of severe long-standing cases the spleen may be palpable. In anaemia due to deficiency of iron the combination of dysphagia, glossitis and anaemia is known as the Plummer-Vinson syndrome or as sideropenic dysphagia (p. 358).

While paraesthesiae may occur, objective signs of disease of the central nervous system are never found in anaemia due solely to iron deficiency. Blood examination shows a hypochromic, microcytic anaemia. The haemoglobin level may be as low as 4–8 g/dl (4–8 g/100 ml), with the red cell count between 3 and $4 \cdot 5 \times 10^{12}/l$ $(3–4 \cdot 5 \times 10^6/mm^3)$, and an MCHC of 26–30 g/dl. Anisocytosis and poikilocytosis are present but not marked. The total and differential white counts show little change from normal. The bone marrow shows a normoblastic reaction.

Diagnosis. The differential diagnosis from other types of anaemia depends on accurate blood examination. When the presence of hypochromic anaemia has been established a search for possible causative conditions must be undertaken. These include bad diet, haemorrhage, obvious or occult from any site, malignant disease, especially of the alimentary tract, tuberculosis and other infections, and the appropriate examination and investigations must be carried out.

Prognosis. The anaemia is often well advanced, e.g. haemoglobin level 7–8 g/dl before significant symptoms are apparent. If untreated the condition follows a chronic course. The importance of the syndrome is not that it is dangerous to life but that it leads to a loss of efficiency and lowered resistance to infection.

Hypochromic Anaemia in Infancy and Childhood

Aetiology. *Prematurity and Low Birth Weight.* At birth the full-term baby has about 300 mg of iron stored mainly in the liver and largely accumulated in the last trimester *in utero.* Hence infants born prematurely have low iron stores and inevitably become anaemic by about the tenth week unless prophylactic iron therapy is given. Premature infants or infants of low birth weight (e.g. twins) are also at a disadvantage as they have a smaller circulating red cell mass and derive a reduced amount of iron from the red cell destruction that occurs in the first 3 months.

Prolonged Milk Feeding. Breast-fed infants and particularly artificially fed infants who are kept on milk alone without supplements of iron-containing foods become anaemic.

Other Factors. These include nutritional anaemia in the mother, infections in infants, and, rarely, intestinal malabsorption as in gluten enteropathy.

Clinical Features. In infants the symptoms of anaemia are in general much less easy to recognise than in adults but anaemia leads to impairment of general health and vitality and an increased incidence of infections.

Hypochromic Anaemia in Pregnancy

Anaemia is commonly found during pregnancy. The fall in the haemoglobin is due to one or a combination of the following three causes:

(*a*) Iron deficiency anaemia present before pregnancy but exaggerated by (*b*) and (*c*); (*b*) the relative increase of the plasma volume compared to the red cell mass which usually occurs in pregnancy; and (*c*) a deficient intake of iron in relation to the increased demands of the growing fetus. This may be aggravated by anorexia or vomiting.

Anaemia due to Loss of Blood

Acute Posthaemorrhagic Anaemia. The sudden loss of a large volume of blood, 1 litre or more, from, for example, trauma or intestinal bleeding, produces the features of acute circulatory failure (p. 192).

The rapid loss of 2–3 litres of blood is usually fatal, whereas an even greater quantity may be lost without causing death if it is spread over a period of 24 to 48 hours. During this period restoration of the circulating blood volume is proceeding by the withdrawal into the blood of tissue fluid. Hence, immediately after a haemorrhage in a previously normal person, the blood count will show normal readings, but some hours later when dilution has occurred the haemoglobin level will have fallen, e.g. after a haematemesis (p. 372). When the circulating blood volume is partially restored, the acute symptoms of shock subside. During convalescence the general symptoms and signs of anaemia may be present. During recovery, red cells are formed more rapidly than haemoglobin and the MCHC falls unless adequate iron is available. New red cell formation is reflected by the appearance of a temporary reticulocytosis of 5 to 10 per cent and there is anisocytosis, poikilocytosis and a leucocytosis. The platelet count may be increased.

Chronic Posthaemorrhagic Anaemia. This results from persistent or repeated loss of small amounts of blood. Frequent causes are menorrhagia, and alimentary bleeding from haemorrhoids, carcinoma, peptic ulcer or ancylostomiasis (p. 907). Alimentary bleeding is also commonly due to aspirin. Persistent blood loss causes a progressive fall in haemoglobin. The clinical and haematological features are similar to those found in chronic nutritional hypochromic anaemia. In addition, the features of the causative disorder will be present.

Prevention of Iron Deficiency Anaemia. This necessitates the regular consumption of a well-balanced diet containing an adequate quantity of the iron-rich foods and the periodic administration of medicinal iron to women during times of increased physiological demands, e.g. pregnancy, lactation and when menstruation is excessive.

In the prevention of iron deficiency anaemia in infants the maintenance of a normal blood level in the mother is desirable. Premature and unduly small infants should be given medicinal iron as a routine. Iron-containing foods should be introduced into the infant's diet by the third to fourth month and thereafter be progressively increased. Following the control of infection, iron should be given if the haemoglobin level is reduced.

Treatment of Iron Deficiency Anaemia. In iron deficiency anaemia, unlike pernicious anaemia and the haemolytic anaemias, there is a depletion of the body's usually considerable iron reserves. In consequence the absorption of iron through the intestinal wall is greatly increased in such patients. The ferrous salts of iron are far more effective in treatment than the ferric salts. A very satisfactory preparation is ferrous sulphate, which should be given in the form of tablets of 200 mg, 1 tablet being taken thrice daily after food. Alternative preparations of iron in pill or tablet form are ferrous gluconate, ferrous succinate and ferrous fumarate. All these preparations are equally effective in treatment, but ferrous sulphate is less expensive. Intolerance to oral preparations of iron is infrequent if the drug is taken only after meals. Proprietary liquid preparations are the most palatable. In the average case the blood level is restored to normal in 4 to 8 weeks. In general, synthetic vitamin preparations need not be prescribed if iron medication is supplemented by a well-balanced diet. In particular, expensive preparations containing iron and folic acid should not be used. Attention should be paid to sites of gross focal infection, and any source of abnormal blood loss controlled. Apparent lack of response to iron therapy usually means that the patient is not taking the iron.

When the haemoglobin is below 4 g/dl it is usually advisable for the patient to be kept in bed. The decision to transfuse red cells should be based more on the clinical state of the patient than on the haemoglobin level.

After restoration of the blood to normal in a patient who has a chronic iron deficiency anaemia it is desirable to continue iron therapy for at least 8 weeks in order to replenish the depleted body stores. Therafter relapse can usually be prevented by an iron-rich diet. The periodic administration of iron may, however, be required in women of the child-bearing age.

Parenteral Iron Therapy. Commercial preparations of iron for injection are available. As a general rule such preparations should not be used except when one or other of the oral preparations of iron mentioned above cannot be tolerated or is found to be ineffective. The parenteral route of administration is suitable for the few patients who are genuinely unable to take iron by mouth because of pain, vomiting and diarrhoea, or who are unable to absorb iron because of some disorder of the gastrointestinal tract, e.g. in the malabsorptive disorders (p. 392). Iron given by injection has been recommended for the treatment of the anaemia of rheumatoid arthritis and for the correction of severe anaemia in the late stages of pregnancy and following major operations.

The recommended single dose of iron-sorbitol is 1·5 mg of iron per kg of body weight given daily. A 2 ml ampoule contains 100 mg of iron. It is assumed that about 250 mg of iron are required to increase the haemoglobin level by 1 g/dl of blood. The preparation is administered by deep intramuscular injection and the total dosage of iron should not exceed 2·5 g. Its use is contraindicated in patients with liver or kidney impairment or in those with active urinary tract infection. Oral iron should be discontinued before starting parenteral iron therapy. Iron-sorbitol should never be given intravenously.

Iron-dextran is seldom given intramuscularly because of local irritation and since it has been shown to cause sarcomatous change in certain animals. It can be given intravenously by what is known as the 'total dose infusion method' in a suitable diluent. Alarming systemic anaphylactic reactions may occur (p. 39).

The treatment of iron deficiency anaemia in infants requires the administration of a liquid iron preparation as well as the introduction of iron-containing food into the diet. The dose should give about 6 mg iron per kg body weight daily. A suitable ferrous sulphate mixture for infants is given in the British National Formulary. Only when parenteral therapy is essential should iron, e.g. iron-sorbitol, be given intramuscularly.

It should be remembered that accidental poisoning from iron can occur if tablets are left within the reach of infants (p. 810).

Hypochromic Anaemia due to Abnormal Utilisation of Iron

SIDEROBLASTIC ANAEMIA. Abnormal utilisation of iron with failure of haem synthesis by the marrow may cause a refractory anaemia. In this rare condition there is the characteristic blood picture of chronic iron deficiency anaemia but a failure of response to iron therapy. The serum iron level is high and the bone marrow contains an excess of stainable iron. Primary sideroblastic anaemia is very rare and sometimes sex-linked. The secondary type may be caused by drugs such as isoniazid or be associated with chronic general diseases. Some cases respond to treatment with pyridoxine (p. 137).

B. Anaemias due to Deficiency of Vitamin B_{12} or Folate— The Megaloblastic Anaemias

A deficiency of vitamin B_{12} or folate results in a change of normal erythropoiesis to a megaloblastic marrow characterised by the presence of pathological nucleated red cells which differ from normoblasts. Early megaloblasts are larger than early normoblasts. While the cytoplasm is deeply basophilic in both, the nucleus of the megaloblast has a much more loosely woven network of chromatin. This essential character is seen in megaloblasts even when haemoglobinisation is taking place. Thereafter disintegration and disappearance of the nucleus occurs. The resulting erythrocyte, called a macrocyte, is larger than a normal erythrocyte, has a full complement of haemoglobin, and hence stains uniformly pink; it tends to be more oval than round in shape. Since a certain amount of normoblastic blood formation is proceeding simultaneously in a megaloblastic marrow, the peripheral blood shows a wide variety of cells of different shapes and sizes. Another feature that is often noted is the presence of giant metamyelocytes in the bone marrow. Megaloblastic anaemia may arise in several ways:

1. By a failure in assimilation of vitamin B_{12} consequent on defective production of intrinsic factor by the stomach. This is the cause of Addisonian pernicious anaemia. A similar result occurs after total gastrectomy and may occur after partial gastrectomy or, occasionally gastroenterostomy. Very rarely there may be an inborn deficiency of intrinsic factor secretion, giving rise to so-called juvenile pernicious anaemia.

2. By an intake of a diet deficient in folate, vitamin B_{12}, or both, leading to nutritional megaloblastic anaemia.

3. By a failure of absorption of folate or vitamin B_{12} as a result of dysfunction, disease, resection or short-circuiting of the small intestine.

4. Where there is a blind or stagnant loop of small intestine containing bacteria which apparently utilise vitamin B_{12}, thus rendering it unavailable to the host. The same may occur in jejunal diverticulosis.

5. In pregnancy and infancy. Sometimes in pregnancy, and exceptionally in infancy, there develops a megaloblastic anaemia which invariably responds to folic acid but may be partially or completely refractory to a cobalamin. In countries where malaria is endemic, megaloblastic anaemia in pregnancy is common and due to the greater susceptibility of the pregnant woman to malaria and the resulting increased haemolysis placing additional stress on the availability of adequate folate. For the same reason infants may also develop folate deficiency anaemia very readily.

6. Infection with the fish tapeworm, *Diphyllobothrium latum* (p. 904). This is

found chiefly in Finland, may lead to megaloblastic anaemia particularly in those predisposed to pernicious anaemia because the worm ingests vitamin B_{12} in the alimentary tract of the host.

7. From the administration of various drugs. There are three main groups, (a) folate antagonists, e.g. methotrexate and pyrimethamine, which interfere with the dihydrofolate reductase system (p. 592), (b) anticonvulsant drugs, particularly phenytoin or primidone, whose method of interference with folate metabolism is uncertain, and (c) cytarabine and certain other agents which interfere with DNA synthesis.

8. Where there is a haemolytic or leukaemic process. The rapidly dividing cells may have an increased utilisation of folate.

Incidence. In Britain most cases of megaloblastic anaemia are due to intrinsic factor deficiency (Addisonian pernicious anaemia), but, in the elderly, nutritional folate deficiency is equally common in some areas. In tropical countries most megaloblastic disease is due to folate deficiency associated with malnutrition, pregnancy and concomitant infection. In contrast Addisonian pernicious anaemia appears to be relatively uncommon in the tropics and in some areas quite rare.

Addisonian Pernicious Anaemia

The name Addisonian pernicious anaemia should be limited to the group of megaloblastic anaemias which is due to a failure in secretion of intrinsic factor by the stomach other than from surgery.

Aetiology. This disease is rare before the age of 30 and affects females more than males between 45 and 65 years of age. The condition is often familial. The gastric mucosa fails to produce the intrinsic factor required for the absorption of vitamin B_{12} from the alimentary tract and there is evidence from the finding of gastric antibodies that an autoimmune mechanism may be responsible for initiating the process (p. 40).

Pathology. In the stage of relapse there is extension of red bone marrow into the shafts of the long bones. This marrow shows megaloblasts but normoblasts may be present. Polymorphonuclear leucocytes and megakaryocytes are diminished in number. Giant metamyelocytes are a common feature. There is evidence of increased blood destruction—including hyperbilirubinaemia and increased deposition of iron (haemosiderin) in the liver, spleen, kidneys and bone marrow. The gastric mucosa is thin and atrophic. In untreated or inadequately treated cases degenerative changes in the posterior and lateral tracts of the spinal cord may be found.

Clinical Features. The onset is insidious and the degree of anaemia is often great before the patient consults the doctor. In addition to the general symptoms of anaemia (p. 597) there may be intermittent soreness of the tongue and occasionally periodic diarrhoea.

On examination the patient generally appears well nourished despite the fact that weight loss is a common feature. The skin and mucous membranes are pale, and in severely anaemic cases the skin may show a faint lemon-yellow tint. The surface of the tongue is usually smooth and atrophic, but sometimes it is red and inflamed. The spleen is seldom palpable. Gastric analysis invariably shows achlorhydia when pentagastrin is injected. The urine is found to contain excess of urobilinogen in the relapse stage. In many cases in relapse paraesthesiae occur in fingers and toes—numbness, tingling, 'pins and needles'. Occasionally there are objective signs of involvement of the posterior and lateral columns of the spinal cord (subacute combined degeneration, p. 740), which may rarely be found before the anaemia. Dementia may also occur.

Examination of the stained blood film shows a macrocytic anaemia. The mean corpuscular volume is raised and the macrocytes appear fully stained. There is marked anisocytosis and poikilocytosis and many cells are oval in shape. Occasionally in severe cases a few nucleated red cells or haemoglobinised megaloblasts are seen in the peripheral blood. Reticulocytes number less than 1 per cent (except during the commencement of remission). There is leucopenia, the reduction involving only the granulocytes, which are mature, some having an increased number of lobes (more than five) in the nuclei. There is thrombocytopenia, which is usually moderate but can be marked and associated with purpura. The serum bilirubin level is raised.

Diagnosis. It should be realised that the term 'macrocytic anaemia' merely signifies that the number of large red cells in the peripheral blood is increased. It can arise from many causes and the bone marrow may be megaloblastic (as in the conditions mentioned on p. 601) or normoblastic (as in some cases of haemolytic anaemia, pancytopenia, hepatic cirrhosis, myxoedema, leukaemia). The term megaloblastic is reserved for cases in which megaloblasts can be demonstrated in the bone marrow or in the 'buffy coat' of the blood after centrifugation. Pointers to causes of megaloblastic anaemia other than pernicious anaemia include the age of the patient, pregnancy, malnutrition, evidence of malabsorption and the administration of anticonvulsant drugs. In addition to marrow biopsy the serum B_{12} and folate levels should be measured. Thereafter treatment can be commenced in urgent cases without obscuring the diagnosis. In pernicious anaemia a test of gastric acid secretion will show achlorhydria, and, in the Schilling test (p. 000), absorption from the alimentary tract of cyanocobalamin labelled with radioactive cobalt will be impaired but will be corrected by the addition of intrinsic factor available commercially from animal sources.

Treatment. *General.* The patient may require to be kept in bed until the haemoglobin is about 7 g/dl. The decision to give a blood transfusion is based on general principles concerning the clinical state of the patient. When the haemoglobin level is so low as to endanger life, e.g. under 4 g/dl, it should be seriously considered. In all types of chronic anaemia of sufficient severity to require transfusion the blood must be carefully matched and should be given very slowly, preferably as packed cells, because of the danger of producing sudden cardiac failure. Frusemide (p. 162) should be given simultaneously by mouth or even intravenously with the packed cells.

Specific. Hydroxocobalamin should be given in a dosage of 1,000 micrograms twice during the first week, then 1,000 micrograms weekly until the blood count is normal. Folic acid should never be used in the treatment of Addisonian pernicious anaemia as it does not prevent the development of neurological complications, and may possibly precipitate them.

Within 48 hours of the first injection of hydroxocobalamin the bone marrow shows a striking change from a megaloblastic to a normoblastic state. Within 2 to

3 days the reticulocyte count begins to rise, reaching a maximum about the sixth day. In some cases the rapid regeneration of the blood depletes the iron reserves of the body so that the MCHC falls below normal. To prevent this occurring ferrous sulphate, 200 mg thrice daily, should also be given soon after the commencement of treatment. A combined deficiency of vitamin B_{12} and iron is recognised by the presence of macrocytosis and hypochromia. It is sometimes referred to as a dimorphic blood picture.

If a patient diagnosed as having pernicious anaemia fails to respond to the parenteral administration of adequate dosage of hydroxocobalamin, this suggests that the diagnosis is wrong or the preparation used is not potent, or the patient is suffering from one of the other types of megaloblastic anaemia, e.g. megaloblastic anaemia of pregnancy or of idiopathic steatorrhoea, which may be partially or completely refractory to hydroxocobalamin. Such cases respond to folic acid.

Maintenance. It is vital that the patient suffering from pernicious anaemia should continue to receive regular doses of a cobalamin for the rest of his life. The dose of hydroxocobalamin usually given is 1,000 micrograms by intramuscular injection every 8 weeks. Theoretically the interval between doses may be longer than this but there is no merit in seeking the minimal effective dose. Blood counts should be done once every year and the assessment should never be made solely on clinical impression or on the haemoglobin level alone.

Prognosis. With the maintenance of a normal blood count by adequate specific treatment the patient remains healthy and has a normal expectancy of life. There is, however, a statistically significant increase in deaths from gastric carcinoma in patients with pernicious anaemia.

Nutritional Megaloblastic Anaemia

This type of megaloblastic anaemia is directly due to the prolonged ingestion of a diet which is deficient in folate, and perhaps vitamin B_{12} and other unknown factors. Such diets are gravely deficient in many nutrients but especially in protein foods, fruit and vegetables. It is of common occurrence in tropical countries, and is very rarely encountered in most areas of Britain although there have been a number of reports of folate deficiency in the elderly, and a few instances of primary deficiency of vitamin B_{12} in immigrant Asian women.

Achlorhydria is not a characteristic feature and lesions of the central nervous system are extremely rare. The peripheral blood shows a macrocytic anaemia unless there is a complicating iron deficiency. The bone marrow is megaloblastic.

Treatment consists of the administration of a well-balanced high protein diet together with folic acid 5–10 mg daily. Injections of hydroxocobalamin alone are frequently ineffective, but it is reasonable to supplement folic acid therapy with injections of hydroxocobalamin. Other vitamins and iron may be required in addition. Maintenance treatment with folic acid is not required if the patient takes an adequate diet.

Megaloblastic Anaemia in Pregnancy

A temporary macrocytic anaemia with megaloblastic reaction in the bone marrow may occur during pregnancy or the puerperium. The factors involved in its causation include increased demands and dietary deficiency, especially of folate and more rarely of vitamin B_{12}.

Cases of megaloblastic anaemia of pregnancy usually respond dramatically to the oral ingestion of 10 mg of folic acid daily. If the anaemia is very severe and is not discovered until close to full term, transfusion of compatible blood is indicated in addition. Folic acid therapy should be stopped after the puerperium when the blood level has reached normal, since the disease is self-terminating. Megaloblastic anaemia may recur in subsequent pregnancies. A co-existing deficiency of iron is frequent, and this leads to a dimorphic blood picture. Iron therapy is indicated in such cases. Since there is biochemical evidence of folic acid depletion in about 20 per cent of pregnant women in Britain and because Addisonian pernicious anaemia is rare in this age group, it is reasonable to give folic acid as a prophylactic in pregnancy. This is even more important in tropical countries. In Britain it is convenient to give 1 tablet of a preparation such as Pregaday (Glaxo) daily for prophylaxis. Each tablet of this contains 350 micrograms of folic acid and 100 mg of elemental iron as ferrous fumarate. Numerous alternative proprietary preparations are available.

Megaloblastic Anaemia in Infancy

This type of anaemia occurs infrequently in infants whose diets are markedly deficient in protein, folate and ascorbic acid, and who in addition are suffering from infections and diarrhoea. Although the disease is very rare in Britain it is being recognised in underdeveloped countries as a complication of protein calorie malnutrition (p. 104). The anaemia responds to treatment with folic acid and ascorbic acid. In gluten enteropathy, anaemia is almost invariably due to iron deficiency, but the occasional case with a megaloblastic anaemia will respond to folic acid therapy. Juvenile pernicious anaemia is a rare disease in which there is lack of intrinsic factor, usually without achlorhydria. It should be treated with hydroxocobalamin.

Megaloblastic Anaemia associated with Haemolytic Anaemia or with Leukaemia

Patients with haemolytic anaemia may develop megaloblastic change in the marrow if for some reason, particularly malnutrition, they are deficient in folate. Folic acid therapy is necessary in megaloblastic anaemia if it is a complication of haemolytic anaemia. In acute leukaemia or in the chronic myeloid form the rapidly dividing white cell precursors may deplete the red cell precursors of folate. Treatment with folic acid may cause exacerbations of an acute leukaemic process and thus necessitate more intensive anti-leukaemic therapy.

Megaloblastic Anaemia associated with the Administration of Drugs

When this form of anaemia is due to drugs which interfere with the dihydrofolate reductase mechanism, treatment should be with folinic acid (p. 592). When caused by anticonvulsants, these can be continued provided that simultaneous folic acid therapy is given.

C. Anaemia due to Deficiency of Vitamin C

Anaemia may be found in association with scurvy (p. 126). It may be normocytic or macrocytic in type but the bone marrow is not megaloblastic unless there is coincidental deficiency of folate or vitamin B_{12}. The administration of vitamin C alone may produce a reticulocytosis and a rapid increase of erythrocytes. When associated with an iron deficiency, iron must also be given.

Although frank scurvy is rare in Britain, subscorbutic levels of vitamin C are not infrequently present in cases of nutritional iron deficiency anaemia, especially in elderly men living alone. The giving of ascorbic acid is however generally unnecessary if a well-balanced diet containing fruit and vegetables is prescribed.

D. Anaemia due to Deficiency of Thyroxine

The anaemia of myxoedema is usually moderate in degree and normocytic or macrocytic in type. Accompanying iron deficiency is not uncommon. The clinical picture may strongly suggest pernicious anaemia, but treatment with hydroxocobalamin is ineffective, except in the rare cases with coexisting pernicious anaemia. It is recognised that pernicious anaemia occurs more commonly in patients with myxoedema and that in both conditions there may be evidence of an autoimmune process (p. 44). In the true anaemia of myxoedema, administration of thyroxine produces a slow improvement in the blood level. Associated iron deficiency must be corrected.

E. Pancytopenia

Primary (Idiopathic) Pancytopenia (Aplastic Anaemia)

This is a rare disease of unknown aetiology. The bone marrow shows a great reduction in all formative elements, and the sample obtained by sternal puncture contains only a few scattered cells in a gelatinous and fatty matrix. The disease may occur at any age but is most common in young adults, or in the elderly.

The clinical features are those of a steadily progressive anaemia with haemorrhage into the skin or from the mucous membranes (due to thrombocytopenia) and fever and necrotic ulcers in the mouth and throat (due to granulopenia). The blood picture is that of a normocytic normochromic anaemia. The reticulocyte count is persistently low. There is leucopenia with progressive diminution in the proportions of granulocytes. The platelet count also falls progressively. The terms 'aplastic' or 'hypoplastic' anaemia are more correctly restricted to cases in which the red cell series is particularly affected. The disease is usually fatal within 3 to 9 months, but complete recovery can occur and cases in childhood may improve spontaneously at puberty.

Secondary Pancytopenia

This may be due to:

1. Idiosyncrasy to certain drugs such as chloramphenicol, phenylbutazone, oxyphenbutazone, indomethacin, sulphamethoxypyridazine, tolbutamide and troxidone, or to certain industrial chemicals and insecticides, chiefly benzol and its derivatives such as trinitrophenol, trinitrotoluene and gamma-benzene hexachloride. It may also result from the use of antimetabolites and cytotoxic drugs which are employed in the treatment of malignant disease.

2. Exposure to X-rays and radioactive substances.

3. Replacement of normal marrow by abnormal cells or fibrous tissue.

There is usually no direct correlation between the dose of a toxic agent and the occurrence or degree of anaemia. Some persons are unduly sensitive. Pancytopenia may develop weeks or months after the cessation of administration of such drugs or exposure to industrial poisons, a point of legal importance in claims for compensation.

Clinical Features. The clinical features and blood changes are similar to those of primary pancytopenia.

The course varies from that of a rapidly progressive fatal condition to a chronic hypoplastic process in which an anaemia of 6–9 g haemoglobin per dl, with a corresponding depression of granulocytes and platelets, may persist for months or years. Complete recovery occasionally occurs, but is rare when chloramphenicol or an analgesic is the causative agent.

Diagnosis of Pancytopenia. The essential haematological findings which serve to distinguish this from other types of blood disorders are: a normochromic anaemia with little anisocytosis and poikilocytosis, absence of reticulocytes or others signs of blood regeneration, granulopenia and thrombocytopenia. A failure to respond to the administration of iron, cobalamin, folic acid and vitamin C strongly supports the diagnosis.

The diagnosis from subleukaemic leukaemia (p. 617) may be very difficult unless the bone marrow is examined. It is important to be sure that the patient does not have megaloblastic anaemia.

Treatment. Since the cause of idiopathic pancytopenia is unknown, all that can be done is to support life by repeated whole blood transfusions and give the patient ample amounts of all known haemopoietic factors such as a cobalamin, folic acid, iron and vitamin C. If bleeding is troublesome platelet transfusions may be of great value. In addition prednisolone 60 mg daily may be tried. A synthetic derivative of testosterone, oxymetholone, has given a good response in some children and adults. It is given orally in a dosage of 4–5 mg per kg of body weight daily. It should be continued for several months, but the dosage should be halved when there is evidence of a remission. Treatment with repeated blood transfusions, oral antibiotics and haematinics must be continued for at least 6 months before being abandoned as recovery occurs in a small proportion of cases.

Bone marrow transplants are being given a trial in some centres. If the cause of secondary pancytopenia can be found and removed the patient may recover provided the bone marrow has not been irretrievably damaged. Injection of dimercaprol (p. 643) should be tried if the condition is due to gold or organic arsenicals. In other respects treatment is the same as for primary pancytopenia.

II. Anaemias due to Excessive Blood Destruction (Haemolytic Anaemias)

Destruction of red blood corpuscles causes anaemia if the degree of haemolysis exceeds the regenerative ability of the bone marrow. The excessive destruction of red cells results in hyperbilirubinaemia with latent or manifest jaundice but without bilirubinuria, hence the name acholuric jaundice. There is, however, excess of urobilinogen in the urine. The continuous demand for new red cells results in a constant reticulocytosis, often over 10 per cent. Thus the essential features of any haemolytic anaemia are persistent anaemia, persistent reticulocytosis, hyperbilirubinaemia and excess urobilinogen in the urine and the faeces.

Haptoglobins are plasma globulins which specifically combine with free haemoglobin to form complexes which are removed by the reticuloendothelial system. When haemolysis occurs the haptoglobins may be used up more quickly than they are produced and estimations of their level can provide an indication of the degree of the haemolytic process. Rarely in cases of severe haemolysis there is free haemoglobin in the plasma and in the urine.

A. Haemolytic Anaemia due to Hereditary Abnormalities of the Erythrocyte

The principal disorders are hereditary spherocytosis, G6PD deficiency (p. 821), haemoglobinopathies, such as sickle-cell disease (p. 822) and thalassaemia (p. 826). G6PD deficiency and the haemoglobinopathies are most common in Negroes and thalassaemia in the Mediterranean area. There has been a rise in the incidence of these disorders in Britain because of an increase in immigration.

Hereditary Spherocytosis (Acholuric Jaundice)

This disease is inherited as an autosomal dominant trait, frequently of variable penetrance (p. 12). The underlying cause is unknown but many of the red cells produced are abnormal in shape, being more nearly spherical than biconcave (microspherocytes). Such cells are unduly fragile and therefore more easily destroyed. This is the fundamental abnormality which is responsible for the clinical and haematological features of the disease.

The symptoms usually appear in childhood but they are often insufficient to cause the patient discomfort. However, moderate pallor and a slight yellow tint in the skin are noticeable. The spleen is invariably enlarged, but is not massive.

Crises may occur at variable intervals with severe anaemia and jaundice and increased splenic enlargement. At such times the patient complains of weakness and breathlessness, which, in severe cases, may be very marked and associated with rigors, fever and vomiting. The mechanism of the crisis is not fully understood, but it may be precipitated by infection.

Between the crises, blood examination shows a moderate normochromic anaemia, e.g. haemoglobin 10 g/dl, red cells $3 \cdot 5 \times 10^{12}/l$. The reticulocyte count is persistently raised—5 to 20 per cent. Stained films show well-filled red cells, the diameter of which is less than normal, but the thickness of which is increased—microspherocytosis. The red cells are unduly fragile in hypotonic salt solution. The serum bilirubin level is usually from 34 to 68 μmol/l (2–4 mg/100 ml). The urine contains excess urobilinogen but no bilirubin. During a haemolytic crisis the red blood count falls rapidly and subsequently the reticulocyte count rises sharply to 40 to 60 per cent or even more. A leucocytosis also occurs. Normoblastic hyperplasia of the bone marrow is found.

The recognition of the existence of a haemolytic anaemia is made on the finding of the characteristic blood picture as described above. The differentiation from other types of haemolytic anaemia depends upon the demonstration of increased fragility of red cells, microspherocytosis, splenomegaly, and especially on the family history of other cases of anaemia and jaundice. Spherocytes may be found in other forms of haemolytic anaemia. If red cells are tagged with [51]Chromate and returned to the patient's circulation, their time of survival will be found to be reduced. The Coombs' test (p. 40) is negative in hereditary spherocytosis.

While many patients lead a normal life and die of old age, others suffer from severe episodes of haemolytic anaemia or cholecystitis secondary to the development of pigment stones in the gall-bladder. Such episodes may end fatally.

Treatment. Splenectomy results in striking and usually permanent improvement both in the symptoms and in the anaemia. All authorities are agreed that operation should be advised when the anaemia causes persistent impairment of health, when severe haemolytic crises have occurred, when other members of the family have died from the disease, or where evidence of cholecystitis and cholelithiasis is present. Opinion differs as to the desirability of operation in mild cases with no resulting disability. The operation should be carried out during a period of remission, and in young children should be deferred until school age. Severe haemolytic crises require treatment by blood transfusion. Blood must be matched very carefully and administered by very slow drip, as gross haemolytic transfusion reactions are common in this disease. Iron and other haematinics are of no value. In this type of haemolytic anaemia treatment with corticosteroids is not indicated.

B. Haemolytic Anaemia due to Infective or Toxic Factors

Haemolytic streptococci, staphylococci and *Clostridium welchii* are the most important micro-organisms which can produce a haemolytic anaemia in man, although such an occurrence is very rare. Malaria is an important cause of haemolysis in tropical countries (p. 836).

Of the numerous agents which on occasion have been reported to cause haemolytic anaemia, mention should be made of the following: arsenic and its derivatives, lead, sulphonamides, potassium chlorate, naphthalene, methyldopa, mefenamic acid, cephalothin and nitrofurantoin.

C. Haemolytic Anaemia due to Erythrocyte Antibodies

The most important examples of anaemia in this group are haemolytic disease of the newborn, autoimmune (acquired) haemolytic anaemia, symptomatic haemolytic anaemia, and paroxysmal haemoglobinuria.

(a) Haemolytic Disease of the Newborn

This disease, previously called erythroblastosis fetalis, occurs in either sex at birth or within the first 2 to 3 days. The first-born child in the family is usually healthy, but in successive children the severity of the disease increases and later children may be born dead. Hydrops fetalis is the most severe form, death occurring *in utero*; icterus gravis neonatorum is a dangerous illness but compatible with survival; haemolytic disease of the newborn is the mildest form.

It appears that in most cases the rhesus (Rh) factor is the sensitising agent or antigen. The majority (85 per cent) of people, men and women, have red cells which contain the Rh antigen, D, and these people are said to be Rh-positive. Some of the children of an Rh-positive father and an Rh-negative mother are Rh-positive, since the factor is inherited as an autosomal dominant. The Rh-negative mother becomes sensitised by the Rh-positive substance contained in the fetal red cells. The maternal agglutinins (antibodies to Rh-positive factor) thus produced penetrate the placental barrier and cause haemolysis of the fetal erythrocytes.

In about 1 pregnancy in 10 the mother is Rh-negative and the fetus Rh-positive.

However haemolytic disease of the fetus is very rare in first pregnancies (provided the mother has not previously been sensitised by transfusion) and, fortunately, sensitisation does not occur as often as might be anticipated even in subsequent pregnancies. Indeed the risk of an Rh-negative woman having a baby with haemolytic disease of the newborn in any pregnancy other than the first one is about 1 in 22.

If a mother is Rh-negative and her husband Rh-positive, the maternal serum must be tested for antibodies between the 32nd and 36th week of each pregnancy. If they are found, delivery should be carried out in hospital. If no antibodies are detected the infant will probably escape the disease, but nevertheless the cord blood should be tested for antibodies. If they are present, preventive treatment can be instituted.

Very occasionally an antigen other than D is responsible for the development of haemolytic disease of the newborn.

It must be remembered that an Rh-negative mother who has had an Rh-positive fetus may be sensitised to Rh-positive blood. If she receives a transfusion and Rh-positive blood is given a haemolytic reaction may occur. Consequently all women of child-bearing age or under and all pregnant women who may require transfusion must have their blood typed for Rh factors as well as for the main blood groups.

Clinical Features. The clinical features of haemolytic anaemia of the newborn are those of severe haemolytic anaemia with oedema and enlargement of the liver and spleen. Clinical jaundice is usually absent for 24 hours after birth. Thereafter deep jaundice leading to kernicterus (p. 733) may occur. The severity of the jaundice is largely due to the immaturity of the fetal liver which is unable to conjugate the large amounts of bilirubin with which it has to deal. The blood picture is very striking. The haemoglobin level, which should normally be about 18 g per 100 ml at birth, falls rapidly. Enormous numbers of nucleated red cells and a reticulocytosis of 10 to 50 per cent are found in the peripheral blood.

In the severe cases the mortality is 70 to 80 per cent without treatment, death occurring within 2 weeks, but with exchange transfusion the mortality is low. Spontaneous recovery occurs in the mild cases.

Treatment. Exchange transfusion should be given to all severely affected infants, as this is the only method of treatment that will overcome heart failure in the very anaemic infant and prevent deep jaundice and kernicterus in others. Delay of even a day may prove fatal and hence early diagnosis is essential. Antenatal prediction from tests of the maternal serum for antibodies gives the infant his best chance. In mild cases simple transfusion will be sufficient, and in some instances no treatment is required.

It is now believed that the most common cause of primary Rh immunisation may be transplacental haemorrhage during the third stage of labour. The likelihood of an Rh-negative woman developing anti-Rh antibodies is related to the number of Rh-positive red cells present in her circulation immediately after delivery. The injection of gamma globulin containing a high titre of anti-D immunoglobulin into the mother shown to have such cells should be carried out within 72 hours of delivery. This will destroy the infant cells that have leaked into the mother's circulation and will prevent the development of haemolytic disease in later babies.

(b) Autoimmune (Acquired) Haemolytic Anaemia

In this form of haemolytic anaemia no family history can be obtained and the fault is believed to lie in the production of autoagglutinins and autohaemolysins which injure the red blood corpuscles (p. 40).

The clinical features are the same as those described for the hereditary type, but the crises are more severe and more frequent and the residual anaemia during remissions of greater degree. Microspherocytosis may not be present and the fragility of the red cells is either normal or only slightly increased. A serological test for immunoglobulin (Coombs' test, p. 40) is positive in acquired haemolytic anaemia, but negative in the hereditary form. It should, however, be realised that the test is not a specific one for the former condition, being positive also in certain uncommon haemolytic disorders, especially in infancy and following the administration of methyldopa.

The prognosis is more serious than in the hereditary form, death in haemolytic crises being more frequent.

It would appear reasonable to try the effect of prednisolone in a dosage of 60 mg daily by mouth for 3 to 4 weeks, and if a remission is induced the dose should be reduced to the lowest that will maintain the patient in remission without inducing adverse effects. Should corticosteroids fail initially or if the disorder is particularly severe, transfusion of carefully matched blood is required but the risks of reactions are even greater than in the hereditary form. If corticosteroid therapy fails, splenectomy should be carried out, especially if excessive blood destruction by the spleen can be shown by radioactive isotope studies to be present. The results are not as satisfactory as in hereditary haemolytic anaemia and when splenectomy and corticosteroids fail, immunosuppressive therapy (p. 49) or thymectomy (p. 50) may have to be considered.

(c) Symptomatic Haemolytic Anaemia

Haemolytic anaemia occurs occasionally in association with a variety of diseases such as chronic leukaemia, lymphadenoma, malignant disease, cirrhosis of the liver and infections such as syphilis and tuberculosis. The underlying mechanism is obscure but autoimmune factors contribute. A cold-antibody type of haemolytic anaemia sometimes occurs as a complication about the third week of an attack of virus pneumonia and may be associated with Raynaud's phenomenon (p. 243). Treatment is that of the underlying condition where possible.

(d) Paroxysmal Haemoglobinuria

This condition, caused by intravascular haemolysis, is found occasionally in association with syphilis or after severe exertion. Paroxysmal nocturnal haemoglobinuria is a rare condition of uncertain cause, occurring during sleep, and differs from these others in that frank haemolytic anaemia is not a feature.

Transfusion with Incompatible Blood

Transfusion with incompatible blood may arise: (1) when the infused red cells are of the wrong main blood group due to careless typing of the bloods; (2) when the bloods of recipient and donor are of compatible main groups but incompatible subgroups. Direct cross-matching of recipient's serum against donor's cells greatly reduces this risk; (3) from the transfusion of Rh-positive blood to a sensitised Rh-negative recipient.

Symptoms usually begin after only a few millilitres of blood have been given, and if the transfusion is immediately stopped there may be no serious consequences. In severe reactions the patient complains of shivering and restlessness, nausea and vomiting, precordial and lumbar pain. There is a cold, clammy skin with cyanosis. The pulse and respiration rates increase and the temperature rises to 38–40°C. The blood pressure falls and the patient passes into a state of shock. There is haemoglobinaemia, and possibly even haemoglobinuria; oliguria may occur with renal failure due to acute tubular necrosis. Jaundice appears after a few hours. In severe cases the anuria persists and uraemia develops, from which the patient may die. In others diuresis occurs even after several days and the patient recovers. In the majority the acute features subside in 24 to 48 hours.

Prophylaxis involves great care in the typing of blood and direct cross-matching before administration. The first 50–100 ml of any transfusion should be given very slowly and the transfusion stopped at once if any untoward symptoms develop. The patient should be under continuous observation during transfusion. This is especially important when an unconscious patient is being transfused.

Treatment of the established reaction involves giving 100 mg of hydrocortisone hemisuccinate intravenously, and initiating the general treatment of peripheral circulatory failure. When acute tubular necrosis occurs the measures recommended for its treatment on page 496 must be instituted at once.

III. Anaemias of Uncertain Origin

Infection. Anaemia, which is mild or moderate in degree and normochromic in type may develop secondary to a severe chronic infection, particularly if fever is present. A mild degree of iron deficiency may be found. The response to iron therapy, both oral and parenteral, is usually unsatisfactory unless the infection is eliminated.

Rheumatoid Arthritis. A hypochromic, normocytic anaemia occurs, resistant to oral iron (p. 643).

Uraemia. In chronic renal disease anaemia is common but the bone marrow remains cellular until renal failure is very marked, when hypoplasia may be found. It is possible that in advanced renal damage there may be deficiency of erythropoietin (p. 690) and also a haemolytic component. The anaemia may be normocytic, microcytic or even macrocytic, and hypochromia may be present.

Hepatic Cirrhosis. Here the anaemia is usually macrocytic or normocytic and the marrow macronormoblastic. If megaloblastic anaemia occurs this is probably due to primary malnutrition; it is found particularly in chronic alcoholics with cirrhosis. The occurrence of iron deficiency anaemia suggests gastric or oesophageal haemorrhage.

Malignant Disease. The causes of anaemia in widespread malignant disease are numerous. They include impaired appetite, malabsorption or blood loss from the alimentary tract and occasionally increased haemolysis. Metastases in the bone marrow may cause a leucoerythroblastic anaemia (p. 596).

Erythrocytosis and Polycythaemia

In these conditions there is an increase in the number of circulating blood cells in response to a physiological stimulus (erythrocytosis) or as a result of a pathological condition (polycythaemia). Leucocytosis and leukaemia are the equivalent terms for the white cell series.

Relative Erythrocytosis

An increase in the haemoglobin percentage and the red cell count is found in the presence of marked dehydration and haemoconcentration, e.g. after persistent vomiting or diarrhoea, traumatic shock, or extensive burns. There is a decrease in plasma volume and in total circulating blood volume, and the haemoglobin and red cell count fall when the dehydration is overcome.

Secondary Erythrocytosis

This most commonly occurs as a physiological response of the erythropoietic tissue to the stimulus of anoxaemia. Hence it is found in persons living at altitudes over 10,000 ft, in chronic pulmonary disease such as emphysema and in congenital heart disease, especially when an arteriovenous shunt is present. Erythrocytosis may also be associated with high levels of erythropoietin, for example in some patients with renal cysts. It may occur occasionally, for reasons unknown, in cases of Cushing's syndrome, hepatoma and hydronephrosis.

The clinical picture is that of the underlying condition. In contradistinction to what occurs in polycythaemia vera, splenomegaly is rarely present. Blood examination shows haemoglobin 16–20 g/dl, red cell count $6 \cdot 0$–$8 \cdot 0 \times 10^{12}/l$ or more. The PCV is correspondingly raised. Leucocytosis and thrombocytosis are usually absent. The total blood volume is increased.

This variety of erythrocytosis is usually beneficial to the course of the underlying condition and thus requires no treatment.

Polycythaemia Vera (Erythraemia)

This is a rare disease occurring in both sexes mostly about middle age. The cause is unknown. There is overactivity of the haemopoietic tissue, with extension of red marrow throughout the long bones. Microscopically the marrow is hyperplastic, with an increase of normoblasts, myelocytes and megakaryocytes. It is believed that the disease represents a proliferative disorder of the marrow which occasionally progresses to myelofibrosis (p. 596) or to chronic myeloid leukaemia (p. 620). These conditions are probably interrelated and, together with haemorrhagic thrombocythaemia (p. 634), are referred to as the *myeloproliferative disorders*.

Clinical Features. The onset is insidious and the patient complains of throbbing headache, dizziness, tinnitus, dyspepsia and fatigue.

In the later stages of the disease, hypertension occurs in about 50 per cent of cases and atherosclerosis is even more common. Owing to the increased platelet count and viscosity of the blood, there is liability to thrombosis. Thus symptoms of peripheral occlusive vascular disease, and vascular accidents, such as coronary thrombosis and cerebral thrombosis, or cardiac failure, may occur. There is also a tendency to haemorrhage from the stomach, urinary tract or uterus.

Physical examination shows a dusky red and cyanotic facies. The spleen is palpably enlarged and firm in about 75 per cent of cases.

Examination of the blood shows haemoglobin 16–20 g/dl, with a corresponding rise in the red cell count and haematocrit reading. The granular white cell count is elevated, and the platelet count is often much increased. The red cells are usually slightly smaller than normal and there may sometimes be a relative deficiency of haemoglobin giving a low MCHC. There is a marked increase in blood viscosity due to the increase in red cell mass which is the total volume of red cells in the body and which can be measured by special techniques. In contrast to what is found in chronic myeloid leukaemia (p. 620) the leucocyte alkaline phosphatase score is normal.

Treatment and Prognosis

1. Venesection. This gives temporary relief, and removal of 500 ml of blood once or twice weekly can be done to bring the PCV down to about 0·54 (54 per cent).

2. Irradiation. A satisfactory method of reducing erythrocyte production is by irradiation of the bone marrow. This may be achieved by the administration of radioactive phosphorus (^{32}P), a single dose of 3–7 millicuries of ^{32}P being given by intravenous injection. Further treatment of this nature will depend upon the response to the first dose.

3. Chemotherapy. Busulphan (p. 620) in an initial dosage of 2–4 mg daily followed by a maintenance dose of 2 mg once or twice weekly has been found effective. It has been suggested that patients treated in this way are less likely to develop acute myeloid leukaemia than after treatment with radioactive phosphorus. The antimalarial drug pyrimethamine is a folate antagonist which may be used if other therapy is not available or is contraindicated.

With modern treatment expectation of life may be normal, but death may occur in a few years from one of the complications, such as the various thrombotic or haemorrhagic episodes mentioned above, or from heart failure. Some cases develop myeloblastic leukaemia and others may terminate as myelofibrosis.

DISORDERS OF THE WHITE BLOOD CELLS AND THE RETICULO-ENDOTHELIAL SYSTEM

Agranulocytosis

Agranulocytosis is a serious disease characterised by marked leucopenia with great reduction in, or absence of, neutrophil granulocytes.

Aetiology

1. In most cases the cause is an idiosyncrasy or sensitisation to, or poisoning by, a variety of drugs. Among these the most important are amidopyrine, chlorothiazide, chlorpromazine, chlorpropamide, imipramine, phenindione, phenylbutazone, oxyphenbutazone, streptomycin, various sulphonamides and thiouracil derivatives. Exposure to insecticides should also be considered.

2. In some cases there is no discoverable cause—idiopathic agranulocytosis.

3. It may follow excessive irradiation or the use of cytotoxic drugs or antimetabolites (p. 619).

4. Agranulocytosis is found as an integral part of pancytopenia (p. 606), leukaemia and some cases of hypersplenism (p. 625).

5. It occurs, rarely, in severe infections.

Pathology. In most cases the bone marrow shows a virtual disappearance of the granular cells and their precursors. In some the marrow contains many early myelocytes, with few mature forms—an arrest of maturation. In the cases in group 4 the appearance of the bone marrow is that of the underlying blood disease.

Clinical Features. There may be a history of exposure to one of the agents mentioned above. The onset may be either sudden or gradual. In the acute and severe cases the condition begins with sore throat, fever and often rigors which are followed by great prostration. There is rapidly advancing necrotic ulceration in the throat and mouth, with little evidence of pus formation. In fulminating cases the patient dies in a few days from toxaemia and septicaemia. In less acute cases there may be a preliminary period of malaise and weakness.

Blood examination may show little alteration in the haemoglobin or red cell count. There is marked leucopenia, usually below $2 \cdot 0 \times 10^9/l$ (2,000 per mm^3), and falling to $5 \cdot 0 \times 10^8/l$ or less. The percentage of granulocytes falls rapidly until none may be found.

A chronic type has been described in which there is a persistent or recurring leucopenia with granulopenia. Rarely the neutropenia occurs in cycles of three weeks (cyclic neutropenia). In such cases the symptoms are chiefly malaise, low grade fever and sore throat often without ulceration.

Prophylaxis. All the drugs mentioned at the beginning of this section should be regarded as potentially dangerous and should be carefully employed. The patient should be warned to report to his doctor if he-feels unwell and feverish or if he develops a sore throat.

Treatment. On the first appearance of sore throat and fever the administration of any of these drugs should be stopped and a white cell count carried out. A blood culture should be obtained and antibiotics should be administered preferably by the oral route, e.g. ampicillin (p. 90), and fresh blood should be transfused. Even the fulminating cases may be saved by these means, but no cure will result unless the formation of granulocytes is resumed. This usually occurs within 2 to 3 days if infection is controlled and the cause has been removed. Should improvement not occur, the patient should be given blood transfusions. Careful nursing in isolation is required with adequate diet and extra vitamins. Regular toilet of the mouth will contribute greatly to the patient's comfort. Dimercaprol injection should be given if agranulocytosis follows the administration of gold salts or organic arsenicals.

Prognosis. In severe cases the mortality is very high, but in chronic or recurring cases recovery is common. Spontaneous resumption of granulocyte formation frequently occurs, especially if the leucotoxic drug is withdrawn, and this gives rise to difficulty in assessing the value of therapy.

Infectious Mononucleosis

(Glandular Fever)

This is a benign acute infective disease most probably due in many instances to the Epstein Barr virus as antibodies to this agent can be found in the serum of patients who have recovered from the disorder. It occurs chiefly in children and young adults of either sex both sporadically or in epidemics. The condition is mildly infectious, the incubation period probably being 5 to 10 days.

Clinical Features. The most common presenting features are tiredness, malaise and generalised pains in muscles, headache, pyrexia and enlargement of superficial lymph nodes. An early sign may be the occurrence of petechial haemorrhages at the junction of the hard and soft palate and this is frequently followed by sore throat with or without exudate. The glandular enlargement may not occur until the third week. A maculopapular rash often appears during the first 10 days in adults. Hepatitis is common. The spleen may be enlarged but seldom extends much below the costal margin. It is soft and not tender. Pain in the right iliac fossa may result from mesenteric adenitis.

There is usually no anaemia and in the early stages the white cell count is frequently normal or low. However in the first few days there may be an increase in the proportion of granulocytes, but thereafter the characteristic increase in non-granular white cells appears, amounting to 60 to 80 per cent of the total white cell count. These include ordinary lymphocytes, ordinary monocytes and 'atypical' lymphocytes (large cells with blue-staining often foamy cytoplasm and nuclei with coarse chromatin, which may be oval, kidney-shaped or have a pseudopodial appearance). The proportions of these cells vary greatly in different cases but immature leucocytes are not present. The total white cell count is commonly $10 \cdot 0 - 20 \cdot 0 \times 10^9/l$ ($10 \cdot 0 - 20 \cdot 0 \times 10^3/mm^3$).

Diagnosis. Heterophile antibodies develop in the serum of patients with infectious mononucleosis and their demonstration forms the basis of valuable diagnostic tests. After the first week of the illness the Paul-Bunnell reaction becomes positive in titres of 1 in 200 or more in over 80 per cent of cases and may remain positive for many weeks. Absorption techniques are necessary to distinguish the specific antibodies of infectious mononucleosis from those of serum sickness which may also cause a positive reaction. The Wassermann reaction also may be falsely positive in infectious mononucleosis. A simple and rapid slide test known as the 'Monospot Test' is now commonly used as a screening procedure in infectious mononucleosis and is quicker and more sensitive than the Paul-Bunnell reaction. It has also been observed that if patients with infectious mononucleosis have been given ampicillin to treat what was thought to be a bacterial throat infection, they develop, in over 90 per cent of instances, a skin eruption due to the drug within 2 to 3 days. The reason is not understood but it is unsafe to give ampicillin as a diagnostic test as laryngeal oedema may occur in some cases.

Differential Diagnosis. During the invasive phase, especially in children, the disease may be confused with the various exanthemata, tonsillitis and diphtheria. Distinction must be made from leukaemia in which there is persistence of the clinical features, including lymph node enlargement, and in which the marrow biopsy is characteristic and the Paul-Bunnell test is negative; and from lymphadenoma in which the lymph node enlargement is persistent and progressive and the peripheral blood does not show the characteristic 'atypical' lymphocytes. The secondary stage of syphilis must also be excluded. In young people, infectious mononucleosis in a milder form may cause general ill-health and be overlooked unless a blood film is examined. In contrast in severe cases there may be features of lymphocytic meningitis or mild encephalitis. It should be noted that in toxoplasmosis

(p. 853), and in cytomegalic inclusion disease, there may be enlargement of lymph nodes and changes in the blood picture similar to those found in infectious mononucleosis.

Treatment and Prognosis. This is symptomatic, the patient being kept in bed during the febrile period. Corticosteroid therapy may be helpful if the constitutional symptoms are severe.

Although recovery is invariable, some patients may be ill for weeks or months with intermittent fever, sweats and debility. Very occasionally rupture of the spleen may occur. Sometimes there is thrombocytopenia or haemolytic anaemia of the autoimmune type.

The Leukaemias

In these disorders there is an abnormal proliferation of the leucopoietic tissues throughout the body which is usually associated with an increase in the number of white blood cells of one type in the peripheral blood, among which immature forms occur. Leukaemia is a progressive and fatal condition causing death from anaemia, haemorrhage or intercurrent infection, though its course may vary from a few weeks to several years.

The cause of leukaemia is not known. The uncontrolled proliferation of cells and the development of foci of leucocyte formation in organs other than the bone marrow, spleen and lymph nodes lead to its classification as a neoplastic disorder. However, the cells show no truly invasive properties and the process appears to start as a generalised cellular disturbance. Chromosomal abnormalities, such as may be produced by exposure to ionising irradiation, can be found in some leukaemic cells and irradiation may be an aetiological factor in the disease. In some animals and birds viruses are known to cause leukaemia and it is recognised that these agents can transform cells of the lymphocyte series. Though the possibility of a viral aetiology of leukaemia in man continues to attract attention, there is no direct evidence that the disorder is caused by such an infection.

The leukaemic process may affect the formation of any one of the granulocyte, lymphocyte or monocyte cell series. In acute leukaemia, of which there are three varieties according to the cell line involved, the disorder pursues a rapidly progressive course with excessive production of the most primitive precursor cells referred to as 'blast' cells. In chronic myeloid and chronic lymphatic leukaemia the overproduction affecting the granulocytic or lymphatic series is a slower and more benign process reflected in the appearance of more mature cells in the blood. The term *subleukaemic leukaemia* (sometimes called *aleukaemic leukaemia*) is applied to any form of leukaemia in which the total white cell count in the peripheral blood is not increased, though the differential blood count may show the presence of immature circulating leucocytes and bone marrow examination is essential to establish the diagnosis. A rare variation of acute myeloblastic leukaemia associated with an extraordinary proliferation of red cell precursors in the marrow and with large numbers of normoblasts in the peripheral blood is referred to as *di Guglielmo's disease* or *erythraemic myelosis*.

Acute Leukaemia

Owing to the similarity in the clinical picture, it is convenient to consider all forms of acute leukaemia together. Acute lymphoblastic leukaemia is in general the most common variety, and is the most frequent type of leukaemia in children. It is the most common cause of death from malignant disease in childhood and in two-thirds of the cases presents in the subleukaemic form. Acute myeloblastic leukaemia and the least common variety, monoblastic leukaemia, occur at all ages. Both sexes are affected. The pathological changes are similar to those found in the chronic forms (pp. 620, 621), but myeloblasts, lymphoblasts or monoblasts predominate in the respective types. The spleen and lymph nodes do not usually become as large as in the chronic forms.

Clinical Features. The disease may begin insidiously but the clinical onset is usually abrupt. There is fever, malaise and a rapidly advancing anaemia. Epistaxis, spongy bleeding gums or other haemorrhagic manifestations, including purpura, are common and are due largely to thrombocytopenia. Sore throat and ulcers in the mouth or pharynx are frequent, due to reduction in normal polymorphonuclear leucocytes. Hypertrophy of the gums is often noted in monoblastic leukaemia. Muscular and joint pains may occur. The spleen and often the liver are enlarged in the later stages. The cervical lymph nodes may be enlarged secondary to pharyngeal sepsis, but in the lymphatic form increase in size of these and other lymph nodes is a common early feature.

Blood examination shows a profound and increasing anaemia of normochromic type. In the myeloblastic and monoblastic varieties normoblasts and increased numbers of reticulocytes are frequently seen in the peripheral blood, due to disturbance of the erythropoietic tissues in the bone marrow by leukaemic infiltration. Thrombocytopenia is common with a prolonged bleeding time. The white cell count may be normal or low but is usually increased to $20–50 \times 10^9/l$. Immature ('blast') cells comprise 30 to 90 per cent of the white cells. Using Romanowsky stains the distinction between the different types of primitive white cells is often difficult, but in acute myeloblastic leukaemia myelocytes and granulocytes, in acute lymphoblastic leukaemia lymphocytes, and in monoblastic leukaemia monocytes, form most of the remainder of the white cells and suggest the diagnosis. The cell type can be easily determined by the use of special cytochemical stains.

The bone marrow shows a marked predominance of the appropriate primitive white cell to the almost complete exclusion of all normal marrow cells.

Diagnosis. In the early stages the condition may be confused with infective illnesses, such as miliary tuberculosis, acute rheumatic fever, and infectious mononucleosis, this last being most important in differential diagnosis. Pancytopenia, agranulocytosis and the haemolytic anaemias may also be simulated. The rapidly advancing anaemia, the eventual enlargement of the spleen, liver or lymph nodes and the finding of immature white cells in the peripheral blood suggest the diagnosis and this is established by marrow biopsy, which shows a large excess of primitive white cells of the appropriate type. The subleukaemic form may give particular difficulty since the total white count is normal or low, but immature cells are to be found in the peripheral blood on careful search or in buffy coat smears, and marrow biopsy reveals the typical picture of acute leukaemia.

Treatment. While there is no known cure for leukaemia there have been great changes in the approach to intensive treatment in recent years. The results have been particularly encouraging in the acute lymphoblastic form in childhood where it now seems possible to achieve cure in an increasing proportion of cases. It must be emphasised that the best results have been obtained in centres experienced in coping with the complex problems of the chemotherapeutic regimes involved. The details of the latter in current use are beyond the scope of this chapter and what follows is a brief account of the types of drugs employed and an indication of the ways in which they may be used.

Mention must first be made of prednisolone which has a specific lympholytic effect in addition to an action on capillaries which reduces the bleeding tendency associated with thrombocytopenia. It is thus a most important drug in the induction of a remission in cases of acute lymphoblastic leukaemia and is given in the other acute varieties when the platelet count is low. Most of the other drugs used in this form of chemotherapy act by interfering with nucleic acid synthesis and they affect not only the dividing leukaemic cells but also normal cells so that severe haemopoietic depression and other serious side-effects can be produced. Mercaptopurine, thioguanine, methotrexate and cytarabine are examples of antimetabolites; vincristine is a plant alkaloid, and daunorubicin an antibiotic, while cyclophosphamide is one of a large group of alkylating agents which also include the nitrogen mustards. These compounds act in various ways to interfere with cell mitosis. Asparaginase is an agent which destroys asparagine on which some leukaemic cells are dependent. Radiotherapy is of no value in acute leukaemia except in the eradication of leukaemic cells in the brain in children.

Supportive treatment of patients with acute leukaemia is important because of the effects of the disorder and the side-effects often induced by chemotherapy. Blood transfusion is given to correct anaemia, platelet concentrates may be required to arrest a bleeding tendency not prevented by prednisolone and antibiotics may be necessary to combat infections associated with pancytopenia and immunosuppression.

The aim in treatment is to induce a haematological remission by destroying the maximum number of leukaemic cells and, when the patient's general state has improved, to attempt to eradicate any remaining leukaemic cells by intensive chemotherapy. Combined drug therapy is always used to attack the cells in different ways simultaneously. Thus in a child with acute lymphoblastic leukaemia, prednisolone and vincristine are given to induce a remission which can be expected in 3 to 4 weeks. Thereafter the aim is to consolidate the remission with intensive chemotherapy, but since many of the drugs used do not cross the blood-brain barrier, cranial radiotherapy is first given along with intrathecal injections of methotrexate to eradicate leukaemic cells in the central nervous system which might survive to cause relapse of the condition. After this cyclic courses combining mercaptopurine, methotrexate and cytarabine are instituted and repeated for up to 3 years, alternating with short reinduction courses. Full remissions of more than 5 years in 60 per cent of cases are being achieved by such measures in special centres with expectation of further improvement as co-ordinated trials of new drug regimes proceed.

Prognosis. The results of treatment in the other varieties of acute leukaemia in children and in all types of adults are at present much less impressive than those indicated above. In the acute myeloblastic and, to a lesser extent, in the acute monoblastic types, daunorubicin has proved valuable in producing temporary ablation of the bone marrow for the purpose of initial treatment. Its use in combination with cytarabine and thioguanine in intermittent short courses has led to prolonged remission in an increasing number of cases. In addition attempts to stimulate immune mechanisms by the injection of irradiated blast cells pooled from similar cases are being employed in some treatment centres.

Chronic Myeloid Leukaemia

The disease occurs chiefly between the ages of 35 and 60 years and is equally common in males and females.

Pathology. There is extension of the marrow through the long bones. The marrow is grey and gelatinous and is crowded with myelocytes and young polymorphonuclear leucocytes. Leukaemic infiltrations occur in the liver, spleen and lymph nodes, and in most organs throughout the body.

Clinical Features. The onset is insidious and the clinical features are very varied. There may be slowly advancing anaemia with loss of weight, dragging discomfort in the left upper quadrant of the abdomen due to the great enlargement of the spleen, and prominence of the abdomen. Attacks of acute left upper abdominal pain may develop when infarction occurs in the spleen. Epistaxis or other haemorrhages may occur in the later stages.

The spleen is found to be much enlarged, occasionally extending across the midline and reaching below the umbilicus. It is firm and smooth and may be tender if infarction has recently occurred. The liver is also enlarged but the lymph nodes are usually of normal size.

Blood examination shows an anaemia of normocytic, normochromic type which increases as the disease progresses. Normoblasts are often found. The white cell count is greatly increased to $50-500 \times 10^9/l$ or more and consists almost entirely of young granulocytic cells, myelocytes and occasional myeloblasts. In the later stages the appearance of an increasing number of myeloblasts indicates the approach of a terminal acute phase. The platelet count is often high initially but thrombocytopenia gradually develops.

Diagnosis. This depends upon the finding of the characteristic blood picture. Marrow biopsy may be required to exclude other conditions causing a leucoerythroblastic blood picture (p. 596). The granulocytes of chronic myeloid leukaemia are deficient in alkaline phosphatase and this is the basis of a staining reaction to differentiate them from normally developing granulocytes. In a high proportion of cases a characteristic abnormality of the 22 chromosome, the Philadelphia chromosome (p. 10), is found in the myelocytes. The relationship to other myeloproliferative disorders is described on page 613.

Treatment. Effective palliative treatment can restore most patients to a period of symptom-free life. The method of choice is by chemotherapy using the alkylating agent, busulphan (Myleran). It is given orally in a commencing dose of 4 mg daily and can bring about a temporary but satisfactory clinical and haematological remission in a high proportion of cases with marked reduction in splenomegaly. Subsequent maintenance dosage, e.g. 2 mg daily, is continued and regulated according to the results of frequent blood examinations and the general state of the patient. It must be emphasised that all such drugs are capable of producing severe haemopoietic depression and their administration requires careful haematological supervision. The too rapid destruction of abnormal white cells may cause a rise in blood uric acid and even uric acid nephropathy.

Allopurinol (p. 650) can be used to prevent this complication. Blood transfusion may be necessary to correct increasing anaemia and in some cases, where there is evidence of haemolysis, corticosteroids may be beneficial. In some centres a trial of splenectomy following the induction of remission is being made in the hope that it may prolong survival by making chemotherapy more effective in subsequent relapses.

Radiotherapy, given as a course of localised splenic irradiation, reduces the size of the spleen and brings about a fall in the abnormal white cell count with a simultaneous improvement of the anaemia and general health. The dosage is controlled by frequent blood examinations and treatment is stopped when the white cell count falls to about $20 \times 10^9/l$ or if the platelet count drops excessively. Further irradiation is needed when relapse occurs, usually after about 9 months, and thereafter courses may be required at shorter intervals.

Prognosis. The disease pursues a chronic course with increasing general features of anaemia. With treatment the average duration of life from the time of diagnosis is about 3 years, though some patients live longer. The terminal acute stage is indicated by the appearance of an increased number of myeloblasts, up to 10 to 15 per cent or more, by marked anaemia and by haemorrhages.

Chronic Lymphatic Leukaemia

This is the commonest variety of leukaemia and occurs much more frequently in males than in females and in the age period 45 to 80 years.

Pathology. There is moderate enlargement of lymph nodes and other lymphoid tissue throughout the body, the normal structure being replaced by a mass of lymphocytes. The spleen and liver are moderately enlarged and show lymphocytic infiltration. The bone marrow becomes progressively infiltrated with lymphocytes, which eventually replace the erythropoietic and myeloid tissue.

Clinical Features. The onset is very insidious and in contrast to chronic myeloid leukaemia the development of anaemia tends to be much slower and the presenting feature is usually the finding of firm rubbery, discrete and painless lymph nodes in the cervical, axillary and inguinal regions. The spleen is palpable but is usually smaller than in chronic myeloid leukaemia. The liver may also be enlarged. Haemorrhagic manifestations are much less common than in the chronic myeloid variety, but in widespread lymphoproliferative disorders there is an increased tendency to recurrent infections due possibly to altered immunity mechanisms.

Peripheral blood examination usually shows a mild but increasing anaemia, though normoblasts are rarely found. Haemolytic anaemia may occur. The white cell count may be greatly increased, up to $500 \times 10^9/l$. Of these cells about 95 per cent are lymphocytes, which are predominantly of the small variety. Lymphoblasts are rare except in the terminal stages. The platelet count is usually low and may fall below $100 \times 10^9/l$.

Diagnosis. When the white cell count is very high the recognition of the disease is easy by examination of a blood film. When the white cell count is below $30 \times 10^9/l$ marrow biopsy is essential. Chronic lymphatic leukaemia must be distinguished from (1) *lymphadenoma* and other forms of lymphoma in which there is no characteristic blood picture and which usually occur in a younger age group;

(2) *infectious mononucleosis*, which has an acute febrile onset, in which the enlarged lymph nodes are soft and may be tender, the proportion of monocytes is increased, the lymphocytes are atypical and the Paul-Bunnell test is frequently positive; and (3) *tuberculous cervical lymphadenitis*, which occurs in young people and in which there is usually no enlargement of lymph nodes in other areas or of the spleen.

Treatment. Elderly patients with chronic lymphatic leukaemia may remain in relatively good health with little or no anaemia for several years. When treatment becomes necessary, or in younger patients, chemotherapy may be used. In general the response in chronic lymphatic leukaemia is less dramatic than in chronic myeloid leukaemia, and increasingly frequent courses of treatment are required. The most satisfactory chemotherapeutic agent at present available is the alkylating agent chlorambucil. The suggested dose is $0 \cdot 1$–$0 \cdot 2$ mg per kg of body weight given daily in tablet form for 2 to 8 weeks depending on the haematological response. Corticosteroid therapy may be of value where there is evidence that haemolysis is contributing to the anaemia. Radiotherapy may also be used in treatment, either as localised irradiation to shrink a large mass of lymph nodes or as splenic irradiation in cases with gross splenomegaly. Allopurinol (p. 650) should be given when a high lymphocyte count is reduced rapidly by treatment.

Prognosis. The course of the disease is more slowly progressive than that of chronic myeloid leukaemia, but death usually occurs within 5 to 10 years of the time of diagnosis. In elderly patients it tends to progress very slowly and may not materially shorten the expectation of life. An increase in the number of lymphoblasts is a grave prognostic sign; it often heralds an acute terminal phase.

The Malignant Lymphomas (The Reticuloses)

These terms are applied to a group of neoplastic disorders affecting the reticuloendothelial tissues and causing lymph node and splenic enlargement without the peripheral blood picture of leukaemia. The progressive proliferation of cells, which may initially start as a localised process, eventually becomes widespread and involves the bone marrow with replacement of normal haematopoiesis. Anaemia and suppression of normal immunity mechanisms occur in the more advanced stages of the disorders. Complex pathological classifications of these diseases are based on the type of reticuloendothelial cell or cells that are responsible for the histological abnormalities seen in biopsies obtained from affected lymph nodes and the diagnosis is established in this way.

Immunological studies using surface marker techniques to identify T and B lymphocytes have been applied to human lymphoproliferative disorders. In many cases of lymphocytic lymphoma the disease represents a monoclonal B cell proliferation as in chronic lymphatic leukaemia. T cell neoplasia appears less common but it is known that T cells form many of the proliferating cells within the nodes of lymphadenoma (Hodgkin's disease) which is a common and important member of this group of disorders. Other malignant lymphomas include lymphosarcoma, reticulum cell sarcoma, follicular lymphoma and Burkitt's lymphoma (p. 827).

Lymphadenoma (Hodgkin's Disease)

This disease is characterised by progressive painless enlargement of lymphoid tissue throughout the body, and anaemia.

Aetiology. The disease occurs in both sexes, chiefly in adolescence and early adult life. The pathogenesis is unknown and the condition is regarded as a form of malignant disease allied to other tumours of the reticuloendothelial system.

Pathology. Microscopic examination of the enlarged discrete lymph nodes shows a replacement of the normal structure by proliferation of reticuloendothelial cells. Giant cells with two or three nuclei are seen, and there may be many eosinophils. The fibrous stroma is often increased. Caseation and necrosis are not found. Infiltration with greyish areas of Hodgkin's tissue causes enlargement of the spleen and liver. The bone marrow, lungs, kidneys and alimentary tract are also frequently involved though deposits are very rare in the nervous system. The type of histological picture gives an important indication of the degree of malignancy of the disease process in relation to treatment and prognosis.

Clinical Features. The disease has an insidious onset, enlargement of one group of superficial nodes usually occurring first. The cervical groups are often involved earliest. The progressive enlargement includes the axillary and inguinal groups and extends to thoracic and abdominal nodes which are occasionally affected first. The nodes are usually painless, discrete and rubbery, and they vary in size from about 2 to 6 centimetres in diameter. The skin is freely mobile over them. Pressure by the node masses and Hodgkin's deposits on neighbouring structures may cause a variety of features such as dysphagia, dyspnoea, venous obstruction, jaundice and paraplegia. The spleen is enlarged and usually palpable; it is firm and painless, and splenomegaly may be the earliest presenting feature. Enlargement of the liver is commonly present.

General features include progressive weakness and loss of weight. Fever is often present, and in some cases is of a low grade irregular type, while in others there are recurrent bouts of pyrexia with the temperature rising to 39°C for several days, alternating with apyrexial periods (Pel-Ebstein fever). Fever is common in cases in which the spleen and abdominal lymph nodes are primarily affected. In many cases there is no fever until the terminal stages. Pruritus is a troublesome symptom in about 10 per cent of cases. Some patients experience discomfort at the site of a lesion, e.g. in bone, a few minutes after drinking alcohol.

Anaemia is usual and progressive. It is commonly normochromic and normocytic and occasionally symptomatic haemolytic anaemia is present. There is no diagnostic change in the white cells. The count may be normal, but it is often moderately increased initially and decreased in the terminal phases when there is frequently accompanying thrombocytopenia. The proportion of granulocytes is usually increased, and 15 to 20 per cent of cases show a moderate eosinophilia. An important diagnostic point is that a lymphocytosis does not occur. Usually marrow puncture fails to reveal any diagnostic features, although occasionally Hodgkin's tissue may be found in the marrow if a trephine needle is used.

Diagnosis. This involves the differential diagnosis of conditions producing enlargement of lymph nodes and of the spleen. The diseases with which Hodgkin's disease are most readily confused are: *tuberculous lymphadenitis*, which is usually confined to the neck, in which the nodes may become matted together, may show caseation and sinus formation, and there is no splenomegaly; *chronic pyogenic lymphadenitis* (chiefly also of the neck), in which the nodes are small and tender, a source of infection can be found, and there is no splenomegaly; *lymphatic* *leukaemia*, in which the examination of the blood and bone marrow reveals the characteristic changes; *infectious mononucleosis*, in which the lymph node and splenic enlargement is transient and the blood examination and a positive Paul-Bunnell test are diagnostic; *other types of malignant lymphoma* which can be distinguished only by microscopic examination of an excised node; *secondary syphilis* with generalised lymph node enlargement, in which the swelling is transient, a skin rash is common and serological reactions are positive; *the anaemia associated with portal hypertension* in which there is splenomegaly but lymph node enlargement is absent.

The diagnosis can be established with certainty only by biopsy of a lymph node. Liver biopsy may provide the diagnosis in cases with hepatic enlargement.

Treatment. Considerable advances have been made in the treatment of this disease with increasing hopes that cure may be achieved in some cases. Clinical classification into four stages according to the degree of involvement at the time of diagnosis is considered in relation to the histological changes shown at lymph node biopsy. The radiological technique of lymphangiography is used to determine the extent of lymph node involvement. In the most favourable cases where the disease is found to be limited to one anatomical site and unaccompanied by systemic symptoms (Stage 1), megavoltage irradiation yields most encouraging results with survival in good health for 10 years or more in about 50 per cent of patients. Even though the spleen is not enlarged in the early stages, splenectomy is now advocated in many centres as part of the initial treatment as histological examination has shown that early changes of the Hodgkin's process may be removed by this procedure. This is still a controversial matter.

In cases where the disease is found to be more widespread at the time of diagnosis more extensive radiotherapy is employed and courses of chemotherapy are used in addition. The latter becomes the mainstay of treatment in the more advanced stages of the disorder when the systemic effects and increasing anaemia render palliative therapy more difficult. As in the acute leukaemias the current trend in chemotherapy is to use courses of combinations of drugs which are more effective than agents used singly. A quadruple therapy course which has produced better remissions in Hodgkin's disease than those previously achieved combines prednisolone with mustine hydrochloride, procarbazine and vinblastine. Again as with the leukaemias the best results are obtained in centres with experience in dealing with such treatment.

Prognosis. The disease is fatal but in many cases is only slowly progressive. The 5-year survival rate in patients with localised disease treated by radiotherapy exceeds 70 per cent, and they may remain free from symptoms for 10 to 20 years. When the disease is widespread the course is fairly rapid over a period of months but intensive chemotherapy may produce long remissions. Histological features are also helpful in assessing prognosis.

Myelomatosis

(Plasma Cell Myeloma)

This relatively uncommon malignant condition is associated with a neoplastic proliferation of abnormal plasma cells in the bone marrow. It appears that these plasma cells arise from a monoclonal B lymphocyte proliferation. Myelomatosis is one of a group of disorders to which the name *paraproteinaemias* is given. They are characterised by an abnormal pattern of immunoglobulins in the peripheral blood produced by the abnormal cells in the bone marrow (p. 37) and seen as a 'myeloma band' on electrophoresis. Certain of these conditions show an increase in the serum content of immunoglobulin M, and the term '*macroglobulinaemia*' is then used. The plasma cells produce local tumours of bone, sometimes solitary at first, but eventually becoming widespread and in this form the condition is known as *multiple myeloma*.

Clinical Features. Myelomatosis occurs in either sex, chiefly after the age of 50 years. A common presenting symptom is back pain due to pressure on spinal nerve roots, and pathological fracture may occur in any bone involved. Vertebral body collapse may give rise to paraplegia. Increasing plasma cell replacement of the marrow is associated with progressive normocytic anaemia, and eventually there is also granulopenia and thrombocytopenia. In the variety known as diffuse myelomatosis the clinical picture is that of progressive marrow involvement without the formation of bony lesions, and, in the rare extramedullary type, soft tissue tumours may occur. There is usually no enlargement of the spleen, lymph nodes or liver. Other features are an undue liability to infections, especially of the respiratory tract, a very rapid ESR and Bence-Jones protein in the urine (p. 37). Precipitation of this protein in the tubules may cause renal failure but this may also result from the amyloidosis which may be associated with the later stages of myelomatosis. Hypercalcaemia is commonly present. The disease is fatal, usually in 2 to 3 years.

Diagnosis. This is based on bone marrow examination which reveals large numbers of plasma cells with a slate-blue cytoplasm and an eccentric, sometimes double, nucleus. Radiological examination of the skeleton may show widespread punched-out osteolytic areas best seen in the skull, ribs, pelvis and vertebrae, and diffuse osteoporotic changes are common. Determination of the electrophoretic pattern of the serum proteins is important and abnormal protein may be demonstrated in the urine.

Treatment. There is no curative treatment but localised irradiation will reduce the severity of bone pain and allow healing of spontaneous fractures. Courses of combined chemotherapy using large doses of prednisolone along with the alkylating agent melphalan repeated at regular intervals have achieved remissions of 2 years or more in cases treated in experienced centres. In cases with anaemia associated with marrow replacement, repeated blood transfusions may prolong life and intercurrent infections should be promptly treated. In the cases with renal failure, with high levels of plasma urate or calcium, corticosteroid therapy is indicated.

Hypersplenism

This term is used to describe the depression of leucocyte and platelet counts in the peripheral blood which is often encountered in a wide variety of conditions in which splenomegaly is a prominent feature, such as portal hypertension (p. 451). The cause of the leucopenia and the thrombocytopenia is not fully understood but it may in part be due to sequestration of leucocytes and platelets in the enlarged spleen. Splenomegaly is extremely common in the tropics for reasons which are discussed on page 839.

Diseases of Lipoid Storage

Examples of these rare disorders are *Gaucher's disease* and *Niemann-Pick disease* which are autosomal recessive conditions characterised by lysosomal enzyme deficiencies. In consequence there is abnormal storage of lipoids in the cells of the reticuloendothelial system, splenomegaly and hypersplenism. There is no specific treatment for these slowly progressive diseases.

HAEMORRHAGIC DISORDERS

Under this heading are included a large number of conditions characterised by an abnormal tendency to bleeding.

The factors concerned in the arrest of haemorrhage are many. They include (*a*) contraction of damaged small vessels, (*b*) the plugging of tears in such vessels by the aggregation of platelets, and (*c*) the coagulation of the blood which is believed to involve a chain of reactions between at least twelve factors.

(*a*) *The Vascular Factor*

Active contraction of capillaries in response to injury constitutes an essential feature of natural haemostasis. This, together with plugging of the bleeding points by platelets, gives time for clotting to occur before the injured vessels reopen.

(*b*) *The Thrombocyte*

An adequate supply of normal platelets is of great importance in arresting haemorrhage. Not only do platelets take an important part in the production of thromboplastin, but they also play a mechanical role in the plugging of bleeding points in vessels. It is also possible that they may play some part in maintaining a normal resistance of capillary endothelium to injury. Even in thrombocytopenic states there are sufficient thrombocytes to initiate clotting.

(*c*) *Intrinsic and Extrinsic Factors concerned with the Coagulation of Blood*

Much of our knowledge of blood coagulation is hypothetical, but all schemes distinguish between an intrinsic system, occurring in the blood, and an extrinsic system which is activated by tissue factors either in laboratory investigations or in the body as a result of tissue injury, particularly in lungs, placenta or brain.

According to Macfarlane's enzyme cascade theory, each clotting factor has an inactive precursor. Once the process of clotting commences, an active enzyme is formed, and this sets the next stage in motion. The intrinsic system of coagulation is illustrated in Figure 12.1.

In the extrinsic system, the activated factor VIII is replaced by tissue factor and by a plasma factor (factor VII).

Within the meshwork of the fibrin clot, red and white cells and platelets are enclosed. The fibrin filaments contract, the clot shrinks and becomes firmer and serum is expressed.

There is also a fibrinolytic mechanism which limits fibrin deposition by dissolving this protein. Plasminogen activator is released from damaged tissues and leads to the production of an enzyme, plasmin, from the inactive precursor, plasminogen, in the blood thus:

$$\text{Plasminogen} \xrightarrow{\text{Plasminogen activator}} \text{Plasmin}$$

$$\text{Fibrin} \longleftarrow \longrightarrow \text{Fibrin degradation products.}$$

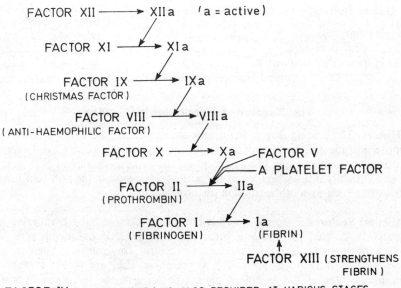

FACTOR IV (CALCIUM IONS) IS ALSO REQUIRED AT VARIOUS STAGES

Fig. 12.1   The intrinsic system of coagulation

Classification of Haemorrhagic Disorders

The following classification is provisional, since in many forms the exact pathogenesis is not fully understood.

A. Due to Defects of the Capillary Endothelium

1. The vascular purpuras.

   (*a*) Infections, e.g. typhus, typhoid, meningococcal meningitis, measles, infective endocarditis, septicaemia, smallpox.

   (*b*) Chemical agents, e.g. aspirin, ergot, frusemide, indomethacin, iodides, phenobarbitone, phenylbutazone, phenytoin, quinine and snake venom.

   (*c*) Anaphylactoid purpura. (Purpura simplex and Henoch-Schönlein purpura).

   (*d*) Metabolic purpura (uraemia, p. 485; hepatic failure, p. 430).

   (*e*) Scurvy (p. 126).

2. Von Willebrand's disease.
3. Hereditary haemorrhagic telangiectasia.

B. Due to Deficiency of Blood Platelets

1. Idiopathic thrombocytopenic purpura.
2. Secondary or symptomatic thrombocytopenic purpura.

C. Due to Defects in the Clotting Mechanism

1. Haemophilia.
2. Christmas disease.
3. Hypoprothrombinaemia.
4. Congenital or acquired fibrinogenopenia.

The Diagnosis of Haemorrhagic Disorders

History. The guiding factors in the assessment of a patient with a haemorrhagic disorder include a knowledge of the sex of the patient, of any history of exposure to drugs or chemicals and of any recent infection. Enquiry should also be made about the family history and about the patient's response in the past to traumatic procedures such as tooth extraction or tonsillectomy.

Clinical Features. Purpura, which is not itself a disease but a manifestation of disease, is defined as bleeding into the skin or mucous membranes. The haemorrhagic spots do not disappear on pressure. Tiny purpuric haemorrhages about the size of a pinhead are known as petechiae. They are usually most prominent in the legs of the ambulant patient because of the increased hypostatic pressure, but even here they may be overlooked if inspection is cursory. Petechiae indicate a deficiency of platelets or a defect of the endothelium. Large purpuric haemorrhages are known as ecchymoses and these may be due not only to platelet or vascular deficiencies but also to coagulation defects. Bleeding into a joint (haemarthrosis) usually indicates a severe coagulation defect such as haemophilia. Bruising is not necessarily an indication of a haemorrhagic disorder as it may readily be induced in many healthy persons, particularly women.

Investigation. The decision about which tests to carry out and the order in which they should be performed depends upon the initial clinical appraisal. A platelet count is usually required but a rough indication of whether gross platelet deficiency exists can be obtained by examination of a blood film stained with cresyl blue. The bleeding time is prolonged in thrombocytopenia and is most reliably estimated by Ivy's method. In the assessment of coagulation defects the blood clotting time is an insensitive measure and is abnormally prolonged only when the coagulation factors are seriously deficient. More specific tests include the one stage prothrombin time (p. 633), and estimations of the quantity of fibrinogen and thromboplastin. A useful rapid qualitative test for fibrinogen deficiency is readily available, whereas laboratory facilities are required for a test such as the partial thromboplastin time which detects coagulation defects too small to lead to prolongation of the whole blood clotting time. Many disorders of coagulation require specialised laboratory investigation.

A. Haemorrhagic Disorders due to Defects of Capillary Endothelium

1. The Vascular Purpuras

In this group of haemorrhagic diseases the lesion usually consists of damage to the capillary walls from the factors noted on page 627. In the types due to infections and chemical agents and in anaphylactoid purpura it is unusual to find qualitative or quantitative changes in the platelets and under these conditions the term non-thrombocytopenic purpura may be used. In a minority of cases of vascular purpura, however, the capillary damage is accompanied by a reduction in the number of platelets, due presumably to the combined effects of the toxic and sensitising factors mentioned above.

In senile purpura and in patients on long-term corticosteroid therapy the defect is not in the capillary endothelium but in the supportive connective tissues, which are atrophic and permit rupture of small vessels by shearing stresses. Large purple haemorrhages appear on the back of the hands and are slowly reabsorbed. This form of purpura is unsightly but benign.

Anaphylactoid Purpura. The various clinical forms of this rare condition are manifestations of an allergic reaction but the antigen is often unknown.

Purpura Simplex is found in association with sensitivity to certain bacterial infections, notably streptococcal. Thus is occurs in rheumatic fever, scarlet fever, etc. Small haemorrhagic spots appear on the limbs or over the whole body. The condition is usually of no significance and calls for no treatment.

Henoch-Schönlein Purpura occurs in children and adolescents. Serohaemorrhagic effusion into the wall of the gut may cause colic and melaena and intussusception may be simulated. Periarticular effusion may cause painful swelling of the joints. Mild fever is usual. Purpura of the skin may or may not be present. The prognosis is good but relapses often occur.

In anaphylactoid purpura other allergic manifestations are sometimes found in addition, such as urticaria or angio-oedema. Acute nephritis is the most dangerous complication when the purpura is secondary to streptococcal infection. The platelet count and the bleeding and coagulation times are all normal. The capillary resistance test may be positive. The diagnosis may present great difficulty if purpura of the skin or mucous membranes is not present.

2. Von Willebrand's Disease

This rare disease that affects both sexes is inherited as a simple Mendelian dominant. The main defect is believed to be an abnormality of the capillaries. The bleeding time is prolonged but the coagulation time and platelet count are normal. In some cases a deficiency of antihaemophilic factor has been demonstrated. The bleeding manifestations include prolonged bleeding from minor injuries and tooth extractions, menorrhagia and haemorrhage from the gastrointestinal tract. Treatment is symptomatic, namely iron and blood transfusions as required.

3. Hereditary Haemorrhagic Telangiectasia

This is a rare hereditary disease transmitted as an autosomal dominant trait. It is characterised by bleeding from multiple telangiectases which consist of localised collections of non-contractile capillaries. It occurs in both sexes and the first and frequently the only symptom may be epistaxis. However haematemesis, haemoptysis or bleeding elsewhere may occur. Telangiectases are not usually prominent till the age of 20 or more and may be found on the face or hands, or in the mucous membrane of the nose or mouth. Treatment of bleeding areas is sometimes difficult, but cauterisation of the nose may be helpful.

B. Haemorrhagic Disorders due to Deficiency of Blood Platelets

Idiopathic Thrombocytopenic Purpura

This is a disease of unproved aetiology characterised by a quantitative deficiency of platelets; in some instances it may be due to an antigen-antibody reaction. The disease occurs most commonly in children and young adults. In children it frequently follows a viral infection.

Intermittent purpura and bleeding may occur in any site, most frequently from the nose, alimentary or urogenital tracts, and such bleeding may be fatal, especially should it occur in the brain or subarachnoid space. The disease is usually a chronic one with remissions and relapses, bleeding tending to occur when the platelet count falls below $40 \times 10^9/l$ (40,000/mm^3). The spleen is not palpably enlarged. The blood shows, in addition to the thrombocytopenia, a hypochromic microcytic anaemia, the degree depending on the amount of blood loss. The bleeding time is much prolonged, e.g. 15 to 20 minutes, and the capillary resistance test is strongly positive during relapse. The coagulation time is normal but the clot formed is soft, friable and retracts poorly.

Treatment. The effects of repeated transfusion of blood and large amounts of prednisolone (60 mg daily) should always be tried before surgery is contemplated. In a high proportion of cases remissions varying in degree and duration can be produced. In the majority of patients, however, cessation of corticosteroid therapy or reduction of dosage to a level which can be tolerated by the patient is usually followed by clinical and haematological relapse. If the bleeding tendency is not controlled or greatly improved by blood transfusion and corticosteroids within 2 weeks, splenectomy should be carried out without further delay. Within a few minutes of the removal of the spleen, the prolonged bleeding time and increased capillary fragility start to improve, to be followed within 24 to 48 hours by a rise in thrombocytes. Although these beneficial haematological effects are not always maintained, at least 80 per cent of cases of idiopathic thrombocytopenic purpura are greatly benefited by splenectomy. In children recovery usually occurs spontaneously or may follow corticosteroid therapy.

Secondary or Symptomatic Thrombocytopenic Purpura

Secondary or symptomatic thrombocytopenic purpura occurs in pancytopenia, leukaemia, hypersplenism, multiple neoplastic deposits in the bone marrow, from excessive exposure to X-rays or radioactive substances, and occasionally in very severe fevers. It may be found in megaloblastic anaemia and in systemic lupus erythematosus. It can follow massive blood transfusion.

Thrombocytopenia may be part of a general pancytopenia following drugs (p. 606). In addition patients may develop thrombocytopenia because of sensitivity to other drugs such as chlordiazepoxide, chlorothiazide, chlorpropamide, frusemide, indomethacin, oxyphenbutazone, certain sulphonamides and tolbutamide. Here the prognosis is much better, provided the drug is withdrawn and transfusion given as required. Platelet concentrates are available in some centres.

The name *onyalai* has been given to a form of thrombocytopenic purpura of unknown origin which occurs sporadically in Africa. Large haemorrhagic bullae on the tongue and buccal mucosa are a conspicuous feature.

C. Haemorrhagic Disorders due to Defects
in the Clotting Mechanism

1. Haemophilia (Factor VIII Deficiency)

Of the various factors in normal plasma concerned with the clotting mechanism, the most important from a clinical point of view is the anti-haemophilic factor (Factor VIII, AHF or AHG), a deficiency of which leads to haemophilia. This factor is normally present in the globulin fraction of plasma.

Haemophilia is a hereditary disorder of blood coagulation characterised by a lifelong tendency to excessive haemorrhage and a greatly prolonged coagulation time. The haemophilia gene is transmitted as an X-linked recessive character (p. 16). It follows that the sons of a haemophilic man do not suffer from haemophilia and do not transmit the trait to their descendants. The daughters of a haemophilic man all carry the trait. Some of the sons of a female carrier suffer from haemophilia. Some of the daughters of a female carrier carry the trait. There is no method of detecting whether any woman of a haemophilic family can marry with impunity. In many instances no family history can be obtained.

Clinical Features. The bleeding tendency is not apparent at birth, but is usually noticed within the first three years. Haemorrhage occurs from the nose, in the mouth or alimentary tract, from the urinary tract, from injuries to the skin, into the muscles, subcutaneous tissue or joints, or after eruption or extraction of teeth, circumcision, tonsillectomy, etc. Some trauma is necessary for the initiation of the bleeding, but often this may be so slight as to pass unnoticed. Injury may in fact cause haemorrhage in any organ, including the brain and spinal cord. There can be repeated haemorrhages into joints without serious after-effects, but organisation of the blood clot may lead to firm ankylosis with marked deformity and crippling.

The coagulation time is usually prolonged and the bleeding time, platelet count and prothrombin time are normal. Anaemia may be a feature depending upon the extent of the bleeding.

Diagnosis. The occurrence of habitual haemorrhage in a male with a family history of bleeding in male relatives or forebears and with the haematological findings described above suggests that the diagnosis is either haemophilia or Christmas disease (p. 632). Occasionally, however, the coagulation time is normal. Such cases can be recognised by more complex laboratory tests, one of the most useful of which is the thromboplastin generation test. Methods are being devised to detect the carrier state in females, but they are not always of positive value. They involve measuring the factor VIII level by a conventional test and also by an immunological method and calculating the ratio of the two. Amniocentesis makes it possible to determine the sex of a fetus and hence decide whether a pregnancy should be terminated. There are haemophilia centres in all regions of Britain at which investigations can be done. The patient is then issued with a card giving necessary information, including the diagnosis and blood group.

Treatment. Even for the most trivial surgical intervention, such as the extraction of a tooth, the patient must be given intravenously, before and after operation, cryoprecipitate, or a special preparation of the globulin fraction of human plasma containing the antihaemophilic factor. Fresh blood is required to replace blood that has been lost. The management of the case requires careful planning by the dentist or surgeon, the physician and the blood transfusion specialist.

When bleeding occurs the patient should be confined to bed. The most widely used form of treatment is with cryoprecipitate which is prepared in a two plastic bag system by collecting blood, centrifuging, transferring the plasma to the secondary pack, freezing it, and thawing at 40°C. At a few transfusion centres suitable concentrates are produced by other methods and superconcentrates are being developed. These must be hepatitis B antigen negative. Some patients can be trained to give themselves intravenous therapy at home.

Local measures consist of the application to the bleeding point (after cleaning away blood and clot) of dressings soaked in substances designed to promote haemostasis. These include Russell's viper venom, adrenaline, fresh whole blood, and preparations of thrombin. Soluble dressings such as gelatin sponge, oxidised cellulose or fibrin foam are useful. Epistaxis may require firm packing of the nose with gauze dressings. Bleeding from tooth sockets can be controlled by packs which may be retained in position by a special dental plate. It may be necessary to give an antibiotic because of infection, particularly in the mouth, but intramuscular injections should be avoided because of the danger of haematoma formation.

A joint which is the site of bleeding should never be opened surgically but should be splinted, lightly bandaged and protected. The same applies to haematomas. Aspiration should be avoided. Most patients obtain relief from the pain due to haemorrhage into a joint if cold packs or icebags are applied. Splinting of the limb should not be continued too long or fibrous ankylosis will result. Analgesics may be required but pethidine and morphine should be avoided because of the danger of addiction and aspirin should not be given in case it leads to a haematemesis.

Prognosis. In some patients the disease is mild, causing little inconvenience. In others it may be very severe, with recurrent joint haemorrhages and troublesome bleeding from minor cuts or after surgical procedures. The whole life of the haemophiliac is coloured by the fear of haemorrhage, particularly into the joints. With modern methods of treatment, the prognosis has improved greatly.

Prophylaxis. Since there is no known cure for the disease, haemophilic men, their sisters and their daughters should be strongly advised not to have children, although, as has already been indicated, amniocentesis now makes it possible to determine the sex of a fetus. In certain instances sterilisation should be considered. Limitation of the risks of bleeding involves the haemophiliac leading a sheltered and careful life with avoidance of trauma, but sufferers from the conditions should not be encouraged to consider themselves as curiosities. Some children with mild haemophilia can attend ordinary schools, but for others education should be provided by the local authority either in the patients' homes or in a school for handicapped children. When the boy reaches the age of 14 or 15 the local Youth Employment Office should be approached to assist in the choice of a career. Regular dental supervision is necessary as a prophylaxis against tooth extraction.

2. Christmas Disease (Factor IX Deficiency)

About one-tenth of the patients with the clinical picture of haemophilia can be shown by special laboratory tests, particularly the thromboplastin generation test, not to have haemophilia but Christmas disease, so-called after the surname of the first patient investigated in Britain. The condition is frequently less severe than haemophilia, but it, too, is a recessive X-linked disease that occurs in males and is transmitted by females. The blood of these patients is not deficient in antihaemophilic factor, but in a different factor, the so-called Christmas factor, which is less labile than the antihaemophilic factor. Local and general treatment and prophylactic measures are the same as in haemophilia, except that preparations of antihaemophilic factor are of no value in the treatment of Christmas disease. At a very few centres, factor IX concentrates are available. Fresh frozen plasma is more commonly used.

3. Hypoprothrombinaemia

This condition is characterised by a deficiency of plasma prothrombin, a tendency to spontaneous and traumatic internal and external haemorrhage, and a prolonged coagulation time.

Prothrombin is formed in the liver from the fat-soluble vitamin K, which is ingested in certain foodstuffs (p. 125) and is also synthesised in the gut by bacterial action. The absorption of vitamin K from the intestine requires the presence of bile salts.

Hypoprothrombinaemia occurs:

1. In *haemorrhagic disease of the newborn*, which appears in about 1 in 800 births. The bleeding tendency is due to an exaggeration of the normal hypoprothrombinaemia which occurs 24 to 72 hours after birth. During this time there is no bacterial formation of vitamin K in the gut. Two to four days after birth, bleeding may occur into the alimentary tract (melaena neonatorum), into the skin or subcutaneous tissue, brain, spinal cord, peritoneal cavity, etc. In some cases so-called birth injuries may be due to bleeding consequent on hypoprothrombinaemia. Spontaneous recovery usually occurs in mild cases, but death may result in severe cases.

In the newborn, especially if premature, water soluble analogues of vitamin K may cause hyperbilirubinaemia and kernicterus (p. 733). Phytomenadione (vitamin K_1) is relatively free from these effects and can be given to the affected baby in a dose of 1 mg intramuscularly. Blood transfusion may also be required.

2. In *gross hepatic disease* bleeding results from impaired synthesis of prothrombin by the liver.

3. In *obstructive jaundice* there is a failure in absorption of vitamin K because of lack of bile salts.

4. In certain *diarrhoeal diseases* such as idiopathic steatorrhoea, fistulae and Crohn's disease there is a failure of absorption of vitamin K.

5. As a result of the administration of *warfarin* or *phenindione*. These anticoagulants, and particularly the former, are employed in the management of venous thrombosis and pulmonary embolism.

Dosage of anticoagulants is controlled by the test commonly referred to as the *one stage prothrombin time*. This is the time taken for plasma to clot under certain standard conditions, but it is a measure of the level, not only of prothrombin, but also of certain other factors. Another test, the *thrombotest*, measures in addition factors IX and possibly X which may also be affected by these anticoagulants. Bleeding can result from factor IX deficiency when the result of the prothrombin time tests suggests that the dosage of warfarin or phenindione is satisfactory.

Treatment consists of the stoppage of the anticoagulant drug, the administration of vitamin K_1, 10 mg by mouth or by intravenous injection, and, occasionally the transfusion of fresh blood, especially if the bleeding has made the patient anaemic.

4. Fibrinogenopenia

A deficiency of plasma fibrinogen, which may be complete or partial, may arise very rarely as a congenital abnormality or as a result of severe liver disease.

Disseminated Intravascular Coagulation. In this condition the entry into the circulation of a tissue thromboplastin starts off the coagulation process. This may occur from amniotic fluid embolism, abruptio placentae, snakebite or septicaemia. There is found to be a low platelet count, a very low plasma fibrinogen and a high level of fibrin degradation products. Generalised bleeding may be serious and yet the treatment, which should be carried out by a specialist, may include the giving of heparin to block further activation of the clotting process.

Thrombocytosis

An increased number of platelets may be found

(a) after haemorrhage and, to a lesser extent, after operation or injury;
(b) after splenectomy;
(c) in myeloproliferative disorders:
   (i) in chronic myeloid leukaemia;
   (ii) in some cases of polycythaemia vera and of myelofibrosis;
   (iii) in a rare primary disease called *haemorrhagic thrombocythaemia* with excessive production of abnormal platelets.

Prospects in Haematology

When the first edition of this book was published a quarter of a century ago, the number of drugs known to produce blood disorders as a side-effect was about 50. Now there are reports of this having been a problem in certain individuals in relation to at least 1,110 drugs, and in most instances the mechanism is unknown. In the future we can expect to see progress in this field of study, but at the same time new therapeutic agents will cause aplastic anaemia, agranulocytosis, thrombocytopenia or haemolysis in man, despite careful screening in animals prior to marketing. It is hoped that a drug will be discovered that will stimulate the hypoplastic marrow.

Research into leukaemia and related disorders is intense and world-wide. The classification of these conditions is unsatisfactory, and study of the ultrastructure of cells may lead to a more logical and universally acceptable nomenclature. It may be that, unexpectedly, the causation of one or more of the forms of leukaemia will become clear in the foreseeable future. It is certain that new therapeutic agents will emerge and that, quite soon, we shall have more precise knowledge of the best combinations to employ in the various members of this group of diseases. Already there are claims for cure in some patients with lymphatic leukaemia, but a number of years must pass before we shall know whether this means total eradication of the disease in those believed to be cured.

In haemophilia and Christmas disease, amniocentesis followed by termination of pregnancy, if the offspring of a haemophiliac is found to be a female, should lead to the condition being less prevalent. If repeated analysis shows low levels of factor VIII in a suspected carrier, this almost certainly confirms the suspicion, but more accurate tests are being sought. The same is true in relation to factor IX in Christmas disease. So far as treatment is concerned, the development of higher potency extracts from human plasma will enable home treatment by self-injection to be more commonly practised.

R. H. GIRDWOOD
JAMES INNES

Further reading:

Alstead, S. & Girdwood, R. H. (1977) *Textbook of Medical Treatment.* 14th edition. Edinburgh: Churchill Livingstone.—For further information about treatment of blood disorders and the use of blood and blood products.

Dacie, J. V. & Lewis, S. M. (1970) *Practical Haematology.* 4th edition. Edinburgh: Churchill Livingstone.—For information regarding investigative procedures.

Girdwood, R. H. (1976) *Clinical Pharmacology.* London: Ballière Tindall.—For information about haematinics, anticoagulants and drugs used in malignant disease.

Nilsson, I. M. (1974) *Haemorrhagic and Thrombotic Diseases.* London: Wiley.

Wintrobe, M. M. (1974) *Clinical Haematology.* 7th edition. London: Kimpton.

Woodliff, H. J. & Herrmann, R. P. (1973) *Concise Haematology.* London: Arnold.

13. Diseases of Connective Tissues, Joints and Bones

In recent years the miscellaneous group of conditions primarily involving the musculoskeletal structures has been the subject of intense study. Much has been learned about their clinical features, course and prognosis. Diagnosis has been rendered more precise by an increasing number of serological and biochemical tests. A wide range of effective therapeutic measures has become available. Extensive study of the pathological changes has revealed that the primary lesion, whether inflammatory or degenerative in nature, involves the connective tissue matrix. The term, 'diseases of connective tissue' would therefore seem more appropriate for this group of conditions than the time honoured 'chronic rheumatic diseases'.

It is convenient to consider first those diseases in which symptoms arise as a result of diffuse inflammatory changes. These include rheumatoid arthritis, ankylosing spondylitis, systemic lupus erythematosus, dermatomyositis, scleroderma, polyarteritis, polymyalgia rheumatica and gout.

Another large group consists of those disorders in which symptoms arise as a result of degenerative changes in connective tissue, and includes osteoarthrosis, intervertebral disc disease and a miscellaneous group of painful syndromes in which the joints themselves do not appear to be involved. There is also a small group of rare inherited disorders of connective tissue such as Marfan's syndrome (p. 241) and others in which the skin is particularly involved.

Diseases of connective tissues are responsible for much temporary or permanent disablement. In 1971, just over one million spells of incapacity among the insured population in Britain were due to 'rheumatic complaints' and caused a loss of productivity of £420 million. Time lost from work amounted to 44 million days. 'Rheumatic complaints' were second only to accidents as regards the number of people affected and second only to bronchitis for the number of days lost. Surveys in general practice suggest that nearly 10 per cent of the work of family doctors is devoted to the diagnosis and treatment of musculoskeletal disorders grouped under the term 'rheumatism'.

Rheumatoid Arthritis

Rheumatoid arthritis can be defined as a chronic polyarthritis affecting mainly the more peripheral joints, running a prolonged course with exacerbations and remissions, and accompanied by a general systemic disturbance. The disease is characterised by swelling of the synovial membrane and periarticular tissues, subchondral osteoporosis, erosion of cartilage and bone and wasting of the associated muscles.

Aetiology. *Age.* The average age at onset is about 40, but the disease may occur at all ages. It is less common before puberty.

Sex. Females are affected two to three times as frequently as males.

Heredity. Although the influence of heredity is not known, a family history of the disease is not infrequently obtained.

Climate. In the past it was believed that the disease was most common in temperate zones and was particularly associated with cold and damp. Whilst the incidence is less in tropical countries a recent survey of the population of a sub-tropical region has shown that rheumatoid arthritis is as common there as in temperate climates, although it tends to be less severe.

Infection. It can be stated that rheumatoid arthritis is not due to invasion of the joints by any organism which can be demonstrated regularly by methods available at the present time, although there is a growing body of opinion that a viable agent may be concerned in initiating the disease.

Autoimmunity. The presence in the serum of abnormal immunoglobulins in a high proportion of patients together with the histological appearances in the synovium and lymphoid tissue have led to the idea that rheumatoid arthritis may be associated with a derangement of the immune response to exogenous antigens or to antigens derived in part at least from the patient's own tissues.

Psychological Factors. Rheumatoid arthritis is sometimes precipitated and often aggravated by emotional disturbances or excessive and long-continued worry and overwork.

In summary, the aetiology of the disease remains obscure, but it may well arise as a result of the interplay of a number of factors, some of which may be genetically determined while others may be of environmental origin.

Pathology. The earliest change is swelling and congestion of the synovial membrane and the overlying connective tissue, which become infiltrated with lymphocytes, plasma cells and macrophages. Effusion of synovial fluid into the joint space takes place during the active phase of the disease. Subsequently, hypertrophy of the synovial membrane occurs. Inflammatory granulation tissue or pannus is formed, spreading over and under the articular cartilage which is progressively destroyed. Later, fibrous adhesions may form between the layers of pannus across the joint space and fibrous or even bony ankylosis may occur. Muscles adjacent to inflamed joints atrophy and there may be focal infiltration with lymphocytes.

Subcutaneous nodules have a characteristic histological appearance. There is a central area of fibrinoid material consisting of swollen and fragmented collagen fibres, fibrinous exudate and cellular debris, surrounded by a palisade of radially arranged proliferating mononuclear cells. The nodule is surrounded by a loose capsule of fibrous tissue. Similar granulomatous lesions may occur in the pleura, lung, pericardium and sclera. Lymph nodes are often hyperplastic and show many lymphoid follicles with large germinal centres. Plasma cells are numerous in the sinuses and medullary cords.

Clinical Features. In many cases the onset is insidious. For a period of weeks or months before the joints are clinically involved the patient may complain of transient articular or muscular pain and stiffness, tiredness and malaise. In less than 10 per cent of cases the onset may be acute with fever and rapid involvement of many joints. Some patients may present with acute episodes of pain in various individual joints before developing polyarticular symptoms. In the typical case the small joints of the fingers and toes are the first to become affected. Swelling of the proximal interphalangeal joints gives rise to the characteristic spindled appearance of the fingers. As the disease progresses it spreads to involve such joints as the wrists, elbows, shoulders, ankles and knees. Only in more severe cases are the hips affected. Involvement of the cervical spine can lead to gross instability of the atlantoaxial and other upper cervical articulations. The temporomandibular and sternoclavicular joints are occasionally involved. Muscular stiffness is a prominent symptom, and it is particularly marked in the morning or after periods of inactivity. As the disease progresses, joint pain and swelling increase and muscular stiffness becomes more marked. Muscular atrophy takes place early and becomes a very prominent feature.

In more advanced cases pain and muscle spasm give rise to flexion deformities in the joints. At first these deformities are correctable, but later, permanent contractures develop and the joints may become completely disorganised. The characteristic deformity in the hands is anterior subluxation of the metacarpophalangeal joints and ulnar deviation of the fingers.

Subcutaneous nodules appear in 10 to 20 per cent of patients. The most common site is the extensor surface of the forearm just distal to the elbow joint. They may also occur over the patella, scapula, sacrum, scalp and along the tendons of the fingers and toes. In severe cases amyloidosis may complicate the later stages of the disease.

Diffuse vasculitis is a common feature of rheumatoid arthritis, especially in patients with nodules and a positive test for rheumatoid factor. Leg ulcers, episcleritis, scleritis, keratoconjunctivitis sicca, pericarditis, pleural effusion and peripheral neuropathy are among the extra-articular manifestations encountered in these circumstances. Rheumatoid arthritis may coexist with coal-worker's pneumoconiosis (p. 331). Amyloidosis (p. 483) may complicate severe cases.

During the active stage of the disease signs of a systemic disturbance are present. Low-grade pyrexia, tachycardia, hypochromic normocytic anaemia, mild polymorph leucocytosis, raised ESR, altered plasma protein pattern (increased globulin and fibrinogen; decreased albumin) and lymphadenopathy are found.

In the early phase radiological examination of the affected joints will show only demineralisation of the bone ends. Later, as the pathological process progresses to involve the articular cartilage, there is narrowing of the joint space and marginal erosions appear. In the late stages, in damaged joints which are still capable of some movement, radiological examination will show the appearance of osteoarthrosis, which arises as a secondary manifestation.

Immunological Tests. The rheumatoid factor is an autoantibody usually IgM, which reacts with IgG. It can be demonstrated if IgG is attached to a particulate carrier such as erythrocytes or latex. The Rose-Waaler (sensitised sheep cell) test is positive in 65–70 per cent of cases of rheumatoid arthritis. It is also positive in 25–30 per cent of patients with systemic lupus erythematosus or scleroderma and in 15–20 per cent of cases of juvenile rheumatoid arthritis. The latex fixation test is simpler and more sensitive but less specific.

Examination of Synovial Fluid. In cases of doubt this may provide valuable information. In rheumatoid arthritis or pyogenic infection the fluid is of low viscosity, turbid, clots on standing and contains many cells. When infection is suspected fluid should be cultured. In gout, uric acid crystals may be seen on microscopic examination. Fluid from traumatic or degenerative forms of arthritis is clear, viscid, does not clot and contains few cells.

Differential Diagnosis. In the average case of rheumatoid arthritis there is usually little difficulty in reaching a diagnosis, but when the disease starts in an atypical manner it will have to be distinguished from the following conditions:

Rheumatic Fever. In this condition the joint pain is of a flitting character. The fever is usually higher and spindling of finger joints is rare. Occasionally subacute rheumatic fever may be difficult to distinguish from rheumatoid arthritis with a febrile onset, but the articular symptoms of rheumatic fever are more likely to be suppressed by full doses of aspirin. The ASO titre (p. 199) will usually be elevated in rheumatic fever.

Gonococcal Arthritis. An acute arthritis with fever may follow a gonorrhoeal infection, but since the advent of antibiotics this complication has become much less frequent. It can be distinguished from rheumatoid arthritis by a history of urethritis preceding the joint symptoms by 2 or 3 weeks. In the majority of cases demonstration of the gonococcus in smears from the urethra, prostate or cervix uteri will confirm the diagnosis. In only about 25 per cent, however, can the gonococcus be cultured from the synovial fluid but the gonococcal complement fixation test is usually positive.

Reiter's Disease. This disease is characterised by acute urethritis or diarrhoea, conjunctivitis and arthritis. The condition may occasionally be difficult to distinguish from rheumatoid arthritis when the syndrome is incomplete. The joint symptoms in Reiter's disease usually clear up completely but in a small proportion of cases the disease becomes chronic and involvement of the spine and sacro-iliac joints may develop. Characteristic skin lesions ('keratoderma blennorrhagica') may be seen.

Acute Pyogenic Arthritis. This is usually monarticular. The joint is acutely inflamed and painful. The signs of a generalised infection, including high fever, are present. Both blood and synovial fluid should be cultured. Occasionally rheumatoid arthritis may be complicated by a superadded pyogenic arthritis which is almost invariably associated with a septicaemia and may be masked by corticosteroid therapy.

Gout. This arthritis in its earlier stages may be confused with the acute episodic variant of rheumatoid arthritis. In the classical case of gout the first joint to be affected is the metatarsophalangeal joint of the big toe. The onset is very sudden, the pain extremely acute, but the attack usually responds dramatically to specific treatment (p. 650), leaving no residual changes in the joint. A high blood urate will usually be found in this disease.

Tuberculous Arthritis. The onset is insidious. Usually only one joint is involved, but occasionally several are affected. The condition is most common in children. In adults tuberculosis of the spine is the most common form. The radiological appearances, demonstration of the organisms in the synovial fluid or biopsy of the synovial membrane will differentiate this condition from rheumatoid arthritis.

Osteoarthrosis. This usually affects the larger joints such as the knees, hips and spine. In middle-aged women, however, osteoarthrotic changes not uncommonly affect the fingers, and care should be taken to distinguish this condition from rheumatoid arthritis. In a typical case Herberden's nodes (p. 652) appear in relationship to the terminal interphalangeal joints. At first these nodes may be painful, but later they subside to leave a firm hard nodule which frequently causes deformity of the distal interphalangeal joint. The ESR is usually within normal limits.

Psoriatic Arthritis. It is now accepted that an erosive arthropathy resembling rheumatoid arthritis may complicate psoriasis. It is characterised by being milder and seronegative. Subcutaneous nodules are absent but the spine and sacroiliac joints are not infrequently affected. In some cases there is involvement of the terminal interphalangeal joints, ridging, thickening, cracking and pitting of the nails.

Brucellosis. This condition may be suggested by a history of a possible source of infection or by an intermittent pyrexia and confirmed by a positive agglutination test (p. 75).

Osteomyelitis. Here pain and tenderness are maximal over the bone rather than the joints.

Treatment. As the aetiology of the disease is unknown, treatment must be directed towards the relief of symptoms, the improvement of the patient's general health and the conservation and restoration of function in the joints damaged by the disease process. In achieving these objectives important measures are rest for the inflamed joints, physiotherapy, analgesics, anti-inflammatory agents, corticosteroids in selected cases, various surgical procedures and a co-ordinated rehabilitation programme.

1. GENERAL MEASURES IN THE ACUTE PHASE. When many joints are swollen and painful and when signs of severe constitutional disturbance, such as fever, anaemia and rapid ESR are present, the patient should be confined to bed until these signs and symptoms begin to subside. This period of general rest may last for several weeks and certain measures must be adopted to prevent unnecessary deterioration in physical efficiency. Attention should be directed to the maintenance of good posture. The mattress should be firm or fracture boards should be inserted beneath it. A back rest with the minimum number of pillows should be in position during the day; at night only one firm pillow should be allowed. A roomy cage with a padded footrest should be placed over the legs and feet; pillows behind knees should be forbidden; after the midday meal the patient should spend an hour resting flat with a small pillow under the lumbar spine. Foot and quadriceps excercises should be performed daily by all patients confined to bed. The general level of physical efficiency should be maintained by the use of suitable exercises. These exercises are designed to have their effect on the groups of muscles in the thoracic, gluteal and abdominal regions. Rest in bed, by the cessation of weight-bearing on the inflamed joints, will go far towards fulfilling the first principle of treatment—the relief of symptoms, as pain and spasm are largely conditioned by movement and weight-bearing. Most patients in the acute phase of the disease will have lost weight and the diet should be of high energy value with ample protein. Additional vitamin concentrates are not necessary if a well-balanced diet containing milk, eggs and fruit is eaten. A liberal supply of milk should be given to ensure an adequate intake of calcium and first-class protein.

2. LOCAL MEASURES IN THE ACUTE PHASE. Experience has shown that the correct treatment of the inflamed joints may be of fundamental importance in controlling both local and systemic symptoms in rheumatoid arthritis. Painful joints should be immobilised in skin-tight plaster of Paris splints. These splints should be maintained in position until the more acute symptoms have subsided. In the past undue emphasis may have been placed on the use of daily active and passive movements at this stage. The symptoms of inflammation subside more quickly if the joints are left at complete rest for a period of 1 to 3 weeks. The danger of joints becoming ankylosed if immobilised in this way has been exaggerated. The principle of a period of complete rest is of particular importance in the treatment of weight-bearing joints. When pain and swelling have subsided the splints are removed for active non-weight-bearing exercises. The patient should be taught these exercises and instructed to perform them frequently throughout the day. The

application of heat before the sessions of exercise is useful in relieving stiffness. When the constitutional symptoms have begun to subside and power has been restored to wasted muscles, the patient is allowed up for increasing periods. Wax baths are beneficial in reducing stiffness in the joints of the hands and feet. Faradic foot baths may be helpful in initiating activity in the intrinsic muscles of the feet. Residual pain may be eased by radiant heat, infra-red rays or shortwave diathermy.

Occupational therapy is of considerable value in restoring manual dexterity and conditioning the patient for a return to productive employment.

3. ANTI-INFLAMMATORY AND ANALGESIC DRUGS. *Aspirin*, the most valuable anti-inflammatory agent for controlling symptoms, apparently acts by inhibiting prostaglandin biosynthesis. Aspirin soluble tablets (B.P.) is the preparation of choice in a dose of 4 to 6 g daily. In severe cases it should be given to the limit of the patient's tolerance. Aspirin may cause gastrointestinal bleeding (p. 371); dyspepsia may be troublesome, in which case enteric-coated tablets should be used. *Codeine phosphate*, 30 mg two to three times a day, can also be prescribed when pain is severe but it may cause constipation. *Paracetamol* is less effective but should be tried when aspirin is poorly tolerated. The dose is 3 to 6 g daily.

Phenylbutazone is effective in controlling symptoms but the dose should not exceed 300 mg daily as toxic effects occur in about one-third of the patients. Most common are nausea, vomiting, rashes and oedema due to sodium retention. Less common but more serious complications include haematemesis, perforation of peptic ulcers, agranulocytosis, thrombocytopenia, aplasia of the bone marrow, haematuria, anuria, chromosomal abnormalities and an increased incidence of leukaemia. An enteric-coated preparation causes less gastrointestinal intolerance. Phenylbutazone should be used only when the response to aspirin has been unsatisfactory and if there is no evidence of gastrointestinal, renal or heart disease.

Other Non-steroid Anti-inflammatory Drugs. These may be tried when aspirin or phenylbutazone is ineffective or contraindicated. Propionic acid derivatives include *mefenamic* or *flufenamic* acid (300–600 mg daily), *ibuprofen* (600–1,600 mg daily) and *naproxen* (500 mg daily). They may cause dyspepsia or peptic ulceration. Naproxen is probably the most effective and best tolerated but the response of the individual varies and it may be necessary to try several drugs in order to determine the most suitable. *Indomethacin* also provides an alternative but has various side-effects including headache, vertigo, depression, nausea, vomiting and gastrointestinal haemorrhage. *Penicillamine* (p. 733) is effective but may cause disturbance of taste, alopecia, thrombocytopenia, proteinuria and rashes. The dose is 125 mg, very gradually increased to 500–750 mg daily but, because of the frequency of side-effects, the drug should be reserved for the more severe cases.

4. CORTICOSTEROIDS. The potent anti-inflammatory properties of corticosteroids are counterbalanced by their adverse effects, especially if used in high dosage on a long term basis. Their use can therefore be justified only if less potentially dangerous therapy is ineffective.

Prednisolone. This drug, or prednisone, with which it is interchangeable, has an optimum daily dose of 10 mg or less. For relieving disabling morning stiffness, 2·5–5 mg at bedtime is often effective. Major adverse effects are very likely to occur in patients having 15 mg or more daily (p 549). To reduce the incidence of dyspepsia and peptic ulceration the tablet should be crushed and taken along with food.

Alternatively enteric-coated and soluble preparations are available which should be used in patients with dyspepsia or with a previous history of peptic ulceration.

A number of other synthetic corticosteroids have also been produced (p. 549) but there is no evidence that they have any advantage over prednisolone which is the drug of choice when corticosteroid therapy is indicated.

Local Use of Corticosteroids. The intra-articular injection of a suspension of hydrocortisone acetate is followed by a reduction of pain and swelling. Duration of relief varies from a few days to 2 to 3 weeks in individual patients, but is worthwhile in over half the cases treated. The dose used varies from 5 mg in the small joints of the fingers to 50 mg in the case of the knee. Repeated injections of corticosteroids at short intervals should be avoided, particularly in the case of weight-bearing joints, as rapid deterioration of the radiological appearances has been noted in the absence of a recurrence of symptoms.

Painful ligamentous attachments, tenosynovitis around the wrist and ankle, and nodules in tendons leading to limitation of movement can also be treated by local injection of hydrocortisone.

Eye drops of hydrocortisone (1·5 per cent solution) are valuable in controlling inflammatory conditions of the eye which occur not infrequently in the more severe cases of rheumatoid arthritis.

Corticotrophin (ACTH). Stimulation of the patient's own adrenal glands by the injection of corticotrophin is as effective as prednisolone by mouth. Stable, long-acting preparations are available, which need be injected only once daily. Side-effects are similar to those which may complicate treatment with prednisolone, but fluid retention and hypertension are more common. On the other hand, dyspepsia and peptic ulceration occur less frequently. The initial dose is 20 units daily. In most cases a satisfactory response is maintained by a dose of between 10 and 20 units daily. Patients can be taught to inject themselves. It is claimed by the advocates of this form of treatment that a remission of the disease occurs in a significant number of patients (15 of 78 patients in one report) which is maintained after the slow withdrawal of the hormone. In contrast, treatment can rarely be stopped in patients who have been on prednisolone for any length of time. The disadvantage of daily injection and the development of resistance to the hormone limits the value of corticotrophin, but it may have a place in the treatment of severe and progressive cases who cannot tolerate prednisolone.

Some of the disadvantages of corticotrophin have been overcome by the introduction of the hormone in synthetic form (tetracosactrin). This is available as a depot preparation and can be injected intramuscularly in a dose of 0·5–1 mg twice weekly. Tetracosactrin should be given under close medical supervision because fatal anaphylactic reactions have been reported (p. 544).

5. GOLD SALTS. Evidence of the effectiveness of gold salts in some cases of rheumatoid arthritis has been provided by a controlled trial conducted under the auspices of the Arthritis and Rheumatism Council. A water-soluble preparation such as Myocrisin, a 50 per cent solution of sodium aurothiomalate, is recommended. Intramuscular injections of 50 mg are given at weekly intervals to a total of 1 g. If there is little or no response after the full course of injections, gold therapy should be discontinued. In other cases, improvement may be maintained by the continued administration of 50 mg every 3 or 4 weeks over a period of many months. Adverse reactions may occur at any time during treatment, dermatitis being the commonest. Thrombocytopenia, agranulocytosis and anaemia may result from depression of bone marrow. Only rarely has evidence of renal or

hepatic damage been recorded.

The most important measure during the administration of gold salts is to impress on the patient the necessity of reporting immediately any untoward symptoms. Before each injection the patient should be asked specifically about pruritus or rash.

Treatment of Toxic Reactions. Dimercaprol combines with heavy metals to form a stable compound which is rapidly excreted in the urine. It is given by intramuscular injection in doses of 3 mg/kg body weight every 6 hours for 3 to 4 days. It should be used if signs of toxicity persist for more than a few days after injections of gold have been stopped. Should agranulocytosis develop, antibiotics should be given in full doses. For more severe reactions prednisolone 15–20 mg daily has proved valuable in controlling symptoms.

6. CHLOROQUINE AND HYDROXYCHLOROQUINE. These anti-malarial drugs are moderately effective in rheumatoid arthritis and may be used as an adjunct to basic treatment. The dose of chloroquine phosphate is 250 mg daily and of hydroxychloroquine sulphate is 400 mg daily. Although these drugs are relatively toxic, they are more acceptable than corticosteroids for long-term use. Side-effects include rashes, gastrointestinal upsets, headaches, mental disturbance and leucopenia. Corneal deposits of the drug may produce disturbances of vision which disappear when the drug is withdrawn. More rarely, permanent visual impairment results from retinopathy. Ideally the eyes should be examined every 3 to 6 months during long-term therapy with these drugs.

7. IRON. The anaemia is resistant to iron given by mouth possibly because iron is deviated to local sites of inflammation. However, in the majority of cases improvement follows the administration of iron by intramuscular or intravenous injection (p. 600). Utilisation may be increased by adding ACTH 10–20 units daily during the course of iron injections.

8. TREATMENT OF MILD CASES. Many patients suffering from rheumatoid arthritis never become severely incapacitated, as the disease frequently runs a subacute course and can be kept under control with anti-inflammatory drugs, physiotherapy and remedial exercises. These patients should remain under observation and measures detailed for the active stage should be started if symptoms become acute.

9. SURGICAL TREATMENT. Orthopaedic surgeons, particularly when working in close collaboration with physicians, have important contributions to make to treatment. In rheumatoid arthritis involvement of extra-articular structures is responsible for much of the disability, particularly in the earlier stages of the disease. Involvement of tendons and their synovial sheaths, at the wrists and in the palm, the growth of nodules in the substance of tendons leading to rupture, compression of the median nerve in the carpal tunnel, inflammation in bursae in relation to joints and contracture of joint capsules can also impair function before significant damage has occurred within the joints. All can be effectively dealt with surgically. At a later stage, when the synovial membrane has become inflamed and hypertrophied, synovectomy in both large and small joints can be followed by local remission of activity for prolonged periods. When cartilage and bone have been eroded and the mechanics of joints disturbed, arthroplasty, arthrodesis and the insertion of prostheses to replace damaged structures play a valuable part in

treatment. Pain in the forefoot, resulting from clawing of the toes and callosities over the eroded heads of the metatarsal bones, can be completely relieved by excision of the heads and necks of all five metatarsals, avoiding much wasteful expenditure on surgical shoes, which rarely control symptoms effectively. When hips have been damaged to an extent that pain is incapacitating, total hip replacement by a number of techniques has been remarkably successful. Prostheses are also available for other joints. Physicians dealing with all forms of arthritis should establish combined clinics with their surgical colleagues to reach decisions as to what should be done and when it should be done and to plan post-operative care and assessment in conjunction with physiotherapists, occupational therapists and social workers.

10. REHABILITATION. When the patient cannot return to a former occupation it will be necessary to suggest a change of employment where less strain will be thrown on the damaged joints. Training schemes are available in special centres in Britain. Rehabilitation and vocational training constitute an essential part of any scheme for the treatment of the chronic arthritic diseases. It cannot be emphasised too strongly that adequate treatment initiated in the early stages enables most patients to return to some form of wage-earning activity. Severe disability can be reduced even in the 25 per cent of cases running a progressive course.

Prognosis. Rheumatoid arthritis usually runs a subacute or chronic course over a period of years. Its progress may be interrupted at any stage, so that no patient with rheumatoid arthritis should be considered as being beyond medical aid. In severe cases the disease progresses by a series of exacerbations and remissions. Each acute attack causes further damage to the joints, deformity and disability and the patient may become completely bedridden. Relapses may be precipitated by a variety of factors such as intercurrent infection, cold, damp, worry, overwork, or excessive use of the affected joints. The outlook so far as life is concerned is good. In some 300 patients admitted to hospital over a period of three years and followed up for an average of nine years, 24 per cent remained fit for normal activities, 40 per cent suffered only moderate impairment of function, 26 per cent were more severely disabled, but only 10 per cent had become helpless cripples. The earlier adequate treatment is instituted, the better will be the prognosis in the individual case.

Juvenile Rheumatoid Arthritis—Still's Disease

In children under 5 years of age, in addition to arthritis, there is often splenomegaly, lymphadenopathy, leucocytosis, pyrexia, rash and involvement of the cervical spine. Although growth may be retarded, the condition is usually self-limiting. In older children rheumatoid arthritis gradually merges into the form encountered in adults.

The treatment of Still's disease is that of rheumatoid arthritis but in addition educational facilities are essential when long-term hospitalisation is necessary. Prednisolone and corticotrophin are effective but their use in treatment is limited by the same considerations already discussed in relationship to rheumatoid arthritis and by the risk of retarding growth.

Felty's Syndrome

The association of lymphadenopathy, splenomegaly and neutropenia with rheumatoid arthritis constitutes Felty's syndrome. Infected skin lesions and septicaemia may occur. Thrombocytopenia is not uncommon. The neutropenia and thrombocytopenia may respond to ACTH if not to corticosteroids, and in some cases splenectomy is undertaken.

Sjögren's Syndrome

Sjögren in 1933 described a group of patients in whom dryness of the eyes and mouth was associated with polyarthritis of the rheumatoid type. Keratoconjunctivitis sicca develops as a result of reduction in the secretion of tears, and xerostomia follows involvement of the salivary glands. Mucus secreting glands of the upper respiratory tract are commonly affected, resulting in recurrent respiratory infections. Not infrequently there is loss of hair and atrophic changes in the nails.

The diagnosis depends on the demonstration of diminished lacrymal secretion and the presence of ulcers on the cornea. The test for rheumatoid factor is positive in the majority of cases. Treatment is essentially the same as that outlined for rheumatoid arthritis. Topical application of hydrocortisone eye drops (1·5 per cent) has proved useful in controlling local inflammation in the eye. Artificial tears (methycellulose drops) may also be required in more severe cases and may be combined with sealing of the lacrymal puncta.

Ankylosing Spondylitis

The disease, a progressive inflammatory arthritis of the spinal articulations, affects persons between the ages of 20 and 40. Males are affected more commonly than females. The disease presents many of the features of an infective process. The ESR may be rapid and low-grade pyrexia is not uncommon in the active phase. However, no specific organism has been isolated and the aetiology of the disease is unknown. The test for rheumatoid factor is negative in virtually all established cases. The histocompatibility antigen HLA-B27 is found in more than 90 per cent of patients with established ankylosing spondylitis, and in early cases the demonstration of this antigen can be a useful diagnostic aid.

Pathology. Biopsy material from cases in which the peripheral joints have been affected shows changes similar to those found in rheumatoid arthritis. Bony ankylosis, however, occurs more frequently in ankylosing spondylitis. Radiological changes are seen first in the sacroiliac joints, which show irregularity of the joint margins. There is an increase in density of the bone adjacent to the joints. Later the sacroiliac joints become ankylosed and the vertebral ligaments show progressive ossification (bamboo spine).

Clinical Features. The onset is often insidious. A history of repeated attacks of backache in a healthy young male should always suggest the possibility of ankylosing spondylitis. Early morning pain and stiffness are characteristic features. As the disease progresses there is increasing stiffness of the whole spine. Involvement of the costovertebral joints gives rise to marked limitation in chest expansion. In milder cases the spine may become rigid without much deformity. In more severe cases kyphosis involving the cervical, dorsal and lumbar spine is not uncommon. Such patients are severely incapacitated, and if the hips become affected they may be rendered helpless. In a small proportion of cases the disease involves the peripheral joints, in which the changes closely resemble those found in rheumatoid arthritis. Iritis occurs in between 25 and 30 per cent of cases and may occasionally be the first sign of the disease. Rarely, aortitis followed by aortic regurgitation develops, usually in the later stages of the disease. Ankylosing spondylitis may be associated with either Crohn's disease or ulcerative colitis.

Differential Diagnosis. Osteoarthrosis of the spine may give rise to pain and limitation of movement. This disease seldom gives rise to symptoms before the age of 50. It is not accompanied by signs of systemic disturbance and the two conditions are readily differentiated by radiological appearances. In osteoarthrosis the sacroiliac joints are rarely involved, the intervertebral spaces are commonly diminished due to degenerative changes in the discs; and exostoses develop at the edges of the vertebral bodies. Protrusion of the nucleus pulposus of an intervertebral disc can also affect young men and present with backache. Scoliosis and sciatic pain are common in protrusion of intervertebral discs and are rare in ankylosing spondylitis.

Treatment. Phenylbutazone is particularly effective in relieving symptoms and is worthy of trial before considering radiotherapy. The dose should not exceed 300 mg daily. Close supervision is required in view of the possibility of toxic effects (p. 641). Indomethacin (100 mg daily) or as a suppository at night and naproxen (500–750 mg daily) may also be effective.

Radiotherapy is the treatment of choice in the active phase of ankylosing spondylitis if the response to drug therapy is unsatisfactory. In early cases the results are excellent and the disease process is apparently arrested. Even in more advanced cases with fixed deformities much benefit may result. The incidence of leukaemia is significantly increased following radiotherapy (3 per 1,000 cases treated); but in active cases this risk is outweighed by the good results obtained. In all cases exercises for strengthening the spinal muscles and mobilising the costovertebral joints should be prescribed. In the more advanced cases a spinal support may be required to maintain reasonable posture. Deformity of the spine may be corrected by the use of serial plaster shells. Where such correction is not possible and where the deformity is marked, spinal osteotomy may allow the patient to regain a reasonable posture. Where the hips have become affected, surgery has now much to offer (p. 643). The general measures described in the treatment of rheumatoid arthritis should be used in the acute phase, but prolonged immobilisation should be avoided. Prednisolone and corticotrophin are effective in ankylosing spondylitis, but their use in treatment is limited by the same considerations already discussed in relationship to rheumatoid arthritis (p. 641).

Prognosis. In early active cases treated by phenylbutazone and radiotherapy the prognosis is good. Even in more advanced cases the combination of general measures, radiotherapy and orthopaedic procedures can do much to restore these patients to a reasonable level of function.

Systemic Lupus Erythematosus (SLE)

This is a disorder in which immune complexes of DNA and anti-DNA produce a vasculitis causing lesions in many parts of the body, particularly the joints, skin, kidneys, spleen, pleura, pericardium, endocardium and nervous system. In some cases a viral infection may induce the autoimmune changes. A number of other factors may precipitate the onset or precede an exacerbation. These include unaccustomed exposure to sunlight, infection and the administration of drugs such as sulphonamides, penicillin, procainamide, isoniazid, anticonvulsants and, occasionally, oral contraceptives.

The incidence of the disease is considerably higher than was thought in the past, due largely to more accurate diagnosis since immunological tests for SLE became available.

Clinical Features. Over 90 per cent of cases occurs in young women and the age of onset is usually between 20 and 40 years. The most common presenting features are fever and an acute migratory arthralgia resembling rheumatic fever. An erosive arthritis of the rheumatoid type is rarely seen. Rashes are common, particularly one of 'butterfly' distribution on the face. Raynaud's phenomenon (p. 243) occurs and there may be dermal infarction and ulceration. Diffuse or local alopecia may occur. The presence of proteinuria, splenomegaly, pleural effusion, pericarditis or endocarditis indicates the diffuse nature of the disease. There is involvement of the nervous system in over one-quarter of the patients. Anaemia, leucopenia or thrombocytopenia may be found and the sedimentation rate is usually rapid.

Although fulminating cases occur, the disease usually runs a more chronic course, periods of activity alternating with remissions of varying length. The presence of proteinuria early in the course of the illness is of serious prognostic significance. Renal failure is the commonest cause of death.

Diagnosis. An antibody to nuclear material, antinuclear factor (ANF), demonstrable by immunofluorescence techniques, is present in the great majority of cases. While failure to detect this factor is against the diagnosis of systemic lupus erythematosus, it can be found in other conditions, notably rheumatoid arthritis. Antibodies to DNA also occur and generally correlate with disease activity and depression of serum complement levels.

Further diagnostic evidence can be obtained by the demonstration of the LE factor in the serum of the majority of cases in the active phase of the disease. This more specific test also depends on the presence of an abnormal immunoglobulin with an affinity for the nuclei of cells. Normal leucocytes, incubated in serum of patients with the disease, extrude nuclear material which is phagocytosed by other leucocytes. These cells, containing amorphous inclusion bodies of altered nuclear material, present a typical appearance on staining. These 'LE cells' are not absolutely diagnostic of systemic lupus erythematosus as they are found occasionally in rheumatoid arthritis, particularly in patients with severe systemic disease.

Treatment. In the presence of acute manifestations prednisolone is the treatment of choice, but large doses may be required (40–60 mg daily). At this dosage the incidence of serious side-effects is high and the dose should be gradually reduced until an effective maintenance level is reached, usually 10–20 mg daily. Care must be exercised in the use of corticosteroids in the presence of renal involvement, as hypertension not uncommonly develops. If the response to prednisolone is unsatisfactory, particularly in severe cases with renal involvement, an attempt may be made to correct the immunological abnormality with other measures such as immunosuppression therapy with azathioprine or cyclophosphamide.

In the subacute or chronic forms chloroquine (p. 643) may be used. It has proved valuable in controlling the lesions of the skin.

Dermatomyositis

This rare disease is characterised by focal or segmental necrosis of voluntary muscles sometimes preceded by infiltration with inflammatory cells. Later there may be an increase in fibrous tissue between the muscle fibres or calcification may occur. Two forms of the condition have been described but intermediate grades also occur:

1. Acute dermatomyositis, most common among children, in which oedema, tenderness, swelling and weakness of the proximal muscles of the limbs are accompanied by fever, leucocytosis and an erythematous skin eruption. A common clinical manifestation is oedema of the eyelids with a characteristic heliotrope discolouration. Involvement of the respiratory muscles may rapidly lead to a fatal termination, but in other cases the acute phase subsides, leaving deformity of the limbs due to contracture of fibrous tissue in the muscles.

2. Chronic dermatomyositis, which runs a more prolonged course, and involves especially the peripheral muscles. Lesions of the skin are not always present and in such cases the term '*polymyositis*' is used (p. 756). This is the type most commonly seen in adults. It may be associated with malignant disease, especially of the gastrointestinal tract.

The diagnosis of dermatomyositis is confirmed by the finding of raised serum creatine kinase, by abnormal potentials on electromyography or by muscle biopsy.

In acute cases the response to prednisolone may be dramatic and even life-saving. Large doses may be required initially (60 mg daily); these are then slowly reduced. In the self-limiting form of the disease, complete withdrawal may be possible. In others maintenance therapy is required (10 mg prednisolone daily). Response in the more chronic cases is usually unsatisfactory. A combination of splints and physiotherapy is used to prevent or correct deformity. Occasionally, calcified deposits may be removed by oral treatment with diphosphonate compounds.

Scleroderma

In this disease the collagen fibres of the dermis first become swollen, then dense and sclerotic, giving rise to contractures and deformities of the joints. Changes are most prominent in the hands and face. The pathology is not confined to the skin. In progressive cases the alimentary tract, lungs, myocardium and kidneys may be affected (*systemic sclerosis*). Blood vessels in the skin and viscera show marked intimal thickening. Intercurrent infection, and cardiac or renal failure are common causes of death. Treatment is unsatisfactory. The corticosteroids are of little value. It is claimed that d-penicillamine (p. 733) can soften the skin in some cases. Every effort must be made to prevent crippling deformities of the peripheral joints by the use of splints and physiotherapy, but care must be exercised in the use of all forms of heat because of the marked impairment of the circulation to the skin.

Polyarteritis

This condition is described on page 242.

Polymyalgia Rheumatica

Polymyalgia rheumatica affects the middle-aged to elderly and women more often than men. The aetiology is unknown but in some cases there is evidence of cranial (giant cell) arteritis (p. 243) and biopsy of the temporal artery may provide confirmation of the diagnosis. Polymyalgia rheumatica is characterised by pain and especially stiffness affecting mainly the muscles of the shoulder and pelvic girdles. It is accompanied by systemic disturbance in the form of mild fever, weight loss, increased ESR and moderate anaemia. Limitation of movement in the shoulders may arise insidiously and persist for several months but usually then subsides without residual disability.

Treatment consists initially of rest and full doses of analgesics. Should improvement not occur within a week or 10 days, and particularly when systemic symptoms are marked, 15–20 mg of prednisolone should be given daily in divided doses. When symptoms are controlled the dose should be gradually reduced, e.g. by 2·5 mg every few days. Complete withdrawal is possible within 4 to 6 months in the majority of cases. When signs of arteritis are present prednisolone should be given at once in doses of 30–40 mg daily and maintained until symptoms are fully controlled. Withdrawal should be even more gradual in these patients.

Gout

Gout is a disease characterised by recurrent attacks of acute pain and swelling at first affecting only one joint, usually the metatarsophalangeal joint of the big toe, later becoming polyarticular. Although primary gout is the result of an inborn error of purine metabolism, it is described in this section because its principal clinical features are connected with the locomotor system.

Aetiology. *Hereditary Factors.* Primary gout is a hereditary disorder. A family history of the disease is obtained in from 50 to 80 per cent of cases.

Age and Sex. Gout is infrequent before the age of 40 and in women.

Diet. In the past it was believed that an excessive intake of foods high in purines was the primary cause of gout. This view is not now accepted, although an acute attack can be induced by a high purine diet in patients predisposed to gout.

Secondary gout may occur as a complication of haematological disorders such as polycythaemia, leukaemia and myelofibrosis, and following administration of drugs, notably thiadiazine diuretics and frusemide.

Precipitating Factors. An acute attack may be precipitated by dietary indiscretions including overindulgence in alcohol and an idiosyncrasy to certain foods. An attack may also be precipitated by injury, excessive exercise, intercurrent infection and surgical operations.

Pathology. Urates are deposited in the articular and periarticular tissues, the extra-articular cartilages of the ears (tophi), and the kidneys. The deposits lead to absorption of bone and give rise to the cyst-like appearances or punched-out areas seen in radiographs. There is an inflammatory reaction in the synovial membrane. As the disease progresses the articular cartilage becomes eroded and thinned. Urates are deposited in the subchondral bone and synovial membrane. Finally the changes of osteoarthrosis appear.

Clinical Features

Acute Form. The metatarsophalangeal joint of the great toe is the first to be affected in over 90 per cent of cases. The onset is sudden; the patient is commonly awakened by excruciating pain; the joint becomes red, swollen, hot and exquisitely tender. The appearances may suggest a pyogenic infection or local cellulitis. Gout should always be borne in mind when these symptoms appear for the first time in a middle-aged male. Pyrexia, a polymorph leucocytosis and a rapid ESR are common accompaniments of the acute attack. After a few days the pain decreases. The skin over the affected joint becomes scaly and itchy. In the early stages of the disease the attacks occur at long intervals. Between attacks the patient is free from symptoms and radiological examination reveals no change in the affected joint. During the acute attack the plasma urate is raised, but may return to normal between attacks, i.e. 0·12–0·42 mmol/l (2–7 mg/100 ml).

Chronic Form. In some patients there is persistent pain and stiffness with deformity of the affected joints. Deposits of urates of a chalky consistency, known as tophi, appear in the periarticular tissues and the cartilages of the ear. Excessive excretion of uric acid may lead to calculus formation and attacks of renal colic. In the late stages atherosclerosis, hypertension and renal failure may complicate the picture. Because of effective modern treatment the chronic form of gout is now rarely seen.

Treatment

ACUTE ATTACK. Phenylbutazone is the drug of choice in doses of 600 mg daily for 2 to 3 days then reduced to 300 mg until pain disappears. Corticotrophin or corticosteroids will be required only in exceptional cases of gout which fail to respond to the administration of phenylbutazone or if this drug is not tolerated (p. 641). Colchicine is highly effective but causes vomiting and diarrhoea. Indomethacin is liable to cause severe headache and gastrointestinal symptoms in the doses necessary to suppress symptoms.

PROPHYLAXIS. *Uricosuric Agents.* Prolonged administration of drugs which increase the excretion of uric acid leads to a diminution in the number of acute attacks, a lowering of the blood urate, a decrease in the size of tophi, and may diminish the incidence of renal damage. The drugs of choice are probenecid in doses of 0·5 g 3 or 4 times daily and sulphinpyrazone in doses of 200–400 mg daily. The incidence of acute attacks during the early stages of uricosuric therapy can be reduced by the administration of colchicine 0·5 mg 3 times daily. Ample fluids should be taken to prevent the deposition of urates or uric acid in the kidney. Since salicylates antagonise the uricosuric action of these drugs, their coincidental use must be forbidden.

Allopurinol. This drug inhibits the enzyme xanthine oxidase responsible for the conversion of xanthine and hypoxanthine to uric acid. Thus the level of plasma uric acid falls and the excretion of its precursors is increased. These are more soluble and have a higher renal clearance rate than uric acid. The serum urate can be reduced to normal levels by a dose of 300–400 mg daily. Allopurinol has been shown to be remarkably free from toxic effects, mild rashes being the most common.

Special indications for the use of allopurinol are:
1. Failure of uricosuric drugs to control gout or intolerance of these drugs, e.g. allergy.
2. Severe tophaceous gout.
3. Recurrent uric acid stones or advanced impairment of renal function.
4. Treatment of leukaemia or malignant lymphomas with chemotherapy, when massive amounts of uric acid may have to be excreted.

DIET. Dietary restrictions are not of primary importance in the treatment of gout except in the presence of obesity. However, if attacks of gout are precipitated by certain wines, spirits or foods rich in purine (sweetbreads, liver, kidney, brain, heart, small fatty fish, fish roe, meat extracts) the offending substance should be excluded from the diet.

OTHER MEASURES. In cases with damaged or deformed joints the physiotherapeutic measures described for the treatment of rheumatoid arthritis should be applied. When tophi have become large or have ulcerated through the skin, they should be excised.

Pseudo-Gout

(Chondrocalcinosis; Pyrophosphate Arthropathy)

In this condition, crystals of calcium pyrophosphate are deposited in cartilage and other articular structures, giving rise to degenerative changes. The cause is unknown but there is a strong familial tendency and the condition is often associated with various other diseases such as hyperparathyroidism and haemochromatosis. Acute episodes which closely resemble true gout occur at intervals. There is no general metabolic disturbance. The synovial effusion contains crystals distinguishable microscopically from uric acid and radiological examination reveals deposits of calcium in the cartilage. Treatment of acute incidents with phenylbutazone, 600 mg daily, reducing the dose as symptoms are controlled, is usually effective. Treatment between attacks is along the lines laid down for osteoarthrosis.

Osteoarthrosis

Osteoarthrosis is characterised by degeneration of the articular cartilage and the formation of bony outgrowths at the edges of the affected joints. Usually only one or two of the larger joints are involved. The condition occurs amongst elderly people of either sex but may appear at any age in a joint which has been damaged by disease or injury.

Aetiology. Osteoarthrosis arises as a result of an exaggeration of the normal ageing process. Degenerative changes are present in the joints of most people over the age of 50 years, but only a few have symptoms. When one joint is particularly affected a history is frequently elicited of an injury to that joint some years before. Malalignment, following fractures of the long bones, often gives rise to osteoarthrosis in adjacent joints. Symptoms are prone to develop in weight-bearing joints and in those joints subjected to excessive strain. Thus, osteoarthrosis of the hips, spine or knees is particularly common in those engaged in heavy labour, and in obese subjects.

Pathology. There is patchy degeneration and splitting of the articular cartilage at the points of maximum weight-bearing, with exposure of the underlying bone, which tends to become denser and harder. New bone is laid down at the edges of the joints, resulting in the formation of osteophytes. Bony ankylosis never occurs, although limitation of movement may be very marked.

Clinical Features. The joints most frequently involved are those of the spine, hips and knees. In the majority of patients the disease is confined to one or two joints. The symptoms are gradual in onset. Pain is at first intermittent and of an aching character, appearing especially after the joint has been used, and relieved by rest. As the disease progresses, movement in the affected joints becomes increasingly limited, at first by muscular spasm and later by the loss of joint cartilage and the formation of osteophytes. There may be repeated effusions into the joints, especially after minor twists or injuries. Crepitus may be felt or even heard. Muscular wasting is always present to a greater or lesser extent. This is an important factor in the progress of the disease, as in the absence of normal muscular control the joint becomes more prone to injury.

Primary generalised osteoarthrosis is a clinically distinct form of osteoarthrosis which occurs mainly in middle-aged females as a familial trait. The terminal interphalangeal joints of the fingers are commonly affected, cartilaginous or bony outgrowths appear on the dorsal aspect of these joints (Heberden's nodes) and may give rise to considerable deformity and at times pain, but little disability. The first carpometacarpal joints, apophyseal spinal joints, the hips, ankles and knees may also be involved.

Radiologically there is characteristically a loss of joint space, and some sclerosis of the articular margins. In more advanced cases osteophytes appear at the bone edges.

Differential Diagnosis. There is usually little difficulty in distinguishing osteoarthrosis from rheumatoid arthritis, in which there is evidence of a general systemic disturbance and characteristically the proximal interphalangeal and metacarpophalangeal joints are involved. It must be borne in mind, however, that in long-standing cases of rheumatoid arthritis and gout, degenerative changes may appear in the affected joints.

Treatment. The pathological changes in osteoarthrosis are irreversible, but much may still be done to alleviate symptoms, especially in the early stages of the disease and if undue stresses and strains can be removed from the affected joints by a change of occupation or transfer to lighter work. The patient may also require to give up unduly strenuous hobbies. The institution of rest periods during the day may greatly alleviate pain and stiffness. The fitting of rubber heels to the footwear may help by reducing jarring and minimising the risk of slipping. In obese patients the most important single form of treatment is to obtain a substantial reduction in weight, especially when the hips or knees are affected. If pain is prominent rest in bed is required, combined with local heat and gentle active exercises and analgesics such as aspirin and codeine. Phenylbutazone (p. 641) may be effective in relieving pain where other measures have failed. It should be used with caution. Hydrotherapy is a useful palliative measure. Where one hip or one knee is dominantly affected, arthrodesis of the joint will provide a stable pain-free joint. Arthroplasty has also been used with success in osteoarthrosis of the hip and knee.

The intra-articular injection of hydrocortisone may be helpful, particularly in the knee (p. 642). Improvement may be maintained by injections given at intervals of 1 to 3 months. Patients should be warned to avoid excessive use of weight-bearing joints during the period following injection.

Miscellaneous Lesions of Connective Tissue

Many people suffer episodes of pain and stiffness of acute or insidious onset for which no obvious cause may be found. The most common sites are the neck, shoulder girdle, spine and gluteal regions. Muscle spasm of reflex origin is a prominent feature and accounts for the stiffness which must be differentiated from limitation of movement due to joint damage. Absence of signs of systemic illness and a normal ESR distinguishes this group of conditions from diffuse diseases of connective tissues.

Certain factors may be of importance in precipitating attacks in susceptible individuals. Exposure to cold and damp has always been suspected as a cause of 'rheumatic' complaints. Unaccustomed physical effort, undue fatigue, minor injuries and poor posture have also been incriminated. Complaints become more common with increasing age. Any reduction in muscular efficiency will render an individual more prone to strain or injury of tendons, ligaments and extra-articular soft tissue structures. Pain arising from such deep structures is poorly located, and referred diffusely to the overlying skin. Probably the most important cause underlying many such complaints is a loss of efficiency of the spinal shock absorbers, the intervertebral discs. Loss of resilience and elasticity occur long before radiological evidence of disc degeneration becomes apparent and the interfacetal joints of the spine are more exposed to strains and sprains. Pain may be referred from the cervical intervertebral joints to the occipital region, shoulder girdle and arm. Lumbago and sciatic pain without signs of root pressure are most commonly due to reduced capacity of the disc system to withstand acute stress or more chronic strain caused by poor posture, flabby muscles or obesity. Occupational factors are of great importance. Sickness absence attributable to 'rheumatic' complaints is much higher among miners, dockers and foundry workers than it is among employees in light industry or clerks.

A stiff, painful shoulder with progressive limitation of movement (*'frozen shoulder'*) may be due to synovitis, rupture of the capsule, subacromial bursitis or a lesion in the muscle complex round the joint, particularly in the supraspinatus. There may be a history of trauma or of unaccustomed use of the joint but often the cause of the lesion is not clear.

Diffuse muscular pain and stiffness is common in certain infections, particularly of viral origin, such as influenza, rubella and measles. Epidemic myalgia (*Bornholm disease*) is due to a virus of the Coxsackie group and is characterised by fever accompanied by intercostal or abdominal pain. The illness may last for 5 to 10 days but occasionally continues for several weeks. Epidemics of stiff neck have also been attributed to a viral infection.

Many anxious and depressed people complain of aches and pains, particularly in the region of the neck, shoulders or lower back.

Clinical Features. Symptoms are variable depending on the underlying cause. Pain is the usual presenting feature and may be accompanied by muscle spasm and limitation of movement. The onset can be acute or insidious. When the condition is subacute or chronic, pain and stiffness are most marked after a period of inactivity and may be eased by moderate exercise. Tender areas may be present, sometimes referred to as myalgic lesions, but such areas of local tenderness can be reproduced by injection of an irritant into deep structures, such as the interspinous ligaments.

Diagnosis. It is essential to carry out a careful clinical examination as many diseases of diverse origin frequently present with musculoskeletal symptoms. Too often a diagnosis of 'fibrositis' is made in patients suffering from osteoporosis, osteomalacia, hyperparathyroidism or metastatic bone disease. Myalgia or myopathy may be an early manifestation of malignant disease. It is also important to distinguish pain and stiffness of psychogenic origin.

Treatment. In all cases the cause must first be sought and, if possible, removed. The vast majority of patients will make a good recovery if treatment is adequate, but inaccurate diagnosis may lead to prolonged incapacity.

In the obese patient the most important measure is to secure a reduction of weight. An endeavour should be made to prevent further attacks by correcting faulty posture and by giving advice regarding the avoidance of chilling and excessive physical fatigue. The treatment of lesions of the intervertebral discs is described on page 748.

When pain is severe full doses of an analgesic will be required. Local symptoms are greatly eased by the application of some simple form of heat by means of a hot water bottle or electric blanket. When areas of acute local tenderness are present, the injection of 2–3 ml of local anaesthetic (1 per cent of procaine) may be followed by marked relief of pain. Injection may have to be repeated once or twice to obtain the maximum benefit. Infiltration should be followed by heat, massage and active exercises. Local pain throws the musculature out of balance, and if this is not corrected postural changes may be produced, causing a recurrence of symptoms.

In certain more chronic cases hydrotherapy provides heat combined with active movement and this is often effective where other measures have failed.

DISEASES OF BONE

Metabolic and Endocrine Diseases

Rickets (p. 119) and *osteomalacia* (p. 123), *osteoporosis* (p. 124), *hyperparathyroidism* (p. 531) and *Cushing's disease* (p. 536) all show an impairment of the composition of bone which is reflected in decreased density on radiological examination and in a liability to pathological fractures.

Infections

Osteomyelitis is most commonly encountered in children under the age of 12. *Staph. pyogenes* is the cause in the majority and in about half of these has its origin in a boil or a superficial staphylococcal infection. Thence there is a haematogenous spread to the metaphyseal region of a long bone. In children the onset is often abrupt with fever, nausea and severe pain at the site of infection. Rarely indolent infections of bone become localised and persist for long periods—the so-called Brodie's abscess. The most effective treatment, particularly early in the disease, is the administration of lincomycin (p. 93).

Tuberculosis may affect the anterior aspects of one or more vertebral bodies and the intervening intervertebral discs. The vertebrae later collapse causing a kyphosis usually in the thoracic region. Tuberculosis of the spine is now uncommon in Britain.

Paget's Disease

(Osteitis Deformans)

The incidence of this common condition of unknown aetiology increases with advancing years; it is seldom seen before the age of 50 years. Histologically and radiologically there is evidence of increased osteoblastic and osteoclastic activity as indicated by areas of increased bone formation and density alternating with areas of rarefaction. The lesions may be found in the pelvis, skull, humerus, spine, femur, tibia or elsewhere. The distribution is characteristically irregular, so that normal bone may be found between affected areas.

Clinical Features. Many patients have no symptoms and the disease is recognised only when radiological examination is made for some other reason. In some, pain occurs and occasionally is severe. The affected areas may be unusually warm on palpation, due to the increased vascularity of the bones. When the skull is involved, headache may be troublesome, and hearing may be impaired from compression of the auditory nerve. Deformity of bones develops when the condition is advanced. Fractures may occur spontaneously or after minor trauma but usually heal normally. Osteogenic sarcoma is an uncommon late complication of the disease.

Rarely the lesions are so widespread and so vascular that they form, in effect, an arteriovenous shunt in the bones. The cardiac output is therefore increased, and heart failure may ultimately occur.

The serum calcium and phosphorus are normal, except during periods of immobilisation, when they may be considerably raised. The serum alkaline phosphatase, which in these circumstances is a measure of osteoblastic activity, may be increased to as much as 725 i.u./l or more.

Treatment. Little can be done to alter the course of the disease. It is liable to be of long duration and is often accompanied by apparent remissions. Symptomatic treatment for pain in the bones or headache may be required, and if fractures occur they should be treated as if the bone were otherwise normal. Calcitonin (p. 530) helps those patients with much pain.

Tumours

Simple tumours and primary malignant disease, such as osteogenic sarcoma, are much less frequently encountered than secondary carcinoma from primary growths, most commonly in the lung, breast, prostate, thyroid or kidney. The first clinical manifestation of the carcinoma may be a pathological fracture or diffuse discomfort which may be dismissed by the doctor as 'rheumatic'. In contrast the patient may be symptomless and yet metastases may be widespread throughout the skeleton and seen on radiological examination as multiple osteolytic or osteosclerotic areas. Myelomatosis may present in similar ways; early diagnosis is important as this condition can be controlled with chemotherapy. Oestrogen therapy or surgery, such as orchidectomy or oophorectomy, may be helpful in the management of metastases from the prostate or breast and local radiotherapy may be a useful palliative measure when pain is a problem, wherever the primary carcinoma may be situated or even if it cannot be identified.

Prospects in Rheumatology

Although the aetiology of the diverse group of connective tissue diseases is still unknown, classification of these diseases has improved considerably and diagnosis is more precise. The outlook for patients afflicted by the articular and systemic manifestations of connective tissue disease is now much brighter than 30 years ago. Intervention by the orthopaedic surgeon has salvaged many patients who hitherto would have been severely and permanently disabled by joint disease. The efficacy of early synovectomy in relieving pain and restoring function is well established and replacement arthroplasties for the hip, knee and finger joints are now commonplace. Continuing collaboration between bioengineers and orthopaedic surgeons will undoubtedly lead to more effective methods of reconstructing joints such as the shoulder, elbow and ankle for which satisfactory prostheses are not yet available. The introduction of artificial lubricants for the treatment of degenerative joint disease may also become a reality in the foreseeable future.

The development of new drugs will inevitably lead to more effective treatment of the connective tissue diseases. The patient with chronic tophaceous gout has already become a clinical rarity following the introduction of the uricosuric agents and allopurinol, while the survival rate in systemic lupus erythematosus has improved considerably since the advent of the corticosteroids. With the sophisticated laboratory techniques now available for monitoring disease activity and detecting early cases, it is likely that the prognosis in systemic lupus erythematosus will continue to improve. The continuing development of non-steroidal drugs with highly specific activity in the prostaglandin system and against other chemical mediators of inflammation will eventually allow more effective control of inflammatory joint disease.

Knowledge concerning the role of genetic, biochemical and immunological factors in the connective tissue diseases is expanding rapidly, and there is some reason to hope that the aetiology of rheumatoid arthritis and allied conditions will not remain undiscovered for another 30 years.

J. J. R. Duthrie
J. N. McCormick

Further reading:

Boyle, J. A. & Buchanan, W. W. (1971) *Clinical Rheumatology.* Oxford: Blackwell.
Copeman, W. S. C. (1970) *Textbook of Rheumatic Diseases.* 4th edition. Edinburgh: Livingstone.
Hollander, J. L. & McCarty, J. R. (1972) *Arthritis and Allied Conditions.* 8th edition. London: Kimpton.
Mason, M. & Currey, H. L. F. (1970) *An Introduction to Clinical Rheumatology.* London: Pitman.

14. Diseases of the Nervous System

THE approach to patients presenting neurological problems must follow a logical course. Clinical examination reveals neurological signs which reflect disordered neural function. The nature and distribution of these signs depend on the anatomical localisation of lesions within the central nervous system. It is a fundamental error to relate particular signs to specific pathological processes. Paralysis of one side of the body, hemiplegia, may equally well arise from a stroke or from a cerebral tumour since both lesions may similarly interrupt motor pathways. It is the history of the neurological illness which indicates the nature of the pathological process involved. A careful chronological assessment of the way in which a neurological disability has developed is essential if a diagnosis is to be made. Attention to the symptoms and signs which indicate loss of function of particular parts of the nervous system then follows for purposes of localisation.

Lesions which suddenly affect the nervous system, cause maximal disability within a few hours and after a static period of days or weeks then show a tendency to improve are usually due to vascular disturbances and sometimes to trauma. Disabilities of insidious onset and slow but inexorable progression are often due to degenerative disorders or to tumours of the central nervous system. A remittent history, wherein episodes of disability are followed by periods of improvement, with later recurrence of symptoms elsewhere in the nervous system, is characteristic of multiple sclerosis. Inflammatory lesions such as infections often develop rapidly, but less acutely than traumatic or vascular catastrophes and the recovery phase is also usually rapid. Some conditions are characterised by paroxysmal short-lived disorders of function, followed by rapid and complete recovery. A history of this type may be due to epilepsy or migraine or to transient ischaemic attacks. These general principles are a useful guide but atypical presentations occur. Sometimes a neoplasm may produce very rapid deterioration and occasionally repetitive, minor vascular lesions give rise to a progressive, 'stepwise' deterioration of function.

Some diseases cause systematised affection of cells or fibres of similar type; these conditions, of which motor neurone disease is a good example, usually result in bilateral and symmetrical dysfunction. Tumours produce progressive involvement of adjacent neural structures causing clinical disabilities which may later be accompanied by symptoms resulting from the occupation of space by the tumour within the confines of the skull or the spinal canal.

A neurological diagnosis is achieved by the integration of all the information gained from the patient's history, the general medical examination and the neurological examination.

Applied Anatomy and Physiology

The Motor System

Movements, whether voluntary or involuntary, are the result of the contraction or controlled relaxation of groups of muscles and never of a single muscle only.

They are effected by contraction of muscles which act as prime movers and reciprocal relaxation of their antagonists. The action of the prime movers is provided with a firm base by contraction of synergists which stabilise the joints, and by appropriate adjustments of posture. The postural adjustments are largely under the control of the extrapyramidal motor system and the vestibular and spinal reflexes. Voluntary movements require the participation of the precentral gyrus of the cerebral cortex ('motor area') and the timing and degree of contraction or relaxation of the muscles of the synergy are coordinated by the cerebellum, especially when a movement involves more than one segment of a limb. The activities of the upper motor neurones from the motor area of the cortex, the extrapyramidal motor system and the cerebellum influence, directly or indirectly, the cells of the anterior horn of spinal grey matter or motor cranial nuclei from which the lower neurone runs to a group of muscle fibres ('motor unit'). Thus the lower motor neurone is the 'final common path' for all efferent impulses directed at the muscle and the groups of anterior horn cells may be considered to 'represent a muscle' in the same sense as the cells of the motor cortex 'represent a movement'. This distinction is vital to an understanding of the signs and disorders of the motor system.

Upper Motor Neurone. The fibres arise from cells in the precentral gyrus ('motor area'). These initiate movements of different parts of the opposite side of the body, the parts being represented in the following order from below upwards—tongue, face, hand, forearm, arm, trunk, thigh, leg, foot and perineal areas with considerable overlap. The cortical area representing movements of each of these parts is proportional to its functional importance rather than to its anatomical size. The projections of the upper motor neurones to the contralateral motor nuclei of the brain stem and anterior horn of the spinal cord are shown in Figure 14.1.

A destructive lesion of the lateral corticospinal tract above its decussation causes a loss of some voluntary movements of part of the opposite side of the body, according to the fibres involved, but automatic associated movements, such as the stretching of a paralysed arm when yawning, may persist and other voluntary or reflex movements using the same lower motor neurones and muscles may be preserved. This is the essential difference between paralysis of upper motor neurone type and that due to a lower motor neurone lesion. For the same reason stretch reflexes are retained but these are usually of heightened activity. This indicates that the pyramidal tract normally carries fibres which are inhibitory to the stretch reflex. The pattern of cutaneous protective reflexes also changes, causing the emergence of an extensor plantar reflex. There are thus two types of disturbance, a negative one due to loss of a particular activity, and a positive one due to the release of lower levels from control. Hughlings Jackson considered this to be a principle of general application in the nervous system and the concept is important in understanding the signs of pyramidal disease. Another type of positive symptom results from irritative lesions (usually incomplete damage to a nerve cell or its fibre) which cause spontaneous activity of the affected neurones. Spontaneous activity in upper motor neurones causes involuntary movements as in focal epilepsy (p. 686).

SIGNS OF A LESION OF THE UPPER MOTOR NEURONE. These are:
 1. Weakness or paralysis of movements of part of one side of the body.
 2. Increase of tone of spastic type. This is characterised by an increased

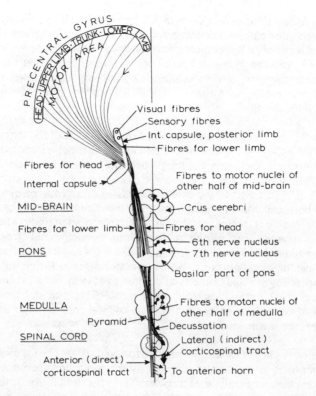

Fig. 14.1 The motor pathways.

resistance to passive movement, which is maximal at the beginning of movement, smoothly sustained, and suddenly lapses as passive movement is continued ('clasp-knife phenomenon'). It occurs predominantly in flexor muscles in the upper limbs and extensor muscles in the lower limbs (the antigravity muscles).

3. Increase in amplitude of tendon reflexes; clonus may be present.

4. Loss of the abdominal reflexes.

5. An extensor plantar response (Babinski reflex).

6. No muscle atrophy apart from slight wasting which may occur as a result of disuse.

7. Normal electrical excitability of the involved muscles (p. 660).

These signs occur with disease involving any part of the upper motor neurone from the cortex down, but the exact level at which the lesion lies may be determined by the upper level of increased reflexes and by associated features.

Cortex. Localised paralyses, affecting for example, one limb only, are characteristic of lesions at the cortical level. The upper motor neurones are spread over a wide area and only very large lesions could cause a hemiplegia. There may be associated evidence of cortical dysfunction such as dysphasia and focal epileptic fits sometimes occur.

Internal Capsule. As pyramidal fibres here are closely packed, a hemiplegia is likely, with involvement of face, arm and leg on the opposite side. There may be hemihypaesthesia and hemianopia from damage to adjacent sensory and visual fibres.

Brain Stem. Lesions in this area are rarely confined to the pyramidal tract. One presentation comprises affection of one or more cranial nerves on the side of the lesion and signs of an upper motor neurone lesion on the opposite side.

Spinal Cord. The pyramidal pathways may be affected bilaterally. The level of the lesion in the cord is often delineated by accompanying lower motor neurone signs or by sensory disturbance or loss of tendon reflexes, which indicate a segmental localisation.

Lower Motor Neurone. Axons emerge from the cells of the anterior horn of the spinal cord and from the nuclei of the motor cranial nerves and pass through the anterior nerve roots to enter a mixed peripheral nerve in which they run to the muscles which they supply. Each lower motor neurone has a terminal branching so that it is distributed to the motor end-plates of a group of muscle fibres. The anterior horn cell, the axon and a group of muscle fibres comprise the motor-unit and each muscle is composed of a large number of such units. The anterior horn cell is activated by impulses from the corticospinal tracts, from the extrapyramidal tracts, and from some afferent fibres of the posterior nerve root responsible for spinal reflexes. The lower motor neurone is thus an integral part of the spinal reflex arc and is the final common pathway for all motor impulses, involuntary or voluntary, directed to a muscle. Normal nutrition of a muscle appears to depend on its contact with the spinal cord through the lower motor neurone since if it is interrupted the muscle rapidly wastes.

SIGNS OF A LESION OF THE LOWER MOTOR NEURONE. The following signs will be present only in those muscles supplied by the particular neurones affected:

1. Weakness or paralysis of muscles. This affects all movements in which they take part whether as prime movers or synergists, voluntary or involuntary, or in reflex contractions.

2. Loss of tone on passive movement (flaccidity).

3. Wasting of the affected muscles which appears within two or three weeks of an acute lesion (atrophy).

4. Absence of reflexes subserved by the affected neurones. Abdominal and plantar reflexes remain normal unless the neurones to the appropriate muscles are damaged and then these reflexes cannot be elicited.

5. Single fibres contract spontaneously when they are no longer influenced by their associated lower motor neurone. This phenomenon, called fibrillation, is detectable by electromyography but is invisible through the skin. Lower motor neurones which are damaged but still able to conduct impulses may give rise to spontaneous contractions of bundles of fibres in the muscles supplied. Such contractions (fasciculation) may be visible, e.g. in motor neurone disease (p. 735).

6. Contractures of muscles due to replacement by fibrous tissue and 'trophic' changes such as dryness and cyanosis of the skin, and brittleness of the nails, partly due to impaired circulation.

7. The electrical excitability of the peripheral nerves and muscles is altered as can be shown by special tests. They may usefully be combined with electromyography to confirm that a weak and wasted muscle is denervated. Lesions of peripheral nerves short of complete interruption may cause slowing of conduction which can be measured by special techniques.

If lower motor neurones are damaged in the cord or nerve roots the muscles and reflexes affected in the ways described above will be those supplied by one or more segments of the spinal cord. If the neurones are damaged more peripherally after they have been redistributed in the nerve plexuses, the paralysis will occur in the territory supplied by the appropriate peripheral nerve and it is probable that there will be similar damage to the sensory fibres with which they are associated in the mixed nerve.

Extrapyramidal System. This is a complex neuronal network, extending from the cortex to the medulla, from which emerge descending spinal pathways whose influence on lower motor neurones modifies voluntary motor activity. Interspersed in this latticework of fibres are areas of grey matter. Some of these are but loose aggregations of nuclei in the reticular formation of the brain stem, but there are also several well defined nuclear masses called the basal ganglia, which include the corpus striatum comprising the caudate nucleus and putamen, the globus pallidus or pallidum, the substantia nigra and the subthalamic nucleus.

There are rich interconnections between the constituents of the basal ganglia and thence via the ventrolateral nucleus of the thalamus to the extrapyramidal areas of the cortex and to the medullary reticular formation. The normal functions of the extrapyramidal system are ill-understood.

SIGNS OF AN EXTRAPYRAMIDAL LESION. *Disturbance of Voluntary Movements.* There is not true paralysis in extrapyramidal disease, but rather slowness of movement and poverty of movement in that spontaneous gestures, changes in facial expression, and associated movements for postural adjustment such as swinging the arm when walking are lost on the side opposite to the lesion.

Disturbance of Tone. Tone may be increased as in parkinsonism or decreased as in chorea. Increase in tone, of extrapyramidal type, has characteristic features. It is present throughout the whole range of passive movement; it affects opposing muscle groups equally; it may be smooth and plastic ('lead-pipe rigidity') or intermittent ('cog-wheel rigidity') which is more common.

Involuntary Movements. There are many varieties but three important types are the tremor of parkinsonism (p. 728), choreiform movements (p. 734) and athetosis (p. 734).

Cerebellum. The cerebellum is the most important part of the nervous system for the coordination of movement and the muscular contractions required to maintain posture. The cerebellum receives impulses from many sources, principally the proprioceptive end-organs, the skin, the vestibular nuclei and the cerebral cortex. The pontine nuclei and the inferior olive relay fibres from the cerebral motor cortex and basal ganglia respectively to the cerebellar cortex of the opposite side. The cerebellar cortex integrates this information about body posture, limb position and motor intention and sends efferent fibres via the cerebellar nuclei to the reticular formation, red nucleus and vestibular nucleus of the opposite side, whence fibres descend to influence motor cells in the anterior horns of the spinal cord; as these descending fibres cross again each cerebellar hemisphere controls the ipsilateral side of the body. Efferent fibres from the cerebellum also ascend to the contralateral thalamus through which the cerebral cortex is influenced. The cerebellum is therefore a great coordinating centre controlling the synergistic action of muscles during voluntary and automatic movements as well as adjusting posture.

SIGNS OF A CEREBELLAR LESION. The effects of disease of the cerebellum are best seen in acute lesions, for in chronic lesions considerable compensation occurs so that the deficit is less than might be expected. A lesion of the cerebellar hemisphere produces all its effects on the same side of the body. The principal effects are:

Muscular Hypotonia. The muscles are flaccid on palpation, show diminished resistance to passive movement and, when an outstretched limb is suddenly displaced, it makes a greater excursion than usual and oscillates before resuming its posture.

Disturbance of Tendon Reflexes. The reflexes are either diminished or pendular as when the knee jerk is followed by a series of diminishing oscillations.

Disturbance of Posture and of Gait. The head may be tilted towards the side of the lesion and the patient leans or may even fall towards that side. His gait is reeling and he tends to stagger to the side of the lesion.

Disorders of Movement. Incoordination, hypotonia and the fact that muscular contraction is unregulated by the muscle spindles cause ataxia which manifests itself in different ways:

1. Dysmetria. Movements are not accurately adjusted to their object, so that the finger may overshoot or fall short of the object it is required to touch. If a movement is attempted with the eyes closed the finger overshoots towards the side of the cerebellar lesion ('past-pointing').

2. Dyssynergia. Movements which involve more than one joint are broken up into their component parts. When severe this leads to decomposition of movement which resembles the jerky movements of a marionette.

3. Intention tremor. A combination of dyssynergia and dysmetria causes faulty correction of the badly directed limb movement so that it approaches the target in a zig-zag manner. The coarse irregular tremor increases as the target is approached. It is not increased when the eyes are closed. The contraction of muscles necessary to maintain a posture may be similarly affected so that tremor at rest occasionally occurs in cerebellar disorders.

4. Dysdiadochokinesis. The arrest of one movement and its immediate replacement with the opposite movement requires accurate coordination of the various muscles of the synergy. Rapidly alternating movements are therefore disturbed and carried out in a clumsy, irregular, jerky fashion.

5. Rebound phenomenon. For the same reason a strong contraction cannot be arrested when resistance is suddenly removed, whereupon the limb shoots beyond the normal range.

6. Disorders of articulation and phonation. Articulation is irregular, slurred and explosive as the volume of sound is poorly controlled. A rarer form of dysarthria is scanning-speech in which the syllables tend to be separated from each other.

7. Disturbance of eye movement. Jerking nystagmus in the horizontal plane is commonly seen. It is a defect of postural fixation involving conjugate gaze (p. 678). In a unilateral cerebellar lesion the movements are greater in amplitude and slower in rate when the eyes are deviated to the side of the lesion.

The Sensory System

Superficial sensation which arises from the skin has four primary components, touch, pain, warmth and cold. *Deep sensations* arising from subcutaneous structures are deep pain, pressure and proprioception which enables the recognition of movements of joints and the position of the parts of the body relative to one another. Vibration is a sensation due to rhythmical stimulation of groups of deep and superficial touch receptors. Some of the afferent impulses carried in 'sensory' nerve fibres do not reach consciousness but convey impulses directly or indirectly to motor neurones for reflex functions or to the cerebellum for purposes of coordination, e.g. many impulses from muscle and tendon receptors. All sensory impulses arise in the sensory receptors or end-organs which are widely distributed throughout the body. It is probable, though debatable, that specialised receptors respond to specific types of stimuli. Stimulation of an end-organ causes impulses to pass along the first sensory neurone to the spinal cord. This neurone has its cell body in a dorsal root ganglion but does not synapse until it reaches a second order neurone in the spinal cord or brain stem. On entering the cord by the posterior nerve root, fibres subserving proprioception, vibration and a proportion of touch sensation turn medially and ascend in the posterior column of the same side to the lower part of the medulla oblongata to synapse with cells in the gracile and cuneate nuclei (Fig. 14.2). From there, the second order neurone crosses to the other side of the medulla and ascends in the medial lemniscus to the main sensory nucleus of the thalamus. Fibres subserving pain, warmth, cold and the remainder of touch sensation synapse in the posterior horn of the spinal cord soon after entering it. Most of the second order neurones cross at the same level, or one or two segments higher, to reach the anterolateral column where they ascend to the thalamus as the spinothalamic tract. Some of these fibres do not cross but enter the ipsilateral spinothalamic tract. As it ascends through the brain stem the tract gradually intermingles with the medial lemniscus and terminates along with it in the main sensory nucleus of the thalamus. Third order neurones, maintaining their functional specificity, are then relayed from the thalamus to the sensory area of the cortex which is situated in the postcentral gyrus.

Areas of the sensory cortex representing the different parts of the body are arranged in a similar manner to the motor cortex. Some appreciation of sensation is possible at the thalamic level but the cortical projection is necessary to allow discrimination of the intensity and pattern of stimulation. From the postcentral gyrus further connections are made with other parts of the cortex, particularly in the parietal lobe where the information derived from superficial and deep sensation is integrated so that judgement of the size, shape, weight, texture and pattern of objects is possible. This sensory information is also integrated with information derived from the special senses to provide a mental picture of the body (body image). This synthesis is mainly carried out in the non-dominant parietal lobe. The corresponding part of the left cerebral hemisphere is important for other mental functions in which recurrent patterns of stimulation achieve the status of symbols and so are used for the receptive and interpretative aspects of speech functions. For this reason it is usually called the dominant or major hemisphere (in some left-handed people speech is mainly represented in the right hemisphere). This important part of the parietal lobe is connected with the lower part of the motor cortex of the same side so that patterns of lip, tongue, respiratory and finger movements may be used to convert ideas into motor symbols, the motor side of speech. An understanding of the link between symbol and meaning requires a knowledge of the physiological basis of the mind which we do not have at present.

Most of the afferent signals entering the central nervous system never reach consciousness. Some are used for spinal reflexes and make contact directly or through interneurones with motor neurones. Other fibres which originate in muscle receptors end at the base of the posterior horn in contact with second order neurones. These neurones turn laterally to the periphery of the cord to ascend in the anterior and posterior spinocerebellar tracts to the cerebellar cortex. Most of these ascend without crossing but some second order neurones cross to the opposite anterior spinocerebellar tract. These fibres carry some of the proprioceptive information required to enable the cerebellum to coordinate limb movements. Still other sensory fibres, which do not carry 'sensation' in the ordinary sense, are extremely important for the maintenance of consciousness. These are collateral branches of the main spinothalamic pathways and of the special sensory tracts which turn medially into the upper part of the reticular formation in the midbrain. Here there is a chain of short neurones with intimate interconnections which also receives neurones from most parts of the cerebral cortex. It is therefore an important integrating centre. At its upper end it communicates with the non-specific nuclei of the thalamus which relay impulses to all areas of the cortex. Activity in this system is considered to be essential for the conscious state and may be important in some mental functions in collaboration with the cerebral cortex.

Disease of the sensory system may be accompanied by positive phenomena such as pain or paraesthesiae due to spontaneous activity or irritation of sensory neurones, or by negative phenomena in which there is loss of the ability to appreciate some modality of sensation (anaesthesia and analgesia). These symptoms occur only with disorders of the first or second order neurones, i.e. from the endorgans to the thalamus. Suprathalamic lesions show certain differences. Paraesthesia may occur with irritative lesions of the sensory cortex but

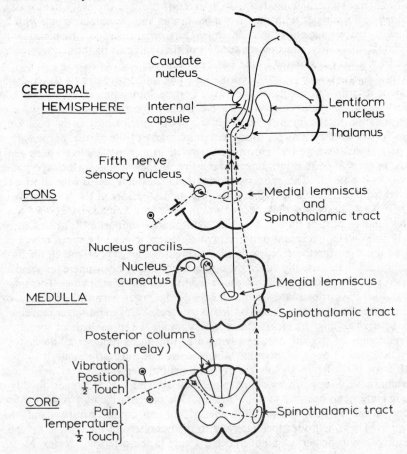

Fig. 14.2 The sensory pathways.

anaesthesia does not. Instead there is a loss of sensory discrimination and of the spatial and quantitative aspects of sensation.

SIGNS OF SENSORY LESIONS. *Peripheral nerve*. With a complete lesion all forms of sensation are lost in the area supplied by the affected nerve, but the zone of anaesthesia may be limited by the fact that neighbouring nerves overlap into its territory, the extent varying from person to person. The resistance of different types of fibres to disease need not be the same so that it is common for one type of cutaneous or deep sensation to be more affected than another and indeed some may be spared. If the afferent fibres of a reflex arc are affected, as the sciatic nerve in the ankle jerk, the reflex concerned is lost. Some neuropathies do not affect individual nerves but rather damage fibres selectively. As a general rule the longest fibres are most susceptible and so the sensory and motor disturbance is first noticed at the tips of all the toes and fingers, irrespective of nerve supply, and spreads proximally as the advancing disease involves progressively shorter fibres. This produces a 'glove and stocking' distribution of sensory loss.

Posterior Root. The different forms of sensation are affected by a posterior root lesion in the same way as for a peripheral nerve but the distribution of the loss follows a dermatome pattern. The overlap from adjacent roots may be so great that no anaesthesia can be detected. When the root is irritated pain and paraesthesia are experienced in the full dermatomal distribution of the root and pain may also be experienced in the deep structures such as muscles and ligaments which are supplied by the root. (These structures do not necessarily underlie the dermatome.) Any reflex subserved by the involved root is also lost, for example, the ankle jerk when the S 1 posterior root is damaged by a prolapsed intervertebral disc.

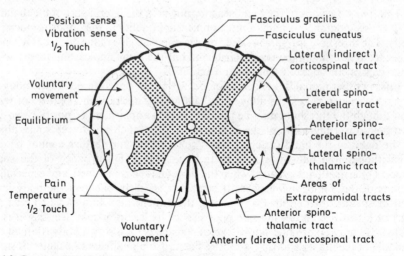

Fig. 14.3 Cross-section of spinal cord.

Posterior Column. A lesion confined to the posterior column of the spinal cord will cause loss of position and vibration sense on the same side, but the sensations of pain, touch, warmth and cold will be preserved (Fig. 14.3). The loss of the sense of position causes sensory ataxia since the patient is unable to control his movements by awareness of the position achieved at each instant. Sensory ataxia differs from cerebellar ataxia in that it is more marked when the eyes are closed, because vision can compensate to a certain extent for loss of proprioceptive information. Thus there is unsteadiness in the finger-nose test which is greater when the eyes are closed but without the marked tremor of cerebellar ataxia. The gait is ataxic and the patient walks with a broad base to give himself a firmer foundation and steps high to make sure that his feet clear the ground which he is unable to feel with certainty. If his eyes are closed he is unable to stand with feet close together without swaying (Romberg's test). Vibration sense is abolished below the level of the lesion ipsilaterally. The same symptoms will be found if the first order neurones of the proprioceptive nerve fibres are damaged peripherally but they will then be associated with other signs of peripheral nerve disease.

Spinothalamic Tract. Lesions of the anterior and lateral spinothalamic tracts in the anterolateral columns of the cord or their continuation through the brain stem cause impairment of the ability to appreciate pain, warmth and cold on the contralateral side of the body below the level of the lesion. Touch is usually modified (it feels 'different') but not abolished because of its alternative pathway in the posterior columns. This is the situation produced by the operation of anterolateral cordotomy for the relief of intractable pain.

Brain Stem. Since the spinothalamic tract and medial lemniscus run close together and eventually intermingle, lesions of the upper brain stem usually affect all forms of sensation on the contralateral side of the body. With midbrain lesions the hemihypaesthesia will extend to the face, but with pontomedullary lesions the second order neurones from the trigeminal sensory nucleus or the nucleus and descending tract of the fifth nerve may be damaged so that sensory loss will be on the same side of the face as the lesion but on the contralateral side of the rest of the body (Fig. 14.2, p. 664).

Thalamus. Lesions of the main sensory nuclei in the lateral part of the thalamus may cause spontaneous pain of most unpleasant quality in the opposite side of the body. The threshold for pain is raised on the opposite side of the body but when it is exceeded the resulting pain is exquisite and has the same unpleasant quality which often causes considerable emotional reaction.

Loss of other modalities of sensation occurs on the opposite side of the body.

Sensory Cortex. Lesions above the thalamus do not abolish any form of sensation though the threshold may be raised. There is impairment of position sense, of two-point discrimination, of the ability to localise touch and to recognise objects in the palm of the hand (astereognosis) since shape and texture cannot be identified though the patient is able to feel the object. Disturbance of the spatial aspects of sensation is greatest when the parietal lobe is involved, and especially in lesions of the 'minor' hemisphere this may cause disturbance of the body image and of spatial orientation. For instance the patient may be unable to recognise part of his own body on the side opposite to the lesion or may feel that it is distorted. He may ignore one side of external space or of his own body (though he is capable of feeling it) and this is most evident if the unaffected (ipsilateral) side of his body, or visual field, is stimulated simultaneously. When presented with this 'perceptual rivalry' his brain 'ignores' the stimulus on the side contralateral to the affected parietal lobe though a stimulus applied to that part alone would be recognised immediately. Lesions of the dominant hemisphere in the region where parietal, temporal and occipital lobes meet (angular and supramarginal gyri) are associated with receptive dysphasia (p. 669). This is a special case of the failure to analyse the temporal and spatial aspects of sensory stimuli.

The Reflexes

Certain functions are economically catered for by the nervous system by means of reflexes, which are short chains of neurones (the reflex arc) connecting a receptor to an effector organ such as muscle or gland, so that an appropriate stimulus invariably leads to a specific response. The quantity but not the nature of the response may be modified by other stimuli or by supraspinal influences from the cortex, extrapyramidal system or the cerebellum. There are two main categories of reflex—postural and protective. The appropriate stimuli for postural reflexes are muscle stretch and vestibular impulses. Protective reflexes are evoked by stimuli to pain receptors. They are usually superficial (cutaneous or corneal); the protective 'spasm' of muscles around a painful lesion is similar in nature.

Tendon (Stretch) Reflexes. A basic postural reflex depends on the stimulation of muscle spindles when a skeletal muscle is stretched. The afferent fibre enters the cord by a posterior nerve root and communicates directly or via a chain of interneurones with the anterior horn cells which control the stretched muscle, thus causing it to contract and so resist the displacement. A sudden tap to a tendon results in a sharp but brief contraction of the muscle. This activity may be increased by certain manoeuvres such as clenching the teeth or pulling the interlocked hands apart. This is termed reinforcement of the reflex and a tendon jerk should not be declared absent until reinforcement has failed to make it visible. The stretch reflex is inhibited by receptors in the tendon if muscle tension rises too high, thus risking the integrity of its fibres. This may happen when the reflex is exaggerated by withdrawal of a normal inhibitory effect of the corticospinal tract (p. 658), so that the contraction is abruptly stopped. This is the mechanism of the 'clasp-knife' response. There are also supraspinal facilitatory and inhibitory influences from the extrapyramidal system and cerebellum so lesions of these systems may abolish the reflexes.

An example of a monosynaptic stretch reflex is a knee jerk. A tap on the patellar tendon activates stretch receptors in the quadriceps muscle giving rise to impulses in first order sensory neurones which pass directly to the lower motor neurones to the quadriceps muscle making it contract. A lesion anywhere along this path will cause loss of the reflex, hence it is important in the localisation of disease to know through which spinal segment each reflex passes. The common tendon reflexes are the brachioradialis or supinator (C 5–6), the biceps (C 5–6), the triceps (C 7), the knee (L 3–4) and the ankle (S 1).

Superficial Reflexes. These are polysynaptic reflexes originating from stimuli to superficial structures. The interneurones may connect with motor neurones at several segmental levels and so the response may be a coordinated movement, usually designed to withdraw the stimulated part from a potentially dangerous stimulus. There are very many of these reflexes, some of which are conflicting. For example, stimulation of the sole of the foot evokes both flexion and extension reflexes. Which reflex will predominate is determined by higher influences. The nature of this influence is unknown but is believed to require the corticospinal (pyramidal) tract and damage to this tract will cause a change in the predominant reflex pattern.

Plantar Reflex. When the outer border of the sole of the foot is stroked in normal people after infancy, there is plantar flexion of the great toe. In 1896 Babinski pointed out that when the upper motor neurone was damaged the same stimulus caused dorsiflexion of the toe. (Anatomically this is described as an extensor plantar response though physiologically it is part of the flexion withdrawal reflex.) When the reflex is well developed it can be elicited from the medial side of the sole of the foot or even from the lower part of the leg and the hallux response is accompanied by dorsiflexion and abduction or fanning of the other toes and even withdrawal of the limb. The fundamental importance of the extensor plantar or Babinski response as a sign of loss of function of the upper motor neurone is widely accepted but it may occur in transient form during temporary states such as coma or after an epileptic fit and need not indicate permanent damage. It is often extensor in normal infants during the first year of life.

Abdominal Reflexes. When the skin on one side of the abdomen is stroked with a pin, there is a reflex contraction of the underlying muscles, a reflex for protection of the viscera. This may be lost on the affected side in disease of the upper motor neurone though the sign is less reliable than the plantar reflex. For instance the abdominal reflexes may be lost early in multiple sclerosis yet retained despite severe pyramidal tract damage in motor neurone disease. The abdominal reflexes may not be obtained on either side in elderly, obese or multiparous patients, and may be lost where operative incisions have severed the nerves concerned. The abdominal reflexes are served in their peripheral course by the intercostal nerves arising from segments T 8 to 12.

Corneal Reflex. A light touch on the cornea provokes a blink of the eyelids on both sides. The afferent path for this reflex is the first division of the trigeminal nerve and the efferent path is the facial nerve. Loss of both corneal reflexes is a valuable indication of a deepening level of unconsciousness from any cause but should be elicited with discretion to avoid accidental damage to the cornea.

Nervous Control of the Bladder and Rectum

Bladder. The nerve supply to the bladder is derived from three sources:

1. Sympathetic, from the first and second lumbar segment via the inferior hypogastric plexus and hypogastric nerves, which relax the bladder wall and contract the sphincters.

2. Parasympathetic, from segments S 2, 3, 4 via the pelvic nerves (nervi erigentes) which contract the bladder wall and relax the internal sphincter.

3. Somatic, from segments S 2, 3, 4 via the pudendal nerves, which contract the external sphincter of the urethra.

Afferent impulses from the bladder wall travel via the pelvic nerves and from the sphincters via the pudendal nerves. Distension of the bladder activates stretch receptors in the bladder wall and stimulates the parasympathetic fibres by means of a reflex arc through the upper sacral segments of the spinal cord; for example in the infant the bladder empties automatically when distension reaches a certain degree. Subsequently two descending pathways from higher levels assume control, one which inhibits the automatic reflex emptying, and the other which relaxes the inhibition when appropriate. The expression of urine is then promoted by contracting the abdominal and relaxing the pelvic muscles.

Interruption of the sacral reflex arc leads to retention of urine. This is accompanied by loss of bladder sensation if the lesion is on the afferent side of the arc, as in tabes dorsalis. Damage to the anterior sacral nerve roots causes an atonic bladder without loss of sensation ('lower motor neurone paralysis'). Lesions in the spinal cord above the sacral segments may damage the inhibitory fibres, causing urgency, precipitancy or incontinence of urine, or damage to the facilitatory fibres may cause hesitancy or retention. If the higher control is completely lost there is a period of retention with overflow from a passively dilating atonic bladder until the sacral reflex begins to function as in infancy, restoring automatic bladder emptying. The bladder is hypertonic ('upper motor neurone paralysis') and may shrink if this is not prevented. Cerebral lesions at the vertex near the motor or sensory areas may also give rise to incontinence or retention, and with frontal lobe lesions the intellectual disturbance may be associated with failure to inhibit reflex emptying.

Rectum. The rectum has a dual nerve supply from the sympathetic (inhibitory) and the parasympathetic (facilitatory) systems. Disturbances of function similar to those in the bladder occur, but are less severe and more transient.

Speech

Speech employs verbal symbols to communicate thoughts and information. Coherent speech requires the formulation of propositions, which are translated into conventional symbols, earlier acquired and readily accessible, which then reach external expression by means of an efficient vocalising apparatus. Disease processes may interrupt this sequence at various levels to produce different types of speech defects.

1. Intellectual Impairment. Speech is deranged as a result of a generalised deficit of intellectual function which prevents the organisation of meaningful propositions. Such a disturbance reflects a diffuse impairment of cortical function which may be a temporary phenomenon in toxic confusional states (delirium) or permanent in dementia.

2. Dysphasia. This comprises disturbances of the symbolic aspects of language and these arise as a result of damage in or near the cortex of the dominant hemisphere. The nature of the defect varies with the site of the lesion. In *expressive or motor dysphasia* the patient can formulate his thoughts in appropriate words (i.e. internal speech is preserved) but is unable to translate them into corresponding sounds. This occurs despite an intact articulatory system and represents a specialised form of apraxia (p. 672) which results from lesions in the posterior part of the inferior (3rd) frontal convolution. Impaired comprehension of language is called *receptive or sensory dysphasia*. The patient fails to understand or carry out spoken instructions. Internal speech is disturbed and hence there is also impairment of the patient's external speech. This is an agnosic deficit (p. 672) and results from lesions of the posterior part of the upper temporal convolutions and the angular gyrus of the parietal lobe.

In clinical circumstances all the speech areas of the major hemisphere are often injured together, which results in combined receptive and expressive dysfunctions. This picture, called 'global or central dysphasia', is usually due to occlusion of the internal carotid or middle cerebral arteries which supply all the regions concerned with speech.

3. Dysarthria. Imperfect articulation of speech is called dysarthria. Precise enunciation of words requires normal function and coordination of lips, tongue and palate. Any abnormality thereof results in slurring and distortion of speech. Dysarthria may be due to mechanical derangements such as cleft palate or ill-fitting false teeth. Lesions of muscles, myoneural junctions, or lower motor neurones of lips, tongue or palate will also result in dysarthria as will upper motor neurone and extrapyramidal affections of these structures.

When normal monitoring of speech is disturbed by deafness, dysarthria may ensue. This is particularly liable to occur when auditory feedback is distorted by impaired hearing in early childhood.

4. Dysphonia. Reduced volume of speech, often accompanied by hoarseness, results from dysfunction of the phonating mechanism. This may be due to weakness of respiratory movements so that air flow across the vocal cords is reduced or to malfunction of the vocal cords. The causative lesion may be in the respiratory musculature, in the peripheral nerves, or in central structures. Thus, for example, bilateral palsies of the recurrent laryngeal nerves cause aphonia. Dysphonia may be part of the picture of a bulbar palsy or it may result from extrapyramidal disease, such as parkinsonism.

The Visual Pathway

The optic nerve carries second order neurones, the first order neurones being very short fibres within the retina. For much of its length it is surrounded by a protrusion of the meningeal membranes into which cerebrospinal fluid can pass, especially if intracranial pressure is raised. For these reasons the optic nerve is liable to suffer from different pathological states than other nerves. The visual pathway is illustrated in Figure 14.4. Sensory impulses from the retinae pass along the optic nerves to the optic chiasma where the fibres from the temporal halves of the retinae continue posteriorly in the lateral angle of the chiasma into the optic tracts on the same side. Fibres from the nasal halves of the retinae decussate so that the optic tract carries fibres from that part of each retina which receives light from the contralateral half of the visual field of each eye (the light rays crossing in the refractory media of the eyes). In the same way the light rays from the upper part of the visual field stimulate the lower part of each retina and the fibres arising there remain inferior throughout their further path to the cortex. The optic tracts continue to the lateral geniculate bodies where the fibres concerned with vision synapse and the impulses are relayed along the optic radiations to the calcarine area of the occipital cortex. The uppermost fibres which carry impulses derived from the superior quadrants of each retina (lower quadrants of visual fields) pass directly through the parietal lobe, whereas the lowermost fibres which relay impulses from the lower quadrants of the retinae (upper quadrants of visual fields) sweep downwards and forwards round the temporal horn of the lateral ventricle in the temporal lobe before passing to the occipital cortex (Fig. 14.4). Throughout the whole of the visual pathway fibres from the various parts of each retina maintain approximately the same relationship with each other.

Some fibres originating in the retina and passing centrally in the optic nerve form the afferent limb of the light reflex arc of the pupils. These bypass the lateral geniculate bodies and pass medially to the superior colliculi of the midbrain where they synapse with neurones which pass to the nuclei of the third cranial nerves on each side. From these nuclei arise the efferent limbs of the light reflex (direct and consensual) to the sphincter muscles of the pupils. No visual stimulus is required for the accommodation 'reflex' of the pupil which is more properly an associated contraction related to the movement of convergence of the eyes. This is believed to involve an unidentified cerebral path and a midbrain nucleus which controls the pupillomotor cells of both third nerve nuclei. This explains the dissociation between the light reflex and the convergence reflex which may occur in neurosyphilis and other diseases.

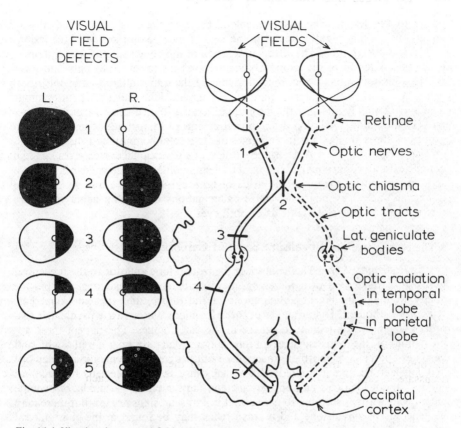

Fig. 14.4 Visual pathways and field defects.

CLINICAL MANIFESTATIONS OF LESIONS OF THE VISUAL PATHWAY

The Optic Nerve. A complete lesion of the optic nerve produces total loss of vision in the affected eye. There is no light reflex, direct or consensual, when that eye is illuminated but both pupils contract normally when the unaffected eye is illuminated. The pupil may be slightly larger in the blind eye. If the lesion is only partial, islands of loss of vision (scotomata) of various shapes occur in the field of the affected eye. When the fibres originating in the macular area are damaged there is a loss of visual acuity (amblyopia) which cannot be corrected by lenses. Direct and consensual light reflexes are depressed or absent when the amblyopic eye is stimulated but the convergence pupil response is unaffected.

The Optic Chiasma. A lesion of the central portion of the chiasma involves the decussating fibres from the nasal halves of both retinae and so gives rise to bitemporal hemianopia. In practice such lesions are rarely symmetrical and hence the degree of involvement of the visual fields of each eye is often unequal. A pituitary tumour first compresses the lower fibres and so the bitemporal hemianopia begins in the superior quadrants, whereas a suprasellar cyst compresses the chiasma from above so that field loss starts in the lower quadrants.

The Optic Tracts. A lesion of an optic tract gives rise to a homonymous hemianopia, the lost half of the field of vision of each eye being on the side opposite to the lesion. The involvement of the two fields is often unequal ('incongruous'), being slightly greater in the field of the eye on the side of the lesion.

The Optic Radiation. The effects of a lesion of the optic radiation depend on its exact site. A lesion of the temporal lobe involves the lower fibres only and gives rise to a homonymous defect involving mainly the upper quadrants of the visual fields. A lesion in the anterior part of the parietal lobe causes a homonymous hemianopia mainly affecting the lower quadrants as it affects fibres from the upper parts of the retinae. A lesion at the posterior part of the parietal lobe, where both groups of fibres are again adjacent, gives rise to a total homonymous hemianopia.

The Occipital Cortex. A destructive lesion of one occipital cortex gives rise to a complete (and congruous) homonymous hemianopia if it is extensive, or to a scotoma which is present in the fields of both eyes. Irritative lesions, as in the ischaemia caused by migraine, cause hallucinations of flashing lights which are referred to the contralateral fields of both eyes.

The Localising Signs of Cerebral Disease

The Prefrontal Lobe. This comprises the frontal lobe anterior to the precentral gyrus. It is concerned with some aspects of psychological reactions, notably the ability to make intelligent anticipations of the future, and the emotional correlations of thought. Disturbances of these functions cause vague psychiatric disorders which are difficult to diagnose in the early stages. The patient loses appreciation of the consequences of his actions, fails to take forethought and becomes apathetic or morbidly facetious. With progressing dementia his memory and intellect become impaired. His social sense is also affected; he becomes careless about his dress and appearance and may micturate in public or become incontinent without seeming to care about it. Physical signs are few but there may be generalised convulsions and a grasp reflex may be found in the contralateral hand. With this reflex, the patient involuntarily clutches at an object which is drawn lightly over the skin of the palm between the index finger and the thumb. The contralateral arm may be ataxic if the frontopontine fibres connecting with the cerebellum are interrupted. Expanding lesions of a frontal lobe may compress the underlying olfactory nerve causing unilateral loss of the sense of smell (anosmia, p. 674). These signs may be missed in a routine examination. It is important, therefore, to search for them when confronted with a patient with early mental changes.

The Precentral Gyrus. Lesions in this region give rise to unequivocal signs. Jacksonian epilepsy (p. 686) occurs and monoplegia (p. 659) readily develops. A lesion such as a meningioma arising from the falx cerebri involving the superior ends of both 'motor areas' may give rise to signs of an upper motor neurone lesion in both lower limbs, the upper limbs being spared. When a lesion in the dominant hemisphere extends forwards from the inferior end of the precentral gyrus it gives rise to dysphasia of expressive type.

The Parietal Lobe. Lesions of this area may also present with Jacksonian epilepsy, but of sensory type, and in addition there is disturbance of the integrative and localising aspects of sensation on the opposite side of the body.

Lesions situated more posteriorly in the parietal lobe may cause:

1. Spatial disorientation—lack of the patient's ability to find his way about.

2. Apraxia—loss of the ability to perform a pattern of movements though the patient understands its purpose and has no motor or sensory deficit.

3. Agnosia—loss of the ability to recognise a previously familiar object though

the patient has good vision and sensation.

4. 'Sensory inattention' or 'perceptual rivalry'—the patient tends to ignore a cutaneous or visual stimulus on the contralateral side presented simultaneously with one on the same side as the lesion, though it is perceived if presented alone. This is most prominent in disease of the non-dominant hemisphere.

5. Receptive dysphasia—lesions of the angular and marginal gyri or the posterior temporal-parietal junction cause receptive dysphasia which may be predominantly for written or spoken speech. There may be specialised types of dysfunction such as the loss of ability to count or to recognise parts of the body such as a particular finger.

6. Homonymous hemianopia—deep lesions in the parietal lobe may involve the optic radiation and so cause a contralateral homonymous hemianopia.

The Occipital Lobe. Irritative lesions cause crude visual hallucinations such as flashing lights, while destructive lesions cause a contralateral homonymous hemianopia.

The Temporal Lobe. Irritative lesions in the posterior temporal lobe may cause visual sensations which are more elaborate than with occipital lobe irritation. Patterns of moving colours or hallucinatory pictures may be experienced by the patient. A similar lesion of the anterior part of the temporal lobe may cause auditory hallucinations (superior temporal gyrus), gustatory and olfactory hallucinations (uncus) or misinterpretations (illusions) of auditory and visual sensations. These are often associated with altered states of consciousness such as dreamy states, automatic behaviour, temporary upsets of memory (*déjà vu*) or brief amnesia. In affections of the dominant hemisphere there may be dysphasia of receptive type (see below). An important sign easily overlooked is a homonymous upper quadrantanopia due to destruction of the lower fibres of the optic radiation which sweep down into the temporal lobe (p. 672).

The Cerebrospinal Fluid

The cerebrospinal fluid (CSF) is secreted by the choroid plexuses in the lateral, third and fourth ventricles. It leaves the ventricular system through apertures in the roof of the fourth ventricle and flows through the cerebral and spinal subarachnoid spaces. It is returned into the venous sinuses by the arachnoid villi. In health, the fluid is clear and colourless. The pressure in the lumbar subarachnoid space with the patient lying on his side is 50–150 mm of cerebrospinal fluid.

The CSF is no longer invariably examined in patients suffering from neurological disease since other methods of investigation may obviate the need for lumbar puncture in such conditions as cerebral tumour. A lumbar puncture should not be performed in the presence of raised intracranial pressure. The CSF provides useful information in a number of conditions and is invaluable in the diagnosis of acute and chronic inflammatory diseases of the nervous system. A large number of polymorphonuclear leucocytes is found in bacterial meningitis and a smaller number in the earliest stages of tuberculous and viral meningitis. A lymphocytosis accompanies viral meningitis and encephalitis, tuberculous meningitis and neurosyphilis.

A rise in the total protein content of the CSF is a non-specific finding in many neurological diseases. Very high values are associated with a complete block within the subarachnoid space, with neurofibromas and with Guillain-Barré polyneuropathy. A rise in the gammaglobulin (IgG) fraction of the CSF protein is a feature of multiple sclerosis, neurosyphilis and connective tissue disorders. A rise in the glucose content of the CSF reflects the hyperglycaemia of diabetes. Glucose is absent or very low in pyogenic meningitis and reduced in tuberculous and carcinomatous meningitis. Appropriately stained smears and cultures of the CSF often define the infecting agent in cases of meningitis.

Hydrocephalus. This term denotes an excessive amount of CSF within the cranial cavity. It may be a consequence of atrophy of the brain parenchyma, which results in passive dilatation of the ventricles; it is then called compensatory hydrocephalus.

Hydrocephalus may, rarely, result from oversecretion of CSF due to a papilloma of the choroid plexus. Much more commonly it is caused by obstruction to CSF circulation or to a failure of absorption. Obstruction may occur anywhere within the ventricular system due to an intraventricular tumour or from extrinsic compression due to a space-occupying lesion or oedema. The ventricular 'narrows' comprising the third ventricle, aqueduct and fourth ventricle are particularly likely to be occluded. Inflammatory exudate may block the foramina in the fourth ventricular roof or occlude the subarachnoid space. Absorption through the arachnoid villi may be prevented by thrombosis of the sagittal sinus.

Of particular interest is normal pressure (sometimes called normotensive or low pressure) hydrocephalus. In this condition the ventricular system is dilated. The dilatation initially results from an obstruction to flow due to trauma, meningitis, or other cause. The initial lesion subsides. It is postulated that the force exerted outwards on the brain is proportional to the surface area of the ventricles. These having been dilated the force exerted on the brain, by fluid at normally innocuous pressure, is increased. The brain atrophies and the conditions for progressive ventricular dilatation and cerebral atrophy are established. Dementia and ataxia result. An operation which reduces CSF pressure by a shunt from a lateral ventricle to the superior vena cava sometimes improves the patient's dementia and ataxia.

DISORDERS OF THE CRANIAL NERVES

The cranial nerves are frequently involved in generalised disease of the nervous system. In addition, there are specific conditions affecting a single cranial nerve.

The First Cranial Nerve

The olfactory nerve arises from olfactory receptors in the nasal mucosa. The fine first order fibres pass through the cribriform plate in the floor of the anterior fossa of the skull. They synapse in the olfactory bulb and second order neurones run to the olfactory area of the brain (the anteromedial part of the temporal lobe) and higher autonomic centres by the olfactory tract which lies under the orbital surface of the frontal lobe. Thus tumours of the frontal lobe may compress it and cause loss of the sense of smell (anosmia) on one side of the nose. The fragile fibres passing through the cribriform plate are readily damaged by head injuries.

The Second Cranial Nerve

The anatomy and central connections of the optic nerve are described on page 670 and the visual field defect caused by a lesion of the nerve on page 671.

Papilloedema. This term describes swelling of the optic nerve head (optic disc). The swelling may be due to obstruction to the venous drainage of the retina. Lesions of the optic nerve itself, some of them inflammatory, may also cause swelling of the optic disc which is usually then referred to as *papillitis*.

The main disorders resulting in papilloedema are:

1. Increased intracranial pressure due to any cause such as cerebral tumour, cerebral abscess, or meningitis. The rise in pressure of the cerebrospinal fluid causes distension of the subarachnoid space round the optic nerve and compresses the veins.

2. Obstruction of the venous drainage from the orbit by thrombosis of the central vein of the retina, cavernous sinus thrombosis or, rarely, an orbital neoplasm.

3. Lesions of the optic nerve such as optic neuritis.

4. Diseases of the retinal arteries such as cranial arteritis.

5. Extracerebral conditions such as malignant hypertension and severe respiratory failure.

The earliest manifestation of papilloedema is engorgement of the retinal veins, followed by an intensified pink colouration of the optic discs and blurring of the disc margin which usually begins on the nasal side. As swelling proceeds the physiological cup is obliterated and the whole optic disc may be elevated. If the papilloedema is severe and particularly when it is of rapid development, there may be accompanying haemorrhages abutting on to the disc (Plate II). If papilloedema is of long standing the disc becomes progressively paler as optic atrophy develops.

Often it is of clinical importance to differentiate the swelling due to raised intracranial pressure from that due to lesions of the optic nerve which present indistinguishable ophthalmoscopic appearances. The visual acuity is usually well preserved when papilloedema is due to raised intracranial pressure whilst optic neuritis usually causes marked loss of visual acuity. Papilloedema due to raised pressure gives rise to early enlargement of the blind spot; chronic severe papilloedema may be accompanied by peripheral constriction of the visual field. Optic neuritis is accompanied by a central scotoma.

Optic Neuritis. This term encompasses inflammatory, demyelinating and some vascular diseases of the optic nerve which, in common, cause loss of vision. In many cases pain in the eye, aggravated by movement and tenderness over the eye, precedes or accompanies the visual disturbance. There is loss of central vision and the direct reaction to light is impaired whilst the consensual light reflex is preserved. When the lesion lies anteriorly in the nerve there may be swelling of the optic disc (papillitis). Where the ophthalmoscopic appearances are normal, the lesion lies posteriorly and is called a *retrobulbar neuritis*.

Optic neuritis is most commonly due to demyelination, itself usually a manifestation of multiple sclerosis, and in this condition recovery of vision within four to six weeks is usual. Rarer causes include vitamin deficiencies, syphilis and toxins, such as methyl alcohol and quinine.

The optic neuritis associated with vitamin B_{12} deficiency and that accompanying excessive smoking of strong pipe tobacco (*tobacco amblyopia*) may have a common pathogenesis. Tobacco smoke contains cyanide which experimentally has been shown to cause demyelination. Hydroxocobalamin, derived from vitamin B_{12}, plays an important part in the detoxication of cyanide. If the intake of vitamin B_{12} is low and cyanide ingestion is high, demyelination of the optic nerve is liable to occur. This is an important observation since tobacco amblyopia may effectively be treated by large doses of hydroxocobalamin.

Optic Atrophy. Loss of fibres in the optic nerve is followed by reactive gliosis and reduced vascularisation. These pathological changes are manifest clinically by pallor of the optic disc and may result from many causes including (a) optic neuritis from the various causes listed above; (b) pressure on the optic nerve by glaucoma, tumours, aneurysms etc.; (c) long-standing papilloedema; (d) thrombosis of the central retinal artery; (e) trauma.

The Third Cranial Nerve

The oculomotor nerve supplies all the external ocular muscles except the lateral rectus and the superior oblique. It also supplies the levator palpebrae superioris, the constrictor of the pupil, and the ciliary muscle. It may be involved in multiple sclerosis, meningovascular syphilis, diabetes mellitus, and cerebral aneurysms which may compress the nerve at several sites. The manifestations of a third nerve palsy are ptosis, diplopia, external deviation of the eye (divergent strabismus) due to the action of the unopposed lateral rectus muscle and defective ocular movement in the directions in which the muscles supplied by the third nerve move the eye. The patient complains of double vision but in a long-standing lesion one of the images is suppressed. A complete lesion of the third nerve also paralyses the constrictor of the pupil; consequently the pupil is large and fails to react to light (by the direct or consensual path) or on convergence.

The Fourth Cranial Nerve

The trochlear nerve supplies the superior oblique muscle. A lesion of the nerve gives rise to defective movement and diplopia which is maximal when the patient attempts to look down with the eye turned inwards. The pupils are not affected. An isolated lesion of the nerve is rarely encountered, as usually there is also involvement of either the third or sixth nerve.

The Sixth Cranial Nerve

The abducent nerve supplies the lateral rectus muscle of the eye. A lesion of the nerve causes diplopia due to inability to abduct the eye, and deviation of the eye medially (convergent strabismus) due to the unopposed action of the medial rectus muscle. The sixth nerve may be involved by pressure from an aneurysm in the cavernous sinus. Downward displacement of the brain stem due to raised intracranial pressure may stretch the nerve causing a lateral rectus palsy. The causal lesion may lie at a distance from the sixth nerve whose involvement in this manner constitutes a false localising sign.

Squint

Squint (strabismus) may be paralytic or concomitant.

Paralytic squint is due to weakness of one or more of the extraocular muscles. Defective movement of the eye can be seen when the patient uses the weak muscle to move the eye, and this usually causes diplopia. The rules for identifying the paretic muscles causing diplopia or squint are:

1. The separation of the images is greatest when the patient attempts to look in the direction to which the paretic muscle should move the eye.

2. In this position, the most peripheral image is the 'false image' from the

affected eye. It is identified by covering one eye with a green glass and the other with a red one.

Concomitant squint ('lazy eye') is due to failure to maintain the correct posture of an eye which is so defective in vision that its image is suppressed by the brain. There is no muscle paresis and both eyes are capable of full movements in all directions. The most common cause is an error of refraction during childhood. If recognised and properly treated with suitable spectacles the squint can be prevented though a 'latent squint' often remains.

Nystagmus

Nystagmus is a series of involuntary, rhythmic oscillations of one or both eyes. It may be manifest in horizontal or vertical planes or as a series of rotations of the eye about its central axis (rotatory nystagmus). The oscillations may be equal in speed and amplitude in both directions of movement (pendular nystagmus) or movement in one direction may be faster than in the other (jerking nystagmus). When there are fast and slow components, the direction of the nystagmus is arbitrarily defined by the direction of the fast component. When severe, nystagmus may be present on looking to the side opposite to the fast component—this is a measure of severity, not an indication of nystagmus to both sides. It may occur spontaneously or be induced in response to a stimulus such as rotation of the head. When testing for nystagmus it is important to keep the visual fixation point within the field of binocular vision. Some normal people show sustained fine jerking nystagmus at the extremes of lateral gaze, especially when fatigued.

Pathological nystagmus results from impairment of the mechanisms controlling conjugate eye movements, namely:

Gaze Mechanisms. Voluntary conjugate movements of the eyes depend on pathways descending from centres in the frontal lobe to brain stem structures which then relay impulses to the nuclei of the extraocular muscles.

Fixation Mechanisms. Reflex mechanisms enable the object of interest continuously to be viewed by the macular area of each eye even when the object is moving. These reflexes are mediated through pathways which run from the eye to the cortex of the occipital lobe and adjacent parietal lobe and to the superior colliculi of the brain stem.

Vestibular Mechanisms. These are reflex adjustments which enable the retinal images to be stabilised, even when the head is being moved in space: they are evoked by impulses arising in the semicircular canals of the labyrinth and these are relayed to the central vestibular systems.

Cerebellar Mechanisms. The cerebellum also participates in the coordination of eye movements, as it does in the coordination of limb movements.

Peripheral Mechanisms. All the above mechanisms need an efficient effector apparatus and hence peripheral lesions of nerve or muscle may also lead to nystagmus.

TYPES AND CAUSES OF NYSTAGMUS

Gaze Nystagmus. This is usually due to lesions of the brain stem. The nystagmus is of jerking type. There is no nystagmus when the eyes are in the central position but it appears on deviation of the eyes laterally. The faster component is always in the direction of gaze.

A special form of gaze nystagmus involves only the abducting eye on conjugate lateral deviation of the eyes. This is called *ataxic nystagmus* and results from lesions of the medial longitudinal bundle in the pontine region. The ocular movements are dissociated. On looking to one side, the abducting eye shows coarse nystagmus. The other eye fails to adduct fully and if it exhibits nystagmus this is of smaller amplitude. This type of nystagmus is common in multiple sclerosis but also occurs in brain stem gliomata and Wernicke's encephalopathy.

Fixation Nystagmus. This type of nystagmus is usually present when the eyes are in the mid position, i.e. gazing straight ahead. A common cause of fixation nystagmus (often called ocular nystagmus) is defective central vision, which usually gives rise to pendular movements. Congenital visual defects produce this type of nystagmus, which may also result from working in very dark environments, as in 'miner's nystagmus'. Rarely fixation nystagmus is associated with diffuse brain stem lesions.

Vestibular Nystagmus. This may arise from lesions of the labyrinth or the vestibular nerve.

1. Disorders of the labyrinth. Imbalance between labyrinthine stimuli from the two ears leads to jerking movements of both eyes. If the lesion involves the end-organs in the semicircular canals or their central connections, nystagmus is precipitated by sudden movements of the head. Lesions of the otolith organs or their central connections cause nystagmus which occurs when the head is in a particular position.

Spontaneous nystagmus is present with acute lesions of the labyrinths but tends to subside in a few days or months. This tendency to adaptation may be seen during testing, as nystagmus, brought on by movement of the head or by caloric stimulation, is not maintained. It may be difficult to elicit again if the test is repeated. It is often associated with vertigo (p. 682) and this is also brief. Cochlear function is usually affected, causing tinnitus or deafness. Labyrinthine nystagmus may be caused by inflammatory diseases (serous or purulent labyrinthitis), degenerative middle ear disease, hypertension, atherosclerosis of the internal auditory artery, head injury and Ménière's syndrome.

2. Lesions of the vestibular nerve. Nystagmus due to lesions of the eighth nerve has the same features as labyrinthine nystagmus. It may be due to an acoustic neuroma or neuronitis (p. 682). The latter is a short-lasting disease.

Lesions of the Central Vestibular Systems and Cerebellum. Spontaneous nystagmus, or nystagmus induced by head position or head movement, may be found with brain stem lesions affecting the vestibular nuclei. Spontaneous nystagmus unaffected by head position and maximal on looking to the side of the lesion is found with some cerebellar lesions. Central nystagmus often occurs without vertigo, but when nystagmus is present it tends to persist and neither the nystagmus nor the vertigo shows the adaptation which is a feature of a peripheral lesion. Central nystagmus and vertigo often occur without cochlear symptoms, and may be associated with other brain stem symptoms, such as diplopia, or with asynergia of the limbs or dysarthria if the lesion involves cerebellar connections. The nature of the nystagmus may be like that of peripheral vestibular lesions, but vertical nystagmus, or nystagmus which affects each eye differently, is always central in origin. It may be caused by multiple sclerosis, vascular lesions such as occlusion of the posterior inferior cerebellar artery, pontine and cerebellar tumours, encephalitis, syringobulbia, or as the result of toxic states of which alcoholism is the most common. Postconcussional vertigo and nystagmus may be peripheral or central in type, and they are often precipitated by a particular posture of the head. Indirect disturbances of the vestibular nuclei may occur when the intracranial pressure is raised. Nystagmus is then a 'false localising sign'.

Nystagmus Due to Muscle Paresis. This common cause of nystagmus is often overlooked. If one or more of the extraocular muscles are weak, then the affected eye will manifest jerking nystagmus when it is moved by the weakened muscles. Thus a partial sixth nerve palsy will result in nystagmus in the affected eye on attempted abduction.

The Fifth Cranial Nerve

The trigeminal nerve has an extensive sensory distribution through its three branches, the ophthalmic, maxillary and mandibular divisions. It supplies the skin of the face (excluding the angle of the jaw), the cornea, the sinuses, the mucous membrane of the nose, the teeth, the tympanic membrane and common sensation (but not taste) to the anterior two-thirds of the tongue. The motor division of the nerve innervates the temporal, masseter and pterygoid muscles which are responsible for the closure and opening of the jaw. The nerve fibres and nuclei may be involved within the brain stem by conditions such as syringobulbia and thrombotic lesions, and the peripheral nerve by localised pressure such as occurs in cerebral aneurysms in the region of the cavernous sinus, and by tumours of the cerebellopontine angle. The ganglion of the nerve may also be involved by herpes zoster, giving rise to the characteristic shingles lesion over the skin of the face and causing ulceration of the cornea when the ophthalmic division is involved.

Trigeminal Neuralgia (Tic Douloureux)

This is a condition of unknown aetiology and without recognised histopathology which usually affects elderly people.

Clinical Features. Pain, usually paroxysmal and of lancinating type is the characteristic feature. The pain is confined to the distribution of the fifth nerve. The maxillary or mandibular divisions of the nerve are usually first involved and spread from one to the other is common but the ophthalmic division is rarely affected. Each paroxysm lasts for only a few seconds but the stab of pain may be followed by a dull ache, or frequent attacks following one another may make the pain appear to be of longer duration. The pain is precipitated by touching localised 'trigger zones' on the affected side of the face. A cold wind blowing on the face, washing the face, chewing or even talking may be sufficient to bring on an attack. Paroxysms may continue for days or weeks, after which a remission of equal or longer duration may follow, but remissions become shorter and less frequent as the disease progresses. The agonising pain commands the patient's full attention. It may provoke a spasm of the facial muscles. No abnormalities of fifth nerve function can be detected on examination.

Diagnosis. When a typical history is volunteered by an elderly patient the diagnosis is obvious. If similar symptoms occur in a young person the possibility of multiple sclerosis needs to be considered. Facial pain, mimicking trigeminal neuralgia may rarely be a manifestation of basilar aneurysm or cerebral tumour, particularly of a neurofibroma of the fifth nerve itself. In these and other instances when the fifth nerve is implicated in disease processes, the pain is often continuous and there are usually signs of fifth nerve dysfunction and there may be associated disturbances of other cranial nerves or neural pathways.

Treatment. Medical treatment should be used in the first instance. Carbamazepine 200 mg thrice daily is the most effective drug. Phenytoin 100 mg three times daily is also useful and may with advantage be combined with carbamazepine. Either or both of these drugs will reduce the frequency and severity of the pain in the majority of patients. Clonazepam (1–2 mg t.i.d.) is a useful alternative. Long remissions may occur. If pain persists and remissions are rare or of short duration it is necessary to interrupt the central passage of pain impulses by injection of phenol or alcohol into a branch of the nerve, if neuralgia is localised, or into the Gasserian ganglion. Section of the sensory part of the fifth nerve or its descending root in the medulla has the disadvantage of requiring intracranial operation but permits sparing of corneal sensation which is difficult to achieve with injection of the ganglion. These procedures secure permanent relief from pain but the face becomes anaesthetic. Loss of sensibility from the cornea demands that special care must be taken to avoid trauma with its danger of subsequent corneal ulceration.

The Seventh Cranial Nerve

The facial nerve innervates the muscles of expression of the face and, through its chorda tympani branch, carries taste fibres from the anterior two-thirds of the tongue. Paralysis of the facial muscles may be due to: (1) lesion of the fibres of the upper motor neurones concerned with voluntary movement, (2) lesion of the fibres of the upper motor neurones concerned with emotional movement, (3) lesion of the lower motor neurones.

1. Upper motor neurone fibres originating in the lower part of the precentral gyrus are distributed to the part of the opposite facial nucleus subserving the muscles of the lower part of the face, and to the parts of the facial nuclei on both sides of the pons which supply the upper parts of the face. Accordingly, a lesion of the upper motor neurones affects more severely the voluntary movement of the lower part of the face, contralaterally. Weakness of the upper part (the orbicularis oculi and frontalis muscles) may occur transiently but is often absent because the lower motor neurones to the upper facial muscles are supplied by upper motor neurones from both hemispheres. The patient is unable to retract the angle of the mouth on command, but in smiling and talking the mouth may move well because emotional movement is controlled by upper motor neurones which are not those concerned with voluntary movement of the face.

2. Upper motor neurones concerned with emotional movement of the face take origin further forward in the frontal lobe and so may be damaged by a lesion which spares the fibres for voluntary movement of the face. Involvement of these fibres is revealed by defective movement of the angle of the mouth when the patient smiles and talks, with preservation of the ability to retract the angle of the mouth on command.

3. Since the lower motor neurone is the final common pathway, complete damage to the facial nucleus or nerve abolishes both voluntary and emotional movements equally in upper and lower parts of the face. Lower motor neurone paralysis restricted to part of the facial muscles can occur only when the lesion is distal to the branching of the nerve, e.g. with disease of the parotid gland, through which the nerve passes, or in leprosy.

The most common cause of damage to the nerve proximal to its branching in the parotid gland is Bell's palsy but it may be damaged by disease of the brain stem, by an acoustic neuroma, or by inflammation during its passage through the middle ear.

Bell's Palsy

This term should be restricted to cases of isolated facial paralysis of unknown cause. Bell's palsy is accompanied by oedema of the facial nerve within the facial canal. It has been suggested that the swelling may be due to a viral infection since minor epidemics of the condition occasionally occur. Swelling within the rigid facial canal results in pressure on the nerve causing paralysis of function and sometimes Wallerian degeneration.

Clinical Features. The condition occurs in both sexes at any age. The first symptom is often an ache in the region of the stylomastoid foramen which may persist for a few hours or 1 or 2 days. A unilateral facial paralysis then develops. The eye on the affected side cannot be closed and the mouth is drawn over to the opposite side so that often it may appear to the patient that there is a spasm of the normal side. Saliva and fluids may escape from the angle of the mouth. Food may collect between the teeth and the paralysed cheek when the patient is eating. The patient often complains that the affected side feels 'numb', but there is no objective impairment of sensation of the skin. In most instances the lesion is distal to the chorda tympani and facial paralysis is the only feature. In a minority of cases when the lesion lies proximal to the chorda tympani there will be loss of taste on the anterior two-thirds of the tongue and diminished salivation. When the lesion is proximal to the nerve to the stapedius, hyperacusis on the affected side is an additional complaint.

Physical examination reveals paralysis of the upper and lower parts of the affected side of the face. The lines of expression are flattened, the patient is unable to wrinkle his brow or whistle or retract the angle of his mouth. He cannot close the eye on the affected side, and on attempting to do so the eyeball rolls upwards. Herpes zoster of the geniculate ganglion is a rare cause of facial palsy and is accompanied by vesicular eruptions on the anterior two-thirds of the tongue and within the external auditory meatus.

Treatment. There is good evidence that ACTH and oral steroids, if given early after the development of Bell's palsy, increase the rate of recovery. Maximal benefit from steroids is obtained if they are given within the first 48 hours of the onset of the palsy. Dexamethasone, 2 mg three times daily for 5 days, is a suitable treatment.

Prognosis. Complete recovery occurs in over 90 per cent of patients; recovery usually starts after 2 or 3 weeks and is complete after 2 to 3 months. Approximately 5 per cent of patients have permanent loss of function and develop facial contractures and involuntary spasms of the facial muscles. Complete recovery is virtually certain if there is any return of voluntary movement within a week after the onset and is probable if recovery of function occurs within a month. A guide to the prognosis is given by electrodiagnostic studies. The facial nerve is electrically stimulated at the stylomastoid foramen and muscle potentials recorded through surface electrodes. If the voltage required to produce a contraction on the abnormal side is more than twice that on the normal side, Wallerian degeneration has probably occurred. This indicates a poor prognosis. However, a good response after stimulation of the facial nerve within a week of the onset indicates that there is merely a conduction block and complete recovery is likely. Recurrence of Bell's palsy is unusual.

The Eighth Cranial Nerve

The auditory nerve has two components, the cochlear nerve which is concerned with hearing and the vestibular nerve which is concerned with the appreciation of the position of the head and its movement in space. It is impossible without special tests to differentiate lesions involving these nerves from lesions confined to their end-organs in the inner ear. Irritative lesions of the inner ear or of the cochlear nerve cause tinnitus, and destructive lesions deafness. Thus, tinnitus may be an early symptom of a neuroma of the eighth nerve (acoustic neuroma) but it is often due to aural causes. The most important destructive lesion of the eighth nerve is an acoustic neuroma, but it may also be damaged in meningitis, and by the toxic effects of streptomycin and kanamycin.

Irritative lesions of the vestibular part of the eighth nerve cause vertigo.

Vertigo

The term 'vertigo' is used by many people to describe a sensation of 'giddiness' or 'dizziness'; these symptoms are common in patients with an anxiety neurosis or with transient general upsets of cerebral function as well as in lesions of the vestibular pathways. For this reason it is convenient to restrict the term 'vertigo' to the description of a subjective feeling of movement of the external environment or of the head. The movement may be rotatory or a feeling of displacement in one direction. Vertigo is always accompanied by a disturbance of balance which usually causes the patient to seek support, and if sudden and severe may throw him to the ground. It often causes a reflex autonomic discharge leading to cold sweating, pallor, nausea, vomiting, and sometimes diarrhoea, bradycardia or even syncope.

The most important causes of vertigo are:

Cerebellar Lesions. Cerebellar lesions may cause vertigo when the cerebello-vestibular connections are involved but this symptom is not invariable.

Brain-stem Lesions. Lesions such as insufficiency of the basilar artery, medullary infarction or syringobulbia may cause severe vertigo when they involve the vestibular nuclei. The vertigo may be produced by particular positions of the head.

Lesions of the Vestibular Nerve. An acoustic neuroma may damage the nerve and cause vertigo. Vestibular neuronitis is a more common cause; it is a benign short-lasting condition of unknown aetiology which may occur in epidemics.

Aural Lesions. Aural lesions of many kinds, including otitis media and Ménière's syndrome, cause vertigo. The labyrinth may be damaged in a head injury and the vertigo may then be most severe when the head is in a certain position, usually backwards and to one side. A similar type of positional vertigo may occur in brief paroxysms. It is a benign condition which may disappear after a few months. The labyrinth may be damaged by mumps and by various toxic drugs such as streptomycin. Quinine and salicylates are also believed to cause vertigo by an action on the middle or inner ear. Hearing is almost invariably affected when the lesion is labyrinthine rather than in the nerve or central connections.

Ocular Lesions. Diplopia may be accompanied by vertigo because the false projection of one image causes confusion regarding position in space.

Ménière's Syndrome

Ménière's syndrome is characterised by recurrent paroxysms of vertigo associated with tinnitus and progressive nerve deafness. The cause is unknown, but the condition is associated with dilatation of the endolymphatic system (hydrops) due to increase in the amount of endolymph. Many patients also give a history of migraine.

Clinical Features. The most common initial symptoms are progressive deafness and tinnitus which are frequently slight at the onset. Sooner or later vertigo occurs and is characterised by suddenness of onset and severity. It may develop so suddenly that the patient may fall, and at the height of the attack he may be unable to stand. There is often accompanying nausea and vomiting, and there may be sweating, weakness and faintness. Deafness and tinnitus may be intensified during the attack which may last for a few minutes to several hours. Examination during an attack shows rotatory nystagmus and ataxia. Between attacks there is only nerve deafness with impaired vestibular function as shown by caloric tests. The frequency of attacks tends to decrease as deafness increases but the disease may last many years.

Treatment. No treatment will abort an episode of vertigo; during severe attacks the patient should lie still and may be helped by an intramuscular injection of 50 mg of chlorpromazine. Treatment is aimed at preventing or reducing the number of attacks. Cinnarizine 15 mg 3 or 4 times daily, prochlorperazine (5 mg t.d.s.), betahistidine (8 mg t.d.s.) and others are used for this purpose. All of these drugs are sometimes effective but none is consistently so. If attacks are frequent and disabling, destruction of the labyrinth by surgery or ultrasonics may be required.

The Ninth, Tenth and Eleventh Cranial Nerves

These nerves are grouped together because isolated lesions of one nerve alone are rarely encountered. The glossopharyngeal nerve (IX) transmits taste and common sensation from the posterior one-third of the tongue and motor fibres to the pharynx; the vagus nerve (X) is the parasympathetic nerve for the viscera of the thorax and upper part of the abdomen and also supplies somatic motor fibres to the soft palate and the larynx; the spinal accessory nerve (XI) supplies the trapezius and sternomastoid muscles. Unilateral lesions disturb their somatic functions but do not appreciably affect visceral function. These nerves or their nuclei may be involved by disease of the medulla such as syringobulbia or in their course across the posterior fossa by neoplasms and basal meningitis. Lesions at the jugular foramen, such as thrombophlebitis of the internal jugular vein following suppuration in the skull or neck, may involve all three nerves as they emerge from the skull.

The Twelfth Cranial Nerve

The hypoglossal nerve supplies motor fibres to the muscles of one side of the tongue. Upper motor neurone lesions cause spastic contraction of the muscle fibres. The tongue is small and pointed but not atrophic. Articulation is defective (spastic dysarthria) especially for the lingual sounds. There is rapid recovery of function after a unilateral lesion of upper motor neurone type, but bilateral lesions cause permanent dysarthria. This may occur in motor neurone disease or in pseudobulbar palsy due to bilateral impairment of blood supply in the internal capsules. Lower motor neurone lesions cause wasting and fasciculation of the affected part of the tongue and, when protruded, the tongue deviates to the side of the lesion. The usual cause is motor neurone disease.

The lower cranial nerves may be involved by carcinoma of the nasopharynx spreading to the base of the skull so otolaryngological examination is necessary. All cranial nerves, but particularly those emerging from the base of the skull, may be affected by bone disease in that area, particularly by Paget's disease.

The Cervical Sympathetic Fibres

The higher centres for autonomic functions in the hypothalamus are connected with some areas of the cortex, notably the orbital surface of the frontal lobe and the insula. From the hypothalamus sympathetic fibres descend through the brain stem and spinal cord to their lower neurones in the small lateral horn of the thoracic region of the spinal cord from which they pass into the anterior spinal roots from T1 to L2. Fibres destined for the head and neck emerge mainly through the first thoracic anterior root, and ascend in the cervical sympathetic chain, reaching their final destination by means of the plexuses in the walls of blood vessels. Stimulation of the cervical sympathetic fibres causes dilatation of the pupil, protrusion of the eye-ball and elevation of the upper eyelid; conversely paralysis of these fibres results in pupillary constriction, enophthalmos and ptosis (*Horner's syndrome*). In addition, sweating is impaired on that side of the face. These signs may occur in lesions of the brain stem such as syringobulbia and thrombosis of the posterior inferior cerebellar artery, in lesions of the cervical part of the spinal cord such as syringomyelia, and in such lesions at the thoracic outlet as bronchial carcinoma at the apex of the lung.

THE EPILEPSIES

(Grand Mal; Petit Mal; Temporal Lobe Epilepsy; Jacksonian Epilepsy; Status Epilepticus)

An epileptic fit may be defined as a brief disorder of cerebral function, usually associated with a disturbance of consciousness, and accompanied by a sudden, excessive, electrical discharge of cerebral neurones. The electrical activity recorded by the electroencephalogram (EEG) is of high voltage relative to the background and results from an unphysiological, hypersynchronous discharge of an aggregation of neurones. The basic mechanism of epilepsy depends on a population of abnormal, hyperexcitable nerve cells. Such susceptible neurones are subject to excitatory and inhibitory influences from other sources. Excitatory chemical transmitters released from connecting nerve terminals tend to depolarize epileptic neuronal membranes; inhibitory transmitters lead to hyperpolarization of membranes. The discharge of the abnormal group of cells is governed by the balance at a given time between these two opposing factors. Acetylcholine is an excitatory transmitter. Gamma-aminobutyric acid (GABA) is an inhibitory transmitter and hence has anticonvulsant properties.

Epilepsy may be classified into two broad groups:

1. *Generalised seizures* in which loss of consciousness is accompanied by generalised, symmetrically synchronous EEG discharges. It has been suggested that generalised fits originate in midline diencephalic areas. Recent work indicates that the site of the abnormal discharge could be in the cortex and the generalised manifestations occur because of rapid spread to brain stem structures leading to loss of consciousness and then to the secondary evocation of bilateral discharges over the hemispheres.

2. *Partial or focal fits* in which consciousness may be retained to some extent. In focal fits the discharge arises in a localised area of the cortex. It may remain circumscribed or spread to adjacent cortical regions, to the opposite hemisphere via the corpus callosum or to the brain stem. In the latter case sequential activation of both hemispheres may result so that a fit, initially focal, may become generalised.

Aetiology. In many, perhaps the majority, of cases, epilepsy arises from causes which at present cannot be identified. This large category of cryptogenic or idiopathic epilepsy includes may cases in which generalised fits first occur in children whose relatives are similarly affected but also includes many other cases without a family history or with atypical fits.

Any intracranial disease may give rise to epilepsy, either as a manifestation of an active pathological process or as sequel thereof. Important causes of 'symptomatic' epilepsy include cerebral tumours, head injuries and cerebrovascular disease.

Fits may occur as a result of disease elsewhere than in the brain. Hypoglycaemia, uraemia, heart block, ingestion or sudden withdrawal of alcohol or drugs are but a few of the conditions which may evoke seizures.

Clinical Features. There are two common varieties of *generalised fit*—grand mal and petit mal.

GRAND MAL. These fits conform to a stereotyped clinical pattern in which several stages may be recognised:

1. A *prodromal phase*, lasting hours or days, may warn the patient that an attack is impending. This is an occasional phenomenon and usually takes the form of a change of mood.

2. An *aura*, which is uncommon in grand mal fits. When it does occur, it is of brief duration and vague nature, usually being no more than an apprehension that a fit is about to occur.

3. The *tonic stage*, which is an invariable part of a grand mal attack. At the onset of this stage the patient loses consciousness and, if upright, falls to the ground. A sustained, tonic spasm of all the musculature occurs and involves the respiratory muscles, so that air is forcibly expired through the partially closed glottis giving rise to a sound or 'cry'. This phase lasts 20 to 30 seconds and during this time respiratory movements are suspended so that cyanosis occurs.

4. A *clonic phase* in which the sustained tonic spasm gives place to interrupted powerful jerking movements of face, body and limbs. The movements of jaw and tongue cause saliva to froth in the mouth. This stage, also, lasts about half a minute.

5. The *stage of relaxation:* After movements cease, the patient lies in a flaccid, comatose state which evolves into normal sleep. This phase often lasts only a few minutes but may be prolonged for half an hour or more.

During the tonic and clonic stages the patient may bite and chew his tongue and may be incontinent of urine and, less often, of faeces. After regaining consciousness there is often a phase of variable duration wherein the patient is confused and may suffer from headache.

PETIT MAL. This term is often used imprecisely. It is best restricted to those cases showing a characteristic EEG pattern, namely bilaterally synchronous spike and slow wave complexes occurring at a frequency of three per second. This pattern occurs with three types of clinical manifestation:

1. The most common variety of attack takes the form of a transient loss of consciousness. The patient interrupts whatever he is engaged in and may stare blankly ahead. The whole episode usually lasts only 10 or 15 seconds, and is so brief and undramatic that it may pass unnoticed. Such 'absences' as they are called, may occur very frequently in childhood. Petit mal invariably starts in childhood but may persist into adult life. Sometimes the attacks cease during adolescence or give place to grand mal fits.

2. Less commonly the brief loss of consciousness is accompanied by myoclonic jerking of the arms.

3. The least common type of attack is the akinetic seizure in which the patient falls to the ground unconscious but recovers consciousness, and is able to rise again, almost immediately.

PARTIAL OR FOCAL EPILEPSY. Since there are many neuronal regions from which epileptic discharges may originate there are many clinical variations of focal fits. Any focal discharge may spread to become generalised, and initially localised clinical disturbances may progress to mimic a grand mal fit. It is important, therefore, to establish the nature of the phenomena which occur at the onset of any form of seizure since these indicate the focal origin.

1. The *temporal lobe* is the commonest site of focal epilepsy. Most characteristic of the clinical manifestations are hallucinations of smell though these are uncommon; hallucinations of taste, hearing or sight also occur. Also indicative of temporal lobe fits are disturbances of memory including the so called *déjà vu* phenomenon. This refers to the patient's sensation of reliving an experience or a feeling of great familiarity with his environment. Sometimes these features are associated with intense emotional or mood changes.

In temporal lobe attacks consciousness is usually disturbed but not necessarily lost. The patient often maintains some contact with the surroundings but feels remote from them, often likening the experience to a dream-like state. Occasionally the patient during this state will carry out well-coordinated and apparently purposeful motor acts, even of a violent or antisocial nature, without any memory of such activity thereafter (automatism).

Temporal lobe discharges do not always give rise to such distinctive clinical features and an EEG may be required in order to reveal the temporal lobe origin of seizures.

2. *Jacksonian epilepsy* is a term best restricted to fits in which clinical disturbance of function, initially confined to a circumscribed part of the body, spreads to involve adjacent areas. There is a relatively slow 'march' of clinical events which reflects the spread of the electrical discharge to nearby cortical areas. Motor seizures usually take the form of involuntary twitching or clonic movements which begin in part of a limb, spread to involve the whole limb, then perhaps the whole of one side of the body or the involvement may even eventually become bilateral. The extent of the spread is highly variable. Consciousness may or may not be lost. Sometimes after recovery from a Jacksonian fit, the parts affected remain paralysed. This is called a *Todd's palsy* and if prolonged for more than an hour or two suggests that there is a structural lesion in or near the cortical representation of the paralysed part.

Diagnosis. The first step is to make a diagnosis of epilepsy. This is essentially a clinical process. Observation of an episode by a trained observer is the best and most certain method of diagnosis, but is rarely possible. A good description by, and cross-examination of, an eyewitness furnishes useful, and often conclusive evidence. The patient's own account of his attacks and the circumstances attendant upon them will sometimes give diagnostic information. The EEG is not a substitute for this type of clinical assessment nor can an EEG, recorded between attacks, alone establish or refute a diagnosis of epilepsy. The EEG may be helpful in supporting a clinical diagnosis and may be of great value in localising a cerebral cause of symptomatic epilepsy.

Note should be made of factors which precipitate attacks. Some patients have fits only during sleep, or when they are pyrexial. Others recognise that certain sensory stimuli, such as flickering light, or emotional disturbances trigger their seizures. A careful and detailed history, including past illnesses and family history, is the key to effective management of patients suffering from epilepsy.

After the diagnosis of epilepsy has been established the next stage is to assess its cause. In practice the most important aspect of this process is to recognise patients whose epilepsy is due to a structural or progressive lesion.

Fits of recent onset, of focal nature, occurring in patients of middle age, would obviously suggest an underlying lesion, perhaps a tumour. Accompanying headache and neurological signs would strengthen such a suspicion.

The history and examination will in most cases furnish pointers to the aetiology of fits and hence to the need for special investigations. An EEG and skull X-rays should be obtained in all cases. Before embarking on more traumatic investigations, such as lumbar puncture or contrast radiography (p. 693) the need for such tests should be appraised in the light of the clinical features. In many instances repeated observation of patients over a period is the most valuable and least distressing course of action.

Treatment. The care of the patient comprises social and psychological as well as pharmacological aspects. The condition, because of folklore and superstition, carries overtones of disgrace. Patients and their relatives and too many of the general public believe that epilepsy bears a stigma. Simple, rational explanations of the nature and causes of seizures should be given to those concerned. Many patients are more socially disabled by feelings of bitterness and agression engendered by society's rejection than by their fits.

Restrictions should be kept to a necessary minimum. Children, in particular, are often in danger of being overprotected by their parents but until fits are well controlled it is unwise for children to cycle on public roads; nor should they swim alone at sea. Unless an epileptic child has a concurrent intellectual deficit he should be educated at a normal school. An adult should be guided into an occupation in which neither he nor the community is put to risk by his propensity to fits. Exposure to moving machinery and work at heights should be avoided. The legal restrictions about driving should be explained to patients. In Britain no one who has suffered from fits may drive a motor vehicle until free of attacks during waking hours for 3 years. Continued treatment with anticonvulsants and the occurrence of nocturnal fits do not debar the patient from driving.

During a fit the patient should be protected from injury. It will rarely be possible to break the fall during a grand mal attack because the warning is too short. The patient should be moved away from fires and sharp and hard objects. A padded gag should be inserted between the teeth if this can be accomplished without force. The incident should be treated with a minimum of fuss. Embarrassment because of public attention is usually the most distressing aspect of a fit from the patient's viewpoint. Factors such as flickering light or other afferent stimuli which are known to precipitate fits should be avoided if possible.

Anticonvulsant drugs will in most cases be needed to control fits. For all forms of epilepsy, phenobarbitone, (30 mg b.d. to 60 mg t.i.d.) is useful. Phenytoin (100 mg t.i.d.) and primidone (250 mg t.i.d.) are of value in the treatment of grand mal fits. Phenytoin may, with advantage, be combined with either phenobarbitone or primidone and any of these three drugs may also be used to treat focal attacks. Drowsiness may occur with all of these drugs. Phenytoin may cause cerebellar ataxia or hypertrophic gingivitis.

Most anticonvulsants are inducers of hepatic enzymes (p. 426) and this can affect not only their own metabolism but that of other drugs. They can also interfere with the metabolism of vitamin D, causing osteomalacia, and of folate, causing megaloblastic anaemia.

Sodium valproate is a drug of recent introduction and considerable interest which differs in chemical structure from all other antiepileptic drugs. It seems to act by inhibiting the enzymatic breakdown of gamma-aminobutyric acid (GABA) and hence increasing its level within the brain. Sodium valproate is useful in the treatment of grand mal epilepsy and is particularly effective in petit mal attacks (200 mg t.i.d. gradually increased, if necessary, to 800 mg t.i.d.). Nausea and vomiting are fairly common side-effects; a temporary loss of hair is a rare complication. Sodium valproate is now probably the drug of first choice for the treatment of petit mal. Ethosuximide (250 to 500 mg t.i.d.) is also effective.

Many other drugs, e.g. carbamazepine and clonazepam, are used in the treatment of epilepsy. There is, however, a real danger of unnecessary treatment as well as of polypharmacy and drug interactions if patients on anticonvulsants are not regularly reviewed and their treatment tailored to their individual needs. An anticonvulsant drug should not be discontinued abruptly as status epilepticus may be precipitated.

Status epilepticus refers to a continuous succession of fits occurring without any period of recovery. It may be fatal if not rapidly controlled. It is more common in childhood or in epilepsy associated with intracranial lesions but may occur in all types of epilepsy if medication is irregular or is suddenly withdrawn.

Treatment should be prompt and energetic since status epilepticus constitutes a grave emergency. An adequate airway and respiration must be maintained and the fits suppressed. Sodium phenobarbitone 200 mg given intramuscularly at 2-hourly intervals or phenytoin 250 mg intramuscularly at intervals of 4 hours are sometimes effective.

In severe cases and in those in which intramuscular treatment has been ineffective, intravenous therapy is required. Two preparations are used. As much as 100 mg of thiopentone or 60 mg of diazepam are slowly injected until fits cease and the corresponding drug is then given by slow intravenous drip for as long as necessary. Both of these drugs are highly effective but should be used in this way only when means of artificial respiration are available.

Narcolepsy

This is characterised by irresistible attacks of sleep from which, however, the patient can be aroused immediately. He may go to sleep at work and several attacks may occur in a day. It is often associated with three other phenomena; *cataplexy*, in which, as a result of a sudden emotion, power is lost from the limbs, though consciousness is preserved; *sleep paralysis*, in which on waking or falling asleep the patient finds himself unable to move though mentally he is wide awake; *hallucinatory states*, in which vivid and terrifying hallucinations occur, often just as the patient is falling asleep. This combination of symptoms may be associated with disease in the region of the hypothalamus. In most cases no abnormality can be demonstrated in the nervous system. Amphetamine sulphate (5–10 mg b.d.) or methylphenidate hydrochloride (10 mg b.d.) reduce the frequency and intensity of narcolepsy. Cataplexy often responds dramatically to treatment with a tricyclic antidepressant such as imipramine (50 mg t.i.d.). However, tricyclics and amphetamines should not be given together. Which drug is used will depend on whether narcolepsy or cataplexy is the patient's principal disability.

CEREBRAL TUMOURS (see Psych. P. 65)

Intracranial tumours account for 2 per cent of deaths at all ages. Neoplasms classified histologically as malignant and benign occur but the implications of these categories differ from those in other sites. Since they grow within the rigid confines of the skull all types of neoplasm may cause disability and death by impinging on and displacing the cranial contents. The clinical features produced by an intracranial tumour depend primarily on its site of origin and its rate of growth. The histological characteristics of tumours offer a guide to rapidity of growth and to the possibility of complete removal.

Pathology. Malignant cerebral tumours rarely give rise to extracerebral metastases but approximately a half of all brain tumours are secondary deposits from carcinoma elsewhere, particularly in bronchus and breast.

Of primary cerebral tumours those derived from glial cells are the commonest. These vary in cellular type, in degrees of malignancy and in rates of growth. An astrocytoma Grade 1 is a slow-growing, infiltrative tumour which may spread widely throughout the brain, sometimes for years, before causing serious disability. A Grade 4 astrocytoma (also called a glioblastoma multiforme) is a highly malignant, fast-growing tumour causing rapid clinical deterioration. Other glial tumours such as oligodendroglioma and ependymoma are graded from 1 to 4 as the degree of malignancy increases. Medulloblastoma occurs most commonly in children, arises usually in the cerebellar vermis, and is almost always highly malignant. The various types of glioma account for a quarter of all cerebral tumours. They can rarely be completely excised.

Meningiomas comprise approximately one-fifth of intracranial tumours. They are almost always benign, encapsulated, attached to the dura and, in the majority of instances, completely removable. Their common sites of origin are the convexities of the hemispheres, the sphenoidal ridges, the suprasellar region and the olfactory groove.

Other less common tumours arise within the cranial cavity. Craniopharyngiomas (p. 510), adenomas of the pituitary gland (p. 510) and neuromas from the sheaths of the eighth and fifth cranial nerves are benign and potentially curable.

Intraventricular tumours are rare but colloid cysts of the third ventricle and papillomas of the choroid plexus can cause raised intracranial pressure and are removable.

Clinical Features. Primary brain tumours occur at all ages with a maximal incidence in the fifth decade. Medulloblastomas are commonest in children.

Acoustic neuromas usually present in the third and fourth decades. Glioblastomas and meningiomas are commonest in middle life. In general brain tumours in children are situated in the posterior fossa and in those over thirty, supratentorial tumours account for 85 per cent of cerebral neoplasms.

Cerebral tumours produce symptoms and signs by their local effects and by causing alterations in intracranial pressure and hydrodynamics.

FEATURES DUE TO LOCAL INVOLVEMENT. The local effects of a tumour on adjacent cerebral tissue may cause paralysis of function and/or excitatory effects. The neural deficits produced by a brain neoplasm are dependent on the site of origin of the tumour. Lesions in the various lobes of the brain can cause the types of dysfunction outlined on pages 672–673. Vascular lesions affecting these same structures cause similar disturbances but those produced by tumours are characterised by the time course of their development. In general the focal disabilities produced by a tumour are of slow onset and are progressive. The rate of this progression is highly variable and depends on the rate of growth of the tumour and its nearness to neural structures whose interruption evokes clinical signs. Occasionally localised oedema in the brain tissue surrounding a tumour will cause a rapid progression of paralytic symptoms and the picture thus produced may mimic a cerebrovascular lesion. Sometimes, too, the initial manifestations of a metastatic tumour are of sudden onset, followed by a period of improvement. Rarely, haemorrhage into a tumour causes an acute presentation of signs and symptoms which resembles a stroke.

In addition to local paralytic effects the infiltration by tumour cells of an area of cerebral cortex often evokes excitatory responses in neighbouring cerebral neurones. Thus a discharging epileptic focus may be a manifestation of a cerebral tumour. The nature of the fit produced is variable and depends on the site of origin of the epileptic discharge and the extent of its propagation. Focal epilepsy beginning in adult life should always suggest the possibility of a tumour.

Headache is a common, but not invariable manifestation of cerebral tumour. The tumour mass tends to distort and exert traction on nearby arteries, venous sinuses or meninges which are pain sensitive structures. Headache is often localised to one area of the cranium and its site offers a rough guide to the location of the tumour. In general headache is felt on the same side as the neoplasm. Tumours which lie in the anterior and middle cranial fossae are often attended by headaches situated in front of a line joining the ears. Posterior fossa tumours usually cause headaches which are felt over the occiput or nuchal area. There are many exceptions to these generalisations. Headache is also caused by an increase in intracranial pressure; its features are discussed below.

FEATURES DUE TO INCREASED INTRACRANIAL PRESSURE. Since cerebral tumours occupy space within the rigid skull they may cause an increase in pressure within the cranium. The liability of tumours to do this varies and several mechanisms may be involved. The mass of the tumour itself, if large enough, will cause a rise in pressure due to relative incompressibility of the brain. Slowly growing tumours may achieve large size before there is any rise in pressure whereas a highly malignant and rapidly growing tumour, though relatively small, may cause early changes. Raised intracranial pressure may also result from obstruction to the flow of cerebrospinal fluid. Subtentorial tumours are particularly liable to do this but even supratentorial lesions may cause obstruction to the foramina of Monro and tumours of the temporal lobe may compress the third ventricle. Tumours lying within the ventricles themselves may cause a sudden rise in intracranial pressure in the absence of focal neurological abnormalities. Increased pressure may also occur as a result of cerebral oedema or from obstruction of the cerebral venous system by malignant tissue impairing the absorption of CSF. Whichever of these mechanisms is operative the end result is a rise in pressure within the skull causing similar clinical features.

Headache is an almost invariable accompaniment of increased intracranial pressure; the pain is felt diffusely over the head and is aggravated by manoeuvres which cause a further rise in intracranial pressure. The headache is intensified by bending, coughing and straining at stool. Such headaches often tend to be particularly troublesome on waking in the morning when the patient is lying flat and to be relieved to some extent when the patient stands upright and moves about since this causes a slight fall in intracranial pressure.

There is often clouding of consciousness, varying in degree from listlessness and drowsiness to deep coma, depending both on the level of the raised pressure and the rapidity of its attainment. During the early stages of this alteration in consciousness there may be behavioural and personality changes with apathy and irritability or withdrawal and inattention predominating.

Generalised epileptic fits are commonly produced by raised intracranial pressure from tumours at any site.

Many patients with increased intracranial pressure complain of dizziness which may take the form of true rotatory vertigo or of sensations of light headedness or unsteadiness. Such feelings of instability are often produced or aggravated by head movement.

Papilloedema is one of the most significant signs of raised intracranial pressure (p. 675). It may be of insidious onset and slow progression but equally often a sudden rise in pressure due to cerebral oedema or obstructive hydrocephalus causes the rapid development of papilloedema attended by haemorrhages radiating out from the optic disc. The amount of visual disturbance produced by papilloedema is variable. Often there is little change in the visual acuity but the production of transient blurring of vision when the patient stoops or bends is characteristic. Swelling of the optic nerve head is usually bilateral but may be unilateral in the early stages. When the underlying lesion has caused optic atrophy in one eye papilloedema occurs only in the other eye. Such is the case sometimes with tumours of the inferior surface of a frontal lobe which compress the adjacent optic nerve causing optic atrophy and as the tumour grows in size raised intracranial pressure supervenes and papilloedema occurs in the other eye; this is known as the *Foster Kennedy syndrome.*

As intracranial pressure continues to rise vomiting occurs and the pulse rate is progressively slowed.

The rise in intracranial pressure does not necessarily occur evenly over the whole of the cerebral contents and sudden alterations in pressure relationships within the skull may lead to displacement of parts of the brain. Large supratentorial lesions may cause herniation of the hippocampal gyrus and the upper brain stem downwards through the incisura of the tentorium. This not only causes damage to the hippocampal gyrus itself but may also lead to compression of the cerebral peduncles, occlusion of the posterior cerebral artery and stretching of cranial nerves, particularly the sixth nerve.

These developments themselves cause signs which may lead to erroneous localisation of the cerebral tumour. They are called false localising signs. Commonest of these is a sixth nerve palsy occurring on the side of the lesion or bilaterally. The third nerve may similarly be involved and occasionally the fourth nerve is also implicated. The cerebral peduncle on the side opposite the tumour mass may be compressed giving rise to pyramidal tract signs on the side of the lesion. Compression of the posterior cerebral artery may lead to a homonymous hemianopia or quadrantanopia. Very rapid downward movement of the brain stem may lead to haemorrhage in the mid brain with coma and death.

Another form of herniation or 'pressure cone' is the downward movement of the cerebellar tonsils so that they impact within the foramen magnum thus compressing the medulla. This may lead to further aggravation of raised intracranial pressure since the onward passage of cerebrospinal fluid into the spinal subarachnoid space is blocked. Such an event is often manifest by loss of consciousness and the rapid development of palsies of the sixth and third nerves with dilatation of the pupil on the side of the lesion being followed by dilatation on the opposite side. Frequently when a medullary pressure cone has occurred the patient takes up a decerebrate posture, at first intermittently. These developments almost invariably lead to death.

Such brain displacements and pressure cones may occur spontaneously because of increased cerebral oedema or some other alteration in cerebral haemodynamics caused by the tumour's growth but are particularly liable to be produced if the closed CSF system is disturbed by lumbar puncture.

Methods of Investigation. The investigation of cerebral tumours should, in most instances, begin with simple and non-traumatic procedures which may obviate the need for more specialised techniques or indicate which would be the more apposite to a particular case.

Plain X-rays. A chest radiograph may reveal a bronchial carcinoma and hence enable the metastatic nature of a cerebral tumour to be inferred.

A straight X-ray of skull will rarely give definitive information about cerebral tumours but should never be omitted since occasionally it will reveal very significant abnormalities. Some slow growing tumours in the brain calcify and hence are visible on a radiograph of the skull. Erosion or thickening of the skull bones may point to an underlying malignant tumour or a meningioma respectively. A calcified pineal gland may be displaced from the midline by a tumour mass. Raised intracranial pressure may give rise to erosion of the clinoid processes which may also result from tumours arising near the pituitary. The pituitary fossa may be expanded by an adenoma therein.

Computerised Axial Transverse Scanning. This is a new and remarkably effective technique of visualising the intracranial contents. The method is tomographic. The head is divided into a series of slices each of which is irradiated by a narrow beam of X-rays. The X-ray tube and detectors face each other in a common frame and scan the head linearly taking 250 readings of the transmissions through the head. At the end of the first scan the system rotates 1 degree and the process is repeated through 180 degrees. A vast number of readings of the transmissions are obtained and processed by a computer. The absorption coefficients of the tissues, through which the X-ray beams pass, vary with the atomic numbers of the constituents and are reflected in variations in the recorded transmitted radiation intensity. The computer provides a numerical print out of the transmission data which is then converted to analogous shades of grey so that it can be presented pictorially on an oscilloscope or television monitor.

The sensitivity of the method enables a clear distinction to be made between grey matter, white matter and CSF within the ventricular system, as well as between pathological changes in the brain. Lesions are seen as alterations of normal density. Increased density is produced by meningiomas, low-grade astrocytomas, calcium in the walls of aneurysms and blood clot. Density is lowered below normal levels in tissue necrosis (e.g. infarction), oedema, cysts and haemorrhage before clotting has occurred. The density of some lesions, notably tumours, may be enhanced by the intravenous injection of substances containing large atoms (such as sodium iothalamate).

The technique is precise and painless and exposes the patient to a relatively low dose of radiation. The equipment is expensive and hence its accessibility is restricted. Computerised axial tomography markedly reduces the need for other potentially painful or hazardous investigations.

Electroencephalography. Abnormally slow waves may localise a tumour in the cerebral hemispheres. Diffuse slowing may arise as a result of raised intracranial pressure from tumours situated above or below the tentorium.

Echoencephalography. Ultrasonic waves are reflected back from midline structures in the brain and displayed on a cathode ray tube. Displacement of these structures can be shown and hence space-occupying lesions can be lateralised. The procedure is simple and rapid in execution and can be carried out at the bedside.

Radio-isotope Encephalography. Isotope-encephalography, also known as 'brain scanning', depends for its effectiveness on a concentration, greater in cerebral tumours than in normal brain tissue, of an isotope (usually technetium) given intravenously. It is particularly successful in outlining meningiomas, less accurate in demonstrating gliomas and least effective in revealing metastatic tumours and those tumours situated in the posterior fossa.

Cerebrospinal Fluid. Lumbar puncture should rarely be carried out if there is evidence of raised intracranial pressure and never in such circumstances unless neurosurgical help is rapidly available. If there is clear evidence of a space-occupying lesion in the brain, examination of the CSF is usually unnecessary and unhelpful. Where a meningitic picture is present and no tumour mass can be demonstrated the diagnosis of carcinomatosis of the meninges may be made by examination of the CSF, whose sugar content is reduced and which may contain tumour cells.

Arteriography. The intracranial vessels, outlined by a radio-opaque dye injected into the carotid or vertebral arteries, may be displaced in the region of a tumour, and the appearance of the vessels may indicate the pathological nature of the lesion. The procedure is relatively safe and does not upset the balance of intracranial pressure as does pneumoencephalography.

Pneumoencephalography. Air injected into the cerebrospinal fluid by lumbar puncture to replace an equal volume of fluid (20–30 ml) may be used as a contrast medium which can be manipulated to the various parts of the ventricular and subarachnoid space by suitable positioning of the head, thus enabling enlargements or displacements of the ventricular system and atrophic dilatations of the cortical sulci to be recognised. In the presence of raised intracranial pressure air is introduced directly into the ventricles through a burr hole in the skull (ventriculography). This diminishes the risk of impacting the brain stem in the foramen magnum but the danger of secondary rise in pressure from expansion of the air is sufficiently great to limit this investigation to a pre-operative procedure. A less risky procedure with special applications is to introduce a radio-opaque medium such as Myodil into the ventricles through a brain cannula.

Diagnosis. It is highly desirable that cerebral tumour be diagnosed before signs of raised intracranial pressure appear. This can be done only if the possibility of a tumour being present is considered in every case presenting cerebral symptoms for the first time and if careful examination, continued observation and, if necessary, special investigations are carried out in suspected cases. The differential diagnosis depends largely on the presenting clinical features which may be headache, epilepsy or manifestations of a focal lesion in a particular area. Other space-occupying lesions such as abscess or subdural haematoma must also be borne in mind.

Treatment. Medical treatment of tumours can never be anything more than temporary or palliative. Medical measures for relief of raised intracranial pressure are often demanded in circumstances when surgery is not available or when the patient's life is threatened before investigation has revealed the diagnosis. This can best be achieved by the administration of dexamethasone 4 mg four times daily, initially given by injection and later by mouth; striking improvement in a patient's conscious level is often produced and sometimes regression of focal disabilities. The use of intravenous hypertonic solutions has largely been supplanted by treatment with dexamethasone but the intravenous administration of 50 per cent sucrose or of a 15 per cent solution of mannitol or of a 30 per cent solution of urea can produce marked but short lived reduction of intracranial pressure.

Cytotoxic drugs, such as cyclophosphamide have been administered either systemically or through a carotid artery for treatment of malignant cerebral tumours. This treatment is still in an experimental stage and at present seems to offer little more than temporary palliation.

The definitive treatment of intracranial tumours is surgical. When possible the whole of a tumour should be excised but complete removal of the tumour depends on a number of factors. The tumour may be inaccessible and thus its exposure may be attended by unacceptable brain damage. It may invade areas where excision of small amounts of tissue may cause major disability as is particularly likely to happen in the brain stem or in areas of the dominant hemisphere.

In general benign tumours such as meningiomas and neuromas offer the best prospects for complete removal without unacceptable damage to vital structures. Meningiomas can usually be totally excised and rarely is there any recurrence. Meningiomas of the olfactory groove, those in the suprasellar area and those over the convexity of the hemispheres have a particularly favourable prognosis. Often, meningiomas of the inner part of the sphenoidal ridge and within the cerebellopontine angles cannot be completely removed but their partial excision results in long continued improvement. Even after a successful removal of a meningioma, a number of patients may develop recurrent fits.

Craniopharyngiomas, though benign, can sometimes be completely removed but often the closeness of the hypothalamus prevents total excision. Pituitary adenomas can usually be extirpated and even when only incomplete excision is possible further visual loss is prevented.

Colloid cysts of the third ventricle and other intraventricular neoplasms can often be removed but sometimes their complete excision is technically very difficult.

Malignant gliomas cannot be removed completely though favourably situated tumours may benefit markedly for a time from partial removal.

Less malignant slow growing tumours such as Grade 2 astrocytomas and oligodendrogliomas, though they can rarely be completely excised, may benefit for many years from partial removal. The prognosis for cystic astrocytoma is particularly good if the cyst is drained and as much as possible of the tumour removed. Medulloblastoma of the cerebellar vermis, found in childhood, cannot be completely excised and surgery produces little improvement.

There is a place for palliative surgery even when complete excision of a tumour cannot be attempted. Partial removal or drainage of a cyst is often of benefit. Decompression and hence relief of raised intracranial pressure may be produced by removing part of the tumour or excising normal brain tissue in the frontal or temporal lobes. Removal of part of the skull vault is also effective in reducing pressure. Internal hydrocephalus may be relieved by a short circuiting procedure in which a drain is placed in one of the lateral ventricles and led into the cisterna magna.

Prognosis. The precise surgical approach and the prognosis for a cerebral tumour can be assessed only in the light of its site, its pathological nature, its blood supply and the degree of disability it causes. Early treatment is particularly important for those tumours which are susceptible to complete removal and which menace life or sight. Early diagnosis of acoustic neuromas and pituitary tumours markedly improves the outlook for their treatment.

Death is inevitable if a cerebral tumour cannot be removed though it may be postponed by palliative decompression; even so, the average expectation of life is less than six months in the case of the more malignant growths. Benign tumours can be removed completely if they grow in an accessible part of the brain as can gliomas, or even a solitary metastatic tumour, when they are in a part of the brain such as the frontal lobe or cerebellum which can be sacrificed with relative impunity.

Headache

Headache is a term which literally describes pain felt anywhere in the head. Custom usually restricts its usage to pains in the region of the cranial vault; facial pain and nuchal aches are excluded, but the lines of demarcation are vague and overlapping.

Headache poses certainly the commonest, probably the most ambiguous and sometimes the most difficult clinical problem in medicine. It has a multiplicity of causes but is produced by relatively few mechanisms. In the vast majority of cases the cause is trivial and reversible but in a few patients headache presages sinister intracranial disease.

Aetiology. The extracranial coverings and arteries are sensitive to pain. Within the cranial cavity there are few pain sensitive structures. The brain parenchyma, pia-arachnoid, ventricular linings and choroid plexuses are insensitive. Pain can be evoked from the venous sinuses, the arteries and the dura at the base of the brain. Displacement and distortion of these structures, particularly if rapid, cause headache. The fifth, ninth and tenth cranial nerves contain pain fibres and direct compression of these nerves produces pain.

Clinical Features. Pain in the head may be due to lesions in nearby structures, such as the eye and ear, causing referred headache, the cranial neuralgias, meningeal irritation, vascular disturbances, traction and distortion of intracranial structures, or to psychogenic causes.

Referred Headaches. Disease of structures in the head may cause pain referred to the cranium. Eye diseases such as glaucoma and iritis cause frontal headache.

Ciliary spasm induced by some errors of refraction may cause pain but 'eye strain' is certainly not a common cause of headache. Nasal and sinus disease causes pain in the malar, nasal and frontal areas which responds to nasal vasoconstrictors. Dental and aural conditions may cause pain spreading far beyond the area of primary pain. Occipital headaches occasionally result from severe cervical spondylosis. An occasional cause of referred headache is produced by a cold stimulus, usually ice-cream, on the soft palate. In some people this evokes a dull, frontal headache (ice-cream headache).

Cranial Neuralgias. The episodic, lancinating pain of trigeminal neuralgia (p. 679) and the continuous, burning pain of postherpetic neuralgia (p. 723), both occurring within the distribution of the fifth cranial nerve, present well-defined and usually easily-recognised entities. Less common is glossopharyngeal neuralgia in which pain, usually of a stabbing character, is felt in the pharynx and deep in the ear. The pain occurs in bouts and may be triggered by swallowing and talking. It responds to treatment similar to that given for trigeminal neuralgia. There are a number of facial neuralgias and pains which present inconsistent and vaguer patterns of affection. Temporomandibular neuralgia arises as a result of derangement of the temporomandibular joint secondary to an alteration of the bite caused by loss of teeth, ill-fitting dentures or habitual overclosure of the jaws because of tension. Pain which varies from a dull ache to intense stabs may radiate from the region of the affected joint to the temporal and frontal areas, the cheek, lower jaw and occasionally to the neck. X-rays usually reveal malocclusion, and a prosthetic device to prevent overclosure of the jaw is a simple and usually effective treatment.

Other types of atypical facial pains of variable characteristics occur, particularly in the elderly. They defy categorisation and some patients present individual patterns of discomfort over long periods which are resistant to all forms of treatment.

Meningeal Irritation. Headache is an almost invariable accompaniment of encephalitis and meningitis. It is probable that meningeal inflammation lowers the pain threshold of the pain-sensitive structures at the base of the brain so that minor mechanical stimuli produce headache. The headache is usually generalised though it may be more intense in the occipital region, is of a continuous aching or boring character and is frequently associated with photophobia and drowsiness. The pain is increased by exertion and even by minor movements of the head; the accompanying pyrexia and neck stiffness usually make the diagnosis obvious.

Blood in the CSF due to subarachnoid haemorrhage produces headaches and neck rigidity similar to those of meningitis, but the pain in this condition is characteristically of abrupt and even explosive onset and may be accompanied by loss of consciousness (p. 705).

Vascular Headaches. Headache may arise from dilation of the intracranial or extracranial arteries. Vascular headaches are almost always described as throbbing in character and are aggravated by head movements. There are many causes. The features of 'hangover' headaches strongly suggest that they are due, at least in part, to a vascular mechanism. Vascular dilation and headache may be a feature of hypercapnia in patients with respiratory failure. Severe arterial hypertension may cause headaches whose occurrence in the early morning may mimic the ache of raised intracranial pressure. Headache may be an accompanying feature in patients with mild or moderate hypertension but usually this is a manifestation of tension in those who know they have high blood pressure and are fearful of its consequences. In the elderly localised temporal headache may be due to cranial arteritis (p. 243).

The commonest form of vascular headache is migraine (p. 698). A migrainous variant, *'cluster' headache*, presents a distinctive picture. 'Cluster' headache is the name given to a variety of vascular headache which is unilateral, intense and brief. Many attacks occur in quick succession during a period of a few hours or a few days, and then there is often a prolonged period of freedom, hence the name 'cluster'. The pain is usually severe and burning in character, primarily involves the frontal region and the eye but often spreads to the face and sometimes to the neck. It occurs most commonly in young males, characteristically wakes patients from sleep and is often accompanied by flushing of the skin, rhinorrhoea and injection of the conjunctival vessels. It is thought to be due to histamine sensitivity and attacks can sometimes be precipitated by the subcutaneous injection of 0·3 mg of histamine. Patients sometimes respond to treatment with antihistamines and to the measures used in the treatment of classical migraine.

Rare causes of vascular headaches include saccular aneurysms (p. 705) and arteriovenous malformations (p. 706).

Headaches Due to Traction on Intracranial Structures. Headaches may occur in the presence of an expanding intracranial lesion such as cerebral tumour or subdural haematoma whether or not there is a generalised rise in intracranial pressure (p. 690).

Traction headache due to reduced CSF pressure may occur after lumbar puncture; patients tend to develop their symptoms when standing or sitting and a recumbent posture produces rapid relief. Traction headaches whether produced by raised or lowered intracranial pressure are usually aggravated by bending, straining at stool and coughing.

Sometimes traction headache may be produced in patients who have raised intracranial pressure, unassociated with a space-occupying lesion, in the syndrome of benign intracranial hypertension.

Psychogenic Headache. Rarely headache may be a feature of psychotic illness such as schizophrenia and it may occur in conversion hysteria. Most commonly, however, psychological headaches are associated with anxiety and depression, and other manifestations of these affective disorders (p. 774) may be present concurrently. Most patients suffering from psychogenic headache describe their pains as of 'pressing' character. Pain tends to be localised to the front of the head or to the vertex or it may involve the whole head. It is usually not prominent on waking in the morning and in most instances tends to get worse as the day wears on. It is often described as severe, continuous and unrelieved by analgesics.

Diagnosis. The diagnosis may offer little difficulty particularly in those patients who present with non-recurrent headache as a manifestation of systemic illness. Most viral and bacterial infections are accompanied by headache of varying severity. Recurrent headaches present the common diagnostic problem since it is necessary to distinguish the common causes such as tension and migraine from those due to intracranial structural lesions. If there are accompanying signs the differentiation is simplified but in the vast majority of instances a carefully taken history is the only clinical guide towards diagnosis and management. A detailed account of the nature, distribution, temporal relationships, aggravating and relieving factors, and associated symptoms should be obtained. In general those headaches described as 'throbbing' or 'burning' are more significant than those of 'pressing' nature. Localised headaches are often more significant than diffuse pain. Headache affecting the occipital or frontal regions is more worrying than pain situated over the vertex. Headaches which prevent sleep or which are present on waking often bespeak an organic cause. Headache which is of recent onset is always more potentially serious than headaches which have been present for many years. Associated features, such as epilepsy or double vision, suggest the presence of an underlying intracranial lesion.

Management. The extent and nature of investigations to be employed are determined by the history. Non-traumatic procedures such as radiographs of chest and skull and computerised axial tomography should precede more traumatic investigations. The taking of a detailed history followed by a meticulous examination will not only help to clarify the diagnosis but will also be therapeutic in patients suffering from psychogenic headache. Reassurance and explanation after careful clinical assessment of these patients is often more effective than treatment with drugs.

Migraine

Migraine is characterised by periodic headaches which are usually unilateral and are often associated with visual disturbance and vomiting.

Aetiology. The condition is believed to be due to a disturbance in the carotid or vertebrobasilar vascular tree. An initial phase of vasoconstriction causes symptoms of local cortical or brain stem ischaemia and this is followed by vasodilatation. These changes affect both intra- and extracranial arteries and it is dilation of the extracranial vessels which causes pain by stretching the pain nerve-endings in the arterial wall. Pain may be prolonged by secondary muscular contraction.

There is a genetic predisposition; approximately three-quarters of patients who suffer from migraine have close relatives similarly affected.

Migrainous attacks may be precipitated by a variety of factors such as menstruation, flashing lights, stress and anxiety. Cheese, chocolate, sherry and red wine are common precipitants and are all rich in tyramine; experimental ingestion of tyramine will often promote an attack. Reserpine, which liberates 5-hydroxytryptamine (serotonin) in the brain, can also cause migraine. It is of interest that some serotonin antagonists are helpful in treatment. The significance of these findings is not yet clear but it seems likely that, in some and perhaps many instances, migraine is mediated by one or more biochemical disturbances.

Clinical Features. The condition usually starts after puberty and continues until late middle life. Headaches occur in paroxysms and are often related to emotional stress. Attacks occur at intervals which vary from a few days to several months. The first symptom is due to vasospasm. This is commonly a sensation of white or coloured lights, scintillating spots, wavy lines, or defects in the visual fields. Paraesthesiae or weakness of one half of the body may be experienced or there may be numbness of both hands and around the mouth. These symptoms may last up to half an hour, and are followed by headache which usually begins in one spot and subsequently involves the whole of one side of the head; this may be the same or the side opposite to the visual or sensory symptoms. The side affected is not constant with each attack and the headache often becomes bilateral. The pain is usually severe and throbbing and is associated with vomiting, photophobia, pallor, sweating and prostration which may necessitate the patient taking to bed in a darkened room. The attack may last from a few hours to several days and it leaves the patient weak and exhausted. In rare cases the cerebral changes may last for several days, particularly if the motor area is involved (*hemiplegic migraine*).

Rare cases of headache resembling migraine are caused by a cerebral aneurysm or angioma ('symptomatic migraine'). In these cases the pain is unilateral and usually associated with focal signs.

Treatment. An attentive physician, a carefully recorded history and a meticulous examination followed by a full explanation of the nature and phenomena of migraine often relieves the patient's anxiety about the possibly sinister significance of his headache. These simple measures are themselves effective therapy as is the physician's continuing interest in the patient's well-being.

Neither the patient's personality nor the stresses and strains of his life can be altered, but such trigger factors as flashing lights and dietary precipitants can be avoided.

If the patient suffers only occasional attacks of headache at intervals of months, it is probably unnecessary to embark on drug treatment. For those whose lives are disrupted by migraine, treatment should include prophylaxis together with appropriate treatment to abort the headaches.

There are numerous prophylactic treatments; all are inconsistently successful. Phenobaritone (30 mg b.d. or t.i.d.), diazepam (2 mg t.i.d.), clonidine (50 µg t.i.d.) and pizotifen (0·5 mg t.i.d.) frequently reduce the frequency of headaches. Occasionally other drugs, such as monoamine oxidase inhibitors and tricyclic antidepressants are helpful. Methysergide, a serotonin antagonist (1 or 2 mg t.i.d.) is sometimes effective but it is prone to produce peripheral vasoconstriction and, rarely, retroperitoneal fibrosis and should be used only in those patients who have not responded to simpler measures and whose attacks are very frequent, severe and disabling.

Treatment of a migrainous episode is based on the use of ergotamine, which should be given as early as possible during the premonitory stages. Ergotamine tartrate (1 mg) held under the tongue is rapidly absorbed and often aborts an attack at its inception. Even more rapid absorption is obtained when ergotamine is administered in aerosol form using an inhaler containing finely divided powder packed under pressure. The powder should be inhaled deeply when the inhaler is activated; in this way 0·3 mg of ergotamine can be administered. The dose may be repeated three or four times at 5 minute intervals at the beginning of an attack. Unfortunately, all the oral methods of administration of ergotamine frequently produce nausea and vomiting. In such circumstances ergotamine suppositories are sometimes helpful and if the patient is capable of giving his own injections ergotamine tartrate (0·5 mg) given subcutaneously or intramuscularly may effectively halt an attack. Too frequent use of ergotamine may, rarely, cause peripheral vasoconstriction. It should not be given during pregnancy, nor to patients suffering from ischaemic heart disease or hypertension.

CEREBROVASCULAR DISEASE

Intracranial vascular lesions are the third commonest cause of death in Western countries. The pithy and commonly used term 'stroke' describes the sudden neurological defect that often ensues. The incidence of strokes of various types is more than 1 per cent in those over 65 years old. In every 1,000 of the population in any one year, two people will suffer an initial stroke and one will die from a stroke. The high morbidity caused by cerebrovascular disease in the elderly is reflected in the large number of hospital beds occupied by such patients.

Despite the prevalence of the problem and its high cost in economic terms as well as human disability, cerebrovascular disease claimed, until recently, less attention and study than some rarer conditions. Diagnoses of 'cerebrovascular accident' or 'stroke' without specification are still common. Such imprecision in assessment leads to vagueness about prognosis and apathy in treatment. Conversely, attempts rigidly to link patterns of clinical disability to blockage of individual cerebral arterial branches have been shown to be simplistic and often misleading as well as therapeutically unrewarding.

Knowledge of the natural history of intracranial vascular disease is still incomplete. Cerebrovascular disease may be due to lesions of veins and capillaries as well as arteries but the latter are much the commonest. Arterial lesions can logically be divided into two main groups: (1) Ischaemic cerebral lesions due to reduced perfusion of brain tissue by blood and often resulting in infarction. (2) Haemorrhagic lesions in the brain or in the spaces between the brain and skull.

This division into ischaemic and haemorrhagic lesions is pathologically justified, but clinical differentiation is often difficult. The definition of factors predisposing to each is hampered by the lack of firm diagnostic criteria. There is an association between cerebrovascular disease and ischaemic heart disease. In those patients who suffer an attack of transient cerebral ischaemia more people die from myocardial infarction than from cerebral infarction. Atheroma and thrombosis are related to both conditions. Despite this association the risk factors of cerebrovascular diseases are not as well understood as those in myocardial ischaemia (p. 212) and there are notable discrepancies between the two. Genetic predisposition, hyperlipidaemia and diabetes seem to be much less important factors in cerebral than in myocardial infarction. Cigarette smoking and obesity have been clearly linked to an increased incidence of coronary arterial disease but not to liability to strokes. Hypertension is a factor which seems strongly to predispose to both cerebral and cardiac vascular disease.

Cerebral ischaemic and haemorrhagic processes, though clinically intermingled, need to be discussed separately.

1. Ischaemic Cerebral Lesions

General Considerations. Approximately a fifth of the cardiac output normally passes through the carotid and vertebral arteries to supply intracranial structures. A reduction in total cerebral blood flow to less than half of normal will impair cerebral function. Cerebral ischaemia may occur when perfusion is locally reduced even when total blood flow to the brain is normally maintained. Factors causing general circulatory impairment as well as local obstructions to blood flow need to be considered in patients suffering from cerebral ischaemia. A reduction in cardiac output due to arrhythmia, a fall in systemic blood pressure, anaemia or polycythaemia may cause or contribute to cerebral ischaemia or infarction.

Occlusion of a cerebral artery usually, but not necessarily, leads to infarction in the tissue it normally supplies. A system of anastomoses and collateral channels affords a safety mechanism. The circle of Willis usually provides wide connecting channels between the two carotid arteries and the vertebrobasilar system. Perforating branches from the major cerebral arteries and from the circle of Willis pass through the brain to anastomose with capillaries derived from other branches of the anterior, middle and posterior cerebral arteries which ramify over the surface of the hemispheres and penetrate through the cortex. A similar anastomosis between centrifugal and centripetal twigs is found in the brain stem where the vertebral and basilar arteries give off penetrating and circumferential branches. At the junctions between their respective areas of supply the anterior cerebral artery anastomoses with the middle cerebral artery which in turn anastomoses with posterior cerebral branches. There are also collateral channels between the internal and external carotid circulations through their orbital branches.

These alternative routes of blood supply to the brain mean that the effects of impaired cerebral flow are determined by complex factors. Reduced cardiac output or systemic hypotension tend first to produce ischaemia in the border zones between the anterior, middle and posterior cerebral arteries. Variations in this pattern occur if, in addition to generally reduced brain perfusion, there is a superimposed local blockage in one of the branches of the three major vessels.

If one internal carotid is occluded in the neck there is an immediate increase in flow through the other carotid artery. Young adults who sustain a blockage within one of the four major arterial trunks may manifest no ill-effects. However, the occlusion of one of these arteries in the neck in the presence of widespread arterial disease (a likely accompaniment in the elderly) may give rise to extensive infarction. The compensatory mechanisms are less effective more distally and occlusion of one of the deep penetrating branches arising from the circle of Willis often produces infarction of predictable extent.

The results of any arterial obstruction depend, in part, upon the rate of its development. Sudden blockage is more likely to produce infarction than is the gradual reduction of an arterial lumen which allows time for the opening up of collateral channels.

Reduced blood flow is often attributed to arterial spasm. Cerebral vasoconstriction occurs in young people and is responsible for transient cerebral dysfunction in migraine and may, in this condition, rarely lead to infarction (p. 698). Spasm also occurs if cerebral arteries are manipulated during operations and as a result of irritation during angiography and after a subarachnoid haemorrhage (p. 705). Ischaemia may result from vasoconstriction due to hypertensive encephalopathy (p. 222) or to the concurrent ingestion of tyramine and monoamine oxidase inhibitors. There is, however, no evidence that arterial spasm plays any significant part in the production of ischaemia in elderly patients suffering from cerebrovascular disease.

Reduced blood flow and arterial occlusion may result from arteritis, from syphilis and perhaps from trauma but atheroma is by far the commonest cause.

Cerebral Atherosclerosis

Atheromatous changes in cerebral arteries are almost invariable findings in people over 60 years old, but even quite extensive atheroma is commonly symptomless. Atheromatous plaques may cause narrowing (stenosis) or may lead to thrombosis and occlusion of arteries. Fibrin, platelet and lipid emboli may arise from such plaques in the proximal vessels including the aorta and be carried distally in the cerebral circulation eventually to impact in small vessels. These mechanisms can cause localised ischaemia or infarction or a generalised, progressive loss of brain tissue.

Clinical Features. Symptoms are rare before the age of 40, and uncommon before 50. The clinical presentations comprise (1) a 'stroke', i.e. the rapid development of focal cerebral dysfunction, due to infarction, (2) a relatively slow, or stepwise, extension of an infarct—sometimes called a stroke-in-evolution, (3) transient ischaemic attacks wherein neural disability presents suddenly and recovers completely within 1 hour, (4) progressive, diffuse loss of cerebral functions. More than one of these patterns may be manifest in a single patient. After a series of transient ischaemic attacks a patient may present with a completed stroke which may also supervene during the course of progressive, diffuse cerebral atherosclerosis.

STROKE. Haemorrhage and occasionally cerebral tumour, as well as infarction, may sometimes be the cause. When due to infarction, there are often premonitory features such as mild headache or malaise during the few days preceding a stroke.

The onset of focal disability may occur at any time. The patient may awake with an established lesion. Very frequently the deficit evolves during a period of 1 or 2 hours. Rarely the maximal level of disability will be attained within a few minutes and occasionally impairment will progress for 1 or 2 days. Loss of consciousness at the onset occurs in a minority of cases though drowsiness is common. Severe headache is unusual. Epileptic fits, sometimes of the focal type, occasionally occur at the beginning or during the extension of a stroke.

The neurological picture presented depends on the site of infarction. The area supplied by the middle cerebral artery is most commonly involved so that a hemiplegia involving the face, arm and leg on the side opposite the lesion is a frequent presentation.

If the paralysis develops very rapidly it may initially be of flaccid type, but spasticity and hyperreflexia are soon manifest and usually are detected from the onset. There may be loss of the visual half fields and hemianaesthesia on the side of the hemiplegia. If the infarct lies in the dominant hemisphere dysphasia may supervene. This familiar stroke pattern reflects the frequency of infarcts in the brain territory supplied by the middle cerebral artery but it should not be assumed that the causal lesion lies within this artery. In more than half of cases presenting this picture the primary lesion lies in the internal carotid artery or in more proximal vessels.

Other clinical presentations occur. An infarct within the area normally supplied by the anterior cerebral artery often causes a hemiplegia in which the leg is weaker than the arm and which may be accompanied by disturbance of micturition, apraxia (p. 672) or motor dysphasia. Lesions in the posterior cerebral territory usually lead to contralateral homonymous hemianopia with macular sparing and occasionally, if the thalamus is involved, diffuse, burning pain on the opposite side of the body. This thalamic syndrome may also result from infarcts in the area served by the anterior choroidal artery.

Approximately a tenth of infarcts involve the brain stem where they are more commonly accompanied by severe headaches than are those within the hemispheres. Vertigo, ataxia and vomiting, double vision and nystagmus are common features. A crossed paralysis, with ipsilateral affection of one or more cranial nerves and contralateral long tract (usually pyramidal) signs are characteristic of brain stem infarction.

STROKE-IN-EVOLUTION. The temporal pattern of a stroke is sometimes extended. Disability usually increases by step-wise progression; sudden deteriorations are interspersed with static intervals. Less commonly there is slow uninterrupted progression; the deficit spreads and intensifies. The full extent of the patient's lesion may not be exhibited for 3 or 4 days; occasionally the disability may extend for 1 or 2 weeks. This type of clinical presentation, which may suggest the diagnosis of a cerebral tumour, is often associated with occlusion of an internal carotid artery.

TRANSIENT ISCHAEMIC ATTACKS. A sudden neural deficit followed, within the hour, by complete recovery of function is called a transient ischaemic attack. A duration of up to 24 hours is accepted by some authorities as a transient ischaemic attack. Most such episodes last only a few minutes. If symptoms persist for more than 1 hour infarction has probably occurred. Symptoms depend on the site of ischaemia. Transient loss of vision in one eye and a hemiparesis or sensory disturbance affecting the contralateral half of the body are due to ischaemia in the carotid territory. Ischaemia affecting the area supplied by the vertebral and basilar arteries may cause vertigo, diplopia, hemiparesis or loss of consciousness.

The duration and frequency of transient ischaemic attacks are variable. Some patients suffer many attacks daily for periods of a week or more; attacks then cease and may not recur for months or years. Other patients have only occasional episodes at intervals of months. The attacks in an individual patient are usually stereotyped, the pattern and duration of dysfunction being repeated again and again.

Many transient ischaemic attacks are due to emboli which arise from atheromatous plaques, are carried distally, lodge in and block small arteries and then break up and disperse. In other cases flow through a stenotic artery may be reduced because of hypotension or reduced cardiac output and may cause transient cerebral ischaemia. Occasionally, in patients suffering from cervical spondylosis, neck rotation leads to pressure on, and reduced flow through, a vertebral artery causing ischaemia in the brain stem.

An uncommon cause of transient cerebral ischaemia is the 'subclavian steal syndrome'. This may arise if the subclavian artery is stenosed proximal to the origin of the vertebral artery. The increased blood flow needed when the arm on the affected side is exercised may be met by blood from the unaffected subclavian artery via the two vertebral arteries. Blood destined for the basilar artery from the vertebral artery on the normal side is syphoned down the other vertebral artery to supply the arm being used. The brain stem is thus rendered ischaemic. Such symptoms as diplopia or ataxia, produced by use of an arm, should suggest the possibility of 'subclavian steal'. A significant difference between the blood pressures measured in each arm, and a bruit audible over the supraclavicular fossa on the affected side, are distinctive signs of the syndrome.

Recent investigations suggest that some episodes labelled as transient 'ischaemic' attacks may be due to small intracerebral haemorrhages.

DIFFUSE CEREBRAL ATHEROSCLEROSIS. Gradual reduction in cerebral blood flow leads to progressive brain atrophy which is reflected in a clinical picture of blunted intellectual function and multiple motor deficits. Increasing dementia may predominate but is usually accompanied by features of bilateral lesions of the pyramidal tracts notably supranuclear bulbar palsy. These defects cause lability of emotional expression, dysarthria and dysphagia as well as a reduction in spontaneity, drive and movement which mimics parkinsonism. In some cases true parkinsonian features accompany bilateral pyramidal signs.

Sudden accelerations of disability, or transient episodes of neural deficit, usually differentiate this type of vascular disease from other causes of progressive cerebral atrophy and dementia.

Cerebral Embolism

The role of cerebral embolism in the production of cerebral ischaemia and infarction is consistently underestimated. Post-mortem studies have shown that at least half of cerebral infarcts can be attributed to embolisation from the heart or from atheromatous plaques in the large arteries in the neck and thorax. Transient ischaemic attacks are frequently the result of emboli from these same sources. The disability produced by the lodgement of an embolus in a cerebral artery may be of very sudden onset. However, in many instances the picture produced by cerebral infarction due to thrombosis and that due to cerebral embolism is indistinguishable in terms of the time course and nature of the neural picture presented. A firm diagnosis of embolism demands evidence of a source of emboli and the presence of multiple sites of impaction. In many cases of cerebral embolism both criteria—and particularly the latter requirement—are absent. Cardiac arrhythmia, particularly atrial fibrillation associated with rheumatic or ischaemic heart disease, may lead to the presumptive diagnosis of cerebral embolism. However, evidence of an embolic source within large proximal arteries is often difficult to obtain.

Direct evidence of embolisation is occasionally provided by ophthalmoscopy. Emboli, composed mainly of platelet aggregations, can sometimes be seen in the retinal vessels of the affected eye during an attack of transient monocular blindness. The likelihood of embolic infarction may be inferred if there is a history of earlier transient ischaemic attacks. The presence of an embolic site is suggested by a bruit localised to the region of the carotid bifurcation.

More cerebral emboli arise in the heart than in any other site. Thrombus following old or recent myocardial infarction is the commonest source of emboli; rheumatic valvular lesions, cardiomyopathy, infective and thrombotic endocarditis and atrial myxoma are other potential causes of cerebral embolism. A large embolus of cardiac origin may block the internal carotid artery at its origin. Smaller emboli often lodge at the trifurcation of the middle cerebral artery. Embolism at these sites is usually followed by thrombosis and complete occlusion.

A meticulous exploration of the possibility of embolic ischaemia should be made in all cases of occlusive cerebrovascular disease since the patient's management may thus be significantly influenced (p. 709).

Arteritis

A completed stroke or multifocal, minor cerebral lesions or a toxic confusional state may be a manifestation of arteritis due to systemic lupus erythematosus or polyarteritis (p. 242). Associated systemic features will usually suggest the diagnosis. Cranial arteritis (p. 243) is a frequent cause of arterial inflammation in the elderly and occasionally the disease causes cerebral infarction.

Cerebral infarction may be the presenting feature of meningovascular syphilis and the possibility should always be considered when a stroke occurs in a relatively young person. Occasionally tuberculous arteritis, associated with meningitis, may cause multiple small cerebral infarcts. Rarely a disabling stroke may be the predominant feature of tuberculous meningitis.

2. Haemorrhagic Cerebral Lesions

Primary Intracerebral Haemorrhage

Intracerebral haemorrhage is strongly associated with hypertension. In severe hypertension there may be a necrotising arteriolopathy and vessels so affected rupture to cause bleeding into the brain. Patients with long-standing hypertension develop hyaline changes in the muscular and elastic arterial layers which give rise to small aneurysms that are also liable to rupture. The penetrating branches of the middle cerebral artery, notably the lenticulostriate arteries, are particularly prone to develop such aneurysms and the majority of intracerebral haemorrhages occur in the region of the internal capsule.

An intracerebral haemorrhage usually presents abruptly when the patient is awake and is prone to occur whilst he is engaged in physical exertion. There may be premonitory severe headache and in over a half of patients there is loss of consciousness, sometimes accompanied by an epileptic fit. Since the internal capsule is so frequently involved, a hemiplegia commonly supervenes and initially may be of the flaccid type. When the haemorrhage is massive and bleeding persists, intracranial pressure is raised; coma deepens and papilloedema develops. Haemorrhages frequently extend into the lateral or third ventricles and sometimes there is rupture through the surface of the brain into the subarachnoid space so that in many cases of initially intracerebral haemorrhage, blood is found in the cerebrospinal fluid. A massive haemorrhage accompanied by loss of consciousness has a grave prognosis; approximately a half of patients die within a few days. Smaller haemorrhages occurring in any part of the brain may present a clinical picture indistinguishable from infarction.

Haemorrhage into the pons usually produces rapid loss of consciousness, pinpoint pupils and periodic respiration; often there is bilateral involvement of cranial nerves and pyramidal pathways. Hyperpyrexia is sometimes a feature.

Cerebellar haemorrhage is frequently of abrupt onset and is usually ushered in by occipital headache, vomiting, vertigo and ataxia. Consciousness is often lost after a few hours at which time the patient frequently develops pupillary constriction and a contralateral hemiplegia.

Subarachnoid Haemorrhage

Haemorrhage into the subarachnoid space results from rupture of a vascular malformation, notably a saccular aneurysm, from trauma, from extension of an intracerebral haemorrhage or from a bleeding cerebral tumour.

The onset of subarachnoid haemorrhage is often marked by severe and sudden headache, which is sometimes followed by impairment or loss of consciousness. There may be focal features whose nature depends on the site of the lesion; diplopia or other cranial nerve lesions, hemiparesis and aphasia occur. Signs of meningeal irritation, i.e. neck stiffness and a positive Kernig's sign, are present. Ophthalmoscopy may reveal unilateral or bilateral haemorrhages between the retina and the hyaloid membrane. The shape of these subhyaloid haemorrhages is determined by gravity so that if the patient is sitting upright the upper border is horizontal. If the subarachnoid haemorrhage is extensive and continuous, papilloedema may occur.

The outlook for subarachnoid haemorrhage due to an extension of intracerebral bleeding is similar to that of the primary condition. If subarachnoid haemorrhage is due to the rupture of a saccular aneurysm bleeding is liable to recur within 6 to 8 weeks.

Saccular Aneurysm. The first manifestation of an intracranial aneurysm is often a subarachnoid haemorrhage, but sometimes aneurysms present focal features before rupture. The nature of these depends on the site of the aneurysm. An aneurysm of the internal carotid artery within the cavernous sinus usually causes pain or paraesthesiae in the distribution of the ophthalmic division of the fifth nerve and a third nerve palsy sometimes accompanied by palsies of the fourth and sixth nerves. Rarely, an aneurysm of the internal carotid artery will rupture into the cavernous sinus, forming a caroticocavernous fistula. This causes severe pain in and around the eye, pulsatile exophthalmos, papilloedema and complete ophthalmoplegia. A loud bruit can usually be heard over the affected eye.

Aneurysm of the supraclinoid part of the internal carotid artery may compress the optic nerve, chiasma or tract leading to impaired visual acuity and a variety of scotomata and visual field defects. These visual disturbances may be accompanied by paralysis of the third nerve.

Aneurysms on the middle cerebral artery tend to present with bleeding, but occasionally their presence will be heralded by focal epilepsy and occasionally by a progressive hemiparesis. Anterior communicating and anterior cerebral aneurysms may compress the optic chiasma from above, resulting in bilateral loss of the inferior part of the visual fields.

Posterior communicating aneurysms often lead to an isolated third nerve palsy. Aneurysms of the posterior cerebral artery often compress the cerebral peduncle and the adjacent third nerve causing an ipsilateral third nerve palsy and contralateral pyramidal signs.

Arteriovenous Malformation. A subarachnoid haemorrhage without antecedent clinical features is the commonest presentation of an arteriovenous malformation. Some present with focal epilepsy accompanied later by progressive focal signs and others cause recurrent localised headaches of throbbing character which superficially may resemble migraine. A bruit can often be heard through the skull overlying a large arteriovenous malformation.

Extradural Haematoma

This is produced by skull fractures involving the branches of the middle meningeal artery. Symptoms usually develop a few hours after the injury. Coma rapidly ensues with an obvious hemiparesis. Later there are signs of tentorial herniation which often rapidly causes death.

Subdural Haematoma

This may occur as an acute complication of a head injury resulting from venous haemorrhage into the subdural space. The picture then resembles that of an extradural haematoma. A chronic subdural haematoma may follow a minor head injury in an elderly person. Often the injury is so slight that the patient has no memory of it. After an interval of weeks or months the patient may present with headache, a confusional state, or the development of focal neurological signs such as hemiparesis. Characteristically, as the subdural haematoma increases in size, there is fluctuation in the level of consciousness, and, later, signs of raised intracranial pressure may be manifest. The progressive picture may closely mimic that of a cerebral tumour.

Diseases of Intracranial Veins and Venous Sinuses

Occlusion of cortical or deep veins or major venous sinuses by thrombosis is the principal lesion which may affect the cerebral veins. The thrombus may be infected or aseptic. The importance of septic venous thrombosis lies not only in the resulting neurological disturbance but also in the possibility of complications such as leptomeningitis, suppurative encephalitis or brain abscess.

Infection may spread to the veins or sinuses from a source of infection on face or scalp, in dental roots, middle ear or air sinuses; it may also complicate fracture of the skull and meningitis. A venous sinus thrombosis may occur during the course of septicaemia.

Phlebothrombosis is relatively rare. It may occur in circumstances similar to those in which deep leg vein thrombosis may be expected (p. 244) and in those suffering from water and salt depletion. Polycythaemia, malaria and, in infants, marasmus may also be responsible.

Occasionally a cerebral venous thrombosis occurs in the puerperium. Such cases are possibly due to alteration in coagulation factors after childbirth but venous emboli from pelvic veins may pass up the vertebral venous plexuses to reach the intracranial venous sinuses. The incidence of apparently spontaneous thrombosis is slightly increased in women using oral contraceptives.

Superior Sagittal Sinus Thrombosis. This may result from extension of infection in the nose or from retrograde spread from the transverse sinus or as a result of septicaemia and meningitis. The sagittal sinus is particularly liable to be affected during the puerperium. Severe headache, accompanied by papilloedema, may be the principal feature. However, in most cases thrombophlebitis spreads to the adjacent cortical veins; the motor or sensory areas of one or both hemispheres may thus be infarcted. Characteristically there is a paraparesis, though often one leg is affected more than the other. Occasionally a hemiplegia results. Less commonly there are hemianopia and aphasia. At the onset there is occasionally a generalised epileptic seizure.

Transverse Sinus Thrombosis. This is usually due to spread of infection from suppurative middle ear disease, mastoiditis and infection of the petrous bone. It is most common in children. The primary symptom is severe pain felt behind the ear and often associated with pain in the neck. Generalised headache and vomiting are common. There may be associated papilloedema and drowsiness.

At the onset there are usually few signs of focal cerebral infarction but extension to involve the superior petrosal sinus and veins draining the lower part of the precentral gyrus may give rise to faciobrachial paresis, hemiparesis or hemianopia, and spread to the superior sagittal sinus may give rise to a paraparesis. Occasionally the thrombosis spreads into the jugular veins, sometimes leading to paralysis of the lower cranial nerves.

Cavernous Sinus Thrombosis. This nearly always follows an infection, e.g. a boil on the face or rarely an infected air sinus. It occasionally occurs as a result of polycythaemia or invasion by carcinoma.

Usually the patient is gravely ill, and before antibiotics were available few patients survived. Headache and fever are marked and there is a neutrophil leucocytosis. Occlusion of the ophthalmic veins causes proptosis, chemosis and oedema of the eyelids. There are almost always complete palsies of the third, fourth and sixth nerves as well as pain in and above the eye and diminished sensation over the forehead. Papilloedema in the affected eye is common. The condition is usually initially unilateral but often becomes bilateral within 2 to 3 days.

Thrombosis of Cortical Veins. Superficial cortical veins may be thrombosed as a result of adjacent infection, trauma or extension of thrombosis within the dural sinuses. Occasionally thrombosis follows a blood-borne infection or polycythaemia. Initially there is usually localised headache or an epileptic seizure followed by focal neurological deficit whose nature depends on the area of cortex involved. Monoparesis or hemiparesis may occur, and sometimes extension of thrombosis to neighbouring veins causes progressive neural disability.

Diagnosis of Cerebrovascular Disease

The diagnosis and assessment of a patient suffering from cerebrovascular disease ideally comprises four stages. Firstly, the nature of the patient's disabilities are defined and the site and extent of the lesion inferred. Secondly, other possible causes of the disturbance of function are excluded. Thirdly, the nature of the vascular pathology is determined. Fourthly, the state of the systemic circulation is investigated and associated diseases delineated.

The time course of a completed stroke will usually suggest the correct diagnosis. Occasionally patients suffering from a cerebral tumour will present with a rapidly developing disability. Multiple sclerosis and demyelinating encephalopathies present acutely but in most instances the age of onset, multiple lesions affecting the spinal cord as well as the brain and a characteristic earlier history will distinguish these conditions from cerebrovascular disease. The progression of a stroke-in-evolution may closely imitate the features of a rapidly growing cerebral tumour.

Transient ischaemic attacks may need to be distinguished from epilepsy and migraine. Consciousness is unimpaired in most transient ischaemic attacks. Migraine rarely presents after the age of 50 years whilst transient ischaemic attacks usually occur after this age. Transient ischaemic episodes are rarely accompanied or followed by headaches.

Progressive, diffuse, cerebral atherosclerosis may be difficult to distinguish from other forms of senile and presenile dementia and the diagnosis should not be made too readily. The occurrence of acute focal disabilities, interrupting otherwise steady deterioration, is in favour of diffuse cerebral atherosclerosis as is circumstantial evidence such as accompanying hypertension, peripheral vascular disease or myocardial ischaemia. In most instances the history and clinical findings will differentiate cerebrovascular disease from other intracranial pathologies. In a minority of instances special investigations will be required to confirm the diagnosis.

The elucidation of the type of cerebrovascular disease is sometimes difficult. It is important rapidly to define those conditions which require life-saving, urgent or specific treatment. The history of trauma and the clinical features are distinctive in extradural and acute subdural haematoma. The diagnosis of chronic subdural haematoma can occasionally be made with confidence on clinical grounds but the possibility of this condition should be considered and investigated particularly in any elderly patient manifesting a progressive cerebral deficit accompanied by headache. Signs of meningeal irritation indicate a subarachnoid bleed which can be confirmed by lumbar puncture. Arteritis will often be diagnosed because of accompanying systemic clinical features and by the results of simple investigations such as a raised ESR, positive ANF, positive serology for syphilis or a CSF leucocytosis.

Finally it is important to attempt to distinguish between patients suffering from cerebral infarction due to thrombosis or embolism and those who have bled into the brain. There are some useful clinical pointers in this differentiation. A history of transient ischaemic attacks favours a diagnosis of infarction rather than haemorrhage. The development of neural disability during sleep is likely to be due to infarction; onset during exertion suggests a haemorrhage. Blood in the CSF obviously indicates intracranial bleeding. A source of emboli is in favour of arterial occlusion rather than rupture. Hypertension is frequently associated with both infarction and haemorrhage but severe hypertension, particularly in young patients, predisposes to haemorrhage. Though these clinical hints are generally valid they do not provide firm criteria for differentiating thrombosis, embolism and haemorrhage.

The cerebral circulation cannot be considered in isolation. In any patient who suffers from cerebrovascular disease the status of heart, blood pressure, blood vessels and blood should be carefully appraised. The heart should be examined clinically, electrically and radiologically to define the presence or absence of arrhythmias, valvular or myocardial lesions and heart failure. Peripheral limb vessels and the arteries in the neck should be palpated and auscultated to detect changes in the walls and the presence of stenoses. Recordings of the blood pressure are mandatory. Abnormalities of the blood, particularly anaemia, polycythaemia and thrombocytopenia should be sought.

The extent to which diagnostic investigations should be pursued depends on individual circumstances and was, until recently, often a matter of fine judgement. The advent of computerised axial tomography has simplified the problems. This technique (p. 692) will not only reveal tumours but in many instances will define the nature of cerebrovascular lesions. Intracerebral bleeding gives high density abnormalities so that even very small haemorrhages are detected. Intraventricular, subarachnoid and subdural haemorrhages are readily distinguished and sequential scanning will monitor the subsequent organisation and resolution of intracerebral haematomas. Ruptured aneurysms can be differentiated from primary intracerebral haemorrhage in almost all instances and the site of the aneurysms predicted with fair accuracy.

Cerebral infarction leads to low density abnormalities which may be detectable within a few hours of onset. Some infarcts are not revealed by computer tomography but even in these cases the confident exclusion of tumours and haemorrhage enables a firm presumptive diagnosis to be made.

Computerised axial tomography is the most useful tool for the investigation of cerebrovascular disease. If this facility is not available other means of investigation are perforce employed but are less informative. The EEG usually shows marked abnormalities after infarction or haemorrhage and serial recordings demonstrate progressive improvement. Similar EEG abnormalities due to tumour persist and become more marked. Echoencephalography may reveal a shift of the midline echo. A marked shift suggests the presence of haemorrhage rather than infarction. Facial thermography may indicate reduction of flow through a carotid artery. Cerebral angiography should be undertaken only if surgery is likely to be required. It should be performed if there is evidence of a tumour, vascular malformation, subdural haematoma or extracranial vascular disease in a young patient which might be amenable to surgical treatment.

Treatment of Cerebrovascular Disease

The management of patients suffering from cerebrovascular disease should be approached in a logical sequence. Initially patients may need to be protected from the dangers of unconsciousness and immobility. The causal lesion should be treated if possible and measures to improve functional recovery instituted. Patients who survive but are left with residual disability need support and rehabilitation. Finally, progression and recurrence of cerebrovascular lesions should, as far as possible, be prevented.

General Measures. An adequate airway should be established in those patients whose consciousness is impaired. The patient's fluid and nutritional intake should be maintained, employing a nasogastric tube or intravenous infusion, if necessary. Pressure sores should be prevented by frequent alteration of the patient's posture, the use of pads and massage of vulnerable areas of skin. Catheterisation may be needed because of urinary incontinence. Rapid cleaning is required by the patient who is incontinent of faeces. Passive movement of limbs should be started early and the patient should be moved from bed and sat in a chair for periods during the day as soon as possible. Intercurrent urinary or respiratory infections should be treated with appropriate antibiotics.

Specific Treatment. A minority of patients have treatable underlying conditions. Those with meningovascular syphilis should be given a course of penicillin (p. 719). Those suffering from temporal arteritis or a connective tissue disorder may need steroids. Polycythaemia or anaemia should be treated appropriately.

Early operation is required for those patients who have bled from a ruptured aneurysm. The neck of the aneurysm should be clipped if this is technically possible. The wall of the aneurysm may be reinforced by plastic or muscle. If such a direct attack is impracticable carotid ligation may reduce the liability to further bleeding from the aneurysm. Surgical drainage of extradural and subdural haematomas usually produces dramatic and rapid improvement.

Stroke. Little can be done to reverse the effects of infarction or haemorrhage. In a very few instances blood flow has rapidly been restored through an occluded carotid artery by surgical removal of thrombus. This is effective only when the affected artery is accessible and when the operation is carried out within a few hours of the onset of symptoms. These conditions very rarely obtain. Treatment is aimed at minimising the extent of brain death. Around the margins of an infarct or haemorrhage there is potentially viable tissue whose function can be restored if an alternative supply of blood is available. To this end a variety of agents have been used. Attempts to provoke cerebral vasodilatation have involved the breathing of high concentrations of CO_2, stellate ganglionectomy and a number of drugs such as papaverine and betahistidine. None has been effective and it is likely that the promotion of generalised cerebral vasodilatation could be harmful by 'stealing' blood from the damaged area. Low-molecular-weight dextran has been employed in the expectation that its effects in decreasing the aggregation of platelets and blood viscosity would improve cerebral circulation. Five hundred ml of a 10 per cent solution of dextran in dextrose is given intravenously as early as possible after the onset of symptoms and repeated at 12-hourly intervals for three days. There is evidence that this treatment reduces the early death rate from severe strokes but there is no long-lasting benefit.

Dexamethasone (4 mg t.d.s.) reduces cerebral oedema and may help those patients with cerebral infarction or haemorrhage who develop deepening coma. There is little evidence that it improves the long-term prognosis. Anticoagulants have no place in the treatment of an established stroke. Thrombolytic agents such as streptokinase are ineffective. There is thus as yet no specific medical treatment available which significantly and consistently improves the outlook for patients who have suffered a stroke.

Stroke-in-evolution. The early use of anticoagulants has been advocated to halt progression in an evolving stroke. There is some evidence that this treatment does help but there is a danger that anticoagulants may cause haemorrhage and before they are used in this situation an intracerebral haemorrhage must be excluded by investigation. There may be a place for the use of low-molecular-weight dextran in the treatment of a stroke of gradual development.

Transient Ischaemic Attacks. There is much evidence to support the use of anticoagulants in transient ischaemic attacks. The treatment seems to reduce the incidence of future strokes. Some would regard this treatment as of still unproven benefit. Recently, treatment with inhibitors of platelet aggregation has been employed. Aspirin 150 mg b.d., dipyridamole 25 mg four times daily or sulphin-pyrazine 200 mg four times daily are used for this purpose. Their efficacy has not yet been fully assessed.

Diffuse Cerebral Atherosclerosis. Little can be done to halt the progress of this condition. Hypertension should be controlled.

Cerebral Embolism. There is general agreement about the value of anticoagulants in embolic cerebral disease. They should be given, probably for life, to patients who have suffered from cerebral embolism, provided other concurrent conditions do not contraindicate their use.

Cerebral Venous Thrombosis. The basis of treatment is the administration of antibiotics. This has markedly improved the outlook for infected thromboses such as occur in the cavernous sinus. Surgical drainage of pus in adjacent sinuses may be necessary. Anticoagulants are unhelpful but treatment with thrombolytic enzymes such as activated human plasmin is under trial.

Rehabilitation. A large number of patients are left with residual deficits as a result of cerebrovascular lesions. Much can be done to mitigate disabilities so that patients can live a largely independent life in the community. Early institution of treatment is essential. In the period immediately following a stroke, passive movements of limbs should be practised. Supervised exercises and encouragement should later aim at the development of mobility. Few, if any, patients, no matter how severe their original hemiplegia, cannot be taught to walk again. Later the patient should be guided into the performance of the activities of everyday living. Modifications of dress, housing, baths, lavatories and kitchen equipment may enable the patient to cope at home.

Throughout the period of rehabilitation communication should be encouraged, using, if appropriate, the skills of the speech therapist. The degree and extent of paralysis is less of a bar to successful rehabilitation than are disorders of perception, spatial disorientation, dysphasia and, particularly, dementia. Active co-operation between physicians, nurses, physiotherapists, occupational therapists, speech therapists and social workers strikingly improves the end result of the physical and social rehabilitation of patients who have had a stroke. The recruitment and education of relatives enables them to continue rehabilitation at home.

Prevention of Recurrence. Some of the treatments outlined above, such as anticoagulant therapy and inhibitors of platelet aggregation, are preventive measures. The most important prophylactic factor is the control of hypertension by appropriate drugs (p. 223). It has been shown conclusively that early, effective and continued reduction of high blood pressure significantly improves the outlook for both occlusive and haemorrhagic cerebrovascular disease.

Prognosis. The prognosis for an individual suffering from a cerebrovascular lesion depends on complex factors. There are some general guidelines. In one well-studied series of strokes the mortality within the first month after infarction was roughly 30 per cent. From proven intracerebral haemorrhage the mortality in the same period was 80 per cent. After a subarachnoid haemorrhage 65 per cent died within 1 month. This investigation emphasised the poor prognosis after large haemorrhagic lesions. Many epidemiological studies have stressed the general tendency of clinicians to overestimate the incidence of cerebral haemorrhage. Data from death certificates suggest that haemorrhage is twice as common as infarction. Careful differentiation of the two types of lesion indicates that infarction is at least five times commoner than haemorrhage and in those over 75 years of age, 20 times more frequent.

Signs of a poor outlook for a stroke, whether due to infarction or haemorrhage, are impairment of consciousness, defects in conjugate gaze and a severe hemiplegia. Of those who survive an initial stroke life expectancy is roughly halved. Approximately 10 per cent suffer a second stroke within 1 year of the first and 20 per cent within 5 years. Many patients who initially present with stroke die from myocardial infarction.

The prognosis in patients who suffer transient ischaemic attacks is difficult to ascertain because of difficulties of definition. A subsequent stroke is to be expected in approximately one-third of patients who have transient ischaemic attacks and is most likely to occur within 3 years of the first attack. In 50 per cent of patients attacks cease within 1 to 3 years of their onset. Transient ischaemic attacks are attended by a worse prognosis (in terms of survival) in people below the age of 65 than in those over this age when compared with the rest of the population.

Much further work is needed to define the factors which influence the prognosis of cerebrovascular disease.

INFECTIONS OF THE BRAIN, MENINGES AND SPINAL CORD

Suppurative Encephalitis and Intracerebral Abscess

Aetiology and Pathology. Direct infections may occur following a compound fracture of the skull or there may be local spread by suppurative thrombophlebitis from an infected ear, paranasal sinus or scalp. Metastatic infections may occur from the lungs or from infective endocarditis.

The initial infection causes a suppurative encephalitis. The pus is slowly localised by a surrounding wall of gliosis which in a chronic abscess may form a tough capsule. Multiple abscesses, communicating or discrete, occur, particularly with metastatic spread.

Clinical Features. There are three main types of presentation:

Acute Encephalitis. Soon after head injury or otitis media (in which aural discharge may be temporarily suppressed) the patient develops headache, vomiting and drowsiness passing to coma. Focal cerebral signs may be present and the temperature is raised.

Subacute or Delayed Encephalitis. Head injury, cranial infection or infected embolism may be followed after weeks or months of apparent recovery by symptoms of encephalitis or of a chronic space-occupying lesion. During the latent interval there may be minor headache, irritability, malaise and intermittent pyrexia. These symptoms should lead to a search for a focal cerebral lesion in patients with infections such as otitis or bronchiectasis.

Chronic abscess. This may follow one of the previous types of onset or there may be nothing to suggest that the lesion is infective. The chronic abscess causes focal symptoms of a cerebral lesion (p. 672) and those of raised intracranial pressure which are indistinguishable from those of cerebral tumour. The temperature is usually normal or even subnormal.

Lumbar puncture may help to confirm the diagnosis but should be avoided if the diagnosis is highly likely and especially if localising signs suggest cerebellar abscess. The CSF pressure may be raised and there is usually an increase in cells with a predominance of lymphocytes. The protein may be raised; the chloride and glucose contents are normal and no organisms are found unless there is also a meningitis. The blood shows a polymorphonuclear leucocytosis and the ESR is often raised, but absence of these findings does not exclude chronic abscess.

The EEG shows certain characteristic changes during the acute stage which may be valuable in diagnosis. As the diffuse encephalitis subsides changes in the EEG may be found which are very valuable for localisation of the abscess cavity or cavities. The radiological signs do not differ from those of cerebral tumour but radiological examination may show a causative lesion in ear, sinuses or chest.

Treatment. Prevention should be the first aim by efficient treatment of otitis media, sinusitis, fractures of the skull and bronchiectasis. Acute suppurative encephalitis is treated by immediate intramuscular injection of benzylpenicillin, 1–2 g followed by 600 mg 4 hourly. Surgical assistance should be sought early and the abscess, localised by EEG and angiography, tapped with a brain cannula for aspiration of pus and instillation of antibiotics. Myodil, a radio-opaque iodine compound, is also instilled so that progress may be followed by serial radiography. Antibiotic medication is subsequently determined by the bacteriological findings. Measures to reduce intracranial pressure may also be required (p. 694). Excision of the abscess cavity may have to be undertaken at a later stage. In view of the high incidence of symptomatic epilepsy all patients should be given phenobarbitone prophylactically after the acute stage for a minimum period of two years.

Spinal Epidural Abscess

This condition usually arises as a metastasis from infection elsewhere, often a boil, which may be so trivial as to be easily overlooked. Pain of root distribution is severe. It develops acutely and is followed by progressive loss of sensation and power in the lower limbs with sphincter disturbance. The signs are those of transverse myelitis (p. 742) but the local root irritation is the clue to the true cause. The temperature may be only slightly raised, but a polymorphonuclear leucocytosis is found in the blood. There may be radiological evidence of localised osteomyelitis of the spine. Paraplegia will become complete and irreversible if treatment is delayed. Large doses of antibiotics such as benzylpenicillin 600 mg 4 hourly should be given immediately and the patient transferred to the care of a neurosurgeon without delay.

Meningitis

Aetiology and Pathology. Inflammation of the pia and arachnoid membranes may be sterile or infective.

Sterile. Blood in the CSF as in subarachnoid haemorrhage causes severe meningeal inflammation (p. 705). Meningeal irritation ('*meningism*') without inflammatory reaction occurs in acute specific fevers, otitis media and pneumonia in childhood. Cellular reaction (lymphocytic) may be associated with symptoms and signs of meningeal irritation in poliomyelitis (p. 722) and acute encephalomyelitis (p. 721). Carcinomatosis of the meninges is a rare cause.

Infective. Formerly the most common meningeal infections were due to meningococcal infection or infection with pyogenic organisms carried in the blood from a distant focus or introduced from without (e.g. an infected ear), or from within by rupture of a cerebral abscess. These types of meningitis have become rare since the introduction of the antibiotics, and for similar reasons, tuberculous meningitis is now seldom seen in Britain. The most common infection is now viral. Rare infections are due to syphilis or to fungi.

The pia-arachnoid is congested and infiltrated with inflammatory cells. A thin layer of pus forms and this may later organise to form adhesions. These may cause obstruction to the free flow of CSF leading to hydrocephalus, or may damage the cranial nerves at the base of the brain. The CSF pressure rises rapidly, the protein content increases and there is a cellular reaction which varies in type and severity according to the nature of the inflammation and the causative organism. The sugar content of the CSF is decreased in bacterial infections and in carcinomatosis of the meninges. If the patient is not kept in electrolyte balance the chloride content may be reduced due to loss by sweating and vomiting.

Clinical Features. Signs of meningeal irritation are present:

Neck Rigidity. The patient complains of neck stiffness and the examiner is unable to put the patient's chin on his chest by passive flexion of the neck. When he attempts to do so the muscle spasm evoked makes the neck so rigid that the head and trunk may be lifted from the bed. Spasm may be so severe, particularly in children, as to cause head retraction.

Kernig's Sign. If the patient's thigh is flexed to 90 degrees from the abdomen, it is then impossible to straighten the knee passively owing to spasm of the hamstring muscles. This manoeuvre stretches the roots of the sciatic nerve which are inflamed at their exits from the spinal theca.

Meningococcal Meningitis

This is described on page 76.

Acute Pyogenic Meningitis

Infection by staphylococci, streptococci, pneumococci or *Haemophilus influenzae* sometimes occurs primarily in the meninges but it is more commonly secondary to infection in the heart, lungs, bones or elsewhere.

Clinical Features. Headache (p. 696) and signs of meningeal irritation are present. A primary focus of infection may be evident. There is no rash and other pyaemic signs are rarer than in meningococcal infection. Bacteriological examination of the cerebrospinal fluid establishes the diagnosis and should be performed without delay.

Treatment. Both sulphonamides and penicillin should be started immediately without waiting for bacteriological confirmation as the treatment can later be modified appropriately. Sulphadiazine 6 g by mouth is given at once followed by 2 g 4 hourly. Benzylpenicillin 6 mg mixed with 10 ml of the patient's CSF is injected intrathecally at the start of treatment but thereafter intramuscular injection is usually sufficient if given in large doses (at least 300 mg every 4 hours). For an infection with *H. influenzae*, the drugs of choice are chloramphenicol and ampicillin initially administered intravenously. Thereafter, for an adult, 2 capsules each containing 250 mg of either drug should be given at 4 hourly intervals. In all types of acute pyogenic meningitis treatment must be continued until the CSF has returned to normal and the temperature has been normal for at least two days.

Tuberculous Meningitis

Aetiology and Pathology. The usual source of infection is a caseous focus in the meninges or brain substance adjacent to the cerebrospinal fluid pathway. The focus arises as a result of spread by the blood stream from a site elsewhere. The condition occurs most commonly shortly after a primary infection in childhood, but people of any age may be affected. The breakdown of the caseous focus may be due to head injury or to any illness causing diminished resistance. Tuberculous meningitis may occur as part of miliary tuberculosis.

The brain is covered by a greenish, gelatinous exudate especially around the base, and numerous scattered tubercles are found on the meninges.

Clinical Features. In children the onset of tuberculous meningitis is so insidious that it may be 2 weeks before the parents realise that the illness is serious. At first there is merely lassitude, loss of interest in toys and in play, unwillingness to talk, anorexia and constipation. Headache, at first slight, gradually becomes worse but meningeal signs may not appear until the third week. In adults the malaise, headache and meningeal signs progress more rapidly though not as quickly as in acute pyogenic meningitis. There may be occasional vomiting. The temperature is intermittently raised to 38°C during the period of ingravescence but remains raised, though rarely to high levels, once meningeal signs appear. The condition then progresses more rapidly, and in untreated cases cranial nerve palsies, hemiparesis or other signs of cerebral damage, hydrocephalus with drowsiness, coma and moderate papilloedema may occur. In miliary tuberculosis choroidal tubercles may be seen in the ocular fundi.

The CSF is under increased pressure. It is usually crystal clear or slightly turbid but, when allowed to stand, a fine clot forms like a cobweb. The fluid contains up to 400 cells per cmm predominantly lymphocytes (the count must be made on a fresh specimen before it forms a clot). There is a slight rise in protein and a marked fall in glucose. Detection of the tubercle bacillus in a smear of the centrifuged deposit from the CSF may be difficult, the clot being the most likely place to find it. Inoculation of CSF into a guinea-pig is valuable for confirming the diagnosis if this cannot be done from smears or cultures of the CSF but as the outcome will not be known for six weeks, treatment must be started without waiting for confirmation.

Diagnosis. As the ill effects of delayed treatment are so serious it is extremely important to diagnose tuberculous meningitis early. It should be considered especially in any patient known to have tuberculosis who develops a persistent headache, perhaps with slight pyrexia in the evening. If there is neck stiffness or choroidal tubercules there should be no hesitation in performing lumbar puncture and evidence of miliary tuberculosis should be sought by radiography of the chest. The differential diagnosis in the later stage is from other infections of the nervous system and is made largely upon the findings in the cerebrospinal fluid.

Treatment. Chemotherapy should be started as soon as the diagnosis is made using one of the regimes described on p. 292, together with pyrazinamide (pp. 292 and 295). All patients should also receive prednisolone, 10 mg four times daily. If subsequent lumbar punctures suggest the development of a spinal subarachnoid block, then hydrocortisone hemisuccinate should be injected intrathecally each day in a dose of 1 mg/kg body weight. If obstructive hydrocephalus develops in spite of treatment with corticosteroids, surgical methods for ensuring continuous ventricular drainage must be adopted. During the acute stage of the illness skilled nursing is essential and measures must be taken to maintain adequate hydration and nutrition.

The intensive regime of drug treatment should be continued for eight weeks and be followed by a continuation phase (p. 294). Prednisolone is then reduced to 20 mg daily and stopped after about three months (p. 295).

Prognosis. Untreated tuberculous meningitis is fatal in a few weeks but complete recovery is the rule with modern treatment if it is started before the appearance of focal signs or stupor. When treatment is started at a later stage the recovery rate is 60 per cent or less and the survivors may be mentally deficient, epileptic, deaf, blind or show some other permanent deficit.

Viral Meningitis

Acute lymphocytic choriomeningitis and other forms of viral meningitis are described on page 720.

Neurosyphilis

An old and frequently reiterated neurological aphorism says that neurosyphilis may mimic any neurological disease. As a corollary it is emphasised that neurosyphilis must be included in the differential diagnosis of all neurological problems.

Neurosyphilis may present as an acute or chronic process and may involve, singly or in combination, the meninges, blood vessels and parenchyma of brain and spinal cord. Though the clinical manifestations produced are diverse certain general observations are pertinent.

Pupillary abnormalities, described by Argyll Robertson, may accompany any neurosyphilitic clinical syndrome. The pupils are small, irregular and unequal. They do not react to light but respond to convergence and show an impaired response to mydriatics. The irises may be atrophied. In relatively few instances will all of these features be present. The complete picture of Argyll Robertson pupils is most frequently seen in tabes dorsalis and is distinctly uncommon in general paresis wherein some pupillary changes occur in about half of the cases. The observation of any discrepancy between the pupillary response to light and convergence even when other manifestations are lacking, should always suggest the possibility of neurosyphilis.

The *Wassermann reaction* is usually positive in neurosyphilis. In general paresis it is almost always so in both blood and cerebrospinal fluid, as it is in about 90 per cent of cases of meningovascular syphilis. In a fifth of tabetic patients, the Wassermann reaction in the CSF is negative and 10 per cent show negative serology in the blood. The FTA and TPI (p. 79) are more specific tests for the detection of neurosyphilis.

Examination of the CSF reveals abnormalities in the vast majority of cases of neurosyphilis. An increase in the cell count, usually lymphocytic and of moderate degree is almost invariably present when the disease is active. A moderate rise in the protein content is usual and the gamma globulin fraction thereof is often increased.

Meningovascular Syphilis

The essential lesion is endarteritis obliterans which may lead to arterial thrombosis and to the formation of a granuloma or gumma. The meninges may be covered by an exudate which damages cranial nerves. Lesions may predominantly affect arteries or meninges or both structures may be involved. Clinical manifestations usually occur within five years of the primary infection.

Intracranial Lesions. Occlusion of a cerebral artery may be due to syphilis which should be considered as a possibility in cases of stroke, particularly when cerebral infarcts occur in young people.

Basal gummatous meningitis may present with cranial nerve palsies. Meningitis over the surface of the hemispheres may give rise to headaches and fits in addition to focal signs of cortical dysfunction. Rarely, a single large gumma may present as a slowly growing cerebral tumour.

Spinal Lesions. Thrombosis of the anterior spinal artery gives rise to lower motor neurone signs at the level of the lesion. Below the affected segments, pyramidal tract disturbance is usually manifest and there may also be impairment of pain and temperature sensation though the latter is often transient.

Thickening of the dura mater in the cervical region—called *hypertrophic pachymeningitis*—gives rise to lower motor neurone lesions in the arms and upper motor neurone lesions in the legs.

Meningitis accompanied by myelitis in the dorsal region causes 'girdle' pains and leads to progressive cord damage.

Parenchymal Disease

GENERAL PARALYSIS OF THE INSANE

The principal pathological changes are seen in the cortex. There is degeneration of cortical neurones giving rise to atrophy, particularly marked over the anterior part of the hemispheres. The meninges are thickened and infiltrated with lymphocytes. General paralysis of the insane usually presents 5 to 15 years after the primary infection. Men are much more often affected than women.

Clinical Features. The initial and most characteristic feature is dementia, often of insidious onset and slow progression. Relatives or workmates usually first recognise the patient's intellectual deficit and later his deteriorating social adaptation. Delusions of grandeur occur only in a minority of cases. Signs of upper motor neurone lesions, usually bilateral and initially mild, are usually present and tremors of the head and lips are often manifest. Less common features include epileptic fits and transient episodes of focal cerebral disturbance such as hemiplegia, hemianopia or dysphasia.

TABES DORSALIS

The primary lesion is a degeneration of first order sensory neurones, central to the dorsal root ganglia, in the lower thoracic and lumbar nerve roots. Obvious macroscopic wasting affects the dorsal columns but all modalities of sensation may be impaired. Males are more often affected than females, usually 5 to 20 years after the primary infection.

Clinical Features. Sensory disturbances are the most common initial symptoms. 'Lightning' pains of severe, lancinating nature occur in paroxysms. They are most common in the legs. Pains radiating around the trunk in a 'girdle' distribution also occur. Paraesthesiae often affect the feet.

Other disabilities may accompany these sensory manifestations or may be presenting features. Ataxia, of sensory type, due to proprioceptive loss is often prominent. Sphincter disturbance, particularly retention of urine, may be accompanied by impotence. Failing vision or diplopia may be symptoms. Perforating, painless ulcers of the feet and swollen, unstable joints (Charcot's joints) are sometimes found. Visceral crises may cause acute symptoms and the disturbance in function of a viscus may point to disease in the affected organ rather than in its innervation. Most common are gastric crises which give rise to abdominal pain and vomiting. Less common are laryngeal crises causing stridor, the strangury of vesical crises and tenesmus due to rectal crises.

The signs of tabes are mostly explicable on the basis of posterior root lesions. Tendon reflexes are lost, due to interruption of the reflex arcs, first at the ankles, then at the knees and later in the upper limbs; hypotonia with resultant hyperextensibility of the joints appears. The pain fibres are affected early with delay in or impairment of the response to pin prick over a characteristic distribution. The classical areas of loss are around the nose, the trunk from the angle of the sternum to the costal margin, the inner border of the forearms and the ring and little fingers, the perineum and the distal part of the lower limbs. Deep pain appreciation is also impaired so that the tendo calcaneus, calf muscles and testes become insensitive to pressure. Vibration and position sense in the feet are also lost early, but light touch is not affected until a later stage. The combination of loss of position sense and hypotonia gives rise to severe ataxia, so that the patient walks on a wide base lifting his feet high and stamping them down in an irregular and forceful manner. Romberg's test (p. 666) is positive. The plantar responses remain flexor, but may be absent as a result of sensory loss.

Bilateral ptosis with compensatory wrinkling of the forehead and Argyll Robertson pupils constitute a typical tabetic facies. Less constant clinical manifestations also include pallor of the optic discs, defects in external ocular movement, distension of the bladder, and trophic changes such as ulcers or painless arthropathy.

Combined Neurosyphilitic Lesions

It is emphasised that the clinical syndromes outlined above represent only the commoner presentations of neurosyphilis. Combinations of pathological lesions also occur and give rise to mixed clinical pictures. Tabetic manifestations sometimes accompany those of general paralysis of the insane and the hybrid (*taboparesis*) may lead to cases of dementia accompanied by ataxia, lightning pains or areflexia; patients presenting with visceral crises may be found to have extensor plantar responses.

Treatment of Neurosyphilis

The essential part of the treatment of neurosyphilis of all types is the injection of procaine benzylpenicillin, 1 g daily for three weeks. The aim of treatment is to arrest the disease and restore the blood and CSF to normal. Further courses of penicillin must be given if symptoms are not relieved, the condition continues to advance, or the CSF continues to show signs of active disease. The first abnormality to regress is the increase in cells but these may not return to normal until three months after treatment has been completed. The elevated protein takes longer to subside and the Wassermann reaction may never revert to normal. Lumbar puncture should be repeated at 6 monthly intervals for 2 years and further courses of penicillin given so long as signs of activity remain. Evidence of clinical progression at any time is an indication for renewed treatment.

Viral Infections

Some viruses have a propensity for invasion of nerve cells and are called 'neurotropic'. The affinity may be specially marked for one type of nerve cell; the zoster variant of the varicella virus particularly involves sensory neurones and the anterior horn cells are vulnerable in poliomyelitis. Though these viruses most commonly invade their sites of predilection they may also sometimes involve the nervous system more widely; the virus of poliomyelitis often gives rise to a meningoencephalitis and the zoster virus may rarely cause motor disability. Many viruses which usually cause diseases of other systems may sometimes implicate the nervous system. The many varieties of echo and Coxsackie viruses, which are common enteric pathogens, fairly often cause neurological disease as well as more widespread manifestations in other systems. The viruses of herpes simplex and mumps, among many others, may occasionally invade the nervous system.

Some neurological diseases, of which encephalitis lethargica is one, are presumed to be of viral origin because of their epidemiological, clinical and pathological features though the causal agent has not been identified.

Neurological disorders are sometimes indirectly associated with viral diseases. In these instances abnormal immunological responses, evoked by the virus, cause damage to neural tissue without any viral invasion of neurones. The demyelinating encephalomyelitis (p. 728) which may follow any of the exanthemata is such an entity.

Slow Viral Infections. There is now interest in the concept of 'slow' viral infections of the central nervous system causing chronic or relapsing neurological disease. Slow viral infections exhibit a long latent period (months or many years) between the initial infection and the subsequent clinical illness which, once manifest, tends to run a protracted course. Two diseases of sheep, scrapie, an invariably fatal encephalopathy and visna, a demyelinating myelopathy, are proven examples of slow virus infections. Evidence for a similar cause of human disease is as yet scanty but there are suggestive findings.

A degeneration of grey matter, most marked in the cerebellum, causing a progressive ataxia, called *kuru*, is a disease which occurs naturally only in the members of one cannibalistic New Guinea tribe. The disease can, however, be transmitted to chimpanzees and there is much evidence to suggest that kuru is a slow viral infection transmitted by the eating of the infected brains of dead tribal members. The rare *subacute spongiform encephalopathy* (*Creutzfeldt–Jakob dis-*

ease) is characterised by dementia, epilepsy, extrapyramidal and motor neurone signs and can also be trasmitted from man to chimpanzees.

A slow viral infection has been adduced as a possible cause of a number of chronic neurological diseases, including motor neurone disease and multiple sclerosis.

Viral Meningitis

Viral infections of the central nervous system such as encephalitis and poliomyelitis may be associated with meningitis. Viral meningitis can also occur alone, without clinical manifestation of parenchymal involvement of the nervous system in acute lymphocytic choriomeningitis and infection by echo or Coxsackie viruses. Thirdly, meningitis may develop as a complication of viral infections primarily involving other organs, e.g. mumps, measles, infectious mononucleosis, psittacosis, herpes zoster and viral hepatitis.

ACUTE LYMPHOCYTIC CHORIOMENINGITIS
(*Benign Lymphocytic Meningitis*)

Aetiology. The virus is believed to be endemic in house mice. It can sometimes be isolated from the CSF of patients and transmitted to mice. There is probably an initial viraemia, and pneumonia may be associated with meningitis. Acute lymphocytic choriomeningitis occurs sporadically or in small epidemics.

Clinical Features. The condition commonly occurs in children and young adults. The onset is acute and evidence of meningeal irritation develops rapidly. Focal neurological signs are usually absent but diplopia and mild papilloedema may be observed. There may be a high pyrexia which gradually drops to normal in 5 to 7 days. The CSF is under increased pressure. It is usually clear but may be turbid as there is an excess of lymphocytes which may persist long after clinical cure. There may be a slight increase in the protein but the sugar and chloride levels are normal.

Differential Diagnosis. In pyogenic meningitis the turbid CSF contains an excess of polymorphonuclear leucocytes and the causative organism can be isolated. Tuberculous meningitis may be difficult to distinguish owing to the technical difficulties of isolating the tubercle bacillus. A normal level of sugar in the CSF is in favour of a diagnosis of acute lymphocytic choriomeningitis. If there is any serious doubt as to the diagnosis, it is better to start treatment for tuberculous meningitis while awaiting further bacteriological reports.

Treatment and Prognosis. There is no specific treatment. The patient is kept at rest in bed on symptomatic measures until the temperature has returned to normal. Complete recovery is the rule in acute lymphocytic choriomeningitis.

Viral Encephalitis

All of the viruses which cause meningitis may also give rise to an encephalitis. Encephalitic features may predominate or a combined picture of meningo-encephalitis may occur. More specific types of viral encephalitis occur in epidemic forms, such as Japanese-B encephalitis (p. 881). Sporadic cases occur fairly commonly but often the causative virus is not isolated though influenza and herpes simplex viruses are fairly frequently implicated.

Pathology. The distribution and extent of lesions vary to some extent with the type of infecting virus. There is usually diffuse damage to cells in the cortex, basal ganglia and brain stem. Inclusion bodies are often present in neurones and glial cells. There is usually infiltration between neurones and in the perivascular spaces by polymorphonuclear cells initially and later by lymphocytes and mononuclear cells. There is accompanying neuroglial proliferation. Herpes simplex encephalitis tends particularly to affect the temporal lobes and in encephalitis lethargica the substantia nigra, mid brain and basal ganglia are most prominently involved.

Clinical Features. An acute onset of headache, often accompanied by fever, is the usual clinical presentation common to all types of viral encephalitis. Disturbance of consciousness, varying from mild drowsiness to deep coma, usually supervenes early and may sometimes advance dramatically. Epilepsy of focal or generalised type is common. A variety of focal signs such as aphasia, hemiplegia or tetraplegia, cranial nerve palsies and sensory disturbances may occur but sometimes there are none. The clinical features usually do not enable a firm diagnosis of the causal agent to be made but some types of encephalitis present distinctive manifestations as follows:

Herpes Simplex Encephalitis. The onset is usually acute and commonly is marked by behavioural disturbance and a confusional state resembling a psychosis. This often lasts 2 or 3 days before other features develop. Fits are very common. Papilloedema and variable focal neurological signs may be present. Progression over a few days to coma is common.

Brain-stem Encephalitis. This is presumed to be of viral origin but the causal agent has not been defined. There is usually an antecedent history of mild upper respiratory infection. The onset, attended by headache, is often marked by double vision and dysarthria. Later there is increasing drowsiness and progressive cranial nerve involvement.

Encephalitis Lethargica. This occured in epidemic form during the 1920s. Its present incidence is difficult to determine. Some believe that it has disappeared but there is evidence that sporadic cases still occur. The illness varies markedly in severity. Headache and double vision may be the only features but sleep disturbances, respiratory tics, pyramidal and extrapyramidal signs may be manifest. Oculogyric crises or parkinsonism may develop during the early stages of the illness or may be a sequel.

Benign myalgic encephalomyelitis. This is a condition which is presumed, though not proven, to be of viral origin. It occurs in closed communities such as schools and hospitals. It presents with pyrexia and diffuse muscle pains, tremors and marked mood disturbances which may recur over long periods.

Subacute sclerosing panencephalitis. This condition is now thought to be due to infection by a myxovirus which is either measles virus or a closely related agent. It occurs in children and adolescents. The onset is usually an insidious intellectual deterioration, apathy and clumsiness accompanied later by myoclonic jerks and other involuntary movements. The EEG is distinctive, showing bursts of triphasic slow waves. As the disease progresses rigidity and dementia supervene.

Rabies. This presents a distinctive clinical picture described on page 882.

Diagnosis. These various forms of viral encephalitis should first be distinguished from other intracranial diseases such as cerebral tumour or abscess, from encephalopathies and from demyelinating encephalomyelitis (p. 728). Thereafter the type of viral infection should, if possible, be determined. The differential diagnosis depends on the nature of the clinical features and the attendant circumstances. When the predominant features are progressive, focal affection of one hemisphere accompnaied by headache and drowsiness the picture may strongly suggest a space-occupying lesion and intensive investigation may be needed to exclude such conditions as cerebral abscess. When the illness is mild, neurological signs indefinite and there are attendant general signs of viral infection the diagnosis will often be made presumptively after the patient improves.

Investigations are more helpful in excluding other lesions than in confirming the diagnosis of viral encephalitis. In a minority of instances the CSF is normal. Usually the CSF pressure and protein content are moderately raised and there is a lymphocytic pleocytosis. The sugar content is normal. The EEG is usually altered. There is a diffuse slowing of the rhythms but the findings are nonspecific except in subacute sclerosing panencephalitis.

Occasionally in herpes simplex encephalitis a cerebral scan will show areas of increased uptake in one or both temporal lobes. This condition is potentially treatable so that it is important to establish the diagnosis when the patient's illness is severe and progressive. In such circumstances a surgical biopsy of the temporal lobe may be justified.

Serological tests and culture may identify the infecting virus but the results of such tests are usually available too late to guide treatment.

Treatment. The management of most cases of viral encephalitis consists of nursing care and the prevention of intercurrent infections. When a positive diagnosis of herpes simplex encephalitis has been made, idoxuridine (p. 95) may be given intravenously; the total dose is 500 mg/kg and this should be given slowly in equally divided doses over five successive days. Alternatively cytarabine may be used; it also acts on viral DNA.

Prognosis. This is highly variable. Most patients survive and may recover completely but persisting focal defects are frequent. A significant number (perhaps 10–30 per cent) die. The outlook is particularly poor in herpes simplex encephalitis and in subacute sclerosing panencephalitis. Brain-stem encephalitis has a good prognosis; complete, if sometimes slow, recovery is almost invariable.

Poliomyelitis

Aetiology and Pathology. The disease is caused by one of three related polioviruses which comprise a subdivision of the group of enteroviruses. It is becoming much less common following the widespread use of prophylactic immunisation by oral vaccines (p. 60). Infection usually occurs through the nasopharynx.

The virus is particularly liable to affect the grey matter of spinal cord, brain stem and cortex and has a particular propensity to damage anterior horn cells especially those within the lumbar segments. There is often accompanying infiltration of the meninges with lymphocytes.

Clinical Features. The incubation period is 7–14 days. At the onset there is usually mild pyrexia and headache which improves after a few days. Many cases do not progress beyond this stage. In other instances, after a period of well-being lasting approximately a week there is a recurrence of pyrexia and headache accompanied by neck stiffness and signs of meningeal irritation. Paralysis may occur later. The extent is variable. Weakness of one muscle group may progress to widespread paresis. Respiratory failure may supervene if intercostal muscles are paralysed or the medullary motor nuclei are involved.

The CSF shows a lymphocytic pleocytosis, a rise in protein and a normal sugar content.

Treatment and Prognosis. In the early stages bed rest is imperative. At the onset of respiratory difficulties a tracheostomy should be performed and intermittent positive pressure respiration instituted.

Epidemics vary widely in their incidence of abortive and nonparalytic cases and in mortality rate. Death occurs from respiratory paralysis. Paralysis is greatest at the end of the first week of the major illness. Gradual recovery may then take place for several months but any muscle showing no signs of recovery by the end of a month will not regain useful function. It is difficult to make a more definite prediction about the extent of permanent disability until three to six months after the onset. Second attacks are very rare.

Herpes Zoster (SHINGLES)

Viral invasion of posterior root ganglia causes pain followed by a rash over the cutaneous distribution of the affected nerve root. The virus is the same as that causing chickenpox, and contacts with one disease may develop the other. In herpes zoster there is a high level of specific antibody in the blood, and this is believed to indicate reactivation of a previous infection by chickenpox virus which has lain dormant in the body. The virus occasionally invades the spinal cord or the brain, giving rise to myelitis or encephalitis. It sometimes involves nerve roots which are the site of another pathological process such as neuroma, metastatic tumours, Hodgkin's disease and leukaemia.

Clinical Features. The first symptom is usually severe continuous pain in the distribution of the affected nerve root. There is often little systemic upset but malaise and pyrexia may accompany the pain, especially in old age. After three or four days the skin in the affected area becomes reddened and vesicles appear. The vesicles dry up over the course of 5 or 6 days leaving small scars. The affected dermatomes may be permanently anaesthetic. Scarring is more severe if the vesicles are secondarily infected. The pain of herpes zoster usually subsides as the eruption fades, but occasionally, especially in old people, it may be followed by a persistent and intractable neuralgia which may last for months or years.

Any dorsal root ganglion may be infected, most commonly those supplying the trunk where two or three adjacent dermatomes on one side only are often involved. Infection of the trigeminal ganglion usually involves the ophthalmic division; the vesicles appear on the cornea and may lead to corneal ulceration with the danger of scarring and impairment of vision (*ophthalmic herpes*).

Segmental muscle wasting may occur sometimes. It may result from involvement of the motor root in the inflammatory reaction, but it is often delayed until a month after the sensory signs, suggesting a delayed allergic reaction. Facial palsy may be caused by infection of the geniculate ganglion spreading to the trunk of the facial nerve.

Diagnosis. Herpes zoster is easily recognised when the rash has appeared but, in the antecedent painful stage before development of the rash, it is frequently misdiagnosed as pleurisy, cholecystitis or a spinal cord lesion. It is important to remember the possibility that herpes zoster may be associated with an underlying lesion of the dorsal root ganglia due to organic disease.

Treatment. Cytarabine (p. 96) may be used in severe or complicated cases. The vesicles should be kept dry with talcum powder. An ointment containing such local anaesthetic as ung. cinchocain co. BPC applied to the site of the rash gives relief in the acute stage. Analgesics may also be required.

The treatment of post-herpetic neuralgia is difficult. Analgesics should be continued, but the more addictive ones, such as morphine, should be avoided. Radiotherapy to the affected root may be advised if the pain proves intractable. Section of the nerve or nerve roots is never successful but section of the spinothalamic tract may be carried out with benefit.

DEMYELINATING DISEASES

Loss of myelin sheaths occurs with many disorders of the central and peripheral nervous systems but there is a particular category with certain clinical and pathological features in common in which loss of myelin is considered to be the primary change and the axis cylinders may be spared or, if affected, are damaged secondarily. The lesions are almost entirely confined to the white matter of the central nervous system. They are initially inflammatory in type but differ from lesions known to be caused by direct viral infection and so they are grouped separately from viral encephalitis.

Multiple Sclerosis

Multiple sclerosis, also known as *disseminated sclerosis*, is the commonest of the demyelinating diseases. It affects about 1 in 2,000 of the population in Britain.

Aetiology. The cause of the disease is unknown but there is much information about its prevalence and about the factors associated with its development. Incidence varies widely in different geographical areas. It is very low in the tropics and high in the temperate zones of both northern and southern hemispheres. Migrants from a high to a low prevalence area have a reduced risk of developing multiple sclerosis. Those who migrate from a low to a high prevalence area are at greater risk than had they remained in their original environment. These effects apply only to those who move before the age of 15 years. Migrants at a later age bear the same liability to the disease as do the people of their country of origin.

The occurrence of multiple sclerosis in close relatives of sufferers is greater than it is in the general population. This increased familial incidence is not of sufficient degree to implicate a primarily genetic causation. Moreover, the prevalence rates of the children of immigrants in low prevalence areas is similarly low whether or not their parents came from high or low risk areas. The epidemiological data suggest that environmental influences are the determining causative factors. Speculation has centred upon three possible aetiologies. These is some evidence to support an autoimmune cause. Other findings suggest the possibility of a viral, possibly a slow viral, infection. Dietary factors, notably the ingestion of saturated fatty acids, may play some part in the development of the disease. None of these hypotheses is proven.

Pathology. The acute lesion consists of a circumscribed area in which the myelin sheaths have undergone destruction while the axis cylinders show only irregular swelling. The plaque has a swollen pinkish appearance as blood vessels are dilated, but there is little infiltration with inflammatory cells. Reactive gliosis follows, so that the chronic lesion becomes a glial scar with a shrunken greyish appearance. The lesions are widely scattered in the white matter of the brain, especially round the ventricles, in the spinal cord, and in the optic nerves. Despite the disseminated distribution there is a tendency for spinal cord and brain stem lesions to occur in symmetrical situations.

Clinical Features. These are diverse. It is impossible to outline a 'typical' history. Characteristic features are a relapsing and remittent course and widespread lesions which result in varied symptomatology.

The first manifestation may occur at any age but onset before puberty or after the age of 60 years is rare. Initial symptoms present between 20 and 40 years of age in the majority of cases. Women are affected about one-and-a-half times as often as men.

Weakness of one or more limbs developing acutely is probably the commonest presentation. Unilateral retrobulbar neuritis is also a frequent mode of onset as are paraesthesiae affecting a limb or felt in a girdle distribution around the trunk. Diplopia, vertigo and ataxia are also common initial features. Less frequent are epilepsy, aphasia, hemiplegia, facial palsy and bouts of facial pain resembling trigeminal neuralgia.

In most instances the symptoms and signs of the initial manifestation recover completely within 1 to 3 months of the onset. A period of well-being follows and after a very variable interval there is a recurrence. In a few instances there is no remission; the initial disability progresses and more widespread deficits develop. A minority of patients suffer three or four further exacerbations during the year following the onset. Another small group remain well for more than 10 years after the first disturbance. In many cases neural deficits recur within 2 years of the first incident. The outlook for the second and subsequent manifestations is variable. Some patients continue to show exacerbations with virtually complete recovery for many years. In other instances successive relapses are attended by diminishing degrees of improvement. Eventually half of the sufferers enter a chronically progressive stage with persisting and increasing disability.

The signs depend on the site of the demyelinating lesion. Pallor of one or both optic nerve heads is common and is particularly prominent over the temporal halves of the discs even in patients who give no history of an earlier retrobulbar neuritis. Patients who develop diplopia show affection of the third or sixth cranial nerves. Nystagmus is often found and is usually of cerebellar or ataxic type. Signs of motor dysfunction are usually found at some stage, particularly involving the pyramidal pathways. The abdominal reflexes are often absent early in the course of the disease and remain so. Pyramidal tract signs in the early stages may be unilateral but usually become bilateral as the disease progresses. Later pyramidal signs in both upper and lower limbs become more marked. Spasticity and paraplegia- in flexion and flexor spasms ensue. In people who develop the disease in middle age the only manifestation is often a slowly progressive, moderate paraparesis without remission but without severe exacerbations.

Cerebellar signs include the staccato, interrupted rhythm of scanning speech, ataxia and intention tremor; they are usually found during the progressive stage of the disease and are especially disabling.

Motor deficits are often temporarily but strikingly aggravated after a hot bath.

Sensory symptoms are almost invariable at some time during the course of the disease. Paraesthesiae of varying type and distribution occur. Objective impairment of superficial sensation is usually less prominent than would be anticipated from the intensity of symptoms. A distinctive symptom is a tingling or 'electric shock-like' sensation which radiates into the arms, down the back, or into the legs when the patient flexes his head. This is sometimes called the 'barber's chair' sign. It is most commonly due to multiple sclerosis but is not diagnostic thereof since it may occur in other diseases of the cervical spinal cord such as compression, syringomyelia or vitamin B_{12} deficiency. Localised muscle wasting, parkinsonian tremor and choreoathetotic movements are rare and it is unusual for the spinothalamic tracts to be involved to such an extent as to cause painless burns and trophic lesions. As the disease progresses sphincter disturbances occur; notably frequency and urgency of micturition.

A number of patients exhibit a sustained euphoria. This is by no means invariable; some patients are fully aware of their disabilities and become depressed. Late in the course of the disease there is often significant intellectual impairment.

Some abnormality in the CSF is present in approximately 70 per cent of patients. The total protein level is normal in the majority of cases and rarely is raised slightly. An increase in the gammaglobulin fraction is the most frequent finding. A mild lymphocytosis occasionally occurs.

Diagnosis. There is no clinical feature or test which is pathognomonic of multiple sclerosis, which may simulate almost any disease of the nervous system. The diagnosis depends on the demonstration of signs indicating multiple lesions and on a history of relapse and remission. The diagnosis may be suspected but cannot be made with certainty after a single episode of demyelination. Sometimes, as outlined above, the course of multiple sclerosis is progressive and the lesion apparently confined to one area in the spinal cord. Furthermore, remissions may occur in other neurological diseases, such as neurosyphilis. In some cases, therefore, the diagnosis of multiple sclerosis is achieved by a process of exclusion. It is important in all patients to eliminate potentially curable conditions. The appropriate investigations and the lengths to which these should be pursued depend on the particular clinical syndrome. In cases of slowly progressive spastic paraparesis a myelogram may be needed to exclude compression of the spinal cord. Syphilis should always be eliminated and the possibility of vitamin B_{12} deficiency will sometimes need to be explored.

Treatment. There is no curative treatment but much can be done to support the patient during the course of his illness. There is evidence that corticosteroids promote more rapid and complete recovery during acute exacerbations. ACTH given initially in a dose of 120 units daily and gradually reduced over a period of 3 to 4 weeks is a suitable regime. It is probable that 2 mg of dexamethasone given orally three times daily for 5 days is as effective as the more prolonged course of ACTH. There is no evidence that the long-continued administration of corticosteroids significantly alters long-term prognosis. When spasticity is severe, baclofen (20 to 60 mg daily in divided doses) is sometimes very helpful. Severe, painful flexor spasms may be relieved by intrathecal injections of phenol in glycerine.

Of prime importance in the management is encouragement and support of patients and their relatives. Regular medical supervision contributes to this end. Patients with motor disabilities should avoid gain in weight. Some physicians advocate a diet low in animal fat supplemented by linoleic acid in the form of 20 ml of sunflower seed oil daily. Periods of physiotherapy help the disabled patient. Assisted and passive movements and walking exercises improve gait as well as the patient's morale. In general the patient should be advised to avoid long periods in bed during intercurrent infections. Pressure sores should be prevented by advice about changes in posture and skin care; should they occur they must be treated early and vigorously in hospital.

The care of the bladder is particularly important. Infections should be treated with an appropriate antibiotic. Male patients suffering from incontinence, urgency and frequency can be relieved by continuous drainage, through a tube attached to the penis, into a portable urinal strapped to the thigh. In some patients bladder neck resection is helpful. Various appliances are now available which help incontinent female patients. A permanent in-dwelling catheter, changed at intervals of a month or two, often makes life more comfortable and helps to prevent pressure sores.

Walking aids such as tripod supports or frames and the provision of wheel-chairs and motor vehicles together with the advice of an occupational therapist may enable the patient to function more easily at home and at work and to enjoy some form of social life. Nurses and social workers should regularly visit the patient at home to help in their care and to ensure that all the help which the community can provide is made available.

Prognosis. This is variable. Multiple sclerosis does not inevitably lead to immobility and a chair-bound or bedridden existence. Approximately 5 per cent of patients die within 5 years of the onset of the disease but a rather larger proportion remain well and retain unrestricted mobility for 20 years. The disease may run a progressive, disabling course, or may be relatively benign. It is not possible to predict the outlook with confidence in any individual patient though there are some useful indicators.

A favourable course often follows when retrobulbar neuritis is the initial manifestation, particularly when it occurs unaccompanied by any other neural deficit. A long gap between the presentation and the next recurrence often presages a fairly good prognosis, and particularly so if both manifestations recover completely. If motor function is only slightly impaired during the early years of the disease, crippling disability is usually long delayed. Repeated episodes of purely sensory deficit with complete recovery point to a benign course. Those whose initial manifestation is relatively late have usually a better prognosis. In those who show the so-called middle-aged spinal form the disease remains confined to a very slow progressive paraparesis.

Males generally seem to be more severely affected than females. An onset in the late teens or early twenties is often attended by a bad prognosis. Incomplete recovery from the initial attack is a sinister feature. Early recurrence, within 6 months of the initial manifestation, also suggests that relapses are likely to be frequent and disability rapidly progressive. Early manifestations of motor disability or brain stem and cerebellar dysfunction usually forecast a poor outlook. However, at any stage of the disease striking improvement may follow sudden deterioration.

Acute Demyelinating Encephalomyelitis

This is a group of related acute disorders occurring without obvious cause or following an upper respiratory infection and certain infectious diseases such as measles and chickenpox or after vaccination. The pathology is probably due to a sensitivity reaction. There are areas of perivenous demyelination widely disseminated throughout the brain and spinal cord.

Clinical Features. The time of onset varies with the different infectious diseases; in measles it is the 4th to the 6th day, and in chickenpox the 5th to the 12th day of the illness. The disease appears on the 10th to the 12th day after vaccination. Headache, vomiting, pyrexia and delirium are common presenting features and signs of meningeal irritation may also be found. Fits or coma may occur. Flaccid paralysis and extensor plantar responses are common but sensory loss is unusual. Cerebellar signs may be present especially when the disorder follows chickenpox. Retention of urine is also a frequent manifestation.

The CSF may be normal or show a small increase of mononuclear cells and protein. The Lange curve shows no characteristic pattern.

Neuromyelitis optica is a restricted form of the disease characterised by massive demyelination of the spinal cord and both optic nerves.

Diagnosis. When the features of an acute encephalitis occur in association with one of the exanthemata or following vaccination the diagnosis should be easy; in cryptogenic cases viral encephalitis (p. 720) and encephalopathy due to causes such as lead (p. 750) or thiamin deficiency (p. 742) must be considered. It may be impossible to distinguish acute demyelinating encephalomyelitis (or especially neuromyelitis optica) from acute multiple sclerosis until the passage of time has shown that remissions and relapses do not occur. Syphilitic myelitis is distinguished by the serological reactions.

Treatment and Prognosis. ACTH 80–120 units by injection or prednisone 60 mg by mouth daily for several days followed by a maintenance dose for 2 to 3 weeks is beneficial. These drugs must be used with caution in chickenpox if encephalitis develops before the rash has subsided as the rash may become confluent and haemorrhagic. The usual care of the paralysed and incontinent patient is required.

The mortality rate is high in neuromyelitis optica and in postvaccinal encephalomyelitis but is low in the postexanthematous cases. If the patient survives, the recovery may be remarkably complete and second attacks are very rare.

DISEASES OF THE EXTRAPYRAMIDAL SYSTEM

In diseases of this system voluntary movement is disturbed, involuntary movements appear and muscle tone is altered.

Parkinsonism

Parkinsonism is the name given to a clinical syndrome comprising impairment of voluntary movement (hypokinesis), rigidity and tremor. Its prevalence is approximately 1 in every 1,000 of the population rising to about 1 per cent in those over 60 years of age.

Aetiology. Parkinsonism is caused by lesions in the basal ganglia and is associated particularly with damage to the interconnecting system between the substantia nigra and the corpus striatum (caudate nucleus and putamen). The nigrostriatal pathways utilise dopamine as a neurotransmitter, and parkinsonism is associated with a dopamine deficiency. The precise pathophysiology and the interdependent biochemical abnormalities in parkinsonism are incompletely defined.

More than a dozen known agents cause the clinical features of parkinsonism. The commonest entity, accounting for perhaps three-quarters of cases, is paralysis agitans (also called idiopathic parkinsonism or Parkinson's disease) which is of unknown origin. It has been suggested that a slow virus infection might cause paralysis agitans. Parkinsonism is a well-recognised and fairly common sequel of encephalitis lethargica and rarely results from other encephalitides caused by such viruses as Coxsackie type B and Japanese B. Parkinsonism is frequently—and usually wrongly—attributed to cerebral atherosclerosis. Many patients suffering from parkinsonism also show signs of cerebral atherosclerosis, but it is probable, in most instances, that the two conditions—both common in the elderly—occur coincidentally. Discrete cerebrovascular lesions affecting the substantia nigra may, very occasionally, cause parkinsonism.

Of the known causes drug-induced parkinsonism is the commonest. Reserpine, α-methyldopa, the butyrophenones such as haloperidol and, particularly, the drugs of the phenothiazine group all may be responsible. Parkinsonism may occasionally follow a single head injury and is often a sequel of repeated head trauma in the 'punch-drunk' syndrome. There are other infrequent causes of parkinsonism, namely cerebral tumours, notably those causing midbrain compression, parasagittal and sphenoidal ridge meningiomas, meningovascular syphilis, carbon monoxide poisoning, manganese poisoning and copper deposition in Wilson's disease.

Pathology. In parkinsonism the most consistent histological change is cellular loss and depigmentation of the substantia nigra. In paralysis agitans the characteristic pathological changes accompanying loss of cells are Lewy bodies (hyaline masses of cytoplasm and sphingomyelin) in the central areas of the substantia nigra. In postencephalitic parkinsonism the cell depletion affects the whole substantia nigra and is usually more severe than in paralysis agitans. Other changes, such as atrophy of the globus pallidus and patchy cortical atrophy, are inconstant.

Clinical Features. Two-thirds of patients first develop symptoms in the fifth or sixth decades. Initial manifestations are usually so slight and develop so insidiously that a gap of 2 or 3 years may elapse between the onset of the condition and its diagnosis. Occasionally the presentation is acute and progression is rapid; this is particularly likely in postencephalitic or drug-induced cases.

Tremor is usually the feature which causes the patient to seek advice. It first involves the fingers and spreads to proximal parts of the arm; it may later extend to the tongue and legs. The tremor is slow and in the earliest stages involves rhythmical movement of the thumb towards the fingers. The fully developed movement comprises a combination of adduction and abduction of the thumb, flexion and extension of the interphalangeal and metacarpophalangeal joints as well as pronation and supination of the wrists. The tremor is present at rest and often is lessened during purposive activity. Stress and embarrassment aggravate the tremor's amplitude. These factors are operative during clinical testing so that requested movements may be accompanied by increased, rather than reduced, tremor. Head tremors are rare in parkinsonism. Tremor may never be present during the course of the condition and often diminishes as rigidity progresses.

Rigidity is usually detectable early. Resistance to passive movement is increased throughout the range of movement of a joint. Concurrent tremor may lead to the 'cog-wheel' phenomenon—a superimposed jerky sensation. Profound rigidity is accompanied by fixed abnormalities of posture. The patient is flexed at neck, hips, elbows and knees. The hands are flexed at the metacarpophalangeal joints and hyperextended at the interphalangeal joints; these deformities, accompanied by adduction of the thumb across the palm, present a characteristic picture.

Hypokinesis, comprising delay in initiation of movement together with paucity, slowness and lack of precision of movements, is the most disabling feature. Of insidious onset it may first be manifest by a gradual reduction in size and legibility of a patient's handwriting. Other fine movements, such as fastening buttons and laces, are impaired, and later feeding and even turning over in bed become difficult. There is often difficulty in rising from a chair and in starting to walk. Loss of normal arm swinging when the patient walks is a very early sign of hypokinesis. Later the gait displays characteristic features. Steps are short and shuffling. Walking is usually slow but is sometimes accompanied by periods of uncontrolled acceleration when walking downhill. This phenomenon, called festination, causes the patient to take ever more rapid, smaller and smaller steps as he chases his own centre of gravity. Falls often result.

Normally pliant emotional movements of the face are slow in starting, reduced in amplitude and prolonged in their accomplishment. Blinking is usually reduced but spontaneous blepharospasm is an occasional feature, particularly in postencephalitic parkinsonism.

Impaired pupillary accommodation is a common finding in all types of parkinsonism. Sustained, involuntary, conjugate deviation of the eyes, usually upwards, called oculogyric crises, may last for minutes or hours; they occur in postencephalitic and drug-induced parkinsonism.

Speech is often affected. Some loss of voice volume is almost invariable. Delayed initiation and dysarthria are common. The cadence is slow; inflection is restricted so that speech becomes monotonous.

Hypokinesis may be overcome for short periods under the influence of a strong emotional drive such as fear or anger. Though the defects in voluntary movement are often striking and disabling, power is well preserved.

Pyramidal tract signs are not found in uncomplicated paralysis agitans, but they may be detected if there is accompanying cerebral atherosclerosis; they commonly accompany postencephalitic and post-traumatic parkinsonism and are found in those rare instances where parkinsonism is due to a cerebral tumour.

Little diagnostic help is afforded by special investigations. Electromyography can confirm the rate of a tremor. Low levels of homovanillic acid (a dopamine metabolite) in the cerebrospinal fluid are found in parkinsonism but the normal range is wide and such estimations are rarely diagnostic in an individual case.

Differential Diagnosis. Physiological tremor often is exaggerated in the elderly. Anxiety, alcoholism and thyrotoxicosis also increase the amplitude of physiological tremor. Physiological tremor is much faster than parkinsonian tremor, tends to occur only in one plane and lacks the abduction/adduction movement of the thumb.

Cerebellar atrophy is of fairly frequent occurrence in elderly patients who manifest intention tremor. Such a tremor is relieved when an affected limb is supported and relaxed and increases as the limb approaches a target.

Depressed and hypothyroid patients are often apathetic and lack normal facial expressiveness so that their appearance may suggest a diagnosis of parkinsonism.

Atherosclerotic dementia, with its attendant apathy, is often associated with increased tone due to bilateral pyramidal signs and may mimic parkinsonism. Other clinical features such as an exaggerated jaw jerk, increased tendon reflexes and spasticity rather than rigidity differentiate this condition from parkinsonism.

Treatment. Ideally, this should be aimed at the cause. The drug-induced condition is the only type which is both relatively common and curable. If the offending drug is discontinued, patients are usually, but not invariably, relieved of parkinsonian symptoms. Removal of a tumour and treatment with penicillin of the rare cases due to syphilis may improve parkinsonian features. In the majority of parkinsonian patients the cause is not known and treatment is designed to ameliorate disability. The most effective treatment now available is a combination of an anticholinergic preparation together with levodopa plus a decarboxylase inhibitor.

Anticholinergic drugs produce modest improvement in parkinsonism. There are a number of synthetic preparations, such as benzhexol hydrochloride (2 mg or 5 mg), benztropine (2 mg) and orphenadrine (50 mg). One of these drugs is introduced in small amounts, such as one tablet twice daily, and the dose is increased until toxic effects of dryness of the mouth or blurring of vision supervene. The dose is then reduced slightly to obviate these effects.

Levodopa has strikingly improved the treatment of parkinsonism. Given by mouth in doses varying from 2 to 8 g (average 5 g) daily levodopa reduces disability in more than two-thirds of patients and is particularly effective in relieving hypokinesis. The drug causes many side-effects, some of which develop early, e.g. nausea, vomiting, and cardiac arrhythmias; these are reduced if the drug is given together with a dopadecarboxylase inhibitor.

More than 90 per cent of an orally ingested dose of levodopa does not reach the brain and is metabolised in extracerebral tissues. Selective inhibition of extracerebral dopadecarboxylase reduces the amount of levodopa required to produce a therapeutic effect and also diminishes the side-effects caused by peripheral breakdown of levodopa. Preparations are available which combine levodopa with extracerebral dopadecarboxylase inhibitors, e.g. 250 mg of levodopa and 25 mg of carbidopa (Sinemet). One such tablet is equivalent in its therapeutic effect to 1 g of levodopa. This combined therapy, like levodopa itself, must be introduced in small amounts (half of a tablet twice daily) and increased gradually by a further half tablet every 4 or 5 days. Another preparation (Madopar) contains levodopa and benserazide in the ratio of 4 to 1; average effective daily doses range between 400 and 800 mg of levodopa in this combination, which is equivalent to five times this amount given in isolation.

The long-term and centrally determined side-effects of levodopa are not reduced by combined therapy. Induced involuntary movements and psychiatric disturbances are very troublesome and may demand reduction or temporary cessation of treatment. Particularly disabling is the so-called 'on/off' effect which develops in patients who have been treated, often with considerable success, for more than 2 years. Manifestations of this phenomenon include unsteadiness of gait, hypotonia, anxiety and, commonly, profound akinesia. These disabilities tend to develop and regress suddenly. Accompanying the 'on/off' effect in some patients and persisting between the acute manifestations are unusual defects in higher cerebral function, including disinhibition, aphasia, apraxia and memory impairment. It seems likely that the frequency of occurrence of these distressing phenomena increases as treatment becomes more prolonged. Their alleviation requires withdrawal of levodopa therapy for several weeks, after which patients will often again tolerate and derive benefit from the drug.

Alternative treatment includes agonists which sensitise dopaminergic receptors. The most useful is bromocriptine (p. 507). An initial dose of 2·5 mg twice daily is gradually built up to 30 to 40 mg daily. The drug may be given alone or in combination with levodopa. Amantadine hydrochloride, an antiviral agent (100 mg b.d.), produces some effects both therapeutic and untoward, resembling those of levodopa but less in degree; improvement is maintained for only a few months in most cases. Other drugs, notably amphetamine and tricyclic antidepressants, have mild antiparkinsonian properties. Monoaminoxidase inhibitors should not be given to patients taking levodopa.

Stereotactic thalamotomy is now rarely employed; however, for those occasional patients whose disability is unilateral tremor unresponsive to medical treatment, it may be helpful.

Prognosis. There are extreme variations in the rate of progression and the degree of disability produced. Twenty per cent of patients suffering from parkinsonism at any given time cannot cope independently with the normal activities of living. The mortality of patients suffering from parkinsonism is three times that of the general population of similar age. Levodopa, though it ameliorates disability, does not affect the progress of the basic pathology. There is some evidence that it slightly increases life expectancy.

Hepatolenticular Degeneration

Aetiology. Hepatolenticular degeneration (*Wilson's disease*) is a rare autosomal recessive disorder of copper metabolism. Copper is normally absorbed in small amounts from the gut as a loose complex with albumin and carried to the liver. There some of it is reexcreted in the bile but a fraction enters the general circulation. In the liver some of the blood copper is transferred to globulin to which it is more firmly bound, forming caeruloplasmin. This copper-globulin is an oxidase enzyme but its physiological role is unknown.

In Wilson's disease copper is absorbed in excess but the transfer from the albumin-bound to the globulin-bound complex is defective, thus the serum caeruloplasmin level is low. Some of the extra copper absorbed is excreted in the urine while the rest is deposited in the tissues, particularly in the brain, liver, kidney and in Descemet's membrane in the eye. These organs may be damaged either by enzymatic poisoning by the heavy metal or by cellular necrosis followed by fibrosis (or gliosis in the brain).

Clinical Features. The biochemical abnormality of Wilson's disease is present from birth, but clinical evidence does not appear until adolescence. There are two main clinical types depending on whether the cerebral or hepatic signs are more evident.

In the cerebral type necrosis and sclerosis of the corpus striatum cause basal ganglion syndromes in adolescence. Most common is choreoathetosis, but parkinsonism may be caused according to the site mainly affected. There is usually cortical involvement leading to progressive dementia in which loss of emotional control is a feature.

In the hepatic type (p. 457) episodes of jaundice, fulminant hepatic failure, active chronic hepatitis or a well-compensated cirrhosis may occur.

In both types copper deposition in Descemet's membrane of the eye causes a golden-brown, yellow or green ring round the cornea. This Kayser-Fleischer ring is pathognomonic of Wilson's disease.

The urine contains excess copper and often excess amino acids. Renal tubular damage by copper may upset excretion of uric acid, sugar and phosphates. Caeruloplasmin is deficient in the blood (p. 432).

Treatment. This disorder was previously progressive and fatal within a few years after the appearance of clinical signs. It can now be arrested by giving copper-binding drugs (chelating agents) which mobilise copper from the tissues and promote its excretion in the urine. The most valuable of these is penicillamine, 300 mg t.d.s. orally. If it is not available or too expensive, dimercaprol (BAL) or disodium calcium versenate may be given but either is a less satisfactory substitute. Hepatic and cerebral symptoms are treated symptomatically with diet and antiparkinsonism drugs.

Siblings should be examined as clinical or biochemical evidence of Wilson's disease may be detected at a stage where treatment, if started promptly and continued throughout life, may prevent the appearance or progression of clinical features.

Kernicterus

Kernicterus is a disorder of the basal ganglia and auditory nuclei occurring in association with neonatal jaundice, particularly in premature infants. It may be caused by haemolytic disease of the newborn (p. 609), but any severe neonatal jaundice may be followed by this complication, and prematurity is more important than Rh incompatibility.

Premature babies have a functional immaturity of the glucuronyl transferase enzyme system of the liver, and as a result of this unconjugated bilirubin formed by haemolysis of any sort is not conjugated. When the infant is born it is deprived of its placental excretion route, and unconjugated bilirubin rapidly accumulates in its blood to toxic levels which depress oxidative metabolism of brain cells, and in particular those of the basal ganglia. The danger decreases rapidly about 10 days after the birth in normal full-term infants when the liver enzyme system matures, but the premature baby is in danger for a longer period.

Clinical Features. Convulsions, coma, opisthotonos and rigidity may be early manifestations but athetoid movements or spastic paralysis, deafness of nuclear type, and mental deficiency may not appear until the baby is several months old.

Prevention and Treatment. Prevention depends on the early detection of haemolytic jaundice, especially in the premature child, and its prompt treatment by exchange transfusion (p. 610). There is no treatment for established kernicterus and the future management is that of the child with cerebral palsy.

Chorea

Choreiform movements are irregular, jerking, ill-sustained and unpredictable, easily recognised when fully developed. In milder forms the condition may seem to be no more than restlessness or fidgeting. Often chorea is accompanied by athetoid movements.

Sydenham's Chorea

Sydenham's chorea (St. Vitus' dance) occurs in adolescents and is commoner in girls. It often follows a streptococcal throat infection. The onset may be abrupt or insidious. Choreiform movements are usually generalised and are accompanied by emotional lability so that often the condition is thought initially to be psychogenic. Pregnancy may precipitate a recurrence of chorea.

Because of the agitation, the patient, in all but the mildest cases, should be admitted to hospital and preferably nursed in isolation. Diazepam or haloperidol should be prescribed. An initial course of penicillin should be given.

Most patients recover within a month, though more prolonged illnesses occur and relapses are common. Since many patients later develop valvular heart disease their future observation and management should be as for rheumatic fever.

Huntington's Chorea

Huntington's chorea is of autosomal dominant inheritance and usually first presents in the thirties. Choreiform movements, often particularly prominent in the face, are accompanied by progressive dementia. The movements may be well controlled by tetrabenazine (50–200 mg/d) which is usually tolerated in this condition. The mental deterioration is untreatable and institutional care may be needed as the disease progresses.

Ballism

Flinging limb movements of wide amplitude are called ballismic movements. They resemble chorea but are much more violent. It is sometimes an arbitrary decision whether one calls movements severe chorea or ballism. Usually they suddenly affect one side of the body (hemiballism or, if less dramatic, hemichorea) as a result of a vascular lesion in elderly patients. Spontaneous improvement usually occurs over a period of weeks and during this time tetrabenazine may mitigate the disability. When hemiballism persists it can effectively be treated by stereotactic thalamotomy.

Athetosis

Athetoid movements are relatively slow, confluent, writhing movements, usually most prominent at the periphery of the limbs. They are often accompanied by choreiform movements and by forced axial rotations of the trunk and neck (torsion dystonia). Athetosis usually results from cerebral hypoxia or trauma at birth or during the neonatal period and from kernicterus. Drug treatment is usually ineffective, though tetrabenazine, haloperidol or diazepam occasionally produce improvement in mild cases. Stereotactic procedures, indicated only in severe disability, sometimes help.

Differential Diagnosis. The involuntary movements of chorea, athetosis and ballism must be distinguished from *tics* which in most cases are not due to organic disease of the nervous system. Tics are usually rapid, repetitive, co-ordinated and stereotyped movements, most of which can be mimicked. Their pattern varies widely but an individual's tic tends to be reproduced faithfully. Common mild tics, including blepharospasm, sniffing, and shrugging movements, may be irritating but rarely need treatment. When well established in an adult they are virtually irremediable. In contrast, many children develop tics, often elaborate facial movements which cause much parental concern but which almost always disappear.

In adults, tics of recent development may be induced by drugs. Amphetamine addiction leads to repeated, rapid chewing movements of the jaws. Complex tongue, mouth, and cheek movements may result from taking phenothiazines or levodopa. Withdrawal of the causal drug usually leads to rapid cessation of the movement.

Spasmodic torticollis is a form of tic which is sometimes regarded as a psychogenic disorder but which may well be due to as yet unidentified changes in the extrapyramidal system. Spasmodic torticollis chiefly comprises involuntary turning of the head to one side and starts most commonly in the thirties. Initially rapid and correctable rotating movements may give place to long-sustained and later to fixed deviation of the neck.

CONGENITAL AND DEGENERATIVE DISEASES

In many diseases of unknown cause, there is clinical and pathological evidence of damage which is confined to a special type of neurone, e.g. motor neurone disease. Although no causative factors have been identified, it seems probable that many of the following disorders will ultimately be classified together as being due to 'biochemical lesions'. The metabolic functions of the neurone are controlled by its cell body but when any gradual failure of any of these processes occurs the effect is first seen at the end of its axon, so that there occurs a progressive 'dying back' of the neurone from its termination towards the cell body, associated with loss of nucleoprotein in the cell (chromatolysis). This will be seen to be the typical feature of the pathology of the congenital and degenerative disorders.

Motor Neurone Disease

This rare disorder is the paradigm of a systematised neurological disease.

Aetiology and Pathology. The cause is unknown. Toxic causes have been adduced (p. 141). Metallic poisoning, particularly by aluminium, has been implicated. As in all progressive neurological disorders autoimmune and slow virus aetiologies have been postulated. The latter possibility at present seems particularly attractive since Creutzfeldt-Jakob disease (p. 719) is of proven slow virus origin and shows some features in common with motor neurone disease.

Loss of motor neurones and gliosis can be demonstrated in the motor cortex, in the motor nuclei of the brain stem and in anterior horn cells of the spinal cord. In the cord, there is also loss of myelinated corticospinal fibres.

Clinical Features. Motor neurone disease is characterised by the insidious onset and uninterrupted progression of combinations of lesions of upper and/or lower motor neurones. The condition is twice as common in males and is rare before 40 years of age. The commonest age of onset is in the sixth decade. Some patterns of evolution are frequently manifest and are usefully categorised because they offer a guide to prognosis.

Progressive bulbar palsy comprises dysarthria, dysphonia and dysphagia. Impaired articulation is usually the earliest feature but difficulty in swallowing, hoarseness and loss of voice volume supervene. There are signs of true, as well as supranuclear, bulbar palsy. Wasting and fasciculation of the tongue are accompanied by spasticity thereof and a pathologically brisk jaw jerk. Features of bulbar palsy eventually develop in the later stages of the other types listed below.

Amyotrophic lateral sclerosis is probably the commonest mode of presentation and is characterised by lower motor neurone signs in the upper limbs and pyramidal tract signs in the legs. Wasting and weakness of the small muscles of the hands, usually the earliest manifestation, are accompanied by spasticity of the legs and extensor plantar responses. Wasting and fasciculation spread to the proximal arm muscles and the leg musculature; increased tendon reflexes in the arms may later indicate involvement of the upper motor neurones.

Progressive lateral sclerosis is an uncommon entity in which progressive paraparesis usually antedates lower motor neurone signs by many months.

Progressive muscular atrophy implicates only lower motor neurones for long periods. It usually presents with foot drop, which is often initially unilateral but eventually becomes symmetrical. Wasting and weakness of the hands, proximal spread of lower motor neurone affection in the limbs and the addition of pyramidal tract affection occur after an interval of years.

Course. These labelled entities are frequently recognised but variant patterns are common. As the disease progresses the pictures of the different categories merge so that the final picture usually includes severe bulbar palsy as well as upper and lower motor neurone signs in all four limbs.

Diagnosis. Some aspects of the clinical features of motor neurone disease, irrespective of the particular type of natural history, are useful in diagnosis. There are no sensory signs. Sensory symptoms, with the exception of pain, are rare. Aches caused by the use of weakened muscles and painful cramps in the legs are fairly common. Paraesthesiae, unless clearly attributable to a coincidental cause, are not a feature of motor neurone disease and their presence should lead to critical reappraisal of the diagnosis. Fasciculations (p. 660) though far from pathognomonic of the condition, are seen almost invariably in motor neurone disease in which they are usually more obvious and more widespread than in any other disease. Though the initial manifestations are commonly unilateral, the affection becomes bilateral, and indeed symmetrical, in the vast majority of instances, within a few months.

In few other conditions do severely wasted muscles subserve pathologically brisk tendon reflexes. This phenomenon, sometimes called tonic atrophy is common to all types of motor neurone disease other than progressive muscular atrophy during its early stages. Defects in external ocular movements and sphincter disturbances are extremely rare. Full awareness and normal intellectual abilities are usually preserved intact throughout the course of the illness. The CSF is almost always normal.

Differential Diagnosis. The conditions which need to be distinguished depend on the pattern of affection presented.

Features of dysphagia, dysarthria and dysphonia resembling progressive bulbar palsy may result from bilateral cerebrovascular lesions within the cerebral hemispheres. The latter condition is characterised by sudden exacerbations due to small strokes and is usually accompanied by dementia (pseudobulbar palsy). Bulbar myasthenia presents similar but usually variable disabilities. An intravenous edrophonium test confirms the diagnosis of myasthenia.

Amyotrophic lateral sclerosis needs to be differentiated from cervical spondylosis, tumours of the cervical cord, syringomyelia and thrombosis of an anterior spinal artery. Sensory features usually distinguish the former three conditions and the last is of sudden onset.

Primary lateral sclerosis may initially be indistinguishable from multiple sclerosis, particularly from the spinal type seen in middle age. The lack of sphincter involvement, the later development of lower motor signs and the normal CSF as well as the progression of the condition usually serve to differentiate motor neurone disease from multiple sclerosis.

The initial foot drop of progressive muscular atrophy may suggest the diagnosis of a prolapsed lumbar intervertebral disc. Sciatica and root sensory loss are absent in progressive muscular atrophy which eventually progresses and extends symmetrically. Some types of predominantly motor polyneuropathy (p. 750) may need to be differentiated from progressive muscular atrophy by investigation.

Though a large number of conditions may be confused with the various types of motor neurone disease they can usually be distinguished by the clinical features and natural history. Three pathological processes which are potentially treatable may closely mimic motor neurone disease and should always be excluded. (i) An occult carcinoma (particularly of the bronchus) may produce systematised motor neurone lesions. A chest radiograph should always be obtained in patients presenting the features of motor neurone disease, and if there are indicative clinical features further investigations should be performed. (ii) Diabetic amyotrophy (p. 782) may resemble motor neurone disease and accordingly diabetes mellitus must be excluded. (iii) Meningovascular syphilis can present a picture similar to that of motor neurone disease and syphilitic serology is an essential investigation.

The CSF should always be examined if motor neurone disease is suspected. Any abnormality therein should intensify the search for an alternative diagnosis.

Treatment. No medical treatment improves the outlook in motor neurone disease. Claims have been made for the efficacy of steroids, amantadine and various mixtures of amino acids but none has been substantiated. Management includes the provision of walking aids and wheel-chairs and the maintenance of morale. Physicians have a duty to support patients and their relatives and to relieve distress in the disease's terminal stages.

Prognosis. Motor neurone disease is inexorably progressive and invariably fatal. Death usually results from pneumonia and respiratory failure and within 2 years of the onset of bulbar palsy. Amyotrophic lateral sclerosis and primary lateral sclerosis are compatible with 4 or 5 years of life from the initial manifestation. Progressive muscular atrophy runs the most prolonged course; death usually occurs in 8 to 10 years from the onset.

The final state, resulting in anarthria, aphagia and widespread limb weakness in a patient fully aware of his state is unbearably distressing for the patient and his family.

The Hereditary Ataxias

This is a group of related hereditary or familial disorders in which the systems of neurones which 'die back' (p. 735) are mainly the spinal and brain stem tracts leading to the cerebellum, the corticospinal tracts, and the optic nerves. Different combinations of these elements form recognisable clinical pictures, which usually 'breed true' in a family, but it may be impossible to differentiate the different types during life. The group forms a link with hereditary disorders of the peripheral nerves such as peroneal muscular atrophy (p. 750) and with neurofibromatosis (p. 739) and these may occur in association with the hereditary ataxias either in one individual or in the same family. Congenital deformities, particularly pes cavus, are also commonly present.

Clinical Features. The onset may be any time from infancy to middle life. Symptoms are slowly progressive. Where cerebellar or spinocerebellar neurones are involved there is progressive ataxia of gait, followed by intention tremor of the arms, dysarthria of explosive type and, in some types, nystagmus. Where the main lesion is in corticospinal tracts there is a hereditary spastic paraplegia. Optic atrophy and loss of bladder reflexes may occur.

Friedreich's ataxia is the most common type, usually familial but occasionally sporadic. Unaffected members of the family as well as the patients may show pes cavus. There is degeneration of the spinocerebellar and corticospinal tracts, and of the posterior columns. There is therefore very severe ataxia. Tendon jerks are lost at an early stage, the ankle jerks first, then the knee jerks but finally all tendon jerks may be absent. Muscle tone is decreased. The plantar reflexes are extensor. Muscle-joint and vibration senses are impaired as the posterior column degeneration progresses. Scoliosis and pes cavus are almost invariable and other congenital abnormalities such as spina bifida and conduction defects in the heart, giving rise to ECG abnormalities, are common.

Diagnosis. The familial history, the presence of pes cavus, and the absence of remissions distinguish these diseases from multiple sclerosis. In Friedreich's ataxia tendon reflexes are absent and there may be electrocardiographic changes.

Onset of cerebellar degeneration in later life is often due to carcinomatous neuropathy (p. 757).

Treatment and Prognosis. There is no specific treatment. Co-ordination exercises and occupational therapy will help the patient to overcome his disability in the early stages but a wheel-chair life becomes inevitable later. Scoliosis and pes cavus may require appropriate appliances or orthopaedic surgery. All diseases of this group are progressive but compatible with a long life.

Syringomyelia

Cavities, filled with fluid and surrounded by glial tissue, lying near to the centre of the spinal cord, are the characteristic pathological lesions in syringomyelia.

Aetiology. Central cavities were thought to result from incomplete fusion of the cord or from the inclusion of abnormal cells within the cord. These explanations may account for some cases, but it seems likely that many cavities represent dilatation of the central canal of the cord. This dilatation often results from increased pressure in the canal associated with congenital malformations of the brain in the region of the foramen magnum. Herniation of parts on the cerebellum through the foramen magnum (*Arnold-Chiari syndrome*) and cysts in this area are found.

The most important aetiological factor is failure of development of the foramina of Magendie and Luschka. Cerebrospinal fluid cannot escape into the subarachnoid space from the fourth ventricle since its roof is imperforate. Pressure rises within the closed ventricular system and is communicated to the central canal of the cord which expands along irregular paths of least resistance. The expanding cavity usually disrupts second order spinothalamic neurones (p. 664), often interrupts the lateral columns and may extend laterally to damage anterior horn cells. Clinical signs predictably reflect the interruption of function of these neural structures which is usually maximal in the lower cervical region.

Clinical Features. Symptoms are of insidious onset, and slow progression. Patients usually present in the third or fourth decade but signs may be detectable much earlier.

Sensory Features. Most characteristic is 'dissociated' sensory loss, i.e. loss or depression of pain and temperature sensation with preservation of the modalities of touch, vibration and position. The patient often recognises this sensory loss and seeks advice because of it. Less commonly, when pain fibres are irritated, pain in the arms is a presenting feature.

Trophic Lesions. Loss of protective sensory functions leads to painless burns and ulcers on the hands and sometimes painless, disorganised joints (*Charcot's joints*) in the upper limbs.

Motor Features. Wasting of the small muscles of one or other hand is often manifest early. Characteristically there are pyramidal tract signs in the legs.

Reflex Changes. Loss of one or more reflexes in the arms is almost invariable. Hyperreflexia in the legs and extensor plantar responses are common.

Associated Skeletal Abnormalities. Kyphoscoliosis, pes cavus and spina bifida are commonly found.

Syringobulbia. Upward extension of the cavities to involve the lower brain stem leads to dissociated sensory loss on the face, palatal palsy, Horner's syndrome and nystagmus.

Investigations should be aimed at defining potentially treatable anomalies around the foramen magnum. Straight radiographs of this area may show bony malformations. Myelography or pneumoencephalography should be performed in order to demonstrate cysts or Arnold-Chiari malformations.

Treatment and Prognosis. Where causative congenital lesions are demonstrated early, surgical treatment is indicated. A variety of procedures have been used. Decompression of the foramen magnum, opening the roof of the fourth ventricle, aspiration of the cavity in the cord and occlusion, by muscle, of the upper end of the central canal, may prevent progression of the disease.

If surgical treatment is not feasible, management is directed toward preventing the patient injuring himself, and relieving pain, when present, by radiotherapy aimed at the cavity. If untreated the condition is slowly progressive, and worsens if the brain stem is involved.

Neurofibromatosis

Neurofibromatosis (*von Recklinghausen's disease*) is an autosomal dominant disorder in which tumours are derived from the neurilemmal sheath of the peripheral nerves, nerve roots or cranial nerves. Cutaneous fibromas, which are pedunculated tumours named *mollusca fibrosa*, are considered to be of similar origin. Tumours such as gliomas, meningiomas and phaeochromocytomas may also be associated with neurofibromatosis.

Clinical Features. A patient may show only one or many of a wide range of cutaneous or of peripheral or central neurological abnormalities. Some of the more comon are *café-au-lait* patches of skin pigmentation, cutaneous fibromas and benign tumours of peripheral nerves which are discrete, movable lumps arranged along lines of nerves. The nerve trunks may be thickened or there may be a diffuse plexiform growth. Solitary neurofibromas may occur on a spinal nerve root or on a cranial nerve, especially the eighth. The tumours may also occur within body cavities, in the eyes and within the bones where they cause cystic change or kyphoscoliosis. New tumours gradually appear throughout life but the progress is slow. Any tumour may become malignant (sarcoma) but the chances of it doing so are small.

Biopsy of a tumour is rarely necessary. With intracranial and intraspinal types the protein level of the CSF is very high, often exceeding 10 g/l (1,000 mg/100 ml). Radiology may show that an internal auditory meatus or intervertebral foramen is widened if it contains a neurofibroma.

Treatment. No treatment is required unless there is cerebral or spinal compression, or sarcomatous change, when operative removal of the tumour is necessary.

NUTRITIONAL NEUROLOGICAL SYNDROMES

As with the hereditary and degenerative diseases, deficiency diseases affect particular types of cells according to their peculiarities of metabolism. The cell bodies are damaged but the neurones tend to 'die back' from the periphery. The most susceptible neurones appear to be those of the peripheral nerves, the longest fibres usually being the first affected as in the polyneuropathies of beriberi, alcoholism and pregnancy (p. 139).

The spinal cord is involved in vitamin B_{12} neuropathy and the mid-brain in Wernicke's encephalopathy (p. 742).

Vitamin B_{12} Neuropathy

(Subacute Combined Degeneration of the Cord)

This disease is characterised by peripheral neuropathy together with progressive degeneration of the posterior and lateral columns of the spinal cord.

Aetiology. The disease is due to deficiency of vitamin B_{12}. It most commonly appears about the age of 50 in patients who are found also to be suffering from pernicious anaemia but it is sometimes the initial manifestation of vitamin B_{12} deficiency. The condition may be produced by the administration of folic acid to patients with Addisonian pernicious anaemia. Vitamin B_{12} neuropathy is rarely found after gastrectomy or other causes of malabsorption of vitamin B_{12}.

Pathology. Degenerative changes develop in the peripheral nerves. Areas of demyelination appear in the lower cervical and upper thoracic regions of the spinal cord, particularly in the posterior columns, the corticospinal tracts and the spinocerebellar tracts. These tracts then demyelinate and subsequently the axis cylinders break down starting from the termination of the tract and spreading towards the appropriate cells of origin. Areas of degeneration may also appear in the cerebral white matter and in the optic nerves.

Clinical Features. The disease usually develops gradually and almost invariably the presenting symptoms are due to peripheral neuropathy, usually tingling paraesthesiae of the toes, spreading later to the fingers. The patient also complains that the extremities feel cold and numb, and he may notice difficulty in holding small objects. Motor symptoms, such as weakness and ataxia, appear later but become severe as the cord is involved.

The physical signs depend on the relative involvement of the peripheral nerves and the posterior and lateral columns. Objective sensory changes are almost invariably present and consist of impairment of all forms of sensation in the distal parts of the limbs ascending in a 'stocking and glove' fashion. Sensory loss may spread on to the trunk where it may show a horizontal border. Tenderness of the muscles, especially of the calves, is commonly found in the early stages of the disease and indicates the presence of peripheral neuropathy. Position sense and vibration sense are commonly impaired. In the majority of cases sensory ataxia is the outstanding feature. In the minority of cases, signs of an upper motor neurone lesion predominate in the lower limbs. The condition of the tendon reflexes depends on the extent of involvement of peripheral neurones. Most commonly the ankle jerks are lost and later the knee jerks, though increase in these reflexes may be found. Primary optic atrophy occurs on rare occasions and, in severe cases, mental impairment is not uncommon.

The CSF is normal. There is usually achlorhydria though free hydrochloric acid may be found in malabsorption states leading to vitamin B_{12} neuropathy. Examination of the blood and sternal marrow shows a macrocytic anaemia with megaloblastic formation. The level of vitamin B_{12} in the serum is low and its uptake from the gastrointestinal tract is impaired.

Diagnosis. The presentation of a patient with symmetrical paraesthesiae in the limbs should always raise the suspicion of vitamin B_{12} neuropathy and evidence of involvement of the posterior and lateral columns of the cord should be sought. The association with glossitis, megaloblastic anaemia and achlorhydria strongly suggests the diagnosis which should be confirmed by estimation of the serum vitamin B_{12} level. Peripheral neuropathy from other causes may present in the same way but without signs of spinal cord involvement. Tabes dorsalis may be confused with vitamin B_{12} neuropathy because of the sensory loss in the distal parts of the limb, absent reflexes and ataxia, but the muscles are less tender than normal, and other signs of syphilitic infection such as the Argyll Robertson pupil and changes in the CSF are commonly found. Multiple sclerosis and myelopathy due to cervical spondylosis may give rise to damage to the posterolateral columns but there are no signs of peripheral neuritis. Combined spinal cord and peripheral nerve lesions may be caused by carcinomatous neuropathy (p. 756).

Treatment and Prognosis. The treatment of vitamin B_{12} neuropathy is that of pernicious anaemia (p. 603), but the dose of hydroxocyanocobalamin should be two or three times as large as is given in uncomplicated cases of pernicious anaemia and this intensive therapy must be continued as long as there is evidence of neurological improvement. Thereafter, regular maintenance doses sufficient to keep the blood normal must be given for the rest of the patient's life.

Untreated subacute combined degeneration of the cord progresses to death within about 2 years. The response to treatment depends on the stage at which it is initiated. If signs are due only to peripheral neuropathy a complete recovery may be expected. Ataxia may improve remarkably. If, however, there is severe damage to the spinal cord, only limited improvement in signs such as spasticity can be anticipated although the progress of the disease can be arrested.

Wernicke's Encephalopathy

This condition, which is due to thiamin deficiency (p. 128), often presents acutely. The cardinal features are disorders of ocular movement, impaired pupillary reflexes, nystagmus and Korsakoff's psychosis (p. 131). The defects of eye movement vary and nystagmus may be of cerebellar or ataxic type (p. 677). The condition may be rapidly fatal or may leave permanent neural deficit. It should be considered in any patient who exhibits any disorder of ocular movement or an acute psychosis, and particularly so in alcoholics and in prolonged vomiting. Immediate treatment with 50 mg of thiamin hydrochloride given slowly intravenously, followed by 50 mg daily, given intramuscularly, will often result in dramatic improvement. Recovery will be complete if treatment is started within a few hours of the onset of treatment and is progressively less complete the longer treatment is delayed.

Other Nutritional Neurological Syndromes

These are described in the chapter on nutritional disorders (p. 138).

Compression of the Spinal Cord or Nerve Roots

Aetiology and Pathology. The more important causes of spinal cord compression are:

1. *In the vertebral column:* crush fracture of a vertebral body; posterior protrusion of an intervertebral disc; secondary carcinoma (from breast, prostate, bronchus or other sites); myelomatosis and tuberculous disease of the spine.

2. *In relation to the spinal meninges:* epidural abscess; tumours (meningioma, neurofibroma; infiltration with lymphomatous and leukaemic deposits); arachnoiditis and syphilitic leptomeningitis (common causes in some tropical countries).

3. *In the spinal cord:* tumours (gliomas, ependymoma and metastatic deposits).

Tumours, disc protrusions and trauma account for the majority of cases of spinal cord compression. It is convenient in practice to divide the tumours into those arising outside the spinal cord (extramedullary), which constitute about 80 per cent, and those arising within (intramedullary).

A space-occupying lesion within the spinal canal may involve nerve tissue directly by pressure, or indirectly by interfering with the blood supply. Oedema from venous obstruction impairs the function of the neurones. Ischaemia from arterial obstruction leads to necrosis of the spinal cord. The earlier stages are reversible but severely damaged neurones do not recover so it is most important to diagnose and treat spinal compression without delay.

Clinical Features. The onset of symptoms of spinal cord compression is usually slow but it may be acute with trauma or metastases, especially if there is arterial occlusion. Pain localised over the spine or in a root distribution is the most common initial symptom. It may be aggravated by spinal movement or by coughing, sneezing or straining at the toilet which cause temporary increase in the pressure of the spinal fluid. Paraesthesiae and numbness or cold sensations may also develop early, especially in the lower limbs. Motor symptoms, which usually appear later, consist of heaviness, stiffness or weakness of a limb. Urgency or hesitancy of micturition, leading eventually to urinary retention is usually a late manifestation.

The signs found on examination vary according to the structures involved. There may be a local kyphosis if there is spinal disease, and local tenderness may be present with vertebral disease or extradural abscess. A bruit may be heard with a stethoscope over the site of a vascular tumour (angioma). Involvement of the posterior roots gives rise to hyperaesthesia and later to sensory loss over the appropriate dermatome. When the anterior roots are affected there are signs of a lower motor neurone lesion at the corresponding level. Interruption of ascending fibres in the spinal cord causes sensory loss below the level of the lesion which may be of superficial sensation or of proprioceptive sense, according to which tracts are mainly involved. Light touch, however, is often affected early. Interruption of descending fibres gives rise to upper motor neurone signs below the level of the lesion and control of the sphincters may be lost. If damage is confined to one side of the cord the *syndrome of Brown-Séquard* results. On the side of the lesion there is a band of hyperaesthesia with below it loss of proprioceptive sense and upper motor neurone signs. On the other side there is loss of spinothalamic sensation (pain, warmth and cold) as fibres of that tract decussate soon after entering the cord.

The distribution of these signs varies with the level of the lesion. Lesions above the fifth cervical segment give signs of an upper motor neurone lesion and sensory loss in upper and lower limbs (tetraplegia); a lesion between the fifth cervical and first thoracic segments gives signs of a lower motor neurone lesion and segmental sensory loss in the upper limbs and signs of an upper motor neurone lesion in the lower limbs; a lesion in the thoracic cord causes a spastic paraplegia with sensory loss having a horizontal upper level on the trunk; a lesion in the lumbosacral cord gives signs of a lower motor neurone lesion in the appropriate segments of the lower limbs and sensory loss. Spinal lesions lower than the first lumbar vertebra cannot damage the spinal cord but may damage the roots of the cauda equina.

Examination of the CSF is of great value but withdrawal of fluid may alter the pressure balance above and below the lesion in the cord and lead to rapid exacerbation of compression. For this reason, if lumbar puncture confirms the diagnosis, the patient should be referred without any delay to a neurosurgeon and if the diagnosis is highly probable on clinical grounds the puncture should be postponed until it is convenient to operate on the patient. Queckenstedt's test may reveal the features of a partial or complete block but a normal result does not exclude the diagnosis. The cell content is normal but there is a great excess of protein and xanthochromia is present (*Froin's syndrome*). Radiological examination of the spine may reveal abnormalities at the site of the lesion but often contrast radiography, after introduction of air or a radio-opaque substance into the spinal canal (myelography), is required.

Diagnosis. Pain, which is so often a presenting symptom of spinal cord compression, may be wrongly attributed to such conditions as pleurisy, cholecystitis or 'rheumatism', but a careful examination will reveal signs of organic nervous disease. It is insufficient to be content with eliciting the tendon reflexes, as motor signs may be delayed long after sensory signs are present. If there is indisputable evidence of spinal cord damage it is essential to decide the site of the primary lesion. A general examination may reveal evidence of disease elsewhere making it likely that the lesion in the cord is secondary to this. A careful search should be made for a primary tumour in another organ, enlargement of lymph nodes, the cutaneous signs of neurofibromatosis and the presence of sepsis which could lead to extradural abscess. An abscess should always be considered if pain is severe and signs of cord disease develop rapidly as immediate treatment is imperative. If the lesion causing compression arose initially in the spinal cord it is necessary to distinguish it from conditions such as multiple sclerosis, syringomyelia, motor neurone disease and subacute combined degeneration. Multiple sclerosis appearing for the first time in middle-aged people may present as a slowly progressive lesion of the spinal cord. The differentiation from spinal cord compression is, however, so difficult and of such importance that there should be no hesitation in seeking expert advice.

Treatment and Prognosis. Surgical relief of the compression is a matter of great urgency since recovery from severe paralysis is unlikely. A delay of even a few hours may be critical in extradural abscess. Exploration is also often required to ascertain the pathological nature of the lesion. If a benign extramedullary tumour is found, it may be removed. In malignant tumours, leukaemic infiltration, and in most intramedullary lesions decompression helps little if at all. Radiotherapy may halt the course of the disease and may be of help in the relief of pain.

Prognosis depends on the severity and duration of the compression before it is relieved. In addition, the nature of the cause must be taken into account. Thus decompression for a malignant lesion may be undertaken though it will be of only temporary benefit.

Paraplegia

Paraplegia may result from many causes, particularly tumours, trauma and other forms of spinal compression, multiple sclerosis, subacute combined degeneration of the cord and, in India, lathyrism (p. 141).

Treatment. This must be directed to the cause but management of the paraplegia itself is most important if complications which may in themselves lead to death are to be avoided. Pressure sores, urinary infections, renal calculi, faecal impaction and contractures are complications which can be prevented. Attention must, therefore, be given to the skin, the bladder, the bowel, the paralysed parts and to the rehabilitation of the patient.

Skin. The skin is liable to be damaged with the formation of pressure sores because of the loss of sensation, diminished blood supply and the immobility of the patient. The patient must be nursed on a specially made rubber mattress and the skin kept dry and clean. Every two to four hours he should be turned and nursed in such a position as will avoid pressure on bony prominences such as the sacrum and heels. This is most easily done by nursing the patient in a Stryker frame. If a pressure sore forms, the patient must not lie on the affected side and scrupulous asepsis must be observed until healing takes place. Skin grafting may be required. Nutrition must be maintained by a well-balanced diet containing adequate amounts of protein, vitamin C and iron. Blood transfusions may be required in individual cases.

Bladder. If retention occurs, aseptic intermittent catheterisation must be carried out. An indwelling catheter may then be inserted and attached to a water-seal drainage bottle. It should be clipped and allowed to drain at regular intervals to establish reflex emptying of the bladder. As the rhythm becomes established the catheter is withdrawn and the patient trained to micturate reflexly at fixed times. Emptying of the bladder should be assisted by manual compression of the lower abdomen by patient or nurse. It is not advisable to give antibiotics prophylactically but if infection develops it must be treated promptly. An adequate consumption of fluid should be ensured. Frequent turning and early ambulation where possible are the best measures for reducing the dangers of urinary stagnation and calculus formation.

Bowel. Constipation must be prevented by suitable diet and laxatives. If it occurs it must be relieved by enemas; otherwise the faeces will become hard and impacted and may require to be removed manually.

Paralysed parts. Spasticity readily leads to the development of flexor spasm and contractures in the limbs. This danger can be reduced by regular passive movement of the limbs and by nursing the patient in such positions as will discourage flexion of the joints. The weight of the bedclothes should be taken from the lower limbs by a cradle to reduce reflex stimulation and prevent drop-foot deformity. If there is no hope of recovery, flexor spasms may be abolished by intrathecal injection of phenol in glycerine or by section of anterior nerve roots.

Rehabilitation. When the cause of paraplegia is not progressive, a great deal can be done by rehabilitation. The patient may learn to walk with calipers or to use a wheel-chair. He may thus be able to care for himself and may even follow a suitable occupation and take part in a variety of recreational activities.

Cervical Disc Herniation and Cervical Spondylosis

Degenerative changes occur in the cervical intervertebral discs in the same manner as in the lumbar region (p. 746) and may lead to herniation. The herniation may affect one disc only, most commonly that between the sixth and seventh cervical vertebrae, or there may be involvement of several discs with secondary osteoarthrosis. The latter changes (cervical spondylosis) are especially liable to interfere with the blood supply to the spinal cord, and thus lead to further damage. Osteoarthrosis in any part of the spine is a common degenerative disorder which often causes no symptoms. The clinical syndromes of acute cervical disc protrusion and chronic cervical spondylosis may occur at different times in the same patient, depending on the anatomical relation of disc protrusions and osteophytic outgrowths to the nerve roots and spinal cord, and on secondary postural or traumatic factors. Acute herniation is usually laterally situated and causes compression of a nerve root. The chronic degeneration of discs is associated with midline herniation and so spinal cord compression may result.

Acute Protrusion of a Cervical Intervertebral Disc. This may occur at any age, usually without apparent trauma to the neck. The patient complains of attacks of pain in the neck often termed 'cricks'. In severe attacks pain is referred to the skin segmental area of one of the lower cervical nerve roots and to the muscles, bones and joints which it supplies. Hyperaesthesia and hyperalgesia may be found in the

affected segment but sensory loss sometimes occurs. Depression of tendon reflexes utilising the affected root is common and lower motor neurone paresis of root distribution is also an occasional finding. The neck is held stiffly, and pain is produced by its movement. The spinal cord is not involved by acute herniation of an intervertebral disc in the cervical region, since this usually occurs in a dorsolateral direction.

Cervical Spondylosis. This term is usually reserved for the disorder resulting from chronic cervical disc degeneration. The highest incidence is in the decade 60 to 70. The symptoms are of two types depending on whether the protrusion is lateral or dorsomedial.

(1) Lateral herniation of discs, with secondary calcification and osteophytes encroaching on the intervertebral foramina, causes radicular symptoms like those of the acute disc syndrome just described, but the onset may be subacute or insidious and involvement of more than one root on one or both sides is common.

(2) Dorsomedial herniation of discs which become calcified results in transverse bars which cause pressure on the spinal cord and on the anterior spinal artery which supplies the anterior two-thirds of the cord. The onset is insidious. Upper motor neurone weakness involves one or more limbs and the legs may be spastic before the upper limbs are involved. Sensory loss is most common in the upper limbs where it has a dermatome pattern but involvement of the spinothalamic tracts may cause disturbance of pain and temperature sensation in the lower limbs, and in some cases muscle-joint sense is also defective. Pain and limitation of movement of the neck are not marked features unless a particular posture causes nipping of a nerve root.

Diagnosis. The acute disc herniation syndrome must be differentiated from other causes of brachial neuralgia (p. 749). If the eight cervical and first thoracic roots are affected by spondylosis the pain may resemble that of myocardial ischaemia. Myelopathy due to cervical spondylosis may resemble tumour of the spinal cord, syringomyelia, multiple sclerosis, motor neurone disease or subacute combined degeneration of the cord. It must be remembered that osteoarthrosis in the spine is common and may accompany any of these diseases. For this reason it may be necessary to confirm the diagnosis by myelography. Radiological examination shows narrowing of the disc spaces and osteophyte formation with loss of the normal cervical lordosis. Oblique views show encroachment by osteophytes on the intervertebral foramina. Queckenstedt's test (p. 743) should be performed while the neck is flexed and extended, as a complete or partial block may be present when the head is in one or other of these positions. The fluid is normal unless its circulation is obstructed, when the protein may be raised.

Treatment. The acute syndrome is treated by rest in bed or by intermittent neck traction followed by immobilisation of the neck in a light metal or plastic collar. Some form of immobilisation should be maintained for at least three months. It is important to watch for progressive cervical cord compression but decompressive surgery is rarely required.

The Lumbago-Sciatica Syndrome

Lumbago is pain in the lower part of the back; sciatica is pain in the distribution of the sciatic nerve. They are not, therefore, disease entities but symptoms and they are often associated.

Aetiology and Pathology. The most common cause is herniation of an intervertebral disc. Other causes are much rarer but important to recognise. They include spinal tumour (neurofibroma and meningioma), ankylosing spondylitis, malignant disease in the pelvis, and tuberculosis of the vertebral bodies or of the sacroiliac joint. Degenerative changes in the intervertebral discs may appear as early as 20 years of age, but herniation is often precipitated by trauma such as twisting the spine, lifting heavy weights while the spine is flexed or during childbirth. The nucleus pulposus may bulge or rupture the annulus fibrosus, giving rise to lumbago by pressure on nerve endings in the spinal ligaments and by producing changes in the joints of the vertebral arches, and to sciatica by causing congestion of, or pressure on, the nerve roots.

Clinical Features. The onset may be sudden or gradual, and may follow closely upon trauma to the back. Attacks of lumbago may precede sciatica by months or years. Lumbago is characterised by sudden severe low back pain when the patient is bending, preventing him from straightening. The sciatic pain is felt in the buttock and radiates down the posterior aspect of the thigh and calf to the outer border of the foot. It is exacerbated by coughing or sneezing which raises the pressure in the spinal subarachnoid space. Paraesthesia and later numbness may be felt over the distribution of the involved nerve root, most often the first sacral. In severe cases, weakness of the calf muscle or foot-drop may occur, according to which roots are involved. The signs associated with prolapse of an intervertebral disc may be divided into two groups.

Signs due to altered mechanics of the Lumbar Spine. Spasm of the sacrospinalis mucles causes flattening of the lumbar curve and scoliosis at the level of the prolapsed disc. Scoliosis increases as pain is felt if the patient tries to touch his toes. He is usually unable to do so as movement of the spine is limited. Tenderness may be found when pressure is applied to the side of the vertebral spines in the region of the affected disc.

Signs due to pressure on the Nerve Root. These depend on the particular root involved. Involvement of the *first sacral* root causes loss of the ankle jerk, weakness of eversion and plantar flexion of the foot, and sensory loss over the outer border of the foot. The glutei may be wasted on the affected side. Involvement of the *fifth lumbar* root causes weakness of dorsiflexion of the toes and sometimes foot-drop. Sensory loss occurs on the dorsum of the foot and the lateral aspect of the leg over the fifth lumbar dermatome. The ankle jerk is not affected. Involvement of the *fourth lumbar* root causes weakness of inversion of the foot and of the quadriceps muscle and loss of the knee jerk. Sensory loss is over the medial aspect of the leg.

A valuable sign of root pressure is limitation of flexion of the thigh on the affected side if the leg is kept straight at the knee (Lasègue's sign).

Diagnosis. The diagnosis is based on the mode of onset of the pain, its aggravation by flexion of the spine, and its relief by immobilisation, as well as on the distribution of the pain and signs of nerve root involvement. Other causes of sciatic pain can be excluded by pelvic examination and by radiological examination of the lumbosacral spine. There may be no apparent radiological change in acute disc herniation, or there may be narrowing of the disc space with osteophyte formation at the margins of the vertebral bodies. Myelography is required only if the diagnosis is in doubt or for purposes of localisation before operation. Intraspinal neoplasm as the cause should be suspected if the CSF protein is raised.

Treatment. The initial treatment in all cases is rest in bed on a firm mattress supported by fracture boards. Rest must be absolute with prohibition of the sitting position. Compromise in this respect and permission to leave bed for toilet purposes are the usual reasons for failure of this treatment. The roots most commonly involved are the first sacral and the fifth lumbar, in which case the patient should be kept supine and no rotation of the spine permitted; but in disc protrusion involving the fourth lumbar root the lateral position with flexion of the hips is best suited to relax tension on the affected root and hence to relieve pain. Bed rest is continued for two to four weeks, after which gradual mobilisation with back-strengthening exercises is carried out over a further period of 10 to 14 days. For middle-aged or elderly patients with chronic residual backache and a tendency to acute attacks of lumbago, a spinal support may be of great value. Cases which do not respond to rest, or in which there have been recurrences, may require surgery.

DISEASES OF PERIPHERAL NERVES

A rational approach to diseases of peripheral nerves should be based on the recognition of their fundamental structure. The cells of origin lie in the anterior horns of the spinal cord and the dorsal root ganglia. Axons represent elongated processes of these cells. They are enveloped by a series of Schwann cells, forming the fatty myelin sheath. Pathological processes which primarily affect cell bodies may first manifest themselves at the distal ends of axonal processes.

Many diseases affect peripheral nerves whose pathological reactions may, however, be grouped under two broad headings:

(1) *Parenchymal neuropathy* where the lesion affects (*a*) nerve cells or their axons, or (*b*) the myelin sheath.

(2) *Interstitial neuropathy* where the pathological process primarily affects the connective tissue or blood vessels of nerves.

Although these rather stereotyped pathological reactions do not lead to distinctive clinical features, a knowledge of the pathological nature of a neuropathy is particularly helpful in assessing its course and prognosis. The clinical classification of peripheral nerve lesions is best based on their anatomical distribution.

Mononeuropathy

This term refers to affection of a single nerve. Trauma is a common cause. Sustained pressure or stretching of nerve occurs in a variety of situations. The radial nerve is commonly implicated as, for instance, in the 'Saturday night' palsy which results from bizarre sleeping postures caused by drunkenness. The ulnar nerve at the elbow and the common peroneal nerve at the head of the fibula are also frequently involved. The signs are those of lower motor neurone paresis and sensory loss in the distribution of the respective nerves. Complete recovery of function in four to six weeks is almost invariable.

Nerves may also be compressed whenever they pass through or near rigid anatomical structures, particularly fibro-osseous tunnels. This type of lesion, called an *entrapment neuropathy*, is one of the most frequent affections of peripheral nerves. *Compression of the median nerve in the carpal tunnel* is the commonest entrapment syndrome. It occurs most frequently in middle-aged women and is then usually unaccompanied by other disease. It may also be a complication of pregnancy, myxoedema, acromegaly or rheumatoid arthritis. The patient complains of pain, numbness, tingling or an 'electric shock' feeling in thumb and fingers supplied by the median nerve, especially after using the hand or in bed at night when it may waken the patient from sleep. There is sometimes objective sensory loss of the radial three and a half digits and there may be weakness and wasting of abductor pollicis brevis and opponens pollicis muscles. The condition is often bilateral. Rest and splinting at night should be tried. Local injection of hydrocortisone is sometimes effective if there is no muscular wasting. Thyroxine therapy relieves the carpal tunnel syndrome in myxoedema. The syndrome occurring in pregnancy usually disappears in the puerperium but may be relieved by the use of diuretics. If these measures are unsuccessful the condition can be relieved by surgical decompression of the nerve in the carpal tunnel.

The lower trunk of the brachial plexus may be compressed at the thoracic outlet, especially if there is a *cervical rib*. Nocturnal pain in the arm and sensorimotor disturbance in the C_8–T_1 distribution are relieved by rest and physiotherapy. Operative treatment is rarely necessary.

The lateral cutaneous nerve of the thigh may be entrapped at the inguinal ligament giving rise to paraesthesiae and pain over the anterolateral aspect of the thigh (*meralgia paraesthetica*).

Mononeuritis Multiplex

In this condition several spinal nerves are damaged concurrently or serially. Clinically signs are limited to discrete neural territories. Leprosy is a common cause of this picture in some geographical areas (p. 856). Polyarteritis, and other connective tissue disorders, diabetes mellitus and sarcoidosis may also give rise to multiple peripheral nerve lesions.

Localised Radiculopathy

Demyelination of a localised group of nerve roots may give rise to *neuralgic amyotrophy*. This condition sometimes follows a vaccination or inoculation and an immunological mechanism may be responsible. It may also occur after infection, injuries or operations.

The patient complains of severe pain over one shoulder girdle, sometimes spreading up the neck or down the arm. Simultaneously, or two or three days later, paralysis develops in the painful muscles. These are usually supplied by the fifth and sixth and less commonly the seventh cervical roots so that the deltoid, spinati, and serratus anterior muscles are usually involved, and frequently also the muscles of the upper arm. The tendon jerks disappear in the affected limb and wasting is rapid. Sensory loss is slight or absent. If present it is usually on the outer aspect of the upper third of the affected arm. The brachial plexus is often tender. Sometimes paralysis of single nerves of the upper limb occurs and occasionally both shoulder girdles are involved. Constitutional symptoms are mild or absent. The CSF is normal or shows only slight lymphocytosis.

Pain usually subsides in one to two weeks. Recovery from paralysis is slow. It usually takes several months, but eventual complete recovery after two or more years is usual. Recurrent attacks of neuritis in the same or the opposite shoulder rarely occur.

Corticosteroids should be tried in neuritis believed to be the consequence of an allergic mechanism. Otherwise treatment is symptomatic and along the lines of those adopted for poliomyelitis.

Generalised Polyneuropathies

In this group of conditions discrete neural affection is not manifest. There is a generalised affection of all nerves. The peripheral nerves show Wallerian degeneration or segmental demyelination. In acute cases little may be found at autopsy since the early changes are biochemical in nature. The most common clinical picture is a symmetrical dysfunction of both motor and sensory nerves first manifest at the distal part of limbs.

Aetiology. There are many causes. Some of the more important are:

Hereditary. Peroneal muscular atrophy; hypertrophic interstitial neuropathy.

Metabolic. Diabetes mellitus; acute intermittent porphyria.

Deficiency. Vitamin B_{12} neuropathy; beriberi.

Poisons. Lead, arsenic, mercury, triorthocresylphosphate (ginger paralysis). In addition many new substances produced for therapeutic and industrial purposes carry this hazard.

Infectious and Toxic or Allergic Reactions. Leprosy (p. 856) is an infection of peripheral nerves. Diphtheria causes toxic neuropathy. Polyneuropathy associated with exanthematous disease and inoculations is probably allergic in nature. Acute post-infective polyneuritis, for long believed to be due to a virus, may have a similar cause.

Malignant Disease. Carcinoma of the bronchus and other tumours may cause polyneuropathy which may be the first manifestation of malignancy.

Clinical Features. Polyneuropathy presents with paraesthesiae and numbness in the periphery of all four limbs, usually starting in the toes; in addition there may be great pain. These symptoms gradually spread proximally as shorter fibres are involved so that the distribution does not follow that of any particular nerve root or peripheral nerve. The patient then has difficulty with fine movements such as fastening buttons because of developing loss of proprioception or he notices that objects feel 'different'. Sensory ataxia may follow; weakness soon becomes apparent starting peripherally and spreading proximally.

Involvement of the autonomic system as in diabetes mellitus may cause impotence, postural hypotension or disturbances of bowel or bladder function.

Examination shows impairment or loss of all forms of sensation, extending from the periphery of the limbs in a 'glove and stocking' fashion. A characteristic feature is that the muscles are often extremely tender to pressure. Damage to the motor fibres causes the signs of a lower motor neurone lesion, especially at the periphery of the limbs, so that wrist-drop and foot-drop may appear. The proximal muscles are later involved and then the trunk and sometimes the face. Respiration may be endangered by paralysis of the intercostal muscles or the diaphragm. Interruption of the reflex arcs causes loss of the tendon reflexes.

There are features peculiar to polyneuropathy due to:

Alcoholism. Pain is usually severe and other evidence of alcoholism may be apparent, such as tremor of the hands, mental impairment or signs of liver disease.

Lead. Lead poisoning causes paralysis of muscles, usually within the distribution of the radial or lateral popliteal nerves, but without involving all muscles supplied by these nerves. It is, for instance, common to find paralysis of the extensor muscles of the wrists and fingers with sparing of the brachioradialis and abductor pollicis longus muscles. Some authorities consider that this is due to local poisoning of muscles rather than true neuropathy. There is no loss of sensation. Other clinical features associated with chronic exposure to lead are anaemia with punctate basophilia of red cells (p. 595) and a blue line on the gums if the patient is not edentulous. If the amount of lead ingested is sufficient to cause poisoning there may be colic and headache and acute or chronic encephalopathy, causing mental changes and epileptic seizures. The clinical picture may resemble that of porphyria.

Acute Post-infective Polyneuritis. (Guillain-Barré syndrome.) This begins with headache, vomiting, pyrexia and pain in the back and limbs. It is caused by inflammation with oedema of the spinal nerves near their formation by junction of the nerve roots. After a variable period of hours or days paralysis appears, beginning usually in all four limbs simultaneously, though sometimes starting in the lower limbs and spreading in ascending fashion. Unlike other types of polyneuropathy, proximal rather than distal muscles in the limbs may be affected. The trunk and respiratory muscles may be involved and also the muscles supplied by the cranial nerves, particularly the seventh. Sensory loss may be confined to the limbs or may spread on to the trunk. Reflexes are lost and sphincter difficulties occur. Death may be caused by bulbar respiratory paralysis.

The CSF shows striking changes, there being a normal cell count but a great increase in protein up to $10 \text{ g}/l$ (1,000 mg/100 ml). If the death from respiratory paralysis is prevented or avoided, the outlook is good, as most cases recover in 3 to 6 months. The evidence for an infective aetology is unsatisfactory. The possibility of an autoimmune mechanism provides a rationale for the use of corticosteroids.

Acute Intermittent Porphyria. This condition may cause a neuropathy similar to that of acute infective polyneuritis. Acute intermittent porphyria is characterised by attacks of unexplained colicky abdominal pain, constipation and psychiatric disturbances, notably confusion and emotional lability. Tachycardia and hypertension are frequent. An attack of acute porphyria may be precipitated by phenobarbitone, oral contraceptives, sulphonamides, pentazocine, methyldopa, chlorpropamide, alcohol and other drugs. The diagnosis is confirmed by the findings of porphobilinogen in the urine (p. 476).

Diabetes Mellitus and *Diphtheria.* These are described on pages 554 and 65.

Diagnosis. Pain in the limbs occurs from causes such as ischaemia or arthritis but will be unaccompanied by abnormal neurological signs. Tabes dorsalis causes lightning pains, absence of the tendon reflexes and sensory loss. The description of the pain however is different, there is decreased rather than increased muscle tenderness and Argyll Robertson pupils are usually present. Acute infective polyneuritis is often mistakenly diagnosed as poliomyelitis but in the latter disease the weakness is asymmetrical, there is no sensory loss and the CSF changes are different (p. 722). Motor neurone disease should not be confused as no sensory loss occurs in that condition. Nevertheless motor neurone disease and polymyositis (p. 756) may be difficult to differentiate from motor forms of polyneuropathy. If lower motor neurone and sensory signs are restricted to the lower limbs the possibility of a lesion of the cauda equina should be considered.

Treatment. Prevention is very important. Any new drug which is liable to cause neuropathy must be used with care and industrial hazards should be avoided by protective clothing, exhaust ventilation and other techniques advised by the industrial medical officer. When polyneuropathy has developed as a result of exposure to a toxic substance the first step is to remove the patient from further exposure. When the cause is nutritional or metabolic the appropriate treatment must be initiated without delay. Thus therapy may be required for beriberi, diabetes or pernicious anaemia. Corticosteroids are indicated for acute 'infective' polyneuritis. Chelating agents, sodium calciumedetate or penicillamine are used in the treatment of lead poisoning.

In severe cases bed rest is essential since the nervous control of the heart may be defective and cardiomyopathy is sometimes associated. The limbs should be supported in the optimum position, and passive movements carried out several times a day. A cage should protect the feet from the weight of the bed-clothes. Respiratory insufficiency may require tracheostomy or institution of intermittent positive pressure respiration (p. 266). When recovery begins, active movements should be carried out under the supervision of a physiotherapist.

Myasthenia Gravis

This condition is characterised by undue fatiguability of certain muscle groups, with incapacity to sustain muscular activity.

Aetiology. The cause of myasthenia gravis is unknown. Muscle fatiguability is due to a failure of transmission at the myoneural junction. The defect may be presynaptic, due to the release of smaller than normal quanta of acetylcholine or perhaps to release of an abnormal transmitter. It may lie postsynaptically and involve a block of the muscle receptors. Recent evidene suggests that both pre- and postjunctional sites are involved. Electron microscopy has now demonstrated that there is a structural abnormality of both the terminals of motor nerves and the endplates of muscle, with widening of the synaptic cleft.

There is evidence of an immunological disturbance. Antibodies against muscle receptors are present in most patients suffering from myasthenia gravis. Antibodies against myosin are also found in those who also have a thymoma (approximately 15 per cent of all cases). The thymus gland contains an excess of germinal centres in all cases of myasthenia. Circumstantial support for an autoimmune mechanism is provided by the association of myasthenia gravis with systemic lupus erythematosus, rheumatoid arthritis, thyrotoxicosis, Hashimoto's disease, pernicious anaemia and diabetes mellitus.

Clinical Features. The disease usually appears between the ages of 15 and 50 and females are more often affected than males. It tends to run a remitting course especially during the early years. Relapses may be precipitated by emotional disturbances, infections, pregnancy and severe muscular effort. The cardinal symptom is abnormal fatiguability of muscles; movement, though initially strong, rapidly weakens. Intensification of symptoms towards the end of the day or following vigorous exercise is characteristic. The first symptoms are usually intermittent ptosis or diplopia but weakness of chewing, swallowing, speaking or of moving the limbs also occurs. Any muscle of a limb may be affected, most commonly those of the shoulder girdle, so that the patient is unable to undertake work above the level of the shoulder, such as combing the hair, without frequent rests. Respiratory muscles may be involved and respiratory failure is a not uncommon cause of death. Asphyxia occurs readily as the cough may be too weak to clear foreign bodies from the airways. Muscle atrophy may occur in longstanding cases. There are no signs of involvement of the central nervous system.

An invaluable diagnostic aid is the increase in muscle strength produced by an intravenous injection of a short-acting anticholinesterase, edrophonium hydrochloride. An initial dose of 2 mg is injected and a further 8 mg given half a minute later if there are no undesirable reactions such as fasciculation, sweating and colic. Improvement in muscle power occurs within 30 seconds of the injection and usually persists for 2 or 3 minutes. Ptosis or defects in eye movements are the most convenient parameters of improvement but diminution of dysarthria or increase of power in the limbs can also demonstrate a response to edrophonium.

Diagnosis. Multiple sclerosis, motor neurone disease and myopathy may all superficially resemble myasthenia gravis. Frequently myasthenic manifestations are first attributed to hysteria. The diagnosis will rarely be missed if its possibility is borne in mind and an edrophonium test carried out in any patient who displays variable muscular weakness in the absence of neural deficit.

Treatment. Treatment is based on the administration of anticholinesterase drugs of which neostigmine and pyridostigmine are the most widely used. The dose of either of these drugs varies between individuals. Fifteen mg of neostigmine given orally four times daily is sometimes sufficient but in some patients 30 mg every 2 hours is needed. Pyridostigmine gives less prompt relief than neostigmine but has a more prolonged action. It is particularly useful when given late in the evening when it preserves muscle power during sleep. Sixty mg of pyridostigmine is equivalent in its effect to 15 mg of neostigmine. Anticholinesterase drugs frequently cause bowel colic and sometimes diarrhoea and excessive salivation. These side-effects may be controlled by propantheline (15 mg t.i.d.) or, on occasion, by the parenteral administration of atropine (0·5 mg). When the patient is unable to swallow and during pre- and postoperative periods neostigmine may be given intravenously (0·5–1 mg hourly). One mg of neostigmine intravenously is equivalent to 15 mg given orally.

There is a danger of overdosage with anticholinesterase drugs, and this is perhaps particularly likely when long acting preparations are used since their effect tends to be cumulative. Excessive dosage of anticholinesterases can cause permanent depolarisation block at the neuromuscular junction. This is sometimes referred to as a *cholinergic crisis*. Warning signs of overdosage are fasciculations, pallor, sweating, persistently small pupils and excessive salivation.

Overdosage can be prevented by 'titrating' the dose according to the reaction to intravenous edrophonium. If the limit of anticholinesterase dosage has been reached then edrophonium will increase muscle weakness. Some muscle groups may be overdosed while others are still responsive to neostigmine. It is, therefore, important to observe the effect of an injection of edrophonium on respiration rather than on ocular or limb movement.

Sudden exacerbations of myasthenia or cholinergic block may require intermittent positive pressure respiration to save life.

Some patients benefit markedly from thymectomy. The operation should always be performed if a thymoma is demonstrated and if disability progresses despite medical treatment. It is particularly indicated if bulbar muscles are involved. The best results follow thymectomies carried out on young women whose disease has been present for less than 3 years.

High dosage steroid treatment is of value in myasthenia gravis, particularly in those who have responded poorly to thymectomy. A daily dose of 1 g of methyl prednisolone is given intravenously for 10 days, followed by gradually reducing doses of oral prednisolone. A few days after the introduction of steroids there is often a marked exacerbation of myasthenia and the treatment should only be carried out in hospital where facilities for artificial respiration are available.

Prognosis. This is variable. Remissions sometimes occur spontaneously. When myasthenic affection is confined to the eye muscles prognosis for life is normal and disability slight. Rapid progression of the disease more than 5 years after its onset is uncommon. Thymectomy, perhaps followed by high dosage steroid treatment, often leads to marked improvement so that disability is minimal and life expectancy normal. When the disease is associated with a thymoma, even though this be removed, the outlook is markedly worsened.

DISEASES OF MUSCLE

Diseases of muscle are not diseases of the nervous system, but as some of their manifestations may be readily confused with neurological conditions some relevant examples are described here. There are obvious exceptions, but it is a useful generalisation that muscular disease affects mainly the proximal muscles of the limbs whereas neuropathic disease (polyneuropathy or motor neurone disease) affects mainly the distal muscles.

Myopathy is a generic term comprising all primary diseases of muscle. It may be subdivided into:

1. Genetically determined myopathy—(a) progressive muscular dystrophy, and (b) myotonic dystrophy.
2. Congenital myopathies.
3. Metabolic myopathies.
4. Inflammatory myopathies or myosites.

1. Genetically Determined Myopathy

(a) Progressive Muscular Dystrophy

This is a group of hereditary disorders characterised by progressive degeneration of groups of muscles without involvement of the nervous system. The wasting and weakness are symmetrical, there is no fasciculation, tendon reflexes are preserved until a late stage and there is no sensory loss. Several clinical types have been described; from a prognostic viewpoint there are three major groups.

Pseudo-hypertrophic type (Duchenne type). This is transmitted by a X-linked recessive gene and occurs almost exclusively in males (p. 16). The disease usually appears within the first three years of life, beginning in the pelvic girdle and lower limbs and later spreading to the shoulder girdle. About 80 per cent of cases show an initial pseudohypertrophy involving the calf muscles, quadriceps, glutei, deltoids and infraspinati. Contractures are common. The affected muscles are larger and firmer than normal, but are nevertheless weak. The weakness gives rise to a characteristic waddling gait, and when rising from the supine position, the child rolls on to his face and then uses his arms to push himself up. Death occurs from inanition or respiratory infection by the middle of the second decade.

Limb girdle type (Juvenile scapulohumeral type of Erb). The gene carrying this disorder is inherited as an autosomal recessive, affecting both sexes. It usually appears in the second or third decade. It starts in either the shoulder or pelvic girdle and later spreads to involve both. The rate of progression is variable; it may be slow, with long periods of arrest, but severe disablement usually occurs within 20 years and the patient does not survive to middle age.

Facio-scapulo-humeral type (Landouzy-Déjerine). This type is inherited by an autosomal dominant gene so that several siblings of both sexes may be affected. It appears at any age, first in the facial muscles and then in the shoulder girdle. After many years the pelvic girdle may also be involved. The disease progresses very slowly with periods of arrest and is compatible with a long life.

The *diagnosis of muscular dystrophy* is readily confirmed by electromyography (EMG) or muscle biopsy. Aldolase, or creatine kinase and other enzymes which are usually intracellular, are increased in the serum, especially in the rapidly advancing Duchenne type. Serum enzyme changes may be found before other clinical signs, enabling early detection of the disease in siblings. Less severe changes of the same type are found in women who carry the abnormal gene of the Duchenne type.

Differential Diagnosis. Progressive muscular dystrophy must be distinguished from acquired myopathies in which treatment is possible or spontaneous remission may occur; these occur alone ('polymyositis', p. 756) or as part of dermatomyositis, endocrine disease or carcinomatous myopathy (p. 757).

Myasthenia gravis shows exacerbations of weakness with effort, and responds to injection of endrophonium or neostigmine.

Diseases of the lower motor neurone from which muscular dystrophy must be distinguished are (*a*) progressive spinal muscular atrophy, (*b*) motor neurone disease which is associated with fasciculation, (*c*) peripheral neuropathy in which there is distal involvement of muscles and sensory loss, and (*d*) residual poliomyelitis which is commonly mistaken for muscular dystrophy, if the history of the acute illness is not known, but the lesions are asymmetrical and not progressive.

Treatment. No effective treatment is known. Deterioration may occur with excessive confinement to bed. Physiotherapeutic and orthopaedic measures may be required to counteract deformities and contractures.

(b) Myotonic Dystrophy

Myotonia consists of slow relaxation of muscles due to hyperexcitability of the muscle cell membrane.

Myotonia congenita (Thomsen's disease) is inherited as an autosomal dominant and appears in early childhood. The only symptom is the slow relaxation of a muscle if it is contracted voluntarily or by mechanical stimulation. The patient may be unable to relax his grasp or to open his eyes if they have been closed tightly. The muscles may be unusually powerful in early life.

Myotonia atrophica (myotonic dystrophy) is also autosomal dominant and appears between the ages of 20 and 30. There is wasting of the facial and temporal muscles, sternomastoids, shoulder girdle, forearms, quadriceps and leg muscles, and all these and the tongue show myotonia after voluntary contraction or after percussion of the muscle. Ptosis is prominent. Unlike most muscular diseases, distal muscles are more severely affected than proximal. There is also cataract, frontal baldness and gonadal atrophy leading to impotence and sterility in men and amenorrhoea in women.

Treatment. There is no treatment for the muscular dystrophy, but if myotonia is troublesome it can be relieved by procainamide, 0·5–1·0 g q.i.d., quinine sulphate 300–600 mg t.i.d., or diphenylhydantoin 100 mg t.i.d.

2. Congenital Myopathies

This group of rare myopathies presents in infancy with muscular weakness and limpness. Serum enzymes tend to be normal or slightly raised. The EMG is usually myopathic. The mode of inheritance is variable. They are named according to the type of structural abnormality found in the skeletal muscle fibres. Most cases are non-progressive or only slowly progressive.

3. Metabolic Myopathies

Thyrotoxic Myopathy. Mild weakness of the proximal muscles of the limbs is a common feature of thyrotoxicosis. In a few patients muscular wasting and weakness predominate, and the other manifestations of hyperthyroidism may not be obvious.

Corticosteroid Myopathy. Weakness of the pelvic girdle may occur in Cushing's syndrome and as a result of treatment with corticosteroid hormones.

Familial Periodic Paralysis. This is characterised by attacks of profound weakness, lasting for several hours and often occurring after exertion or after a heavy carbohydrate meal. In the common variety the attacks of weakness are accompanied by a fall in the serum potassium level.

4. Polymyositis

This group of muscle diseases is characterised by damage to muscle fibres accompanied by the interstitial infiltration of inflammatory cells. Clinically, muscle weakness and wasting may be patchy and may be accompanied by muscular pain and tenderness. Dermatomyositis is described on page 648. Often the diagnosis can be made with certainty only by a muscle biopsy. When a myositic picture presents in middle age it may be associated with occult carcinoma. Some cases of myositis respond to treatment with corticosteroids.

Neurological and Myopathic Complications of Carcinoma

Cerebral invasion or spinal compression may be the presenting feature of a metastasis from an unsuspected primary neoplasm or may augment the disability already caused by tumours arising elsewhere in the body, particularly in bronchus and breast. More than half of all cerebral tumours are secondary deposits and this high incidence emphasises the need for a careful search for a primary neoplasm in those patients who present with an intracranial space-occupying lesion.

Neurological complications may arise at a distance from a primary carcinoma in the absence of metastases. The relationship between the underlying malignant process and the neurological manifestations remains obscure in most instances. Neural disturbances may occur at any stage during the development of the primary lesion and frequently antedate the symptoms directly attributable to the carcinoma by weeks or months and occasionally by as much as two or three years. At the time of neurological presentation the primary carcinoma often cannot be defined even by radiological techniques. Nor does the course of the neurological complication consistently parallel the development of the carcinoma. Immunological mechanisms, conditioned nutritional deficiencies and the direct effects of toxins produced by tumours have all been adduced as explanations of attendant neurological dysfunction but there is little supporting evidence for any of these hypotheses. Investigations have suggested the possibility that tumours may produce an alteration in protein metabolism which in turn interferes with the synthesis of enzymes and hence causes neural dysfunction. It is likely that progressive multi-focal leucoencephalopathy (below) results from viral infection when immunological responses are impaired by malignant disease.

The neurological features evoked by distant carcinoma are protean; they may affect singly, or in combination, muscles, peripheral nerves as well as central neural structures and the brain. The syndromes presented are most conveniently categorised anatomically.

Myopathy, Myositis and Myasthenia. A proximal weakness of late onset, usually first affecting the legs may be due to a lesion of muscles secondary to a distant carcinoma. Histologically the muscles may show changes of a non-specific myopathy or there may be collections of inflammatory cells, characteristic of polymyositis. Sometimes the myopathic weakness is markedly exacerbated by exertion producing a myasthenic syndrome. Weakness and fatiguability usually most often affect the legs, and less commonly the arms; bulbar and ocular affections are uncommon in contrast to myasthenia gravis. Fatiguability of muscle may sometimes be improved by an intravenous injection of edrophonium hydrochloride but this response is inconstant and is often poorly sustained. The electromyographic picture in these carcinomatous myasthenic syndromes differs from that produced by myasthenia gravis. Guanidine 40–50 mg/kg body weight sometimes improves muscle power in carcinomatous myopathy.

Peripheral Neuropathy. Peripheral neuropathy is probably the commonest of the distant neurological complications of carcinoma. Clinically the neuropathy is usually of mixed sensory-motor type (p. 750). The cerebrospinal fluid protein content is often raised. Much less commonly a pure sensory neuropathy may be manifest, almost always in association with a bronchial carcinoma of oat-cell type. Pathological lesions in this rare condition are mainly situated in the dorsal root ganglia where there is degeneration of the sensory neurones.

Spinal Cord Affection. Carcinomata may produce a picture which resembles motor neurone disease with loss of anterior horn cells, accompanied sometimes by upper motor neurone signs. Uncommonly this picture, which mimics amyotrophic lateral sclerosis, may be accompanied by a bulbar palsy. Necrosis affecting the cells and the tracts of the spinal cord, maximal in the thoracic segments, is a rare complication of carcinoma.

Subacute Degeneration of the Cortical Layers of the Cerebellum. This is an uncommon manifestation of distant carcinoma. Ataxia, affecting upper and lower limbs, is a consistent presenting feature; dysarthria too is often found but nystagmus is present in only a minority of cases.

Encephalopathy. This has occasionally been found in patients suffering from carcinoma particularly of the bronchus, breast and uterus. The most common presentation is an insidious and progressive dementia with memory disorder and sometimes mood disturbance. These psychiatric and mental symptoms may occasionally be accompanied by features of brain stem involvement such as double vision or bulbar palsy and often there are accompanying pyramidal tract signs.

Progressive Multifocal Leucoencephalopathy. This rare disease does not seem to occur as an independent state but occurs late in the course of an antecedent disease, e.g. reticulosis or carcinoma. The pathological findings comprise widely disseminated demyelinating lesions in the brain together with distinctive changes in the glial cells suggestive of invasion by one of the papova group of viruses. It is a condition of rapid and progressive nature usually leading to death within a few weeks or months of its being manifest. The clinical picture varies widely. Hemiparesis is the commonest disability but dysphasia, dysarthria, and hemianopia are also frequent. Dementia may occur, as may convulsions.

Treatment. The treatment of the neurological complications is that of the primary lesion. Improvement, and occasionally complete remission, of a myasthenic-myopathic syndrome may occur with removal of the primary tumour but this is by no means invariable. Carcinomatous motor neurone disease often tends to halt its progress despite the fact that the primary carcinoma continues to grow. Clearly the treatment for the underlying malignancies is imperative but the response of the neurological complications is unpredictable.

Prospects in Neurology

Exciting changes are in prospect. Traditionally neurology has depended on precise localisation of lesions whose pathology could often be determined only by uncomfortable or hazardous investigations. The aetiology of many conditions was unknown and treatment was restricted. In diagnostic, aetiological and therapeutic fields advances are in progress.

Computerised axial scanning (p. 692) has revolutionised diagnostic neurology. It is analogous to the advent of chest radiography in respiratory medicine and provides information of comparable precision to the neurologist. It is now possible to visualise the intracranial contents through the skull without danger to patients. The diagnosis of tumours is simplified. Definition of cerebral haemorrhages and infarcts not only aids diagnosis but sequential monitoring will provide a firm basis for the clarification of the natural history of cerebrovascular disease. When the equipment is more widely available computerised tomography will become a screening tool for patients suffering from epilepsy and headache, leading to early diagnosis of causal lesions. The use of higher resolution scanning, thinner sections scanned and contrast enhancement will enable very small lesions, such as intracranial aneurysms, to be demonstrated. It is possible now, using the body scanner and contrast enhancement, to visualise the spinal cord. Within the near future the diagnostic applications will be extended to cord lesions.

The discovery of slow viruses has suggested possible aetiologies for a number of neurological conditions. There is already some evidence, albeit incomplete, of such a cause for multiple sclerosis, motor neurone disease, and paralysis agitans. Proof of a viral origin for these conditions may not be established and no therapeutic agents are yet available for the treatment of slow viruses. It is, however, encouraging that the search for causal factors is active and that many diseases, depressingly labelled 'degenerative', may be found to have external, definable aetiologies.

The manipulation and alteration of neurotransmitters offers hope of new treatments. Dopaminergic treatment of parkinsonism is already successful and the enhancement of cerebral GABA concentration by sodium valproate (p. 688) opens a new approach to the treatment of epilepsy. Further advances in this field, particularly in the treatment of extrapyramidal disorders, spasticity, epilepsy and migraine, are imminent.

C. MAWDSLEY
J. A. SIMPSON

Further reading:

Matthews, W. B. & Miller, H. (1975) *Diseases of the Nervous System.* 2nd edition. Oxford: Blackwell.—A concise, readable account of neurological disorders intended for undergraduates.

Walton, J. N. (1975) *Essentials of Neurology.* 4th edition. London: Pitman Medical.—A short but authoritative textbook, designed for undergraduates and packed with accurate information.

Brain, Lord & Walton, J. N. (1977) *Diseases of the Nervous System.* 8th edition. London: Oxford University Press.—See next reference.

Elliot, F. A. (1971) *Clinical Neurology.* 2nd edition. Philadelphia: Saunders.—Both of these are comprehensive texts written for postgraduate students but they are suitable reference works for undergraduates.

Jennett, W. B. (1977) *An Introduction to Neurosurgery.* 3rd edition. London: Heinemann.—A succinct and clearly written introduction to surgical neurology.

Adams, R. A. & Sidman, R. L. (1968) *Introduction to Neuropathology.* New York: McGraw-Hill.—Though it deals in considerable detail with pathological processes this book is particularly valuable because of its extensive discussion of the correlation of pathological lesions and clinical features.

15. Psychiatry

PSYCHIATRY is the study and treatment of disorders of the mind. The mind, or psyche, is usually defined as the part of the person consisting of the thoughts, the feelings and the function of willing. Psychiatric disorder, therefore, can be viewed to occur whenever there is an impairment of thinking (cognition), feeling (affect) or willing (volition). In a paranoid reaction, for instance, the patient wrongly thinks he is being persecuted by an ill-intentioned acquaintance; in depressive psychosis the patient is incapacitated by a persistent feeling of intense gloom; and in schizophrenia some patients are inactive, ineffectual and lacking in volition.

Psychiatry is the proper concern of all doctors, not only of psychiatrists. Only a small proportion of the psychiatric illness in the community is seen and can be treated by psychiatrists. In a country as well doctored as Britain only 1 in 20 cases of psychiatric illness is treated by psychiatrists. The epidemiological evidence makes it clearly evident that the great proportion of psychiatric morbidity falls in the clinical domain of non-psychiatrists: general practitioners mainly but also physicians, surgeons, obstetricians and gynaecologists. Neurologists should also be singled out, for they treat many psychiatric patients. Another reason for requiring all doctors to be psychiatrically informed and skilled is that psychiatric disorder and physical illness frequently occur in the same patient.

It follows that the priority is to ensure that psychiatric knowledge and skills, and professional attitudes appropriate to adequate provision of psychiatric care, are part of the clinical equipment of all doctors.

Knowledge. In this area all doctors need to know the symptoms, signs and syndromes in psychiatry, and they should all be aware of the psychological, pharmacological and physical treatments that are effective in psychiatric illness.

Skills. The basic skills are the ability to take a psychiatric history and to examine the mental state; such technical competence enables the doctor to elicit the clinical features of psychiatric disorder presented by the patient. Interviewing is the chief tool of all doctors, and when doing *psychiatric interviewing* four distinct interviewing approaches are available:

1. The *descriptive approach* is akin to medical history-taking and examination and leads to syndrome identification. As in other branches of medicine, it is appropriate in psychiatry to think in terms of disease entities, that is, to assume that the patient is suffering from a particular disease with its specific aetiology, pathology, signs and symptoms, which can be elicited by history-taking and examination.

2. The *analytical approach* enables the doctor to elicit any relevant complexes or pathogenic ideas of which the patient may be partially unaware; Charcot, the nineteenth century French neurologist who was the first modern doctor to treat emotional disorder with individual psychotherapy, spoke of a 'psychic lesion' and described '. . . those remarkable paralyses which have been designated psychical paralyses, paralyses depending on an idea, paralyses by imagination'. He gave the

name 'dissociation' to the process by which distressing thoughts, memories or ideas disappeared from awareness, and then reappeared in disguised form as a dream or a physical symptom. The minor psychiatric disorders are usually associated with bodily discomfort and patients naturally consult their doctors about these complaints; many medical-sounding names have been coined, like anorexia nervosa or globus hystericus or cardiac neurosis. As a result it is easy to assume that each such diagnostic term refers to a separate disease process. Here, however, the 'disease-orientated' model can be misleading. In addition to their symptoms, patients suffering from these conditions can also be found to have disturbances in the relations with people close to them. These self-defeating patterns of behaviour in personal relationships have been learned by life experience; the early life of the neurotic or psychosomatic patient has included some painful, frustrating or damaging experiences which disturbed his peace of mind and continue to interfere with his performance. Moreover, the minor psychiatric disorders differ from diseases for being biographically meaningful. We can often understand why that person became ill in that way at that particular time as we come to understand the course of his life and to comprehend his dilemma in relation to the people of importance to him. A psychoneurosis, in this sense, symbolises a personal predicament of the patient.

3. A third interview procedure is the *interpersonal approach* in interviewing, the doctor now exploring a patient's significant interpersonal relationships; much psychiatric illness, as we shall see, accompanies difficulties the patient currently has in his associations with the people most important to him.

4. Finally, the *phenomenological approach* is the method whereby the doctor, by an effort of imagination, uses his own life experience to enable him intuitively to grasp what the patient is suffering; such empathic perception of the patient's present predicament in living calls on the clinician to attempt a feat of fellow-feeling by which he can extend his understanding of the patient derived from the other three approaches.

Professional Attitudes. Three habits of mind, or mental sets, are relevant to psychiatric work, in addition to those clinical attitudes which are necessary for the practice of medicine in general. First, the clinician needs, for purposes of comprehensive interviewing, to surrender temporarily the relative detachment and authority appropriate to the practice of internal medicine, and instead to adopt a more receptive, less directive, clinical style: much of the patient's experiences relevant to the psychiatric illness are locked up in the patient and get disclosed only if security, trust and some hope of being helped can be aroused in the patient. A paranoid patient who believes that there is a plot against him may conclude the doctor is part of the plot, unless by warmth and encouragement the doctor reassures the patient and brings him out of himself; a phobic patient may consider her fear of open spaces too ridiculous to disclose to the doctor, especially if already that doctor seems abrupt and critical.

Michael Balint wrote, in *The Doctor, His Patient, and the Illness* (1968), that medical training handicaps many clinicians for psychological work. He had in mind that when a person becomes a doctor he sets aside to some extent the innate perceptiveness, readiness to be informed by the patient and to be led by him into unexpected avenues. The question-and-answer interviewing technique in medicine, and the professional status as the expert who knows what course the clinical discussion should take, often constrains the patient. The 'small but necessary personality change' the doctor has to make, for purposes of psychiatric interviewing, is to be more passive, less decided in advance about matters to be explored and more ready to receive private disclosures from the patient. Indeed, at first the patient often imparts a 'cover story', a version of his illness and his personal troubles which he hopes will not offend the doctor; only when he confirms for himself that the doctor is not censorious and remains open to receive further revelations will the patient give utterance to more distressing facts.

The second professional attitude of importance in psychiatric work is related to a skill which has already been indicated. The doctor must practice minimal intervention himself and allow the patient to be the more active.

Third, the doctor doing psychiatric work requires an orientation of self-scrutiny, reflecting constantly on the impact he is having on the patient and asking himself whether he is influencing the patient as he had intended. A readiness continuously to study his own personality in clinical action and the responses he makes to his patients enables the doctor progressively to increase his knowledge about the life experiences of others, his skills for alleviating personal distress, and his capacity for gaining self-knowledge. The doctor's personality is his chief clinical tool. It is always in his personal capacity that the psychiatrically ill patient will respond to him, over and above the clinical expertise he exercises when engaged on the exploration, diagnosis and management of any disorder of the patient's mind or personality.

Diagnostic Decision-making

When he is examining a patient for psychiatric disorder, the doctor's first consideration is to question whether the patient may be suffering from a psychosis, one of the serious disorders to which the term 'insanity' used to be applied. The psychoses are the serious illnesses which interfere with a patient's perceptions, thinking and feelings so profoundly that, at times, what he says to his fellow-men no longer makes sense to them and he is regarded as insane. The doctor scans the

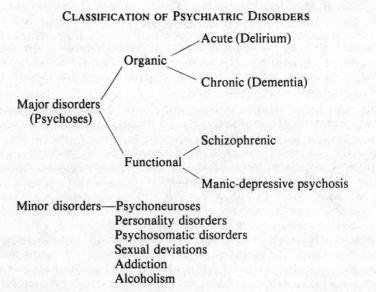

CLASSIFICATION OF PSYCHIATRIC DISORDERS

Major disorders (Psychoses)
- Organic
  - Acute (Delirium)
  - Chronic (Dementia)
- Functional
  - Schizophrenic
  - Manic-depressive psychosis

Minor disorders—Psychoneuroses
Personality disorders
Psychosomatic disorders
Sexual deviations
Addiction
Alcoholism

Mental handicap (mental retardation)

understanding he has obtained by means of history-taking and examination of the mental state, perhaps augmented—when the patient is uncooperative—by information from a relative or other informant. He judges whether the syndrome presenting indicates an illness of psychotic quality and severity. Syndrome identification is of course possible only if the doctor has knowledge about the signs and symptoms of the two main classes of psychoses; the organic psychoses due to cerebral impairment, and the functional psychoses presumed to be related to an as-yet undiscovered disturbance of cerebral biochemistry.

The Major Disorders (The Psychoses)

Organic Psychoses. In these organic brain syndromes the functioning of the brain is impaired either by a physical lesion (trauma, tumour or infection) or by a toxic or degenerative process. Organic brain syndromes when acute are known as *delirium*. Examples are the toxic confusional states occurring with brain trauma, cerebral anoxia, infection, or intoxication with barbiturates, amphetamines or alcohol.

The chronic psychoses, where an irreversible brain lesion has occurred, are the *dementias*. The most common are those associated with ageing—cerebral atherosclerosis and senile psychoses. Mild degrees of dementia make the patient forgetful, easily confused, irritable and emotional; more severe dementia results in disorientation, gross loss of memory and deterioration in personal habits.

Functional Psychoses. These are the major psychiatric illnesses occurring without brain disease or impairment. It is postulated that a neurophysiological or neurochemical aetiology will be found, resulting from the operation of complex causes. The two most common forms are *manic-depressive psychosis*, in which the principal symptom is a profound disturbance of the patient's mood, and the *schizophrenias* in which the patient's thoughts become bizarre and disorganised, so that he loses contact with his fellows and with his surroundings.

The Minor Disorders

The second step in the decision-making progress towards a psychiatric diagnosis, having excluded the presence of psychosis, is for the doctor to determine whether the patient suffers from a minor psychiatric disorder. The following forms of minor disorder are differentiated:

The Psychoneuroses. The doctor considers that the evidence he has obtained indicates that psychiatric illness is present, of minor degree. Again, clinical recognition of one of the forms of psychoneurosis depends on the doctor knowing the signs and symptoms of each syndrome and of being able to elicit the relevant clinical data from the patient. The psychoneuroses are the most common forms of psychiatric illness encountered in general medical practice. They are subdivided into *anxiety neurosis, hysterical neurosis, obsessive neurosis, phobic neurosis* and *depressive neurosis*.

Personality Disorder. This term is used to describe patients whose personalities differ markedly from the normal population.

The third diagnostic rule, after the presence of possible psychosis and of psychoneurosis has been considered, is to make an appraisal of the personality of the patient. An individual's personality is regarded as normal if his actions and reactions are not grossly different from customary behaviour in society; when a personality is diagnosed as disordered, the implication is that the person deviates observably in behaviour, presenting a type of abnormal personality which is well recognised clinically. The abnormal personality manifests in recurrent disturbance in relationships with other people. In addition to their social difficulties, such people have traits (e.g. hostility, passivity) not found to the same degree in the personalities of normal people. Patients with moderate degrees of personality disorder are distressed by their inability to get on constructively with others and often seek treatment; otherwise they do so when they are further disabled by psychoneurosis or psychosomatic illness. Those with gross degrees of disorder (sociopathy) interfere disruptively in the lives of their relatives and associates and may come into conflict with the law; they may not regard themselves as abnormal and reject any efforts to treat them.

It is by no means unusual, indeed it is usual, for psychiatric illness and personality disorder to coexist. When the associated illness is of psychotic dimensions, the symptoms may so distort behaviour that a reliable estimate of the pre-illness personality will be possible only after recovery from the insanity. When the illness is a neurotic reaction, however, functioning personality remains sufficiently intact for a personality diagnosis to be made at the same time as the illness is appraised.

Psychosomatic Illnesses. These are the extremely common illnesses (such as some cases of asthma, peptic ulcer, dermatitis, ulcerative colitis, etc.) which emotional factors help to precipitate or to prolong.

Sexual Deviation. People not conforming sexually to the prevailing norm most often consult (or are brought to) their doctor only when their abnormality has become seriously disturbing to their relatives or has put them into conflict with the law. Some, however, are themselves distressed by their deviation and may on occasion need psychiatric treatment for complicating psychiatric disorder, such as a depressive illness or paranoid reaction. Now that sexual relations between consenting adult males is no longer a crime in many countries, homosexuals are less vulnerable socially.

Drug Dependency (Addiction). An addict is physically or psychologically dependent on a drug which he uses repetitively, and suffers distressing side-effects when deprived of it.

Alcoholism. An alcoholic is an excessive drinker who is unable to stop although to do so has become necessary because of health impairment, marital strife or difficulties at work.

Mental Handicap

A final diagnostic decision is to be clear about a patient's *intellectual status*; also included in the field of psychiatry is *mental subnormality*, present from birth or an early age, unlike psychiatric illnesses which supervene after a more or less normal psychological development. In intelligence defect present from infancy two categories are distinguished.

Mild mental retardation (I.Q. 50 to 70). Although the intelligence level is below normal (I.Q. 85 to 115), the child may benefit from teaching and social training.

Severe mental retardation (I.Q. 49 and below) refers to those so handicapped that they require very considerable attention and support and are incapable of leading an independent existence. The most common single cause of severe subnormality is Down's syndrome (p. 9). A definite cause of subnormality is found only in a minority of cases, and then various clinical conditions can be responsible, e.g. phenylketonuria, cretinism, etc. Patients who are mentally subnormal may also suffer from other mental illnesses. They may, for example, become depressed or schizophrenic, but when this happens the symptoms of their mental illness will be modified by their basic handicap of mental retardation.

Personality Development

Personality is socially acquired, given its genetic basis, over the course of time. The individual arrives at an adult psychological state after passing successively through a series of maturational stages. A baby is born into a human family, which provides immediate social support and responses. From the start the baby's 'personality' consists of the totality of his actions, but also of the reactions he makes particularly to the caring parent. At first the baby is helpless and receptive, dependent utterly on succour; such total care occurs as a result of nurturing impulses in the mother, fostered from the first days by the relationship and the interactions which develop in the nursing couple. The baby's cries, its smiles after some weeks, its need of nourishment and the relative satisfaction or distress deriving from its alimentary experiences, its fear of strangers from 8 months, all combine to bring out the protectiveness of the parental family. During this *oral stage*, the baby is perforce relatively passive; its needs are for care and nourishment.

During the *anal stage*, from 9 months to 18 months of age, the infant comes to gain sphincter control and to become more socialised as a member of the human family in other ways also, starting to learn the language and its usage, and coming to grasp the rules of the parental household.

The *genital stage* extends from 18 months up to 6 years of age. One of its characteristics is that the child now has sufficient awareness of family interactions and social norms to want to become informed about such matters as the difference between the sexes, where babies come from and how they are made; boys begin to imitate and assimilate aspects of their father's behaviour and character, while girls also become less concentrated in their attachment to the mother; they can show the most intense affection for their fathers, a passion that apparently needs recognition and an affectionate response for proper personality growth.

During the *oedipal phase* (as this period is called in the psychoanalytic literature), the child is often intensely frustrated by his diminutive size, puny powers and subservience to the powerful parents at a time when perception, knowledge and mastery of his environment evolve rapidly as his physical and mental abilities develop.

At 6 years, the child enters the *latency period*, which will last to puberty. He is socially obliging, very actively adapting to school life and is becoming increasingly an independent personality, able to be away from the parents for substantial portions of the day. If the parents are not seriously deficient as culture carriers, through neurotic illness or crippling social handicaps, the child now comes closely to grips with the norms, the roles, the sterotypes and the obvious and prevailing values in his culture. He is extremely impressionable, as advertisers on television well know, eager to add to his personality and experience by observing and borrowing from the behaviour and ideas of others.

At *puberty* the child's personality can enter a period of relative flexibility, when he may be given 'a second chance' and can set aside some trait patterns and in their place substitute new attitudes and beliefs; with the bodily and sexual changes of this period come demands for new orientations and relationships; a special requirement is for a friend. Children, just before entering their teens, either do succeed in achieving a close friendship or else they may suffer from a sense of unpopularity or loneliness.

The early teens are the period when *identity formation* either occurs or else fails to happen when identity diffusion will result. Then the youngster continues in a state of not knowing what he wants to be, what his capacities and potential allow him to aim for. The boy may be timid and lacking in confidence, or compensatorily brusque and hostile; the girl may inwardly bewail her female state, be perturbed at having menstrual periods and feel uncertain and wretched in social relationships especially as these relate to the future prospect of being courted. When identity formation does occur successfully, the young person decides on life goals and works towards them more or less hopefully, while feeling common cause with enough age-mates to be a member of a group.

At about 18 years, the late adolescent becomes capable of *intimacy*, able to regard the welfare of another loved person as no less important than his own. Young adulthood follows, with the capacity for *generativity*, with the intention and the potential to provide responsibly and reliably for others.

When the question of psychological normality of a patient is at issue, this chronological and subjective progression through biographical epochs has to be borne in mind. Psychological theory holds that each of these different stages is not obliterated by the one succeeding it but, like layers of an onion, one developmental phase superimposes the challenges (and the person's solutions to them) over and around the earlier solutions achieved. The residues of past developmental periods persist to give individuality to the person. When particularly upsetting setbacks (psychologically traumatic experiences) are encountered, a *fixation* may result, the person not negotiating oral, or anal, or genital challenges but instead remaining unduly preoccupied with the issues of that earlier life epoch. Often the facts about the psychic trauma are not remembered, as when a small child is parted from his parents for a surgical operation he does not comprehend. Jean Piaget was a pioneer in discovering the stages of unrealistic thinking characteristic of the successive phases in the child's intellectual development. Only at 13 years does logical thinking become possible. Thus each of the psychosocial phases described above takes place in parallel with magical, prelogical modes of thought. This knowledge makes it clearer why there are infantile psychic remnants in the thinking of many disturbed adults. Although knowledgeable about sex, a girl can fear she is pregnant despite intercourse not having occurred; a man can be distressed that he 'caused' the death of his mother by behaving harshly to her when she was terminally ill. Thinking that departs from reality or distorts it is often related to early demands which the child found unmanageable, or to distress which was intolerable emotionally at that time of life, such as the loss of a parent through death, or the family breaking up.

The adult, when handicapped by a persistence of immaturity, need not constantly manifest distortion of thinking or feeling in his behaviour. Only when a fresh set-back occurs in adult life may he decompensate in behaviour and *regress* to act in extreme variance from his everyday demeanour, with dependency and passivity (as when confronted by major surgery), or with obstinacy or hostility.

Mechanisms of Defence

As a consequence of excessive strains occurring early in life with which the personality was insufficiently mature to cope, the person can make use of psychological devices, 'mental tricks', to alter the inner environment or the surrounding reality and create an illusion of safety and predictability. A girl, unable to clarify sexual issues at the age of 5 years, perhaps denied a reassuring relationship with a kindly father, may use *denial* excessively: there are women who remain unaware of their sexual impulses and behave like school-girls forever: 'pregenital' personalities, some writers name them. A person may *overcompensate*: a timid, insecure boy setting out to acquire the outward characteristics of a tough male when he reaches adulthood. A boy who copes with upsetting homosexual desires at puberty by means of *repression*, in later life can be in greater emotional difficulty should he use the mechanism of *projection*: if psychotic, such a man may have an auditory delusion that other people are alleging he is a homosexual. A sexually deprived single women, using the same mechanisms, may be profoundly distressed, in the course of a paranoid reaction, by her erroneous beliefs that neighbours view her as sexually promiscuous: her own suppressed wishes are not admitted to her awareness but are exteriorised so that she believes others falsely suspect her of immorality.

There are other psychological mechanisms in the range of distortions and evasions to which troubled people can have recourse in extremity. By *reaction formation* we imply that an individual gives forth the opposite of facts he cannot acknowledge about himself: the son dominated by his father becomes not a domineering adult himself, but a timid, ingratiating, subservient adult—perhaps hen-pecked by an intimidating wife. However, such a man can change character drastically (the 'return of the repressed' is a term applied) and turn on his oppressor; the bedroom is the commonest setting for matrimonial murder when the victim is the wife; the husband dies most often in the kitchen.

Of course, psychological defence mechanisms rarely present so dramatically, and for clinical purposes more precise observation of smaller cues is required. We all use defence mechanisms at times of great stress: the surgeon's matter-of-fact manner is sometimes seen as necessary suppression of sympathetic emotions which could impair his competence, and his *selective inattention* to pathetic life circumstances may be altogether appropriate in an emergency. A civilian disaster is not the time for anguish over the human condition, if one is a surgeon with an operation to carry out. The defences which a person assumes psychologically, therefore, can be of much social value to others. A latently homosexual youth leader may be a boon to a neighbourhood—until his *sublimation* no longer serves, perhaps if he drinks excessively and loses his customary mental controls. School teachers and clergymen who interfere sexually with boys are in this category, and some doctors who become sexually involved with patients. In the course of clinical work, we judge a patient to assess whether he or she is spontaneous and unconstrained, or whether in contrast the patient when troubled denies mental conflict and imaginatively but unknowingly distorts surrounding reality in order to gain psychological relief.

Psychological Normality

In common with medical practice generally, individuals are often considered psychiatrically normal if no evidence of disorder is clinically evident. An epidemiologist doing a population survey may use an *empirical definition of normality* and regard as normal everybody who has not seen a psychiatrist nor consulted a general practitioner for any nervous ailment during the preceding year.

Another concept of normality at times invoked is an *ideal norm*, conveying an aspiration towards a desired state of well-being (such as is expressed in the preamble to the World Health Organisation constitution), devoutly to be wished but not to be found in this world: 'Health is a state of complete physical, mental and social well-being and not merely the absence of disease or infirmity'.

Psychiatrists occasionally write about normality, or aspects of it, in such inspirational terms that only too evidently they are not describing people as they are but as they would be, if a theoretical schema or 'mental health' blueprint were to become actual.

The third concept is a *statistical norm*, implying the state of most people contained in the community of which the patient is a member. In this sense, without straining after the ideal, we can indicate features characteristic of psychiatric normality in mature adults. Each of these can be readily identified, especially when the doctor has additional background information from prior acquaintance with the patient or members of his family.

A person who has successfully negotiated the sequence of stages in personality development is *appropriately autonomous*; he can manage his own affairs and tasks without undue reliance on others and can be depended on to meet obligations and to discharge responsibilities appropriate to his occupation, social circumstances and interests. The statement that a mature person can work, love and play perhaps reflects this capacity for autonomy.

A second feature of normality is *accurate self-perception*, the person not overestimating nor belittling his abilities. A third characteristic is correct *reality-testing*, the environment being perceived in an undistorted way. A fourth feature is *adjustment*, the person taking things as they are and making the best of them. The final two qualities of maturity are *integration* (relative coherence of the parts of the personality in contrast to gross self-contradictions), and *achievement*, the person using his skills and interests in such a way that his efforts are productive.

Incidence of Psychiatric Morbidity

In Britain serious psychiatric illness is relatively infrequent: about 1 in 200 of a general practitioner's adult patients is likely to suffer from severe depressive illness in the course of a year; the incidence of schizophrenia is much less, but since this illness runs a long course the cases tend to accumulate. The overall prevalence of schizophrenia, as shown by community surveys, is just under 1 per cent. As people grow older the occurrence of organic psychoses due to disease of the brain becomes increasingly common. The frequency of minor forms of psychiatric illness, such as neurosis, personality disorder and psychosomatic disorders, is very much greater. Careful counts have shown that minor psychiatric illness occurs every year in no less than 14 per cent of the patients on a general practitioner's list: if one includes cases in which psychological factors significantly influence coexisting physical complaints, the count rises to over 40 per cent.

Patients with emotional disorders tend to consult their doctors more often than patients with physical diseases and complain of a wider variety of symptoms. As a result, they are often referred to a succession of clinics for specialist investigation and commonly undergo minor or major surgery without avail. This involves a waste of both doctors' and patients' time, which could be avoided if the psychological disorder had been recognised and treated at an earlier stage. It is therefore necessary for all doctors to include a psychiatric appraisal as part of the clinical examination of his patients. This is a skill which has tended to be neglected in the past, but in medical schools where clerkships in psychiatry are provided, medical students have shown themselves rapidly able to acquire the necessary technical skills.

The Psychiatric Examination

It must be emphasised that attention should be paid to the patient's emotional state not only when a frank psychiatric illness is suspected, but in the course of any thorough clinical examination. Psychiatric disturbances can be elicited while taking the history and while examining the patient's mental state. The procedure for conducting these two aspects of the psychiatric examination are described in *Clinical Examination* (p. 798) and will be indicated only briefly here.

The Psychiatric History. Taking a psychiatric history is one of the chief clinical skills in psychiatry. The technique differs from history-taking in general medicine, being rather less directive, the doctor to a greater extent, perhaps, allowing the patient to raise apparently unconnected subjects and expand in directions initiated by the patient rather than the clinician. In general medicine the doctor may have a course of enquiry which he wants to have pursued; this is also so with psychiatric history-taking, but inevitably the patient will have personal information to give which may be unexpected. Hence the clinician is well advised to be especially receptive and to encourage disclosures which the patient initiates. The following topics need to be explored in the course of taking the history:

(i)   The date of the examination and the reason why the patient is seeking help.
(ii) The complaints and the patient's detailed account of the present illness.
(iii) The patient's parental family: an account of father, mother, each brother and sister (with the patient's birth order in the sibship), and the home atmosphere.
(iv) The personal history, including early childhood; schooling and other education; sexual development and experience; work record; friendships; marriage.
(v)   Previous illnesses, physical and psychiatric.
(vi) The personality before illness, with an account of the patient's interests, social activities, traits and such information about subjective and introspective experiences as the patient can provide.

Taking the history is the first therapeutic step. Psychological treatment begins the moment that the patient and doctor meet. The doctor's attitude to the patient and to his illness are powerful therapeutic factors which operate immediately. If history-taking is done patiently, thoroughly and objectively the patient feels interest is being taken in his case and that his problem is being understood. A spontaneous account of the illness by the patient should be encouraged. Too systematic an approach to the history often results in a mass of facts being obtained, but the real problem, from the patient's aspect, is entirely overlooked.

Examining the Mental State. As the interview proceeds, the doctor already is observing the patient's current mental functioning. The examination of the mental state is carried out in a systematic manner, paying attention in turn to the separate aspects of observable behaviour which disclose the state of mind.

Appearance and Behaviour. The appearance of the patient may be immediately informative, a dejected posture suggesting depressive illness: if the gestures the patient makes are tense and restless, clues may be provided which guide the doctor to enquire after further evidence of anxiety.

Mood. Whether the patient feels cheerful or depressed, confident or fearful, suspicious or bewildered, will become evident when the doctor asks the appropriate questions. 'How do you feel in yourself?' may be enough, but many patients need some help before they can unburden themselves of fears, anxieties or feelings of intense unhappiness. Some patients are ashamed to mention some emotional disturbances, such as a phobia, unreasonable intense anxiety experienced in certain settings, e.g. in open spaces. The patient may show a lack of emotional response; a very marked lack of rapport should also alert the doctor to the possibility that the patient may be schizophrenic.

Thought Processes. The way a patient thinks is evident in the patient's talk, which may be abnormal through incoherence, changes of topic, or bewildering shifts from one topic to another: all these can be features of schizophrenia. The patient may speak very rapidly, with puns and rhymes, as occurs in mania. Talk may be laboured, slow and flat and indicate a depressive state. Repetitive thoughts characterise obsessional psychoneurosis, an important feature of which is an *obsession*, a persistent idea which the patient cannot get rid of; the repetitiveness may be extremely distressing even when the patient recognises the idea as absurd—e.g. a girl may ponder whether she could be pregnant, although she knows perfectly well she has not had sexual intercourse.

Perceptions of Environment. The doctor next ascertains if the patient's perceptions are accurate. He may be unduly sensitive to glances or chance remarks. He may suffer from *illusions*, misinterpretations of sensations arising from real stimuli: a patient with delirium tremens may misinterpret furniture as menacing persons. *Hallucinations* are sense perceptions, such as visions, which occur in the absence of any kind of external stimulus. *Delusions* are false beliefs, such as that one is being slowly put to death, to which the patient adheres even when demonstrably wrong; a man with a hypochondriacal delusion, e.g. a depressed patient convinced he has venereal disease, persists in his morbid notion despite evidence to the contrary. A schizophrenic may be firmly of the belief that he has changed sex. These are signs of major illness.

Intellectual Functions. While listening to what he tells us, we can at the same time pick up clues about the patient's intellectual level from his choice of words and from the ease or difficulty with which he expresses himself. If there is reason to suspect that he may be intellectually impaired, one can test his general information by posing simple questions, such as asking him to name the Prime Minister, the capitals of the larger countries in Europe, or to perform simple sums of mental arithmetic. The best clues to mental retardation, however, are given by the patient's scholastic record and by the type of job which he has been able to perform in adult life. We note whether he knows the date and time of day, and recognises where he is and to whom he is talking: this tests his orientation for time, place and person. Impairment of mental function is commonly shown by inability to concentrate, to 'take things in', and hence to remember recent events. This may become apparent during the interview or it may be elicited by asking the patient to remember a name and address or a telephone number and then asking him to repeat it after an interval of 1 or 2 minutes. The final step in the mental state examination is an assessment of the patient's degree of insight into his condition; that is, does he recognise that he is ill or is he wrongly convinced that it is his environment and his fellows that are at fault?

When the history has been taken and an examination of the mental state completed, a thorough *physical examination* should be carried out and, following this, appropriate investigations when required. Such intervention needs to be handled well. Investigations which are necessary must be carefully planned, and quickly executed, and then a halt must be called. The pernicious habit of 'just having one more test' must be avoided as it undermines the confidence of the patient in the certainty of the diagnosis; the practitioner must be able to decide how much evidence is required to elucidate the nature and the cause of the disorder and, having obtained it, he must act upon it.

Diagnosis and Formulation. The doctor is now in a position to make a formal *diagnosis*, deciding from which psychiatric syndrome the patient suffers, i.e. whether the patient's illness falls in the general class of neurosis, personality disorders, functional psychosis or organic mental illness.

The next step is the *formulation*, a brief statement in which the doctor summarises his understanding of the disorder and the person suffering from it, including the main setbacks or conflicts with other people, in the sequence in which they occurred.

The Psychoneuroses

The first syndromes of psychiatric illness to be described are those which are most frequently encountered within general medical practice, namely the psychoneuroses.

There are two conditions to be met before the doctor can regard an illness as psychoneurotic. First, one of the typical syndromes (to be described below) must be in evidence. Second, the person must have experienced a recent setback, usually a disturbance in his relationship with a person or persons important to him. Often, when the first condition applies, the doctor may need to act on the basis of his clinical diagnosis without having elicited the biographical corroboration, but he must know that the omission exists and needs to be remedied, otherwise serious mistakes can happen. A casualty officer, an experienced, firm doctor, had a young athlete brought in who had begun coughing and breathing strangely at the end of a race he had failed to win. The casualty officer treated the boy as hysterical (a conversion reaction) at first kindly and supportively, but later quite authoritatively and even harshly—once slapping the boy's face in an effort to interrupt his agitation and dramatically laboured breathing. He missed the finding, made at post-mortem, of bits of apple in the boy's throat.

The setback preceding the onset of psychoneurotic illness need not be a gross one. However, it will be highly charged emotionally, in the context of the patient's biography, sometimes fitting as a key does into a lock with an earlier similar setback. It then seems understandable that the recent miscarriage of a relationship (the dynamic 'cause', or the process event) has disorganised the adaptation of a person previously sensitised by an earlier emotional trauma (the 'predisposing' cause). A woman who becomes ill with psychoneurosis when afraid that she may be deserted on discovering that her husband has become attracted to another woman may be found by further questioning to have lost her loved father through his death before her teens. The threat of the present loss is more understandably distressing in relation to the earlier deprivation.

Psychoneurosis, one of the 'minor' disorders, is an illness taking the form of one of the well-described syndromes in this category of disability: anxiety neurosis, hysterical neurosis, obsessional neurosis, reactive depressive illness, or phobic neurosis.

With all these characteristic syndromes the patient will be only partially disabled, many aspects of personality and social competence being unaffected. Hospitalisation is usually not needed. The man or woman can often cope with work and household responsibilities, and hence be treated as an out-patient. Reality testing is not impaired in any gross way, i.e. the misperceptions of the human and material environment characterising psychotic illness do not occur. The patient has only partial energy available for everyday activities.

There is a great amount of psychoneurotic illness in every community, for psychoneurosis is much the most common psychiatric disorder. Many individuals will be mildly disturbed and may not need medical treatment. The presence of a psychiatric syndrome does not of itself necessarily require intervention. A man with a fear of heights is not disabled if he works on the ground in a community made up of low houses; the same man who moves for postgraduate work to New York, for example, where he may have to attend seminars in skyscrapers, can become seriously impaired. On the other hand, flying phobia developing in any member of airplane personnel is instantly incapacitating.

Given the much greater amount of psychiatric disability in all countries than there are facilities for treatment, the doctor may consider that he will treat those psychoneurotic patients in whom there is both a clinical syndrome and also fairly conspicuous incapacity. The presence of psychoneurosis of itself does not necessarily call for treatment. Subjective distress on the patient's part is the indication that therapeutic intervention is needed.

Not all patients, of course, will accept with equanimity a diagnosis of psychoneurosis when their preferred concept of their illness is a physical one. This will often be evident from the initial reluctance with which some patients accept advice for psychiatric referral. A sickness of one's body is not regarded as a matter for which one is culpable (although Samuel Butler in *Erehwon* fancifully developed the opposite notion—that physical illness could be one's own fault). In contrast, a disturbance of one's mind could be regarded as an affliction of one's very self, and therefore a weakness in one as a person. The early neurologists, such as Head and Holmes, in discussing the body schema or body image, indicated the extent to which a person regards his body as somehow intermediate between the self and the outside world.

It has been demonstrated that the higher the social class of the patient, the more prepared he is to accept a psychiatric diagnosis. The same correlation between socioeconomic disadvantage and somatisation is evident in transcultural psychiatric studies: in the East and in Africa, patients in much greater numbers than in developed countries present psychogenic illness in the form of physical complaints. Indeed, as university health service experience with medical and other students has shown, even sophisticated patients often tend to complain first about somatic symptoms such as headache or stomach discomfort (and many doctors are more receptive about physical illnesses), and only afterwards proceed to relate a personal problem or to describe emotional distress.

The most important clinical rule is the need not only to elicit any psychoneurotic syndrome which may be present, but also to uncover the intrapersonal subjective tension preceding the onset of the illness; it usually consists of an upset in an important personal relationship (e.g. with a wife, another relative or a work associate).

A final point should be made about the diagnostic process, which is confusing to some doctors. Frequently, a patient with psychoneurosis is found to present more than one psychoneurotic syndrome. For instance, an emaciated amenorrhoeic girl refusing to eat and preoccupied with thoughts of food is also found to perform ordinary actions in sequences of five steps—such as rising from a chair in five different procedures: hands on the arm rests, extend elbows, etc.; the girl also is compelled to wash herself frequently and to want multiple baths each day. In such a mixed disorder, the primary diagnostic emphasis is given to the most prominent symptoms and the other aspects of the clinical picture are specified descriptively. In the case cited, an appropriate diagnosis would stress first the hysterical psychoneurotic syndrome, i.e. anorexia nervosa, adding that the primary syndrome is accompanied by obsessional features.

Anxiety Neurosis

Anxiety is a state of fear, occurring with a feeling of inner tension and somatic manifestations such as tense muscles, sweating, tremor and tachycardia. Anxiety neurosis is the most common form of psychoneurosis. Although anxiety is a symptom of many psychological disorders, in this syndrome it dominates the clinical picture and other symptoms are but minor features of the total illness.

Aetiology. Hereditary factors play a part, although a relatively small part, in the genesis of anxiety neurosis, manifestations of anxiety being found in 15 per cent of parents and siblings of patients, which is more than in the population as a whole (5 per cent). Twice as many women as men are affected.

In addition to the genetic trait, even more important aetiologically are emotionally disturbing experiences during the early formative years. These traumatic experiences need not be highly distressing nor need they be single events such as early loss of the mother. An isolated trauma is therefore not to be expected as a frequent predisposing cause in early life. More often it is found that the patient's early years were attended by prolonged insecurity. For example, a parent may have been so burdened by problems that the child felt unloved, if not unwanted; a brother or sister may have seemed to get preferential treatment; or a mother's own exaggerated anxieties may have imparted an excessive timidity to her child, profoundly undermining the child's self-confidence.

This emotional trauma may not be apparent for several years, particularly if the experiences of school life and early adolescence prove free of alarming or painful incidents: but a setback in early adult life may precipitate adult emotional illness. Painful events, such as a bereavement, a reverse in a love affair, disappointment in one's career, being obliged to contend with disagreeable or frankly hostile people at work, or being involved in prolonged domestic strife, may cause a vulnerable individual to succumb to feelings of anxiety which interfere materially with his ability to cope with the day-to-day routine. The adult setback will often be found to have been similar in quality to the earlier childhood emotional trauma.

Clinical Features. The illness may take many forms. It may occur as an acute anxiety attack, often severe in intensity, appearing against a relatively normal background, or a chronic anxiety state, present since adolescence in mild degree, but subject to periodic exacerbations occurring at the time of social setbacks, disappointments in close relationships, or work stresses.

The outstanding feature of the illness is anxiety, with its accompanying feeling of inner tension and unpleasant anticipation. Sometimes the anxiety is fear of a potential danger but often it is a diffuse dread. (A *phobia* develops when the anxiety is associated with a specific form of activity such as travelling in a bus or train, and so much may this be dreaded, that the patient is eventually house-bound through being unable to travel at all.) The fear and foreboding fluctuate in intensity, being sometimes a mild feeling of tension or nervousness, at other times a state of panic, in which the patient may be overwhelmed by a feeling of terror, which is no less disturbing because he is unable to say just what it is that makes him so afraid.

This state of anxiety gives rise to other symptoms. The ability to concentrate is impaired and decisions are difficult to make. There may be a continuous state of restlessness or extreme irritability. The patient may fear becoming insane or committing suicide though, in fact, both are extremely rare in anxiety neurosis. Preoccupation with bodily functions and fear of serious illness (*hypochondriasis* and *cancerphobia*) are frequently manifested. Continued stress exhausts the patient and, lacking energy and perseverance, he may no longer be able to carry on with his work.

Somatic symptoms are also prominent. There is a general tenseness of muscles, with hyperactivity, especially the hands. A fine tremor of the fingers is present and profuse perspiration, especially of the palms and forehead, is common. The pulse rate is raised, the blood pressure labile and overactivity of plain muscle is commonly manifest by frequency of micturition or of defaecation. Breathing is often rapid and feelings of nausea and flatulence occur; headaches of tension type, dizziness and unsteadiness are frequent. The patient sleeps badly, finding it difficult to get off to sleep and being easily disturbed. Appetite is poor, and loss of weight may be a pronounced feature. Disturbances of menstruation are common.

Not uncommonly the patient omits mention of his distressing emotional state and complains to the doctor only of the somatic accompaniments of anxiety; unnecessary special investigations can be initiated or diagnostic errors made if the doctor omits to ask about the state of the patient's mood.

Diagnosis. Medical illnesses that produce symptoms resembling those of anxiety neurosis include cardiac arrhythmias, angina pectoris, hyperthyroidism, pheochromocytoma and parathyroid disease.

It is scarcely surprising that some patients who know that they suffer from physical disease, e.g. diabetes, angina, peptic ulceration, renal failure or other forms of chronic disease, undergo episodes of severe anxiety which is in part at least related to the real threat to their lives. These patients with psychological complications of organic disease have to be distinguished from those who are crippled by an unjustified conviction that they have just such diseases (hypochondriasis). Not only will there be a negative physical examination, but when the patient has been helped to give free expression to his fears a positive diagnosis of the anxiety neurosis syndrome can be made.

Differentiation from other psychiatric illnesses is less difficult. Though hysterical, obsessive or depressive symptoms may be present in an anxiety state, the diagnosis can usually be made on the totality of the picture: anxiety often occurs in attacks and its accompanying somatic manifestations dominate the clinical presentation. It is rarely difficult to distinguish an acute anxiety state from a case of depressive psychosis with severe agitation and restlessness.

Treatment. When the formulation of the case indicates that emotional factors are prominent, some form of psychotherapy is required; the patient needs an opportunity for exploration and clarification, and for gaining greater insight into the nature of his difficulties. Simply informing the patient that there is nothing wrong with him, or that he must pull himself together, is useless. Even telling the patient that his difficulties are psychological and indicating the emotional problems in his life is unlikely to be of benefit, because although he may acquiesce verbally, his emotional tension will not be thereby lessened.

A series of interviews, for which periods of at least half an hour or longer should be set aside, are needed when the patient is encouraged to talk about his difficulties. Initially, the discussions should be allowed to proceed in any direction the patient desires; subsequently, aspects of his problems which come to seem relevant may be suggested by the doctor as themes for more detailed discussion. The error that is commonly made with this form of psychotherapy is for the doctor to talk too much and give advice. In order that the patient may achieve a better knowledge of himself, it is essential that he should do most of the talking, the doctor saying little, but maintaining an attitude of interest and expectation. If the patient's flow of talk is arrested, encouragement can often be given, without diverting him from his present theme. Thus, if he says, 'I found the job far too much for me', and then becomes silent, after giving him ample time to resume spontaneously, the doctor may say, 'You found the job far too much for you?', which starts the patient off again. The effect of this approach is first that the patient feels better for having talked to someone about his troubles. A second effect is that frequently the patient comes to grasp more accurately the nature of his problems, and will, at that stage, often accept suggestions and interpretations which, if given earlier, would have been rejected. What emerges is that the patient is having difficulties with a person of importance to him: a spouse, a parent, or an employer, for example, and that he needs to improve his management of the relationship. He may be too dependent on his wife, too docile to his parent, or too subservient to his employer—in which case his interviews should encourage greater assertiveness.

When the psychological disorder takes the form of somatic symptoms and fear of bodily disease is prominent, it is not sufficient simply to tell the patient that there is no evidence of organic pathology. It is necessary to let him know that his distress and his symptoms are recognised as genuine and need exploration. It is often possible to use events in the patient's own experience to illustrate the influence of emotion on bodily functions. Many people can recognise what it feels like to be sick with excitement, to be aware of a pounding of the heart in moments of fear or to experience frequency of micturition when keyed up before an examination. Patients are further helped when they can go one stage further, to confront the painful situation and to master it, e.g. the patient can say to his employer that he considers he is being exploited and his abilities insufficiently recognised. When this is done, there is commonly an immediate, even if temporary, relief from the distressing symptom, together with a sense of accomplishment which encourages the patient to persevere with further efforts of self-discovery.

The use of drugs to obtain reduction of distressing mood disturbance is often a necessary preliminary to effective psychotherapy. A very anxious patient will not be able to concentrate sufficiently to benefit more than partially from clarification of conflicts discussed during an interview. Diazepam and chlordiazepoxide are effectively anxiety-reducing drugs (p. 795). The phenothiazines, though widely used, are more likely to give rise to lethargy or drowsiness but thioridazine can be of value when the patient is both fearful and restless.

In the treatment of all forms of neurotic illness it is important to decide what can best be done, within the limitations of resources for treatment and in the circumstances of each individual patient. For example, one may recognise that a patient has shown a life-long pattern of minor phobias and proneness to worry but that recent events in his personal life have caused one particular phobia (such as the fear of going into crowded places) seriously to interfere with his normal activities. Here, the principal aim of the treatment should be limited to helping him to master the presenting symptom.

Behaviour therapy is a form of psychological deconditioning or desensitisation, often effective when a single disabling phobia, such as agoraphobia (fear of open spaces) or a specific phobia (e.g. of dogs, air journeys, public speaking, etc.) constitutes the clinical picture. Explorative psychotherapy, which calls on the patient to take stock of his relationships with people close to him and to modify some of his habitual patterns of behaviour towards them, is more time-consuming and aims to produce personality change as well as relief from the symptoms of the illness.

Brief psychotherapy focuses upon recent events in the patient's personal experience and explores their emotional significance for him. By this method, many patients can be helped to reconstitute the way of life which, for the particular person, represents normal mental health.

Hysterical Psychoneurosis

Hysterical psychoneurosis is a protean group of disorders, common in all branches of medicine. Essentially a hysterical neurosis consists of the production of the symptoms or signs of a 'physical' illness by a patient for some personal purpose, without his being fully aware of his motive in doing so. Familiar examples are sudden 'blackouts' or 'loss of memory' by which a patient evades a particularly painful or embarrassing occurrence.

Aetiology. Heredity is even less important in the development of hysterical neurosis than it is in anxiety neurosis, and plays but a minor role in its aetiology. Environment, by contrast, provides those situational factors which precipitate the development of hysterical symptoms. Lack of emotional security in the early years can encourage and prolong a state of child-like dependency. The lack of development of confidence to tackle practical difficulties makes a person rely on others to solve his problems and such a person may later react with hysterical illness.

During the First World War hysterical symptoms occurred more frequently among 'other ranks' than among officers, who were more subject to anxiety neurosis. Gross hysterical symptoms occur frequently in association with educational and intellectual disadvantage, and are a particularly common occurrence in developing countries.

Conversion Hysterical Neurosis. This type of psychoneurosis includes the illnesses in which the patient presents with a physical lesion, such as sudden blindness, or paralysis of one or more limbs, or total loss of sensation in a part of the body. Neurological examination will often reveal that the disability does not correspond to the anatomical areas served by motor or sensory nerves: instead, the lesion illustrates the patient's own idea of what it is like to lose the power of his right hand, or to be unable to walk. In many cases, the patient has acquired a concept of a particular affliction as a result of seeing someone who was similarly handicapped. The form the symptom takes may be determined by identification with another person, as when the daughter, after her mother's death, develops the symptoms of her mother's last illness.

The grosser forms of conversion symptoms are not so common today as they were a generation ago, but still occur particularly commonly as a complication of injuries where a compensation award enters the picture. A striking feature of conversion is that although the patient may be quite severely incapacitated by his symptoms, he appears remarkably unconcerned about them. This is because the disability due to the illness has in fact intervened to remove a cause of anxiety, so that the patient feels strangely relieved, although he is not aware of the reason for his being so calm.

The list of conversion hysterical symptoms and signs is extensive, for there are few clinical features which may not be encountered in this protean disorder. Some features, however, occur more commonly than others and may be arbitrarily divided into two groups, sensory and motor. *Sensory symptoms* may be of the special senses, such as blindness and deafness, or in the somatic sphere, when cutaneous and deep sensibility in their various forms are lost. The sensory loss does not obey anatomical or physiological laws but follows the patient's concept of disability. Cutaneous sensory loss may have a sharp horizontal upper margin on the limb. In monocular blindness, the patient may on occasion see with his 'blind' eye. There may also be positive sensory symptoms such as headache, pain, tinnitus and so on.

Motor symptoms consist of aphonia, mutism and paralysis and rigidity of movements. Positive clinical features in the motor sphere consist of tremors, tics and explosive utterances, spasm of ocular muscles, abnormal faints and fits. These fits may vary from simply falling to the ground as in syncope, to bizarre attacks with wild movements of arms and legs. Carpopedal spasm and other manifestations of tetany may result from hysterical hyperventilation.

Dissociative hysterical neurosis. The second type of hysterical psychoneurosis includes the numerous altered states of awareness, such as faints, fits, amnesias, trances, twilight states and forms of multiple personality. A fugue state is one in which the patient wanders away from home in a condition of altered awareness. Hysterical stupor, when the patient lies motionless showing no reaction to the environment, is sometimes seen; in pseudodementia (seen on occasion in a prison setting) the patient behaves as if insane.

Anorexia Nervosa. In this condition patients aim to achieve emaciation, or more accurately to become very slim and to stay so. Anorexia nervosa is often classified with the hysterical psychoneuroses. Frequently preoccupied about food, the patient stubbornly seeks to lose weight. The determination to diet is a disorder of motivation. Exertion of the will, so that over-riding priority is given to becoming thin, is the chief feature of the disorder. It often follows teasing about being plump.

Young girls are mainly affected. If questioned suitably, they often reveal preoccupations (sometimes so distorted as to reach delusional proportions) that they may be pregnant. They have other fears relating to sex, sometimes following misinformation by parents; however, these girls also give evidence of great fear at growing up and accepting mature feminine responsibilities. They are often in a hostile relationship with their mothers. Frequently there have been upsetting life experiences, such as separation from or death of a parent. In addition to dread of sexual development, girls with anorexia nervosa often show athletic preoccupations and are overactive physically. Amenorrhoea at times precedes marked emaciation. The usual mood state is cheerful high spirits, but depression can occur. Sometimes eating orgies occur, after which the patient feels extremely guilty and in advanced stages of the disorder may induce vomiting. Patients usually show unconcern about their physical deterioration and reject treatment, which often has to be very firmly advised and provided.

In-patient psychiatric treatment with psychotherapy to achieve emotional maturation is necessary, in addition to correction of the eating disorder.

Diagnosis of Hysterical Psychoneurosis. This can be the most difficult in medicine. Three steps are required: the first is to identify the psychoneurotic syndrome on the basis of its characteristic symptomatology, as described above. Only after such positive diagnosis need the second step be taken, should any doubt still exist, to demonstrate that there is no organic disease which can account for the symptoms and signs. Only rarely do special physical investigations or laboratory tests need to be carried out to exclude an organic illness. Error in diagnosing hysterical psychoneurosis would be infrequent, however, if the diagnosis were not made until the third step was also taken: this consists of discovering what disappointment or setback preceded the development of symptoms. The precipitating cause of a hysterical illness is usually an emotionally charged experience or setback, the unpleasant consequences of which the patient cannot face, and so excludes it from consciousness and escapes from the situation by means of symptoms.

If evidence of previous hysterical breakdowns can be uncovered, the diagnosis is more secure. It should be kept in mind, however, that the stress of organic disease may provoke a superadded hysterical reaction in a person so disposed. An axiom worth remembering is that alleged hysterical neurosis appearing for the first time in a stable person in middle life has almost always an organic basis.

Treatment. This may be a difficult problem. Removal of a symptom can often be achieved by a prolonged interview in which intense persuasion is used; but if the precipitating situation is unaltered, relapse is usual. The method may be justified, however, in certain circumstances as when aphonia prevents discussion, or when loss of memory in hysterical amnesia prevents the patient from communicating his identity or revealing the events which precipitated his illness.

The principles described for psychotherapy in the treatment of anxiety neurosis are also relevant in hysterical psychoneurosis. When hysterical personality disorder is also present, special aspects of management become necessary, as described on page 785.

Obsessional Neurosis

An *obsession* is a constantly recurring thought which the patient recognises as his own, but of which he tries to rid his mind because it is foolish or repugnant. In spite of his efforts to dismiss the thought, it persists in returning so that in the end he becomes tormented by it. A *compulsion* is a similarly insistent urge to perform, or to repeat, some act which the patient consciously repudiates as meaningless or troublesome; he struggles against the urge, but finds himself experiencing very acute anxiety, which is allayed only by his giving in and performing the compulsive act.

Obsessive-compulsive symptoms may occur as episodes of illness in otherwise normal individuals. They may become aggravated during an episode of psychiatric illness. Sometimes obsessions and/or compulsions are the outstanding, if not the only, symptoms of which a patient complains. In this condition the patient, although perfectly lucid and in contact with his environment, may be severely handicapped by the unrelenting pressure of his unwelcome thoughts and impulses. The illness is also remarkable in that a person almost incapacitated by obsessional symptoms can appear normal to the external observer, until he discloses his appallingly repetitive thoughts.

Aetiology. Obsessive-compulsive neurosis is often found in the children of parents who are similarly affected, but it is not clear whether this is due to transmission of a hereditary predisposition to the disorder. Many observers believe that the meticulous, rigid routine imposed by such parents is more conducive to obsessional neurosis in the child than the hereditary endowment itself.

Environmental factors, other than the influence of obsessive parents during the formative years, appear to contribute less to the causation of obsessional neurosis than is the case with the other syndromes of neurosis.

Clinical Features. Obsessions may be arbitrarily divided into ideas, impulses and ruminations. The *ideas* consist of thoughts, images (often obscene) and strings of words and phrases, which constantly recur to the patient despite resistance to them, and recognition that they are absurd and meaningless. The *impulses* are urges to some act such as killing offspring, or jumping under a train, or to less fearsome activities like laughing at sorrow or arranging objects in a certain set manner. Fears of some act may accompany impulses. A fear of knives develops from an impulse to use them for murderous ends. Likewise, a patient may not be troubled by obscene thoughts but rather by the fear that he may have such thoughts; he fills his mind with neutral thoughts lest obscenity should intrude. The idea representing an obsessive impulse keeps on invading the patient's consciousness. *Ruminations* comprise the practice of constantly turning over problems in the mind, seeking an answer to a question. Religious scruples are of this order, when the patient has repeatedly to examine and re-examine his conscience, uncertain as to whether he has offended or not.

These symptoms are often intermingled one with another, and may be of all degrees of intensity. Sometimes they are merely a nuisance, not interfering seriously with life, but preventing enjoyment and causing tension. In other cases they become so severe as to arrest all activity and make the ordinary daily round an impossible task. Thus a patient, who was a house painter, stood for three hours, unable to paint over a crack on the wall until he had the 'right' thoughts in his mind. Another patient, a housewife, spent all her time washing her hands for fear they should be contaminated, and so was unable to do her housework.

When the obsessions are severe they cause great anxiety and tension, the patients becoming increasingly agitated as they fight against the compulsion. In addition, they frequently become depressed, since life becomes so difficult and escape from the obsessions seems to be impossible. Suicide is, however, relatively uncommon except when depressive symptoms complicate the illness.

Diagnosis. This does not present great difficulty providing there is adherence to the exact criteria of the definition given at the beginning of this section. There must be the feeling of compulsion and, most important, the patient must recognise it as senseless or absurd and resist it. Delusions must be distinguished from obsessions: a patient does not feel his delusions are silly, but firmly believes in their truth. Similarly, such schizophrenic symptoms as feelings of compulsion or direction by some unknown force should not be confused with those of the obsessive-compulsive, who knows that the thoughts and impulses, however unwelcome, are his own thoughts and impulses. When the severity of such symptoms shows very marked fluctuation, a coexisting recurrent depressive illness should be suspected.

Treatment. The obsessional neurotic does not respond well to treatment, but often the condition is self-limiting, at least in its acute phases. The patient should be encouraged by being given the assurance that his doctor knows that his irrational, obscene or murderous thoughts are not indicative of his true nature. He should be encouraged to avoid situations which foster the development of the obsessions and should diversify his interests as much as possible. The best antidote for obsessive ruminations is for the patient to keep busy with practical tasks which demand his attention.

Depressive Psychoneurosis

This type of depressive illness is at times also named '*reactive*' or '*psychogenic*'; characteristically the morbidly depressed state comes on after a personal setback. This often takes the form of a loss of a person important to the patient, for example through death or separation as occurs with a divorce or a broken engagement. Careful exploration will show that the recent disappointment reflects one that occurred earlier in the patient's life. A typical example is the onset of depressive neurosis after a woman is left by her husband, and further interviewing discloses that she had lost a beloved father as a child. When the illness corresponds to an abnormal grief response after the death of a significant person, the term 'bereavement reaction' is sometimes used.

Only occasionally is psychiatric hospitalisation called for, the patient often responding well to out-patient psychotherapeutic interviews.

It may be confusing but it is nevertheless of the greatest importance to emphasise that admixtures of reactive and endogenous symptoms are extremely common. The clinical task is to scrutinise any case of depressive illness to determine the presence and amount of any component of 'endogenicity', i.e. so-called biological features including loss of energy, sleep disturbance, loss of appetite, constipation, impairment of libido, and—in severe cases—gross self-blame. In such mixed states antidepressant drugs are indicated, and good practice calls for a combined psychotherapeutic and pharmacological approach.

Admixtures of depressive symptoms with anxiety reaction occur frequently; some neurotically depressed patients are hypochondriacal in addition. Depressive reactions with endogenous features also commonly develop after physical illnesses, such as influenza, often causing prolonged depression.

Phobic Neurosis

These widely prevalent illnesses consist of unjustified fear which is firmly related to a precise stimulus, either a place or an object. The patient may be appallingly terrified at being in a supermarket, a bus, an open space (agoraphobia), or a closed place (claustrophobia). Fear of flying can be a nuisance to a housewife and may deter the family from taking overseas holidays, a major handicap to a business executive, and an occupational disaster to a pilot or other member of air crew.

The phobic place or object can be so innocuous as to seem ridiculous, and dreading ridicule the patient may not be able to summon the courage to disclose the affliction to the doctor. Direct questioning may be needed to explore cues which are offered, such as a patient never coming to the surgery unless accompanied by one of her children or by a neighbour.

Phobias can at times be referred to parts of the body, hence the use at times of such terms as 'cardiac neurosis' and 'cancerphobia'.

Patients can be terrified that they may have an urge to urinate when a toilet may not be accessible; when afflicted with this syndrome, patients know exactly the locus of every public lavatory in their neighbourhood.

The subjective benefit to the patient of suffering from a phobic state (rather than, say, an anxiety reaction or an obsessional illness) is that life can be perfectly manageable as long as the phobic stimulus is avoided. A person with a dog phobia need only find a dogless route to work, if one exists.

Antianxiety medication can assist such patients greatly, in association with interviewing which encourages the patient to 'go against the phobia', to enter into as many social occasions as possible. A requisite of treatment is that the doctor should comprehend the terror experienced by the patient (often related to childhood traumatic experience) and avoid a belittling response even when the patient's fear is grotesquely unjustified. A form of treatment which has a high rate of success, *behaviour therapy*, is based on devising for the patient a hierarchy of experiences relating to the phobic object or situation, in which increasing exposure is gradually built up, always avoiding excessive anxiety. Someone with a dog phobia may look with the doctor or clinical psychologist at canine pictures, starting with a benign species and coming at length to an Alsatian; then real dogs can be introduced to the interview, first a docile, aged pet and perhaps later quite daunting beasts encountered on a walk can be approached with due circumspection. A phobic pilot's behaviour therapy may in part occur in a stationary aircraft.

Personality Disorders

In every large community there are a number of people who do not conform to the prevailing norm. Statistically speaking, a person can be outside the range of normal either by being exceptionally gifted or by being so grossly underendowed as to be an eccentric or a social misfit; but it is the latter who are more likely to come to medical attention.

The personality disorders began to gain notice only late during the development of psychiatry as a medical discipline; they have been recognised increasingly as the out-patient responsibilities of psychiatrists have extended, and as psychiatric units have developed in general hospitals. The diagnostic differentiation between psychiatric illness and personality disorder is the more necessary because very often the two coexist. Indeed, clinical convention has it that hysterical psychoneurosis commonly supervenes in individuals with hysterical personality, obsessional neurosis in those with obsessional personality disorders, etc. In addition to their presentation with psychotic illnesses and psychoneuroses, people with abnormal personalities often appear clinically with psychosomatic disorders and may be chronic hospital attenders. Abnormal personalities may not enter the medical ambit at all, but be encountered in penal settings. Still others may continue unrecognised in the community and only escape anonymity when widespread screening of the population occurs, as in wartime when obligatory intake to the armed forces exposes all adults to clinical scrutiny.

The association between the different types of psychiatric illness and the various forms of abnormal personality is now recognised as a more complicated problem than the earlier statements of the position suggested.

The central feature of abnormal personality is some degree of persistent abnormality of behaviour which is frequently, but not necessarily, antisocial in its manifestations. The abnormality varies considerably in degree, ranging in severity from schizoid and hysterical people who are often valuable if somewhat unstable members of the community, to psychopaths who are socially destructive.

Obsessional Personality Disorder

The obsessional person gives scant regard to the emotional aspects of a situation or an interaction. He is rigid rather than flexible, overattentive to details rather than to the wider scope of an event or encounter, and prefers to have everything predictable and orderly. He often appears officious, sometimes so pedantically that he can be comical, and not only controls himself excessively but also attempts to dominate others. He appears to behave in an excessively egotistical manner, and responds in an overriding way when involved in a venture calling for co-operation. He is overcareful, methodical, liking things cut-and-dried, concerned with neatness and orderliness. He can be very meticulous, punctual and overorganised, to the extent of becoming uncomfortable and even upset if his routines are disturbed by any unexpected development. He has a set of fixed standards and points of view, from which he can deviate only with great difficulty. He is uninfluenced, therefore, by the wishes, needs, opinions or views of other people.

The meticulousness and preservation of sameness extends to the person's mode of dress, which can be scrupulously neat. He can be overconscientious, paying greatly excessive attention to minutiae. He may work compulsively, and be unable to make use of opportunities for relaxation. Such a person, in consequence, can be of particular usefulness in a bureaucratic post calling for scrupulous concern with details. He may be highly obstinate when faced by any requirement that he should deviate from his straight and narrow path.

At times such a person appears to leave some loophole, so that the conformity, inhibition and rigidity is waived in some context or other. The precise, neat youngster, who must have everything in place, may for example permit himself to have his clothes cupboard in disorder, or may periodically forget thrift to overspend in a foolish self-indulgence which rationally is at odds with his habitual miserliness.

The gross form of the disorder is easy to recognise. The milder forms may be less obtrusive, and may be particularly evident only at times of pressure, as when an examination is looming for a youngster or when a house-proud woman has relatives coming to stay in her home.

Schizoid Personality Disorder

The schizoid person is essentially solitary. He is aloof in his loneliness, detached and distant from other people. He has few close relationships, and may be much more preoccupied with some impersonal activity in the realms of electronics, physics, mathematics or engineering. Often the engrossing venture is a personal fad or invention, which may be of negligible application in ordinary life, but may be pursued with a single-minded devotion inappropriate to a mere hobby or interest.

Cold, quiet and shy, the person's abnormality may already have been apparent early in childhood, from an inability or disinclination to mix, and a preference for solitary pursuits. The lack of friendships may have been upsetting to the parents; as the person grows up, he can himself be distressed by his incapacity for any intimacy in his associations with others.

The person may appear odd, eccentric, gawky, and in his awkward isolation may appear as a figure of fun. He may seem excessively secretive. Schizoid people are often solitary workers, who cannot function satisfactorily in a team. Bookish, reserved, out of touch with others, relatively blind to social cues, their personal lives may appear barren. However, this remote exterior may belie the strong emotions which some schizoid people cannot express. Others find a vehicle for their private feelings, and may keep a diary, or indulge in day-dreaming, or succeed in establishing some relationship in which the expression of emotion is allowed.

The schizoid person is at times mistrustful, seeing slights where none is intended. He is rigid and brittle. He has little empathy with other people, and so remains unaware of their intentions, feelings and wishes. When he attempts to appraise others intuitively, he is often wildly wrong, thereby complicating his already attenuated relationships. He can be made profoundly uncomfortable when well-meaning but misguided mentors or doctors attempt to have him mix more, or urge him to become intimate with another person, perhaps another isolate as lacking in interpersonal skills as himself.

Suspicion can become the prevailing response to others, the person believing that he is being exploited, misused or disparaged. Some clinicians would differentiate this development separately, diagnosing such a personality as paranoid.

Hysterical Personality Disorder

People of this type can be identified on the basis of a constellation of behaviours: they seek to please and influence others; they crave attention; they are insincere; and they are given to excessive displays of emotion.

An hysterical person appears to be exploitative, with an eye always on the other person. She talks for effect, not to convey any honestly felt intention. One feels her need for appreciation, and her readiness to express herself with that aim in view. She plays up in order to evoke a response, and that response is one which she has already 'decided' to elicit.

Psychiatrists probably over-diagnose this type in abnormal women, attaching the label very much less often to men. The person is showy, histrionic in manner and dress, with a quality of spuriousness and exaggeration, even theatricality, in what she does. The exhibitionism appears intended to impress others, even to shock them. Speech is superficial, with plentiful hyperbole ('heavenly', 'ghastly'), which only heightens the effect of shallowness. Women of this type suffer from sexual timidity and frigidity, the more distressing to them because their frequently seductive manner and provocative dress invites advances with which they cannot cope; hysterical men also have difficulty in establishing a close relation with one woman, and may seek intimacy in a series of attachments of short duration.

Sociopathy

The sociopath suffers from the most severe form of abnormal personality. Because of his serious defect in the capacity for feeling, he is often described as 'affectionless'. Lacking in conscience he has great difficulty in realising that other people are harmed when he behaves antisocially. Loveless, indifferent and destructive, he cannot form satisfactory relationships, and major failures repeatedly occur in his marriage, his work and his social life. He comes into conflict with the norms, customs and laws of his community, not learning from his failures, however catastrophic; already present from an early age, his social ineptitude is persistent, leading him chronically to be in trouble. Many sociopaths are superficially likeable and charming, and initially mislead well-meaning people whom they subsequently disappoint and mortify.

Impulsiveness is usually evident, the sociopath dismaying those associated with him by uncontrolled, often destructive outbursts in the absence of sufficient provocation. Such precipitate and deplorable action has been spoken of as 'short circuit reactions', to indicate that often the person is aware of the buildup to the outburst, and will often admit that after the aggressive or destructive episode he feels calmer and relieved of tension.

The sociopath does not show ability to modify destructive behaviour reactions, or to learn from even drastic setbacks; he may be punished repeatedly for the same unacceptable behaviour, and yet continue it; the individual's antisocial patterns are often monotonously repetitive. Kleptomania, gambling, or physical assaults may each be associated with excitement which the sociopath seeks and indulges repeatedly; the antisocial behaviour can be seriously destructive to others, as in cases of sadistic attacks on children or of pyromania.

The lack of regard for the possible consequences of his actions is also impressive, the sociopath appearing not to care about the outcome, and scant in his consideration even of persons on whom his welfare depends. He disregards his obligations to others: it is on this account that the Mental Health Act (England and Wales) of 1959 described the sociopath's conduct as 'seriously irresponsible'. The lack of concern amounts often to callousness.

His social relationships are shallow and transient. He is not loyal to individuals or to groups. He has poor judgement of situations, and often lies his way out of complications. He is indifferent to the welfare of others. He requires immediate satisfactions, not being able to postpone gratifications; he seeks instant excitement or relief of discomfort, and may misuse drugs or alcohol so that secondary addictions are common. Swindling and deception are frequent features.

Two types of sociopathy are distinguished:

Aggressive Sociopath. The hostility displayed in attacks on other people, damage to property, thefts and fraud may bring the sociopath to legal attention.

Passive Sociopath. A person of this type is seriously inadequate and cannot adapt to social requirements; he is chronically inept, passive and dependent. Many are placid and responsive; others are cold, withdrawn and apathetic. They may exist as aimless drifters, to be found in places where hobos congregate. Even if supported in a family or protective environment such as a half-way house or hostel, such people may be sufferers from drug addiction or alcoholism.

Management Implications

The chief medical relevance of personality disorder, in terms of the doctor–patient relationship, is that patients respond to the clinician in accordance with their particular personality deviation. For this reason, diagnosis of the personality type permits the doctor to plan management realistically, so that he does not expect a degree of co-operativeness which the patient is not equipped to provide. In addition, he will be better able to predict the patient's pattern of behaviour in the future.

For example, the long-term management of a patient with an hysterical personality disorder has much in common with that of a frightened or petulant child. It consists in convincing her that you are on her side, even while refusing to comply with some of her requests. Treating a patient with such a personality disorder is often a test of nerve; in the face of dramatic protestations and apparently alarming social crises, one must quietly but firmly insist upon facing the painful realities from which the hysteric has taken flight. If one has succeeded in gaining her confidence, helplessness and distress will sometimes disappear with dramatic suddenness, but all too often they are replaced by subsequent turmoil. The hysterical patient finds it difficult to abandon the defences against alarming feelings which she has been using since her early adolescence. In addition these patients are especially prone to develop an emotional dependence upon their doctor, which must be recognised and brought to their attention kindly but firmly. The family doctor can give helpful advice to other people in the patient's immediate environment, warning them that hysterical symptoms only become aggravated if too much attention is paid to them, and encouraging them to avoid entering into the hysteric's pattern of self-deception. It is usually much easier for the onlookers than for the patient herself to see the real motivation of her symptoms, but of course, it is no use simply *telling* her—she has to discover for herself why she behaves in the way she does.

The achievement of a long-term cure of an hysterical personality disorder is a formidable task since it requires the patient to mature emotionally. Not surprisingly, both patients and their doctors often tacitly agree not to attempt it. Instead, the doctor may concentrate upon dealing with the most pressing difficulties of the patient's immediate predicament and may settle for her remaining a somewhat demanding and dependent patient. In that case, the goal for each consultation can be to ensure that the patient departs calmer and with more self-esteem than when she arrived. The doctor helps the patient discover some modifiable aspect in a problem which she had considered insoluble.

Alcoholism and Drug Dependence

Alcohol. Alcoholics are often brought reluctantly to their doctor by close relatives who can see more clearly than the patient how seriously his life is being interfered with by his addiction. These unwilling patients are particularly difficult to treat; but the prospect is very different when the patient himself is distressed by his dependence and is anxious for change.

Addiction to drugs or to alcohol represents a form of psychological dependence and indicates that the patient has been unable to attain adequate satisfaction or self-esteem in his personal life. Addictions to drugs and to alcohol are associated with a high risk of suicide. The underlying lack of self-confidence is often so deep-seated that prolonged treatment and rehabilitation is necessary once the drug or alcohol has been given up. Alcoholism is a serious health problem in Britain, and more especially in Scotland. In 1968 mental disorders due to alcoholism were responsible for 26 per cent of male admissions to Scottish mental hospitals. It is an insidious condition, because the enjoyment of alcohol is socially accepted and even encouraged. The process by which an occasional drinker becomes an excessive drinker, and finally dependent on drink can be gradual; acquaintances, and even friends, are reluctant to draw attention to a man's excessive drinking because the alcoholic is notoriously liable to take offence. Here, however, doctors have a clear responsibility because often an intercurrent illness, chronic dyspepsia or haematemesis, or even a street accident will bring the patient to medical care, and a carefully taken history (especially if supplemented by information from others in the patient's family) will reveal the increasing dependence upon alcohol. Sometimes an unexpected hospital admission, interrupting a sustained high intake of spirits, results in the onset of *delirium tremens* which compels attention to the seriousness of the drinking problem. This is characterised by gross peripheral tremors, great restlessness, confusion, misidentification of people and places and delusional ideas. These delusions may be agreeable but much more often they are threatening or even terrifying, especially when accompanied by hallucinatory visions. Because of these complications, hospital admission may be necessary when starting to treat an alcoholic.

Treatment of Alcohol Addiction. This consists initially of 'drying out', which often calls for hospital admission. Withdrawal symptoms can be controlled by phenothiazines, diazepam, haloperidol (p. 796) or chlormethiazole (heminevrin). The last is an hypnotic related to thiamin. It is probably the drug of choice in severe alcohol withdrawal syndromes including delirium tremens. In these circumstances it should not be used for longer than 1 week because of the danger of dependency. Parentrovite intravenously may also be of value.

The next phase of treatment, once the patient is abstinent, is to explore with him by means of a series of interviews, his personal and other problems which require attention. Psychiatric assistance is needed if obvious psychological disorder is apparent once the drinking has stopped. Those abstinent alcoholics who consider themselves in danger of relapse can ensure their sobriety by taking Antabuse (disulfiram) 0·5 g daily, or Abstem (citrated calcium carbimide): when on these drugs, the patient will have an unpleasant reaction after taking only a small amount of alcohol.

The main requirement of treatment is that the alcoholic should become totally abstinent. Many alcoholics are active and valuable members of society and can maintain this necessary abstinence if given appropriate medical supervision.

Morphine. Addiction is seen in doctors, nurses, pharmacists and dentists, and at times in patients who become addicted through therapeutic use. The desired euphoric effect can be achieved by subcutaneous injection, but as tolerance grows intravenous injections are used ('main lining'). Hypodermic tattooing of the skin, thrombosed veins and pinpoint pupils are indications of the condition.

Heroin. Addiction is increasing rapidly in incidence, and many addicts are young people. The drug has a marked euphoriant effect; it acts quickly and its desired action also dissipates quickly. The abstinence syndrome is particularly unpleasant. Many addicts cannot be cured, and their management then is by supplies of the smallest dose of the drug preventing the withdrawal symptoms, or by substitution of methadone in place of heroin.

Cocaine. Those addicted to cocaine take the drug in the form of snuff or in-travenously. The most well-known toxic symptom is formication, the sensation of insects crawling under the skin. Use occurs mainly in those addicted also to heroin, the effect of cocaine alone being unsatisfactorily brief. By the Drug Addiction Act of 1968 issue of heroin and cocaine is limited in Britain to named doctors, usually psychiatrists in designated treatment centres.

Lysergic Acid Diethylamide (LSD). This is used mainly by young people. Taken by mouth, it has dramatic effects lasting about 6 hours. Illusions occur, colour is intensified, mood changes include euphoria, awe or anxiety, a curious blurring between the individual and his environment is experienced, and phantasy thoughts, flight of ideas and delusions serve to heighten the mystical nature of the 'trip'. Proponents of the drug as a 'mind expander' sometimes overlook the serious hazards; these include psychotic reactions with paranoid delusions which can last many weeks, and non-psychotic reactions chiefly terror; both can result in self-injury or suicide. A bad LSD experience can be cut short by chlorpromazine, used intramuscularly in severe cases.

Cannabis (hashish, marihuana, 'pot'). This is also used very commonly by the young, sometimes only a few times; there is no evidence that occasional use is harmful. At first the user feels 'high', and then drifts into a peaceful, drowsy state heightened by unusual mental images. Skin flushing, rapid pulse and dilated pupils may convey that a person has taken cannabis, usually by smoking a 'reefer'. Many addicts use more than one drug.

Barbiturate. Many middle-aged or elderly women come to rely upon a nightly dose of sleeping tablets and some of them find that if they take two or three during the day, this helps to calm their nerves. Gradually, they begin to show the signs of chronic barbiturate over-dosage: slight ataxia, absent-mindedness amounting at times to confusion as to time and place, slurred speech and tremor of the fingers. A sudden cessation of barbiturates can be followed by a major epileptic fit. A patient cured of one addiction, e.g. alcoholism, may start using another drug, e.g. barbiturate, which he erroneously regards as innocuous.

Amphetamine. This drug, formerly used in the treatment of obesity and still used for narcolepsy, soon came to be abused, particularly by teenagers, either alone or combined with barbiturate ('purple hearts') to provide a rapid lifting of the spirits and feeling of well-being. The use of amphetamine readily gives rise to a psychological dependency, when the daily dose taken can increase vastly, tolerance developing with continued use. The amphetamine addict has an imp.es-sion of increased mental and physical drive and competence. He also shows restlessness, irritability and excitability. Amphetamine can give rise also to an acute psychotic reaction with auditory and visual hallucinations and delusions of persecution. These features can be clinically indistinguishable from those of paranoid schizophrenia, but they clear up in about 3 weeks time after withdrawal of the drug. Since the Misuse of Drugs Act (1971) amphetamines are listed as controlled drugs in Britain, special regulations applying to prescribing.

Sexual Deviation

Sexual deviants are people who are unable to obtain physical and emotional satisfaction in normal sexual intercourse, but can do so only in ways which to a greater or less degree are socially condemned. Practices which alarm, threaten or injure other persons, such as exhibitionism, paederasty (having sex with immature partners of either sex) or sadism (deriving sexual pleasure from inflicting pain) are still regarded as antisocial and are punishable by law. On the other hand, public opinion has become somewhat more tolerant of abnormal practices which do not interfere with other people. This change of opinion found expression in the Sexual Offences Act, 1967, which, for the first time in British history, excluded homosexual acts, carried out in private by consenting adults, from any legal sanction.

Most forms of deviant sexual behaviour, such as homosexuality, transvestism (deriving gratification from wearing the clothing of the opposite sex) and fetishism (when the person becomes sexually stimulated by parts of the body not usually experienced as erotogenic—e.g. the feet—or by articles of clothing or other objects) seem to be the result of distorted experiences at the stage of development when boys and girls learn their sexual role. These deviant forms of gratification often prove very resistant to change. If the patient suffers because of them—and many sexual deviants appear to be rather content with their lot—treatment often has to be limited to damping down the intensity of the sexual drive, e.g. by the administration of oestrogens, or to helping the patient (and perhaps also his spouse) to accept his peculiarity.

Psychosomatic Disorders

These are the group of physical illnesses which are caused in part by psychological factors or, when present, are maintained by psychological factors. Examples of such conditions are many cases of peptic ulcer, bronchial asthma, various forms of dermatitis and colitis. The implication of this term is that tension arising from a long-standing emotional conflict can induce changes in bodily function (e.g. excessive secretion of gastric juice; bronchospasm) which, when repeated over a period of time, can in turn lead to actual tissue damage.

For many years, attempts have been made to delineate particular personality types associated with different forms of psychosomatic illness. A review of this literature, however, fails to reveal a specific type of personality in relation to each of these disorders. Instead, psychosomatic subjects tend to be characterised by relatively constant emotional elements, the chief of which are dependency, anger, fear, which appear to be most harmful when they are denied conscious expression. Repressed dependency needs have been particularly associated with peptic ulcer and ulcerative colitis, repressed anger with asthma and hypertension. Individual cases, however, when studied in depth, are not easily fitted into any common mould. Modern psychosomatic theory has, therefore, retreated to the more general observation that all psychosomatic patients have long-standing problems in the control of their own internal emotional homeostasis, and in the conduct of their relationships with people who matter in their private lives. It is probable that genetic factors, which have endowed some of us with a particularly vulnerable organ or organ system, will dictate both the occurrence of a psychosomatic illness (which often indeed coexists with neurotic symptoms) and the choice of the organ which is affected.

Treatment of the emotional disturbance and disregard of the local physical factors, or vice versa, will seldom lead to benefit for the patient, and an assessment must be made in each case of the relative importance of these two factors, so that whichever appears to have the greater aetiological significance can be the main target for therapy. The general practitioner is often in the best position to know the unrealised ambitions, the frustrations at work or at home, or the marital unhappiness which may form the background to the patient's illness. A knowledge of the family history may also reveal that hereditary predisposition plays a part in determining the physical form of the illness, as in migraine, for example.

Functional Psychoses

Depressive Illness

Depression is a mood which all of us experience from time to time, usually as a result of some distressing circumstance. In contrast, patients suffering from depressive illness complain of a prolonged dejected state. Those whose depressed mood set in after some particularly unfortunate experience usually have a depressive neurosis of the type described above. Patients suffering from the more serious condition of depressive psychosis seem to have become ill for no reason they can identify, their low spirits and subjective misery causing them to feel altogether different as people.

Clinical Features. In addition to a mood varying from mild depression to black despair the manifestations are: insomnia of a type characterised by early waking after 2 to 3 hours sleep; diurnal variation of mood, in which the depression often lifts considerably towards evening; slowness of thought, and inability to make decisions; ideas of guilt, unworthiness and self-blame which are often delusional in intensity, i.e. they are impervious to reasoned argument or demonstration of their falsity; and various somatic manifestations such as loss of appetite, loss of weight, amenorrhoea, occipital pressure headache, backache, constipation, retardation of physical activity (more rarely aimless over-activity or agitation), and hypochondriacal delusions. Such a patient may sit bowed and immobile on the edge of a chair obviously in the depths of misery, weeping silently, wringing his hands and answering questions in slow monosyllables; but in the earlier stages the physical appearance is less striking and the diagnosis depends on the doctor's ability to elicit the symptoms described above.

Such patients are suffering from *endogenous depressive illness.* They are often people who have been subject previously to mood swings or people who have overscrupulous, rigid personalities following too strict upbringing and who develop depression particularly in later middle age (involutional melancholia). Endogenous depressive illness may be precipitated by physical diseases such as influenza, pyelonephritis and infective hepatitis, and may sometimes be the first symptom of cerebral disease, such as general paresis or cerebral atherosclerosis, but more often, as its name suggests, it arises without detectable external influences. Endogenous depressive illness is commoner in patients of middle age or older, but certainly does occur in the young and also in children.

Such patients often find meeting people a painful ordeal and prefer to suffer alone. It must be remembered that both profound, endogenous illness and also relatively less serious reactive depressive illness may be precipitated by external events, particularly those which impart a sense of loss, separation or disappointment. The difference in their manifestations is largely a matter of the intensity of the suffering involved, but some very depressed patients are prevented, by the illness itself, from revealing the full extent of their suffering. Their self-deprecation and sense of unworthiness may make them believe that they deserve to suffer and their feelings of guilt may make them reluctant to disclose the full intensity of their feelings. Many severely depressed patients are afraid that they are 'going mad', and many are frightened, as well as ashamed, at their own suicidal thoughts. Some doctors, out of a mistaken fear of adding to their distress, may connive in these patients' attempts to avoid mentioning these painful topics; but in fact, so far from harming the very distressed patient, it often brings a measure of solace if he is helped to give expression to these deep-seated fears. One should not, therefore, hesitate to help him put them into words. The fear of insanity can often be relieved by a frank discussion of the illness, accepting its severity but indicating its likely favourable outcome; thoughts of suicide have to be evaluated differently according to whether they have been fleeting and resisted, or constant and insistent.

Treatment. The first task after diagnosing endogenous depressive illness is to proceed without delay to treat the patient with one of the potent antidepressant drugs (p. 797). One has to bear in mind, however, that these drugs do not take effect until after some 6 to 14 days.

Severe endogenous depressive illness, especially when associated with restlessness and agitation, with delusions of unworthiness and preoccupation with thoughts of death, is an extremely distressing condition and fraught with risks of suicide, especially when the patient states that his mind has been dwelling upon a particular method of killing himself. Such cases should be admitted to psychiatric care in hospital. Electric shock therapy, administered under intravenous anaesthesia and modified by muscle-relaxant drugs may be indicated if the patient's suffering is not relieved after antidepressant medication for 2 to 3 weeks.

As a general rule, it is wise to postpone any practical decisions about business, change of work or domestic matters until the patient has regained his normal frame of mind. Once the patient's mood has responded to drug or other physical methods of treatment, it is essential to review his personal circumstances with him and to help him make plans to cope with the difficulties which may have precipitated his illness. Moreover, the patient may need to know that the psychosis sometimes takes a recurring form and that he must come for examination if there is any recurrence of depressive symptoms. Suicidal risk is often greatest at the onset of depressive psychosis (or when treatment begins to relieve the depression and reduce the accompanying psychomotor retardation).

Manic Illness

In manic-depressive psychosis the patient, apart from depressive attacks, can suffer from morbid elation and hyperactivity. He looks excessively cheerful, speaks rapidly, shifting from one idea to another, often joking, teasing, making puns and paying poor attention to his environment. He is overconfident, overoptimistic and overimportant. He may suffer from grandiose delusions and behave in an extravagantly spendthrift way. He usually does not realise he is ill, and may react with violence if crossed or restrained. Failure to diagnose mania can have very serious consequences for a patient, who can run up vast debts or jeopardise his social position drastically by ill-judged, embarrasing or boisterously inappropriate and undesirable behaviour. Treatment is discussed on page 798.

Schizophrenia

Schizophrenia is the illness with symptoms corresponding most closely to the popular conception of the madman. These patients are likely, at least during the acute phase of their illness, to experience hallucinations (most commonly, in the form of threatening or unfriendly voices) and to express bizarre delusions with little or no appreciation of why it is that their ideas are unacceptable to those around them. Both delusions and hallucinations may occur in other forms of mental illness, such as severe depression, mania, or delirium, but certain features are especially suggestive of schizophrenia. These include (1) *passivity feelings*, in which the patient is convinced that his actions are controlled by some alien power, (2) *thought insertion* and *thought broadcasting*, in which he feels that other people put thoughts into his mind, and are able to read his thoughts and (3) *paranoid delusions* in which he believes that he is surrounded by hostile forces which watch him and secretly intervene to do him harm. Patients with depressive illness may also develop paranoid ideas, but these are coloured by their all-pervading feelings of guilt. For example, a depressed patient may believe that he is being watched by secret police because they have found out that he has committed a terrible crime. The paranoid schizophrenic, on the other hand, is quite sure that it is his unseen enemies who are the villains of the piece, and he their innocent victim. These patients tend to have little insight into the fact that they are ill and in need of treatment. When their behaviour is becoming alarming, it may be necessary, in their own interests, to admit them compulsorily to hospital. The application is made by the patient's nearest relative supported by two medical recommendations by the patient's family doctor and a psychiatrist. The patient's case must be reviewed after 28 days. In many cases he will continue in hospital voluntarily. A mentally ill patient who is a danger to himself or others may also be admitted compulsorily as an emergency for 3 days in England and Wales and 7 days in Scotland. This certificate is signed by only one doctor and can be used when the patient is already in hospital.

These are the more florid manifestations of schizophrenia. Milder signs are less easy to recognise, because they merge into the peculiarities of everyday living. These include instances of unexpected rudeness or tactlessness, abrupt and inexplicable behaviour with a marked withdrawal from ordinary social contacts. Such persons may be considered awkward or unsociable and it is only when they reveal quite bizarre ideas, shout back at their hallucinatory voices, or otherwise behave in a conspicuously strange manner, that one realises that they are not merely eccentric, but mentally ill.

Treatment. The advent of the phenothiazine drugs (p. 795) has very significantly changed the prognosis of schizophrenia but it should be remembered that even before there was any specific drug treatment for this illness, many cases made a spontaneous recovery from the acute stage of the psychosis in the course of 3 to 9 months. Even now, the new drugs offer symptomatic relief of the patient's delusions, hallucinations and alienation from reality, rather than a radical cure of this little-understood disease. There is abundant evidence that the way in which the patient is treated, both in hospital and in the community, will influence both his degree of recovery and the probability of a subsequent relapse.

Putting it briefly, it may be said that schizophrenic patients do badly if they are allowed to withdraw too completely from social contacts and practical activities; but they also do badly if they are involved in emotionally demanding relationships, to which they are unable to respond. Many, if not most, schizophrenics must be regarded as having particularly vulnerable personalities and many emerge from the acute stage of their illness with some residual defects ('end states'). They are best able to cope with their handicap if they can be helped to come to terms with their limitations. These patients are not necessarily intellectually impaired—they may be highly intelligent—but they are seldom able to cope with positions of responsibility, particularly when they are required to supervise, or interact with other people. Hence, they do best in tasks in which they can work on their own, with only rather formal contacts with their fellows.

In recent years, the psychiatric hospitals have discharged the great majority of their schizophrenic patients back to the community and to the care of their general practitioners. The latter can best help them by ensuring that the patients take their prescribed course of drugs for at least the first year or two after discharge. Long-acting phenothiazines, such as fluphenazine ethanate and fluphenazine decanoate can be given by injection each 2 to 4 weeks; an anti-parkinsonian drug is then also needed. The doctor should be ready to enlist the help of a community nurse or of a social worker if his patients appear to be having difficulties either at work or in their domestic relationships.

Organic Psychoses

Psychiatric symptoms may arise in the course of physical illnesses which either primarily or secondarily affect the brain. The occurrence of delirium during the course of febrile illnesses or the mental symptoms of general paresis are two well-known examples. It is important to recognise certain mental symptoms which occur in organic mental syndromes, since their presence should lead to the search for physical factors which may not otherwise have declared themselves. The organic psychoses can be divided into two groups: *delirium*, which is an acute disorder, and *dementia*, which is a chronic disorder. Generally speaking the acute form is potentially recoverable, being the result of temporary effects on the brain from toxic processes or disorders of metabolism, while the chronic form is the expression of more severe and progressive tissue changes in the brain and is thus not reversible. The mental symptoms of each of these organic syndromes are not specific to the causative disease and will be the same whatever may be the underlying physical disorder producing the delirium or dementia.

Delirium

This acute syndrome may be produced by such varied conditions as drug intoxication (alcoholism, LSD), infections (encephalitis, smallpox, typhoid fever), trauma to the brain, electrolyte imbalance and metabolic disorders (hepatic failure, uraemia), vitamin deficiency (Wernicke's encephalopathy), and cerebral hypoxia (heart failure). In addition to the physical symptoms appropriate to the disorder in question there are often found slurred speech, tremor, nystagmus, diplopia and sluggish pupillary reactions. The characteristic mental symptoms are: insomnia and restlessness; disorientation; impairment of memory and of ability to grasp the significance of a situation; hallucinations, particularly in the visual sphere; ideas of persecution (paranoid ideas); and a feeling of fear or terror. All the symptoms and particularly the level of consciousness are variable. The patient when undisturbed may appear deeply asleep, but quite weak stimuli may rouse him to a state of restlessness varying from simple tossing and turning to such activities as aimless searching in the bedclothes or repeated carrying out of motions associated with his occupation. He may appear orientated for time and space and be able to recognise visitors at one moment, only to be quite confused soon after. The patient will often give the easiest answer to a question without regard to the truth and may supplement his faulty memory and perception by invention (confabulation), as when he describes in detail a large meal which he says he has just had, when in fact he has eaten nothing. Visual hallucinations are characteristic of delirium, and are usually vivid and may be terrifying. Many are based on illusional misinterpretations of objects seen in the room; thus patterns on the wallpaper may become an advancing army of hideous and menacing reptiles. Hallucinations of other senses may occur. Doubt and suspicion are readily induced by the impaired mentality leading to misinterpretations and may blossom for a short time into transient and rather ill-defined delusions of persecution. Such an acute organic syndrome is commonly precipitated by withdrawal of alcohol or of barbiturates, from patients who have become habituated to taking them in substantial amounts. When the syndrome is due to alcoholism it is known as delirium tremens, but its features do not greatly differ from those of delirium from other causes.

The course and prognosis of delirium depend, of course, on the underlying physical disease, and treatment of this in most cases clears up the mental symptoms completely. Sometimes, however, delirium may be an episode in a progressive dementia or the herald of a serious psychosis.

Treatment. The use of intramuscular injections of chlorpromazine has transformed the management of acute delirium, enabling the majority of patients to be cared for in a side-room of the medical or surgical ward where their primary disease is being treated. In all these conditions the patient can be helped by explanations and friendly support; patients who are frightened and bewildered tend to regress to a state of childlike dependency and welcome a firm reassurance from someone whom they are willing to trust. They cannot, however, be kept calm if staff changes expose them to many strange faces or if they are bewildered by too many novel events. Some patients have catastrophic reactions following operations on the eyes, when they must submit to being blindfolded for some time, and others have reacted adversely to the accompaniments of cardiac resuscitation or renal dialysis. These acute psychoses contain an element of panic.

Dementia

This chronic organic syndrome may be caused by a wide variety of diseases of the brain. The most common of these is cerebral atherosclerosis, and other important causes include cerebral trauma, inflammations (neurosyphilis, encephalitis), multiple sclerosis, intoxications and deficiency disorders (chronic alcoholism, pellagra, vitamin B_{12} deficiency), prolonged hypoglycaemia, carbon monoxide poisoning, cerebral neoplasm, and a group of degenerative disorders including Huntington's chorea and senile dementia. It will be seen that some of these conditions (encephalitis, alcoholism, vitamin deficiencies) may also cause delirium. The cerebral changes brought about at first by these factors result in delirium and can be reversed by treatment, but if they are allowed to continue unchecked too long, permanent cerebral damage occurs, giving rise to dementia.

The clinical picture of dementia varies to some extent with the cause, the previous personality of the patient, the age of onset, and the rate of progression, but in all cases the mental symptoms are seen to involve the intellect, memory, emotions and behaviour, although the actual degree of impairment depends on the factors mentioned above. Insomnia is often an early symptom and may lead to nocturnal restlessness and confusion as the disease advances. Judgement and reasoning are involved early, and the disability caused by this will depend on the extent to which these faculties are utilised in the patient's daily life and work; it will be more noticeable in a barrister than in an unskilled labourer. Impairment of memory is the most prominent finding, particularly in relation to recent events, and in the later stages this may combine with defective perception to produce disorientation in space and time. Impairment of higher control leads to emotional instability and outbursts of violence or sexual aberrations at variance with the patient's previous character. There may be wide fluctuations of mood with euphoria or depression but finally, as mood flattens, the patient sinks into apathy. Delusions are common, and may be either centred on the patient himself, when they are grandiose or self-condemnatory and hypochondrial according to the mood, or centred on others, when they tend to be paranoid. As the structure of the personality disintegrates, the patient neglects his appearance, becomes lax in personal cleanliness, and careless incontinence occurs. Focal neurological signs may be found, e.g. dysphagia, apraxia, agnosia, hemiplegia, and epileptic attacks, either focal or generalised.

Psychiatric Disorders in the Elderly

In today's medical practice, the care of the elderly plays an increasingly large part. Geriatricians and general practitioners have learned to cope with the multiple minor ailments and chronic handicaps which beset old age. In the realm of psychiatry, too, it has been increasingly realised that old people do not merely suffer from progressive loss of memory and intellectual powers. Even those who show signs of cerebral atherosclerosis, with a succession of minor cerebrovascular accidents, often show fluctuations in their mental capabilities and at times they are themselves acutely aware of the reduction in their mental and physical powers and become correspondingly depressed. Severe depressive illness is common in the elderly and this responds well to active antidepressant treatment. It is a most serious clinical omission to fail to recognise depressive illnesses in the elderly, who may be incapacitated by such superadded psychiatric disability, but become able to cope again when relieved of the morbid gloom and apathy.

What is also not widely appreciated is the fact that episodes of neurotic illness, with anxiety states, phobias, hysterical symptoms or compulsions are also encountered in this age group, and are no less amenable to simple psychotherapy than at other ages. In the after-care of these older patients it is important to remember that social isolation is an important threat to their mental well-being. This becomes even more important when physical disability or deafness further restricts their opportunities of making contact with other people. Here voluntary agencies as well as local authority welfare and preventive services can do useful prophylactic work, but the family doctor is often in the best position to recognise when an ageing (and perhaps recently bereaved) patient is in special need of help.

Elderly patients easily develop delirium, and then adapt poorly to sudden changes of scene and bewildering happenings. It is helpful for them if they can be visited by only a few nurses and doctors who take pains to identify themselves; their sick-room should be well lit and they should be encouraged to keep a few treasured possessions on their bed-side table. Since patients with even very slight clouding of consciousness are prone to misunderstand what is happening round about them, any changes of routine or new procedures should be explained to them in advance, in simple terms and if necessary more than once.

The Uses and Misuses of Psychotropic Drugs

The consideration of the details of drug treatment in psychiatric disorder is kept to the end of this chapter in order to guard against the misleading idea (which pharmaceutical advertising literature may convey) that for every psychiatric syndrome there is a specific medicinal remedy. Used wisely, psychotropic drugs can do a great deal to reduce the distress of psychiatrically disturbed patients and they can be used in conjunction with psychotherapy. During the past 25 years, one of the most striking changes in morbidity in Britain as in other advanced societies, has been a conspicuous increase in the incidence of attempted suicide, particularly cases of self-poisoning (p. 799). More than 80 per cent of these patients had swallowed overdoses of medicines prescribed by a doctor, the most common classes of drug being the barbiturates, the tranquillisers and the antidepressants. These figures can be variously interpreted, but they demonstrate very clearly the danger of relying upon drugs to solve the problems of emotionally disturbed patients.

No attempt will be made in this chapter to discuss all the psychotropic drugs, of which new variants are being introduced every year. However, Table 15.1 gives the pharmacopoeial and trade names and usual doses of drugs in the principal categories which have been frequently recommended.

Hypnotics. The sedatives are useful for patients who sleep poorly. The drugs which are most commonly misused are barbiturate sleeping tablets either alone or in combination with amphetamine (p. 787). EEG studies have shown that when normal subjects take as little as 200 mg of sodium amylobarbitone nightly for 1 week and then stop, their sleep pattern remains disturbed for several nights before reverting to normal. Patients who have become dependent on sleeping tablets thus have some justification for being reluctant to do without them, because they will be very likely to experience broken sleep and troubled dreams for up to 2 weeks before they can re-establish a natural sleep routine. Barbiturates provide effective sedation, but no longer should have pride of place in the treatment of either insomnia or anxiety. Chloral hydrate is of particular value for elderly patients in doses of 0·5—1 g. The sedative nitrazepam has the merit of being remarkably safe. The best policy is to regard insomnia as the symptom of some underlying disturbance and to restrict its treatment to short courses, emphasising to the patient that it is preferable, in the long run, to tolerate a number of sleepless nights rather than to become dependent on a habit-forming drug. On the other hand, sleeplessness can add seriously to the distress of a psychiatrically ill patient, and relief of insomnia may better enable him to tolerate his other symptoms.

Tranquillisers. Tranquillisers are drugs which allay a variety of symptoms, such as acute anxiety, restlessness, agitation, without sedating the patient, who remains alert and in touch with his surroundings but is no longer so oppressed by his symptoms. There are four main categories of tranquillisers:

1. The *phenothiazines*, e.g. chlorpromazine, thioridazine; 2. The *butyrophenones*, e.g. haloperidol; 3. The *benzodiazepines*, e.g. chlordiazepoxide, diazepam, oxazepam; 4. *Meprobamate*.

The phenothiazines are principally used in the treatment of schizophrenia. Chlorpromazine and thioridazine are in general use, 150—1,000 mg being given each day in divided doses during the acute stage of the illness. A suitable

Table 15.1 Summary of psychotropic drugs

Designation	Dose Range (in 24 hours)	Trade Name
Sedatives		
Chloral hydrate preparations		
Dichloralphenazone	650 mg tabs—one or two at night	Welldorm
Barbiturates		
Amylobarbitone sodium	60 mg tabs—one to three at night	Sodium Amytal
Butobarbitone	100 mg tabs—one or two at night	Soneryl
Quinalbarbitone sodium	50 mg tabs—one or two at night	Seconal
Pentobarbitone sodium	50 mg capsules—one or two at night	Nembutal
Phenobarbitone	30 and 60 mg tabs—30–120 mg at night	Luminal
Benzodiazepine derivative		
Nitrazepam	5 mg tabs—5–10 mg at night	Mogadon
Methaqualone		
Methaqualone	250 mg tabs—one at night	Melsedin
Methaqualone with diphenhydramine (25 mg)	250 mg tabs—one at night	Mandrax
Tranquillisers		
Phenothiazines		
Chlorpromazine	50–150 mg daily*	Largactil
Thioridazine	50–150 mg daily*	Melleril
Promazine	50–250 mg daily	Sparine
Trifluoperazine	3–12 mg daily	Stelazine
Prochlorperazine	10–15 mg daily	Stemetil
Butyrophenones		
Haloperidol	4·5–13·5 mg daily	Serenace
Benzodiazepines		
Chlordiazepoxide	10–16 mg daily	Librium
Diazepam	6–40 mg daily	Valium
Oxazepam	45–90 mg daily	Serenid-D
Meprobamate	400–1,200 mg	Equanil
Antidepressants		
Tricyclic Drugs		
Imipramine	75–225 mg daily	Tofranil
Clomipramine	75–225 mg	Anafranil
Trimipramine	75–225 mg daily	Surmontil
Amitriptyline	75–225 mg daily	Tryptizol
Monoamine Oxidase Inhibitors		
Phenelzine	45–90 mg daily	Nardil
Mebanazine	5–30 mg daily	Actomol
Tranylcypromine	10–20 mg daily	Parnate

* Larger doses of this drug are used in the treatment of schizophrenia (see text).

maintenance dose for a schizophrenic in remission is 100 mg 3 times a day. Chlorpromazine is also given by intramuscular injections (50–100 mg) in order to control states of delirium or over-excitement. An important side-effect to remember is its tendency to lower the blood-pressure; patients should be warned against the occurrence of moments of dizziness when they get up quickly from a sitting position. Because this tendency is more marked with elderly patients, they should be given smaller doses. A long-acting phenothiazine, fluphenazine decanoate, can be given intramuscularly on a maintenance basis for schizophrenics treated as out-patients who are unreliable with oral medication. All the phenothiazianes can have adverse extrapyramidal effects, and anti-parkinsonian drugs (e.g. orphenadrine hydrochloride 50–100 mg 3 times daily) may also have to be taken. Restlessness and dystonia of the jaw and neck can occur.

The *diazepines*, which have replaced barbiturates as the antianxiety drugs of choice, particularly diazepam 6–40 mg daily and chlordiazepoxide 10–60 mg daily which relieve the distress of acute anxiety, and *meprobamate* 400–1,200 mg daily can be used to give symptomatic relief to patients whose anxiety is accompanied by feeling 'keyed up' and unable to relax. Small doses of chlorpromazine or thioridazine (up to 150 mg daily) can also be used for this purpose. Prescription of diazepines should be avoided in the first trimester of pregnancy; there is some indication of a higher incidence of cleft-lip and cleft-palate.

The latter drugs can be particularly helpful in tiding a neurotic patient with anxiety over an especially difficult period of subjective distress. They do not, however, do anything to resolve the causes of the patient's symptoms, and unless this is altered either through psychotherapy or through a significant change in his personal circumstances, the symptoms will tend to recur and the patient may find himself becoming dependent on his palliative drug.

Antidepressants. There are two principal groups of antidepressant drugs:

1. *Tricyclic drugs* (e.g. imipramine, amitriptyline and trimipramine).
2. The *monoamine oxidase inhibitors* (e.g. phenelzine, mebanazine and tranylcypromine).

1. Tricyclic drugs (p. 796) are indicated for the treatment of severe depression of the endogenous type, with symptoms of disturbance of sleep, appetite and energy. In order to be effective, they have to be given in sufficient dosage, which may be from 50 to 75 mg three times a day. Tricyclic drugs give rise to some disagreeable side-effects. Imipramine may make the patient feel even more on edge and restless during the first few days, and it may also cause some difficulty in micturition. These drugs have an atropine-like effect on the eyes, causing difficulty in focussing. Amitriptyline tends to make some patients feel uncomfortably drowsy, and causes dryness of the mouth. These side-effects usually recede with continued use and become quite easily tolerated once the patient begins to experience a lifting of his mood and a return of his former energy, which usually becomes apparent after 6 to 10 days. A course of these drugs should be taken for 3 to 6 months, because if they are stopped too soon the symptoms of depression may recur.

2. The monoamine oxidase inhibitor (MAOI) drugs (p. 796) are especially helpful in the treatment of 'atypical' depressions or prolonged phobic symptoms, occurring in patients with good previous personalities. The action of MAOI drugs is associated with an accumulation of catecholamines in the brain and other tissues of the body; hence patients should be warned not to partake of substances

rich in tyramine (such as cheese, Bovril, Oxo or Marmite, chianti and some types of beer) because these may interact with the drug to provoke a hypertensive crisis, with splitting headaches and a risk of subarachnoid haemorrhage. The MAOI drugs also potentiate other drugs, including pethidine, opiates, barbiturates, phenothiazines, amphetamine and alcohol, all of which should be avoided while a patient is taking this form of antidepressant.

Mention must also be made of the treatment of manic-depressive illness with *lithium carbonate*. Lithium is effective in controlling manic states. The patient needs to be in hospital at the start of treatment. It may also prevent the recurrence of manic attacks when used as maintenance therapy, in doses of 750–1,500 mg per day, out-patients returning for weekly estimation of plasma lithium.

Endogenous depressive illness, once of gloomy prognosis, is now eminently treatable, and with appropriate care few such patients become chronic hospital inmates any longer.

H. J. WALTON

Further reading:

Anderson, E. W. & Trethowen, W. H. (1973) *Psychiatry*. 3rd edition. London: Baillière, Tindall and Cassell.
Balint, M. (1968) *The Doctor, his Patient and the Illness*. 2nd edition. London: Pitman Medical.
Forrest, A. (Ed.) (1973) *Companion to Psychiatric Studies*. 2 vols. Edinburgh: Churchill Livingstone.
Silverstone, T. & Barraclough, B. (1975) *Contemporary Psychiatry*. Ashford, Kent: Headley Brothers Ltd. and the Royal College of Psychiatrists.
Slater, E. & Roth, M. (1970) *Clinical Psychiatry*. 3rd edition. London: Baillière, Tindall and Cassell.
Walton, H. J. (1976) *Clinical Examination*, ed. Macleod, J. 4th edition. Edinburgh: Churchill Livingstone.—For a detailed description of the psychiatric examination.

16. Acute Poisoning

ACUTE poisoning presents a very common and urgent medical problem. Its incidence is steadily rising and now at least 15 per cent of all adult emergency admissions to hospitals in Britain are suffering from poisoning (Fig. 16.1). Accidental poisoning in the home is also very common, especially in young children. A major factor in this rise in poisoning is the increased prescribing and therefore availability of drugs which all too often are left carelessly within reach of the

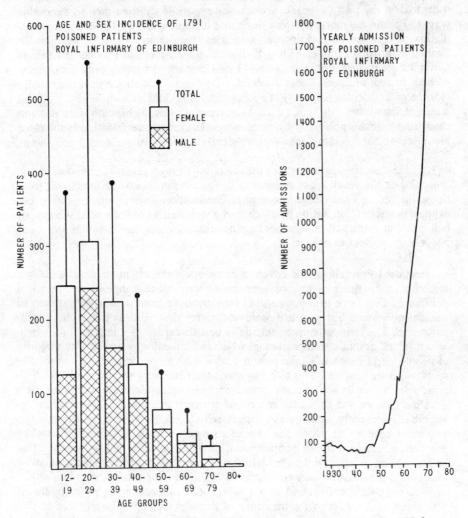

Fig. 16.1 Age and sex incidence and annual admission rate of poisoned patients to Royal Infirmary of Edinburgh.

toddler or provide the means for the impulsive overdosage. On the other hand, due to strict controls, the rate of poisoning in industry and agriculture remains low despite the introduction of many and varied toxic substances. The deaths in Britain from all forms of poisoning amount to about 4,000 per annum.

This chapter deals with the clinical features, diagnosis and management of acute poisoning. Food poisoning is discussed on pages 69–71. Only brief reference is made to industrial and agricultural poisons and none to poisoning by ionising radiation.

Classification of Acute Poisoning

Acute poisoning can be described as either accidental or intentional.

Accidental Poisoning. Death from accidental poisoning has increased almost three-fold in the past 30 years, women being more likely than men to die in this way. In Britain the mortality from this cause is approximately 15 per million population whereas in other European countries there is considerable variation. In Scandinavia, for example, with a highly developed medical service, the rate is about 20 per million, but in Italy and West Germany the rate is only about 9 per million. Except in children it is doubtful if the official statistics reflect the true incidence of accidental poisoning. For example, it is difficult to believe the official statistics that more adults die each year from accidental barbiturate poisoning than from suicidal poisoning by these drugs. Inaccurate certification is the most likely reason for the large numbers apparently dying from accidental poisoning.

SUBSTANCES INVOLVED IN ACCIDENTAL POISONING. Death from accidental poisoning is the result most commonly of (a) carbon monoxide inhalation from domestic gas or fumes from incomplete combustion from stoves or motor car exhaust pipes, or (b) ingestion by children of a wide variety of household substances (e.g. paraffin or bleach), medicines (e.g. aspirin, tricyclics, antihistamines or iron) and, rarely, poisonous berries.

Intentional Poisoning. This covers a broad spectrum of causes ranging from a minority of patients who are determined on self-destruction, i.e. 'suicidal poisoning', to a large group who until recently have been designated 'attempted suicidal poisoning' but who are more accurately described as indulging in 'self-poisoning'. The term 'attempted suicide' is best discarded as it implies a motive to an act of self-administered poisoning, which is frequently incorrect. The majority of people who deliberately take poison do not wish to die; in fact, they often take steps to ensure that measures to bring about their recovery will be available. 'Self-poisoning' is usually a conscious, often impulsive act, undertaken to manipulate a situation or a person to secure redress of circumstances which have become intolerable. Frequently relatives and society rally to the help of the unfortunate victim and the situation which has caused so much distress is rectified. Mistakes, however, do occur through misjudgement of dosage or of a failure to ensure that help would be to hand, and an act which was committed merely to draw attention to a particular situation may end in death. Self-poisoning often occurs in a setting of poverty and alcoholism and with a background of a broken home in childhood. The alarming increase in the incidence of acute poisoning is largely due to self-poisoning which accounts for approximately 90 per cent of all adult poisoned patients admitted to hospitals. This type of behaviour is commoner in countries which enjoy a highly developed welfare state and now constitutes a major social problem. This is the case particularly in areas of dense conurbation and is less marked in small town and rural communities.

Under the heading of intentional poisoning, in addition to suicidal and self-poisoning, homicidal poisoning must also be included.

SUBSTANCES AND METHODS USED IN INTENTIONAL POISONING. *Self-poisoning*. Almost any substance may be taken for self-poisoning, but during recent years there has been a change in the type of drug used. Statistics show that whereas ten years ago 60 per cent of admissions were due to barbiturate poisoning, this figure is now only 10 per cent. Their place has been taken by tricyclic antidepressants, 13 per cent, and the benzodiazepines, 30 per cent. Salicylate poisoning, frequently encountered in younger people, amounts to 10 per cent. Carbon monoxide, previously often the choice of the elderly, is now uncommon.

Combinations of drugs are taken frequently and alcohol also may be involved. This gives rise to problems in assessment of the severity of poisoning and in treatment; chemical analysis may also be rendered more difficult.

Suicide. The methods adopted for deliberate self-destruction vary from country to country and between the sexes. In Britain the most common method employed by women is drugs and the second drowning. In males the first choice is by self injury, such as hanging or strangulation and the second choice poisoning with drugs. In America, where firearms are more readily available, this is the first choice by males but only the second by females. Poisoning by drugs is the first choice of females. In Britain and the United States coal gas has largely been replaced for domestic use by natural gas which is in itself not toxic; this has resulted in a steep decline in the use of gas for suicidal purposes and as a cause of accidental poisoning. Despite this decline the total incidence of poisoning has not fallen.

Diagnosis of Acute Poisoning

Information Service. With the increasing frequency of accidental and intentional poisoning it is important to determine whether the substance ingested is noxious. In Britain and Eire a Poisons Information Service is available to doctors telephoning one of the following numbers:

Belfast: Royal Victoria Hospital. Tel. 0232 40503.
Cardiff: Royal Infirmary. Tel. 0222 33101.
Edinburgh: Royal Infirmary. Tel. 031-229 2477.
Eire: Jervis Street Hospital. Tel. Dublin 45588.
Leeds: General Infirmary. Tel. 0532 32799.
London: Guy's Hospital. Tel. 01-407 7600.
Manchester: Booth Hall Children's Hospital. Tel. 061-740 2254.

Information can be obtained immediately regarding the ingredients of a substance; the approximately fatal dose of a poison and the best method of treatment can be discussed with a physician trained in clinical toxicology.

Differential Diagnosis. In Britain acute poisoning is the most common cause of unconsciousness, in the absence of head injury, in a patient between 15 and 50 years. The diagnosis of acute poisoning is usually made on the history obtained from relatives or friends, from circumstantial evidence, such as finding tablets at the bedside and from a prompt physical examination with special reference to the degree of unconsciousness and circulatory and respiratory failure. In addition, a decision should be reached as to whether the poison has been swallowed, inhaled or absorbed from the skin. Few poisons produce diagnostic clinical features, but the smell of coal-gas, the hyperpnoea and sweating of salicylate poisoning, the markedly depressed respiration and pinpoint pupils of opiate poisoning are helpful diagnostic features on occasions. Treatment should not be delayed by spending excessive time in attempting to identify precisely the poison involved, since there is seldom a specific antidote and the essential immediate treatment of poisoning is dependent on the application of well established basic therapeutic principles. Every hospital, nevertheless, should have some aid to the identification of capsules and tablets which are commonly used in poisoning. For this purpose coloured diagrams are available. The marking of tablets with the name of the manufacturer, code letters and numbers has been introduced to a limited extent and has proved of value in identification. Laboratory analysis of gastric aspirate, blood or urine will confirm the diagnosis. Qualitative and quantitative estimation of paracetamol, salicylate, alcohol, iron, tricyclic antidepressants and barbiturate (with identification as to whether short, medium or long acting) should be readily available. These results, however, seldom influence management but confirm the diagnosis and may be of value for medico-legal purposes.

General Therapeutic Measures

MAINTENANCE OF RESPIRATION. A clear airway is essential. This can be ensured by removal of dentures, vomitus, foreign bodies and excess mucus: the patient should be turned on his side to prevent the tongue falling backwards and to avoid aspiration of vomitus and mucus. An oropharyngeal or cuffed endotracheal tube may have to be inserted to maintain a free airway. Artificial respiration is required if respiration is depressed, using preferably the method of expired air resuscitation (p. 188). Oxygen should be given through an oronasal mask (p. 265). Prophylactic antibiotics to 'protect' the lungs are not recommended, but any infection which develops should be treated.

REMOVAL OR INACTIVATION OF THE POISON. It cannot be emphasised too strongly that it is very important that the poison must be eliminated as quickly as possible. The first-aid treatment is often the responsibility of the general practitioner in the patient's home while awaiting the arrival of an ambulance. Patients with gassing must be removed to fresh air as quickly as possible. When a liquid or solid poison is in contact with the patient's clothes these must be removed at once and any poison on the skin must be washed off to prevent absorption. When the poison has been swallowed conscious patients should be given activated charcoal prior to transfer to hospital. A decision as to whether emesis and gastric aspiration and lavage be also undertaken will depend on three factors: (a) the substance ingested, (b) the state of consciousness of the patient, and (c) the length of time since the poison was ingested.

(a) NATURE OF SUBSTANCE INGESTED. The only contraindication to inducing emesis or passing a stomach tube is the knowledge that paraffin oil (kerosene) or other petroleum distillates have been swallowed, as the entry of even a small quantity of these substances into the lungs will lead to a severe pneumonia. Great care must be exercised in passing a stomach tube in corrosive poisoning, in alcoholics, in patients who have had gastric surgery and in the very young and elderly, but the benefits from gastric aspiration and lavage outweigh the potential dangers of perforating the oesophagus or stomach.

(*b*) LEVEL OF CONSCIOUSNESS. The second factor to be considered is the state of consciousness. Fully conscious patients should be made to vomit by putting one's finger into the throat; if unsuccessful syrup of ipecacuanha (15 ml followed by 200 ml of water) is an effective emetic, especially in children. Its limitations are that there is an average delay in the onset of its action of about 18 minutes. When these measures are impracticable as in a hysterical patient, apomorphine hydrochloride 5 mg may be given intramuscularly. It is a powerful emetic but unfortunately it can produce hypotension, dangerous collapse and persistent vomiting. These effects can, however, be antagonised by administering naloxone 0·4 mg intravenously, followed if necessary 3 minutes later by 0·8 mg by intravenous injection.

In a semiconscious patient emetics are to be avoided in view of the danger of aspiration pneumonia, but gastric aspiration and lavage can be employed provided the cough reflex is still present. Gastric lavage in the deeply unconscious patient without this reflex is a highly dangerous procedure unless the lungs can be protected by the insertion of a cuffed endotracheal tube.

(*c*) TIME SINCE INGESTION. The third factor to be considered is the time which has elapsed since the ingestion of the poison. If four hours have passed since ingestion very little or no recovery of the drug will be achieved by undertaking emesis and gastric lavage; if it is known that the poison was taken less than four hours previously aspiration and lavage must be done. In salicylate poisoning, because of the almost inevitable pylorospasm which prevents the drug from leaving the stomach, it is never too late to undertake these procedures and large amounts of salicylates may be recovered up to 24 hours after ingestion. In the case of tricyclic drugs a worthwhile recovery may be achieved up to 12 hours after ingestion. In other forms of poisoning, provided the two factors already discussed have been considered, gastric aspiration and lavage should be undertaken if less than 4 hours have elapsed since the drug was consumed.

Technique of Gastric Aspiration and Lavage. With the foot of the bed raised about 0·5 m and the patient lying on his left side a wide-bore Jacques rubber stomach tube, English gauge 30, should be passed. A gag may be necessary to prevent biting on the tube. When the tube has been inserted, its position in the stomach is verified by aspiration of stomach contents or by blowing a little air through it and auscultating over the abdomen when a bubbling sound will be heard. Aspiration is best achieved by lowering the funnel to which the stomach tube is attached, to a level well below the patient's head. Aspiration is advisable prior to lavage as initial lavage will drive some of the stomach contents into the duodenum and promote absorption. When no further material can be aspirated repeated careful lavage with tepid water should be undertaken, using the same apparatus and no more than 300 ml for each single washout. Lavage should be continued until the returning fluid is clear which may necessitate a total volume of 40 litres. Except in the specific instances shown in Table 16.1, little is achieved by employing lavage fluid other than water.

On occasions, after lavage, some further impairment of consciousness may occur; hence, except in iron poisoning, the value of leaving fluid in the stomach may be outweighed by the dangers of subsequent aspiration pneumonia if the patient has had no cuffed endotracheal tube inserted. However, with this possibility in mind and provided that no delay in further treatment is occasioned by the preparation of solution, the following may be left in the stomach after lavage: 100 ml milk on account of its demulcent properties in corrosive poisoning; the chelating agent, desferrioxamine, in acute iron poisoning (p. 810). It is frequently recommended that on completion of gastric lavage for salicylate poisoning a solution of sodium bicarbonate should be left in the stomach. In the authors' opinion this is not advisable. Although the bicarbonate counteracts the irritation of the gastric mucosa and when absorbed may help to promote excretion of salicylate by rendering the urine alkaline, its presence in the stomach encourages further absorption of salicylate.

If considerable absorption has occurred the patient may be gravely ill, hence measures to enhance elimination of the poison may be required. These can only be carried out in hospital because of the technical skill and special apparatus required; they include diuresis; forced diuresis (p. 807), peritoneal dialysis, haemodialysis, and exchange transfusion.

In recent years attempts have been made to develop safer ways of increasing removal of toxic substances from the body. The most promising of these is the use of haemoperfusion through ion-exchange resins or charcoal. An effective and safe technique is the use of charcoal coated with synthetic acrylic hydrogel. More detailed studies are required before this form of treatment can be fully assessed.

ANTIDOTES. It is widely but erroneously believed that for each toxic substance there is a specific antidote. There are, in fact, no antidotes for the majority of substances producing poisoning. In about 2 per cent of instances, however, certain pharmacological antagonists are of value. An example is naloxone for opiate poisoning which, with others, is mentioned in Table 16.1.

MANAGEMENT OF ACUTE CIRCULATORY FAILURE. This is described on page 193. The foot of the bed should be raised. Warmth should be applied but sweating must be avoided. Acute circulatory failure may also require treatment by infusion of dextran, plasma or whole blood. Oxygen therapy (p. 264) should always be given.

MANAGEMENT OF HYPOTHERMIA. A rectal thermometer which records low temperatures is required for the accurate assessment of hypothermia. Since it reduces the oxygen demands of the tissues, hypothermia is not a deleterious feature unless below 35°C, when it may cause further hypotension, produce sludging of the blood and confusion and coma.

In general, active reheating should be avoided, and all that is necessary is to prevent further heat loss by nursing in an ambient temperature of 26°C. If the core temperature is less than 32°C, active reheating is indicated and hydrocortisone (100 mg) is given intravenously every 6 hours.

TREATMENT OF CONVULSIONS. These should be controlled with the intramuscular injection of 15 mg of diazepam and/or 200 mg of sodium phenobarbitone.

Psychiatric Assessment

As most instances of poisoning in adults are deliberate acts of self-poisoning it is very important that all patients, whether suffering from 'accidental' or intentional poisoning, should be assessed by a psychiatrist. Self-poisoning is often an important feature of various psychiatric disorders, and depression in particular. Even if there is no major psychiatric disturbance the techniques of psychiatry are well suited for unravelling the underlying situation. It is greatly to the benefit of the patient if the initial psychiatric interview takes place as soon as possible after the act before the patient and his relatives have time to discuss the event and thereafter present the same rationalised and often false picture. The incidence of repeated acts of self-poisoning has been shown clearly to be reduced by early psychiatric consultation.

Barbiturate Poisoning

While barbiturates are used less often now for intentional poisoning, they are still a major cause of death due to poisoning. They cause similar clinical features and require management based on the same principles as many other hypnotic drugs commonly taken in overdosage.

Clinical Features. In poisoning of moderate to severe degree there may be:
Impaired Consciousness. The degree of impairment will vary and is best expressed by the following classification: Grade 1, response to vocal commands; Grade 2, maximal response to minimal painful stimulation; Grade 3, minimal response to maximal painful stimulation; Grade 4, total unresponsiveness to maximal painful stimulation.
Hypotension. Hypotension is produced mainly by the toxic action of barbiturate on the heart and smooth muscles of the blood vessels. The heart rate is normal or only slightly increased.
Respiratory Depression. Both the rate and depth will be depressed. The clinical assessment of the degree of respiratory depression is very difficult. It can be measured with Wright's spirometer; a minute volume of expired air of less than 4 litres indicates severe depression necessitating immediate measures to improve ventilation. Precise assessment of respiratory function can be achieved by measurement of arterial blood gases.
Abnormal Reflexes. Diminution or absence of the tendon reflexes varies and is not a good measure of the severity of the poisoning nor is the size of the pupils nor the presence or absence of the light reflex.
Oliguria or Anuria. Urinary output may be severely reduced owing to a number of factors such as hypotension, anoxia, a central antidiuretic effect, and a toxic action of barbiturate on the renal tubular cells.
Hypothermia. See page 804.
Skin Lesions. Bullous lesions occur in 6 per cent of cases not only on the pressure bearing areas but also on the hands and feet. The initial lesion is a slightly raised patch of erythema with a sharp outline which may proceed to bullous formation. Bullous lesions are most helpful in differentiating poisoning from other causes of coma.
Raised Blood Level of Barbiturate. The longer acting barbiturates produce higher levels than do the shorter acting preparations, e.g. in a patient severely poisoned with phenobarbitone the level may reach 15 mg per 100 ml whereas with a medium acting preparation such as amylobarbitone, the patient may show features of poisoning of a similar degree when the blood level is only 5 mg per 100 ml. It should be remembered that high blood levels with few features of poisoning may be found in epileptics and others habituated to the drug. This

emphasises that assessment of the severity of poisoning must be based on clinical features and not on blood levels. Pre-existing liver disease may exaggerate and prolong the toxic effects of barbiturates.

Additional Features of Poisoning with other Hypnotics. In methaqualone and diphenhydramine (Mandrax) poisoning, hyperreflexia, papilloedema and acute pulmonary oedema occur with, on occasions, a disturbance of the clotting mechanisms. In glutethimide (Doriden) overdosage sudden periods of apnoea and considerable variation in the conscious level may be prominent.

Complications. The complications can be deduced from study of the above list of clinical features. Briefly they are: (1) acute respiratory depression; (2) hypostatic and aspiration pneumonia; (3) severe shock; (4) anuria; (5) fluid and electrolyte imbalance with acid-base disturbance; (6) withdrawal fits and psychoses on recovery of consciousness.

The following complications are the direct effects of treatment: (*a*) aspiration pneumonia from injudicious gastric lavage; (*b*) pulmonary oedema from overloading of the circulation during forced diuresis; (*c*) the hazards associated with haemodialysis and peritoneal dialysis; (*d*) convulsions, cardiac arrhythmias and psychoses from analeptic drugs which should never be used.

Treatment. This is based on the adoption of basic therapeutic principles to maintain respiration (p. 802), support the circulation (p. 804), correct electrolyte imbalance (p. 153) and prevent further absorption of the drug by removal of poison from the stomach. In poisoning producing a mild or moderate impairment of consciousness sometimes no additional medical treatment is required but under careful nursing supervision the patient should be left to sleep off the effects of the drug. In the severely poisoned patient, treatment in hospital includes assisted respiration (p. 266), measures to combat shock and dehydration (p. 193) and possibly measures for enhanced elimination of barbiturate from the body. These subjects are discussed under general therapeutic measures (p. 802) and in other chapters of this book. There is no specific barbiturate antagonist.

Prognosis. As a result of effective treatment the mortality rate for patients suffering from barbiturate poisoning admitted to a well equipped and staffed hospital has fallen from 25 per cent to 1 per cent in the past 25 years.

Benzodiazepine Poisoning

This group of drugs comprising nitrazepam, diazepam and chlordiazepoxide is now taken in overdosage more frequently than barbiturates. However the effects are very different; the ingestion of as many as 100 tablets of nitrazepam will produce no more than a deep sleep from which the patient can be roused. No hypotensive effects occur and only very rarely is there any depression of respiration. No medical treatment other than supervision is indicated.

Poisoning by Tricyclic Antidepressants

These include amitriptyline, imipramine and trimipramine. The effects in overdose include dryness of the mouth, fixed dilated pupils, sinus tachycardia with bizarre arrhythmias, hypotension, marked irritability with hyperreflexia, ataxia, hallucinations, convulsions and loss of consciousness. The dangerous effects are those on the heart and to a lesser extent the convulsions. Intensive supportive therapy is required with antirrhythmic drugs (p. 192) as indicated. Convulsions will be controlled with diazepam, 15 mg intravenously, together with phenobarbitone 200 mg intramuscularly. Physostigmine salicylate (1–3 mg) given by slow intravenous injection is an effective antidote for both the central nervous and cardiac effects.

Salicylate Poisoning

The patient is almost always conscious, hence simple questioning regarding consumption of salicylates will usually prevent the condition from being misdiagnosed as diabetic ketoacidosis or a severe infection, especially of the respiratory tract. Salicylates are often taken in compound tablets with codeine and phenacetin but the important acute toxic ingredient is the salicylate.

Clinical Features. A moderately to severely poisoned patient may have roaring in the ears, deafness and blurring of vision. There may be restlessness and sweating from the stimulant effect of the drug and an increased metabolic rate. The drug also has a direct stimulant effect on the respiratory centre increasing the depth and rate of ventilation, producing a lowering of the Pa_{CO_2} and a respiratory alkalosis. There may be epigastric pain and vomiting; the combination of loss of gastric contents, hyperventilation and profuse sweating leads to severe dehydration and a reduced urinary output.

The serum potassium, despite dehydration, will be low as a result of the initial respiratory alkalosis. The latter may be replaced by a metabolic acidosis, especially in children. Proteinuria may occur and renal tubular casts and cells may be found in the urinary deposit. A purple colour will appear on dipsticks used for the detection of phenylketonuria (Phenistix).

Plasma Salicylate. A level of 50 mg or more per 100 ml indicates severe poisoning.

Complications. Profound disturbances of acid-base equilibrium, especially when associated with impaired consciousness, are to be regarded as a very serious feature and may herald sudden death, but the underlying mechanism is not fully understood.

Despite the tendency for salicylates in therapeutic dosage to cause gastric erosion and hypoprothrombinaemia, haematemesis very rarely occurs and blood-stained gastric contents evacuated by lavage are seldom seen.

Although protein and renal tubular cells are often present in the urine during the acute stage, permanent renal damage has not been recorded.

Treatment. Moderate to severe salicylate poisoning is best treated in an adult by gastric aspiration and lavage (p. 803) which should never be omitted irrespective of the time that has elapsed since the drug was taken.

Salicylate can best be eliminated from the body by *forced alkaline diuresis.* The urine must be rendered alkaline since a rise in urinary pH from 6 to 7·7 increases the excretion of free salicylate tenfold. For this purpose the following should be mixed together and given intravenously at a rate of 2 litres hourly for 3 hours:

Saline (0·9 per cent)	0·5 litre
Dextrose (5 per cent)	1 litre
Sodium bicarbonate (1·26 per cent)	0·5 litre
Potassium chloride	3 g

Table 16.1 Some features and treatment of poisoning by less common agents

Poison	Signs and Symptoms	Treatment
Amphetamine group.	Excitement. Flushing. Tremor. Fits. Insomnia. Psychoses. Tachycardia. Hypertension.	1. General measures. 2. Chlorpromazine, 100 mg intramuscularly. If forced diuresis is indicated the urine must be rendered acid.
Corrosives.	Stains and burns of corners of mouth and chin. Burns of fauces. Pain. Shock.	1. General measures. 2. Gastric lavage with care. 3. Neutralise acid or alkali.
Cyanides and hydrocyanic acid.	Odour of bitter almonds. Shallow breathing. Pink colour of skin and mucosae. Shock. Widely dilated pupils.	1. General measures. 2. Cobalt edetate (Kelocyanor) 300 mg in 20 ml intravenously over one minute. 3. If no recovery in one further minute, repeat 300 mg cobalt edetate. 4. If ingested, gastric lavage with 25 per cent sodium thiosulphate.
Dinitro-ortho-cresol weedkillers.	Yellow skin. Severe sweating. Thirst. Fatigue. Tachycardia. Tachypnoea. Raised temperature.	1. Wash skin. 2. Sedatives. 3. Reduce temperature.
Domestic bleach.	Burning sensation in mouth and fauces. Gastroenteritis.	Gastric lavage with sodium thiosulphate 0·1% if symptoms severe.
Opiates.	Depressed respiration. Pinpoint pupils. Pallor. Vomiting. Coma.	1. If ingested gastric lavage with very dilute pot. permanganate— 1 in 10,000. 2. Naloxone 0·4 mg intravenously and 0·8 mg repeated intravenously 3 minutes later, if required. In heavy overdosage larger quantities may be necessary. 3. Keep under observation and repeat naloxone if necessary.

Table 16.1— (continued)

Poison	Signs and Symptoms	Treatment
Organophosphorous compounds.	Cold. Sweating. Constricted pupils. Salivation. Twitching. Convulsions. Slow pulse. Bronchospasm. Acute pulmonary oedema. Diarrhoea.	1. Remove contaminated clothes and wash skin. 2. General measures. 3. Atropine 2 mg intravenously and repeat 1 mg intravenously to maintain 'atropinisation'. 4. Pralidoxime (P_2S) 1 g in 5 ml water intravenously. Repeat in 1 hour.
Paracetamol (=Acetaminophen in U.S.A.)	Nausea, vomiting, vague upper abdominal pain. Hypotension. Hypoglycaemia. Bleeding. Renal failure. Delirium. Acute liver failure may develop a few days after ingestion and carries a high mortality.	1. General measures. 2. In moderate or severe poisoning (over 20×500 mg tablets paracetamol) within 6 hours of ingestion, cysteamine hydrochloride $2 \cdot 0$ g intravenously over 10 minutes, followed by three 400 mg doses in 500 ml of 5% dextrose infused over 4, 6 and 8 hours to reduce and even prevent liver necrosis. 3. Intravenous glucose to correct hypoglycaemia and maintain hydration.
Paraffin and petroleum distillates.	Vomiting and diarrhoea. Pallor. Cough and dyspnoea.	1. Do NOT wash out stomach (p. 802) 2. Antibiotics if aspiration has occurred.

If forced alkaline diuresis cannot be undertaken or in the rare event of not achieving a diuresis, peritoneal dialysis or haemodialysis will be required.

Prognosis. The mortality from salicylate poisoning is 1 per cent if effective forced diuresis is employed.

Carbon Monoxide Poisoning

Although poisoning by this gas carries by far the highest mortality both in and out of hospital, the incidence of coal gas poisoning is diminishing throughout the world. The amount of carbon monoxide in domestic coal gas in Britain has been reduced and the danger will be averted by the use of natural gas which is not in itself toxic. Natural gas can however produce carbon monoxide when incomplete combustion occurs through, for example, the burning of natural gas in unsuitable appliances. Natural gas may also be harmful by simply displacing oxygen in a closed space.

The smell of coal gas is usually evident but may be absent if the gas coming from a broken pipe has seeped through a layer of earth. It is unusual to encounter a deeply comatose patient in hospital because victims who reach that stage usually die at the site of poisoning.

Since the carbon monoxide in coal gas combines so strongly with haemoglobin to form carboxyhaemoglobin, which is 210 times more stable than oxyhaemoglobin, the clinical features are those of varying degrees of hypoxia. These include disorientation or coma, varied arrhythmias, severe hypotension and heart failure. Respiration is usually rapid and deep. The tendon reflexes are increased and the plantar responses may be extensor; the pupils may be dilated. Skin pallor is common but patchy erythema and even bullae may develop.

By itself the percentage saturation of carboxyhaemoglobin is not a reliable indication of severity nor a good prognostic index. It is about 30 per cent for moderate poisoning and about 50 per cent for severe poisoning, provided there is no associated anaemia.

Treatment. The basic necessity is to remove the patient immediately from the source of gas and, without any delay, apply assisted respiration if indicated. Oxygen should be given. Admission to hospital is essential, resuscitative measures being maintained during transportation. The dangers of hypoxia, especially to the cardiac muscle, must be remembered and all patients with moderate or severe poisoning should be observed carefully for several days until it is certain that the heart has escaped damage. Acute cerebral oedema may be promptly reduced by the rapid infusion of mannitol (p. 694). The hyperbaric oxygen chamber is of limited value in the treatment of carbon monoxide poisoning because of the time which usually elapses before the patient reaches hospital.

Acute Poisoning in Children

Accidental poisoning in children under 4 years of age is an all too common event. Two-thirds of the enquiries dealt with by the Poisons Information Service are about children who have taken a substance which may be noxious. Analysis of the enquiries has shown that whilst sugar coating and colouring of tablets are frequently attractive, an unpleasant odour or taste does not prevent toddlers from sampling a substance. Domestic bleaches and detergents are amongst the most common substances consumed; fortunately they are relatively innocuous and, apart from symptomatic treatment for the irritant effects on the alimentary tract, require no particular management. Poisoning by drugs can be serious in children, especially when salicylate, tricyclic or iron have been ingested. Most of the clinical features of salicylate poisoning resemble those already described in adults but it should be remembered that children are especially susceptible to the severe acid-base disturbance which occurs in this form of poisoning and which may develop at blood levels of salicylate which are not considered dangerous in adults. Exchange transfusion is a valuable therapeutic procedure in severe salicylate poisoning in little children.

Poisoning with iron salts which formerly carried a high mortality, is now effectively treated with the chelating agent, desferrioxamine, given via the gastric tube, intramuscularly and by intravenous infusion. Speed is essential in starting treatment which may be summarised in dosages appropriate for adults which will require adjustment according to the age of the child:

1. An intramuscular injection of 2 g of desferrioxamine is given immediately.

2. Gastric lavage is performed with appropriate volumes of a solution of desferrioxamine (2 g) in 1 litre of warm water, following which 5 g of desferrioxamine in 100 ml of water or saline is left in the stomach.

3. This is followed by an intravenous infusion of desferrioxamine in saline, dextrose or blood. The amount should not exceed 15 mg/kg body weight/hour up to a maximum of 80 mg/kg in 24 hours.

4. Full supporting therapy for convulsions, shock, acidosis, blood loss and electrolyte disturbance is essential.

Tricyclic antidepressants are often prescribed to children for enuresis. Acute overdosage of these drugs, therefore, is common in children and is more liable to cause dangerous arrhythmias than in adults. Appropriate antiarrhythmic drugs should be given (p. 192), and physostigmine (p. 807) is an effective antidote.

Industrial and Agricultural Poisoning

It is sufficient to record that lead (p. 750), cyanide (p. 808), mercury, beryllium (p. 328) and cadmium are potential causes of industrial poisoning. In agriculture many highly toxic weedkillers, including paraquat and the dinitro-ortho-cresol group and the insecticides belong to the organophosphorous compounds have been developed in recent years. They have been responsible for only a small number of cases of acute poisoning in Britain owing to adequate and effective legislation for controlling their use. In some countries, however, they have caused many deaths each spring.

A. A. H. Lawson
Henry Matthew

Further reading:

Matthew, H. & Lawson, A. A. H. (1975) *Treatment of Common Acute Poisonings.* 3rd edition. Edinburgh: Churchill Livingstone.

17. Tropical Diseases and Helminthic Infections

In this chapter those diseases are described which are limited to the tropics or are commoner there than in temperate regions. Some, such as malaria and amoebiasis, are frequently seen in Britain in immigrants, visitors and returned travellers. As parasitic worms are prevalent in the tropics all common helminths are described, including the ubiquitous threadworm. A few infections are also included which do not occur in the tropics but which are related to tropical infections and have not been described elsewhere in this book.

Before presenting individual diseases, consideration is given to the patterns of disease in tropical and developing countries, as they may differ materially from those encountered elsewhere. It will be seen that ill health in the tropics does not consist only of a battle between human hosts and pathogens. It is important that the health problems of the world should be widely appreciated and that doctors should be reliably informed, whether or not they propose to work in the tropics.

The diseases described have been grouped according to the aetiological agents in the following manner:

Protozoa, e.g. malaria, amoebiasis, visceral leishmaniasis (kala azar), African trypanosomiasis (sleeping sickness).
Bacteria, e.g. leprosy, cholera, anthrax, plague.
Spirochaetes, e.g. yaws, relapsing fever, and *Spirillum,* i.e. rat-bite fever.
Viruses, e.g. yellow fever, dengue, rabies.
Chlamydia, e.g. lymphogranuloma inguinale, trachoma.
Rickettsia, e.g. typhus fevers, Q fever.
Helminths: (*a*) flukes, e.g. schistosomiasis.
　　　　　　　(*b*) tapeworms, e.g. hydatid disease.
　　　　　　　(*c*) roundworms, e.g. threadworms, ascariasis, hookworms, filariae.
Fungi, e.g. histoplasmosis.
Arthropods, e.g. scabies.
Snakes and Marine animals, e.g. adders, jelly fish.
Vegetable toxins, e.g. argemone poisoning.

Study of the diseases named above would give the British student a sound introduction to tropical medicine. The other infections described in this chapter should be considered as opportunity arises.

Specific measures for the prevention of each disease are emphasised. Tables of vaccinations and prophylactic measures advised for travellers are given on pages 933 and 934, and a map of the world on page 935 indicates the main hazards to be encountered in different regions. The more difficult problem of how to raise the general standard of health in the tropics is discussed on pages 932 to 936.

PATTERNS OF DISEASE IN TROPICAL AND DEVELOPING COUNTRIES

Patients in the tropics suffer from disorders of all the major systems and psyche, as they do in temperate and developed countries. In tropical countries, however, the aetiological factors may be different, especially in the case of infectious disease which still represents the greatest problem. The genetic constitution of patients in many parts of the world makes them resistant to certain conditions and predisposes them to others. The battle against acute disease is often a single episode in a long campaign against chronic infection and malnutrition. Clinical patterns of illness in the tropics, therefore, differ in many ways from those in temperate zones. Although the principles of diagnosis and treatment will be the same, multiple pathologies and diagnoses are the rule rather than the exception and treatment may need to be modified in the light of the background factors.

The Background to Diseases in the Tropics

Genes and Race. The best example of genetically determined disease is sickle-cell anaemia (p. 822) in which homozygous producers of haemoglobin S become anaemic and often die in infancy. The heterozygous carrier of haemoglobin S, on the other hand, is healthy and enjoys a measure of protection against the severe complications of malaria. Other examples of racially determined responses to disease are seen in leprosy, which is worse in Caucasians and Mongolians than in Negroes, and in tuberculosis, the pattern in Indians differing from that in Europeans.

Nutrition and Agriculture. The presence or absence of malnutrition depends on the availability of food, its cost and the correctness of its use. Traditional practices and taboos may limit the use of available food, e.g. the banning of eggs and milk in pregnancy. Malnutrition impairs both the cellular and humoral components of the immune response and predisposes children to infection which further drains the body's nutritional reserves and retards growth. Moderate degrees of undernutrition are much commoner than the gross malnutrition syndromes and may be overlooked.

Dietary toxins are found in some areas and produce conditions such as tropical ataxic neuropathy from cassava in Africa (p. 140), veno-occlusive liver disease from seneccio alkaloids in Jamaica and elsewhere (p. 458) and hepatoma from aflatoxin in badly stored nuts and cereals (p. 819).

Infections. Acute infectious diseases, especially malaria, measles and gastroenteritis, still account for the high infant mortality in some parts of the tropics where up to 40 per cent of children die before the age of 5 years. Acute infections, may precipitate the syndromes of malnutrition, which may then be complicated by further infection, for example measles leading to kwashiorkor and cancrum oris.

Many of the decimating diseases of the past are now controlled by vaccination (smallpox and yellow fever), vector control (malaria and sleeping sickness) and general improvement of living standards (plague and relapsing fever), but in several instances control is imperfect and the disease reappears as, for example, malaria in Sri Lanka and relapsing fever among refugees. Other epidemic diseases such as cholera in Asia and meningococcal meningitis in Africa remain largely uncontrolled and still kill hundreds of thousands of people annually.

Chronic infections may tax the physiological reserves of vital organs, such as the liver or kidneys in schistosomiasis, the heart in trypanosomiasis cruzi

(Chagas' disease), the lungs, bones and lymph nodes in tuberculosis, the bone marrow reserves of iron in ancylostomiasis, and of folate in malaria, the small bowel in strongyloidiasis and the muscles in leprosy. These organs may then fail prematurely if the demand, imposed on them by work, pregnancy or additional disease, increases. Such infections produce chronic ill health in millions of children and even more so in adults. Tuberculous lymphadenopathy is very common and may involve superficial nodes in all areas or be limited to deep nodes and then be a cause of undiagnosed fever. Very often the degree of suffering is not sufficient to take people to hospital, even if one is available, but the ceaseless pruritus and gradually failing vision of onchocerciasis, the persistent diarrhoea of schistosomiasis mansoni and the immobilising cellulitis of the guinea worm are other examples of conditions sufficiently debilitating to reduce performance, deepen poverty and lead to malnutrition. These chronic infectious diseases are enormous economic burdens on the nation as well as on the patient and his family.

Epidemiological factors determine the distribution, prevalence, incidence and endemicity of a disease, especially if it is infectious, and so affect its pattern in the community. Endemic malaria, poliomyelitis and viral hepatitis affect the indigenous children, who either die or become immune so that adults do not suffer from these diseases. Non-immune adults, such as tourists, invading soldiers or refugees are, however, fully susceptible unless specifically protected. Particular requirements of organisms, vectors, hosts or intermediate stages of parasites make rabies a sporadic disease, meningococcal meningitis a disease of the Sudan savanna, cholera an Indian riverine disease, onchocerciasis a rural disease. Chagas' disease a poverty disease and hookworm primarily a farmer's disease. Cooking and eating habits determine the prevalence of paragonimiasis, clonorchiasis and tapeworm infection.

Immunity and Autoimmunity. The natural immunity of animals to some human infections such as smallpox, which has only man for its host, enables this disease to be abolished, whereas the eradication of yellow fever is prevented by the susceptibility of monkeys to it. Natural immunity of individuals may possibly explain why some people do not suffer certain infections, but immunity acquired in childhood is a more usual explanation. *Mycobacterium leprae*, for example, commonly causes subclinical but immunising infections in children living in an endemic area, so that clinical disease is seen mainly in teenagers and young adults who fail to become immunised.

Most human infections are terminated or controlled by an efficient immune response. When the response is inefficient the organism multiplies unchecked, causing either death or chronic disease as in lepromatous leprosy or onchocerciasis. Immunity is usually accompanied by hypersensitivity, which often causes more damage than the organism itself, as in tuberculoid leprosy or hepatosplenic schistosomiasis. Sometimes the immune response seems to be inappropriate, as in the tropical splenomegaly syndrome of chronic malaria (p. 839), or to be grossly exaggerated, as with the macroglobulinaemia of trypanosomiasis (p. 851). In sharp contrast with their commonness in temperate countries, autoimmune diseases are rarely encountered in the tropics.

Variations within the Tropics. As well as the gross but general differences between patterns of disease in tropical underdeveloped and temperate developed countries, there are many variations within the tropics. A certain condition may be present in only one climatic belt, continent or even community, but be very important there; examples are loiasis in the West African rain forest, Chagas' disease in South America and kuru among the Fore people of New Guinea. Individual infectious and parasitic diseases are considered later in the chapter; their distribution throughout the world is shown on a map on page 935.

GEOGRAPHICAL INFLUENCES ON DISEASES OF THE MAIN SYSTEMS

Cardiovascular Disease

Acclimatisation to a hot, humid environment demands a 20 per cent increase in cardiac output and later an increase in plasma volume. A diseased heart is less able to acclimatise. The ECG pattern of normal individuals in Africa and other tropical countries commonly shows changes in the ST segments and T waves.

Rheumatic heart disease is worldwide, especially where there is overcrowding due to urbanisation and industrialisation. Just as important in children and young adults in parts of East and West Africa, Sri Lanka and Southern India, Brazil and Colombia is endomyocardial fibrosis (p. 229). Infective endocarditis is often secondary to skin sepsis but is no more common than in temperate climates whereas pericarditis is much more frequent and is usually either pyogenic or tuberculous. Chagas' disease, which accounts for 10 per cent of all necropsies in Brazil, is an outstanding cause of myocarditis; other causes in the tropics are African trypanosomiasis, typhoid fever, diphtheria, rickettsial infections and acute schistosomiasis. Cardiomyopathy is due to alcohol in parts of Africa and to thiamine deficiency in parts of South-east Asia and Southern Africa. In some countries congestive cardiomyopathy is a common cause of heart failure as is anaemia due to hookworms, sickle-cell disease or kwashiorkor.

In some rural tropical communities blood pressure does not increase with age. The 'normal' blood pressure is usually lower than in temperate communities, essential hypertension is rare and pregnancy hypertension less common, but in other areas the opposite is true. Atherosclerotic and especially coronary heart disease is virtually unknown in many rural populations, whose plasma cholesterol levels are low and fibrinolytic activity high. Cor pulmonale is also rare in the tropics except where schistosomiasis is highly endemic.

Other forms of arterial disease are rare, but primary arteritis of the aorta, which can affect any of its major branches and of which the Takayasu syndrome (p. 243) is an example, is relatively common in Japan, South-east Asia and parts of Africa. In East and Central Africa an arteritis of unknown origin causes peripheral gangrene.

With the exception of tropical phlebitis, venous diseases such as haemorrhoids, varicose veins and deep vein thrombosis with its complication of pulmonary embolism are rare in the tropics.

Tropical Phlebitis

This phlebitis, of uncertain origin, was first described in East Africa but is now known to occur throughout tropical Africa. Vascular granulation tissue containing fibroblasts, endothelial cells and giant cells is laid down, especially in the middle coat of the vein, but extends outside the wall of the vein which becomes thrombosed. Thrombosis of the splenic vein may cause necrotic infarction and liquefaction in the spleen.

When the affected vein is large, there will be a marked reaction in it with pain along its course, followed by local swelling and enlargement of the veins and tissues distal to the lesion. It may be possible to palpate the affected vein as a hard, cord-like structure. There is usually a febrile reaction during the acute stage. The venous lesion gradually resolves and the circulation is re-established. When the diseased veins are small, the symptoms and signs are slighter. Tender thickenings of one or several superficial veins may be palpated. They usually resolve in a few weeks.

Treatment is symptomatic. The value of anticoagulants has not been determined.

Respiratory Disease

Acute respiratory infection is the commonest cause of childhood death all over the world, especially where measles is still prevalent. Most adult respiratory diseases in the tropics are also due to infection. Pneumococcal pneumonia and tuberculosis are commonest, followed by histoplasmosis in parts of South America, paragonimiasis in South-east Asia, filariasis (pulmonary eosinophilia) in India and the pulmonary complications of hepatic amoebiasis and schistosomiasis. Chronic bronchitis is rare in most rural areas, although common in North and Central India and parts of New Guinea where it is attributed to allergy to fungi growing in roof thatch. Asthma is uncommon in much of the tropics.

Diseases of the Alimentary Tract and Pancreas

Diarrhoea is the second commonest cause of death in childhood the world over and the most frequent in infancy in countries of poor hygiene if the mother is not breast feeding. In adults, infectious disorders are the most important causes of alimentary disease, especially acute gastroenteritis, giardiasis, typhoid and other salmonelloses, ileocaecal tuberculosis, amoebic and bacillary dysentery, schistosomiasis mansoni and, in some countries, tropical sprue (see below). In underdeveloped countries the rural diet is rich in hand-milled grain fibre (bran) which is not only nutritious in vitamins, protein and iron and helps protect against deficiency diseases such as beriberi, but also makes a bulky soft stool which is passed two or three times daily. This bowel habit is associated with a virtual absence of appendicitis and diverticular disease. Other diseases which are rare in the tropics include Crohn's disease and ulcerative colitis. Cholecystitis is infrequent except as a complication from biliary flukes. The prevalence of peptic ulcers varies greatly between different regions.

In certain parts of the tropics calcifying pancreatitis is common and may be related to protein deficiency associated with a highly alkaline vegetarian diet. It occurs in children and young adults and in many instances is not associated with the consumption of alcohol.

Tropical Sprue

Tropical sprue may be defined as malabsorption of two or more unrelated substances occurring in a patient in the tropics, in the absence of other intestinal disease or parasites.

The name sprue was given by the Dutch in Java to a prevalent form of malabsorption, the manifestations of which resemble those of gluten-induced enteropathy (p. 394). The aetiology of sprue is unknown but its prevalence in certain well-defined tropical countries and indeed localities, and its epidemiological pattern, suggest that an infective agent may be involved in its production. In established sprue the jejunal contents are grossly overpopulated with aerobic enterobacteria which seem to play a role in maintaining the disease. Sprue is not due to gluten or any other demonstrable sensitivity and there is usually no evidence of preceding malnutrition, but folate deficiency, as in pregnancy, may precipitate the disease. Not all cases necessarily have the same aetiology, which may account for occasional reports of sprue from Africa and elsewhere where the disease is not usually encountered. It occurs mainly in Asia, including Sri Lanka, Southern India, Malaysia, Indonesia, Hong Kong and China, some Caribbean Islands, Puerto Rico and parts of South America. Sprue has been recognised in European residents in Asia and in indigenous tropical populations, both in their own surroundings and when living away from their homes. There is also an epidemic form in Southern India around Vellore. It is a common problem among travellers returning to Europe overland from India and Nepal.

Pathology. The pathological changes closely resemble those of gluten enteropathy, although they tend to be less advanced. The jejunal villi are blunted or, rarely, absent and there is a subepithelial infiltration with plasma cells and lymphocytes. Mild changes in the jejunal mucosa are common in asymptomatic indigenous peoples, without malabsorption, throughout the tropics (*tropical enteropathy*). In severe cases the abnormality is also found in the ileum. These changes are associated with malabsorption of fat, protein, carbohydrate and vitamins and the presence of diarrhoea which may lead to depletion of water, electrolytes, iron and calcium.

A macrocytic anaemia is common in sprue and in many cases megaloblastic change is present in the bone marrow due to folate deficiency. Vitamin B_{12} deficiency takes longer to develop and is encountered only in sprue of many weeks' duration.

Clinical Features. The condition can be mild or severe. Although the onset may be acute and occur within a few weeks of arrival in the tropics, it is more often insidious with increasing lassitude, mental apathy and depression, loss of weight, anorexia and flatulence. Remissions and relapses are a characteristic feature. Initially or after some weeks a watery explosive diarrhoea occurs which in some cases appears to have been precipitated by a gastrointestinal infection or by dietary or alcoholic indiscretion. Later, up to 10 stools may be passed daily, especially in the morning or during the night. Defaecation is urgent and often follows meals. The stool is bulky, frothy, pale and fatty, loose, foul-smelling and floats in the lavatory pan and is difficult to flush away. Vomiting may occur with nausea, abdominal distention and borborygmi. The tongue becomes sore, first at the tip and edges, the discomfort being increased by smoking or taking hot spicy food; later it becomes fiery red in colour, fissured and painful, the whole mouth and throat feel sore and there may be difficulty in swallowing. Nocturnal urinary frequency and amenorrhoea have also been noted.

In the untreated chronic disease there is much loss of weight. Abdominal distension, pallor and generalised pigmentation appear. The skin becomes coarse and dry (follicular keratosis) possibly due to deficiency of vitamin A. Fever is uncommon unless associated with severe megaloblastic anaemia or with superadded infection, often of the urinary tract. Continued malabsorption of vitamins of the B complex leads to glossitis, cheilosis and angular stomatitis. Bleeding haemorrhoids may be a feature and complicate the appearance of the stools. Loss of fluids and electrolytes may lead to severe dehydration, muscular weakness and cramps, and lack of vitamin D and calcium to osteomalacia and tetany, but bone changes are less than in gluten enteropathy. Hypoproteinaemic oedema may be a feature of the chronic disease. Peripheral neuropathy is very rare.

Diagnosis. The clinical features and the history of residence in an area noted for tropical sprue will suggest the correct diagnosis if care is taken to recognise the early and the mild cases as well as the late presentations. Evidence of malabsorption is obtained by estimation of the faecal fat excretion, by the d-xylose absorption test and the Schilling test of B_{12} absorption. Haematological changes start early; macrocytosis suggests folate deficiency and precedes the onset of frank megaloblastic anaemia. Serum or erythrocyte levels of folate are low. Anaemia may also be hypochromic from defective absorption of iron. Intestinal anatomy is assessed by radiology using a non-flocculable barium preparation for the meal and by intestinal biopsy. The histological appearance is that of partial villous atrophy and neither this nor the radiological signs are specific for tropical sprue but merely indicate that a malabsorption syndrome is present. Differential diagnosis is from other forms of steatorrhoea. Additional causes in the tropics are infections of the intestine with *Giardia intestinalis*, *Strongyloides stercoralis* or *Capillaria philippinensis*. Intestinal hurry as part of an allergic response in the early stages of ancylostomiasis may suggest the onset of sprue. Early symptoms of sprue may erroneously be attributed to amoebiasis or neurosis.

Treatment. Complete rest in bed is required initially for the severely affected patient. Dehydration and potassium deficiency must be corrected. Tetracycline, 1 g daily in divided doses for 28 days, will usually reduce diarrhoea and improve absorption. In addition folic acid, 5 mg daily (10 mg intramuscularly in severe cases), is given as this seems in many patients to improve absorption as well as to relieve symptoms due to folate deficiency. If the bone marrow is megaloblastic there is a brisk haematological response with reticulocytosis and reversion to a normoblastic appearance. Serial jejunal biopsies have shown that in recent cases the jejunal mucosa soon returns to normal. Such a patient can continue to live in the tropics and remain well. It has not yet been established whether to give a small prophylactic dose of folic acid daily to prevent a relapse in patients remaining in the tropics or to administer folic acid only if a relapse occurs. Some patients suffering from long continued chronic sprue may not respond to folic acid because of deficiency of vitamin B_{12}. These patients should be given intramuscular injections of hydroxocobalamin, 1,000 µg twice in 1 week, followed by a dose of 250 µg once a fortnight for 6 weeks in addition to folic acid. Anaemia is corrected and the danger of developing subacute combined degeneration of the spinal cord is avoided. If hypochromic anaemia due to iron deficiency is present, ferrous sulphate must be given. Vitamin K may be required because of bleeding. A multivitamin preparation containing 10 mg thiamin, 5 mg riboflavin and 50 mg nicotinamide twice daily should be prescribed for a few weeks. Tetany necessitates the giving of calcium and magnesium parenterally and vitamin D by mouth.

Complicated diets are no longer advised but the diet initially should be bland

and appetising, limited in fat and carbohydrate and high in protein. Because of their high content of folate and other vitamins the importance of liver, meat and green vegetables in the diet after recovery must be stressed. Folic acid supplements should always be given to women who have had sprue should they become pregnant. Often, after apparently successful treatment, mild diarrhoea and flatulence may persist. These are usually due to secondary hypolactasia and respond to a lactose-free diet.

Diseases of the Liver

Liver disease is a serious cause of disability and death throughout the tropics and subtropics. The microscopic structure of liver from a normal person in tropical Africa differs from that in a European. The hepatocytes are irregular in size and staining and frequently contain more than one nucleus. Portal tracts are infiltrated with mononuclear cells and a variable degree of fibrous tissue. Black pigment may be present in Kuppfer cells or portal tracts. These changes probably reflect the insults to which the liver is exposed in the tropics, including protein and vitamin malnutrition, alimentary infections and toxins, and systemic infections notably malaria and schistosomiasis. The effects of protozoal and helminthic infections on the liver are discussed on page 458.

In most areas where hygiene is poor, type A viral hepatitis is endemic and especially affects children. Cirrhosis of the liver and hepatoma are common in adults and a relationship has been postulated with hepatitis B virus which is extremely common in some parts of Africa where the prevalence exceeds 10 per cent of the population. There is also increasing evidence incriminating aflatoxin isolated from badly stored groundnuts and grains as a cause of cirrhosis and hepatoma.

Diseases of the Kidney and Urinary System

Schistosomiasis haematobium, which is the commonest cause of haematuria in endemic areas, may grossly damage the bladder and ureters. Skin infection with streptococci is a frequent precursor of acute glomerulonephritis. Pyelonephritis is common and in males often follows a gonococcal stricture of the urethra. *Plasmodium malariae* is an important cause of the nephrotic syndrome in children. Lepromatous leprosy (p. 857) may also involve the kidneys. Bancroftian filariasis is a frequent cause of orchitis, epididymitis and hydrocele in endemic areas. areas.

Diseases of the Blood and Blood-forming Organs

Anaemia in the Tropics

In many tropical countries anaemia is common and often severe. This is largely explained by the high frequency of protozoal, helminthic and bacterial infections and the prevalence of malnutrition. It cannot be emphasised too strongly that the aetiology of anaemia in the tropics shows great variation from one country to another, and from one area to another, and effective management can only follow the clear appreciation of local patterns of disease, nutrition and social custom.

Iron Deficiency Anaemia. Ancylostomiasis (p. 907) is a major cause of iron deficiency anaemia. Each worm ingests between 0·03 and 0·15 ml of blood daily; hence the loss of blood in a heavy infection of over 1,000 worms is large and anaemia develops rapidly after the iron stores are exhausted. Folate deficiency may complicate the anaemia if the dietary intake is inadequate for the demands of increased red cell formation. The anaemia responds rapidly to iron but will relapse unless the worms are also eliminated.

Megaloblastic Anaemia. Although Addisonian pernicious anaemia occurs in all races, it is relatively uncommon in tropical countries where megaloblastic anaemia is much more frequently due to nutritional deficiency of folate or vitamin B_{12}. The requirements of both these substances are increased during growth, pregnancy, infections, including malaria, and when there is increased red cell formation as in haemolytic anaemia. In this respect the available body store of folate, being very much smaller, is more vulnerable to depletion than that of vitamin B_{12}, hence most instances of megaloblastic anaemia in the tropics are due to folate deficiency.

Haemolytic Anaemia

The various types of haemolytic anaemia which occur in temperate climates are also encountered in tropical countries. Haemolytic anaemia in the tropics is frequently due to malaria. In addition two types of genetic abnormality resulting in haemolytic anaemia are also particularly common, namely deficiency of the enzyme glucose-6-phosphate dehydrogenase, and the haemoglobinopathies. Haemolysis also occurs in acute bartonellosis and may be caused by the venom of certain snakes.

Haemolytic Anaemia due to Malaria. Malaria is always accompanied by haemolysis and in a severe or prolonged attack very considerable anaemia may ensue. Generally the degree of anaemia is related to the severity of the parasitaemia but the destruction of red cells is always in excess of that due to parasitised cells and sometimes considerably so. During an acute attack of malaria the reticulocyte count may be low but as the patient recovers a brisk outpouring of young red cells occurs. Recuperation may be embarrassed by deficiency states, especially of folate and iron, or by other infections. Where these occur anaemia will be more severe and prolonged.

Immunity to malaria is greatest where the infection rate is highest and lowest where there is a low rate of infection or the patient is non-immune. Furthermore acquired immunity may be prejudiced by pregnancy, prolonged antimalarial therapy, splenectomy, lymphoma and allied disorders. Splenomegaly and anaemia diminish with increasing immunity but are universally found in young children.

Although there are many other important causes of enlarged spleens in the tropics, the 'tropical splenomegaly syndrome' is now attributed to an exaggerated immune response to malaria (p. 839). Whatever the cause, splenomegaly is commonly associated with dilutional anaemia and reduced red cell survival. Where the dilutional factor predominates, the reticulocyte count is usually low and the only therapeutic measure which will raise the haemoglobin significantly is splenectomy or treatment that reduces the spleen size. Iron and folic acid supplements and other haematinics have little or no effect. Red cell mass estimation solves the problem of the anaemia by demonstrating a near normal or normal red cell mass and plasma volume estimations demonstrate a greatly increased plasma volume.

Splenectomy in patients exposed to malarial infection should be done with caution and only if life-long prophylaxis against malaria can be ensured. Otherwise disastrous levels of parasitaemia can develop and the patient die of cerebral malaria.

It should be noted that the tropical splenomegaly syndrome may complicate splenic enlargement associated with other disorders. For instance, patients with chronic lymphatic leukaemia may present with gross splenomegaly which together with the associated anaemia may be greatly improved by long-term antimalarial prophylaxis.

Glucose-6-Phosphate Dehydrogenase Deficiency

Glucose-6-phosphate dehydrogenase (G6PD) is the first enzyme in the hexose monophosphate shunt of the Embden Myerhof glycolytic pathway from which red cells derive most of their metabolic energy. The function of the hexose monophosphate shunt is to service the enzymes glutathione reductase and glutathione peroxidase which protect the red cell against damage due to oxidation. In the absence of G6PD this protective mechanism is crippled and certain drugs in sufficient concentration can seriously injure the red cell.

It is now known that the deficiency is inherited as an X-linked recessive disorder and has a high frequency among Negroes. In West and East Africa about 20 per cent of males (hemizygotes) and about 4 per cent of females (homozygous for the abnormal gene) are affected. A small number of heterozygous females are also deficient of G6PD. A similar deficiency occurs in Caucasian and Mongoloid races where it is usually more severe. *Favism* (haemolytic anaemia from ingestion of the broad bean, *Vicia faba*) is due to deficiency of G6PD of the severe Caucasian variety. In Negroes the activity of the enzyme is about 15 per cent of normal, whereas in the others it is often less than 1 per cent with consequently greater clinical effects. Recently some hitherto unexplained cases of haemolytic disease of the newborn in Caucasians have been found to be due to the same defect. Yet other types of G6PD biochemically different from the above may be associated with congenital nonspherocytic haemolytic disease and have been found in persons of pure British ancestry. In these cases it is important to realise that splenectomy is valueless.

Many drugs in common clinical use, e.g. 8-aminoquinolines, antimalarials, sulphonamides, sulphones, nitrofurantoin, naphthaline and vitamin K, are capable of precipitating haemolysis in individuals with this defect. Infections may also potentiate the haemolytic action of drugs such as acetylsalicylic acid, chloramphenicol, chloroquine, and phenacetin.

Persons with G6PD deficiency normally enjoy good health but are liable to haemolysis if any of the incriminated drugs or foods is ingested. However, it must be emphasised that the haemolytic effect is related to the dose and will not be clinically detectable if the amount does not exceed a critical level. It is thus often possible to employ doses which are not toxic. The anaemia, when it occurs, may be rapid in onset, becoming obvious between 2 and 10 days after exposure to the precipitating agent and may be sufficiently severe to cause haemoglobinuria as well as the other classical signs of haemolysis. In the Negro type of deficiency only cells of a certain age and over are involved so that the haemolysis is to some extent self-limiting even when the offending agent is continued. Young red cells do have some G6PD activity and remain viable until their enzyme complement decays when they become susceptible to haemolysis. Since in the Caucasian variety the enzyme deficiency is much more severe, destruction tends to be more disastrous. Anuria is an infrequent but serious complication.

Diagnosis. This can be confirmed by estimating the G6PD activity of the red cell. This may not be entirely accurate if there is a considerable reticulocytosis. A number of screening tests are also available such as the ascorbate cyanide test of Jacob and Jandl which monitors the whole glutathione regulating system of which G6PD is a fundamental part and spot tests employing either the reduction of soluble tetrazolium compounds to insoluble purple formazan or the fluorescence of NADPH which is a biproduct of G6PD activity. This last test can be performed on aged blood or blood collected on filter paper and dried. The Jacob and Jandl test has the advantage of being cheap. These tests should always be performed alongside normal controls.

Treatment. This is by removal of the toxic agent. Recovery is usually rapid but if the anaemia is severe, transfusion of red cells with a normal enzyme complement may be required. Thereafter the patient should be advised to avoid drugs which may precipitate the disorder.

The Haemoglobinopathies

The haemoglobinopathies can be classified into three subgroups. In the first there is an alteration in the amino acid structure of the polypeptide chains of the globin fraction of haemoglobin, commonly called the abnormal haemoglobins, although some function as normal variants. In the second subgroup the amino acid sequence is normal but polypeptide chain production is impaired or absent for a variety of reasons; these are the thalassaemias. In the third subgroup there is the persistence of haemoglobin, normal in early life, namely haemoglobin F, into adult life. The hereditary persistence of high fetal haemoglobin is a benign condition and can be advantageous to persons carrying the haemoglobin S gene with which it is allelomorphic.

SICKLE-CELL ANAEMIA

Sickle-cell anaemia has been recognised among Negroes and to a lesser extent in other races since the beginning of the century. It is caused by the presence of the abnormal haemoglobin S.

Abnormal haemoglobins are caused by amino acid substitutions in their polypeptide chains. These in turn reflect mutations in the structural genes controlling the production of these chains. There are four loci for these structural genes, all on autosomal chromosomes, active in postnatal life. They are designated alpha, gamma, beta and delta and are responsible for the production of the three main haemoglobins seen after birth, namely haemoglobins F, A and A2. Each of these haemoglobins contain in common two alpha chains and their differences reflect the possession of two gamma chains in the case of haemoglobin F, two beta chains in the case of haemoglobin A, and two delta chains in the case of haemoglobin A2. Thus the globin fraction of these three types of haemoglobin may be written $\alpha2\gamma2$, $\alpha2\beta2$ and $\alpha2\delta2$, respectively. Each chain in the globin fraction carries one haem moiety in its folds. It is convenient and practical to represent normal adult haemoglobins by the capital letter A and the abnormal haemoglobins by S, C and E and so on. As there are now well over 200 haemoglobin variants known, the letters of the alphabet do not suffice and for some years new variants have been given names, often of the towns or districts in which they were discovered. Sickle-cell haemoglobin is the most important but haemoglobin C, D, and E are also significant in some parts of the world, particularly when inherited along with haemoglobin S or with beta thalassaemia (p. 826).

Modern nomenclature includes a statement of the site of the amino acid substitution and the substituting amino acid. Thus sickle haemoglobin may be defined as

$$\text{Hb S } \beta^{\text{6GLU} \to \text{VAL}} \quad \text{or} \quad \text{Hb S } \beta^{\text{A3GLU} \to \text{VAL}}$$

The second is more accurate since it defines the helix or bend in which the substitution occurs.

Control of haemoglobin synthesis is inherited from both parents. Thus a normal adult can be depicted as having the haemoglobin genotype AA, sickle-cell trait by AS and sickle-cell anaemia or homozygous haemoglobin S disease by SS. The inheritance when both parents have sickle-cell trait can be shown thus:

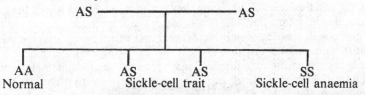

| AA | AS | AS | SS |
| Normal | Sickle-cell trait | | Sickle-cell anaemia |

The patient with sickle-cell trait is relatively resistant to the lethal effects of falciparum malaria in early childhood. The high incidence of this deleterious gene in equatorial Africa is thus explained by the selective advantage for survival it confers in an environment of endemic falciparum malaria. Surprisingly, patients with sickle-cell anaemia do not have a greatly increased resistance to falciparum malaria.

Pathogenesis. When haemoglobin S is deoxygenated, the molecules of haemoglobin polymerise to form pseudo-crystalline structures known as 'tactoids'. These distort the red cell membrane and produce characteristic sickle-shaped cells. The polymerisation is reversible when reoxygenation occurs. The distortion of the red cell membrane, however, may become permanent and the red cell 'irreversibly sickled'. The greater the concentration of sickle-cell haemoglobin in the individual cell, the more easily tactoids are formed, but this process may be enhanced or retarded by the presence of other haemoglobins. Thus haemoglobin C participates in the polymerisation more readily than haemoglobin A, whereas haemoglobin F strongly inhibits polymerisation. In sickle-cell anaemia most of the red cells contain haemoglobin S and little else and are very prone to sickle even *in vivo* under normal conditions. This happens particularly in those parts of the microvasculature which are sinusoidal and where the flow is sluggish. Sickle cells increase blood viscosity, traverse capillaries poorly and tend to obstruct flow, thereby increasing the sickling of other cells and causing cessation of flow. Thrombosis may follow and an area of tissue infarction result causing severe pain, swelling and tenderness (pain crisis). In addition these cells are phagocytosed in large numbers by the reticuloendothelial system, thus reducing their life span considerably.

Clinical Features. The two major problems are chronic anaemia due to reduced red cell survival and episodes of tissue infarction.

Anaemia. Problems do not arise until the fourth month of life when haemoglobin F production gives way to haemoglobin containing beta chains. The anaemia is haemolytic in type, severe, the haemoglobin seldom rising above 10 g/dl and averaging approximately 8 g/dl. Secondary folate deficiency is common and exacerbates the anaemia. When persistent, growth retardation and delayed puberty may occur. Episodes of increased sequestration and destruction of red cells occur, sometimes for no apparent reason and may lead to a swift fall in haemoglobin with rapidly enlarging spleen and liver. Transient hypoplasia of red cell production associated with infections is also liable to have exaggerated effects (aplastic crisis). The chronic anaemia is reponsible for fatigue, reduced exercise tolerance, increased susceptibility to infection, cardiomegaly, leg ulcers and cholelithiasis. Hyperplasia of the marrow in the first year of life expands the marrow cavity producing bossing of the skull, prominent malar bones and protuberant teeth.

Infarction crises are characterised by episodes of severe pain and these punctuate the patients' lives. Commonly they occur in bones and spleen but no tissue is exempt. In the infant they classically affect the fingers and toes, producing large fusiform swellings (dactylitis). Metacarpal and tarsal bones may be affected and residual stigmata of shortening of digits due to epiphyseal involvement may occur. At any age mesenteric infarction may produce acute abdominal emergencies difficult to distinguish from cases requiring laparotomy. The renal papilla is another site of trouble and infarction may give rise to painless haematuria. In adults aseptic necrosis of the head of the femur is a disabling complication.

Precipitating factors include dehydration, chilling and infection, but sometimes the attacks occur spontaneously. The onset is usually rapid, the pain excruciatingly severe in the first 24 hours, thereafter abating over the next few days. Fever, increasing jaundice and malaise are frequent concomitants and, if persistent, may suggest the establishment of infection in the infarcted site. Salmonella osteomyelitis is common.

Pregnancy is hazardous unless careful antenatal care is provided and towards the end of pregnancy infarctive crises in the bones may liberate large amounts of fat and bone marrow emboli which cause diffuse microembolism of the lungs with pulmonary infarction, cor pulmonale and even death. These complications may also be seen in the less severe haemoglobin SC disease.

Diagnosis. Sickle-cell anaemia should always be suspected in a patient who has had symptoms of anaemia since infancy and who belongs to a race which may be affected. In areas where sickle-cell anaemia is common, it should be considered in the differential diagnosis of many disorders. Patients must be adequately screened before major surgery and bloodless field surgery should never be employed, because infarction of the entire limb below the tourniquet may occur.

Microscopic examination of the stained blood film will show some sickle-shaped red cells in patients with sickle-cell anaemia but these are not seen in patients with sickle-cell trait. The presence of haemoglobin S can be confirmed by the demonstration that the red cells will sickle within 20 minutes when mixed on a glass slide with a freshly prepared 2 per cent solution of sodium metabisulphite under a cover slip. Controls should be set up at the same time. Alternatively solubility tests may be employed. If neither of these is available, a small drop of blood diluted in saline may be incubated under a sealed cover slip overnight when sickling will occur. A positive result indicates the presence of haemoglobin S but does not distinguish between sickle-cell trait, sickle-cell anaemia, haemoglobin SC disease, sickle-cell thalassaemia, etc.

When suspected, the diagnosis should always be confirmed by electrophoretic analysis of the haemoglobin and, if necessary, by a family study to demonstrate the inheritance. In this way true sickle-cell anaemia can be differentiated from other diseases in which haemoglobin S is combined with thalassaemia or some other abnormal haemoglobin such as C or D.

Treatment. There is no known method of changing the genetic constitution of an individual and therefore no means of curing this disease. Management is therefore aimed at alleviation of the symptomatology and the promotion of a life-style that will minimise the ill effects of the disorder. Basically this consists of the elimination of infections such as malaria and life-long antimalarials should be taken, if necessary. The patient should avoid becoming chilled or dehydrated. Regular folic acid supplements (5 mg daily) should be prescribed to support the greatly increased erythropoietic activity. Improvement of socioeconomic circumstances is of considerable importance to the underprivileged and will go a long way to alleviating the unfortunate effects of this disease. However, acute episodes will occur whatever is done and these should be managed as follows.

Anaemia. Exacerbation of the chronic haemolytic anaemia is commonly associated with infections and these should be eliminated. The patient should be adequately hydrated but transfusion with red cell concentrate used only in exceptional circumstances. Most patients are habituated to a haemoglobin level of about 8 g/dl and should be transfused only when the haemoglobin drops below 5 g/dl. Clearly the circumstances in individual cases will vary so that transfusion may be needed at higher levels. Diuretics should be avoided unless cardiac failure supervenes when they should be used with caution.

Tissue Infarction Crises. The pain caused by these crises can be extremely severe and the clinician is strongly tempted to use powerful analgesics. However, as the episodes will be recurrent, this should be avoided if at all possible and simple non-addictive analgesics such as aspirin, paracetamol and codeine used. Water and electrolyte depletion should be corrected as quickly as possible. Antibiotics will be necessary if there are infective complications such as osteomyelitis.

Prevention. Many lines of prophylactic therapy of *in vivo* sickling have been tried but even those with a theoretical hope of success have proved disappointing. Sodium bicarbonate orally in large doses may help in altering blood pH but cannot be given for very lengthy periods. High doses of urea orally prove unacceptable to the patient and unrewarding in clinical practice since it is necessary to maintain the patient at uraemic levels. Cyanate therapy is also unacceptable.

Prognosis. It is probable that in Africa without medical attention few children with sickle-cell anaemia survive to adult life. With full medical facilities and improved social and economic circumstances many patients survive and, although subject to recurrent ill health, lead a fairly normal life but are unlikely to reach old age.

OTHER SICKLE-CELL DISEASES

Sickle-Cell Trait. Most patients who are carriers of the sickle gene lead healthy lives. However, under certain circumstances they may be liable to sickling. These include bloodless field surgery and flying at altitudes over 15,000 feet (4575 m) if pressurisation is inadequate. In addition these patients are liable to attacks of painless haematuria due to infarction of the renal papillae.

Haemoglobin SC Disease. This disorder behaves like a mild variety of sickle-cell anaemia. Episodes of infarction crises are less frequent and anaemia is either absent or less severe. Aseptic necrosis of the femoral head, retinal thrombosis and painless haematuria are not uncommon complications.

Pregnancy is the main hazard as the same complications already mentioned under sickle-cell anaemia occur. Treatment of these should be by heparinisation and if necessary by premature induction of labour or delivery by Caesarean section. Heparin should be administered by continuous intravenous infusion and the dose adjusted to give thrombin times between 2 and 4 times that of the control sample. Another risk is that the symptomatology may mimic closely that of pregnancy hypertension but the treatment as for the latter may be lethal. Sedatives should be avoided. Careful antenatal and postnatal care are required and folic acid supplements will be needed and also iron supplements if the patient is deficient.

Haemoglobin C Disease. This is a benign haemoglobinopathy which, in its homozygous form, is not associated with much morbidity but may cause megaloblastic anaemia in pregnancy and considerable splenomegaly in adult life. It requires no specific treatment other than folic acid supplements in pregnancy.

THALASSAEMIA. Thalassaemia is an inherited impairment of haemoglobin synthesis, in which there is partial or complete failure to synthesise a specific type of globin chain. The exact nature of the defect is not yet understood but it is probable that a number of different faults occur along the pathway which translates the genetic information into a polypeptide chain. The gene itself may be deleted. Beta chain synthesis is most commonly affected. When the abnormality is heterozygous, synthesis of haemoglobin is only mildly affected and little disability occurs. When the patient is homozygous, synthesis is grossly impaired and severe anaemia results.

Beta Thalassaemia

Failure to synthesise beta chains (β-thalassaemia) is the commonest type and is seen in highest frequency in the Mediterranean area. Heterozygotes have what has been called *thalassaemia minor*, a condition in which there is usually mild anaemia and little or no clinical disability. Homozygotes (*thalassaemia major*) are unable to synthesise haemoglobin A and, after the neonatal period, have a profound hypochromic anaemia associated with much evidence of red cell dysplasia and increased red cell destruction. Haemoglobin F ($\alpha 2 \gamma 2$) production normally ceases in the neonatal period, but because of the severe anaemia some production persists to provide much of the circulating haemoglobin. Thus these patients attempt to supply their requirements with haemoglobins that normally comprise only 3 per cent of the total. At best they usually manage little more than 30 to 50 per cent of the normal adult complement of haemoglobin.

Clinical Features. The anaemia is crippling and the possibility of survival for more than a few years without transfusion is poor. Bone marrow hyperplasia early in life may produce head bossing, prominent malar eminences and other changes giving a Mongoloid appearance. The skull X-ray shows a 'hair on end' appearance and general widening of the medullary spaces which may interfere with the development of the paranasal sinuses. Development and growth are retarded and folate deficiency may occur. Splenomegaly is an early and prominent feature. Hepatomegaly is slower to develop but may become massive especially if splenectomy is undertaken. Transfusion therapy inevitably gives rise to haemosiderosis. Cardiac enlargement is common and cardiac failure in which haemosiderosis may play a part is a frequent terminal event.

It is not within the scope of this chapter to detail the great variety of clinical manifestations of thalassaemia which present a broad spectrum of disease. It is clear that there are several types of β-thalassaemia; for further study the reader is referred to publications dealing with this subject in greater detail (p. 829).

Diagnosis. Thalassaemia minor is often detected only when iron therapy for a mild hypochromic anaemia fails. The demonstration of microcytes, increased resistance of red cells to osmotic lysis and a raised haemoglobin A2 fraction together with evidence of the same abnormalities in other members of the family establishes the diagnosis. In contrast haemoglobin A2 levels are diminished in iron deficiency states.

The diagnosis of thalassaemia major is made by the finding of profound hypochromic anaemia associated with evidence of severe red cell dysplasia, erythroblastosis, and the absence or gross reduction of the amount of haemoglobin A, raised levels of haemoglobin F and evidence that both parents have thalassaemia minor.

Treatment. Transfusion is the mainstay in the treatment of homozygous β-thalassaemia and if possible the haemoglobin levels should be maintained between 10 and 12 g/dl. The intraperitoneal route may be used in young children to conserve veins. Iron therapy is strongly contraindicated but folic acid supplements should be given. Attempts to remove iron by the administration of chelating agents such as desferrioxamine should be employed but fail to keep pace with the iron deposition from transfusion therapy until the patient has been transfused with over 100 units of red cells when the level of iron overload becomes considerable and chelating agents more effective as a result. Splenectomy may be required for mechanical reasons or for hypersplenism. The later this can be done the better. Intercurrent infection must be treated vigorously with appropriate antibiotics.

ALPHA THALASSAEMIA

The reduction or absence of alpha chain synthesis is found mainly in Southeast Asia. There are probably at least two inherited abnormalities, one associated with severe, and the other with mild inhibition of alpha chain production. Heterozygotes of either abnormality are at little disadvantage since α-chain production is adequate. A slight excess of gamma chain production at birth may form tetramers γ4 (haemoglobin Bart's) and this can be demonstrated by electrophoretic techniques. The combination in the patient of a mild and a severe α-thalassaemia disorder results in a deficiency of α chain production which is less than absolute, so that some normal haemoglobin is formed. There is an excess of beta chains and these form tetramers β4 (haemoglobin H) and this may explain the syndrome of haemoglobin H disease. The inheritance of the severe α-thalassaemia abnormality from both parents is incompatible with life and such offspring are stillborn (hydrops foetalis).

Burkitt's Lymphoma

There a relationship between the incidence of this tumour and climatic factors of temperature and rainfall, and it has been postulated that the high incidence in certain areas may be associated with changes in the lymphoreticular system caused by persistent malaria. It is suggested that an ubiquitous virus, possibly the Epstein-Barr virus, evidence of which can be found in almost all patients with this tumour, tends to produce neoplastic change in patients whose immunological status has been affected by chronic malaria.

Pathology. The tumour is a malignant lymphoma of poorly differentiated lymphoblastic type. The histological pattern is of uniform masses of immature lymphoid cells, interspersed with many large clear histiocytes with poorly staining cytoplasm which create the typical 'starry sky' pattern.

Clinical Features. In Africa this tumour has a peak incidence between the ages of 4 and 8 years. Relatively few cases occur after puberty. The most frequent presenting feature is a tumour of the mandible or maxilla. The first clinical sign is usually loosening of the molar and pre-molar teeth which eventually become displaced, distorted and lost as the tumour grows. Tumours of the maxilla may present as exophthalmos due to early invasion of the orbit. The eye may eventually be totally destroyed and at this stage it is difficult to distinguish this tumour from a retinoblastoma. A particularly characteristic feature is the tendency of the tumours in the jaws to be multiple and it is not uncommon for all four jaw quadrants to be involved simultaneously.

The second commonest clinical presentation is an abdominal tumour, usually caused by involvement of the kidneys, adrenals, ovaries, liver or abdominal lymph nodes. Involvement of the kidneys, adrenals and ovaries is often bilateral.

The third commonest presenting feature is paraplegia which is of sudden onset, flaccid from the outset and associated with incontinence of urine and faeces, without radiological evidence of vertebral collapse.

Other sites characteristically involved in this multifocal tumour are the long bones of the limbs, the thyroid and salivary glands, the testes and the heart. Bilateral massive tumours of the breasts sometimes develop in young adult women. Spread to the bone marrow occurs relatively late in the disease.

The rarity of peripheral lymphadenopathy is particularly characteristic.

Treatment. This tumour is unusually sensitive to a large range of cytotoxic drugs and to radiotherapy. As the tumour is probably always multifocal, systemic chemotherapy is preferred. The best results to date have been obtained with cyclophosphamide and orthomerphalan. The former is given in single large doses of 30 to 40 mg/kg body weight repeated on one or more occasions after recovery of marrow depression. The latter is given in one or two doses of 1·1 to 1·4 mg/kg. A more extensive regime using multiple drugs has been used with success in resistant tumours. Intracranial involvement, recognised by the presence of tumour cells in the CSF, should be treated with methotrexate or cranio-spinal irradiation. The latter is practiced prophylactically in some centres. In some clinics in Africa prolonged survival rates of over 30 per cent have been reported.

Further reading about blood diseases in the tropics:

Beutler, E. (1971) *Red Cell Metabolism, A Manual of Biochemical Methods.* New York: Grune & Stratton.

Girdwood, R. H. (1973) *Blood Disorders due to Drugs and Other Agents.* Amsterdam: Excerpta Medica.——One chapter of this book is devoted to a review of glucose-6-phosphate dehydrogenase deficiency and related problems.

Lehmann, H. & Huntsman, R. G. (1974) *Man's Haemoglobins*. Amsterdam: North Holland Publishing Company.—This book provides a wide-ranging review of all aspects of the subject, including evolutionary, historical as well as biochemical and clinical aspects.
Weatherall, D. J. & Clegg, J. B. (1972) *The Thalassaemia Syndromes*. 2nd edition. Oxford: Blackwell.—In this book the author provides a very detailed description and discussion of the genetic and clinical aspects of the thalassaemias as well as a more brief review of the abnormal haemoglobins.

Metabolic, Endocrine and Connective Tissue Disorders

The prevalence of fluorosis is high in some areas (p. 114). Diabetes seems to be common throughout the tropics, but with few cardiovascular complications. The prevalence of other endocrine disorders is less certain.

Autoimmune disease is rare in most tropical countries. The incidence of dermatomyositis, scleroderma, lupus erythematosus and rheumatoid arthritis is low. Acute tropical polyarthritis, of obscure aetiology, is a common self-limiting disorder. Reiter's syndrome is frequent in Africa and causes much disability.

Tropical Myositis (*Pyomyositis*)

The cause of myositis in the tropics is uncertain. Abscesses explored early are sterile but later the pus may contain staphylococci or streptococci. It has been thought that in some instances 'tropical phlebitis' may precede pyomyositis but the latter occurs frequently in New Guinea where tropical phlebitis is not encountered. Most cases of pyomyositis occur in tropical Africa, South America and South Pacific Islands.

Pyomyositis starts with fever and painful induration of one or more of the large muscles, mostly in the lower limbs. The indurated area subsequently suppurates and a large abscess may form and be associated with a swinging temperature and leucocytosis. The affected area is swollen, hot and tender. When the pus is superficial, fluctuation can be detected.

Diagnosis is usually not difficult although meningitis or peritonitis may be simulated. The differential diagnosis includes Calabar swellings (p. 915), sparganosis (p. 904), scurvy and an underlying osteomyelitis. Staphylococcal pyaemia of other origin is characterised by numerous small abscesses.

When an abscess has formed, it should be incised, the pus evacuated and antibiotics given appropriate to the bacteria cultured.

Neurological and Psychiatric Disease

Infections still cause most of the neurological disease throughout the tropics. Common are pyogenic and tuberculous meningitis, rabies and arthropod-borne viral encephalitis, malaria, tetanus, poliomyelitis, trypanosomiasis in Africa, bartonellosis in Peru, cysticercosis and hydatid disease and in the Pacific eosinophilic meningitis. Leprosy is the commonest cause of peripheral neuritis in the world and Chagas' disease of systemic autonomic neuropathy. Tuberculoma is a frequent and amoebic abscess a rare cause of an intracranial space-occupying lesion. In some tropical communities cerebrovascular accidents and trauma are becoming the chief causes of neurological disease.

Certain diseases, such as tabes dorsalis, multiple sclerosis, parkinsonism and vitamin B_{12} neuropathy are rare.

There are several syndromes, due to dietary deficiencies or toxins, which are locally important. These include beriberi in the poorer areas of South-east Asia, Wernicke's encephalopathy among the Bantu in Southern Africa and pellagra among maize eaters.

Tropical ataxic neuropathy may be caused by cyanide (p. 140). Causes of spastic paraplegia in the tropics include lathyrism (p. 141) in India and the horn of Africa, Burkitt's lymphoma (p. 827) in African adolescents, schistosomiasis in Africa and, commonest of all, spinal tuberculosis. On the Pacific island of Guam is found the world's highest incidence of amyotrophic lateral sclerosis and parkinsonism associated with dementia which together account for 20 per cent of all adult deaths among the Chamono people.

The prevalence of psychiatric diseases in the tropics is similar to that in temperate countries, but some of the precipitating factors and symptom-complexes are different. Included among the causes of organic confusional states are alcoholism, meningitis, syphilis, malaria, trypanosomiasis and typhoid fever. Functional psychoses present in the same ways as in temperate countries, but acute emotional disturbances, especially in Africans, often present with schizophrenic features such as hallucinations and paranoia; the prognosis is good. Neuroses are especially common in people from underdeveloped countries who are suddenly moved to a strange environment. Symptoms are often florid and usually hysterical, the patient having little understanding of their cause. Fear, implanted by witchcraft may have profound effects and, in addition, the subject may have been made to swallow potent poisonous charms.

Malignant Disease

Patterns of malignant disease vary greatly between different communities. Some tumours are rare—for example, carcinoma of the colon in Africa and Asia—and some extremely common locally. Hepatoma is frequent in parts of Africa and in the Singapore Chinese. Carcinoma of the mouth is the commonest cancer in India and Sri Lanka and carcinoma of the nasopharynx is frequent in Kenya and among Chinese in South-east Asia.

Kaposi's sarcoma, or idiopathic multiple haemorrhagic sarcoma of the skin, is a multifocal malignancy composed of new blood vessels and large spindle cells. It presents as firm, bluish-brown nodules in the skin, usually on the limbs. Its incidence is high in parts of tropical Africa.

DISORDERS DUE TO CLIMATE

Exposure to Strong Sunlight; Solar Keratosis; Acclimatisation to Heat; Prickly Heat; Heat Exhaustion; Tropical Anhidrotic Asthenia; Heat Hyperpyrexia; High Altitude Acclimatisation and Deterioration; Mountain Sickness; Cold Injury

Exposure to Strong Sunlight

Sunburn is caused not by the heat of the sun but by ultraviolet light. The skin of those with fair complexions and red hair is especially sensitive to strong sunlight. Natural tolerance to the sun may be won by gradual exposure which enables the skin to acquire protective pigmentation.

Short periods of unaccustomed strong sunlight produce only erythema and itchiness of the affected area of skin. Should, however, the exposure be prolonged, acute pain and oedema with vesicles and bullae soon develop. These local changes are accompanied by malaise, headache and nausea. Severe cases may suffer from prostration and even acute circulatory failure. When a large area of skin has been damaged, this may interfere seriously with sweating and predispose to heat hyperpyrexia (p. 833).

No treatment is needed for mild sunburn, but for severe cases rest in bed in a cool room is required with sedatives to relieve the pain. Shock and dehydration must be corrected. Large blisters should be pricked. Calamine lotion containing 0·5 per cent crystal violet should be applied to intact skin. Antihistamine drugs given by mouth help to relieve pruritus.

Some protection is afforded by face powders and creams containing para-aminobenzoic acid which absorbs ultraviolet light.

Solar Keratosis

After prolonged residence in the tropics atrophic patches are liable to develop on exposed parts of the body especially in those with fair skins. The backs of the hands, the neck and the forehead are most commonly affected. These areas may later develop small patches of hyperkeratosis which occasionally progress to the formation of squamous cell carcinoma. This process is most severe in albinos.

The skin should be protected as far as possible from the sunlight by clothing and creams. Hyperkeratotic areas can be removed by the application for one week of 5 per cent fluorouracil ointment under an occlusive dressing.

Acclimatisation to Heat

In cool climates heat production in the body is balanced by loss from the surface chiefly by radiation and convection. The hypothalamus controls the superficial circulation and produces vasoconstriction or dilation as required for the conservation or loss of body heat. When the atmospheric temperature is above that of the body evaporation of sweat is all-important in the maintenance of a stable body temperature, assisted to a minor degree by insensible loss through the skin and lungs.

Acclimatisation to heat is an essential preparation for workers exposed to excessive heat in certain industries in cool climates as well as for people who live in the tropics. This can be achieved by undertaking exercise daily under artificially produced or natural hot weather conditions for 10 to 14 days. The total volume of circulating fluid increases and compensates for the expanded vascular bed; this is accompanied by a diminished pulse rate and an increased cardiac output. Salt excretion by the kidneys and in sweat is reduced, mainly as a result of increased production of aldosterone. The sweat glands also become more active, responding more rapidly and efficiently to any increase in body temperature; consequently the rise in body temperature in response to exercise diminishes. With these adjustments the individual is better able to work and remain well under conditions of high atmospheric temperature provided an adequate intake of water and salt is maintained.

Heat syncope (fainting, p. 172) occurs in people dressed in unsuitable clothes in a warm atmosphere with poor air circulation, at exercise or on suddenly standing up.

Prickly Heat

Many Europeans living in the tropics, especially when humidity is high, suffer from prickly heat. This arises from blockage of sweat ducts within the prickle cell layer of the epidermis so that sweat escapes into the epidermis and causes severe irritation. The lesions consist of numerous minute papules, surrounded by erythema which become vesicular or pustular. The pus is sterile, although scratching may lead to secondary pyogenic infection. The lesions are most numerous in parts of the body in close contact with clothing.

The principles of treatment are to reduce sweating to a minimum and to overcome the blockage of the sweat ducts. If the patient can be transferred to a cool environment such as an air-conditioned room, the blocked ducts become patent within a week or two. In severe cases, when artificial cooling cannot be maintained, the application of anhydrous lanoline will restore the patency of the ducts.

In prevention it is important to prevent blocking the sweat ducts. Therefore maceration of the skin by sweat or liquid applications, excessive washing and irritation from clothing (either by friction or a chemical contaminant) must be avoided. The use of a bland soap containing hexochlorophane is advocated. Dusting powders should only be lightly applied. Clothing must be loose fitting, changed frequently and thoroughly rinsed after washing. Controlled tanning of the skin with sunlight may help acclimatisation. Obese patients must lose weight. Curries, condiments and alcohol, which cause sweating should be avoided.

Heat Exhaustion

Heat exhaustion is often brought on by a period of great heat or by extra effort under conditions of hot weather, when the patient has not taken enough fluid and salt to balance the increased loss by sweating. The amount of fluid lost as sweat during a working spell under these conditions may be as much as 6 or even 8 litres and even in persons fully acclimatised to heat this may entail a loss of approximately 2 g sodium chloride per litre of sweat. Ill-health, especially gastrointestinal disturbances with vomiting and diarrhoea, will increase the risk of heat exhaustion.

There are usually warnings which should be recognised. These include headache, giddiness, loss of appetite, nausea, muscular cramps, especially of the legs and feet, and personality changes—irritability and lack of co-operation. If the disorder is recognised at this early stage, removal to a cool atmosphere and cool water to drink, with added salt, will restore the patient to normal.

In an established case of heat exhaustion the patient is distressed and anxious, with a pale sweating skin, rapid weak pulse and low blood pressure, and often complains of cramps. Although the skin is cool, the rectal temperature may be slightly raised (the 'cold moist man', cf. p. 833). Dehydration is usually marked but when limited to loss of extracellular fluid there will be no thirst and consequently a considerable degree of water depletion may exist without producing any symptoms.

In severe cases it is usually not possible to give the required amount of fluid and electrolytes by mouth. Intravenous infusion of saline is therefore needed (p. 154). Initial and maintenance treatment should be carried out in a cool place until convalescence is complete. When heat exhaustion is not recognised and treated, the patient may pass into a condition of heat hyperpyrexia (p. 833).

Tropical Anhidrotic Asthenia

The majority of patients with this disorder have suffered from prickly heat. This has left extensive areas of skin, especially on the trunk and limbs, incapable of sweating properly. The condition develops insidiously towards the end of the hot weather, with headache, giddiness, lack of energy, diminished sweating and often marked polyuria, the dilute urine containing chloride. A rise of body temperature is common and may occasionally reach hyperpyrexia.

Prolonged treatment is needed. The patient must live in a cool climate until the skin has recovered and sweating has returned to normal; this may take several months.

Heat Hyperpyrexia (Heat Stroke)

This occurs in those exposed for considerable periods to unusually high atmospheric temperatures, independent of exposure to direct sunlight. Unacclimatised people are more liable to suffer, but a prolonged period of very high temperature may affect even those who are fully acclimatised, including the local inhabitants. The disorder is always associated with cessation of sweating, and then the body temperature may reach 42° to 43°C or even higher. Predisposing factors are those which interfere with the production and evaporation of sweat—unsuitable clothing and poor working conditions with little air movement, heavy work in conditions of high temperature and humidity. Diffuse lesions of the skin, especially if treated with oily preparations and protective coverings, may inhibit sweating and induce hyperpyrexia. Individuals with congenital absence of sweat glands or with cystic fibrosis are particularly vulnerable. Hyperpyrexia may follow heat exhaustion when dehydration leads to cessation of sweating.

Pathological and Clinical Features. The most important changes are in the central nervous system. There is general congestion of the brain with increased pressure of the cerebro-spinal fluid. Microscopic examination may show degeneration of nerve cells, particularly in the hypothalamic region and base of the brain.

In *primary hyperpyrexia* the onset is usually dramatic with no warning in a person who appears to be neither dehydrated nor deficient in salt, but occasionally the patient may have noticed that perspiration had become much less. He may have retired to rest feeling quite well and be found in coma a few hours later. Loss of consciousness may be preceded by prodromal signs of cerebral irritation. On examination a dry burning skin is found (the 'hot dry man'). When the temperature, which must always be taken rectally, reaches between 41° and 42°C unconsciousness supervenes and without energetic treatment the mortality rate can be 50 per cent. Hyperpyrexia may be complicated by acute circulatory failure, hypokalaemia or acute renal or hepatic failure. Haemorrhages are a frequent feature.

In cases of *secondary hyperpyrexia* the early symptoms are those of heat exhaustion or tropical anhidrotic asthenia. If the patient is not treated, the temperature continues to rise and the state of hyperpyrexia supervenes.

Diagnosis. Heat hyperpyrexia is likely during any prolonged period of unusually hot atmospheric conditions. Any patient with an unduly high temperature and dry skin should be treated as such a case, care being taken to exclude other diseases, especially *P. falciparum* malaria. Lumbar puncture will exclude meningitis and at the same time will relieve the increased cerebrospinal fluid pressure characteristic of heat hyperpyrexia.

Treatment. The aim is to reduce the temperature as quickly as possible in order to prevent permanent damage to vital structures. This is done by loosely wrapping the patient in a cool wet sheet and promoting evaporation by fanning, or by immersion in a bath of cold water. Parenteral antimalarial therapy (p. 840) should be given concurrently if malaria is a possibility. As the temperature falls, provided that the brain has not been irreparably damaged, consciousness returns. Cooling should be stopped when the rectal temperature has fallen to 39°C, otherwise the temperature, which goes on falling, may reach excessively low levels. As anoxia is frequently present oxygen should be given. Chlorpromazine (50 mg) should be administered and an adequate airway maintained. When return to consciousness is delayed, lumbar puncture and withdrawal of excess fluid may help. Intravenous hydrocortisone may be life saving in the presence of circulatory failure. Potassium deficiency should be corrected and severe haemorrhage controlled by blood transfusion. For the treatment of acute renal or hepatic failure see pages 496 and 446. During convalescence control of body temperature will remain unstable.

When hyperpyrexia is secondary to heat exhaustion, dehydration is usually severe. Therefore, in addition to reducing the high temperature, adequate water and salt replacement is essential.

Depending on the duration and degree of hyperpyrexia, the patient may recover completely, be left with residual brain damage or fail to respond to treatment.

Prevention of Ill-effects of Heat. Careful selection should be made of those required to work under hot atmospheric conditions. General physical fitness, youth and mental stability are important. Fever, gastrointestinal upsets, alcoholic excess and lack of sleep all predispose to ill-effects of heat. It is highly important that the skin should be healthy and that sweating should be normal.

When the atmospheric temperature is very high, leading to excessive sweating, even the fully acclimatised require to take extra fluid and salt. A daily intake of up to 15 litres of cool drinking water and 30 g of sodium chloride per person may be needed to prevent water and salt depletion. Advice and encouragement is required if such large amounts of fluid are to be taken. The extra salt is taken with food and in the drinking water, but it can, when necessary, be supplied in enteric coated tablets. A total of 30 g of sodium chloride is supplied by adding 3 flat teaspoonfuls of salt or 18 enteric coated tablets, each containing 650 mg of salt, to the normal daily intake of fluid and food.

In addition, everything possible should be done to improve working conditions by arranging for a free circulation of air and for a reduction of high temperature and excessive atmospheric humidity by air-conditioning. Clothing should be light and loose fitting. Hard or prolonged manual work should not be undertaken when atmospheric conditions are exceptionally unfavourable. Off-duty living conditions should be made as cool and comfortable as possible.

High Altitude Acclimatisation and Deterioration

The partial pressure of atmospheric oxygen decreases with altitude. Physiological acclimatisation starts at about 7,000 ft (2,110 m) and most people feel the need to acclimatise by about 12,000 ft (3,650 m). Pulmonary ventilation and perfusion increase, plasma volume decreases and renal excretion of bicarbonate increases. The first two changes serve temporarily to maintain arterial oxygen tension until erythrocyte production raises the haemoglobin and haematocrit. Above 14,000 ft (4,270 m) heart rate and cardiac output increase and pulmonary artery pressure rises. Physically fit young people acclimatise best and do better with each ascent. Lowlanders, however, never attain the performance of highlanders. Lack of acclimatisation is shown by increased respiration, Cheyne-Stokes respiration, mild headache and irritability, easy fatiguability and sleeplessness.

Acclimatisation continues successfully up to 17,500 ft (5,330 m) above which arterial oxygen saturation falls to 70 per cent and physical performance starts to decline. Short bursts of work can be undertaken, but at the risk of the production of an exaggerated lactic acidosis. Prolonged residence above this height causes anorexia, weight loss, decreasing mental and physical capacity and increasing susceptibility to infection. There are no permanent human habitations above 15,000 ft (4,575 m).

Mountain Sickness

Acute mountain sickness is experienced by people who go up too high too quickly; some suffer at 8,000 ft (2,440 m), others reach 19,000 ft (5,795 m) without trouble. The earliest symptoms are headache, nausea and vomiting, followed by lassitude, muscle weakness, breathlessness, cyanosis, dizziness, rapid pulse and insomnia. The symptoms are probably due to intracellular oedema and may herald the onset of two severe, possibly fatal complications: pulmonary oedema (p. 196) and, less commonly, cerebral oedema. Paradoxically the robust young man is prone to pulmonary oedema, probably due to overconfidence. Cerebral oedema causes drowsiness, confusion, fits and coma. Its presence may be confirmed by the detection of papilloedema. Retinal haemorrhages also occur. These complications are prevented by ascending gradually and are treated by descending rapidly and by giving oxygen if it is available. Frusemide (40–120 mg), or morphine (15 mg) is helpful for pulmonary oedema, and acetazolamide (250 mg) for cerebral odema. Venous thromboses, which may lead to pulmonary embolism, may afflict the partially acclimatised; they are due to increased viscosity of blood and are prevented by adequate hydration and exercise.

Chronic mountain sickness is due to alveolar hypoventilation and chronic hypoxia and may affect highlanders as well as acclimatised lowlanders. It causes cyanosis, cardiac failure, pulmonary hypertension and neuropsychiatric symptoms. It is treated by taking the patient down to sea level.

Cold Injury

Cold affects the body adversely by causing frostbite or accidental hypothermia.

Frostbite. Dry cold, below 0°C, freezes poorly insulated tissues such as fingers, especially in people exercising at altitudes where oxygen demand is high and availability low. The warning sign is intense pain in fingers or feet. Superficial frostbite causes blistering of skin, and deep frostbite necrosis of tissues leading to gangrene. Frostbite is treated by rapidly rewarming the whole patient with good insulation and hot drinks, and by warming the affected part in water at 40°C.

Accidental Hypothermia. This can be due to sudden immersion in a cold pond or sea, or to gradual but steady heat loss from exposure or from evaporation off the wet clothes of a poorly clad hill walker on a rainy day. The old and the sick become hypothermic if they are not well insulated at night. Clinical features and treatment are described on page 804.

Further reading about disorders due to climate:

Clark, E., *et al.* (1975) *Mountain Medicine and Physiology.* London: Alpine Club.
Edholm, O. G. & Bacharach, A. L. (1965) *Exploration Medicine.* Bristol: Wright.
Leithead, C. S & Lind, A. R. (1964) *Heatstress and Heat Disorders.* London: Cassell.

DISEASES DUE TO PROTOZOA

Malaria; Amoebiasis; Intestinal Flagellates and Ciliates; Giardiasis; Balantidiasis; Leishmaniasis; Trypanosomiasis; Toxoplasmosis

Malaria

Human malaria results from infection by *Plasmodium falciparum*, *P. vivax*, *P. ovale*, *P. malariae* and rarely other species. The infection may be acquired wherever there are human hosts carrying the parasites and a sufficiency of suitable anopheline mosquitoes, together with conditions of temperature and humidity which favour the development of the parasite in the mosquito. Malaria may also be transmitted by transfusion or inoculation of infected blood.

Hippocrates recognised periodic fevers, characteristic of malaria, together with splenomegaly in people who lived near marshes. Romans, attributing the disease to *bad air* arising from marshes, drained them and reduced the incidence of malaria by unwittingly abolishing breeding places of mosquitoes. Some African languages associate mosquitoes, fever and the spleen but it was not until 1880 that Laveran first demonstrated the causative plasmodium. In 1897 Ronald Ross showed that a similar infection in sparrows was transmitted by mosquitoes and shortly afterwards Italian workers demonstrated that human malaria was similarly acquired. The bark of the cinchona tree, from which quinine is derived, was introduced from Peru into Europe in 1632 and was soon adopted by Sydenham for the treatment of malaria, then endemic in Britain. Drainage of the Fen country led to the disappearance of endemic malaria from Britain, except for small outbreaks after each world war.

As the result of WHO sponsored campaigns of prevention and more effective treatment, the incidence of malaria has been greatly reduced, particularly in the Indian subcontinent. The eradication of the disease is, however, not yet in sight and some resurgence of the disease has occurred. As a result of increased travel and neglect of chemoprophylaxis 750 cases were imported into Britain in 1975 of which 174 were due to *P. falciparum* with five recorded fatalities.

Pathogenesis. The female anopheline mosquito becomes infected when it feeds on human blood containing gametocyctes, the sexual forms of the malarial parasite. The further development and multiplication of the parasite is as shown in Fig. 17.1. The development in the mosquito takes from 7–20 days. Sporozoites disappear from human blood within half an hour, but after $6\frac{1}{2}$ days in *P. falciparum* malaria $8\frac{1}{2}$–11 days or occasionally longer for the other species, a greatly enhanced number of parasites, 'merozoites', leave the liver and invade red cells where further cycles of multiplication of parasites take place resulting in the release of merozoites into the plasma in sufficient numbers to produce fever. Each

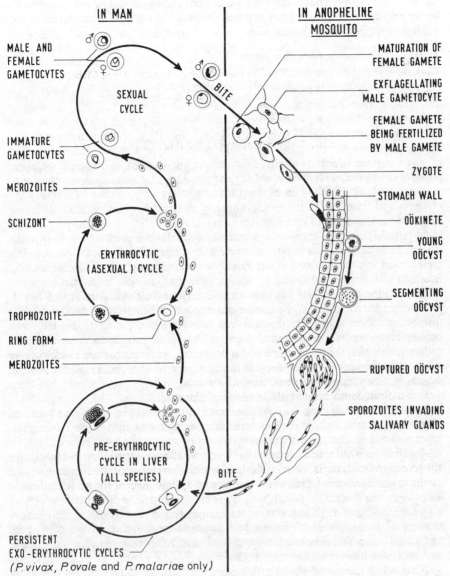

Fig. 17.1 Life cycle of malarial parasites. Adapted from Cruickshank, R. Duguid, J. P. Marmion, B. P. and Swain, R. H. A. (1973) *Medical Microbiology*. Edinburgh: Churchill Livingstone.

cycle in the red cells takes 48 hours in the case of *P. vivax* and *P. ovale* and results in a 'tertian' fever, the temperature rising on alternate days; *P. malariae* takes 72 hours resulting in a 'quartan' fever, while the cycle in *P. falciparum* takes rather less than 48 hours, is less well-synchronised and produces a more constant fever. Most antimalarial drugs are effective chiefly in the asexual cycle in the red cells, hence *P. vivax*, *P. ovale*, and *P. malariae*, by persisting in the liver, may later cause relapses when they leave it and invade red cells. *P. falciparum* has no persistent exo-erythrocytic phase but recrudescences of fever may result from multiplication in the red cells of lingering parasites which have not been eliminated by inadequate treatment and immune processes.

In severe falciparum infections the infected red cells are sequestered in deep capillaries, especially in the brain, kidney and bowel, impairing the function of these organs.

Clinical Features. Malaria is first described as it occurs in the non-immune adult, falciparum malaria (see below) being the most dangerous form. The interval from the time of biting by the infected mosquito to the onset of detectable fever varies but is often about a week or 10 days for *P. falciparum* infections and somewhat longer for the other species. Occasionally an apparent primary attack of vivax malaria occurs months after the patient has left the tropics, and suppressive drugs may delay the onset for as long as a year after stopping the drug.

Vivax malaria. In many cases vivax malaria starts with a period of several days of continued fever before the development of classical bouts of fever on alternate days. The malarial paroxysm has three clinical stages: first a cold stage, followed by a hot stage, which ends in a sweating stage. In the cold stage or rigor the patient feels intensely cold and shivers, and frequently his teeth chatter. The temperature is already elevated and rapidly reaches its height, e.g. 40°C. Vomiting is often troublesome and headache severe. After half an hour or so, the hot stage is reached; the patient feels burning hot and may be delirious. After 1 to 6 hours, profuse perspiration starts, the temperature drops and the patient becomes comfortable and falls asleep. He will feel reasonably well on the next day, but fever subsequently recurs on alternate days. Usually the spleen and, especially in children, the liver become palpable and tender, but the absence of detectable splenic enlargement does not exclude malaria. Herpes simplex, usually round the mouth, is a common accompaniment of malaria.

P. ovale infections are similar to those of *P. vivax*.

P. malariae malaria is usually associated with mild symptoms and bouts of fever every fourth day. With this infection parasitaemia may persist for many years without producing any symptoms.

P. falciparum infections, especially primary attacks, are more insidious and dangerous than other forms of malaria. The fever in this variety is prolonged and irregular and does not usually rise to quite so high a level as in the other forms. Sometimes the patient, although very ill, remains afebrile with a heavy infection. The cold, hot and sweating stages are seldom found, but vomiting and severe headaches occur. A severe haemolytic anaemia develops (p. 820), often with associated haemolytic jaundice. In uncomplicated cases only the ring stage of the parasites and later the gametocytes are found in the peripheral blood, whereas with the other species all stages of the parasites occur in the circulating blood. A patient with falciparum malaria, apparently not seriously ill, may suddenly develop complications which render his condition grave. Children may die rapidly without any special symptoms other than fever. In pregnancy immunity is impaired, a severe macrocytic anaemia commonly develops and abortion from parasitisation of the maternal side of the placenta is frequent. Congenital malaria is rare.

A *mixed infection* with more than one species of malaria parasite may occur, therefore the demonstration of *P. vivax* does not exclude the possibility of a *P. falciparum* infection and vice versa.

Complications of Falciparum Malaria. *Cerebral malaria* is the most urgent complication and is manifested either by the rapid development of coma, usually without localising signs, or by hyperpyrexia or acute mental changes. It is very rare for there to be an increase of cells in the cerebrospinal fluid. Impaired capillary function in the kidneys may produce acute renal failure and in the gastrointestinal tract vomiting or symptoms mimicking dysentery.

Blackwater Fever. This is brought about by a rapid intravascular haemolysis and is invariably associated with a chronic falciparum malaria, most commonly in those who have taken antimalarial treatment irregularly but is uncommon in indigenous races. The haemolysis may be quite unexpected and very extensive, destroying many uninfected as well as parasitised red cells. The attack is not infrequently provoked by administering quinine or by fatigue. The colour of the urine varies from dark red to almost black, depending on the amount of intravascular haemolysis. Acute renal failure may follow.

Relapses. These are characteristic of vivax, ovale and malariae malaria and are due to persistence of the exoerythrocytic form of the parasite in the liver. Immunity eventually overcomes the infection, and relapses seldom occur longer than two years after the patient has left the malarious area.

Endemic Malaria. The manifestations of malaria in unprotected indigenous residents, as the result of immune reactions, show considerable variation according to the degree of endemicity and the age of the patient. In areas of hypoendemicity little immunity is acquired, epidemics of malaria are liable to occur and the disease does not differ materially from that in non-immunes. In mesoendemic areas malaria is frequent but only seasonal. Repeated infections lead to anaemia, considerable enlargement of spleen with the danger of its rupture from a minor blow, and chronic ill-health with bouts of fever. The growth and development of children may be retarded and *P. malariae* infections may cause immune-complex nephritis and the nephrotic syndrome. In hyperendemic areas malaria transmission takes place throughout the year, but with seasonal increases, and adults develop considerable immunity. Although they will have palpable spleens and occasional parasitaemia, malaria causes only occasional short bouts of fever. In holoendemic areas malarial transmission is intense throughout the year and adults do not suffer from the infection, a condition called 'premunity', and enlargement of the spleen does not usually persist but in these areas the tropical splenomegaly syndrome (see below) may be found. In hyperendemic and in holoendemic areas malaria takes a toll of older infants and young children. The regular taking of antimalarial drugs prevents the manifestations of chronic malaria but may impair the development of immunity. Individuals with the sickle-cell trait or deficient in G6PD are relatively resistant to falciparum malaria (p. 823).

Tropical Splenomegaly Syndrome. In some hyperendemic areas gross splenomegaly is associated with an exaggerated immune response to malaria and is seen, unexpectedly, in adults who have high antibody titres to malaria and low parasitaemias. The condition, which is commoner in females and in certain racial and family groups is characterised by enormous overproduction of IgM, levels reaching 3 to 20 times the local mean value. Much of the IgM is aggregated with other immunoglobulin or complement and precipitates in the cold, *in vitro*. The IgM aggregates are phagocytosed by fixed reticuloendothelial cells, in the spleen and the Kupffer cells in the liver, and the demonstration of this by immunofluorescence in a liver biopsy section is diagnostic. Light microscopy of the liver usually shows sinusoidal lymphocytosis. Lymphocytosis of blood and marrow may arise and be confused with leukaemia.

Diagnosis. If a patient is in a malarious locality or has recently left such an area, malaria should be considered. A history of periodic fever, perhaps associated with an enlarged spleen and anaemia, is very suspicious. Well-stained blood films, thick and thin, should be examined and repeated if necessary. *P. falciparum* parasites may be very scanty. Especially in those who have recently taken ineffective doses of an antimalarial drug parasites may be difficult to find.

Treatment. GENERAL. The patient should be put to bed and encouraged to drink fluid freely. Aspirin or paracetamol is useful for the relief of headache. When dehydration is marked and vomiting troublesome, intravenous fluids may be necessary.

SPECIFIC THERAPY. The drugs of choice are the 4-aminoquinolines, chloroquine or amodiaquine. The usual course of treatment is 600 mg of the effective base base (4 tablets) followed by 300 mg base in six hours then 150 mg base twice daily for 3 to 7 more days. In some areas, especially in South-east Asia and Central America, *Plasmodium falciparum* parasites showing some resistance to 4-aminoquinolines may be encountered. If the response to chloroquine is not good, then quinine dihydrochloride 650 mg three times daily for 2 days should be given, followed by a single dose of sulfoxine 1·5 g combined with pyrimethamine 75 mg. To ensure that there will be no relapse in vivax, ovale and malariae malaria other drugs are subsequently required (see below). Proguanil and pyrimethamine alone act too slowly for effective use in the treatment of overt malaria in non-immune subjects. Small doses of antimalarials may be adequate for indigenous residents of endemic areas.

Treatment of Complicated P. falciparum malaria. Patients with 'cerebral malaria' or other severe manifestations are medical emergencies. The immediate intravenous administration of chloroquine or quinine is indicated, the drug being given very slowly to avoid peripheral circulatory failure or acute encephalopathy, taking at least 10 minutes to give the full dose. Quinine is particularly indicated if a chloroquine-resistant infection is at all likely. Ampoules of chloroquine in aqueous solution containing 200 mg in 5 ml are available and 200–300 mg should be given and repeated, if necessary, after 4 to 6 hours. The dose for quinine dihydrochloride is 500 mg, dissolved in at least 10 ml of isotonic saline, and repeated, if necessary, after 12 hours. Severely ill patients may need cautious intravenous saline, and blood transfusions may be required to combat severe anaemia. The results of prompt treatment are very gratifying. Corticosteroids in selected cases may be beneficial but their value has not been fully established. In less fulminating cases intramuscular chloroquine gives excellent results. If in the treatment of a comatose patient return to consciousness is delayed, lumbar puncture is indicated to exclude coexisting bacterial meningitis. Oral treatment should replace parenteral as soon as the patient's condition allows.

The dose of parenteral chloroquine for small children must not exceed 5 mg per kg body weight and intravenous or intramuscular quinine may be safer. Intramuscular quinine is painful and liable to cause tissue necrosis; nevertheless for both children and adults it may be life-saving. Quinine hydrochloride is less irritant than the dihydrochloride.

Treatment of Blackwater Fever. This depends on the amount of blood which has been destroyed. When there has been severe haemolysis leading to a marked degree of anaemia, circulatory and renal failure may ensue and blood transfusion is urgently needed to replace the destroyed red blood cells and to restore the circulation. Corticosteroids are of value in preventing further haemolysis. It is very important that physical and mental rest should be secured; good nursing and sedatives are of great value. Sufficient fluid must be given by mouth, or intravenously if necessary, to ensure a urinary output of more than a litre in 24 hours. Careful records of fluid intake and output must be kept and appropriate treatment should be instituted if features of acute renal failure develop (p. 496). To prevent a recrudescence of falciparum malaria a short course of chloroquine should be administered after the condition has stabilised.

TREATMENT OF TROPICAL SPLENOMEGALY SYNDROME. Splenomegaly and the associated anaemia, which is due to haemodilution and haemolysis, usually resolve over a period of months of continuous treatment with proguanil 100 mg daily, which should be continued for life to prevent relapse. Complicating folate deficiency is treated with folic acid 5 mg daily.

Occasionally splenectomy may be indicated because splenomegaly persists and causes mechanical difficulties, because of hypersplenism (p. 625) or because of dilutional anaemia (p. 820). However, splenectomy in such patients may be associated with greatly increased susceptibility to malarial infection thereafter, if lifelong prophylaxis is not included in their treatment.

It must be remembered that the tropical splenomegaly syndrome may complicate splenic enlargement associated with other disorders, such as chronic lymphatic leukaemia, and that treatment must be directed at all the conditions present.

RADICAL CURE OF MALARIA DUE TO *P. vivax*, *P. malariae* and *P. ovale*. While relapses can usually be prevented by taking one of the antimalarial drugs in suppressive doses over a period of months, radical cure can be ensured only by a course of one of the 8-aminoquinolines, which destroy these parasites in their exoerythrocytic phase in the liver, together with or following a course of chloroquine or amodiaquine. Primaquine is probably the least toxic of the 8-aminoquinolines; each tablet contains 7·5 mg of base; a course of two or three such tablets taken daily for 14 days produces a high percentage of cures. The patient must, however, be under medical supervision for this period as haemolysis may develop. This is relatively frequent in Negroes, affecting those whose erythrocytes are deficient in glucose-6-phosphate dehydrogenase. Cyanosis due to the formation of methaemoglobin in the red cells is frequent but not dangerous. Relapses after leaving endemic areas can be prevented by an alternative regime of 10 weekly doses of chloroquine, 300 mg base, with primaquine, 45 mg base (six tablets). Mild diarrhoea on the days of treatment is usually the only side-effect.

Causal Prophylaxis and Suppression. So far no drug is known which will destroy the sporozoites injected by the mosquito. Clinical attacks of malaria can, however, be prevented by drugs which attack the pre-erythrocytic form ('causal prophylaxis'), or by drugs which act on the parasite after it has entered the erythrocyte ('suppression'). Both proguanil and pyrimethamine destroy the pre-erythrocytic stage of *P. falciparum*; they also act on the asexual erythrocytic forms of all species of human malaria parasites. Consequently they give reliable protection against clinical attacks of malaria if started on entering a malarious region. These two drugs also inhibit further development of the falciparum gametocytes in the mosquito. The adult dose of pyrimethamine is one tablet (25 mg) once a week; for a child up to 6 years $\frac{1}{4}$ tablet (6·25 mg) and from 6 to 12 years $\frac{1}{2}$ tablet (12·5 mg) weekly is adequate. It has an attractive flavour, and some children who have obtained access to the drug have died from an overdose. The suppressive dose of proguanil for adults is 1 or 2 tablets (each containing 100 mg) daily; children aged 1 to 5 years require $\frac{1}{2}$ tablet and under 1 year $\frac{1}{4}$ tablet. Proguanil is a valuable drug for preventing clinical attacks of malaria as it is almost free from side-effects. In addition, since it is taken daily, the routine is unlikely to be forgotten.

Local strains of *P. falciparum* resistant to these two drugs are occasionally encountered; the higher dose of proguanil, namely 2 tablets may then be effective, or chloroquine prophylaxis can be substituted in an adult dose of 300 mg base weekly. Children aged 6 to 12 years require 150 mg and under 6 years 75 mg base weekly. Occasional toxic side-effects include slight visual disturbance. Pyrimethamine 75 mg with sulfadoxine 1·5 mg once weekly should be used where chloroquine resistance is prevalent.

Prophylactic drugs are ineffective unless taken in the required dose with the utmost regularity. These drugs should be begun on the day of arrival in a malarious area and to ensure eradication of *P. falciparum* infection should be continued for four weeks after departure.

Prevention. Control of anopheline mosquitoes especially by the spraying of houses with an insecticide such as DDT has greatly reduced or abolished the risk of malaria in many areas. However, unless eradication is complete, all visitors and non-immune residents should take regular prophylactic or suppressive drugs as detailed above. Sleeping at night under a mosquito net or in a wire-screened and sprayed house, will give freedom from the nuisance of those mosquitoes which bite only in the dark and may also reduce the likelihood of acquiring some mosquito-borne viral infections.

Further reading about malaria:

Hall, A. P. (1976) The treatment of malaria. *British Medical Journal,* 1, 323.
Maegraith, B. G. (1974) Malaria. In *Medicine in the Tropics,* ed. Woodruff, A. W. Ch. 2, pp. 27–73. Edinburgh: Churchill Livingstone.

Amoebiasis

Amoebiasis is due to infection by *Entamoeba histolytica*. This potentially pathogenic amoeba is propagated between humans by its cysts, 10 microns or more in diameter. Another amoeba, *E. hartmanii*, is non-pathogenic, as is *E. coli* which is also harboured at times in the human intestine. The association of amoebae with dysentery was first recorded by Lambl in 1859. Liver abscesses were well known to Hippocrates and their association with dysentery was noticed by Galen, stressed by Annesley in India in 1828 and confirmed by the finding of amoebae in them by Koch in 1883. Leonard Rogers in 1912 showed that injections of emetine hydrochloride were effective in both intestinal and hepatic amoebiasis.

Pathogenesis. Cysts of *E. histolytica* survive well outside the body and are ingested in water or uncooked food which has been contaminated by human faeces. In endemic areas lettuce is a common vehicle of infection. The disease is rarely acquired in Britain. In the colon the vegetative forms, 'trophozoites', emerge from the cysts. While they remain free in the colon the condition is symptomless but under certain circumstances invasion and ulceration of the mucous membrane of the large bowel takes place causing the symptoms of amoebic dysentery. The lesions are usually maximal in the caecum. They may, however, be found as far down as the anal canal. Tiny elevations are produced in the mucosa. These soon break down, producing flask-shaped ulcers varying greatly in size and surrounded by healthy mucosa. Amoebae may find their way into a vein and be carried to the liver where they multiply and cause hepatocellular necrosis ('amoebic abscess'). The liquid contents at first have a characteristic pinkish colour which later may change to chocolate brown and finally to yellow or green. Amoebic ulcers only rarely penetrate through the muscular coat of the colon. A large vessel may sometimes be eroded, and severe intestinal haemorrhage result. A localised granuloma, 'amoeboma', presenting as a palpable local thickening of the bowel wall and causing a filling defect on radiography, is a rare complication. It responds well to antiamoebic treatment; it is therefore important that it should not be mistaken for a carcinoma. Cysts may continue to be passed in the faeces when the disease is inactive.

Clinical Features. The incubation period varies from 2 weeks to many years, but is usually several months after the first possible exposure to infection. *Intestinal amoebiasis,* or *amoebic dysentery* usually runs a chronic course with grumbling pains in the abdomen and two or more rather loose stools a day. Periods of diarrhoea alternating with constipation are a frequent feature. Mucus is usually passed, sometimes with streaks of blood, and the motions often have a very offensive odour. On palpation of the abdomen there may be tenderness along the line of the colon, usually more marked over the caecum and pelvic colon. The right iliac pain may simulate acute appendicitis, and if an operation is performed the amoebae may cause ulceration of the wound and surrounding tissue. Perforation, when it occurs, is usually in the region of the caecum. Particularly in the aged, in the puerperium and with superadded pyogenic infection of the ulcers there may be more acute bowel symptoms, with very frequent motions and the passage of considerable quantities of blood and mucus, thus simulating bacillary dysentery. Bacillary and amoebic dysentery may occur together, the bacillary infection probably lighting up latent amoebiasis.

Hepatic amoebiasis is a common complication of the bowel infection, and the possibility of this condition must always be remembered in anyone who has lived in the tropics or subtropics. Early symptoms may be local discomfort only and malaise; later a swinging temperature, sweating and an enlarged tender liver and pain in the right shoulder are characteristic, but symptoms may remain vague and signs minimal. In particular, the less common abscess in the left lobe may not be diagnosed. There is usually a neutrophil leucocytosis and a raised diaphragm with diminished movement on the right side may be demonstrated radiographically. When hepatic amoebiasis is diagnosed early, before appreciable abscess formation, the response to emetine, metronidazole or chloroquine is very rapid. A large abscess may penetrate the diaphragm and rupture into the lung from where its contents may be coughed up. Rupture into the pleural cavity, the peritoneal cavity or pericardial sac is less common but more serious and necessitates aspiration or drainage.

Diagnosis. The signs and symptoms of intestinal amoebiasis are often vague. A careful naked-eye examination of a freshly passed motion should be made. If mucus is found, a small piece should be selected and examined at once under the microscope. It should be kept at body temperature so that the *E. histolytica* may retain its motility. Such active amoebae are readily recognised; they are about 30 microns in diameter, with a clear ectoplasm and a granular endoplasm, and usually contain red blood cells. Pseudopodia containing clear ectoplasm are protruded and retracted. Movements cease very soon if conditions are not favourable. Macrophages seen microscopically in the stool of patients with bacillary dysentery are sometimes mistaken for amoebae. Sigmoidoscopy may reveal typical ulcers. A scraping from one of these should be examined for *E. histolytica*. Ulcers may, however, be present in the bowel only above the reach of the sigmoidoscope and so escape detection. In chronic amoebiasis a number of stools may need to be examined before cysts are found.

An amoebic abscess of the liver is suspected from the clinical and radiographic appearances described above. If the site of an hepatic abscess is not obvious clinically, radioisotope or ultrasonic scanning may be employed to demonstrate it. The fluid from an amoebic abscess of the liver usually has a characteristic appearance but only rarely contains free amoebae.

Serological tests are becoming increasingly available. The combined results of an indirect immunofluorescent antibody test and a gel diffusion precipitin test are highly accurate in supporting the diagnosis of hepatic amoebiasis and slightly less so in invasive intestinal amoebiasis.

Treatment. The symptoms of active intestinal amoebiasis are quickly controlled in all but the most severe cases by oral metronidazole, 800 mg three times daily for 5 days, or emetine hydrochloride 60 mg daily, subcutaneously for a few days. To make a radical cure more likely diloxanide furoate 500 mg should then be given orally for 7 to 10 days. Four weeks after the course the patient should report for test of cure.

Early hepatic amoebiasis responds quickly to treatment by parenteral emetine, oral chloroquine or metronidazole, a therapeutic response confirming the diagnosis. A standard course of treatment consists of subcutaneous injections of emetine hydrochloride 60 mg daily for 4 days, followed by chloroquine, 300 mg base, twice daily for 2 days followed by half this dose for 14 days. After treating the hepatic infection eradication of amoebae from the bowel is required (see above). In areas of high endemicity very satisfactory results have been obtained, even after recognisable abscesses have formed, by massive doses (2·4 g) of metronidazole on two successive days and subsequent additional oral amoebicides may not be necessary. If the liver contains an abscess causing a persistent local swelling or continued fever, aspiration, repeated if necessary, or surgical drainage is required in addition to the chemotherapy. If culture of the 'pus' indicates that there is secondary bacterial infection, treatment will be required with an appropriate antibiotic.

Prevention. Personal precautions against contracting amoebiasis in the tropics and subtropics consist of not eating fresh uncooked vegetables or drinking unboiled water.

Further reading about amoebiasis:

Stamm, W. P. (1976) Amoebiasis: a neglected diagnosis. *Journal of the Royal College of Physicians of London*, **10**, 294–298.

Intestinal Flagellates and Ciliates

The only pathogenic intestinal protozoa of importance other than *Entamoeba histolytica* are the flagellate, *Giardia intestinalis*, and the ciliate, *Balantidium coli*. When the infections are active the vegetative forms are recognised on microscopic examination of the stools, or the cyst form of *G. intestinalis* during an inactive phase. Giardia may also be found on examination of jejunal juice or mucus.

Giardiasis

This infection is worldwide but commoner in the tropics. It particularly affects children in endemic areas, tourists and inmates of mental hospitals. The flagellates attach to the mucosa of the duodenum and jejunum and cause inflammation or partial villous atrophy. Recurrent attacks of urgent diarrhoea with abdominal discomfort and explosive loose pale stools are characteristic. There may be evidence of malabsorption. Lethargy, flatulence, abdominal distension, duodenal pain and nausea are frequent; vomiting may occur. Metronidazole 2 g as a single dose is given daily, after breakfast, for 3 days and the course should be repeated 1 week later. Patients should be warned not to drink alcohol nor drive a car or operate dangerous machinery while taking the drug. Children under 4 years are given one-quarter of the adult dose, from 4 to 8 years half the adult dose, preferably in a palatable suspension.

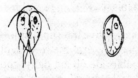

Fig. 17.2 *Giardia intestinalis*. Vegetative and cystic forms.

Balantidiasis

Balantidium coli affects pigs and occasionally man, in all countries, among those who attend pigs. This ciliate may cause local or extensive ulceration of the mucosa of the colon but often lives free in the lumen. Thus the infection may be symptom-free or frequent stools containing blood and mucus may be passed.

Therapeutic success may be obtained from tetracycline 500 mg four times daily for 10 days with the addition of ascorbic acid. Metronidazole, 1 g daily for 5 days, may be used but it is claimed that better results are achieved by nimorazole (Naxogin) 500 mg daily for 5 days.

Leishmaniasis

This group of diseases is caused by protozoa of the genus *Leishmania*, conveyed to man by female sandflies in which the flagellate (promastigote) forms of leishmania develop. The genus is named after William Leishman who in 1902 identified the parasite in the spleen of a soldier from Calcutta. In man the leishmaniae are found in reticuloendothelial cells in oval forms known as amastigotes or Leishman-Donovan bodies (Fig. 17.3). Leishmaniasis may take the form of a generalised visceral infection, kala azar, or of a purely cutaneous infection, known in the Old World as oriental sore. In South America cutaneous leishmaniasis may remain confined to the skin or metastasise to the nose and mouth.

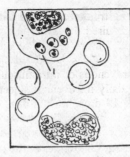

Fig. 17.3 [1]Amastigotes (Leishman-Donovan bodies) seen in smear from bone marrow, spleen or skin.

Visceral Leishmaniasis

(*Kala Azar*)

Kala azar is caused by *Leishmania donovani* and is prevalent in the Mediterranean and Red Sea littorals, Sudan, parts of East Africa, Asia Minor, mountainous regions of Southern Arabia, eastern parts of India, China and South America. In India, where the disease is epidemic, man appears to be the chief host but in many areas, including the Mediterranean area, dogs and foxes are the main reservoirs of infection. Here the disease is endemic and occurs chiefly in childhood or in tourists. In Africa various wild rodents provide the reservoir. Transmission, normally by sandflies, has also been reported to follow transfusion of infected blood.

Pathology. Multiplication, by simple fission, of leishmaniae takes place in reticulo-endothelial cells in various organs, especially the liver and spleen, which becomes greatly enlarged, and in the bone marrow. There is usually a marked progressive granulocytopenia, the leucocyte count falling below $2 \cdot 0 \times 10^9/l$, and a slowly progressive anaemia. There is a great increase of gamma globulin which is mainly IgG. Successful chemotherapy reverses these changes; only rarely does appreciable fibrosis of the liver follow.

Clinical Features. The incubation period is usually about 1 or 2 months but up to 10 years has been recorded. The onset is usually insidious with a low grade fever, the patient remaining ambulant, or it may be abrupt with sweating and high intermittent fever, sometimes showing a double rise of temperature in the 24 hours. The spleen soon becomes enlarged, often massively. Hepatomegaly is less marked. If not treated, the patient will become anaemic and wasted, frequently with increased pigmentation especially on the face. Lymphadenopathy is common and rarely is the only abnormality. After recovery dermal leishmaniasis sometimes develops. It may present first as hypopigmented or erythematous macules on any part of the body and later a nodular eruption may appear, especially on the face. In macular lesions intracellular amastigotes are scanty; in nodules they are more abundant.

Diagnosis. This is established by demonstrating the parasite in stained smears of aspirates of bone marrow, lymph node, spleen or liver, or by culture of these aspirates. Antibody is detected by immunofluorescence or complement-fixation early in the disease. The leishmanin skin test is negative.

Treatment. The response to treatment varies with the geographical area in which the disease has been acquired. In Asia the disease is readily cured, but in the Sudan and East Africa it is more resistant. Sodium stibogluconate, a pentavalent antimony compound, gives good results. A solution containing 100 mg/ml is available for intravenous or intramuscular use. A suitable course of treatment for an adult is 10 daily intravenous injections of 600 mg repeated, if necessary, after an interval of 14 days up to a total dosage of 12 or even 18 g.

The diamidine compounds, pentamidine isethionate employed as in trypanosomiasis (p. 851) and 2-hydroxystilbamidine isethionate, have been found useful in some areas where the disease is resistant to treatment with antimony compounds. The dose of 2-hydroxystilbamidine for an adult is 250 mg intravenously daily for 10 days; the course may be repeated after an interval of 14 days up to a total of 7·5 g given over a period of 2 months. Side-effects such as fever, rigors and headache are not uncommon with this treatment but can be relieved by giving 10 mg of mepyramine maleate three times a day during the course. Amphotericin B (p. 920) is also effective.

The results produced in each case must be assessed by careful observation of physical and laboratory findings, and treatment repeated as required. For the treatment of post-kala azar dermal leishmaniasis the same drugs are used as for visceral leishmaniasis but the response is slower, and intermittent treatment for months may be needed.

Prevention. In an endemic area where they are the reservoir infected or stray dogs should be destroyed. Sandflies should be combated (p. 881). Early diagnosis and treatment of human infections reduces the reservoir and controls epidemic kala azar.

Cutaneous Leishmaniasis of the Old World

(*Oriental Sore*)

Cutaneous leishmaniasis, which is caused by *Leishmania tropica* is a widespread zoonosis in the tropics and subtropics. It is conveyed from many different animals to man by sandflies.

Pathology. On inoculation the parasites are taken up by dermal histiocytes in which they multiply and around which lymphocytes and plasma cells accumulate. With time, the histology becomes more tuberculoid and the overlying epidermis crusts and may ulcerate centrally. Healing is accompanied by subepidermal fibrosis.

Clinical Features. The incubation period is from 2 weeks to 5 or more years but usually is from 2 to 3 months. Lesions, single or multiple on exposed parts of the body, start as small red papules which increase in size and over which a crust may form. Tiny satellite papules are characteristic. Untreated the lesions will heal or will progress to form a rounded ulcer with well-defined indurated raised margins and a granulomatous base. Such a lesion may be up to 10 cm or more in diameter. A seropurulent discharge exudes which may dry and form an adherent scab. Pain is not a feature and general symptoms are usually absent. Sometimes, instead of an ulcer, a fungating nodular mass develops. Occasionally leishmaniae spread from the sore and give rise to nodules in the course of the lymphatics with enlargement of the related nodes. Untreated the ulcer lasts about a year. Healing produces a thin depressed, mottled scar. Cutaneous leishmaniasis may occur in a persistent relapsing form (leishmaniasis recidivans) having a histology indistinguishable from that of cutaneous tuberculosis.

Diffuse cutaneous leishmaniasis occurring in Ethiopia and Venezuela is probably attributable to a defective host reaction to the parasite. The initial papule spreads locally and blood borne cutaneous lesions, which do not ulcerate, are widespread. The lesions contain numerous amastigotes within macrophages.

Diagnosis. The appearance of a typical lesion in a patient from an endemic area suggests the diagnosis. Leishman-Donovan bodies can be demonstrated by inserting a dry needle into the margin of the ulcer, curetting the edge or making a skin slit smear (p. 859) and staining the material obtained with Giemsa's stain or culturing it. The Leishmanin skin (p. 849) is positive except in diffuse cutaneous leishmaniasis. Serology is negative.

Treatment. In the event of secondary infection the crust should be removed by the application of moist dressings and the exposed surface then kept clean. In addition it may be necessary to administer an antibiotic orally. The local application of heat with infra-red rays or hot water may accelerate healing.

Unipolar coagulation diathermy has replaced earlier methods of inducing an inflammatory reaction to expedite cure.

When the lesions are multiple or in a disfiguring site it is better to treat the patient by parenteral injections of pentavalent antimony compounds such as sodium stibogluconate as prescribed for visceral leishmaniasis (p. 847). Some lesions are relatively resistant and require prolonged antimony therapy.

Diffuse cutaneous leishmaniasis responds to antimonials in Venezuela but not in Ethiopia and tends to relapse. Cure can usually be achieved by a prolonged course of amphotericin B (p. 920) or of pentamidine isethionate (p. 851) given once or twice weekly to minimise toxicity; weekly tests of the blood glucose are required to detect the early signs of drug-induced diabetes.

Prevention. In addition to those prophylactic measures described under visceral leishmaniasis against animals and sandflies, a lasting immunity can be achieved by deliberate inoculation of a living culture of *L. tropica*. This produces an ulcer, but the site chosen for the inoculation is one normally covered by clothing so scarring does not cause undesirable disfigurement. This procedure does not protect against visceral leishmaniasis for which no effective vaccine has been prepared.

Cutaneous Leishmaniasis of the New World

In South and Central America leishmaniasis is caused by *L. braziliensis*, *L. mexicana* and *L. peruviana*. They occur in hot, moist, forest regions and are conveyed to man from a variety of animals by several species of sandflies. The disease can be separated into three types. There is the 'espundia' of Brazil caused by *L. braziliensis*. Secondly there is the 'chicleros ulcer' or 'bay sore' attributable to *L. mexicana* found in Mexico, Guatemala and Honduras among gatherers of chicle, used for making chewing gum. The third variety is the disease occurring in the Peruvian Andes, known as 'uta' and caused by *L. peruviana*.

The infections are endemic in Central America, parts of Mexico and the north of South America.

Pathology. The microscopic appearances of the skin lesions may be similar to oriental sore but are not always characteristic. The mucocutaneous lesions begin as a perivascular infiltration; later endarteritis may lead to destruction of the surrounding tissues (see below).

Clinical Features. In the classical espundia of Brazil and surrounding regions the initial papulopustular cutaneous lesions may be single or multiple and affect especially the face, ears, elbows and knees. Mucosal lesions either accompany the skin lesions or appear some years later. The nasal mucosa becomes congested and later all tissues of the nose ulcerate except for the bone. The lips, soft palate and fauces may be invaded and destroyed leading to terrible suffering and deformity. Secondary bacterial infection is a common aggravating factor. The other New World lesions are self-healing and do not metastasise.

Chicleros ulcer affects the ears and may last many years, eroding the pinna. The lesions of uta are often multiple and papillomatous rather than ulcerative.

Diagnosis. This depends on the history and clinical appearance, confirmed by demonstration of the protozoon in smears, culture or histological section. As parasites are not easily found the Leishmanin test is of value. In this an antigen prepared from a culture of leishmaniae is used and 0·1 ml of this is injected intradermally. A positive case will show erythema and induration at the site of the injection after 48 hours. Not all cases of espundia give a positive reaction.

Treatment. Purely cutaneous disease may be successfully treated by sodium stibogluconate given as recommended for visceral leishmaniasis (p. 847) but in established espundia amphotericin B (p. 920) may be necessary.

African Trypanosomiasis

(Sleeping Sickness)

African sleeping sickness is caused by trypanosomes conveyed to man by the bites of infected tsetse flies of either sex. The disease is acquired only in Africa between 12° N and 25° S. There are two trypanosomes which affect man, *Trypanosoma* (*Trypanozoon*) *brucei gambiense* conveyed by *Glossina palpalis* and *G. tachinoides* and *T.(T.)b. rhodesiense* transmitted by *G. morsitans*, *G. pallidipes*, *G. swynnertoni* and also *G. palpalis*. Gambiense trypanosomiasis has a wide distribution in West and Central Africa reaching to Uganda and Kenya; rhodesiense trypanosomiasis is found in parts of East and Central Africa. *G. palpalis* is found only on or near the shady banks of lakes and streams; *G. tachinoides* travels farther afield. *G. swynnertoni* is limited to Tanzania and, in common with other vectors of rhodesiense sleeping sickness, flies across open country covered with scrub. In these areas wild animals are found commonly to be affected by other species of trypanosomes, notably *T.* (*T.*)*b. brucei*. These trypanosomes thus affect man indirectly by reducing greatly the grazing areas on which cattle can survive, thereby reducing supplies of milk and meat, prime requirements for the prevention of protein malnutrition. *T.(T.)b. brucei* has not been distinguished morphologically or antigenically from *T.(T.)b. rhodesiense* but only the latter is pathogenic for man. On epidemiological grounds it appears that there is undoubtedly a reservoir of infection of *T.*(*T.*)*b. rhodesiense* in wild animals and, at times, in cattle. Experimental transmission of *T.*(*T.*)*b. rhodesiense* to man from a bushbuck has been achieved but this does not establish that this animal is the most important reservoir host. There is also evidence that at times *T.*(*T.*)*b. gambiense* may be harboured by cattle.

Pathological and Clinical Features. Even during an epidemic of try-panosomiasis, only a low percentage of tsetse flies are infected. A bite by a tsetse fly is frequently painful but, if trypanosomes are introduced, the site of the bite may again become painful and swollen about 10 days later. The lesion is sometimes described as a 'trypanosomal chancre'. Trypanosomes can be recovered from it. Within 2 to 3 weeks of infection the trypanosomes invade the blood stream. In gambiense infections the disease usually runs a slow course with irregular bouts of fever and enlargement of lymph nodes. These are characteristically firm, discrete, rubbery and painless and are particularly prominent in the posterior triangle of the neck. Sometimes during these early weeks transient circinate erythematous eruptions can be seen, particularly on the front or back of the chest and especially if the patient has a white skin. Bouts of fever lasting a week or more recur over a period of months and tachycardia persists in the apyrexial intervals. The spleen and liver may become palpable. Varying degrees of chronicity may be encountered and signs and symptoms may be few. After some months, in the absence of treatment, the central nervous system is invaded. This is shown clinically by headaches and changed behaviour, insomnia by night and sleepiness by day, mental confusion and eventually tremors, pareses, wasting from inanition, coma and death. The earliest proof of invasion of the nervous system is an increase of protein and cells in the cerebrospinal fluid. The histological changes in the brain are similar to those found in viral encephalitis but trypanosomes are scattered in the substance of the brain and large mononuclear (morula) cells are a feature. The cytoplasm of these cells is eosinophilic and contains globules of IgM; the nucleus is oval, eccentric and deeply stained.

In rhodesiense infections enlargement of the lymph nodes is not a prominent feature. Fever is higher and more constant than in gambiense infections, so that within a few weeks the patient is usually severely ill and may have developed pleural effusions and signs of myocarditis or hepatitis. The clinical manifestations of involvement of the nervous system may not be obvious but within a few weeks of infection the cerebrospinal fluid will be abnormal and in the untreated case death ensues from toxaemia or heart failure. If the illness is less acute, drowsiness, tremors, and coma may be prominent.

Diagnosis. In any febrile patient from an endemic area trypanosomiasis should be considered. In rhodesiense infections the trypanosomes can often be detected by microscopic examination of a wet blood film. Agitation of red cells by the trypanosomes is seen and staining of thick and thin blood films, as for the detection of malaria, will reveal trypanosomes (Fig. 17.4). Where necessary concentration methods, e.g. with centrifuged citrated specimens of blood, should be used. In the earliest stages of gambiense infections the trypanosomes may be seen in the blood or from puncture of the primary lesion but it is usually easier to demonstrate them by puncture of a lymph node. Using a medium sized dry needle, the node, held between finger and thumb, is punctured and the node moved on the needle and the material aspirated and examined in a similar way to the blood. Animal inoculation and culture

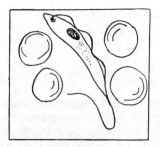

Fig. 17.4 Trypanosome in blood film.

on a special medium can also be employed. A complement-fixation test has been used to detect relapses of *T.(T.)b.gambiense* infections. In the cerebrospinal fluid trypanosomes are best found after centrifugation in glucose-phosphate buffer. The cell count and protein content, are increased and the glucose diminished if the central nervous system is affected. Except in cases with undoubted established neurological abnormalities, lumbar puncture should be deferred until the first dose of a trypanocidal drug has been given. This will reduce the risk of implantation of trypanosomes into the cerebrospinal fluid, by the lumbar puncture needle. Very high levels of serum IgM or the presence of IgM in the cerebrospinal fluid are suggestive of trypanosomiasis.

Treatment. If treatment is begun early, before the brain has been invaded, it will be curative. For this purpose either suramin, diminazene aceturate (Berenil) or pentamidine isethionate may be used, the last named being employed only for gambiense infections. After the nervous system is affected an arsenical, e.g. melarsoprol, will be required as it alone penetrates into the brain.

Suramin, is usually given intravenously. An initial trial dose of 200 mg is given to test for sensitivity. This is followed on the next day by 1 g dissolved in 10 ml of distilled water repeated at intervals of 3 to 5 days to a total dosage of 5 to 10 g. Children are given proportionate doses. Toxic effects include dermatitis, nausea, vomiting, peripheral neuritis and nephritis. The urine should be examined before each injection and the drug discontinued if red cells and casts appear.

Pentamidine isethionate is less toxic than suramin. It is rather painful when administered intramuscularly but, as there may be sudden collapse from a rapid fall in blood pressure when the drug is used intravenously, this route is not recommended. The intramuscular dose is 3 to 5 mg/kg body weight to a maximum of 250 mg dissolved in 5 ml distilled water, on alternate days for 10 injections.

Berenil. Good results have been obtained in early cases by giving three doses, each 5 mg/kg body weight, intramuscularly at intervals of 2 days.

Melarsoprol is a chemical combination of the trivalent melarsan oxide and dimercaprol. It is presented as a 3·6 per cent w/v solution in glycolpropylene and is administered intravenously. Although a toxic drug, it has proved highly efficacious in advanced rhodesiense infections, which were formerly fatal, and for other resistant and relapsing cases. The main danger is encephalopathy due to a Jarisch-Herxheimer reaction following the death of many trypanosomes. Before commencing treatment with melarsoprol the patient's general condition may be benefited by a few preliminary injections of suramin or Berenil. The initial dose of melarsoprol is assessed on the patient's general condition rather than on his weight. Patients who are severely ill may at first only tolerate as small a dose as 0·5 ml and the initial dose must never exceed 2 ml. Further injections are given on the second and third days. The maximum dose is 3·6 mg/kg body weight, i.e. 5 ml for a man of 50 kg. There then follows a rest period of 1 to 2 weeks followed by a second series of three injections. If the initial dose was very small, additional courses may be required during the next 4 or 5 weeks. The total dosage aimed at is 30 ml. Melarsoprol should only be given under strict medical supervision.

Melarsonyl potassium is a water-soluble derivative of melarsoprol suitable for intramuscular injection. It is less toxic than melarsoprol. The daily dose is 4 mg/kg body weight administered as follows. As a test for sensitivity a half dose is given, followed by three successive full daily doses. For intermediate and late cases, after an interval of 7 to 10 days a further four daily doses are given. Good results have been obtained in gambiense trypanosomiasis. It is not a fully reliable drug for rhodesiense infections.

Nitrofurazone is liable to produce undesirable side-effects including haemolytic anaemia in those whose red cells are deficient in G6PD but is occasionally successful. It should be used only when all other drugs have failed. The adult dose is 500 mg orally three times daily for 10 days.

Prevention. Against *T.(T.)b. gambiense* a single intramuscular injection of 250 mg pentamidine gives protection for six months because of the slow excretion of the drug. As the protection against *T.(T.)b. rhodesiense* is less sure and shorter in duration, chemoprophylaxis is not advised in rhodesiense areas as the infection may be masked until a late stage is reached. In such areas it is safer to have no protection but to ensure early recognition of the 'trypanosomal chancre' and to have the blood examined at monthly intervals or whenever there is any fever. Prompt treatment will then be curative.

American Trypanosomiasis

(*Chagas' Disease*)

The cause of Chagas' disease is *Trypanosoma cruzi* transmitted to man from the faeces of a reduviid bug in which the trypanosomes have a cycle of development before becoming infective to man. The bugs are liable to fly down from the ceilings of primitive houses on to the faces of those sleeping below. Infected faeces from the bug are rubbed in through the conjunctiva, mucosa of mouth or nose or through an abrasion of the skin. Dogs and cats are the most important hosts in nature although many wild and domestic animals may harbour the infection. Acute illness has also followed transfusion of infected blood.

The trypanosomes travel by the blood stream and develop into amastigote forms in the tissues. These multiply in the myocardium causing pseudocysts in the muscle fibres and also in the nervous system, giving rise to the changes described below. Chagas' disease occurs widely in South and Central America.

Clinical Features. The entrance of *T. cruzi* through an abrasion produces a dusky-red firm swelling with enlargement of regional lymph nodes. A conjunctival lesion is more characteristic; the unilateral firm reddish swelling of the lids may close the eye and constitutes 'Romana's sign'. Young children are most commonly affected. Evidence of a generalised infection soon appears, with the temperature rising to 40°C and lasting for 2 weeks or more. There may be generalised lymphadenopathy and enlargement of the spleen and liver. Neurological features include insomnia, personality changes and signs of meningo-encephalitis. Chronic infections frequently damage Auerbach's plexus with resulting dilatation of various parts of the alimentary canal, especially the colon and oesophagus. Dilatation of the bile ducts and bronchi are also recognised sequelae. Invasion of the myocardium causes a cardiomyopathy (p. 229) as indicated by cardiac dilation, arrhythmias and partial or complete heart block. Tachycardia may persist for months.

Only infants die readily from the acute infection, death being caused in the first few days of the illness by encephalitis or a few weeks later by myocarditis or overwhelming infection. In those who survive the acute phase the trypanosomes often persist, causing a chronic illness from which the patient recovers slowly. Chronic infections are difficult to diagnose because there may be no apparent site of entry and there may have been no acute phase. Chagas' disease is being increasingly recognised, in endemic areas, as a cause of cardiomyopathy, responsible, on occasion, for sudden death particularly in adult males during exercise.

Diagnosis. A history of residence in an endemic area with suggestive symptoms indicates the need for a search for *T. cruzi* in the blood or for the amastigote forms in other tissues. Trypanosomes are often scanty in the blood but may be recovered by culture or xenodiagnosis. In the latter method infection-free, laboratory-bred, reduviid bugs are fed on the patient and subsequently the hind gut or faeces of the bug are examined for parasites. Complement-fixation and fluorescent antibody tests have also been used in diagnosis. In acute cases a positive result can be expected but in chronic infections the results are less reliable.

Treatment and Prevention. Nifurtimox, a nitrofurantoin, given orally, is proving successful in treatment. The dosage, which has to be carefully supervised to minimise toxicity while preserving parasiticidal activity, is: under 10 years, 15–20 mg/kg body weight; 10–17 years, 12·5–15 mg/kg for 90 days; over 17 years, 8–10 mg/kg for 120 days. Cure rates of 80 per cent in acute disease and 90 per cent in chronic disease are claimed. Temporary side-effects include anorexia, nausea, vomiting and epigastric pain; insomnia, headache, vertigo and excitability; myalgia and arthralgia.

Preventive measures should include improved housing and destruction of reduviid bugs by spraying of houses with lindane (gamma BHC).

Toxoplasmosis

Toxoplasmosis is caused by *Toxoplasma gondii*, a small protozoon. It is probable that human infection after birth results from the ingestion of cysts excreted in the faeces of infected cats. Transmission from mother to foetus causes congenital toxoplasmosis. Human toxoplasmosis is worldwide.

Pathology. In the congenital form the organism is widespread in the central nervous system, eyes, heart, lungs and adrenals. If the infant survives, the parasite soon disappears from most organs except the central nervous system and retina. The brain shows large areas of necrosis with cyst formation and patchy calcification; the spinal cord may be similarly affected. In the acquired disease the organism commonly invades lymph nodes and spleen and less commonly liver and myocardium.

Clinical Features. The manifestations in congenital infections are mainly cerebral. There may be hydrocephalus or microcephaly associated with convulsions, tremors or paralysis with resultant contractures. Radiological examination may show patches of calcification in the brain. Microphthalmos, nystagmus and chorioretinitis are common. The cerebrospinal fluid is often xanthochromic with increased protein and mononuclear cells. An enlarged liver, jaundice, diminished thrombocytes and purpura may also be found. Congenital infections are usually fatal, and if the child survives he is usually gravely incapacitated.

In acquired infections symptoms are more variable. Many are symptomless. In the acute form there may be pneumonitis with fever, cough, generalised aches and pains, profound malaise, inconstantly a maculopapular rash and rarely jaundice and myocarditis. In the more chronic infections, often afebrile, there may be only enlargement of the lymph nodes with a lymphocytosis showing atypical mononuclear cells similar to those present in infectious mononucleosis. Toxoplasmosis is recognised as a cause of chorioretinitis and uveitis in adults.

Diagnosis. In congenital toxoplasmosis the neurological signs and symptoms suggest the diagnosis. The mothers from whom the infection is transmitted have symptomless infections. Serological tests are of value. Antibodies detectable by fluorescence or the dye test appear early in the disease and persist for years. Complement fixing antibodies are late to appear and decline more quickly. A rise in titre indicates active infection. Antibodies may not be detectable in adult ocular toxoplasmosis. Biopsy material from a lymph node may yield the *Toxoplasma* on culture or by inoculation of a laboratory animal, or show characteristic histological changes.

Treatment. A combination of a sulphonamide 1 g 6-hourly and pyrimethamine 25 mg daily for 2 weeks should be administered in all active cases. If the infection is symptom-free, and there is no possibility of pregnancy ensuing, treatment is unnecessary.

DISEASES DUE TO BACTERIA, SPIROCHAETES AND SPIRILLA

1. *Bacterial; Granuloma venereum; Bartonellosis; Melioidosis; Leprosy; Mycobacterial Ulcer; Cholera; Anthrax; Plague; Tularaemia; Chancroid.*
2. *Spirochaetal: Yaws; Endemic (non-veneral) Syphilis; Pinta; Relapsing Fevers.*
3. *Spirillal and Streptobacillus: Rat-bite Fever(s).*
4. *Mixed spirochaetal and bacterial: Tropical Ulcer; Cancrum Oris.*

Granuloma Venereum

Granuloma venereum is a widely spread venereal disease due to *Donovania granulomatis*, characterised by intracellular Donovan bodies, 1 to 2 microns in size, demonstrable in the endothelial and mononuclear cells of the lesion.

Pathological and Clinical Features. At the margin of the lesion there is infiltration of the superficial portion of the corium and of the papillae by lymphocytes and mononuclear cells in which Donovan bodies can be demonstrated. Extensive fibrous tissue is formed especially in lesions of long standing.

The incubation period varies, from a few days to 3 months. The primary lesion is a small nodule or papule in the skin or mucous membrane of the external genitalia, which progresses to form a superficial serpiginous ulcer spreading peripherally. Autoinfection of an opposing surface also extends the spread. Moist warm areas of the body, particularly the flexures of the thighs, the perineum and gluteal cleft, are especially vulnerable. The face and mucous membrane of the mouth may also be affected. Untreated, the lesions may continue for years, spreading at the periphery and leaving an unhealthy scarred area which tends to break down.

Fibrosis may lead to scarring and stenosis of the urethra, anus or vagina. The lymph nodes, however, are not affected, and constitutional symptoms are slight or absent. A few cases of generalised infection have been reported.

Diagnosis. A chronic superficial spreading ulcer in the genital region without any enlargement of the lymph nodes should suggest the disease; the detection of Donovan bodies is diagnostic.

Treatment. Streptomycin 1 g daily for 7 to 14 days intramuscularly or tetracycline for 10 days orally is the treatment of choice. Surgery may be needed to alleviate the effects of scarring.

Bartonellosis

(Carrión's Disease, Oroya Fever, Verruga Peruana)

This disease is caused by a small organism, *Bartonella bacilliformis*, transmitted by sandflies. It is prevalent in narrow hot valleys on the western slopes of the Andes at heights between 2,000 and 10,000 ft (600–3,000 m), in Peru, Ecuador, Bolivia, Colombia and Chile.

Pathological and Clinical Features. In the acute form of the disease, Oroya fever, there is severe haemolysis. Bartonellae are present in large numbers in the erythrocytes and also in the endothelial cells lining small blood vessels. In the later stage of the disease, verruga peruana, cutaneous nodules form, microscopically resembling haemangiomas but containing scanty bartonellae in the endothelial cells.

After an incubation period of 14 to 21 days Oroya fever develops with a sudden rise of temperature to 40°C and rapid haemolysis, accompanied by pains in muscles and joints, nausea, vomiting and diarrhoea, delirium or coma. The spleen and liver are enlarged and tender. Untreated the mortality in the acute form of the disease, especially prevalent in children, is over 90 per cent. Secondary infection by salmonellae is a frequent cause of death. In those who survive, the bartonellae disappear and the destroyed red cells are rapidly replaced. Cultures of the blood taken over a period of months may, however, continue to yield the organisms.

The cutaneous form, verruga peruana, usually follows 30 to 40 days later. The eruption consists of crops of cherry-red haemangioma-like cutaneous nodules 2 to 10 mm in diameter. They are distributed peripherally on the head and limbs and occasionally on the mucosa of the mouth and pharynx. This stage is never fatal, the lesions healing in 2 to 3 months.

Diagnosis. This is suggested by the clinical picture in an endemic area and is confirmed by the demonstration of bartonellae in the erythrocytes, blood cultures or skin lesions.

Treatment and Prevention. In the early febrile stage penicillin, streptomycin or tetracycline for five days give good results. Blood transfusions, fluids and electrolytes may be urgently required. If the anaemia is megaloblastic hydroxocobalamin or folic acid should be given (p. 592).

The use of insecticides, insect repellants and suitable protective clothing is advisable for personal protection.

Melioidosis

Melioidosis is caused by *Pseudomonas pseudomallei*, a micro-organism closely related to *Ps. mallei*, the cause of glanders, which is a rare disease of horses and grooms. *Ps. pseudomallei* is found in puddles following recent rain which suggests it may be saprophytic in nature. Observations suggest that many infections are acquired through abrasions of the skin. Diabetics and patients with severe burns are particularly vulnerable to infection.

The disease has been increasingly reported from the Far East and Malaysia but also from Africa, Australia and elsewhere.

Pathological and Clinical Features. A bacteraemia is followed by the formation of abscesses in the lungs, liver and spleen. In more chronic forms multiple abscesses also recur in subcutaneous tissue.

In the majority there are high fever, prostration and signs of pneumonia, with enlargement of the liver and spleen and sometimes dysenteric symptoms. A chest radiograph resembles that of acute caseous tuberculosis.

Diagnosis. The disease may be suspected from the clinical and radiographic appearances, and, in acute cases, blood culture or culture of the sputum may yield *Ps. pseudomallei* which can also be recovered from abscesses in the more chronic disease. Except in fulminating infections antibodies, which are common also to those produced in glanders, may be detected by agglutination and complement-fixation tests. A haemagglutination test is more sensitive and is specific for *Ps. pseudomallei*.

Treatment. Prompt treatment, without waiting for cultural confirmation, with tetracycline 3 g daily or carbenicillin in large doses daily, has cured some early cases and these antibiotics or a sulphonamide as indicated by sensitivity tests assist recovery from more chronic infections. Abscesses should be drained.

Leprosy

Leprosy is a chronic granulomatous disease caused by *Mycobacterium leprae*, an acid- and alcohol-fast bacillus. The earliest recognisable descriptions of leprosy are found in Indian records dated about 600 B.C., and somewhat later in China and Japan. The disease may have spread to Europe with the armies of Alexander the Great returning from India in 326 B.C. King Robert the Bruce died from leprosy in Scotland in 1329. Danielssen and Boeck gave the first accurate clinical description of leprosy, in Norway, in 1847 and Hansen identified the bacillus in 1873. Leprosy is one of the most seriously disabling and economically important diseases of the world and it is estimated that 20 million people are affected. Growth of *Myco. leprae* in artificial media has not yet been confirmed but thymectomised and irradiated mice, and the armadillo, are proving useful models of the disease. Local multiplication of the organism in the foot-pads of mice is proving a most useful technique for demonstrating the identity and viability of *Myco. leprae* and the existence of drug-resistant strains, for the screening of drugs, for the effect of BCG vaccination, and for the study of cell-mediated immunity. The mode of entry of *Myco. leprae* into the body has not been conclusively proved; it is generally assumed that the organism may pass through damaged skin or respiratory mucosa. The incubation period is usually between 2 and 5 years.

The disease is common in tropical Asia, the Far East, tropical Africa, Central and South America, and in some Pacific Islands. It is still endemic in southern Europe, North Africa and the Middle East.

Pathology. The organisms show a predilection for nerve tissue, skin and the mucosa of the upper respiratory tract. The reaction of the host to their presence varies widely. The early infection, usually transient and self-healing, is called 'indeterminate'. The histological appearances in it are non-specific, and consist of groups of round cells diffusely scattered in the dermis. If the infection does not heal it develops into one of the determinate types, whose features reflect the balance between the host cell-mediated immune response and bacillary multiplication.

In *tuberculoid leprosy* there is a marked cellular response, indicative of vigorous cell-mediated immunity, around nerves, sweat glands and hair follicles. Organisms are scanty, and found mainly in the vicinity of terminal nerve endings in the dermis. They are seen only after prolonged search or by the use of concentration techniques. Lymphocytes, histiocytes and epithelioid cells, some coalescing to form giant cells, are grouped in tubercles but without caseation. The cellular infiltration may extend to and through the subepidermal zone. Tuberculoid leprosy is probably non-infective.

In *lepromatous leprosy*, the infective form of the disease, organisms are present in great abundance in the dermis, eventually replacing the normal architecture. They are mainly grouped in 'globi', which are large macrophages, often showing foamy degeneration, containing 50 or more organisms, and are found in nerve tissue, the erectores pilorum muscles and the endothelial cells of blood vessels; rarely in the cells of the epidermis itself. They are carried in the blood stream to distant and deep organs including muscles, lymph nodes, bone marrow, spleen and Kupffer cells of the liver. Nephritis and amyloidosis are common late complications.

In lepromatous leprosy there is no cell-mediated immunity to *Myco. leprae*. Histology shows the absence of lymphocytes and epithelioid cells, the lepromin test is negative and *in vitro* tests of cellular hypersensitivity are negative.

Between these two 'polar' types of leprosy, there is a spectrum of diverse intermediate manifestations grouped under the terms 'borderline' or 'dimorphous'. The host reaction varies from the near-lepromatous to the near-tuberculoid; it may vary also from time to time in the same patient. *Myco. leprae* are demonstrable in varying numbers. The differing tissue response is usually paralleled by the reaction in the lepromin test which determines sensitivity after 4 weeks to an intradermal injection of a sterilised extract of lepromatous tissue. Positive reactions are obtained in tuberculoid leprosy, negative responses in lepromatous leprosy and negative or weak positive responses in borderline leprosy. This test is of no value in establishing the diagnosis of leprosy since positive results are also found in many normal people, but it is useful in helping to classify patients.

The most serious results of leprosy infection are peripheral neuropathy and its sequelae. The principal mixed nerve trunks of the limbs and face may be severely damaged in their superficial course. The damage is due to cellular reaction to degenerating leprosy bacilli, rather than to the presence of living organisms.

Any determinate form of leprosy may undergo an acute exacerbation or reaction which is caused by an episode of acute allergic inflammation. In lepromatous disease the reaction, Lepra reaction type 2, is due to vasculitis which follows the deposition of immune complexes. In borderline and tuberculoid disease the reaction, Lepra reaction type 1, is due to a sudden increase in cellular hypersensitivity. Borderline reactions are often followed by a shift in the patient's position in the disease spectrum, either towards the tuberculoid pole (upgrading) or towards the lepromatous pole (downgrading).

Clinical Features. The disease usually becomes manifest insidiously, although occasionally it does so more abruptly. The most common first symptom is a small but persistent area of impaired sensation. In other cases the first noticeable feature may be macules, which are usually hypopigmented and erythematous.

The macule of indeterminate leprosy is an inconspicuous lesion 2 to 3 cm in diameter, situated anywhere on the body, exhibiting slight pigmentary and sensory changes. This lesion usually heals spontaneously.

Borderline or *dimorphous leprosy* may present as annular lesions of bizarre shape with ill-defined outer margins, or by plaques and succulent lesions more raised at the centre than at the periphery. Nerve lesions are more numerous than in tuberculoid disease. Borderline disease is immunologically unstable. If the patient's defences succeed in controlling the infection, the disease will upgrade to tuberculoid and heal, but with severe residual disability. If the defences fail the disease downgrades to lepromatous and the complications of extensive bacillary multiplication are added to those of widespread nerve damage. In either event the patient is liable to undergo reactions.

Tuberculoid leprosy is characterised by one or a few solitary lesions in skin and peripheral nerves. Skin lesions are macular or raised as plaques or as rings whose flat centres indicate central healing. The lesion is hypopigmented in dark skins, coppery in pale skins, with a well-defined margin. Its surface is dry, often scaly, and usually anaesthetic unless the lesion is on the face. Lesions are of almost any size and occur anywhere on the body, especially on outer surfaces of arms, legs or buttocks. The nerve twig supplying the skin lesion or a large peripheral nerve at one of the sites of predilection may be enlarged; the ulnar nerve above the elbow, median above the elbow or at the wrist, radial at the wrist, common peroneal in the popliteal fossa, posterior tibial around the medial malleolus, and great auricular across the sternomastoid muscle.

The main complications of tuberculoid leprosy follow from nerve damage. Sensory loss permits trauma from pressure, friction, burns and cuts, the effects of which are intensified if there are abnormal pressures from contractures following muscular paralysis. Autonomic nerve damage causes dry skin which cracks easily and heals slowly. Secondary bacterial infection in an anaesthetic, unprotected limb leads to cellulitis, osteomyelitis and gross tissue destruction which produces the deformities with which the disease is still, so unnecessarily, associated. A combination of fifth and seventh cranial nerve damage exposes an anaesthetic cornea to trauma and sepsis, so the eye easily becomes blind.

Tuberculoid leprosy tends spontaneously to heal slowly, often without residual disability. Sometimes its course is punctuated by a reaction and occasionally it downgrades into the borderline part of the spectrum.

Lepromatous lesions of the skin are described as they progress from early to late, as being macular, infiltrative, diffuse or nodular. Lepromatous macules are numerous, hypopigmented and erythematous. They differ from tuberculoid macules in that they are small, widely scattered on the body, usually symmetrically, and with margins that merge imperceptibly with normal skin. Sensation in them is not impaired. They are often inconspicuous except to the trained eye. As the disease advances, the macular lesions become infiltrated and succulent; in advanced lepromatous leprosy nodular lesions appear, especially on the ears and face, and eyebrows are lost. A less common manifestation of lepromatous leprosy is diffuse symmetrical thickening of the skin, often with thickened lobes of the ear, producing 'leonine facies'.

Clinical evidence of nerve damage appears relatively late in lepromatous leprosy. Anaesthesia and anhidrosis are first detected in the dorsal aspects of the forearms and lower legs, later in a 'glove and stocking' distribution and eventually over the trunk and face, although the palms, soles, axillae and groins may be spared. Muscular weakness results from bacillary infiltration as well as from nerve damage.

The testes may be destroyed and gynaecomastia ensue. The mucous membranes of the nose, mouth and trachea may ulcerate; necrosis of the cartilage and bones may result in late deformities of the phalanges and of nose and oral cavity and loss of the upper incisor teeth. Adjacent lesions may spread into the eye but, more commonly, this is infected through the blood stream. The most frequent lesions in the eye are miliary lepromata on the iris and superficial punctate keratitis, but any part of the eye may be affected although the retina only very rarely.

Reactions. Untreated lepromatous leprosy gradually gets worse. Reactions may be defined as episodes of acute inflammation in pre-existing lesions of leprosy. Sometimes a reaction is the first clinical manifestation of the disease. One-half of patients with lepromatous leprosy and one-quarter with borderline lepromatous disease will be likely to suffer type 2 lepra reactions at some time during the course of their disease, most commonly in their second year of treatment. These reactions are characterised by fever and the appearance of crops of painful roseolar papules or nodules, called 'erythema nodosum leprosum', which may necrose and discharge sterile pus, before subsiding. In addition deeper subcutaneous nodules, iritis, orchitis, lymphadenitis, nerve pain and tenderness, and oedema of hands and feet may develop. Such reactions may threaten eyes and nerves and a succession of them may be extremely debilitating.

Reactions in borderline disease, especially in patients near the tuberculoid pole, are common. They occur spontaneously or possibly are the result of overenergetic or erratic treatment with dapsone. Skin and nerve lesions become acutely inflamed, painful and tender. Nerve function is rapidly lost, irretrievably so unless the reaction is promptly treated. Rarely lesions in the skin ulcerate and nerves caseate.

Diagnosis. Leprosy at or near the lepromatous pole is diagnosed by demonstration of *Myco. leprae* in material obtained by a skin-slit smear. The skin over a lesion and of each ear lobe is pinched between finger and thumb, incised with the point of a scalpel and the exposed dermis scraped with the flat of the blade. The tissue juice obtained, which must be free of blood, is smeared on a microscope slide and stained by a modified Ziehl-Neelsen's method. Nasal mucus may also contain the organisms in lepromatous leprosy and this is a good indication of infectivity. *Myco. leprae* are less readily demonstrable in skin smears in borderline disease in the centre of the spectrum and are undetectable in tuberculoid disease.

In borderline, and especially tuberculoid disease, the cardinal signs of leprosy are enlarged nerves and anaesthesia. Nerves are usually enlarged at sites of predilection asymmetrically and irregularly: they may be tender. Loss or diminution of sensation, or misreference (the inability to locate accurately the site stimulated) may be detected in a skin lesion or in the distribution of a large peripheral nerve. Biopsy of the skin is seldom necessary.

There are virtually no other diseases with enlarged peripheral nerves; familial hypertrophic neuritis and primary amyloidosis are rare. A peripheral nerve may become thickened by a neuroma or as the result of trauma. Sometimes leprosy presents as a mono- or polyneuritis without skin lesions. Very rarely a nerve biopsy may be required.

Treatment. To enable treatment to be carried out successfully it is important to win the confidence and collaboration of the patient.

SPECIFIC CHEMOTHERAPY. *Dapsone*, which is bacteriostatic for *Myco. leprae*, cheap, safe and taken orally, is the drug of choice.

In lepromatous leprosy, which should be treated for life, there is a steadily increasing problem in that *Myco. leprae* becomes resistant unless dapsone is given regularly in relatively large doses. As it is now recognised that there is no danger of dapsone precipitating a type 2 lepra reaction, the drug should be given in a dose of 100 mg daily throughout. This dose produces a blood level about 100 times the minimal inhibitory concentration of dapsone for *Myco. leprae*. In the few patients who cannot tolerate this, the dose is halved. The patient is rendered non-infectious in a few weeks but clinical improvement may not be apparent for months nor complete resolution for years.

In indeterminate and tuberculoid leprosy, which usually heals spontaneously, dapsone 50 mg daily, for 5 and 3 years respectively, is adequate. In borderline disease the essential of successful treatment is close supervision to ensure prompt recognition and management of reactions. Dapsone is given in a dose of 25 or 50 mg daily, and continued for twice as long as there is clinical evidence of active disease, usually 5 to 10 years. In most of the countries where leprosy is endemic patients are widely scattered and medical facilities scarce, so that leprosy is managed by paramedical staff at out-patient clinics held weekly. Under these circumstances it is probably wise to start with dapsone in a supervised dose of 25 mg weekly, increasing gradually over 6 months until a dose of 300 mg weekly is reached; this dose is then maintained for the appropriate time. Children under 5 years are given one-fifth of the adult dose and from 5 to 12 years half the adult dose. Toxic effects, whch are rare with the doses currently used, include anaemia, dermatitis, hepatitis and psychosis.

Thiambutosine is a satisfactory substitute for dapsone. The dose is 500 mg daily for a fortnight increasing by 500 mg fortnightly to a maximum of 2 to 3 g daily, but drug resistance may occur after 2 years.

Rifampicin (p. 292) is the only bactericidal antileprotic drug. It is given in a dose of 600 mg daily for 6 weeks for adults and 10 mg/kg body weight for children. It has the advantage of rendering the lepromatous patient non-infectious in a few days but clinical improvement is not more rapid than with dapsone. It is important to give dapsone additionally in order to prevent the emergence of resistance to rifampicin. Despite its potency, rifampicin does not kill all the bacilli in a lepromatous patient and lifelong treatment with dapsone is still necessary. It is not yet known whether rifampicin given with dapsone will prevent the emergence of dapsone resistance. The high cost of rifampicin prevents its use in most tropical countries.

Clofazimine is as effective as dapsone, although its prolonged or excessive use may cause abdominal pain and tenderness and will inevitably stain the patient's skin brick red or black. It is given in a dose of 100 mg thrice weekly and is of particular value in starting treatment in patients with borderline disease because of its anti-inflammatory properties (see below).

TREATMENT OF REACTIONS. In type 1 lepra reactions, in borderline or tuberculoid disease, dapsone is continued or changed to thiambutosine or clofazimine. Reactions causing pain or tenderness in nerves are treated with corticosteroids, such as prednisolone in a dose of 40–80 mg initially, followed by 20 mg daily for a few days until the inflammation is settling, then tailing off the drug over 2 weeks. Clofazimine, starting under steroid cover, is useful in borderline reactions in a dose of 100–300 mg daily, but many light-skinned patients object to it. Milder reactions, limited to skin lesions, are treated with aspirin 600 mg and chloroquine 150 mg base three times daily or an organic trivalent antimonial, such as stibophen in a dose of 2 ml intramuscularly on alternate days for six doses.

Type 2 lepra reactions in lepromatous patients respond rapidly to thalidomide in a dose of 100 mg four times daily. This drug must *never* be given to premenopausal women because of its disastrous teratogenic effects. If thalidomide is unavailable or contraindicated, the less potent anti-inflammatory drugs are used; reactions threatening nerve damage or extensive skin ulceration or orchitis require systemic corticosteroids. Iritis is a dangerous complication and can usually be managed by local measures, namely the instillation of 1 per cent hydrocortisone drops or ointment (or the subconjunctival injection of a depot preparation of methyl prednisolone), and the twice daily instillation of 1 per cent atropine drops.

MANAGEMENT OF NERVE DAMAGE. In the event of acute paralysis complicating reactional neuritis, the affected limb is splinted, exercised passively each day until function begins to return when active exercises can be added. A patient with an anaesthetic limb must be taught to accept the limitations it imposes, to adjust his life accordingly, to inspect that limb daily for trauma or infection and to learn how not to damage it. Tarsorrhaphy helps protect an exposed anaesthetic cornea. Secondary sepsis is treated with appropriate antibiotics and osteomyelitis and its sequelae are managed in the most conservative manner possible. Patients with plantar ulcers are confined to bed, or given crutches or a walking plaster until healing is complete.

GENERAL MANAGEMENT. In Britain as in many other countries, the disease is notifiable. In endemic areas isolation is impracticable and unnecessary as dapsone renders the patient non-infectious so quickly: elsewhere voluntary isolation of lepromatous cases for a few weeks is desirable. Good nutrition and control of intercurrent disease are important. Initial treatment in a hospital may have medical and educational advantages, but psychological, social and economic disadvantages have to be considered in each case. In many countries the stigma of leprosy is still strong and prejudice against its sufferers may wrongly impose severe additional problems.

Prevention and Control. In endemic areas the disease is commonest among intimate contacts of patients, and children and young adults are especially susceptible. Studies of leprosy that have recently been introduced make it clear that *Myco. leprae* is easily spread and that two-thirds of contacts undergo subclinical immunising infections within 2 years of exposure. Of the small proportion of contacts (about 1 per cent) that develop clinical disease only about 2 per cent will be lepromatous. It is at the moment impossible to identify this small group at risk and logical prophylaxis is impossible. No specific vaccine is available. BCG is of some value, especially in Africa, and should be given to all children contacts of lepromatous patients. Dapsone, in a dose of 5 mg daily, may be given for 2 years to infant contacts of lepromatous patients. Neither measure is a substitute for 6 monthly examination of contacts.

Mass prophylaxis is impossible, but mass treatment and follow-up of all cases identified during a population survey reduces deformity and lowers the incidence of leprosy. With improvement of socioeconomic conditions the disease tends to disappear.

Further reading about leprosy:

Browne, S. G. (1974) *Leprosy in the Bible.* London: Christian Medical Fellowship.
Bryceson, A. D. M. & Pfaltzgraff, R. E. (1973) *Leprosy for Students of Medicine.* Edinburgh: Churchill Livingstone.

Mycobacterial Ulcer

This condition, first accurately described in Australia and New Guinea, then named Buruli ulcer from its frequency in the Nile valley of Uganda, is caused by *Mycobacterium ulcerans*. The epidemiology is unknown but the known foci of infection are consistent with the hypothesis that the environment in swamps following unusual flooding of rivers is of aetiological importance. It begins as a single small subcutaneous nodule situated commonly on the leg or forearm. The skin over the centre of the nodule ulcerates and, untreated, the ulcer extends to involve a progressively large area. Histologically there is much necrosis of subcutaneous fat and *Myco. ulcerans* are abundant in the necrotic tissue in the base of the ulcer.

If suspected before ulceration, the nodule should be excised and healing readily follows. Ulcers require to be excised and skin grafted. Antimycobacterial chemotherapy is disappointing.

Cholera

Cholera, an acute disease of the gastrointestinal tract, is caused by the contamination of food or drink by strains of *Vibrio cholerae*. There are different serotypes named Inaba, Ogawa, Hikojima and also the biotype El Tor (serotype Ogawa), which since 1961 has become widespread throughout the Far and Near East and appears to be displacing the classical *V. cholerae* from most areas and in 1970 spread to Africa. Sporadic infections imported by travellers have appeared in European countries, including Britain, and infection from eating shell-fish has been proved. Formerly thought to be of low pathogenicity, its virulence is now found to be equal to that of other strains. These disease-producing vibrios have to be distinguished from the many non-pathogenic cholera-like vibrios. The most important endemic foci of cholera are in the lower reaches of the Ganges and Brahmaputra rivers. *Vibrio cholerae* usually disappear from the stools of patients within a week of convalescence but exceptionally they may persist up to a month after the acute attack and El Tor vibrios rarely continue to be excreted for years. The disease appears to be maintained in endemic areas by very mild infections in a population with a considerable resistance to it.

Pathology. Cholera vibrios multiply in the lumen of the small bowel and are non-invasive. They secrete a powerful exotoxin (enterotoxin) which stimulates the adenyl cyclase-adenosine monophosphate pathway of the mucosa, resulting in an outpouring of normal alkaline, small bowel fluid. Severe dehydration follows rapidly even though absorption of fluid by the bowel is hardly impaired. There may be acidosis and depletion of sodium and potassium with attendant complications, of which renal failure is the most important.

Clinical Features. After an incubation period of a few hours to 5 days severe diarrhoea without pain or colic, followed by vomiting, usually begins suddenly. Fluid gushes effortlessly from the bowel and stomach. After the faecal contents of the gut have been evacuated the typical 'rice-water' material is passed. This consists of clear fluid with flecks of mucus. In severe cases an enormous quantity of fluid and electrolytes is rapidly lost. This soon leads to intense dehydration with agonising muscular cramps. The skin becomes cold, clammy and wrinkled and the eyes sunken. The blood pressure falls, the pulse becomes imperceptible, and the urine output falls. The patient, however, usually remains mentally clear. Unless fluid and electrolytes are replaced the patient may die from acute circulatory failure within a few hours. With proper treatment, however, improvement is rapid. Rarely anuria persists and may lead to death.

Although this is the classical picture of cholera, the majority of infections cause only a mild illness with slight diarrhoea. Occasionally a very intense illness, 'cholera sicca', occurs in which the patient is overwhelmed by the infection and the rapid loss of fluid into the dilated bowel kills the patient before typical gastrointestinal symptoms appear.

In children under 12 years of age the mortality is higher (15 to 17 per cent) than in adults (4 to 6 per cent). Pulmonary oedema, febrile reactions to therapy, pyrexial convulsions and encephalopathy, tetany, meteorism, hypoglycaemia, hypernatraemia, acidosis and water retention and frequently malnutrition are believed to be the adverse factors in paediatric practice. Over-hydration may cause pulmonary oedema.

Diagnosis. During a cholera epidemic the diagnosis is usually easy. It is, however, important that an atypical case should be recognised early so that the outbreak may be brought rapidly under control. Microscopic examination of the stool may detect the typical cholera vibrio, and culture of the stool or a rectal swab on special media is used to isolate and identify the organism. Other diseases such as acute bacillary dysentery, viral enteritis, *P. falciparum* malaria, food poisoning and certain chemical poisons may produce symptoms like those of cholera. Cholera is notifiable under the International Health Regulations.

Treatment. The chief aim in treatment is to maintain the circulation and prevent renal failure by replacement of water and electrolytes; the earlier this is started, the better is the prognosis. A quick clinical assessment of the patient's state of dehydration is made from the appearance of the patient, the pulse, blood pressure and skin turgor. In severe cases or when there is vomiting, fluids are given intravenously. A large needle is plunged into a large vein; the femoral vein can always be quickly found and the fluid is run in as fast as possible until pulse and blood pressure return. The rest of the estimated deficit is replaced more slowly. If intravenous fluids or apparatus are unavailable, a nasogastric tube is passed and fluid is poured in remorselessly. Vomiting usually stops once the patient is rehydrated and fluid should then be given orally every hour. Patients can be made to drink up to 500 ml hourly. The quantity of fluid required is calculated every 8 hours from the output of urine, stool, vomit and estimated insensible loss which may be as much as 5 litres in 24 hours in a hot humid climate. Total fluid requirements can be in excess of 50 litres over a period of 2 to 5 days. Accurate records are essential and are greatly facilitated by the use of a 'cholera cot' which has a reinforced hole under the patient's buttocks beneath which a graded bucket is placed. The ideal solutions are shown in Table 17.1.

Table 17.1 Ideal Solutions for Treatment of Cholera

	Intravenous			Oral	
	g/l	mmol/l			g/l
Sodium chloride	5	Na 133	Commercial salt		
		Cl 98	(NaCl)		4·2
Potassium chloride	1	K 98	Potassium chloride		1·8
		Cl 98	or citrate		2·7
Sodium bicarbonate	4	HCO₃ 48	Sodium bicarbonate		4
or acetate	6·5		Glucose		20

For intravenous use sodium acetate has the advantage of stability on autoclaving. Sodium lactate and sodium bicarbonate are acceptable alternative sources of alkali, but are not stable and must be sterilised separately and added after autoclaving. Other satisfactory fluids include Ringer lactate (B.P.) or Hartman's solution and Darrow's solution, in which case supplements of potassium are given as 10 mmol/l of intravenous fluid or 2–4 g potassium chloride or citrate three times daily by mouth. Isotonic saline is better than nothing but every 2 litres should be alternated with 1 litre of isotonic sodium lactate (18·7 g/l) or bicarbonate (14 g/l) and added potassium. The presence of glucose in the oral fluid has been shown to promote electrolyte absorption.

The use of correct fluids for replacement has done away with the need for estimation of plasma electrolytes or specific gravity. In children, the elderly, the anaemic and those with underlying heart disease overvigorous intravenous rehydration readily causes pulmonary oedema. Children require most careful attention to fluid balance. Ringer lactate is the fluid of choice and it is important that the oral fluid contain glucose. Renal failure is managed in the usual way (p. 496).

Three days' treatment with tetracycline 250 mg 6 hourly or furazolidine in a single dose of 400 mg reduces the duration of excretion of vibrios and the total volume of fluid needed for replacement.

Prevention and Control. Personal prophylaxis means strict personal hygiene. Water for drinking should come from a clean piped supply or be boiled. Flies must not be allowed access to food. Vaccination with a killed suspension of *V. cholerae* is given in two doses of 0·5 and 1·0 ml 1 to 4 weeks apart but it should not be relied upon to give full protection.

In an epidemic, control of water sources and of population movement are most important. Mass vaccination with a single dose of vaccine and mass treatment with tetracycline are valuable. Disinfection of infective discharges and soiled clothing, the therapeutic use of tetracycline and scrupulous hand washing by medical attendants reduces the danger of spread from treatment centres. It is an international requirement for travellers passing through endemic zones to be in possession of a certificate of vaccination which becomes valid 6 days after the first dose and lasts 6 months.

Anthrax

Anthrax is a disease of domestic animals which become infected by inhaling or ingesting spores of *Bacillus anthracis* passed in faeces. Grazing lands remain infective for years which makes it necessary to bury infected carcasses deeply to avoid contamination of the soil.

Anthrax in man is an occupational disease of farmers, butchers and dealers in hides, animal hair and wool and handlers of bone meal from endemic areas. In primitive conditions, where skins are used as sleeping mats, for clothing or for carrying water, and where diseased cattle are eaten, anthrax is endemic.

Pathology. The primary lesion in man may be in the skin, nares, pharynx, larynx, lung or intestinal tract, from any of which sites the infection may spread to lymph nodes and lead to a bacteraemia and infection of spleen, lungs, meninges and brain. The microscopical changes are those of haemorrhagic inflammation with areas of necrosis and interstitial oedema. There is a neutrophil leucocytosis of the blood and infiltration in the tissues without abscess formation.

Clinical Features. The incubation period is usually 1 to 3 days. When the infection is acquired from a skin or hide or from handling or slaughtering an animal, a cutaneous lesion indicates the portal of entry. This usually takes the form of a 'malignant pustule' on an exposed part of the body, commonly the face. It begins as an itching papule which enlarges and forms a vesicle filled with serosanguineous fluid surrounded by gross oedema. The lesion is relatively painless and accompanied by slight enlargement of regional lymph nodes. The vesicle dries up to form a thick black 'eschar' surrounded by blebs. Occasionally there are multiple lesions. In endemic areas patients may exhibit only slight constitutional symptoms but in non-immune persons high fever and toxaemia are usual and if the sufferer is not energetically treated an overwhelming bacteraemia may prove fatal. Occasionally there may be no localised pustule but only oedema.

When infected meat is eaten, an ulcer with much surrounding oedema may be seen in the pharynx or more commonly the infection causes a severe gastroenteritis which frequently terminates fatally. Some people, usually of an older age, escape unscathed after eating infected meat, presumably because of previously acquired immunity.

Those who acquire the infection by inhalation, 'wool-sorters' disease', may develop an acute laryngitis or a virulent haemorrhagic bronchopneumonia. Anthrax may also present as meningitis.

Diagnosis. The appearance of a cutaneous lesion and the environmental and occupational history should suggest the diagnosis. A stained smear of fluid taken from the edge of a malignant pustule demonstrates the organism, which may be confirmed in an atypical case by culture and pathogenicity tests in mice, rabbits or guinea-pigs. *B. anthracis* is also recoverable from laryngeal and pulmonary anthrax and from the CSF in meningitis. If a group of people who have feasted on an animal which has sickened and died are taken abruptly ill with fulminating gastroenteritis, anthrax should be suspected.

Post-mortem examination is not to be lightly undertaken because of the risk of spreading the infection. *B. anthracis* may be cultured from the faeces. Suspected animal products can be investigated by the use of anthrax immune serum.

Treatment and Prevention. Effective treatment consists of giving penicillin to which *B. anthracis* is usually susceptible or tetracycline in combination with streptomycin, in full doses, for 3 to 5 days. In the presence of urgent symptoms, if an anti-anthrax serum of known potency is available it should be administered intravenously, in a dose not exceeding 50 ml.

The disease is controlled in cattle by slaughter and deep burial of the diseased animal, by the administration of prophylactic antiserum to healthy animals at risk and by annual immunisation with attenuated cultures. Imports from endemic areas should be subject to strict control and sterilisation. A vaccine is used to protect laboratory workers.

Plague

Plague is a disease of great historical interest. In Old Testament times, when the Philistines were afflicted by a lethal disease, associated with inguinal swellings, they made offerings of golden mice. In 543 A.D. the Justinian pandemic occurred. In the fourteenth century, as the Black Death, it caused widespread havoc throughout Europe, followed by further serious outbreaks during the next three centuries. In 1664–1665, 70,000 of London's 460,000 inhabitants died of plague. The causative organism, *Yersinia pestis*, is named after its discoverer, Yersin, who isolated it in Hong Kong in 1894. In 1905 Glen Liston in Bombay proved its transmission to man by bites of fleas from infected rodents. Now the urban disease is largely eliminated but outbreaks still occur, notably in Vietnam and East Africa, arising from infections in wild rodents which may remain healthy but whose fleas may start an outbreak by spread to domestic rats or directly to hunters. In man the bacteraemia may cause pneumonitis with the expectoration of *Y. pestis*. Thus the infection may be spread from man to man by aerosols, the condition then being called 'pneumonic plague'. This condition can also be caused by the accidental inhalation of a laboratory culture or dust containing viable organisms from infected rodents or fleas.

Pathology. Rarely a vesicle with surrounding cellulitis is evident at the site of the flea-bite. The more usual initial lesion is acute inflammation in and around the lymph nodes regional to the site of entry of the organisms. The nodes are haemorrhagic and surrounded by oedematous haemorrhagic cellular tissue. *Y.*

pestis are numerous in and around the infected nodes. This regional lymphadenopathy is the basis of the clinical description 'bubonic plague'.

Signs of a haemorrhagic septicaemia are seen in all fatal cases, with subpericardial and meningeal haemorrhages. There may be haemorrhagic foci of consolidation in the lungs, enlargement of lymph nodes and spleen and multiple small necrotic foci in the liver. In some severe cases there may be little or no swelling of regional lymph nodes; these are the cases clinically presenting as 'septicaemic plague'. In deaths from 'pneumonic plague' the signs are those of acute congestion in one or more lobes of the lungs and evidence of generalised haemorrhagic septicaemia. Patients treated with antibiotics may develop pulmonary abscesses before recovery takes place. *Y. pestis* are numerous in all affected organs.

Clinical Features. The incubation period is short, 3 to 6 days, but less in pneumonic plague.

Bubonic Plague. The most common site of the bubo, made up of the swollen lymph nodes and surrounding tissue, is one groin but, according to the site of the biting by the flea, the bubo may instead be axillary, cervical, epitrochlear or popliteal. The onset is usually sudden with a rigor, high fever, dry skin and severe headache. Soon aching and then also swelling at the site of the affected lymph nodes begin. Some cases are relatively mild but in the majority signs of toxaemia rapidly increase, with a rapid pulse, dilated heart and mental confusion. The spleen is usually palpable.

Septicaemic Plague. Those not exhibiting a bubo usually, but not invariably, deteriorate rapidly. Pneumonia and expectoration of blood-stained sputum containing *Y. pestis* may complicate bubonic or septicaemic plague.

Pneumonic Plague. The onset is very sudden with cough and dyspnoea. The patient expectorates copious blood-stained frothy, highly infective sputum, becomes cyanosed and rapidly deteriorates. Crepitations and rhonchi are heard in the lungs but there are no signs indicating consolidation.

Diagnosis. Early diagnosis is urgent. A report of deaths among rats or of human infection should alert all medical personnel. Especially under these circumstances a bubo, with no evident local pyogenic cause for it, must be punctured, using a dry syringe and needle. Staining a smear of the aspirate with methylene blue will show the characteristic bipolar appearance of the organisms. For confirmation the aspirate or blood can be cultured. A leucocytosis distinguishes septicaemic plague from typhoid fever; blood culture is usually necessary to establish the diagnosis although occasionally the organisms can be seen in a stained blood film. The sputum of a patient with pneumonic plague contains *Y. pestis*. Serological tests show increasing titres of antibodies in convalescence. Plague is notifiable under the International Health Regulations.

Treatment. Streptomycin is the drug of choice in the treatment of plague. The first dose should be 1 g intramuscularly, followed by 500 mg every 6 hours until the temperature has been normal for 24 hours, after which 1 g should be given daily for a further 6 days. Excellent results have been achieved with this course of treatment, especially when it is started early in the disease. Tetracycline has proved to be almost as effective as streptomycin; the initial dose should be given intravenously. The adult oral dose is 1 g every 6 hours for 48 hours or longer, depending on the response. After improvement the dose is reduced to 2 g daily and continued for a further 14 days. In pneumonic or severe septicaemic plague a combination of tetracycline and streptomycin is administered, intravenously if necessary, or co-trimoxazole in full doses. The bubo should not be incised unless rupture is imminent. With antibiotic treatment it is uncommon for suppuration of buboes and ulceration to develop.

Prevention. There are two main types of vaccine, the killed vaccine given in two or three doses, and one containing live avirulent organisms requiring one dose only. Both vaccines cause fever. Booster doses are required after 3 to 6 months.

Prophylaxis against bubonic and septicaemic plague largely depends on preventing biting by fleas carrying plague. This can be achieved in the case of the domestic rat by preventing its access to food and by the use of poisoned bait. Insecticides have revolutionised antiflea measures. Powders containing 1·5 per cent Dieldrin or 2 per cent Aldrin applied to floors and blown into rat holes kill all the fleas and remain active for 9 to 12 weeks. The insecticide chosen should be one to which the local fleas are known to be susceptible.

Unvaccinated contacts should be protected by tetracycline or by intramuscular streptomycin, 1 g daily, or a sulphonamide such as sulphadimidine 3 to 6 g daily for a week. Patients expectorating *Y. pestis* should be isolated and those attending them should weak masks, protective gowns and gloves.

Further reading about plague:

Ziegler, P. (1969) *The Black Death.* London: Collins.

Tularaemia

Tularaemia is an infection due to *Yersinia tularensis* transmitted to mammals and birds by the bites of infected blood-sucking flies and ticks. Man may be accidentally infected in a laboratory or while skinning infected wild rabbits or hares. In Norway lemmings are another source. The micro-organisms enter through dermal abrasions, the conjunctiva or mouth. Contaminated water, infected meat and the bites of infected arthropods are less common sources of human infection.

The disease is found in the Americas, Japan, the USSR, and most European countries.

Pathological and Clinical Features. Focal areas of necrosis occur especially in lymph nodes, spleen, liver, kidneys and lungs. There may be cutaneous, oral or ophthalmic lesions when infection is by these routes.

The incubation period is from 1 to 10 days. There is a sudden onset of high fever followed by sweating and prostration. After some early remission of the fever, the temperature rises again after a few days and remains elevated for 10 to 15 days but in severe infections there may be no early remission and the fever may last continuously for 3 or 4 weeks. There is a moderate neutrophil leucocytosis. The spleen is sometimes palpable. About 2 days after the onset a lesion develops in the conjunctiva of one eye or in the skin at the site of an abrasion if the organisms have entered in this way. Such a site is swollen and painful and accompanied by enlargement of the regional lymph nodes. When the mouth has been the portal of entry a buccal ulcer or inflamed tonsils may be found. Pleuropulmonary and pericardial inflammatory lesions result from inhalation of the organisms or from haematogenous spread. Lymph nodes may remain enlarged for months.

Diagnosis. The organism may be isolated by repeated blood culture or guinea-pig inoculation. An intradermal test using killed *Y. tularensis* may be positive as early as the third day and positive agglutination and complement-fixation tests after 10 to 12 days. Antibodies produced by brucellae may also agglutinate suspensions of *Y. tularensis*.

Treatment and Prevention. Intramuscular streptomycin 1 g daily for 7 days or tetracycline 250 mg 6 hourly for 2 weeks is usually curative.

Masks should be worn in the laboratory and gloves should be used when skinning rabbits and hares in endemic areas. Adequate cooking renders infected meat safe for eating.

Chancroid

(*Soft Sore*)

This is an important and common venereal disease of the tropics, presenting usually in males since the condition in females is asymptomatic, and difficult to recognise. The causative organism, *Haemophilus ducreyi*, a Gram-negative bacillus, is 1 to 2 microns in length and is seen in pairs, chains or arranged like fish in shoals. Invasion of the lesions by pyogenic organisms is common.

Clinical Features. The incubation period is 2 to 3 days, but may occasionally be longer. The initial lesion is a small red papule on the mucous or skin surfaces of the genitalia or on the surrounding skin. In a few days painful necrosis, ulceration and purulent discharge appear, and a well-demarcated surrounding zone of erythema develops. Frequently the lesions are multiple from auto-inoculation and are seen in all stages of development. The inguinal lymph nodes may enlarge, soften and suppurate. Malaise and fever may accompany the local signs.

Diagnosis. Differentiation is required from syphilis, lymphogranuloma inguinale, granuloma venereum and genital herpes. Scraping or aspiration of material from the lesion may reveal the *Haemophilus* which is, however, often overgrown by secondary invaders. Aspiration of a lymph node may be more successful. Autoinoculation of fluid from the lesion on the scarified forearm produces a swelling in which biopsy will demonstrate a recognisable histology. A skin test using a commercial vaccine (e.g. Dmelcos) is also available.

Treatment. It is important not to mask or miss associated syphilis; therefore only local cleansing with saline should be undertaken and an oral sulphonamide administered until four dark-ground examinations have failed to reveal *Treponema pallidum*. Thereafter excellent results will be obtained with tetracycline or streptomycin. Serological tests to exclude latent syphilis should be carried out 3 months after the completion of the course of treatment.

Yaws

Yaws is a granulomatous disease mainly involving the skin and bones and caused by *Treponema pertenue*, morphologically indistinguishable from the causative organisms of syphilis and pinta. The three infections induce similar serological changes and possibly some degree of cross immunity. Organisms are transmitted by bodily contact from a patient with infectious yaws through minor abrasions of the skin of another person, usually a child. Infection is most likely to take place in huts at night when the temperature and humidity are high and families use communal sleeping mats.

Yaws is still to be found among backward indigenous people. Areas of infection exist in Mexico, Panama, the Northern parts of South America, West Indies, Central, East and West Africa, the Pacific Islands, Malaysia, Burma, Thailand (uncommonly in India and Sri Lanka), and also in Indonesia and the Far East, including China where it extends into temperate zones. The mass campaigns by the World Health Organisation in 1950–1960 treated over 60 million people and eradicated yaws from many areas.

Pathology. At the site of the inoculation a proliferative granuloma develops containing numerous treponemata. This primary lesion is followed by eruptions, the most characteristic being multiple papillomatous lesions of the skin with a histology similar to the primary lesion. In addition there may be hypertrophic periosteal lesions of many bones with underlying cortical rarefaction. All these lesions of 'early yaws' heal without appreciable scarring or deformity unless there has been secondary infection. After a variable interval 'late yaws' may develop, characterised by destructive lesions which closely resemble the gummata of tertiary syphilis and which heal with much scarring and deformity.

Clinical Features. The incubation period is 3 to 4 weeks. The primary lesion or 'mother yaw' is usually on the leg or buttocks. The secondary eruption usually follows a few weeks or months later, sometimes before the primary lesion has healed. The most typical are the so-called papillomata, often very numerous, consisting of exuberant tissue covered with a whitish-yellow exudate, and more prolific in the moist flexures and around the mouth. There may be successive crops of lesions. The subject, usually a child, may remain active and unconcerned except for the irritation of the sores and of the flies which they attract. These lesions are highly contagious. Sometimes a pathologically similar lesion erupts through the palm or sole, when walking becomes painful. The resultant gait has given rise to the description, 'wet crab yaws'. The bones of all the fingers distal to the carpus, except the terminal phalanges, particularly in children, may rarify and be surrounded by periosteal deposits. There may be a swelling of a long bone and also of the nasal bones (goundou). The distorted tibia may remain as the 'sabre tibia' but most of the lesions of early yaws will eventually subside. Healing is much more rapid after the administration of penicillin.

Latent yaws. Following the spontaneous resolution of 'early yaws' serological changes may persist, to be followed by further manifestations of 'early yaws' or, after an interval of as much as 5 to 10 years, by the tertiary lesions of 'late yaws'.

Late yaws. Solitary or multiple nodular lesions develop. They ulcerate and spread superficially and also, in places, penetrate deeply into the underlying tissue. In this way gross disfigurement may be caused with distressing ulceration and deformity. The lesions tend to heal with scarring in one part while the ulcer is extending in another. In addition, in radiographs, localised areas of rarefaction may be shown in long bones with surrounding periostitis. Clinically these present as localised swellings of bones over which tissue may ulcerate giving a picture resembling the gummatous ulceration of tertiary syphilis. Lesions in the hand, skull, nose and palate are common. Gross mutilation making the nose and mouth one open cavity ('gangosa') is one of the most tragic results still compatible with life. Other late lesions include hyperkeratosis with fissuring of the palms and soles 'dry crab yaws', hydrarthrosis, bursitis and juxta-articular nodules consisting of painless, firm, subcutaneous fibrous deposits about the elbows, hips and knees.

Unlike tertiary syphilis, yaws does not affect the internal viscera or the cardiovascular and nervous systems.

Treatment and Prevention. Long-acting penicillin is highly effective. Very good results follow the intramuscular administration of 750 mg of procaine benzylpenicillin on two occasions at an interval of 1 week. For a mass campaign a single dose of 750 mg is given to all active adult cases and 375 mg to latent cases and contacts, which in areas of high endemicity include the whole of the remainder of the population. Proportionate doses are given to children. A second survey and campaign of treatment should follow within a year to detect and treat relapses and missed cases. Tetracycline 1 to 2 g daily for 5 days is as successful as penicillin, but the cost and technical difficulties of ensuring that the drug is taken daily make it suitable only for the treatment of patients under supervision.

With improved housing and increased cleanliness the disease disappears. In few fields of medicine have chemotherapy and improved hygiene achieved such dramatic success as in yaws.

Endemic (Non-venereal) Syphilis

In certain tropical countries, where lack of hygiene prevails, this treponematosis occurs as a family disease, the lesions of which show a close resemblance to those of venereal syphilis. This condition has many local names notably bejel in Arabia and sivvens when formerly it was endemic in Scotland. The causative organisms are regarded as modified strains of *Treponema pallidum*, with which they are morphologically identical but biologically distinct.

Congenital infections are extremely rare and sexual transmission unusual. The common mode of infection is through an abrasion, the disease being transmitted from one child to another and occasionally from a child to a parent. Sometimes it spreads in a closed community by the use of common drinking vessels and possibly mechanically by flies. The poor social conditions in which the disease prevails are similar to those where yaws is found but the clinical lesions resemble those of juvenile syphilis.

In contrast to venereal syphilis the primary lesion is rarely seen, except when a child has inoculated the nipple of the mother during suckling, in which case the lesion presents as an ulcerative papule without regional adenitis. The secondary and tertiary lesions include all the common types of skin and bone manifestations of syphilis but the typical papillomatous lesions of yaws are infrequent. In addition, 'mucous patches' in the mouth, due to superficial ulceration, are common and are often the first sign of endemic syphilis but they are very rare in yaws. Visceral and neurological lesions are absent or rare. The usual serological tests give identical results with venereal syphilis and yaws.

Treatment. The disease responds to treatment by penicillin in the same way as veneral syphilis (p. 79). In the social conditions in which it is found the treatment of choice is usually a long-acting penicillin. Prevention depends on the development of improved social and economic conditions and the mass treatment of affected communities with penicillin.

Pinta

Pinta is a clinical and geographic variant of endemic syphilis caused by the related organism *Treponema carateum*. It is endemic in localised areas in Central and South America and in some West Indian and South Pacific Islands.

The incubation period is 14 to 20 days. There is a primary scaly papular lesion on an exposed part, usually the leg. The lesion enlarges slowly, up to 10 cm in diameter and is surrounded by smaller papules. Regional lymph nodes enlarge and like the primary lesion contain treponemata. The second stage is manifest 5 to 12 months later and consists of a generalised eruption of macules and miliary papules, 'pintids', pinkish and slightly scaly. Most of these heal but others coalesce and form hyperpigmented patches, commonly on the face and exposed parts. The secondary lesions may persist for years and may be accompanied by hyperkeratosis of palms and soles. In the tertiary stage the affected patches become atrophic and depigmented and in some cases extensive white areas result. In the second and tertiary stages there are serological changes closely resembling those of syphilis but no cross immunity.

Treatment is by a long-acting penicillin (p. 871).

The Relapsing Fevers

The relapsing fevers are a group of diseases due to infections by spirochaetes of the genus *Borrelia* transmitted by lice or soft ticks. The louse-borne *Borrelia recurrentis* infects only man and is not transmitted from a louse to its progeny. This disease appears in epidemics particularly during wars or famine when refugees are crowded together in conditions under which infestation with the human body-louse is frequent and an infected louse is introduced. It may accompany louse-borne typhus. The disease is endemic in Ethiopia from where recently recorded epidemics have probably arisen. Epidemics occur in hot as well as in cold climates.

Bor. duttoni, the cause of tick-borne relapsing fever, is transmitted by various species of the genus *Ornithodoros*. Ticks live for years and once infected remain infective for life and convey the infection, transovarially, to the offspring. Tick-borne relapsing fever is thus an endemic disease.

Louse-borne Relapsing Fever

Lice cause itching. Borreliae are liberated from the infected louse when it is crushed during scratching which also inoculates the borreliae into the skin.

Pathology. The borreliae multiply in the blood, where they are abundant in the febrile phases, and invade most tissues especially the liver, spleen and meninges. Hepatitis causing jaundice is frequent in severe infections and there may be petechial haemorrhages in the skin, mucous membranes and serous surfaces of internal organs.

In the pyrexial phases free borreliae are demonstrable in the blood. Thrombocytopenia is marked and liver function is impaired. The urine frequently contains protein and sometimes there is frank haematuria.

Clinical Features. After an incubation period varying from 2 to 12 days there is a sudden onset of fever. The temperature rises to 39·5° to 40·5°C and is accompanied by a rapid pulse, headache, generalised aching, injected conjunctivae and frequently a petechial rash, epistaxis and herpes labialis. As the disease progresses, the liver and spleen become tender and frequently palpable and jaundice is common. There may be severe serosal and intestinal haemorrhage. Mental confusion and meningism may occur. The fever ends by crisis between the fourth and tenth day, often associated with profuse sweating, hypotension, circulatory, and cardiac failure. There may be no further fever but, in a proportion of cases, after an afebrile period of about 7 days there may be one or more relapses which are usually milder and less prolonged. In the absence of specific treatment mortality may be as high as 40 per cent, especially among the elderly and malnourished.

The organisms are demonstrated in the blood during fever either by dark ground illumination of a wet film or by staining thick and thin films.

Treatment and Prevention. The problems of treatment are to minimise the severe Jarisch-Herxheimer reaction which inevitably follows successful chemotherapy and to prevent relapses. The safest treatment is with procaine penicillin 200 mg intramuscularly followed the next day by 0·5 g tetracycline. Tetracycline alone is effective and prevents relapse, but gives rise to a worse reaction. Doxycycline, 200 mg once by mouth, as an alternative to tetracycline has the advantage of being curative also for typhus, which often accompanies epidemics of relapsing fever.

Treatment is followed within a half to 3 hours by a chill or rigor, a brisk rise of temperature to 40–42°C, tachypnoea, tachycardia and often cough, confusion, distress, delirium and, occasionally, convulsions and coma. This phase is rapidly followed by the first phase of profound hypotension and vasodilatation which may last from 8–12 hours and may be complicated by cardiac failure. The patient must be confined strictly to bed for 48 hours after treatment, carefully observed and managed as complications demand. Tepid sponging for fever over 41°C, careful attention to hydration, preferably by mouth, and prompt treatment of cardiac failure are required.

The patient and his clothing and all contacts must be freed from lice as in epidemic typhus (p. 893).

Tick-borne Relapsing Fever

This disease, due to *Borrelia duttoni*, is conveyed by a variety of ticks and its endemicity is governed by the presence of the vector. In the Mediterranean area *Ornithodoros tholozani* is responsible; in the Middle East, Iran, Afghanistan and India and in the New World there are other vectors. These ticks can become infected from rodents or bats as well as by congenital transmission and man is only an incidental host. In Central and East Africa, however, *O. moubata* is the vector and man is probably the only important mammalian host. The disease in these areas is thus confined to old camp sites, old houses and their immediate surroundings, infested with *O. moubata* infected from man or by congenital transmission. *O. moubata* lives in dried mud floors and the cracks of the walls of huts plastered with mud.

The pathological changes resemble those of louse-borne relapsing fever but with late neurological lesions.

Clinical Features. These are similar to those of louse-borne relapsing fever. The febrile bouts, although severe, last usually only for 3 to 5 days and the apyrexial periods may also be shorter. Relapses are, however, more frequent and may be as numerous as 10. Iritis and neurological complications, including cranial nerve palsies, optic atrophy, localised palsies and spastic paraplegia, may develop during these later relapses.

The methods used in diagnosis are similar to those for louse-borne relapsing fever. *Bor. duttoni* are, however, scantier in the peripheral blood but laboratory animals are readily infected.

Treatment and Prevention. As many strains are resistant to penicillin, tetracycline 1 g daily for 7 days is given and the course repeated after an interval of a week. Except for the Jarisch-Herxheimer reaction, good results follow a single dose of 200 mg doxycycline.

Ticks can be killed by lindane (gamma BHC) applied to the inside of the walls, floors and across the entrance to houses.

Rat-bite Fevers

There are two rat-bite fevers, one caused by *Spirillum minus*, the other by *Streptobacillus moniliformis*. The latter in addition to being transmitted by a rat-bite has also occurred as an epidemic due to infected milk (Haverhill fever) and in other cases also there has been no known contact with rats or mice. Both infections are worldwide in distribution.

Pathological and Clinical Features. The manifestations of both fevers are very similar. In *Sp. minus* infection (Sodoku) the wound usually heals. After 5 to 21 days it suddenly becomes inflamed, indurated, purplish and painful; it may ulcerate and this stage is accompanied by lymphangitis, regional lymphadenitis, leucocytosis, splenomegaly and fever. After a week the local and general reactions subside but recur after a further few days. Periods of fever lasting 24 to 48 hours are followed by a rapid fall of temperature and, without treatment, febrile bouts may continue to recur for weeks and the patient becomes anaemic. A macular or maculopapular dusky red rash, sparse over the trunk and extremities, appears during the febrile phases. In contrast to streptobacillus fever arthritis is not common.

In streptobacillus fever the incubation period is 1 to 5 days. The bite usually heals well but occasionally an abscess forms in the wound. Regional lymphadenopathy is not marked. The general symptoms resemble those of *Sp. minus* infections but there is frequently painful arthritis and it is unusual to have recurrences of fever after the initial bout which only lasts 48 to 72 hours. Sometimes painful swollen joints may be accompanied by a remittent fever suggesting sepsis.

Diagnosis. *Sp. minus* can be demonstrated in the exudate from the inflamed bite or in fluid aspirated from a lymph node, either by examination under darkground illumination or by inoculation intraperitoneally into an uninfected mouse. Blood similarly inoculated into mice or guinea-pigs will yield *Sp. minus* in the peritoneal fluid 5 to 14 days later. The serum yields false positive serological tests for syphilis. In *Strep. moniliformis* infections specific seroagglutinins are demonstrable after 10 days. A titre of 1 in 80 or a rising titre is considered diagnostic but the serological tests for syphilis are negative. The organism can be recovered from the blood or, more easily, from an effusion into an inflamed joint, by culture on media containing serum or ascitic fluid or by intraperitoneal inoculation of mice.

Treatment. Both infections are readily cured by penicillin, streptomycin or tetracycline.

Tropical Ulcer

The aetiology of tropical ulcers is still in doubt. Predisposing factors are minor injuries occurring in the presence of undernourishment, poor hygienic surroundings and debilitating diseases. The bacillus *Fusobacterium fusiforme* and the spirochaete *Borrelia vincenti* can usually be demonstrated in the ulcer, but the part they play in its production is uncertain. The disease is widely distributed in tropical countries.

Pathological and Clinical Features. The edges of the ulcer are raised, thick, oedematous and infiltrated with neutrophils. In the early stages the ulcerated area is covered with necrotic skin, and the underlying tissue shows fibroblastic proliferation. Staphylococci and streptococci are usually present in addition to *F. fusiforme* and *Bor. vincenti.*

The initial lesion of a tropical ulcer is a bleb filled with sanguineous fluid. It may be painful and itchy with some constitutional upset. Soon the bleb ruptures, and a green-grey moist slough is exposed which rapidly spreads in the skin and subcutaneous tissue up to a diameter of 5 cm or more. In a few days these tissues slough and liquefy releasing an offensive discharge. After about a week there is usually no further spread and the necrotic tissue separates, exposing an ulcer. In a chronic ulcer the edges are raised and slope sharply. The damage may be limited to the skin and superficial fascia, but in severe cases deep structures, e.g. tendons, nerves, blood vessels and periosteum, may be invaded. Bone is rarely affected. Tropical ulcers generally affect the parts of the body exposed to trauma, especially the lower third of the leg and the foot. The ulcer is usually solitary.

General constitutional effects of a tropical ulcer are slight, and adenitis is not found except as a result of secondary infection.

The ulcer heals slowly with a tissue-paper-like scar which breaks down easily. Big ulcers lead to scarring and deformity. Carcinoma (epithelioma) usually of relatively low malignancy sometimes arises in the edge of a chronic tropical ulcer.

Treatment and Prevention. Rest in bed with elevation of the affected part and a generous diet with adequate proteins are important. Local treatment consists in thorough cleansing of the ulcer with hypertonic magnesium sulphate. Procaine penicillin (300 mg i.m.), or tetracycline 2 g daily for 7 days gives good results. In very chronic cases, after cleansing and treatment with antibiotics, excision of the ulcer and scar tissue may be required, to be followed by skin grafting.

Ambulant treatment, with the ulcerative area supported with strips of adhesive plaster, may be effective when rest cannot be enforced. The dressing is changed at intervals of about 5 days.

Where tropical ulcers are a risk, abrasions should be cleansed and covered. The provision of a good diet, washing facilities and a first-aid service have abolished tropical ulcers from labour forces on well-run estates.

Cancrum Oris

Cancrum oris is now rarely observed except in poorly nourished children in the tropics. It is characteristically preceded by an infective illness, especially a severe attack of measles. The pathology is that of a rapidly developing gangrene, beginning inside the mouth and penetrating through the lips and cheek resulting in severe disfigurement. Untreated it frequently causes death. However, with or without treatment, gangrene becomes demarcated and ulceration follows. *Fusobacterium fusiforme* and *Borrelia vincenti* are frequently found in the ulcer.

Penicillin or sulphonamides are highly effective in arresting the disease. The gangrenous areas should be irrigated with saline or a solution of glycothymol and gauze pads soaked in Eusol should be applied to raw surfaces. In the acute stage parenteral fluids, usually including blood are needed. Food and vitamins are best supplied through a nasogastric tube. Subsequently skilled plastic surgery may do much to overcome the hideous defects. Prevention depends on improved nutrition and hygiene in the community and control of acute infectious diseases.

DISEASES DUE TO VIRUSES, CHLAMYDIA AND RICKETTSIAE

1. *Viral: Yellow Fever; Dengue; Sandfly Fever; Kyasanur Forest Disease; Japanese B Encephalitis; Rabies; Lassa Fever; Marburg Disease; Haemorrhagic Fever with Renal Syndrome.*
2. *Chlamydial: Lymphogranuloma Inguinale; Trachoma.*
3. *Rickettsial: Typhus fevers; Q Fever; Rickettsial pox; Trench Fever.*

1. Diseases due to Viruses

In addition to rabies and the cosmopolitan diseases such as poliomyelitis, measles, influenza and smallpox which are transmitted by direct contact, faecal contamination, or by aerosols, there are, in the tropics, a large number of viruses pathogenic to man which are arthropod-borne, known by the abbreviation 'arboviruses'. The majority give rise to a febrile illness of brief duration, following which there is partial or complete immunity against further attacks. Some, in the non-immune, may be neurotropic, giving rise to encephalitis of varying severity. Others, notably yellow fever, may show viscerotropic activity, although it is now recognised that many mild cases of yellow fever occur without appreciable impairment of hepatic or renal function.

On recovery from a viral illness antibodies are demonstrable in the sera. Arboviruses are divided into groups on the basis of their antigenic behaviour.

Group A arboviruses cause Eastern, Western and Venezuelan equine encephalitis; Chikungunya, O'nyong-nyong and Semiliki Forest fevers. All these are conveyed by mosquitoes.

Group B arboviruses cause yellow fever, dengue, Japanese B encephalitis, West Nile, St Louis and Murray Valley fevers conveyed by mosquitoes, and those of Kyasanur Forest disease, diphasic meningoencephalitis, Russian spring-summer fever, louping-ill and Omsk haemorrhagic fever, conveyed by ticks.

Group C arboviruses are limited to South America.

The remaining arboviruses are placed in a number of small groups or are at present ungrouped. Of particular importance are the viruses causing sandfly fever.

There are over 80 arboviruses known to affect man. Within each group viruses produce certain antibodies common to other members of the same group. This is of considerable interest as there is evidence that after several attacks by members of the same group there may be protection against the remainder. This phenomenon may contribute to yellow fever being often mild or subclinical among the indigenous people of an endemic area.

Although the clinical manifestations in an endemic area may be sufficiently characteristic for a fairly reliable diagnosis to be made of such diseases as dengue, sandfly fever and Kyasanur Forest disease, a certain diagnosis rests upon the isolation of the virus in the early stage of the disease by inoculation of laboratory animals or fertile eggs, or by the demonstration of a significant increase in titre of antibodies in sera taken during and after the illness. Moderate increases or the presence of antibodies in a single specimen are not diagnostic of an individual virus since antibodies may be common to a group of viruses.

The accurate elucidation of an infection requires the assistance of a specialised laboratory to which blood and sera should be sent in a thermos flask packed with ice. The identification of the virus may be a laborious and lengthy procedure but may prove to be of extreme importance, as for example, when the outbreak of Kyasanur Forest disease was differentiated from yellow fever.

Prevention of diseases due to arboviruses at present rests mainly on the control of the vectors, but an efficient vaccine against yellow fever is available.

Other viruses than those which are arthropod borne cause rabies, Lassa fever, Marburg disease and haemorrhagic fever with renal syndrome.

Yellow Fever

The arbovirus of yellow fever is transmitted to man by the bite of an infected Aedes mosquito. The virus is in man's blood for 2 days before the onset of fever, for the first 4 days of the fever and exceptionally for longer. The mosquito becomes infective for man 10 to 20 days after ingesting blood containing the virus and remains infective for its life which may be as long as 7 months.

Yellow fever is a human disease but there is a reservoir of infection in primates and other forest animals. In urban areas the vector is *Aedes aegypti* and here it is a disease limited to human beings, the virus being conveyed from man to man by this mosquito. *A. aegypti* breeds in small collections of water in the vicinity of human dwellings. Urban yellow fever is endemic especially in Western and Central Africa, but the areas where it is a risk are much more extensive, stretching from the Atlantic Coast south of the Sahara to the Red Sea and Indian Ocean, and south to Angola and Zambia. Yellow fever is also endemic in the jungles of Panama and South America with the exception of Uruguay and Chile. In forests the virus is conveyed between monkeys by mosquitoes living among the tree tops. Man becomes infected by felling trees and being bitten by the mosquitoes. In Africa monkeys may raid plantations near to forests and *Aedes simpsoni*, present in these rural areas, may become infected by biting the monkeys which are carrying the virus, and later infect man. Life-long immunity is conferred by the disease and babies born to immune mothers are protected for 2 to 4 months. The rarity of overt disease among indigenous people in endemic areas and the results of serological studies suggest that many people acquire immunity from subclinical infections with this and other related arboviruses.

Pathology. The main lesions are found in the liver and kidneys but haemorrhages take place into many organs. If the disease has not been rapidly fatal the tissues will be jaundiced. The liver is often normal in size. Degenerative changes in liver cells are widespread but maximal in the mid-zonal region where fatty degeneration is intense. Usually, 'Councilman bodies', may be seen (p. 439). An acidophilic intranuclear mass also may be detectable, the 'Torres inclusion body'. In addition to haemorrhages under the capsule, the kidney shows the changes of acute tubular necrosis.

Clinical Features. The incubation period is from 3 to 6 days. A mild attack consists of a short fever accompanied by proteinuria, with little or no jaundice. In those who have no prior immunity the classical attack falls into three phases, the initial fever, a period of calm and a subsequent period of reaction or intoxication. In very severe attacks the third stage is reached without the brief apyrexial calm interval. Viral activity ceases at the end of the first stage, the pathology and clinical features of the third stage being the result of hepatic and renal dysfunction which are the usual causes of death in yellow fever. The onset of the fever is sudden, sometimes with a rigor. The fever is highest on the first day and then declines. There are severe supraorbital headaches, backache and pains in bones. The face is flushed, the conjunctivae injected and the tongue is coated and edges are red. The patient becomes prostrated; vomiting may be pronounced and the vomit may contain bile or altered blood. If vomiting persists the prognosis is grave. There is increasing epigastric pain, mental irritability and photophobia. The pulse rate falls more quickly than the temperature, and bradycardia is marked by the third day. This disproportion between pulse and temperature is very characteristic. There is a persistent leucopenia. The urine contains protein in increasing quantities and, later, casts appear and the volume of urine decreases. At the end of four days the temperature reaches normal and the second stage, the period of calm, is reached. Recovery may now take place without further fever.

In more serious cases the third stage, the period of intoxication, follows after a few hours, the temperature rising but the pulse still remaining slow. Jaundice becomes pronounced and the liver palpable and tender. The urine contains bilirubin and red cell casts. There is bleeding, sometimes profuse, from gums, nose, stomach, intestine and urinary tract; petechiae, conjunctival haemorrhages and ecchymoses in the skin may appear. The patient remains mentally clear and anxious until near death, which is only briefly preceded by coma. The pulse rate increases rapidly in the late stages. In fulminating infections the patient dies within a few days of the onset. Death rarely occurs in those who survive for 12 days. In some outbreaks meningo-encephalitis has been a prominent feature. In non-fatal cases convalescence is without incident and there is no residual detectable damage to the kidneys, liver or heart.

Diagnosis. In an endemic area fever, leucopenia and proteinuria with or without jaundice should suggest the possibility of yellow fever. Blood, sent in the early stages to a laboratory equipped to investigate viruses, may yield the virus, and tests on sera taken early and late will show the presence of increasing antibodies. These results will only be of value in making a retrospective diagnosis, which is, however, important on public health grounds. Similarly the establishing of the cause of death by histological examination of the liver may be of the utmost importance. The disease is notifiable under the International Health Regulations.

Treatment. There is no specific antiviral agent. The patient should be nursed under a mosquito net for the first 4 days of the illness because the blood is infectious. When vomiting is troublesome dehydration should be corrected by intravenous glucose saline and blood transfusions should be given if blood loss is severe. Acute renal failure is treated as described on page 496.

Prevention. A single vaccination with the 17 D nonpathogenic strain of virus, available at internationally recognised centres, gives full protection for at least 10 years, the period of validity of the vaccination certificate. Ten days after vaccination adequate antibodies are present in the blood and the certificate of vaccination becomes valid. The vaccine does not produce appreciable side-effects in adults, unless they are allergic to egg protein, when desensitisation may be necessary. There is a slight risk of encephalitis following the vaccination of young children; so, if at all possible, vaccination should not be carried out in infants under 9 months of age. When vaccination against both yellow fever and smallpox is required, that for yellow fever should precede smallpox vaccination by at least 21 days, but in an emergency both may be given at the same time in opposite arms. No ill-effects have as yet been observed from vaccination during pregnancy.

Only travellers possessing valid certificates of vaccination against yellow fever are allowed to proceed from an endemic area to 'receptive areas', by which is meant countries free from the disease but in which the potential vectors exist. In this way the disease has not yet entered Asia. As an additional precaution mosquito control of airports should be maintained. The urban disease can be eradicated by the abolition of the breeding places of *Aedes aegypti*, by the use of residual insecticides in houses and by mass vaccination in endemic areas. If susceptible mosquitoes are present and the virus persists in animals in adjacent forests there remains a risk of an outbreak of yellow fever among the unvaccinated.

Dengue

Six antigenic variants of the dengue arbovirus have been described. It is transmitted to man chiefly by the mosquito *Aedes aegypti*, but other species of this genus are also vectors. Man is infective to the vector 18 hours before the temperature rises and for at least 3 days after the onset of symptoms. The mosquito can transmit the disease 8 to 12 days after feeding on a patient suffering from dengue and remains infective for life.

The disease is a risk in many tropical and subtropical countries, especially in coastal areas. It is most prevalent during the hot season when the mosquitoes are numerous. One attack usually gives immunity for about 9 months and after several attacks a considerable degree of permanent immunity is attained. Some cross-immunity exists between dengue and other members of the B group of arboviruses, including the virus of yellow fever.

Clinical Features. The incubation period is usually 5 to 6 days. The disease varies considerably in its clinical severity. It may be a sharp illness with marked constitutional symptoms and signs lasting for 7 to 10 days or a milder disease resembling sandfly fever. A prodrome of malaise and headache for 2 days may precede the acute onset, characterised by fever and intense generalised aches and pains especially severe in the orbital and periarticular areas. Painful movement of the eyes, photophobia, conjunctival injection and lachrymation, nausea, vomiting, anorexia, prostration, insomnia and depression are often features of the disease. In severe cases the temperature may remain elevated for 7 to 8 days. An afebrile interval lasting 24 to 48 hours may intervene at the end of the third day when symptoms subside temporarily, to be followed with a recurrence of symptoms and a further febrile period of a day or two ('saddleback fever'). The pulse rate is often slow compared with the temperature, and bradycardia may continue well into convalescence. Groups of superficial lymph nodes, usually the cervical, may be enlarged. Leucopenia is present throughout the illness.

A rash may appear, especially during the second febrile period. It is morbilliform but the colour resembles that of scarlet fever. It usually begins on the dorsum of the hands and feet and spreads up the arms and thighs to the trunk. After the temperature has fallen, depression and prostration often persist.

Since 1956 there has been a series of outbreaks of dengue in South-East Asia, sometimes in association with the Chikungunya virus, in which the disease has been complicated by shock and haemorrhage, with a variable mortality among indigenous children, but reaching 10 per cent of those ill enough to be admitted to hospital. The condition is sometimes called dengue haemorrhagic fever. Disseminated intravascular coagulation and complement activation which leads to vascular damage are thought to be triggered by hypersensitivity to the virus.

Diagnosis. This is usually easy in an endemic area when a patient has the characteristic symptoms and signs. However, mild cases may resemble other viral diseases and a severe attack may be mistaken for anicteric yellow fever, but the absence of urinary changes will help to differentiate it. The virus can be recovered from the blood or its presence inferred from a rising titre of antibody.

Treatment and Prevention. There is no specific treatment. The severe pains can be relieved by aspirin or paracetamol, but occasionally opiates are required. Blood transfusions and corticosteroids are indicated in the haemorrhagic varieties.

The patient is nursed under a mosquito net. Breeding places of Aedes mosquitoes should be abolished and the adults destroyed by insecticides (p. 879).

Sandfly Fever

This fever is caused by a small group of closely related arboviruses transmitted by the sandfly *Phlebotomus papatasii* and by other species of this genus. No animal reservoir is known. Man is infective to the vector for 24 hours before and for 24 hours after the onset of the fever. The sandfly can transmit the disease about 7 days after biting an infected person and remains infective for life.

This infection is endemic around the Mediterranean and eastwards into India, Burma and China, especially during the hot dry season. One attack confers immunity for only a few months, so repeated reinfections are necessary to maintain protection. There is no cross-immunity between dengue and sandfly fever.

Clinical Features. After an incubation period, usually of 3 to 4 days, the onset is sudden with a rapid rise of temperature. The symptoms and signs are very similar to those of dengue (p. 879). The fever, however, is usually of shorter duration, up to 3 days, and there is no rash.

In an endemic area the general course of the illness suggests the diagnosis, but a blood film should always be examined to exclude malaria. The virus can be recovered from the blood and antibodies detected.

Treatment and Prevention. Treatment is on the same lines as for dengue.
Sandflies are extremely sensitive to insecticides and combined with the use of repellants useful protection is obtained. The ordinary mosquito net sprayed with an insecticide will keep out the tiny sandfly.

Kyasanur Forest Disease

The arbovirus responsible for this disease, caused a fatal epizootic in monkeys in the Shimogo district of Mysore State. It has been shown by immunological tests to affect about 10 per cent of the rural human population in that area. The vectors are Ixodid ticks increased numbers of which had been introduced by the grazing of cattle in the area. This disease, first encountered in 1957, is of great interest as it was at first feared to be an outbreak of yellow fever in Asia and illustrates how changing pastoral activities may lead to unexpected outbreaks of human disease.
The chief pathological lesions are found in the liver and kidneys.

Clinical Features. The disease in man may be mild with only a short febrile attack or it may be a severe illness with fever lasting for over a week with great prostration and generalised pains in muscles. Mucosal surfaces may bleed. Some patients may relapse after 9 to 21 days when fever, jaundice and signs of meningeal irritation may ensue. In fatal cases death is usually due to liver failure.

Treatment and Protection. The patient requires careful nursing; no specific treatment is known. A prophylactic vaccine has been prepared.

Japanese B Encephalitis

This arbovirus is transmitted to man by the bites of infected culicine mosquitoes which have fed on infected animals or birds, notably nestling herons. Pigs and other domestic animals are important sources of infection acting chiefly as amplifiers of the virus brought to them by mosquitoes. The virus is widespread in the Pacific Islands from Japan to Guam, in the Philippines, Taiwan, Borneo, Malaysia and Singapore. In endemic areas, although serological surveys indicate a high incidence of subclinical infection, only sporadic cases may be encountered. Nevertheless, devastating epidemics, with a high mortality rate, have occurred.
Inflammatory and degenerative changes are found in the brain.

Clinical Features. Many infections are subclinical but overt disease may occur at any age, although children are particularly susceptible. With the development of encephalitis the patient experiences a very severe headache, fever, often with rigors, and vomiting. The physical signs are those of meningoencephalitis, namely, neck rigidity, congestion of the optic fundi, imperfectly reacting pupils, muscular twitching and tremors; and, in severe cases, progressive coma, muscular rigidity and cranial nerve palsies. In some cases only signs of meningitis are present. The cerebrospinal fluid is under raised pressure and an increase of cells and protein appears within several days. The acute illness may last from a few days to 2 weeks or longer. Convalescence is prolonged and tedious. Persistent neurological damage is a feature only in children and after prolonged illness in adults. The mortality rate in overt disease varies from 15 to 40 per cent.
The virus has only rarely been recovered from the blood or cerebrospinal fluid

but in fatal cases may sometimes be obtained from the brain. Increasing titres of specific antibodies in the blood is the usual basis for diagnosis.

Treatment and Prevention. There is no specific treatment and the value of corticosteroids has not yet been established. Skilled nursing and aids for the patient in coma, may be life-saving.

The elimination of breeding places of the vector mosquitoes, the control of piggeries, and the use of insecticides, where practicable, should be instituted. There is no effective vaccine or other antiviral agent available.

Rabies

This dread disease was recognised by Aristotle in 300 B.C. and was described by Celsus and Galen. In 1885 Pasteur achieved the triumph of protecting a boy, Albert Meister, by administering a vaccine. Meister subsequently served as janitor at the Pasteur Institute until the German occupation in 1940. Rabies is caused by a bullet-shaped member of the rhabdoviruses. The virus, which causes an encephalitis, affects a wide range of animals and is conveyed by bites and licks on abrasions or on intact mucous membranes. Transmission by aerosols in confined spaces has also been demonstrated. In Europe the maintenance host is the fox and in recent years the disease has spread from Poland westwards through Germany and has progressively penetrated through France. Man is most frequently infected from dogs but cats and other animals may be responsible. In the U.S.A. skunks are an important host and may infect man, while in Central and South America vampire bats also cause death of domestic animals and occasionally man. Insectivorous bats only rarely convey the infection.

Clinical Features. The incubation period, during which the virus is spreading centripetally along axons to the brain, varies in man from a minimum of 9 days to many months but is usually between 4 and 8 weeks. Severe bites, especially if on the head or neck, are associated with short incubation periods. Although only a proportion of people inoculated with the virus develop the disease, once it is manifest it is almost invariably fatal. At the onset there may be insidious fever and a return of pain or paraesthesia at the site of the bite. After a prodromal period of from 1 to 10 days, during which anxiety may be increasingly evident, the characteristic fear of water, responsible for the alternative name of 'hydrophobia', becomes evident in many cases. Although thirsty, attempts at drinking provoke violent contractions of the diaphragm and other inspiratory muscles and thereafter the sight or even the sound of water may precipitate these distressing spasms and attacks of fear. Delusions and hallucinations may develop accompanied by spitting, biting and maniacal behaviour, with lucid intervals in which the patient is acutely anxious. Sedatives may considerably modify this ordeal. Cranial nerve lesions, such as are common to other forms of encephalitis, may be evident and hyperpyrexia frequently develops. Death ensues, usually within a week from the onset of symptoms.

In a small proportion of cases there is an ascending paralysis without mental excitement and these patients survive, on average, 12 days. This type is particularly associated with bites from vampire bats.

Diagnosis. During life the diagnosis is usually made solely on clinical grounds but rapid immunofluorescent techniques of corneal impression smears or skin biopsies and isolation of the virus have been successfully employed.

Treatment. Two cases of probable rabies treated by tracheostomy and modern methods of maintained respiration have survived but usually only palliative treatment is possible once symptoms have appeared. The patient should be sedated with diazepam 10 mg 4–6 hourly, supplemented by chlorpromazine 50–100 mg, if necessary. A gastrostomy is the kindest way to give fluids and food. Particularly if there is doubt as to the diagnosis or if the patient has previously received a course of prophylactic vaccine the possibility of recovery should be entertained.

Prevention. Initially the wound caused by the bite should be thoroughly cleansed, preferably with an ammonium detergent, and surgical debridement should be carried out but tight stitching should be avoided. Rabies can usually be prevented if the subject is treated early in the incubation period. In order to ascertain if the person is at risk it is important, if possible, not to kill a suspected animal but to keep it under observation in isolation under restraint. A rabid dog will usually die within 5 days; if it survives for 10 days it was almost certainly not infective at the time of isolation. If it dies, a positive immunofluorescence test or the demonstration of Negri bodies in its brain confirms the diagnosis. Human saliva may contain the virus, therefore those attending the patient may be at risk, although interhuman spread is very rare.

To obtain maximum protection, particularly after severe bites, it is necessary to give hyperimmune animal serum 40 i.u./kg body weight intramuscularly and, if possible, an equal amount infiltrated around the wound. Human antirabies immunoglobulin 20 i.u./kg similarly administered is preferable, if it is available. Ideally the serum should be given within 48 hours of the bite, but it may still be of value up to 2 weeks later. Concomitantly, a course of antirabies vaccine must be started. The Semple-type vaccine, containing the killed virus, is potent and still the most readily available effective vaccine. Its use is, however, associated with a risk of a serious neuroparalytic disorder among 1 in 1,600 recipients. It is for this reason that the vaccine should be given only if there is a real risk of rabies and the vaccine should be stopped if the suspected dog survives. The vaccine is given subcutaneously in the anterior abdominal wall, 5 ml daily for 14 days, with booster doses at 10, 20 and 90 days subsequently.

A duck egg vaccine carries a much reduced risk of neuroparalysis (1 in 30,000 recipients) but it is less reliably potent. It may be indicated if the antibody response can be measured and for booster doses. Recently a vaccine has been developed containing killed virus cultivated in human diploid cells; it has the advantage of freedom from neural elements and may be administered in doses of 0·1 ml intradermally. Duck egg and human diploid vaccines are of use in protecting veterinarians and others at risk prior to known exposure to the virus.

During the administration of the Semple-type and duck egg vaccines antihistamines may reduce local tissue reactions. A systemic reaction may herald a neuroparalytic disorder. The vaccine should be stopped, unless the risk of rabies is very great, and corticosteroids given; they appear to ameliorate the neurological reaction which may otherwise take the form of an ascending paralysis, an encephalomyelitis or a polyradiculoneuritis of varying degree.

Human rabies is an infrequent disease even in endemic areas. Its fearful manifestations, however, justify stringent attempts being made to prevent its spread. In endemic areas household dogs should have a yearly dose of a Flury canine (live) vaccine. Importation of all animals into uninfected countries, such as Britain, should be strictly controlled, with isolation of dogs in quarantine kennels for a minimum of 6 months. Vigilance and appropriate measures of control over infected maintenance hosts, such as the fox, are urgently required where areas of endemicity are extending.

Further reading about rabies:

Symposium on Rabies (1976) *Transactions of the Royal Society of Tropical Medicine and Hygiene*, **70**, 175–205.
WHO Expert Committee on Rabies (1973) *Technical Report Series*. World Health Organization, **523**, 6th report.

Lassa Fever

This disease, first observed in 1969, is now known to be due to an arenavirus (containing RNA), a group which also includes the viruses responsible for Argentine and Bolivian haemorrhagic fevers. Recognised outbreaks have so far been limited to West Africa, including Nigeria, Liberia and Sierra Leone. The mode of spread is unknown but case to case transmission in hospital and the presence of the virus in the pharynx and urine is consistent with inhalation of aerosols or infection through abrasions. A reservoir of infection has been demonstrated in rodents by isolation of the virus.

Clinical Features. The disease has the general features of a viral infection, high fever, intercostal myalgia, bradycardia, a low blood pressure and leucopenia. Adherent yellow exudates on the pharynx are particularly characteristic. The fever lasts between 7 and 17 days. In severe cases shock and electrolyte imbalance develop. Mortality rates of overt infections have varied from 36 per cent to 52 per cent but mild and subclinical infections also occur.

The virus has been isolated in special laboratories from serum, pharynx, pleural exudate and urine but diagnosis will usually be established from 'paired sera', the later specimens being taken 6–8 weeks after the onset of infection.

Treatment and Prevention. Isolation and general supportive measures, preferably in an intensive care unit, are required. There is no proved specific therapeutic measure. The administration of convalescent immune plasma has been followed by recovery and is therefore recommended for prophylaxis after accidental exposure to infection.

Marburg Disease

In Marburg, West Germany, in 1967 a severe infectious illness broke out among laboratory workers who had handled tissues from a batch of green monkeys imported from Uganda. The causative agent is a virus, as yet unclassified. In 1976 outbreaks of the disease occurred in Sudan and Zaïre. The natural reservoir of the disease is not known nor is its usual mode of spread, but man-to-man transmission can take place. In these outbreaks the mortality has varied from 25 per cent of treated patients to over 90 per cent in the untreated, but successive human passage seems to reduce virulence.

After an incubation period of 5 to 9 days, the illness presents suddenly with fever, severe myalgia and diarrhoea. By the fourth or fifth day the fauces become inflamed and a bright red, follicular rash appears on the extensor surfaces of the limbs; it spreads to the trunk and face, becomes maculopapular and finally confluent and livid. There may be lymphadenopathy. About the sixth day, in severe cases, bleeding associated with thrombocytopenia starts usually in the gastrointestinal tract. The virus also attacks the brain, kidneys and lungs. Fatal complications, often between the sixth and tenth days of the illness, include haemorrhage, secondary infection, encephalitis, renal failure and pneumonia.

Treatment consists of supportive measures, replacement of blood and the management of complications. Immune plasma may be beneficial if given at an early stage. No vaccine is available.

Haemorrhagic Fever with Renal Syndrome

This disease, formerly called epidemic haemorrhagic fever, is attributable to a virus, although confirmation of its successful isolation is still awaited. Outbreaks occurred in Manchuria and Korea and it, or a similar disease, has been reported from Scandinavia and Soviet Russia. There is a close association with small mammals, in particular bank voles, and it has been established that man becomes infected by aerosols without the intervention of an arthropod vector.

The main changes arise from increased capillary fragility. Thus there are widespread internal haemorrhages and escape into the tissues of fluid rich in protein.

Clinical Features. After an incubation period of 12 to 16 days there is a sudden onset of high fever. After about 5 days the temperature falls, and the second or toxic stage begins; haemorrhages now take place into the skin and from mucous membranes. The urine contains red cells, casts and a large amount of protein. Anuria may threaten. The leucocyte count, low in the early stages, is now much increased, at first with primitive granulocytes and later with primitive lymphocytes, the picture resembling that of leukaemia. The platelet count is diminished and there is a prolonged bleeding time. Death may ensue in this stage but in favourable cases convalescence begins towards the end of the second week, with a plentiful flow of urine of low specific gravity, free from protein and casts. This polyuria may continue for some months. Full recovery is usual but very slow.

In an endemic area the diagnosis is suggested by the characteristic clinical signs and the successive changes in the blood.

Treatment. The disease is managed symptomatically. Oliguria and anuria are treated as advised for acute renal failure (p. 496).

2. Diseases due to Chlamydia

Lymphogranuloma Inguinale

Lymphogranuloma inguinale (venereum) is caused by a member of the *Chlamydia* group which also include the causative organisms of psittacosis-ornithosis and trachoma (p. 886). The disease is venereal and is widely distributed in the tropics, especially in seaports.

Pathology. The primary herpetiform lesion is small and very superficial. The infection passes from the primary lesion to the regional lymph nodes and there causes proliferation of monocytes and lymphocytes and giant-cell formation at numerous foci within the nodes. Untreated, these foci necrose to form multiple small abscesses. Associated with these changes there is a marked connective tissue proliferation in and around the lymph nodes.

Clinical Features. An evanescent genital lesion appears 1 to 4 weeks after infection. The adjacent lymph nodes enlarge. A single node on one side of the groin is usually affected first, but soon other nodes become inflamed and matted together. The infection may spread to the other groin and occasionally to the pelvic lymph nodes. The affected nodes are tender, and adhere to the underlying tissues and to the overlying shiny purplish inflamed skin. Enlargement of the lymph nodes above and below the unyielding inguinal ligament produces the characteristic 'groove sign'. Thick glairy fluid is eventually discharged through the skin by numerous small sinuses. Healing is very slow and often associated with marked scarring.

Sinus formation from pelvic lymph nodes damages surrounding structures with extremely serious and disabling results. Fistulae may form between the rectum, vagina and urethra, and ulcerative proctitis may cause stricture of the rectum. In the female obstruction to the lymphatics may lead to elephantiasis of the external genitalia, a condition called 'esthiomene'. Associated with the adenitis there may be fever, prostration and loss of weight.

Diagnosis. Antigen for the intradermal 'Frei' test, marketed as Lygranum, is a suspension of the organisms grown on the yolk-sac of the chick embryo. In a positive case 24 hours after an intradermal injection of $0 \cdot 1$ ml antigen, a papule exceeding 6 mm in diameter will develop and usually persist for 2 to 3 weeks. The same antigen can be used for the complement-fixation test. Both these tests are positive within 2 to 6 weeks of the development of the adenitis and remain positive for years. There are cross-reactions with ornithosis and trachoma.

Treatment. Rest in bed is important. Many cases respond well to 4 g sulphadimidine daily in divided doses for 14 days. Alternatively tetracycline 2 g daily for 14 days may be used.

Inguinal nodes may require aspiration but should not be incised. When extensive sinuses have formed, complete excision of the mass of inguinal nodes may be required. Severe pelvic complications and rectal stricture require surgery.

Trachoma

Trachoma, recognised since the time of Ancient Greece and Egypt, is a specific communicable keratoconjunctivitis, usually of chronic evolution, caused by an agent belonging to the *Chlamydia* group, and characterised by follicles, papillary hyperplasia, pannus and, in its later stages, cicatrisation. The infecting microorganism is named the trachoma and inclusion conjunctivitis (TRIC) agent. In endemic areas young children are particularly vulnerable to infection. Transmission is usually by contact or from fomites in unhygienic surroundings and some infections occur during birth from the infected genital passages.

Vast numbers of people suffer from trachoma in the hot dry dusty areas of the subtropics and tropics but it is also present in Southern Europe, and among immigrants in Britain. The disease varies markedly in incidence and in severity in different geographical areas.

Pathology. The infection lasts for years and may be latent over long periods. Recrudescence may result from secondary bacterial infection or from reinfection by the agent itself. The conjunctiva of the upper lid is first affected with combined vascularisation and cellular infiltration, pannus, spreading to the upper cornea and later to other areas producing corneal opacity and impairment of vision. Cicatricial deformity of the upper tarsal plate is an early feature. Entropion, trichiasis, ectropion and corneal scarring are late results.

Clinical Features. The onset is usually insidious and infection may not be apparent to the patient. Early symptoms of conjunctival irritation or smarting may be ignored. Watering, stickiness and blepharospasm may be noticed. In underdeveloped areas, unless discovered on surveys, the condition may not be reported until vision begins to fail.

The ophthalmic appearances are described in 4 stages (WHO):

Stage I. Immature follicles are seen on the upper tarsal conjunctiva including the central area and early corneal changes are usually present.

Stage II. Well developed mature soft follicles are present with papillary hyperplasia. Pannus and corneal infiltrates extend from the upper limbus.

Stage III. Some or all of the signs of stage II exist with scarring developing, usually from necrosis of follicles.

Stage IV. The follicles and infiltrates of stage III have been replaced by scar tissue and the disease is no longer infectious although further changes in the scars may follow. The degree of scarring varies from minimal involvement to trichiasis, entropion, corneal opacities and gross impairment of vision.

Trachoma may also present as an acute ophthalmia neonatorum with secondary bacterial infection.

Diagnosis. Differentiation from inclusion conjunctivitis (blenorrhoea) may be clinically impossible, and in some countries no clear separation can be made. The conjunctivitis of adenovirus, herpes virus and Newcastle disease may closely resemble trachoma. Clinically an early ptosis due to deformity of the upper tarsal plate and appreciation of the characteristic follicular conjunctivitis on eversion of the lids may be helpful. Vascularity and cellular infiltration may be seen using the slit lamp before being visible to the naked eye. Intracellular inclusion particles (Halberstaedter-Prowazek bodies) are demonstrated in conjunctival scrapings by iodine or immunofluorescent staining. TRIC agent may be isolated in the developing chick embryo or in cell culture.

Treatment and Prevention. Local ophthalmic ointment or oily drops of 1–3 per cent tetracycline may be used twice daily for 3 months. In mass therapy in endemic areas such topical application twice daily for 3 to 6 consecutive days each month for 6 months has given good results. An oral sulphonamide, daily for 3 weeks is a useful addition to treatment. Deformity and scarring of the lids, corneal opacities, ulceration and scarring require surgical treatment, after control of local infection.

Personal and family cleanliness should be improved. Proper care of the eyes of newborn and of young children is essential. The finding of a case, particularly in a child, should lead to examination of the whole family. Population surveys should lead to discovery and treatment of asymptomatic infections. Trachoma clinics are required in highly endemic areas.

3. Diseases due to Rickettsiae

Rickettsiae are natural inhabitants of the cells of the intestinal canal of arthropods. Some species may parasitise higher mammals including man. Rickettsiae are intermediate between viruses and bacteria and require living cells for their multiplication. Infection is usually conveyed to man through the skin from excreta of the arthropods but in some biting vectors saliva is infected. Transovarian infection in arthropods to the next generation occurs except with *R. prowazeki* and *R. mooseri*, the causes respectively of louse- and flea-borne typhus. The Weil-Felix reaction, which is the non-specific agglutination by the patient's serum of the strains of organisms Proteus OX 19 or OXK, helps in the differentiation of human infections (Table 17.2).

Table 17.2 Weil-Felix reaction

Disease	Vector	Weil-Felix Reaction	
		OX 19	OXK
Epidemic typhus	Louse	+++	negative
Endemic typhus	Flea from rat	+++	negative
Rocky Mountain spotted fever	Tick	+	negative
Other forms of tick typhus	Tick	+	variable
Scrub typhus	Larval mite	negative	+++
Q (Query) fever	None or tick	negative	negative
Rickettsialpox	Mite from mouse	negative	negative
Trench fever	Louse	negative	negative

Although rickettsialpox and trench fever have not been found in the tropics they are included here to complete the group.

Pathological and Clinical Features. Rickettsiae are characteristically parasites of the vascular endothelium, especially of capillaries and other small vessels, producing lesions in the skin, central nervous system, heart, lungs, kidneys and skeletal muscles. Endothelial proliferation, associated with a perivascular reaction (nodules of Fraenkel) may cause thromboses and small haemorrhages. In epidemic typhus the brain and in scrub typhus the cardiovascular system and lungs are particularly attacked.

The rash in epidemic, endemic and scrub typhus is at first central, but in tick typhus it starts peripherally. In Q fever only a sparse rash is occasionally seen. An eschar often shows the site of the bite in tick and scrub typhus and in rickettsialpox, but not in epidemic and endemic typhus or in Q fever.

The common clinical findings in this group of diseases are fever, severe prostration, mental disturbance and often a rash. The diagnosis can be established by the Weil-Felix reaction in epidemic, endemic and scrub typhus and by complement-fixation and agglutination tests using antigen from the specific *Rickettsiae* in all infections. *Rickettsiae* can be isolated in specialised laboratories by inoculation of laboratory animals or fertile eggs.

Epidemic Typhus Fever

Louse-borne or epidemic typhus is caused by *R. prowazeki* and is transmitted by infected faeces from the louse of man, usually through scratching the skin, or sometimes by inhalation. Patients suffering from epidemic typhus infect the lice, and these leave the patient if he is febrile. In conditions of overcrowding the disease may spread rapidly. During interepidemic periods the disease may be maintained by inapparent or latent cases ('*Brill's disease*') or perhaps by infected fleas and rats.

Clinical Features. The incubation period is usually 12 to 14 days. There may be a few days of malaise but the onset is more often sudden with rigors, frontal headaches and pains in the back and limbs. The temperature rises for 2 or 3 days, constipation is constant, and bronchitis usually distressing. The face is flushed and cyanotic, eyes congested, and the patient soon becomes dull and confused.

The rash appears on the fourth to the sixth day and often resembles measles. In its early stages it disappears on pressure but soon becomes petechial with subcutaneous mottling. It appears first on the anterior folds of the axillae, sides of the abdomen or back of hands, thence on the trunk and forearms. The neck and face are seldom affected.

During the second week symptoms increase in severity. Sordes collect on the lips, and the tongue, dry and brown, becomes shrunken and tremulous. The spleen becomes palpable, the pulse feeble and the patient stuporous and delirious. If the patient recovers, the temperature falls rapidly at the end of the second week and convalescence ensues. In fatal cases the patient usually dies in the second week from general toxaemia, cardiac or renal failure or pneumonia.

Common complications are bronchopneumonia, parotitis, venous thrombosis and gangrene. In endemic areas, e.g. Ethiopia, indigenous people may suffer relatively mildly.

Diagnosis. The clinical features may be almost diagnostic especially when there is an epidemic of the disease. In mild cases of the disease, however, clinical symptoms and signs may be much less distinctive. In the Weil-Felix test agglutination of Proteus OX 19 over 1/200 is usual after the seventh day; a rising titre is of particular diagnostic value. The complement-fixation test with a killed suspension of *R. prowazeki* gives reliable results and differentiates it from flea-borne typhus.

Treatment. This is described on page 892.

Endemic Typhus Fever

Flea-borne or 'endemic' typhus is caused by *R. mooseri*. Man is infected when, by scratching, he introduces the faeces or contents of a crushed flea which has fed on an infected rat. Deaths are rare in human infections, so morbid changes have not been studied in detail.

The incubation period is 8 to 14 days. The symptoms resemble those of a mild louse-borne typhus. The rash may be scanty and transient.

The Weil-Felix OX 19 is positive as in louse-borne typhus and the specific complement-fixation test using *R. mooseri* antigen is positive by the ninth day.

Tick-borne Typhus Fevers

ROCKY MOUNTAIN SPOTTED FEVER

The causal organism, *R. rickettsi*, transferred by the bite of ticks, carries disease to rodents and dogs and on occasion to man when brought into contact with these animals. It is widely distributed in western and south-eastern States of the U.S.A. and also in South America.

The vascular changes are similar to those in epidemic typhus. In addition, haemorrhages and gangrene of the genitalia, ears and digits sometimes occur and there may be bronchopneumonia and enlargement of the spleen and liver.

Clinical Features. The incubation period is about 7 days. There may be an eschar at the site of the bite, with enlargement of the regional lymph nodes. Symptoms closely resemble those of louse-borne typhus. The rash appears about the third or fourth day, at first like measles, but in a few hours the typical maculopapular eruption appears. Each day it becomes more distinct and papular and finally petechial. The rash first appears on the wrists, forearms and ankles, spreads in 24 to 48 hours to the back, limbs and chest and lastly to the abdomen where it is least pronounced. The fully developed rash often affects also the palms, soles and face. Petechiae may appear in crops. Cutaneous and subcutaneous haemorrhages of considerable size may appear in severe cases. Complications are as in louse-borne typhus. Untreated, the course of the disease may be mild or rapidly fatal.

Diagnosis. There may be a history of a bite by a tick. The character of the rash, appearing first at the periphery, is helpful. The rickettsiae can be isolated from the blood (p. 888). The Weil-Felix reaction is not of much help. Agglutination and complement-fixation tests using *R. rickettsi* antigen are positive in the second week.

Treatment. This is described on page 892.

OTHER FORMS OF TICK-BORNE TYPHUS FEVER

The causal agents of African tick-borne typhus are *R. conori* and a substrain *R. conori pijperi*. They cause typhus in South and East Africa, the reservoir hosts being dogs and rodents. 'Fièvre boutonneuse' of the Mediterranean is similar, as is also the infection in Queensland where *R. australis* is the causal organism. Infected ticks may be picked up by walking on grasslands or dogs may bring the ticks into the house. An eschar and lymphadenitis are usual. A maculopapular rash may cover the trunk and limbs and affects the palms and soles. There may be delirium and meningeal signs in severe infections but recovery is the rule except in the debilitated. There are no haemorrhages into the skin. Positive results are obtained in the Weil-Felix test in the majority of cases but may be only to a low titre.

Scrub Typhus Fever

Mite-borne or 'scrub' typhus is caused by *R. tsutsugamushi* transmitted by the bite of infective larval mites, such as *Leptotrombidium* (*Leptotrombidium*) *akamushi* and *L.* (*L.*) *deliense*. It occurs in the Far East, Assam, Burma, Pakistan, India, Indonesia, S. Pacific Islands and Queensland.

Pathological and Clinical Features. The pathology is similar to that of louse-borne typhus, but lesions in the lungs are more prominent. A primary eschar shows mononuclear infiltration, vasculitis, and epidermal necrosis.

The incubation period is about 9 days. In most cases an eschar, starting as a small papule, becomes a small rounded or oval ulcer up to 10 mm in diameter surrounded by a red indurated area. Multiple eschars are common. The associated lymph nodes are often enlarged.

The onset of symptoms is usually sudden with headache, often retro-orbital, fever, malaise, weakness and cough, occasionally with diarrhoea. The conjunctivae become injected. In severe cases the general symptoms increase, with apathy and prostration. A rash often appears on about the fifth to the seventh day, as reddish macules on the front and back of the chest and on the abdominal wall. In 24 hours it becomes a maculopapular rash which soon appears on the face, neck, arms, palms, legs and soles and fades by the fourteenth day. The temperature rises rapidly and continues as a remittent fever with sweating until it falls by lysis about the twelfth to the eighteenth day. The fever and rash are frequently associated with generalised enlargement of lymph nodes which are firm, elastic, discrete and painless.

Cough and headaches are troublesome and mental change may be striking. By the tenth day the patient is prostrate, lethargic and querulous, distressed by cough and often deaf. The pulse, slow at first, becomes rapid in severe cases, and peripheral circulatory failure frequently precedes death. There are often signs of pneumonia. The sputum may be frothy and streaked with blood. Radiological changes in the lungs, when present, are similar to those found in viral pneumonia. In patients progressing to recovery the temperature falls by lysis, but convalescence is often slow and tachycardia may persist for some weeks.

Diagnosis. In endemic areas diagnosis is often possible on the clinical findings of fever, severe headache and congested conjunctivae. An eschar, rash, enlarged lymph nodes and mental changes give further assistance.

Isolation of rickettsiae by intraperitoneal inoculation of blood into mice during the first week is diagnostic. The Weil-Felix reaction with Proteus OXK starts after the seventh day and reaches a maximum 2 weeks later. Complement-fixation and agglutination tests using *R. tsutsugamushi* antigen are positive after the second week.

Treatment. This is described on page 892.

Q (Query) Fever

This disease occurs throughout the world and its causative organism, *Coxiella burneti*, differs sufficiently from other rickettsiae to be placed in a separate genus. Ticks of several genera are vectors and these convey the infection to many wild animals and to large domestic animals. These organisms are resistant to drying and so lend themselves to dissemination by air. Man becomes infected by inhaling or ingesting infected dust, rarely, if ever, by the bite of a tick. Dried genital discharges, milk and urine from infected animals appear to be important sources of infection amongst meat handlers and agricultural workers. Infected straw and other packing material have also been incriminated. Infections have been acquired in laboratory and autopsy rooms.

Clinical Features. The incubation period is 7 to 14 days. The onset is sudden with fever, sweating and malaise, cough, retro-orbital pain and anorexia. The temperature rises from 39° to 40·5°C with daily remissions, to fall to normal after 4 to 15 days. The pulse is slow, prostration often marked, and a cough is often present about the fifth or sixth day with scanty sputum, occasionally bloodstained. Pains in the chest are frequent, but physical signs are minimal. The spleen is sometimes palpable and occasionally a sparse rash is present. Radiographs usually show patchy homogeneous ground-glass areas of consolidation, single or multiple, usually towards the base of the lungs. These usually resolve in about 10 days. With the fall of temperature convalescence is usually rapid and complete. Hepatitis, encephalitis, myocarditis and persistent endocarditis (p. 207) are rare complications.

Diagnosis. The clinical symptoms resemble those of viral pneumonia or of septicaemia. The Weil-Felix test is negative but, with a specific antigen from *C. burneti*, antibodies can be demonstrated in the second week and are maximal in the fifth or sixth week. The organisms can be recovered from the blood.

Treatment. This is described below.

Rickettsialpox

This disease is due to *R. akari*, transmitted from the domestic mouse by a mite. It appears to be restricted to New York and Philadelphia where mice are now adapted to live in communal rubbish chutes of apartment houses.

The first lesion starts as a deep-seated papule which gradually enlarges to form a rounded or oval vesicle. This eventually shrinks to a black eschar which separates after 1 to 2 weeks. The regional lymph nodes are usually enlarged. About a week after the appearance of the first lesion fever, sweating and backache begin quite suddenly and continue for about a week. The typical rash appears within the first 4 days of the fever. The lesions are red maculopapules later forming vesicles at their centres. They soon dry to form black crusts which are shed after a few days leaving no permanent scars. There is no special site for the lesions, but they avoid the palms and soles. The patient is never seriously ill.

The rickettsiae can be isolated from the blood during the acute stage. The complement-fixation test with *R. akari* is positive.

Trench Fever

Trench fever is caused by *R. quintana* and is spread to man by louse faeces. It was prevalent in the First World War in the trenches when troops were verminous and again in the Second World War in the USSR.

The incubation period is 10 to 20 days. The onset is sudden with headache, severe pains in trunk and limbs. The temperature rises sharply and remains continuously raised for 5 to 7 days. Occasionally the fever is intermittent. Febrile relapses are common, usually at intervals of 5 to 6 days. Three to four such bouts may be expected. An erythematous rash, usually macular or papular, may appear on the trunk on the second day of the fever and last only 1 day. The spleen is usually palpable. In chronic relapsing cases fatigue is often marked and convalescence prolonged for several months.

Treatment of the Rickettsial Diseases

Antibiotics. The various fevers due to rickettsiae vary greatly in severity but all respond to broad-spectrum antibiotics. Tetracycline is given in a dose of 250 mg 4 times daily. In severe infections the dose is 500 mg 4 times daily for the first 3 days. The fever usually settles within 2 or 3 days. As there is a tendency to relapse tetracycline should be continued for 5 to 7 days after the patient is afebrile. In endemic areas good results have been obtained in louse-borne typhus by a single dose of 100 mg doxycycline.

General Management. The patient suffering from louse- or flea-borne typhus is a danger to others unless he has been disinfested.

When the temperature is high, i.e. over 41°C, cold sponging gives great comfort. If headache is intense and fails to respond to aspirin or codeine, lumbar puncture should be performed to relieve the increased intracranial pressure and to detect any concomitant bacterial meningitis. Delirium may need to be controlled by sedatives while awaiting the effects of specific chemotherapy. Pneumonia may be a serious feature in scrub typhus and oxygen may be needed. Convalescence is usually protracted especially in older people.

Prevention. For louse- and flea-borne typhus and in trench fever steps should be taken to get rid of all lice and fleas and their faeces. An insecticide powder can be insufflated into the undergarments of those at risk without their undressing. To prevent flea-borne typhus food stores and granaries should be protected from rats. Rats and their fleas must be destroyed.

Attendants on patients with louse-borne typhus should wear protective clothing smeared with an insect repellent such as dimethylphthalate (DMP). The patient should be washed, and an insecticide applied all over, especially to the hairy parts. His clothing should be immersed in disinfectant before being sterilised.

To guard against tick-borne typhus dogs should be regularly disinfested of ticks with forceps and should not be allowed to sleep in bedrooms. Protection of the legs when walking through grasslands may reduce the risk of picking up infected ticks. The early removal of ticks and cleansing the site of the bite are also important.

Mite-borne typhus is acquired when man enters scrub country in endemic areas. Protection against the larval mite can be secured by wearing suitable clothing, the inside of which has been smeared once a week with a mite-repellent such as DMP. Mites can be destroyed by aerial spraying of infected areas with Aldrin or Dieldrin, repeated every 3 months.

Active Immunisation. Those likely to be at risk can be protected by vaccines prepared from killed cultures of strains of *R. prowazeki*, *R. mooseri* or *R. rickettsi* cultured in eggs. Three doses each of 1 ml should be given subcutaneously at intervals of 7 to 10 days and booster doses of 1 ml should be given at 6-monthly intervals or yearly.

So far no protective vaccine is available against mite-borne typhus.

DISEASES DUE TO HELMINTHS

Infections caused by the commoner helminths, or worms, are described in this section, grouped according to the three zoological classes which parasitise man; 1, trematodes or flukes, 2, cestodes or tapeworms and, 3, nematodes or roundworms. Much morbidity is caused in the tropics by helminths, many of which may be found in people even years after leaving the tropics.

The only prevalent parasitic helminth of humans in Britain is the nematode *Enterobius (Oxyuris) vermicularis* or threadworm. Other worms which may be acquired in Britain include the roundworms, *Ascaris lumbricoides, Toxocara canis, Trichuris trichiura* (whipworm) and *Trichinella spiralis*. The beef tapeworm is also still endemic in Britain and rarely *Echinococcus granulosus* causing hydatid disease and *Fasciola hepatica*, an endemic fluke infecting sheep, are acquired by man.

Helminths invading tissues usually provoke an eosinophilia. A creeping eruption or 'larva migrans' is caused when the larva of *Ancylostoma braziliensis* (p. 908) travels in the skin and similar but more quickly moving lesions, 'larva currens', are caused by *Strongyloides stercoralis* (p. 909). Visceral larva migrans is associated with *Toxocara canis* (p. 906) and the larvae of *Gnathostoma spinigerum* (p. 911) provoke allergic swellings.

1. Diseases due to Trematodes (Flukes)

Schistosomiasis; Liver Flukes; Paragonimiasis; Fasciolopsiasis

Schistosomiasis (Bilharziasis)

Schistosomiasis was endemic in ancient Egypt (1250 B.C.) but became a serious problem in the nineteenth century after perennial irrigation was instituted. It is one of the most important causes of morbidity in the tropics and is being spread by irrigation schemes.

There are three species of flukes of the genus *Schistosoma* which commonly cause disease in man, *S. haematobium*, *S. mansoni* and *S. japonicum*. *S. haematobium* was discovered by Theodor Bilharz in Cairo in 1861 and the genus is sometimes called *Bilharzia* and the disease bilharziasis. Certain other animal species, *S. intercalatum*, *S. bovis* and *S. matthei* rarely affect man. When the ovum is passed in the urine or faeces and gains access to fresh water, the ciliated miracidium inside it is liberated and, if a suitable freshwater snail is available, it soon penetrates this intermediate host. In the snail the miracidium develops into large numbers of fork-tailed cercariae which are then liberated into the water where they may survive for 2 to 3 days. These cercariae can penetrate the skin if there is only a thin film of water next to it, or the mucous membrane of the mouth of their definitive host, man; after passing to the lung they migrate to the portal vein where they mature. The male worm is up to 20 mm in length and the more slender cylindrical female, usually enfolded longitudinally by the male, is rather longer (Fig. 17.5). Within 4 to 6 weeks of infection they migrate to the venules draining the pelvic viscera where the females deposit their ova. Whereas the eggs of *S. haematobium* are laid chiefly in the walls of the bladder and rectum, the eggs of *S. mansoni* and *S. japonicum* are deposited mainly in the lower bowel wall.

Pathology. Penetration of the skin by the cercariae may produce a papular eruption which may later become vesicular. A similar cutaneous eruption may

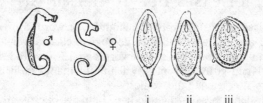

i ii iii

Adults (× 2½)   Ova (× 250)

Fig. 17.5 Schistosoma. i. *S. haematobium*, ii. *S. mansoni*, iii. *S. japonicum*.

follow invasion of the skin by cercariae of non-human schistosomes. During the migration of the immature schistosomes transitory lesions may be produced, including areas of pneumonia. At this stage there is usually an eosinophilia but the count falls progressively after the disease is established. In a heavy schistosomal infection ova may be found widely distributed in many tissues, including the central nervous system, liver, lungs, heart and even the skin, but each species has a special territory for maximum egg deposition (see below). After the egg has escaped from the vein, a granuloma forms around it. This consists of epithelioid cells, fibroblasts and giant cells surrounded by a zone of plasma cells and eosinophils. When the egg is near a mucosal surface, aided by the cytolytic enzyme excreted by the miracidium, it may be discharged into the bowel or bladder. If, however, the ovum is retained in the tissues the miracidium soon dies and the egg then either disintegrates or becomes calicified, and fibrous tissue forms at the site. The degree of fibrosis depends on the intensity of the infection and the length of time the patient has been exposed to re-infection. In endemic areas the immune response to an established infection may limit re-infections.

Clinical Features. The first indication of infection, especially when it is heavy, may be tingling and itching of the part which has been exposed to water containing cercariae. This lasts for 1 or 2 days and may be succeeded, after a symptom-free period of 3 to 5 weeks, by allergic manifestations such as urticaria and eosinophilia and by fever, aches in the muscles, abdominal pain, splenomegaly, headaches, cough and sweating. Patches of pneumonic consolidation may be present. These allergic phenomena (*Katayama syndrome*) may be severe in infections with *S. mansoni* and *S. japonicum* but are rare with *S. haematobium*. Often the patient does not notice or recall them. After 1 or 2 weeks these features subside and for 2 or 3 months after the infection there may be no further symptoms until the deposition of eggs causes fresh ones to develop. The symptoms then depend on the intensity of the infection and the species of the infecting schistosome.

Diagnosis and treatment. These are discussed on page 898.

Schistosoma haematobium

This species of schistosome affects mainly the urinary bladder and the genitalia. The egg is easily recognised by its terminal spine. Man is the only natural host. *S. haematobium* is highly endemic in Egypt, the east coast of Africa and the adjacent islands and occurs throughout most of Africa, in Iran, Iraq, Syria, Yemen, South Arabia, Lebanon and Israel. It also occurs in Turkey, Cyprus and in solitary foci in Portugal and the Maharashtra State of India.

Pathology. The urinary bladder and ureters are characteristically affected. The earliest changes in the mucosa are hyperaemia and petechiae, followed by small granulomata enlarging to form small papillomata but large granulomata may develop in young people. Sloughing may leave an ulcerated surface with associated fibrosis. Calcification of dead ova produces, in intense infections, 'sandy patches' especially towards the base of the bladder and around the ureteric openings. The lower third of the ureter, including its entrance into the bladder, is liable to stenosis causing partial obstruction to the passage of urine. The capacity of the bladder is greatly diminished. Increased intravesical pressure alone or combined with ureteric obstruction produces hydronephrosis or pyonephrosis and extensive renal damage and uraemia. Calculus formation and pyogenic urinary infections may ensue. Carcinoma of the bladder in relatively young males is of common occurrence in some areas of high endemicity of *S. haematobium*. Eggs may be deposited in the urethra, with sinus formation, in the seminal vesicles, vagina, cervix and Fallopian tubes, and this along with superadded pyogenic infection may lead to serious pelvic complications. The rectum may be involved, also the liver (periportal fibrosis), though less severely than in *S. mansoni* infections. Deposition of ova in the pulmonary arterioles may lead to pulmonary hypertension and cor pulmonale. These lung changes are especially frequent in combined infections with *S. haematobium* and *S. mansoni*. Discrete granulomas in the lung may be large enough to be visible radiologically. Ova may also be carried to the central nervous system, skin and elsewhere.

Clinical Features. The characteristic early localising symptom is usually painless, terminal haematuria with or without frequency of micturition. The haematuria is usually increased by exercise. Frequency of micturition follows when the disease is long established due largely to the contracted fibrosed or calcified bladder. These symptoms, constant by day and night, may be very distressing. Pain is often felt in the iliac fossa or in the loin, passing down to the groin. In advanced cases pyelonephritis, hydronephrosis or pyonephrosis may be accompanied by hypertension or end in uraemia. Disease of the seminal vesicles may lead to haemospermia. In females there may be fibrosis of the ovaries, occlusion of the Fallopian tubes and vaginitis or cervicitis, and schistosomal lesions may be mistaken for carcinoma. Intestinal symptoms may result from lesions in the bowel wall.

The severity of *S. haematobium* infection varies greatly, and many with light infections suffer a minimum of discomfort. However, as the adult worms can live for 20 years or more and progressive lesions may develop treatment should always be given, unless impaired renal function makes treatment dangerous.

Schistosoma mansoni

This species of schistosome affects particularly the large bowel. Man is the only natural host of importance although the infection is also found in baboons. *S. mansoni* is endemic in the Nile Delta and Libya, Southern Sudan, East Africa continuing as far south as the Transvaal and in West Africa from Senegal and Gambia to Cameroun, throughout Zaïre and also Arabia. It is also found in South America in Venezuela, Brazil and in the West Indian Islands of the lesser Antilles, Puerto Rico and Dominica.

Pathology. The adult worms reach the tributaries of the inferior mesenteric vein, and the female deposits eggs chiefly in the submucosa of the large bowel, producing early lesions similar to those caused in the bladder by *S. haematobium*—congested spots, granulomata and later papillomata. The papillomata in the bowel exceptionally become very large and pedunculated. They are most numerous in the lower part of the large bowel but may extend throughout its length. Occasionally a segment of the bowel wall becomes infiltrated and thickened but malignant change is very uncommon. In long-standing severe infections rectal polypi may prolapse, and secondary pyogenic infection may create faecal fistulae. Eggs may be deposited throughout the body, in the mesenteric nodes, the small intestine and the subperitoneal tissues. In heavy infections the liver receives many eggs from the portal vein. This, in combination with toxic products from the adult schistosomes, may cause periportal fibrosis (pipe-stem cirrhosis). In the early stage the liver is enlarged, firm, smooth and painless, but later it shrinks. The surface shows little or no irregularity. In advanced cases fibrosis leads to portal hypertension and ascites. The spleen is often slightly enlarged early in the disease, due to reticuloendothelial proliferation, but with the development of hepatic fibrosis and portal hypertension the spleen may become very large and extremely hard. Pulmonary vascular lesions may be marked and lead to cor pulmonale. Eggs may reach the central nervous system and cause a granulomatous space-occupying lesion, the cord being the most usual site. A reversible nephrotic syndrome has been described.

Clinical Features. The symptoms during the invasion by the cercariae and development of the adult worms have been described (p. 895). Depending on the intensity of the infection, symptoms due to deposition of eggs emerge after a period of 2 months or longer. The characteristic localising symptoms are abdominal pain and frequent stools which contain blood-stained mucus. On palpation of the abdomen thickened infiltrated loops of the bowel may sometimes be detected. Where the mucosa of the lower bowel is severely affected, rectal polyps may prolapse during defaecation. Hepatosplenomegaly occurring early in the disease is reversible but in severe cases the liver becomes fibrotic and the spleen enlarged and hard, portal hypertension and ascites may develop and the patient dies of haematemesis, hepatic failure or secondary infection. Jaundice is not a frequent feature of this disease. Where infection is light no inconvenience may be experienced and the infection may be discovered only on routine examination of the stool. Other complications of *S. mansoni* infection include paraplegia from a lesion of the cord and, as described under pathology, cor pulmonale. In highly endemic areas the mortality from this disease is considerable.

Schistosoma japonicum

S. japonicum infects particularly the portal drainage of the small intestine and upper part of the large bowel. The adult worm parasitises, in addition to man, the dog, rat, field mouse, water buffalo, ox, cat, pig, horse and sheep. *S. japonicum* is prevalent in the Yangtse-Kiang basin in China where the infection is a major public health problem. It also has a focal distribution in Japan and occurs in the Philippines, Celebes, Laos, Thailand, Vietnam and the Shan States of Burma.

Pathology. The histopathology of *S. japonicum* lesions is similar to that of the other schistosome diseases in man. As this worm produces more eggs the lesions tend to be more extensive and widespread. The small intestine and upper part of the large bowel are most affected, and hepatic fibrosis with splenic enlargement is usual. Deposition of eggs in the central nervous system, especially in the brain, causes symptoms of cerebral irritation or compression in about 5 per cent of infections.

Clinical Features. The clinical features of schistosomiasis due to *S. japonicum* resemble those of very severe infection with *S. mansoni*. Abdominal pain and diarrhoea may be marked, and hepatic and splenic changes are usually early with ascites and the development of the superficial abdominal collateral venous circulation. Haematemesis and melaena may follow rupture of varicose veins in the stomach and oesophagus. Neurological symptoms include Jacksonian epilepsy, hemiplegia, blindness and terminal coma. Evidence of compression of the cord may also be found.

The morbidity and mortality rate in *S. japonicum* infections is greater than from either of the other species.

Diagnosis of Schistosomiasis. A history of residence in an endemic area with symptoms as described will indicate the need for a careful investigation. In *S. haematobium* infection the terminal spined egg can usually be found by microscopical examination of the last few drops of urine, especially after exercise. The eggs may also be found by microscopic examination of the stool or of a fragment of unstained rectal mucosa removed through a proctoscope. In a case of some duration a radiograph may show calcification in the wall of the bladder while intravenous pyelography may show stenosis or dilatation of the ureters, reduction in capacity of the bladder, or hydronephrosis. Such changes are found commonly in endemic areas and have been shown to be frequent even in children, in whom large intravesical granulomata are common. In a heavy infection with *S. mansoni* or *S. japonicum* the characteristic egg can usually be found in the stool. When, however, the infection is light it may be necessary to repeat the examinations over a number of days. Cystoscopy or sigmoidoscopy may enable the diagnosis to be made from the macroscopic appearance. Otherwise biopsy specimens should be removed and examined for ova.

A complement-fixation reaction, using an alcoholic extract of fresh livers of *Planorbis boissyi* heavily infected with cercariae of *S. mansoni* as antigen, has proved of value in diagnosis, especially in the early stages of infection.

The bowel symptoms of *S. mansoni* and *S. japonicum* infection may be very like those associated with intestinal amoebiasis or with a neoplasm of the large bowel, so steps should be taken to exclude these. There may be concomitant bacillary dysentery.

Treatment of Schistosomiasis. The object of specific treatment is the killing of the adult schistosomes or, failing this, at least a significant reduction in egg laying. The latter is still of considerable value to the individual patient and in mass treatments of a community the spread of infection by snails is reduced. Even in endemic areas reinfection is not inevitable. In the presence of extensive liver damage no drug is safe and established portal hypertension will not be benefited by chemotherapy.

Niridazole, 25 mg/kg body weight daily, orally, for 7 days is highly effective in haematobium schistosomiasis but rather less so in mansoni schistosomiasis. The drug colours the urine brown but the only serious occasional side effect is a temporary psychosis, especially liable to occur if the liver is diseased.

Stibocaptate, a combination of a trivalent antimony compound and dimercaprol, is given intramuscularly in a dose of 8 mg/kg body weight daily, on alternate days or spaced as tolerated, for a total of 5 doses. It is rather more effective than niridazole and dimercaprol reduces the toxic effects of antimony (see below).

Hycanthone in a single dose (3 mg/kg body weight, i.m., maximum 200 mg), has now been widely used and produces good results. Serious hepatotoxic effects are rare. The drug sometimes causes vomiting but it is dangerous to administer a phenothiazine (e.g., chlorpromazine) because of the synergistic toxic effects of the drugs on the liver.

Sodium antimonyl tartrate was for many years the standard drug and is still probably the most effective, particularly for japonicum schistosomiasis. For other infections it is no longer indicated because of the need for caution in its intravenous administration and its occasional dangerous cardiotoxicity. The total dose required is 2 g, given as 18 or more separate injections spaced over 3 to 6 weeks as tolerated, beginning with a dose of 30 mg and gradually increasing to 120 mg each.

Newer drugs are under investigation.

Surgical aid may be required to deal with residual lesions but large vesical granulomata usually respond well to chemotherapy. In cases of chronic *S. haematobium* infection, ureteric stricture and the small fibrotic urinary bladder may require plastic procedures. For rectal papillomata removal by diathermy or by other means may give the patient considerable relief. Granulomatous masses in the brain or spinal cord may call for neurosurgery if the manifestations do not yield to chemotherapy. For portal hypertension, splenectomy or a portocaval shunt may have to be considered, but results are poor.

Prevention. This presents great difficulties, and so far no really satisfactory means of controlling schistosomiasis has been established. If the ova of the schistosome in the urine or faeces are not allowed to contaminate fresh water containing the required snail host, then the miracidia will soon cease to be infective.

In a primitive country bore-hole latrines can easily be constructed but the great difficulty is to persuade the people always to use them. In the case of *S. japonicum*, moreover, there are so many hosts besides man that the proper use of latrines would be of little avail. Mass treatment of the population helps against *S. haematobium* and *S. mansoni* but this method has so far had little success against *S. japonicum*.

Attack on the intermediate host, the snail, presents many difficulties. The most important snail hosts of *S. haematobium* are species of the genus *Bulinus and Planorbarius*. In the case of *S. mansoni*, species of the genus *Biomphalaria, Australorbis* and *Tropicorbis* are the chief intermediate hosts. If an attempt is made to kill these snails by draining away the water in which they live they may preserve themselves by burrowing into the mud. In the Far East snails of the genus *Oncomelania* are the important intermediate hosts. They are very resistant to drying. Many molluscicides have been introduced into streams and canals in an attempt to destroy these snail hosts but so far without much success, although the costs involved have been balanced by increased efficiency at work on some well-managed estates.

Personal Protection. Contact with infected water must be avoided. Accidental immersion or contact should be followed by a shower. Water free from snails, stored for 3 days, will usually contain no living cercariae, but exceptions to this rule have been reported.

Liver Flukes

Table 17.3 sets out the main features of the diseases caused by flukes which infect the bile ducts of man (p. 900).

Paragonimiasis

(*Endemic Haemoptysis*)

There are several species of the flukes of the genus *Paragonimus* which may affect man, the commonest being *P. westermani*. The adult worms measuring

Table 17.3 Diseases caused by flukes in the bile ducts

Disease	Clonorchiasis	Opisthorciasis	Fascioliasis
Parasite	*Clonorchis sinensis*	*Opisthorcis felineus*	*Fasciola hepatica*
Other mammalian hosts	Dogs, cats, pigs	Dogs, cats, foxes, pigs	Sheep
Mode of spread	Ova in faeces into water	As for *C. sinensis*	Ova in faeces on to wet pasture
1st intermediate host	Snails	Snails	Snails
2nd intermediate host	Freshwater fish	Freshwater fish	Nil (encysts on vegetation)
Geographical distribution	Far East, esp. S. China	Far East, esp. N.E. Thailand	Cosmopolitan incl. Britain
Pathology	*Esch. coli* cholangitis, liver abscesses, biliary carcinoma	As for *C. sinensis*	Toxaemia, cholangitis, eosinophilia
Symptoms	Often symptom-free, recurrent jaundice	Jaundice	Obscure fever, tender liver, may be ectopic subcut. fluke
Diagnosis	Ova in stool or duodenal aspirate	As for *C. sinensis*	As for *C. sinensis* also immuno-fluorescence
Treatment	Hexachloroparaxylol 300 mg/kg daily for 3 days or chloroquine 600 mg base daily for 14 days	As for *C. sinensis*	Bithionol 30 mg/kg daily for 10–15 days (formerly chloroquine or emetine hcl. used)
Prevention	Cook fish	Cook fish	Avoid contaminated watercress

10×6 mm live in small cysts in the lung and elsewhere. If a pulmonary cyst ruptures, the sputum of the patient contains ova, some of which may be expectorated and the others swallowed and passed in the faeces. From these eggs the larval worms emerge in water and seek the first intermediate host, a freshwater snail. Larvae emerging from the snail enter freshwater crabs or crayfish. If man or certain other mammals eat these crustacea raw or inadequately cooked, infection takes place. Human infections are most frequent in the Far East but there are also endemic foci in South America, Cameroun, Nigeria, Somalia and India.

Pathological and Clinical Features. The adults lie in cysts up to 1 cm in diameter, containing reddish brown fluid, situated chiefly in the lung. There are seldom more than 20 such cysts present. In heavy infections cysts may also be present in the pleural or peritoneal cavities, in the brain, muscles, skin or elsewhere.

The first symptoms are usually those of slight fever, cough and the expectoration of sputum streaked with blood. Occasionally there are bouts of frank haemoptysis with severe pain in the chest. Increasing signs in the chest may simulate pneumonia or pulmonary tuberculosis and the latter frequently is a coexistent infection. When the parasites lodge in the abdomen there may be symptoms of enteritis or hepatitis. If they settle in the abdominal wall they may produce sinuses with a discharge through the skin. Development in the central nervous system may cause signs of cerebral irritation, encephalitis or myelitis. The disease may be very chronic and the adult worms may survive for 20 years.

Ova may be found on microscopic examination of the faeces, sputum, or a discharge. The radiological appearances of affected lungs are variable but the lesions are usually situated close to the pleural surfaces. Extrapulmonary lesions are diagnosed in life by biopsy.

Treatment and Prevention. Antibiotics are useful to combat secondary pyogenic infections. The specific drug is bithionol given in a dose of 50 mg/kg body weight daily in three divided doses on alternate days. In all, 10 to 15 days of treatment are required and the results are encouraging. Lesions localised to or maximal in one lobe of a lung may be treated surgically.

In an endemic area crab or crayfish should not be eaten unless adequately cooked. Immersion of crustaceans in wine or brine does not kill the parasites.

Fasciolopsiasis

Fasciolopsis buski is the largest fluke to infect man. The adults, 2–7·5 cm long, inhabit the small intestine of man, pigs and dogs. It is common in Central and S. China and amongst Chinese in S.-E. Asia. The infection is spread from ova passed in the faeces into water. The intermediate hosts are snails. Man becomes infected by ingesting metacercariae encysted on water plants, particularly when he uses his teeth to peel them.

Light infections are symptomless. Heavy infections give rise to epigastric pain and loose motions. Very heavy infections may be fatal. The diagnosis is made by detecting ova or adult worms in the faeces. Tetrachloroethylene as prescribed for hookworms (p. 908) is effective treatment. Prevention is by the proper disposal of faeces. Edible water plants can be made safe by immersing them in boiling water.

2. Diseases due to Cestodes (Tapeworms)

Taenia saginata; Taenia solium and Cysticercosis; Echinococcus granulosus; Diphyllobothrium latum; Diphyllobothrium mansoni; Dipylidium caninum; Hymenolepis nana

Cestodes are ribbon-shaped worms which inhabit the human intestinal tract. They have no alimentary system and absorb nutrients through the surface. The anterior end, or scolex, is provided with suckers for attachment to the host. From the scolex arises a series of progressively developing segments, the proglottides, which when shed may continue to show active movements for some time. Cross-fertilisation takes place between segments. Ova, present in large numbers in mature proglottides, remain viable for weeks and during this period they may be consumed by the intermediate host. The larvae liberated from the ova pass into the tissues of the intermediate host, and the human disease is acquired by eating undercooked beef infected with *Cysticercus bovis*, the larval stage of *Taenia saginata* (beef tapeworm), undercooked pork containing *Cysticercus cellulosae*, the larval stage of *T. solium* (pork tapeworm), or undercooked freshwater fish containing larvae of *Diphyllobothrium latum* (fish tapeworm). Usually only one adult tapeworm is present but up to 10 have been reported. The adult worm produces little or no intestinal upset in human beings, but knowledge of its presence, by noting segments from it in the faeces or on underclothing, may distress the patient. The life-cycles of *Hymenolepis nana, Diphyllobothrium mansoni* and *Dipylidium caninum* are different (see below).

Taenia saginata

This worm may be several metres long. The scolex, the size of a pin head, has four suckers; mature segments contain a central-stemmed uterus with 15 to 20 lateral branches which are easily seen if the segments are left in water for 24 hours (Fig. 17.6). The ova of both *T. saginata* and *T. solium* are spherical and indistinguishable microscopically. The thick outer shell has radial striations and the ovum contains six hooklets. It is about the size of a threadworm ovum.

Infection with *T. saginata* occurs in all parts of the world, including Britain.

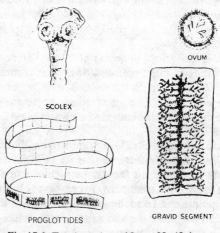

Fig. 17.6 *Taenia saginata (Ovum 30–40μ)*

Diagnosis. The patient usually notices segments on underclothing or in stools. The segments should be identified (as above). Ova may also be found in the stool.

Treatment and Prevention. The drug now used is niclosamide. Before any food is taken in the morning, 2 tablets of the drug, each containing 0·5 g, are chewed and swallowed with a little water. One hour later a further 2 tablets are similarly taken. There are no side-effects and the worm is nearly always successfully destroyed.

Prevention depends on efficient meat inspection or the thorough cooking of beef.

Taenia solium and Cysticercosis

T. solium, the pork tapeworm, was formerly cosmopolitan in distribution but is now rare except in Central Europe, Ethiopia, South Africa and in certain regions of Asia. It is not so large as *T. saginata*, and the uterus has less than 14 lateral branches. The scolex has, in addition to suckers, two circular rows of hooklets anterior to the suckers. The adult worm is found only in man following the eating of undercooked pork containing cysticerci. *Human Cysticercosis* results from ova being swallowed or gaining access to the human stomach by regurgitation from the intestine harbouring an adult worm. In the stomach the larvae are liberated from the eggs, penetrate the intestinal mucosa and are carried to many parts of the body where they develop and form cysticerci. The most common locations are the subcutaneous tissue and skeletal muscles; when superficially placed they can be palpated under the skin or mucosa as pea-like ovoid bodies. Here they cause few or no symptoms; however cysts may also develop in the brain. About 5 years later the larvae die; in the brain the tissue reaction may cause epileptic fits, obscure neurological disorders, personality changes and occasionally internal hydrocephalus. After death of the larvae in muscles the cysts calcify and this enables them to be recognised radiologically. In the brain, however, much less calcification takes place and in this situation calcified larvae are only occasionally demonstrated radiologically. Epileptic fits starting in adult life should suggest the possibility of cysticercosis if the patient has lived in an endemic area. The subcutaneous tissue should be palpated and radiological examination of the skeletal muscles for calcified cysts must be made and repeated after intervals of 6 months if at first negative.

Diagnosis. As in the case of *T. saginata* (see above), identification of a segment enables the diagnosis of *T. solium* to be made.

Treatment and Prevention. *T. solium* can be removed by filix mas administered as follows. After a 48-hour period of bowel preparation by fluid diet and saline aperients morning and evening 2·5 ml of a fresh extract of filix mas in capsules or as an emulsion is given at 6 a.m. and again at 6.15 a.m. and 6.30 a.m.; an appropriately smaller dose is given to a child. The patient takes only sips of water until 7 a.m. when for an adult 60 ml (2 fl oz) of saturated sodium sulphate solution is given. If the scolex is not passed by 9 a.m. a soap and water enema is administered. Food can be offered as soon as the scolex is seen or by 9.30 a.m. in any case. All motions are scrutinised to detect the scolex. Further experience is required before niclosamide can be confidently recommended for *T. solium* as disintegration of a segment might possibly release viable ova with the risk of cysticercosis.

Treatment of cysticercosis of the brain is essentially the same as for idiopathic epilepsy; sedatives and anticonvulsants should be given to tide the patient over the period until the reaction in the brain has subsided. Most patients treated on these lines make a good recovery. Operative intervention is seldom indicated.

Prevention of *T. solium* infection consists in having pork well cooked before consumption. Cysticercosis is avoided if food is not contaminated by ova or segments and if there is no regurgitation of gravid segments or ova from the duodenum into the stomach as may occur from vomiting in a patient harbouring an adult *T. solium*. Great care must be taken by nurses and others to avoid contaminating the hands with ova from the patient.

Echinococcus granulosus (Taenia echinococcus)

(Hydatid Disease)

This is the smallest tapeworm of medical importance. The larval stage, a hydatid cyst, usually occurs in sheep and cattle. Dogs, by ingesting these cysts, are the most important definitive hosts, and a man, after handling a dog, may swallow ova excreted by the dog. The embryo is liberated from the ovum in the small intestine and gains access to the blood stream; it develops most frequently in the liver, but sometimes in the lung or elsewhere. The resultant cyst grows very slowly.

In man a hydatid cyst is typically acquired in childhood and it may, after growing for some years, cause pressure symptoms. These will vary, depending on the organ or tissues involved. In nearly 75 per cent of patients with hydatid disease the right lobe of the liver is invaded and contains a single cyst. In others a cyst may be found in the lung, brain, orbit or elsewhere. The diagnosis depends on the clinical and radiological findings in a patient who has lived in close contact with dogs. Intradermal (Casoni), complement-fixation and immunofluorescent tests may give useful support to the diagnosis.

Treatment. When the cyst is causing pressure symptoms, surgical removal of the cyst and its laminated membrane is required. A significant advance utilises cryotherapy; this prevents spillage of cyst fluid which can cause fatal anaphylaxis or disseminate the disease. A steel cone is frozen on to the organ overlying the cyst. The cyst membranes and contents are then removed through the cone and 0·5 per cent silver nitrate solution is applied to the cavity, followed by irrigation with isotonic saline. Cysts in a long bone usually necessitate amputation.

Diphyllobothrium latum

This tapeworm is relatively common in Finland and the Scandinavian countries but is also acquired from rivers and lakes of many other countries, including some in Africa and Asia. The ova are excreted in the faeces of an infected man or other fish-eating animal. The larval stages take place first in a small freshwater crustacean, *Cyclops* or *Diaptomus* which in turn is swallowed by a fish. The infections are usually symptomless. Occasionally there are signs of allergy and in a small percentage of cases a megaloblastic anaemia develops, the worm competing with the host for vitamin B_{12}. The diagnosis is made by finding ova in the stool and treatment is by niclosamide as for *T. saginata*.

Diphyllobothrium mansoni (Spirometra erinacei)

The adult worms are harboured by cats and dogs. The second larval stage, a sparganum, is occasionally found in the subcutaneous tissues of man. The Masai in East Africa probably become infected by ingestion of the first intermediate host, a *Cyclops*, from well water and the patient presents with a painful swelling usually in the lower limbs. In the Far East ocular *sparganosis* arises from the migration of a sparganum from a split frog applied as a traditional poultice. Sparganosis also occurs in the U.S.A. Surgical removal is required. The exact species can be established only by feeding the removed sparganum to an uninfected cat or dog.

Dipylidium caninum

Dipylidium caninum is a short tapeworm of dogs and cats. The ova are passed in the faeces and the larva has to undergo development in a flea or louse before being swallowed by the definitive host. Children are occasionally infected by picking up and ingesting an infected flea from a dog. The diagnosis is made by finding segments or ova in the stools. Treatment, in appropriate doses for a child, is as for *Taenia saginata.*

Hymenolepis nana

This dwarf tapeworm is unusual in not requiring an intermediate host. It is a common infection in children living in insanitary conditions in the tropics and subtropics. Except for an eosinophilia no signs or symptoms are present except in the presence of numerous worms, when enteritis and allergic phenomena may be encountered. The diagnosis is made by recognising the ova in the faeces. Treatment is by niclosamide as for *T. saginata.*

Further reading about hydatid cysts:

Saidi, P. & Nazarian, I. (1971). Surgical treatment of hydatid cysts. *New England Journal of Medicine,* **284,** 1346.

3. Diseases due to Nematodes (Roundworms)

Enterobius vermicularis; Ascaris lumbricoides; Toxocara canis; Ancylostomiasis; Larva Migrans; Strongyloidiasis; Angiostrongylus; Trichuris trichiura; Trichinella spiralis; Gnathostomiasis; Anisakiasis; Filariases

Enterobius vermicularis (Threadworm)

This helminth is common throughout the world, including Britain. It affects children especially. The sexes are separate, the male being 2–5 mm long and the female 8–13 mm (Fig. 17.7). After the ova are swallowed, development takes place in the small intestine, but the adult worms are found chiefly in the colon.

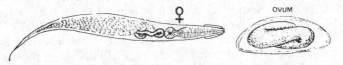

Fig. 17.7 *Enterobius vermicularis (Ova 55 × 25μ)*

The gravid female worm lays fully developed ova around the anal orifice, and her movements in this region are responsible for intense itching, especially at night. The ova are often carried to the mouth on the fingers of the child and so reinfection takes place. In female patients the genitalia may be invaded. The adult worms may be seen moving on the buttocks or in the stool. Ova are detected by applying the adhesive surface of cellophane tape to the perianal skin in the morning. This is then examined on a glass slide under the microscope.

Treatment. Piperazine salts are effective remedies administered with senna. The adult dose is 10 g of the combined preparation containing 4 g of piperazine phosphate; children under 6 years are given 5–7·5 g. The drug is given in a single dose but should be repeated if the infection persists. Other effective anthelmintics are viprynium embonate, mebendazole and pyrantel embonate. Success is more likely to be achieved if the whole family is treated simultaneously, particularly as symptomless infections may be present in adults. Prevention of reinfection is most important. Nails should be kept short, biting of nails forbidden and the hands washed carefully, especially before meals.

Ascaris lumbricoides

This is a large, pale yellow roundworm 20–35 cm long, something like an earthworm, but not segmented. The sexes are separate and the ovum is easily recognised under the low power lens (Fig. 17.8).

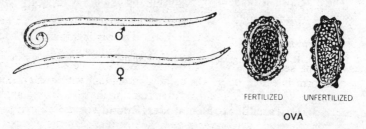

FERTILIZED   UNFERTILIZED

OVA

Fig. 17.8 *Ascaris lumbricoides (Ova 60 × 45μ fertilised; 90 × 40μ unfertilised)*

Man is infected by ingesting food contaminated with ova containing developed embryos. The larvae escape from the ova in the duodenum and find their way to the lungs where they develop further. After invading the alveoli they then ascend the bronchi and trachea and are swallowed, thus entering the small intestine where they reach maturity. In heavy infections, such as occur in the tropics, migration of many larvae through the lung may cause a helminthic pneumonia, with cough, haemoptyses, urticaria and eosinophilia (Löffler's syndrome, p. 305). Symptoms due to adult worms may be absent or consist of nausea, colicky abdominal pain and irregular motions. Sometimes a worm is vomited or passed *per rectum*. In children with severe infections a tangled mass of worms may cause intestinal obstruction. Many worms competing with the host for nourishment may contribute to malnutrition. Other complications include blockage of the bile or pancreatic duct and obstruction of the appendix by adult worms. The diagnosis is made by finding ova in the faeces or by observing an adult worm. A solely male infection is usually revealed only after the giving of an anthelmintic to a patient with an unexplained eosinophilia. Occasionally the worms are demonstrated radiographically by barium.

Treatment. Piperazine salts are easily administered and effective and should be given as recommended for threadworms. Levamisole in a single adult dose of 120 mg (40 mg up to age 3 years) is an effective alternative. The worms may not be passed until several days later.

Toxocara canis

This is a common intestinal ascarid of dogs. The eggs are passed in the animal's faeces. Children who are in close contact with infected dogs are particularly liable to ingest ova of *Toxocara canis*. Larvae, liberated in the stomach, then migrate through the body and may cause allergic phenomena such as asthma, eosinophilia and also splenomegaly ('visceral larva migrans'). The worms do not usually mature in the human host. Occasionally a granuloma develops around a dead larva in the eye and causes an obstruction to vision, resembling a neoplasm.

A skin test using an antigen derived from *T. canis* is employed for diagnosis. The larval worms can be killed by diethylcarbamazine (9–12 mg/kg body weight daily for 3 weeks). Granulomata may require surgical treatment.

Ancylostomiasis

(*Hookworm Infection*)

Ancylostomiasis is caused by parasitisation of the small intestine with *Ancylostoma duodenale* or *Necator americanus*. The adult hookworm is a greyish-white nematode about 1 cm in length (Fig. 17.9). The egg is thin-shelled and oval, slightly smaller than that of *Ascaris lumbricoides* and when passed in the faeces 2 to 8 lobes may be seen in the yolk. In warm moist soil the larvae develop and reach the filariform infective stage. On coming in contact with human skin they penetrate it and are carried to the lungs. After entering the alveoli they ascend the bronchi, are swallowed and develop in the small intestine, reaching maturity in 4 to 7 weeks after infection. The larvae may also enter through the mucous membrane of the mouth. Man is the only host.

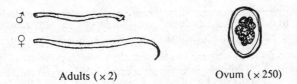

Adults (× 2)   Ovum (× 250)

Fig. 17.9 *Ancylostoma duodenale.*

Hookworm infection is widespread under insanitary conditions in the tropics and subtropics and occurs in certain mines in Europe. *A. duodenale* is endemic in the Far East and Mediterranean coastal regions and is also present elsewhere in Africa. *N. americanus* is endemic in West, East and Central Africa and Central and South America as well as in the Far East.

Pathology. At the site of entry the larvae may cause a minor inflammatory and allergic reaction. When infection is heavy, reaction to the passage through the lungs may cause a patchy inflammation accompanied by eosinophilia. In the small intestine the worms attach themselves to the mucosa by their buccal capsule and withdraw blood. The mean daily loss of blood from one *A. duodenale* is 0·15 ml and for *N. americanus* 0·03 ml. The degree of iron and protein deficiency which develops depends not only on the load of worms but also on the nutrition of the patient and especially on his stores of iron. In those on an adequate diet regeneration of red blood cells may keep pace with blood loss so that no anaemia may result. In the early stage of infection a considerable eosinophilia commonly occurs.

Clinical Features. In a well nourished person with a light established infection there may be no symptoms. At the time of infection hookworm dermatitis (ground itch) may be experienced, usually on the feet. An itchy erythema appears first and soon develops through papules and vesicles to the pustular stage. In a heavy infection the passage of the larvae through the lungs may cause a cough with blood-stained sputum, associated with patchy pulmonary consolidation (an example of Löffler's syndrome). When the worms have reached the small intestine, vomiting and epigastric pain, like that of a duodenal ulcer, may ensue. Sometimes frequent loose stools are passed, the condition then resembling early sprue or giardiasis. In the undernourished, especially when there is a heavy infection, a severe iron deficiency anaemia and hypoproteinaemia may develop with a puffy face, oedema of the extremities and a distended abdomen, sometimes with ascites. Tachycardia and breathlessness and signs of cardiac failure are present in those with severe anaemia. In children mental and physical development may be retarded. Infection with *A. duodenale* usually causes severe symptoms more readily than does infection with *N. americanus*. Untreated heavy infections in the poorly nourished are responsible for many deaths, especially in childhood.

Diagnosis. The characteristic egg can be recognised in the stool either by microscopic examination of a smear of the faeces directly or after concentration. The oedema with anaemia has to be differentiated from that due to kwashiorkor, heart failure or nephritis. Hookworms may be present without being the chief agents responsible for symptoms and signs produced by concomitant associated disease. If hookworms are present in numbers sufficient to cause anaemia, tests of the stool for occult blood will be positive and ova will be present in large numbers. Pulmonary symptoms similar to those present in the invasive phase of an-cylostomiasis may also be produced by the larvae of *Ascaris lumbricoides*, or *Strongyloides* passing through the lungs.

Treatment and Prevention. Specific medication should be given early in the morning when the patient has fasted overnight. A well-established drug is tetrachloroethylene which is given orally. The dose is 0·1 ml/kg body weight with a maximum of 4 ml. The drug has usually to be given on two or more occasions not more frequently than on alternate days. Tetrachloroethylene rapidly deteriorates in warm climates and so must be stored in a cool dark place.

Bephenium hydroxynaphthoate, containing 2·5 g base, as a single dose, is an alternative drug with few side-effects. No preparation or purgation is required. It is more expensive than tetrachloroethylene and is not as effective for *N. americanus* as for *A. duodenale*.

Levamisole in a single dose of 3 tablets each of 40 mg after a light breakfast, moderately effective against *A. duodenale* but less so against *N. americanus*, is a further alternative.

Anaemia associated with hookworm infection responds well to oral iron. When it is severe enough to cause heart failure blood should be transfused slowly, with frusemide 20 mg in each unit.

The population should be educated in the use of properly constructed latrines. Mass treatment of the entire population by tetrachloroethylene or bephenium hydroxynaphthoate may help bring the disease under control but can be costly. The nutrition of the population should be improved. Where practicable the use of shoes should be encouraged.

Hookworms causing Larva Migrans

Ancylostoma braziliensis and A. caninum are intestinal parasites of dogs with a similar life cycle to *A. duodenale*, but in man they cause a creeping eruption or larva migrans. A larva penetrating into human skin, being in the wrong host, is unable to leave the skin and mature. It burrows between the corium and stratum granulosum and progresses irregularly at about 1 cm in 24 hours. The skin at the advancing end is erythematous and the older part of the burrow discoloured and scaly. The patient experiences considerable discomfort from itching. The larva may remain active for some weeks. Treatment by freezing the advancing end with ethyl chloride spray is not always successful, even when frequently repeated. Thiabendazole orally in a dose of 50 mg/kg body weight for three doses at intervals of 12 hours usually succeeds.

Strongyloidiasis

Strongyloides stercoralis is a very small nematode (2 mm × 40 microns) which parasitises the mucosa of the upper part of the small intestine in large numbers. The eggs hatch in the bowel and appear in the faeces as rhabditiform larvae which in moist soil moult and become the infective filariform larvae. These, on entering the tissues of man, undergo a development cycle similar to that of hookworms. In the intestine a few rhabditiform larvae develop into filariform larvae which may then penetrate the mucosa or the perianal skin and lead to auto-infection. Man is the chief natural host, but dogs and cats may also be infected.

Strongyloidiasis is worldwide in the tropics and subtropics and is especially prevalent in the Far East.

Pathology. There may be a dermatitis at the time of entry of the larval worm, similar to that which may accompany invasion by hookworm larvae. In the intestine the female worm burrows into the mucosa and sets up an inflammatory reaction; with very heavy infections the mucosa may be severely damaged leading to malabsorption. Granulomatous changes, necrosis, and even perforation and peritonitis may also occur. Eosinophilia is common in the early stages and may persist. Actively motile larvae are found in the faeces and occasionally in the sputum. Immunosuppressive factors or drugs, such as corticosteroids, may lead to fatal systemic strongyloidiasis.

Clinical Features. An itch may be produced during invasion of the skin. Pulmonary symptoms and signs similar to those of ancylostomiasis may also occur. With slight infections there will be no intestinal symptoms, but in more severe cases abdominal pain and diarrhoea may be produced, which is on occasions severe; urticaria, anaemia, weakness and emaciation may also be present as well as signs of malabsorption, ileus or volvulus. Penetration of the skin about the anus or the intestinal wall by filariform larvae may lead to extremely itchy, linear, urticarial skin reactions. These usually subside in a few hours but tend to keep on recurring. The eruptions may extend 3 or 4 cm in an hour. This rapid progress has led to the term 'larva currens' being used rather than 'larva migrans' or creeping eruption. In addition there are frequently urticarial weals or less well defined areas of erythema.

Diagnosis. Intestinal symptoms and characteristic eruptions should suggest *S. stercoralis* infection. Eosinophilia is usually present. Motile rhabditiform larvae can be seen in the faeces, occasionally in the sputum, urine or bile. Excretion of them is intermittent so repeated examinations may be necessary. In ancylostomiasis, ova, not larvae, are found in a fresh stool.

Treatment. Thiabendazole given orally in a dose of 25 mg/kg body weight twice daily for 2 to 4 days, according to its tolerance, produces a high percentage of cures. Urticaria may recur and a second similar course of thiabendazole may be required.

Angiostrongylus

Angiostrongylus cantonensis, a nematode affecting the lung of rodents, has a larval stage in molluscs and freshwater shrimps. In the Far East and the Pacific, where infected crustacea are eaten or infected slugs on vegetables are inadvertently swallowed, the larvae may cause a serious eosinophilic meningitis and immature worms may be found in the cerebrospinal fluid.

Trichuris trichiura (Whipworm)

Under unhygienic conditions infections with whipworm are common and they are occasionally acquired in rural districts in Britain. Man is the only host. The ova are passed in stools and infection takes place by the ingestion of earth or food contaminated with ova which have become infective after lying for 3 weeks or more in moist soil. The adult worm is 3–5 cm long and has a coiled anterior end resembling a whip (Fig. 17.10). Whipworms inhabit chiefly the caecum but occasionally also the lower ileum, appendix and colon. There are usually no symptoms, but intense infections in children may cause persistent diarrhoea or rectal

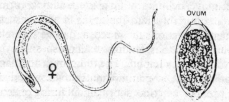

Fig. 17.10 *Trichuris trichiura* (*Ova 50 × 22 μ*).

prolapse. The diagnosis is readily made by examining the stools under the low power of the microscope, when the ova are seen. In heavy infections adult whipworms are found in the anal canal. Treatment is by oral mebendazole in doses of 100 mg twice daily for 3 days.

Trichinella spiralis

This parasite of rats and pigs is transmitted to man by eating partially cooked infected pork, usually as sausage or ham. Symptoms result from invasion of the body by larvae produced by the adult female worm in the small intestine and from their encystment in striated muscles. Outbreaks have occurred in Britain as well as in other countries where pork is eaten. Polar bear meat is another source.

The clinical course of trichinosis depends largely on the number of larvae. If there are only a few worms present there may be no symptoms but many worms may cause nausea and diarrhoea 24 to 48 hours after the infected meal. Soon, however, these symptoms are overshadowed by those associated with larval invasion, namely fever and oedema of the face, eyelids and conjunctivae. Invasion of the diaphragm may lead to pain, cough and dyspnoea; involvement of the muscles of the limbs, chest and mouth causes stiffness, pain and tenderness in the affected muscle groups. Pyrexia may reach 40°C with daily remissions. Larval migration may cause acute myocarditis and encephalitis. An eosinophilia is usually found after the second week. An intense infection may prove fatal, but in those who survive complete recovery is the rule.

Diagnosis. This may be difficult but the disease may be suspected from the clinical picture. It is not uncommon for a group of persons who have eaten infected pork from a common source to develop symptoms about the same time. When suspected, biopsy from the deltoid or gastrocnemius after the third week of symptoms may reveal encysted larvae. Precipitin and intradermal tests are also helpful.

Treatment and Prevention. If diagnosed very early anthelmintics may remove some of the adult female worms from the gut. Corticosteroids are of considerable value in controlling urgent symptoms. Thiabendazole, 50 mg/kg body weight, on two successive days, acting as a larvicide, has been used successfully to relieve persistent pain in muscles.

Pigsties should be kept free from rats. Efficient food inspection or thorough cooking of pork and sausages prevents the disease.

Gnathostomiasis

Gnathostoma spinigerum is a nematode of dogs and cats. In the Far East the third stage larva is acquired by man eating inadequately cooked infected fish or by swallowing water containing infected *Cyclops*. Then the immature worm usually migrates to the subcutaneous tissue where it causes recurrent swellings. The geographical distribution of this infection distinguishes it from loiasis in which similar 'Calabar' swellings are a feature. The full grown adult worm, which may be as long as 3 cm, may develop in man. When the worm, usually single, is visible through the skin it can be removed surgically. During migration in the deeper tissues the worm may cause injury to the brain, kidney, lung, eye or other organs. Eosinophilia is usually pronounced. Diagnosis is easy when the adult worm is visible. Otherwise serological tests are performed. Treatment is not satisfactory but some success has been obtained with bithionol used as for paragonimiasis.

Anisakiasis (Herring Worm Disease)

Anisakis marina is an ascarid which parasitises herrings and other marine animals. Human infections occur in Holland and Japan from the consumption of raw herrings. An eosinophilic granuloma forms in the intestine and may give rise to colic, fever and intestinal obstruction. An indirect haemagglutination test has been used for diagnosis. Surgery may be required.

Filariases

A number of different nematodes of the family *Filariidae* affect man. The adults are thin worms varying from 2 to 50 cm in length and the larvae or microfilariae are easily visible under the low power of the microscope, being about 250 microns long. The mature females are viviparous. The adults of the species *Wuchereria bancrofti* and *Brugia malayi* inhabit and tend to block lymphatic vessels. Adult filariae of the species *Loa loa* wander in the subcutaneous tissue and cause 'Calabar' swellings. The adults of *Onchocerca volvulus* may be surrounded by fibrous tissue in subcutaneous nodules but it is their larvae which cause a dermatosis and sometimes serious lesions in the eye. The larvae of *Dipetalonema streptocerca* may produce a similar but milder dermatosis but *Dipetalonema perstans* and *Mansonella ozzardi*, the larvae of which circulate in the blood, are non-pathogenic. The microfilariae have distinguishing morphological appearances (Fig. 17.11). It should be noted that the microfilariae of *Wuchereria, Brugia* and *Loa* are sheathed, the remainder unsheathed. Filarial infections are commonly associated with a marked eosinophilia.

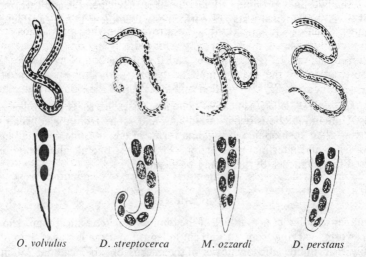

Fig. 17.11 Microfilariae (×250). Second and fourth rows show tails (greatly enlarged).

Bancroftian filariasis

Wuchereria bancrofti is conveyed to man by the bites of infected mosquitoes of a number of different species, the most common being *Culex fatigans*. The adult worms, 4 to 10 cm in length, live in the lymphatics of man, and the females produce microfilariae which at night circulate in large numbers in the peripheral blood. As *Culex fatigans* bites at night the nocturnal periodicity of the microfilariae, first demonstrated by Manson in 1877, facilitates the spread of the infection. In some of the Pacific islands there is a non-periodic strain of *W. bancrofti* maintained by mosquitoes which bite in the day-time. When not circulating in the peripheral blood, the microfilariae are chiefly in the capillaries in the lungs. The infection is widespread in tropical Africa, the North African coast, coastal areas of Asia, Indonesia and Northern Australia, South Pacific Islands, West Indies and also in North and South America.

Pathology. The microfilariae do not harm the human host. Light infections may remain symptomless but are likely to be associated with an eosinophilia. In more intense and repeated infections the presence of mature worms in the lymphatic vessels and nodes lead to allergic inflammation around the lymphatics. These cellular changes are associated with attacks of lymphangitis and lead to temporary lymphatic obstruction. Eventually, after repeated attacks, in some of which secondary bacterial infections may play a part, permanent obstruction of a main lymphatic trunk may be produced. Progressive enlargement of the limb or region below the obstruction then follows with thickening and fibrosis of the tissues.

Clinical Features. After an incubation period of not less than 3 months the first manifestations are bouts of fever accompanied by pain and tenderness along the course of inflamed lymphatic vessels over which there is cutaneous erythema. In addition there may be some scattered urticaria. Inflammation of the spermatic cord, epididymitis and orchitis may be caused by lymphangitis. After a few days the fever abates and the symptoms and signs subside. Further attacks are likely to follow and temporary oedema from obstructed lymphatics tends to become more persistent, and some enlargement of regional lymph nodes may remain. The lymphatics draining the lower limbs, the scrotum and the upper limbs are those most frequently affected, mainly or only in one site in any one individual with the formation of superficial lymph varices and the production of hydroceles. Permanent obstruction of the main lymphatic trunks of a limb causes progressive enlargement, coarsening, corrugation and fissuring of the skin and subcutaneous tissue, with warty superficial excrescences, until a leg resembles that of an elephant. The name 'elephantiasis' is thus applied to this condition which may also occur in an upper limb, the scrotum, vulva or breast. The scrotum may reach an enormous size, a weight of 20 kg or more being attained in some who remain ambulant. Obstruction of the abdominal lymphatics may lead to chyluria or chylous ascites. The interval between infection and the onset of elephantiasis is usually not less than 10 years, after which the condition tends to be slowly but remorselessly progressive, although minor degrees may persist unchanged. Gross elephantiasis develops only in highly endemic areas.

Diagnosis. In the earliest stages of lymphangitis the diagnosis is made on clinical grounds, supported usually by an eosinophilia and sometimes by a positive complement-fixation or intradermal test. After about a year from the time of infection microfilariae appear in the blood at night and can be seen moving in a wet blood film or a sample of lysed blood passed through a microfilter and identified in stained blood smears. They are usually present in hydrocele fluid which may on occasion yield an adult filaria. With the establishment of permanent elephantiasis it becomes unusual for microfilariae to reach the blood stream and eventually the adult worms may die but the lymphatics remain obstructed. Shadows of calcified filariae may sometimes be demonstrable by radiography. An initial exaggeration of symptoms following the administration of the specific drug, diethylcarbamazine, is indicative of a filarial infection.

Non-filarial elephantiasis, usually affecting only one lower limb, occurs in certain geographical areas which are free from filariasis. It is attributed to damage to lymphatics by chemicals absorbed from soil derived from volcanic rocks.

Complement-fixation test. This is a group reaction given by all pathogenic filariae. The antigen is usually prepared from *Dirofilaria immitis* or *Setaria cervi*, filariae of animal origin. This test is positive in only a proportion of cases but is rather more reliable, when positive, than an intradermal test using antigens of the same origin.

Treatment. Diethylcarbamazine, given orally, has a rapid destructive effect on microfilariae and a slower action against adult filariae. The dosage is up to 9 to 12 mg/kg body weight daily in three divided doses for 21 days. The full dosage should, however, only be reached slowly, starting with 50 mg (one tablet) and doubling daily if no untoward allergic responses ensue. This course may be repeated twice at intervals of 4 to 6 weeks. To control allergic phenomena antihistamines or corticosteroids may be required. Treatment with diethylcarbamazine, given early in the disease, produces cure and may lead to some amelioration in the more recently established cases of elephantiasis. In longstanding elephantiasis plastic surgery, preferably after preliminary radiological investigation of the lymphatics, is indicated. Great relief may be obtained by removal of excess tissue but recurrences are probable unless new lymphatic drainage is established. Tight bandaging, or bed rest with suspension or raising of the affected part, by reducing the swelling, will give temporary relief and may be desirable as a pre-operative measure.

Prevention. In endemic areas treatment of the whole population with diethylcarbamazine, 100 mg for adults (50 mg for children) three times daily for 7 days, has reduced but not eliminated the infection. Children are given such a course on starting and just before leaving school. This mass treatment should be combined with control of the vector by insecticides (p. 842). Personal protection is obtained by the wearing of protective clothing and the use of insect repellents. Where the vector is a night-biting mosquito wire-screening of the house or the use of mosquito nets prevent infection. Early chemotherapy prevents later elephantiasis.

Brugia filariasis

Brugia malayi resembles *W. bancrofti* closely. The microfilariae usually exhibit nocturnal periodicity but a semiperiodic form, which may affect man, commonly infects animals. A similar filaria, *Brugia pahangi*, is found chiefly in animals but has been transmitted to man. It, or a similar filaria, may be responsible for some cases of tropical pulmonary eosinophilia. The vectors of *B. malayi* are mosquitoes mostly belonging to the genus *Mansonioides*. *B. malayi* is found in Indonesia, Borneo, Malaysia, Vietnam, South China, South India and Sri Lanka.

The pathology, clinical manifestations, treatment and personal prophylaxis are the same as those recorded for *W. bancrofti* except that elephantiasis is usually limited to the legs. A selective weed-killer, phenoxylene, has been used with success to rid ponds of the water hyacinth upon which the larvae of *Mansonioides* are dependent.

Loiasis

Loiasis is caused by infection with the filaria *Loa loa*. The adults, 3 to 7 cm long, parasitise chiefly the subcutaneous tissue of man. The larval microfilariae circulate harmlessly in the peripheral blood in the day-time, in contrast to the nocturnal periodicity of *W. bancrofti*. This led Manson in 1895 to postulate that the vector would be a fly biting by day, such as *Chrysops*, species of which are now known to convey the infection. A morphologically similar parasite infects monkeys but is not readily conveyed to man. Loiasis may be acquired in West Africa, Zaïre and Angola. It is endemic only in and around equatorial rainforests.

Pathology. The adult worms move about in the subcutaneous tissues and other interstitial planes. Usually there is little evidence, apart from an eosinophilia, of a reaction of the host's tissues but from time to time a short-lived oedematous swelling (a 'Calabar' swelling) is produced, presumably around an adult worm. Calcified dead worms are occasionally seen on X-ray. Encephalitis has been attributed to microfilariae of *Loa loa* on rare occasions.

Clinical Features. The incubation period is commonly over a year but may be as short as 3 months. The infection may be symptomless. The first sign is often a Calabar swelling. This is felt as an irritating tense localised swelling which is painful if it is near a joint. The swelling is generally on a limb; it measures a few centimetres in diameter but sometimes is more diffuse and extensive. It usually disappears after a few days but may persist for 2 or 3 weeks. A succession of such swellings may appear at irregular intervals, often in near-by sites. Sometimes there is some urticaria and pruritus elsewhere. Occasionally a worm may be distinctly seen wriggling under the skin, especially of an eyelid and may cross the eye under the conjunctiva, taking many minutes to do so. When an adult worm is moving in retro-orbital tissues severe unilateral headache resembling migraine is experienced.

A reliable history of the crossing of the eye by a worm or of characteristic Calabar swellings in one who has resided in an endemic area enables a clinical diagnosis to be made. This will usually be supported by an eosinophilia. The demonstration of microfilariae of *Loa loa* in the blood (or the recovery of an adult from the skin or eye) establishes the diagnosis. The filarial complement-fixation test is positive in 80 per cent of infections and the intradermal test is usually positive. These are not specific for loiasis. Calabar swellings may be simulated in gnathostomiasis.

Treatment and Prevention. Diethylcarbamazine (p. 914) gradually increased to a dose of 9 to 12 mg/kg body weight daily and continued at that dosage for 21 days is curative. Treatment may precipitate a reaction characterised by fever, malaise, joint and muscle pain and rarely encephalitis.

Protection is afforded by siting houses away from trees and by having dwellings wire-screened against the fly. Protective clothing and repellents are also useful. Mud flats where *Chrysops* is breeding should be treated with Dieldrin or other chemicals to destroy the larvae and pupae. Treatment of the population with diethylcarbamazine will diminish the infective rate of the potential vector.

Onchocerciasis

Onchocerciasis is the result of infection by the filaria *Onchocerca volvulus*. The adult female may be as long as 50 cm, the male being much shorter. The infection is conveyed by flies of the genus *Simulium* which inflict a painful bite. In West Africa the vector is *S. damnosum*, in Northern Nigeria also *S. bovis* and in East Africa and Zaïre *S. neavei*. The flies breed in rapidly flowing well aerated water, the larvae being attached to submerged vegetation and rocks. The larvae of *S. neavei* may be attached to crabs and mayfly nymphs. Adult flies bite during the day-time both inside and outside houses. Man is the only known definitive host.

Onchocerciasis is endemic in well defined areas throughout tropical Africa, in Southern Arabia and also in South Mexico and Guatemala. It is estimated that over 20 million people are infected. In parts of West and Central Africa it affects the whole adult population and blindness rates of 10 per cent are common, reaching in some parts of Ghana 35 per cent. Because of onchocerciasis huge tracts of fertile land lie virtually untilled.

Pathology. Infective larvae of *O. volvulus* are introduced into the skin by the bite of an infected *Simulium*. The worms mature in 2 to 4 months and live for up to 17 years. A group, including at least two intertwined living adult worms of different sexes, may become surrounded by fibrous tissue and a firm subcutaneous nodule, an 'onchocercoma', results. In these nodules, in the tissues around, and widely distributed in the skin, innumerable microfilariae, discharged by the female *O. volvulus*, move actively and may invade the anterior part of the eye. Live microfilariae elicit little tissue reaction, but dead microfilariae may cause severe allergic inflammation.

Clinical Features. No evidence of the infection, except for an eosinophilia, may be present for periods ranging from 9 to 24 months. The first sign may be the accidental discovery of one or more nodules which are sometimes soft but more usually firm. They are subcutaneous but are sometimes attached to underlying bone or to overlying skin. Common sites are around the pelvis or around joints or the ribs and on the head. They vary in number and size and are painless. None may be evident. The commonest manifestation is a persistent irritating dermatosis, at first localised but gradually spreading and appearing also in multiple sites. In unpigmented skins this is seen as an erythematous rough maculopapular rash, often with excoriations following irresistible itching. In chronic infections the skin becomes inelastic, wrinkled and, in places, depigmented. Massive infiltration of the skin of the groin may cause it to hang down in a fold (hanging groin) and localised lymphatic obstruction may produce an elephantoid condition of the skin of the perineum and scrotum.

In endemic areas the damage done to the eyes by microfilariae has earned the disease the name 'African River Blindness'. Lesions of the eye are more likely to be severe in areas of high endemicity. Early features are photophobia and conjunctival injection. The cornea may soon show interpalpebral 'snowflake' deposits and later there may be a sclerosing keratitis, or chronic iridocyclitis with ciliary injection, synechiae, glaucoma and cataract. Posterior segment changes of choroidoretinitis and optic atrophy are an important cause of blindness in some areas.

Diagnosis. The finding of nodules or characteristic lesions of the skin or eyes, in a patient from an endemic area, associated with eosinophilia, is suggestive. Aggravation of the dermatosis after treatment with diethylcarbamazine supports the diagnosis. A certain diagnosis may be made by removal of a nodule and the demonstration of adult worms and unsheathed microfilariae within it. A skin snip or shaving, repeated if necessary from calf, buttock and shoulder, placed in saline or water and examined under the low power of the microscope, usually reveals the microfilariae. Microfilariae can also sometimes be seen moving in the anterior chamber of the eye examined with a slit-lamp or identified in a conjunctival snip. A filarial complement-fixation test is positive in about 50 per cent of infections and the intradermal test in a much higher proportion. These are not specific for onchocerciasis (p. 914).

Treatment and Prevention. Any nodules detected should be removed.

Diethylcarbamazine (p. 914) rapidly kills the microfilariae and this causes an allergic reaction for the first few days of treatment. The itch increases, eye lesions are aggravated and there may be accompanying fever with pain in the joints. Other reactions include hypotension and respiratory distress. Only a small dose should be given initially, 0·5 mg/kg body weight on the first day, this being gradually increased as the drug is tolerated until, if possible, a dose of 12 mg/kg body weight is reached. This dose should be continued for 17 to 21 days. An antihistamine, such as chlorpheniramine maleate, may alleviate mild reactions but corticosteroids, locally as drops to the eyes and systemically, are needed to control severe reactions. Ideally the patient should be in bed for the first 24 hours of treatment.

Adult worms are killed by suramin (p. 85), the intervals between intravenous injections of 1 g should be 5 to 7 days and the maximum total dose 6 g. In endemic areas where reinfection is inevitable, and in patients with little or no eye involvement, repeated courses of diethylcarbamazine or long-term suppression with 100 mg weekly may be preferred to the potential toxicity of suramin.

Mass treatment is impossible at present. The fly can be destroyed in its larval stage by the application of Dieldrin to streams or the adult flies can be attacked by spraying this insecticide on vegetation near streams. Dimethylphthalate applied to skin or clothing will repel simulia for several hours. Long trousers or skirts and sleeves discourage the fly from biting.

Dipetalonema streptocerca

Microfilariae and adult worms of this parasite have been identified in the skin of man and chimpanzees in Ghana and Zaïre. The intermediate host and vector is the midge *Culicoides grahami*. The microfilariae may produce a mild dermatosis of the trunk, usually less irritating than the dermatosis of onchocerciasis. This filariasis also responds to a course of diethylcarbamazine (p. 914).

Dipetalonema perstans

Dipetalonema (*Acanthocheilonema*) *perstans* is a filarial parasite of man which is usually non-pathogenic. In endemic areas microfilariae of *D. perstans* are commonly found in the peripheral blood in which they circulate both by day and night. The adults inhabit chiefly the retroperitoneal and perirenal tissues and have been found in the pericardial sac. The intermediate hosts are *Culicoides austeni* and *C. grahami*. This filaria is found throughout equatorial Africa as far south as Zambia, also in Trinidad and parts of northern and eastern South America.

D. perstans has never been shown to cause disease but it may be responsible for a persistent eosinophilia and occasional allergic manifestations. It has been suspected of causing effusions into serous cavities and cardiomyopathy. *D. perstans* is resistant to diethylcarbamazine and the infection may persist for many years. A combination of mebendazole 100 mg twice daily combined with levamisole 100 mg daily has been reported to be effective.

Mansonella ozzardi

This filaria of man is non-pathogenic and is found in the West Indies and central and northern parts of South America. The adults inhabit the mesentery and subperitoneal tissues. The microfilariae circulate in the blood. The intermediate hosts are species of *Culicoides*. Diethylcarbamazine is ineffective.

Tropical Pulmonary Eosinophilia

Tropical pulmonary eosinophilia is attributable to an infection with a filarial worm such as *Dirofilaria* or *Brugia pahangi*, which is unable to mature in man. Alternatively it may be an unusual host reaction to *Wuchereria bancrofti* or *Brugia malayi*. The disease is found in many tropical regions including India, Sri Lanka, Malaysia, China, Philippines, Australia, South America and uncommonly in Africa. Its clinical features and treatment are discussed on page 306.

Dracontiasis

(*Guinea Worm Infection*)

The female *Dracunculus medinensis*, which measures over a metre in length, lives in the interstitial and subcutaneous tissues of man for 12–18 months. The male worm, which is rarely seen, is only 2·5 cm long and dies earlier. Man is infected by ingesting a small crustacean, *Cyclops*, which inhabits the bottom of wells and ponds and which contains the infective larval stage of the worm. When the cyclops is ingested by man the mature larvae penetrate the intestinal wall and migrate through the connective tissue of the host. After 9 to 18 months the fully mature female seeks the surface of the skin where a vesicle is raised, soon ruptures and exposes the anterior end of the worm. The distended uterus then ruptures and discharges its larvae externally. The worm is attracted to the surface by cooling, hence the larvae are likely to be expelled into water and to be ingested by a cyclops. Man is the most important host but *D. medinensis* has been found in dogs and cats.

The disease can be extremely disabling and is especially liable to affect farmers at the beginning of the rains and thus seriously interfere with planting. It is found in West, Central and East Africa, the Sudan, Arabia, Iran, Turkey, Pakistan,

Central India, Burma, the Caribbean Islands and the northern parts of South America.

Clinical Features. When mature the adult may sometimes be felt beneath the skin. Some hours before the head of the worm emerges from the skin there is usually some local redness and tenderness. There may also be general allergic symptoms, erythema, giant urticaria, nausea, vomiting and diarrhoea. These symptoms usually subside as soon as the vesicle has ruptured and the larvae begin to be discharged. This is usually complete in 3 to 4 weeks, after which the worm is often spontaneously extruded and healing takes place. The vesicle commonly appears in the lower part of the leg or in any area which has been kept moist and relatively cool. If the worm dies or is broken during extraction there may be a marked allergic inflammation. Secondary infection is common and causes severe cellulitis, septicaemia, aseptic or pyogenic arthritis. Tetanus is a well recognised complication. Multiple infections may occur and reactions around aberrant worms may cause serious lesions, exceptionally spinal cord compression.

Diagnosis is usually easy from the appearance of a vesicle, the protusion of a worm and the recognition of the discharged larvae. A radiograph occasionally shows calcified worms.

Treatment and Prevention. Traditionally the protruding worm has been extracted by winding it out gently over several days on a sterile match stick. Although reports vary, niridazole in doses of 25 mg/kg body weight daily in 2 divided doses for 10 days or thiabendazole 50 mg/kg on 2 successive days may relieve symptoms and aid the extraction of the worm. Antibiotics and prophylaxis of tetanus are required for secondary infection.

The provision of a satisfactory water supply would eradicate the infection. Where this is impracticable, wells and ponds may be protected or treated chemically.

DISEASES DUE TO FUNGI
(Mycotic infections)

Histoplasmosis; Mycetoma; Blastomycoses; Chromoblastomycosis; Sporotrichosis; Cryptococcosis; Coccidioidomycosis; Rhinosporidiosis; Superficial Mycoses

Histoplasmosis

Histoplasmosis is caused by *Histoplasma capsulatum* (*Darling*) which adopts a yeast-like morphology in its parasitic phase but is a filamentous fungus of soil at other times. A variant, *Histoplasma duboisii*, is found in parts of tropical Africa (p. 921). The spores of *Histoplasma* remain viable for years in the soil in which the fungus actually grows, and infected dust, when inhaled, conveys the disease. Occasionally infection passes through the buccal or intestinal mucosa or through the skin. The disease attacks dogs, rats and mice, and the fungus multiplies in soil enriched by the droppings of chickens, pigeons and bats. The infection is thus a hazard for explorers of caves.

Histoplasma capsulatum

This is found in all parts of the United States of America, especially in the East

Central States, and less commonly in Latin America from Mexico to Argentina, in Europe, North, South and East Africa, Nigeria, Malaysia, Indonesia and Australia.

Pathological and Clinical Features. The parasite in its yeast phase multiplies like leishmaniae mainly in reticulo-endothelial cells and produces areas of necrosis in which the parasites may abound in enormous numbers. From these foci the blood stream may be invaded leading to metastatic lesions in the liver, spleen and lymph nodes. Pulmonary histoplasmosis may produce pathological changes similar to those of tuberculosis.

Infection is usually carried to the lung in the first place by inhalation of dust containing spores. Probably 90 per cent of pulmonary infections are benign producing no symptoms, but a more severe infection may closely simulate pulmonary tuberculosis, including the production of a primary complex with enlarged satellite lymph nodes, multiple small discrete lesions and occasionally cavity formation. Areas of calcification are characteristic of the more benign forms of this disease. Lesions of the skin or mucosa may be found on the rare occasions when infection has entered that way and are common in disseminated histoplasmosis which is characterised by enlargement of the liver, spleen and lymph nodes, irregular pyrexia, anaemia and leucopenia. Addison's disease may be produced by caseation in the adrenals. Endocarditis is rare. When the mucosa of the mouth and gastrointestinal tract become infected, the predominant symptoms may be vomiting and diarrhoea. Occasionally the central nervous system is invaded. The severity of the symptoms of histoplasmosis varies from, in the majority of cases, a slight fever of short duration, like influenza, to a severe and prolonged pyrexial illness which ultimately proves fatal.

Diagnosis. In an area where the disease occurs, histoplasmosis should be suspected in every obscure infection in which there are pulmonary signs or where there are enlarged lymph nodes with or without hepatosplenomegaly. Material obtained by biopsy from a lymph node or the lung should be stained to show the intracellular *H. capsulatum*. It can also be demonstrated by culture or by animal inoculation. Radiological examination in long standing cases may show calcified lesions in the lungs, spleen or other organs. In the more acute phases of the disease single or multiple soft pulmonary shadows with enlarged tracheo-bronchial nodes may be revealed. An intradermal test is carried out with a 1 : 1,000 dilution of a standardised histoplasmin antigen. This gives a positive reaction in most patients with either active or healed infections but is usually negative in the rapidly progressive form of the disease. Complement fixing antibodies are detected within 3 weeks of the onset of an acute primary infection and increase in titre as the disease progresses. Precipitating antibodies may also be detected.

Treatment. Specific treatment with amphotericin B is indicated only in severe infections. The dosage is 0·5 mg/kg body weight, in 500 ml of 5 per cent glucose given intravenously over a 6-hour period, gradually increasing to a maximum of 1·0 mg/kg body weight. Daily treatment is necessary at first in seriously ill patients but later, as improvement sets in, it can be decreased to 3 times a week. If badly tolerated the dosage may have to be reduced. Side-effects are malaise, anorexia, nausea, fever, headache and venous thrombosis. These can be controlled to a considerable extent by the addition of 10 mg prednisolone to the intravenous solution. Renal and hepatic function tests should be done during the course of treatment. Amphotericin B may have to be continued for up to a month or longer, depending on the clinical response. Recovery from generalised histoplasmosis is rare but co-trimoxazole has been used successfully.

Histoplasma duboisii

This fungus, first isolated in Ghana, is considerably larger than the classical *H. capsulatum*. It is found in Ghana, Uganda, Nigeria, Senegal, Sudan and Zaïre.

This disease differs in several ways from *H. capsulatum* infection. The bones, skin, lymph nodes and liver develop granulomatous lesions or cold abscesses resembling tuberculosis, but the lungs are seldom involved. The visceral form with liver and splenic invasion is often fatal, while ulcerative skin lesions and bone abscesses follow a more benign course.

Radiological examination may show rounded foci of bone destruction sometimes associated with abscess formation. Multiple lesions of the ribs are common but the bones of the limbs may also be involved.

The disease is treated in the same way as *H. capsulatum* infections. A solitary lesion in bone may require only local surgical treatment.

Other Mycoses

Mycetoma

(*Madura Foot*)

In 1842 Gill of Madura in India described the condition which became known as Madura Foot. In 1860 Carter gave to this swelling, of fungal causation, the name 'mycetoma'. This clinical condition, which is not confined to infections of the foot, may be produced by members of two groups of organisms classified as *Maduromycetoma (Eumycetoma)* and aerobic *Actinomycetecea*. A feature common to both groups is the formation by the fungus of grains, with characteristic colours, ranging from 60 microns to 3 mm in diameter. The incidence of different species appears to be related to climate, being especially high when an arid hot season ends in rains. The term 'mycetoma' is here used in this restricted sense, although some authors have used the term for other granulomatous lesions caused by fungi. The more common species of fungi causing mycetoma, as defined above, are shown in Table 17.4 (p. 922). The fungus can be identified by the microscopic appearances of the tissue and grains and confirmed by culture.

Nocardia asteroides resembles *N. caviae* (Table 17.4) but causes nocardiosis, a fungal infection involving mainly the lungs; grains are not produced.

Pathological and Clinical Features. The lesions may occur in any part of the body but as the fungus is usually introduced by a thorn they are most common in the foot and leg in those who walk bare-footed. At the site of implantation the mycetoma begins as a painless swelling. Unless totally excised at an early stage, or in some species effectively treated by chemotherapy, the mycetoma grows and spreads inexorably and eventually penetrates bones. The histology is that of a chronic granuloma with a fibrous stroma and cyst-like spaces in which lie the characteristic grains. The loose cellular tissue is infiltrated with leucocytes, small round cells and giant cells. Nodules develop under the epidermis and these rupture revealing sinuses through which mucopus containing the coloured grains is discharged. Some sinuses may heal with scarring while fresh sinuses appear

Table 17.4 Fungi causing mycetoma

Species	Type of Grains
Maduromycetoma (*Eumycetoma*)	
Madurella mycetoma	brown or black (big)
Madurella grisea	black or brown (big)
Phialophora jeanselmei	black
Allescheria boydii	white or yellow (big)
Cephalosporium falciforme	white or yellow
Actinomycetecea	
Streptomyces madurae	white, yellow, red (big)
S. somaliensis	white or yellow (big)
S. pelletieri	red (small)
Nocardia caviae	yellow
Nocardia brasiliensis	white, yellow (very small)

elsewhere. There is little pain and usually no fever, but progressive disability. Secondary pyogenic infection does not usually penetrate far down the sinuses, possibly because of antibiotic activity of the fungi.

Madurella mycetomi grows in fascial planes and avoids the muscles until a very late stage; it does not affect nerves and tendons. Although pigment may be carried to regional lymph nodes, it is exceptional for the fungus to reach the nodes unless there has been surgical interference. When the lesion is in the scalp, the skull may be affected but the dura mater appears to be an effective barrier. Apart from involvement of bones by a spreading mycetoma, intra-osseous lesions may be found in the metaphysis of a long bone, especially at the upper end of the tibia and sometimes there may be an encapsulated periosteal mass.

Nocardia brasiliensis often affects the skin of the back. It is seldom localised and may spread widely.

Streptomyces somaliensis and *S. pelletieri* also spread insidiously and early invade muscle. As in the case of *S. madurae* they also readily reach regional lymph nodes.

Extensive damage of bones may be caused in any of these infections.

Treatment. The difference between *Maduromycetoma* and *Actinomycetecea* is crucial in that there is no drug of proven efficacy for the former. Amphotericin B is apparently inactive *in vivo*, though not necessarily *in vitro*, against both *Maduromycetoma* and aerobic actinomycetes that cause mycetoma. Sporadic successes with griseofulvin against the *Maduromycetoma* have been reported, but the results have been mostly disappointing and up to the present maduromycetoma requires to be surgically removed. Mycetoma has a strong tendency to recur locally unless the excision has been adequate or the amputation high enough. The treatment of actinomycetoma is more hopeful. Dapsone (100 mg t.i.d.) frequently cures infections due to *Nocardia* species. Sulphonamides also have some value. It is important to give the drugs for many months. There are reports of the successful treatment of actinomycetoma due to *Streptomyces* species with dapsone, sulphonamides and broad spectrum antibiotics but there have also been many failures. Perhaps the most promising drug is co-trimoxazole. Nevertheless, many cases still require surgical removal.

Blastomycoses

North American Blastomycosis is caused by *Blastomyces dermatitidis*. It also occurs in Africa. This infection may give rise to cutaneous lesions, especially of the face. Systemic infection begins in the lungs and mediastinal lymph nodes and resembles pulmonary tuberculosis. Bones, the central nervous system and the genito-urinary tract may also be affected. Parenteral treatment with 2-hydroxystilbamidine (p. 847) or amphotericin B (p. 920) has achieved much success. Co-trimoxazole may also be effective.

South American Blastomycosis (*Paracoccidioidomycosis*) is caused by *Blastomyces brasiliensis*. Mucocutaneous lesions occur early. Involvement of lymphatic nodes and the lungs is prominent and the gastrointestinal tract may also be attacked. Prolonged treatment with oral sulphonamides or amphotericin B or 2-hydroxystilbamidine may be curative.

The diagnosis and differentiation of blastomycosis is established by culture of the fungus from the pus expressed from the lesion, or in systemic infections from the sputum. Complement-fixation reactions and intradermal tests aid diagnosis.

Chromoblastomycosis
(*Mossy Foot*)

True mossy foot is a fungal infection and is to be distinguished from the warty excrescences which accompany the chronic lymphatic obstruction of elephantiasis and also from Madura Foot or mycetoma. Chromoblastomycosis is due to certain species of *Cladosporium*.

These fungi are acquired on splinters from decaying timber and give rise to a warty condition of the foot and also rarely affect the face, upper limbs, vulva and brain. The diagnosis is confirmed by the recognition of dark brown spheroid bodies 4 to 8 microns in diameter in biopsy specimens or by culture.

Iodides up to 3 g daily and calciferol 1 to 2 mg weekly should be given. This is combined, when necessary, with surgical removal of local lesions but relapse is common. Amphotericin B by local infiltration is now considered the best treatment.

Sporotrichosis

Sporotrichosis is caused by *Sporotrichum schenckii*. The infection occurs throughout the world and is prevalent in Central and Southern Africa. It causes swellings resembling gummata or a chancroid type of ulcer and affected lymphatic vessels may be thickened and palpable as a chain of nodules. Uncommonly dissemination takes place into lungs, bones, the central nervous system and elsewhere. The fungus can be cultured from discharges or biopsy material.

Potassium iodide up to 10 g daily should be given orally until some time after apparent clinical cure. A solution containing iodine in the proportions of 1 g iodine, 10 g potassium iodide in 500 ml of water should be injected into the lymph nodes. Widely disseminated infections respond to amphotericin B (p. 920).

Cryptococcosis

Cryptococcosis is caused by *Cryptococcus neoformans*. It occurs in India, California, Central United States and elsewhere and causes local gummatous-like tumours and granulomatous lesions of the lung, bones, brain and meninges. The cerebrospinal fluid often contains the fungus when the nervous system is affected.

The diagnosis is made by serological tests, biopsy, culture or recognition of spores in the cerebrospinal fluid.

Amphotericin B should be given intravenously and, in disease of the nervous system, intrathecally. It has been suggested from experimental work that a low thiamine diet and gamma globulin injections may be a useful supplementary measure. Some cases of cryptococcal meningitis have been cured by oral 5-fluorocytosine, 100 to 200 mg/kg body weight given daily until the cerebrospinal fluid remained normal. Surgical removal of local pulmonary lesions is essential to prevent spread to the brain. Recovery may be assessed by serological changes.

Coccidioidomycosis

Coccidioidomycosis is caused by *Coccidioides immitis*. This infection is found in Southern United States, and in Central and South America. The disease is acquired by inhalation. In 40 per cent of cases it affects the lungs and lymph nodes. Rarely it may be carried by the blood stream to the bones, adrenals, meninges and other organs. Infected sputum dribbling on to the chin produces a characteristic skin lesion. In 60 per cent of cases the infection is asymptomatic. Infections, including subclinical attacks, are followed by immunity.

The fungi grow readily on culture media but as they are highly infective, diagnostic investigations are usually limited to intradermal, complement-fixation and precipitin tests.

Some localised pulmonary lesions can be successfully treated by surgery. Amphotericin B is the only other treatment which may be beneficial.

Rhinosporidiosis

Rhinosporidiosis is caused by *Rhinosporidium seeberi* and occurs in South America, India, Sri Lanka, East Africa and elsewhere. This organism forms a cyst which on rupture discharges spores which spread by lymphatics to connective tissue. It produces polypi in the nose and localised swellings on the cheek and elsewhere. The characteristic sporangia and spores are recognised on histological examination of the tumour-like tissue but the organism has not yet been cultured. Treatment consists of excision and intravenous pentavalent antimony (p. 847) or amphotericin B (p. 920).

Superficial Mycoses

Mycoses affecting the skin are cosmopolitan and include *Tinea versicolor* and dermatophytosis (ringworm infection). *Tinea imbricata*, characterised by multiple concentric rings, is a common cause of severe pruritus in some Pacific Islands and in South East Asia. It responds to griseofulvin.

Infection of the scalp by *Trichophyton schoenleinii* produces a mass of creamy white material with an offensive odour, the lesion being known as favus. It is treated by epilation and powerful topical fungicides or griseofulvin.

DISEASES DUE TO ARTHROPODS

Crab Louse Infestation; Scabies; Tick Paralysis; Tungiasis; Spider Bite; Scorpion and Bee Stings; Myiasis; Porocephalosis

Mosquitoes, flies, ticks, lice, fleas, winged bugs and mites are the vectors of a variety of diseases as set out in the preceding sections. The following conditions due to uninfected arthropods also deserve mention.

The crab louse, *Phthirius pubis,* infests the pubic hair, other hairy parts, the eyelashes and the hair above the brow of children, causing itching. Gammabenzene hexachloride 1 per cent should be applied to the body and liquid paraffin to the eyelashes.

Scabies is due to the mite *Acarus scabei*; it is common in the tropics but may be mimicked by onchocerciasis. It causes itching, initially between the fingers or on the buttocks or penis where the mite burrows, and later all over the body. Scabies is treated by a single application of gammabenzene hexachloride 1 per cent to the whole body below the neck or by three daily applications of benzyl benzoate 15 per cent.

Tick Paralysis. Fatal poisoning rarely results from absorption of the venom in the saliva of certain hard ticks, when such a tick remains attached to the head or neck for some days causing a flaccid paralysis and failure of respiration. If the tick is removed in time, recovery ensues.

Tungiasis is due to infestation with *Tunga penetrans* (the chigoe or jigger flea). Originally found in tropical America it is now widespread in Africa. Man and pigs are important hosts. The pregnant female flea burrows into the skin, especially about the toes and soles, but fingers and other parts of the body may be invaded. The flea then grows as large as a pea and is packed with eggs which are subsequently discharged on to the surface of the body. Untreated, the site of infestation may irritate and become inflamed but the chief danger is from secondary pyogenic infection or tetanus. The chigoe and egg sac should be removed with a sterile needle, after which a mild antiseptic ointment is applied. Massive infestations, such as may be seen in neglected children and in senile persons, may be treated by immersing the feet in a bath of an aqueous solution containing benzene hexachloride powder 5 per cent and cetrimide powder 0·8 per cent.

Spider Bite

The venom of certain spiders is dangerous to man. One of them is the 'black widow' spider. The adult female is glossy-black with crimson hour-glass markings on the ventral aspect of the abdomen. In South Africa the 'button' spider is also poisonous as is the 'funeral web' spider in Australia. Many other poisonous arachnids are found in different parts of the world. With the bite venom is injected and causes severe local pain followed by redness and swelling. Pain is intense, first in the adjacent muscles but spreading rapidly to all voluntary muscles, especially the flexor groups, causing severe spasms. Contraction of the pupils, salivation and sweating are common, and in severe cases the patient may suffer cardiovascular collapse. Rigidity of the abdominal muscles may simulate an acute abdomen. Later the site of the bite may slough.

Treatment. The bite should be cleansed. Local incision and suction may remove some of the venom. Where a specific antivenom is available this should be injected into the muscles near the bite. If convalescent serum is available it may be tried. A good response may be obtained to an injection of atropine. Corticosteroids are of value. For the relief of muscle spasm 10 to 20 ml of 10 per cent calcium gluconate can be given slowly intravenously. Antibiotics should be used against secondary pyogenic infections.

Scorpion and Bee Stings

SCORPION STINGS

There are many genera of scorpions found in the tropics and subtropics. Paired poison glands are situated in the terminal segment of the flexible jointed tail which is curved dorsally over the scorpion's body before striking.

Clinical Features. There is a single puncture wound at the site of the sting. Intense local pain is felt immediately, and a red oedematous weal, sometimes haemorrhagic, soon appears. Children particularly show severe general symptoms which include sweating, salivation, nausea, vomiting and depression of respiration and may die. From S. India and Jordan occasional deaths of adults also are reported and recent observations point to disseminated intravascular coagulation resulting in defibrination and haemorrhages as the cause of death. In Trinidad stings of the scorpion *Tityus trinitatis* frequently cause acute pancreatitis from which recovery is usual.

Treatment. Pain can be relieved by immersing the part in water as hot as the patient can tolerate, or by the local injection of xylocaine and adrenaline. If antivenom is available a child should be given 5 ml of the serum intramuscularly near the sting as early as possible. When required, general treatment for shock is given. In severe cases with proved disseminated intravascular coagulation intravenous heparin is indicated.

BEE STINGS

A bee sting is always painful and in those who have become sensitised an anaphylactic reaction may result in rapid death. In the majority of fatal cases there has been a severe reaction to a bee sting on an earlier occasion. Desensitisation may be practised with some degree of success. Emergency treatment of anaphylactic shock consists of 0·5 ml of adrenaline injection given intramuscularly followed by an intravenous injection of hydrocortisone hemisuccinate 100 mg. Anyone who has sustained a severe reaction should, however, be furnished with the means of self-administering a subcutaneous injection of 0·5 ml of adrenaline injection in an emergency and should also carry a drug such as isoprenaline, 10 mg of which placed under the tongue produces rapid stimulation of the sympathetic nervous system. Less severe symptoms may be relieved by an antihistamine. Severe envenomation from multiple stings causes shock, local tissue necrosis, intravascular haemolysis and acute nephritis. As they continue to release venom the 'stingers' of the bees should be removed from the skin by scraping with the blade of a knife.

Myiasis

Myiasis is an infestation of various tissues of man by the larvae of flies.

Cutaneous Myiasis. A common cause of cutaneous myiasis is *Cordylobia anthropophaga* (Tumbu fly) which lays its eggs on laundry spread on grass. The larvae penetrate the skin and produce lesions like boils.

Another cause is *Dermatobia hominis* which deposits its eggs on the ventral surface of the abdomen of other *Diptera*, especially mosquitoes. When the mosquito bites man or other animals, the warmth of the body stimulates the emergence of the larva. It burrows through the mosquito-made wound into the subcutaneous tissue and grows, causing a rounded swelling with a central orifice through which it obtains air. After reaching maturity it escapes. A drop of thick oil, such as liquid paraffin, usually brings the larva out in search of air and facilitates its removal. Occasionally the common warble fly (*Hypoderma bovis*) may infest man. *Auchmeromyia luteola*, the Congo floor maggot, imbibes blood through the skin, dropping off when disturbed.

Myiasis of Wounds, Sores and Cavities. The larvae of many flies including *Callitrogra hominivorax* (Screw worm), *Wohlfahrtia*, *Calliphora*, *Lucilia*, *Sarcophaga* and *Fannia* may infest necrotic tissue in open wounds or ulcers and occasionally invade living tissue. Chronic tropical ulcers and necrotic tissue from leprosy or tertiary yaws of the nose and pharynx may be invaded. *Chrysomya bezziana* is a myiasis-producing fly which is found in Africa, India and South Vietnam. It may penetrate the nasal sinuses and cause great destruction. *Wohlfahrtia magnifica* is the only specific myiasis-producing fly known to infest man in Europe.

The application of 10 per cent chloroform in a light vegetable oil is the treatment of choice for infested wounds.

Intestinal Myiasis. In the tropics especially, vague digestive disturbances or abdominal cramps with diarrhoea and vomiting may be caused by dipterous larvae in the intestinal canal. The eggs or larvae are ingested with food, but it is also possible for flies to deposit eggs on the skin around the anus whence the larvae may crawl into the rectum, vagina or even up the urethra and reach the bladder. Species of the genera *Fannia* and *Sarcophaga* are most frequently encountered. When larvae are swallowed they are passed in the stool or vomited. All fly larvae found in the stool have not necessarily been passed from the bowel as in tropical climates flies' eggs deposited in faecal matter rapidly hatch out into larvae. Occasionally larvae of *Aphiochaeta* or *Megaselia* may pupate in the bowel and live flies escape from the anus with the stool.

An aperient is usually all the treatment that is required.

Aural Myiasis. When there is an aural discharge, *Callitrogra hominivorax*, *Sarcophaga*, *Calliphora* and *Fannia* may be attracted to the ear and aural myiasis result. The nasal cavities and eyes may also be infested, and serious destruction result. Instillation of 10 per cent chloroform in a light oil kills the larvae.

Ocular Myiasis. The maggot of *Oestrus ovis* sometimes infests the human eye. The egg may be deposited in the eye of someone tending sheep, even without the fly alighting. A stinging sensation is felt, followed, as the larva develops, by severe pain in the eye. A drop of cocaine is required so that the lids can be opened to allow extraction of the maggot.

Porocephalosis

This name is given to invasions of the body by 'tongue worms', degenerate arthropods of which *Armillifer armillatus, A. moniliformis* and *Linguatula serrata* occur in man. Adult *Armillifer* parasitise the trachea and bronchi of snakes. Man is infected by ingesting ova on uncooked vegetables or by eating snakes. The condition is usually symptomless in man but calcified nymphs may be seen in radiographs of the chest and abdomen.

Halzoun is the name given in the Middle East to a form of acute dysphagia and laryngeal obstruction, due to pharyngitis and oedema of the larynx, which is believed to be due to the ingestion of nymphs of *Linguatula serrata*. These may be obtained by eating the raw liver of goats or sheep but more commonly from the accompanying inadequately cooked lymph nodes of goats. Foxes and dogs are the definitive hosts and wild rodents, goats or sheep, the intermediate hosts. Antihistamines and a local anaesthetic spray are suggested for treatment.

DISEASES DUE TO VENOMOUS SNAKES AND MARINE ANIMALS

Snake Bite; Jellyfish Stings; Stings from Cone Shells; Stinging Fish; Poisonous Fish

Snake Bite

Poisonous snakes belong to five families.

1. *Colubridae*, many of which are non-poisonous, include the Opisthoglypha which are poisonous but only rarely dangerous to man because the grooved fangs are the most posterior teeth in the upper jaw. Examples are tree snakes.

2. *Elapidae* have forward grooved fangs. The fangs are fixed in the upper jaw below or in front of the eyes. The nostrils are lateral and there are large scales over the head. The family includes cobras, kraits and mambas.

3. *Hydrophidae* are poisonous sea-snakes; they have an eel-shaped tail and rather flattened body. Sea-snakes are found along the shores of the Indian and Pacific oceans and are mostly poisonous. The most common dangerous species is *Enhydrina schistosa. Laticauda colubrina*, the banded sea snake or 'coral snake' is poisonous but not aggressive.

4. *Viperidae* are true vipers, including Russell viper and adders. At rest the long canalised fangs lie along the palate pointing posteriorly but during the act of biting they are rotated forward.

5. *Crotalidae* include the pit viper (pit between the nose and the eye) and the rattlesnake.

Pathology. The venoms of *Viperidae* and *Crotalidae* are cytolytic and haemolytic causing swelling and necrosis of tissues spreading from the site of the bite, often with some intravascular haemolysis, or else they cause intravascular coagulation and haemorrhages. The venoms of most *Elapidae* are powerfully neurotoxic, but that of the Asian cobras (*Naja* spp.) is also cytolytic. The venoms of the spitting cobra, (*Naja nigricollis*) and of the *Colubridae* are cytolytic. *Hydrophidae* venom contains a myotoxin which causes necrosis of muscle.

Clinical Features. It is estimated that less than half of those bitten by a potentially lethal snake develop systemic poisoning, but the victim is nearly always acutely anxious. The important signs of systemic envenomation are for *Viperidae* and *Crotalidae*, hypotension, blood-stained sputum and, later, non-clotting blood, for *Elapidae*, ptosis and glossopharyngeal palsy and for *Hydrophidae*, general myalgia and, later, brown or red urine from myoglobinuria.

Bites of *Viperidae* and *Crotalidae* and the Asian cobras give rise to severe pain and early swelling locally and oozing of blood-stained serum from the fang punctures. In severe poisoning extensive swelling of the limb may ensue with discolouration and blistering followed by superficial necrosis and sloughing. Secondary bacterial sepsis is uncommon unless meddlesome incisions have been made or dressings applied prior to sloughing. Systemic involvement exceptionally leads to rapid cardiovascular shock but, more commonly, to bleeding from the lung and into tissues with the danger of death from anaemia or heart failure. In the majority slow healing of the bitten part ensues.

The neurological effects of envenomation from *Elapidae* are usually manifest within 2 hours (exceptionally up to 10 hours) of the bite. They consist of drooping eyelids, incoordinate speech, unsteady gait and difficulty in respiration, progressing in the untreated to generalised paralysis. There may be little, if any, swelling at the site of the bite.

Fishermen dragging nets ashore in muddy water, at or near a river mouth, are the usual victims of bites by *Hydrophidae*. Bathers and paddlers are seldom attacked. The bite on ankle, foot, wrist or hand is felt as a sharp prick but thereafter is painless, inconspicuous and without local swelling. Symptoms of envenomation appear within 1 hour and consist of pain and stiffness, initially in the muscles of the neck, back and proximal parts of the limbs but rapidly becoming generalised. Passive movements provoke intense pain. Later, in severe poisoning, trismus, ptosis and external ophthalmoplegia may appear. Three to six hours after the onset of poisoning, the urine contains myoglobin and protein. Death may result from extensive paresis leading to respiratory failure or from renal failure. If poisoning is less severe, the victim survives but muscle weakness may persist for months.

Treatment. The following first-aid measures can be carried out by untrained personnel. First determine, if possible, whether the bite is of a poisonous snake by killing, examining and retaining the snake, if it can be done safely, and by searching the bite for fang punctures. Reassure the patient and give a mild sedative. Keep the patient at rest and apply a constricting ligature such as a handkerchief above the wound sufficiently firmly to retard the flow in the veins but not to stop the arterial circulation. The ligature must be released for 1 minute in every 30. Venom on the surface of the wound should be wiped away gently with a cloth or washed away with water. The bitten part should be immobilised as for a fracture.

The further treatment depends on the type of venomous snake.

In Britain the only naturally occurring poisonous snake is the adder, *Vipera berus*. If there is a swelling surrounding the bite the victim should be closely observed in hospital for 24 hours, but usually no specific treatment is indicated. If, however, there is persistent or recurrent hypotension, or rarely haemorrhages, it will be necessary to give an infusion of the specific Zagreb antivenom, now available from Regent Laboratories Ltd., London (telephone 01-965-3637). The contents of 2 ampoules are given in isotonic saline during 20 to 30 minutes and repeated if there is by then no clinical improvement. Adrenaline must be ready in case of anaphylaxis.

In other countries if there is evidence of systemic envenomation from a land snake or if local swelling is marked or spreading up the tissue, specific or polyvalent antiserum should be given in an intravenous infusion. Except in extreme urgency, 0·2 ml of the antiserum should be injected subcutaneously to test for serum sensitivity and the patient observed for 15 minutes. If a severe reaction occurs desensitisation is attempted by giving repeated small doses subcutaneously. Information accompanying antivenom is often incorrect. Usually 100 ml (e.g. 10 ampoules) diluted in 200 to 300 ml isotonic saline should be infused. In severe neurotoxic poisoning, this should be repeated within 1 hour, if improvement is not manifest. If blood remains incoagulable, antivenom is repeated every 6 hours. If the antivenom was appropriate for the species of snake involved the effects on systemic manifestations are dramatically beneficial. No dressing should be applied to the bitten part and unless there are signs of systemic poisoning it is doubtful if antivenom is of material value.

Those bitten by sea-snakes should be given similar first-aid treatment, being kept at rest and transported by stretcher to hospital. If more than 1 hour elapses after the bite without the appearance of signs of toxicity only reassurance is required. If there is clear evidence of systemic poisoning specific antiserum should be given intravenously, preferably after testing for anaphylaxis. Acute renal failure may be treated successfully by renal dialysis.

General measures. Shock should be combated by rest, warmth and fluid by mouth or intravenously, and blood should be transfused when indicated. Respiratory weakness following an elapine bite will benefit from oxygen and respiratory paralysis by mouth-to-mouth breathing or by the intratracheal method. Bacterial infection is more likely in *Viperidae* and *Crotalidae* bites, and here penicillin, tetanus toxoid or antitoxin and anti-gas gangrene serum may be advisable.

Diseases due to Marine Animals

Jellyfish Stings. Various jellyfishes, notably the Portuguese man-of-war, *Physalia,* cause lesions in the skin and general reactions in man. The long filamentous tentacles hanging from its under surface contain glands which release a toxin when they come in contact with the human skin. Linear reddish-brown weals are produced in the affected areas of skin. Excruciating local pain is felt, and general symptoms may follow, including profuse sweating and severe griping abdominal pains. Very occasionally a patient dies within a short time of being stung by a jellyfish, in which case one of the *Cubomedusae* (sea-wasps or box-jellies), *Chironex fleckeri* or *Chiropsalmus quadrigatus* is probably responsible.

'Irukandji stings' affects bathers in the sea off N.E. Australia at certain seasons. They are caused by minute Carybdeid (simple sea-wasps). Acute poisoning develops in a few minutes characterised by violent abdominal and generalised pains, vomiting and prostration. The victim appears seriously ill for a few days but always recovers.

Treatment. Methylated spirits or other alcohol should be applied to the stung parts. Dry sand or powder should then be applied and the tentacles and slime scraped off. Resuscitation may be required. An antivenom for sea-wasp stings is available in Australia.

Stings from Cone Shells (Conidae). There are many varieties of cone shells. The occupant is often poisonous and can give a sting causing death by respiratory paralysis.

Stinging Fish. The stonefish (*Synanceja trachynis*) is the most deadly of the stinging fish and it can easily be mistaken for a piece of coral. Along its back are 13 large spines each containing paired poison sacks. The poison causes great pain and swelling at the sites of the stings and may cause death from respiratory paralysis. The poison is destroyed by the application of hot water and an antivenom is available.

Poisonous Fish. There are a number of fish which may be poisonous to eat. Examples are the pufferfish (*Tetraodontidae*), porcupine fish (*Diodontidae*) and boxfish (*Ostraciontidae*). In general, fish covered with hard plates or spines may be poisonous, and the skin and liver, in particular, are dangerous to eat.

Further reading about venomous snakes and marine animals:

Read, H. A. (1974) In *Medicine in the Tropics*, ed. Woodruff, A. W. Ch. 33, pp. 541–548. Edinburgh: Churchill Livingstone.

DISEASES DUE TO VEGETABLE TOXINS

The deleterious effects produced by the ingestion of aflatoxin (p. 819), unripe cassava (p. 140) and bush teas (p. 458) have already been mentioned. In addition, argemone and ackee poisoning merit consideration.

Epidemic Dropsy

(*Argemone Poisoning*)

This disease is due to the use of mustard oil contaminated with the seeds of a poppy weed, *Argemone mexicana*. The weed grows commonly in mustard crops and contains a toxic alkaloid, sanguinarine. This substance interferes with the oxidation of pyruvic acid, which accumulates in the blood and tissues of the patient. Epidemic dropsy occurs in groups of people partaking of the same food, especially curried rice prepared with contaminated mustard oil.

Epidemic dropsy is encountered in India, especially in Bengal, Bihar, Orissa, Madhya Pradesh and Uttar Pradesh. Cases have also been noted among Indian expatriates in Fiji.

Pathology. There is dilation of the smaller arterioles and of capillaries, especially those of the skin, heart muscle and uveal tract. New blood vessels in the deeper layers of the skin and mucosa may form haemangiomata on the cutaneous and mucosal surfaces. Deeper organs and tissues show widespread vascular dilation and oedema.

Clinical Features. The onset may be gradual or acute, affecting a group of people taking the same diet. A period of ill-health with nausea, vomiting and diarrhoea often precedes the onset of the oedema which appears first in the legs and feet and is accompanied by symptoms and signs of cardiac failure which may be fatal, and fever. An erythematous mottling of the skin may follow the oedema, and haemangiomatous tumours up to 1 cm in diameter may appear in the skin or mucosal surfaces. Glaucoma is a serious complication.

Treatment and Prevention. Cardiac failure is treated in the usual way. A high protein diet must be given and all contaminated mustard oil excluded. Improvement is often slow and convalescence protracted. Surgical treatment is usually required to relieve increased intraocular tension.

Steps should be taken to prevent contamination of mustard crops with the weed *A. mexicana*. A test can be carried out to detect this contaminant in mustard oil.

Vomiting Sickness of Jamaica

(*Ackee Poisoning*)

This illness is attributed to eating unripe fruit of a common West Indian and South American tree, *Blighia sapida*. The mature fruit is wholesome but unripe fruit is believed to contain hypoglycin, a water-soluble toxin, which blocks gluconeogenesis in the liver.

Only children from 2 to 5 years of age who are undernourished are affected. The first symptom is vomiting, and after an interval this is followed by drowsiness, going on to convulsions and coma. In the late stages of the illness there is marked hypoglycaemia.

If started early, continuous intravenous glucose can bring about recovery. Without treatment the mortality rate is high.

Advice to Travellers

A pamphlet, *Notice to Travellers*, published by Her Majesty's Stationery Office, London, gives a list of vaccinations currently obligatory for travellers. Much useful advice is given by Turner, A. C. (1973) *Travel Medicine*, Edinburgh: Churchill Livingstone, from which Tables 17.5 and 17.6 are taken. In addition, it is very important that all visitors to the tropics and subtropics should take prophylactic antimalarial drugs regularly from the first day of travel and continue until 4 weeks after returning to a non-malarious area. Details are given on page 841. Neglect of this advice has been responsible for fatalities. Yellow fever vaccination is available at recognised centres in Britain, see *Notice to Travellers*.

A map illustrating the distribution of disease is shown in Fig. 17.12 (p. 935).

PROMOTION OF HEALTH AND PREVENTION OF DISEASE

In Tropical and Developing Countries. A survey of patterns of disease in the tropics and developing countries was made on pages 812–830 and methods of prevention of individual diseases have been discussed. The promotion of health and the prevention of disease is, however, related to fundamental principles sometimes far removed from medical therapeutics and prophylactic measures for individual diseases.

Whereas obesity is a major problem in affluent communities, undernutrition and malnutrition are dominant in underdeveloped countries. Adequate nutrition depends primarily on preserving the fertility of the soil and making good use of its vegetable products and, if customs permit, of the animals which are themselves dependant on the vegetation. Preservation or construction of water supplies is also a fundamental need and afforestation and contour terracing may help to prevent the land becoming denuded by floods. Only if a poor country can become richer

Table 17.5 Vaccinations required under International Health Regulations

Vaccination	Where required	How long before valid	Length of validity	Minimum age	Other comments
Smallpox	In general everywhere outside Western Europe, U.S.A. and Canada. Always required when arriving from an infected area	Primary vaccination 8 days. Revaccination immediate	3 years	Usually 1 year. However some countries no minimum age limit	Preferably 3 weeks apart from yellow fever. Otherwise at the same time but in different site
Cholera	Always entering and *transitting* Pakistan, India, Burma. Also some other countries in Middle and Far East and since 1970 some countries in Africa	6 days	6 months	Usually 1 year. However some countries no minimum age limit or less than 1 year	A few countries require 2 injections at 1 week interval
Yellow Fever	Central Africa 15°N to 10°S. Central America, northern border of Panama State to 15°S but including Bolivia and excluding part of eastern Brazil and Panama Canal	10 days	10 years	Usually 1 year. A few countries have no minimum age limit or less than 1 year	Preferably 3 weeks apart from smallpox. Otherwise at the same time but in different site

Table 17.6 Medically recommended immunisations

Inoculation	Where advised	Course programme	Validity	Minimum age advised	Other comments
Typhoid Paratyphoid (TAB)	Everywhere except Northern Europe	Intradermal injection. 4–6 weeks between 1st and 2nd, 6–12 months between 2nd and 3rd	Booster injection every 3 years	2 years	Can be combined with tetanus as TABT
Tetanus	Everywhere	Frequency as above but subcutaneously. Combined with TAB: frequency as above but intradermally	Booster injection every 3–5 years	NIL	Can be combined with TAB as TABT
Poliomyelitis	Everywhere	3 oral doses at monthly intervals	1 Booster dose every 5 years; if over 5 years 2 doses are recommended	NIL	Not at same time as yellow fever
Plague	Vietnam, Laos, Khmer Republic, Ethiopia. Possibly Pakistan and India. Essential for overlanders	2 injections at 10–20 day intervals, 3rd 6 months later	6 months	1 year	Preferably not at same time as TAB and typhus
Typhus	Vietnam, Laos, Khmer Republic, Ethiopia. Possibly Pakistan and India. Essential for overlanders	2 injections at 7–10 day intervals. 3rd 6 months later	1 year	1 year	Preferably not at same time as TAB and plague
Gamma Globulin for type A Hepatitis s	Countries where sanitation is poor	1 injection	4–6 months	NIL	Necessity for repetition after 6 months is arguable

Malarial prophylaxis (mandatory) see page 841.

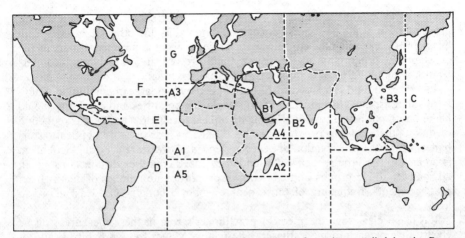

Fig. 17.12 Geographical distribution of disease (Based on information supplied by the Ross Institute of Tropical Hygiene, London)

	Area												
	Africa					Asia			Pacific	America			Europe
Disease	A1	A2	A3	A4	A5	B1	B2	B3	C	D	E	F	G
Malaria	††	††	*	†	*	†	†	††	†	†	*		
Schistosomiasis	†	†	*	††	*	*	1	†		†		*	*
Trypanosomiasis 2	†	†	–,*		*					†			
Leishmaniasis	*	3,†	3,*	†	*	†	†	*		†			*
Cholera 4	*	*	*	*		*	††	†					
Amoebiasis	†	†	†	†	†	†	††	††	†	††	†	*	*
Typhoid	†	†	†	†	*	††	††	††	*	†	†	*	*
Smallpox				5†									
Leprosy	††	††	†	††	*	*	††	††	†	†	*	6,	6,
Onchocerciasis	††	†		†	7,*	*				7,*			
Bancroftian and Brugia filariasis	††	††		†			†	††	††	†	*		
Paragonimiasis	*						8,*	††	8,*				
Opisthorciasis and Clonorchiasis								††	†				

* endemic
† highly endemic
†† very highly endemic

1 Small foci in B2, near Bombay and Madras
2 Sleeping sickness in A, Chagas' disease in D
3 Visceral in A2, cutaneous in A3, both in other areas
4 Situation varies with gradual spread of seventh pandemic
5 Eradication of smallpox in prospect, vaccination requirements vary
6 Only a few small residual foci in F and G
7 Yemen only in B1, north of equator in D
8 Nepal and Ceylon in B2, Korea in C

can sustained improvement in health be expected. More efficient agriculture and animal husbandry will tend to lead to improved health and economy; further progress may follow the utilization of mineral resources and the development of productive industries and tourism. Much help has been given in starting these processes by outside agencies but in order that lasting benefit should accrue it must be accompanied by better education. It is of paramount importance that the people concerned must themselves be fully convinced of the value and practicability of the projects and desire their benefits. Progress may be slow when improvements in health necessitate changes in food habits and other traditional practices, and will be maintained only when projects become an integral part of the development programme of the country and are operated largely by local personnel. Training of local nationals is, therefore, essential.

Increases in food supplies may be outstripped by increases in population. Family planning is, thus, a priority in many developing countries and emphasis should be laid both on the successful bringing up of healthy children and on the reduction of the population. Any progress can be vitiated by war or other political disturbance, hence the preservation of peace and law and order are crucial. Alcoholism is an enemy too little recognised in underdeveloped countries. It affects people in all socioeconomic groups and causes a disproportionate number of deaths from road accidents, frequently of those people whom a country can least afford to lose.

It will be clear that the medical practitioner's role in these measures will be chiefly that of an informed adviser. The relative values to community health of money spent, for example, on improved schooling as compared with eradication of malaria may be very difficult to assess, yet governments with limited resources have frequently to decide between such priorities. It has been shown in some areas that the provision of a protected water supply is the most economical way of improving health. Irrigation schemes may be essential to increase the areas of fertile land but expert advice may be required to prevent the spread thereby of malaria, schistosomiasis and onchocerciasis. The eradication of onchocerciasis and animal trypanosomiasis would lead, but at great expense, to the conversion of vast tracts of unused fertile land to pastoral and agricultural use.

In developing countries the provision of curative measures, which may also be important factors in prevention, involves the same principles as in affluent societies but their application is modified by the limitations of available finance and personnel. Priority should be given to measures which will improve the health and prospects of children and wage earners. In order to reach the scattered rural population a chain of health centres, under 5-year-old clinics and peripheral aid posts have proved of great value. At the health centres maternity and child welfare have priority and at all levels health education is actively pursued. Immunisation of children and, in the case of tetanus, of expectant mothers also, may do much to reduce mortality rates. Domicilary visits from the centres increase the contact with outlying homesteads. The vulnerability of small children to gastroenteritis underlines the importance of education in cleanliness and the provision of pure water supplies, but may also necessitate the provision of local facilities for rapid rehydration.

Making the best use of medical auxiliaries is essential if the health services are to be made widely available. Peripheral clinics have to be related to district and central hospitals from which some degree of supervision can be exercised and to which patients can be referred if transport is available. Minimal curative medicine is carried out at the peripheral clinics, but preventive measures must be seen to be related to curative medicine, otherwise little support for them will be forthcoming. The provision of specialised care, even in the central hospitals, should not be out of proportion to the general standard of medical care and medical education should include experience in both categories. Political pressure to divert effort and money into prestige units should be resisted.

In Disaster Situations. If earthquakes, floods, drought or other disasters strike an area help from outside is urgently needed to maintain food supplies and to prevent the spread of disease from sudden impairment of hygiene. In these circumstances international and charitable agencies do much to supply short-term relief but much remains undone and an even distribution of food and medicines is rarely achieved. When the disaster is war, earthquakes or volcanic eruptions it may be difficult and dangerous to get supplies to the stricken areas.

In Developed Countries. The term 'developed' is used to denote wealthy communities, mainly industrial. It is not intended to imply that the acquisition of more material possessions is necessarily a desirable goal or that the way of life in developed societies does not contain defects, some of which are deleterious to health.

National and local government bodies assume the responsibility for ensuring the availability of adequate food supplies, education, housing, health services and the prevention of environmental pollution but the family doctor plays an important role in encouraging people to make full use of preventive services. Genetic counselling, immunisation programmes and the early recognition and treatment of disease, the provision of vitamins C and D for young children, iron and folate for expectant mothers and financially subsidised school meals do much to ensure a good beginning in the building of a healthy nation. Where local mineral deficiencies exist, fluoridation of water to prevent dental caries and iodized salt to prevent goitre have proved their value.

The medical profession must continue to seek improvement in the working conditions in mines and factories, to identify industrial hazards and to draw attention to the special needs of persons in stressful occupations and repetitive work on mass production assembly lines.

Screening for disease can be carried out readily by the family doctor and can be supplemented by the use of mass miniature chest radiography. Malignant disease of the breast, cervix and uterus can be detected at a very early stage, if apparently healthy young women are examined regularly. For those in the middle years of life, medical reviews, at intervals of no longer than 2 years facilitate the early recognition of disease such as hypertension, diabetes and malignancy.

The needs of the elderly must be met by prophylactic measures such as the use of vitamins C and D, the assessment and treatment of the multiple disabilities frequently overlooked in this age group, social support and community services for the isolated and the provision of suitable accommodation for those requiring continuing care.

For patients of all ages it is the doctor's duty to encourage healthy living habits in matters such as regular physical exercise and diet with emphasis on an energy value appropriate to the needs of the individual, moderation in the intake of saturated fat (p. 947) and an ample content of coarse fibre. There must be a constant awareness of the dangers of tobacco smoking, of excessive consumption of alcohol and of the abuse of drugs by patients and their overprescription by doctors. Much can be done to promote mental health by doctors listening patiently to patients and thus helping individuals to contend with their problems while also detecting those at risk from psychiatric disturbances.

In all communities, there should be continuing demands for improvement in housing standards and in food hygiene. In many societies the morbidity and mortality from road traffic accidents is rapidly increasing. In urban areas there are growing problems in regard to corruption, crime, violence, baby and wife battering, rape and drug abuse. But there are much greater hazards. Man has now the capacity to destroy himself not only with nuclear weapons but by using up the natural resources of the planet so fast and by polluting his environment so thoroughly that he is in danger of precipitating his own doom. Everyone, especially doctors, economists, agriculturists and statesmen, is involved in this challenge and their response to it is vital.

N. C. ALLAN
A. D. M. BRYCESON
F. J. WRIGHT

Further reading about the promotion of health and prevention of disease:

Davey, T. H. & Wilson, T. (1971) *Davey and Lightbody's Control of Disease in the Tropics.* 4th edition. London: H. K. Lewis.
Djukanovic, V. & Mach, E. P. (Eds.) (1975) *Alternative Approaches to Meeting Basic Health Needs in Developing Countries. A Joint UNICEF/WHO Study.* Geneva: WHO.—(Barefoot doctors, etc.—practical approaches to providing health care in rural areas of developing countries.)
King, M. (1966) *Medical Care in Developing Countries.* Nairobi: Oxford Press.
Morley, D. (1973) *Paediatric Priorities in the Developing World.*—Obtainable at low cost from Institute of Child Health, 30 Guildford Street, London WC1.
Ninth Report of the Joint FAO/WHO Expert Committee on Nutrition (1976) *Food and Nutrition Strategies in National Development.* WHO Tech. Rep. Ser. No. 584. Geneva: WHO.

Further reading about parasitology and tropical diseases:

Standard textbooks.
Craig, C. F. & Faust, E. C. (1970) *Clinical Parasitology.* 8th edition. Philadelphia: Lea & Febriger.
Wilcocks, C. & Manson-Bahr, P. E. C. (1972) *Manson's Tropical Diseases.* 17th edition. London: Ballière, Tindall and Cassell.
Woodruff, A. W. (1974) *Medicine in the Tropics.* Edinburgh: Churchill Livingstone.

18. Appendices

DIETS

The diet sheets that follow have been constructed to illustrate the quantitative and qualitative aspects of diets required for the treatment of obesity and diabetes mellitus. The quantities given in a standard diet sheet will obviously require some modification in relation to the size, age, sex and occupation of the patient. In the dietetic treatment of most diseases it is unnecessary to weigh accurately the amounts of the different foods eaten. Under these circumstances sufficient accuracy will be secured by the use of household measures as illustrated in Diet 1 and by the terms 'small', 'medium' or 'large' helping for meat, fish or chicken. A small helping weighs approximately 1 to 2 oz (30–60 g), a medium helping 2 to 3 oz (60–90 g) and a large helping 4 oz (120 g) or more.

The qualitative content of the diet, i.e. the actual food consumed, will vary widely. The examples detailed here are suitable for persons whose food habits are those of the Western world. If they are to be effective therapeutically, diet prescriptions must be carefully adapted to take account of national, cultural and local eating habits.

The subcommittee on Metrication of the British National Committee for Nutritional Sciences of the Royal Society recommended in 1972 that kilojoules should be used in place of kilocalories. 1 kcal = 4·184 kJ, so that the calorie conversion factors (heat of combustion; available energy) for carbohydrate, fat, protein and alcohol are 16, 37, 17 and 29 kJ/g. Useful practical approximations are:

$$950 \text{ kcal} = 4000 \text{ kJ}$$
$$1450 \text{ kcal} = 6000 \text{ kJ}$$
$$2850 \text{ kcal} = 12000 \text{ kJ}$$

DIET 1

LOW CALORIE (ENERGY) DIET
suitable for adults with

OBESITY

(with or without diabetes)

Approximately: Protein 60 g, Carbohydrate 100 g, Fat 40 g, Energy 1,000 kcal (4,184 kJ)

Early morning   Cup of tea, milk from allowance,* if desired.

Breakfast   1 egg or 1 oz (30 g) grilled lean bacon (2 rashers) *or* cold ham *or* breakfast fish.
⅔ oz (20 g) white or brown bread, *or* exchange, with butter from allowance.
Tea or coffee, with milk from allowance.

Mid-morning   Tea or coffee, with milk from allowance, or 'free' drink from Group A3.

* *Allowance for day:*   ½ pint milk (300 ml) with the cream poured off the top. (The use of whole milk will increase the caloric content of this diet to approx. 1,100 kcal.)
½ oz (15 g) butter or margarine. (Cut a ½ lb packet into 16 equal portions, each portion = ½ oz.)
Exchanges for ⅔ oz (20 g) bread (½ slice from a large cut loaf):
2 cream crackers.   { 1½ of any }   1 potato (the size of a hen's egg).
2 water biscuits.   { crispbread. }   1 portion of fruit (from list below).
                                        1 triangular oatcake.
Exchanges for 1⅓ oz (40 g) bread (1 slice from a large cut loaf):
4 cream crackers.   { 3 of any }   2 potatoes (size of hen's egg).
4 water biscuits.   { crispbread. }   2 portions of fruit (from list below).
                                        2 triangular oatcakes.
Fruit to be taken as part of diet at lunch or evening meal:
1 piece of fresh fruit, i.e. apple, pear, orange, peach or medium sized helping of fruit stewed without sugar.

Mid-day meal Clear soup, tomato juice or grapefruit, if desired.
Small helping, 2 oz (60 g) lean meat, ham, poultry, game or offal *or* 3 oz (90 g) white fish (steamed, baked or grilled) *or* 1 egg *or* 1 oz (30 g) cheese.
Salad or vegetables from Group A1 as desired.
1⅓ oz (40 g) bread (white or brown) *or* exchange, with butter from allowance if desired.
1 portion of fruit from list below.
Tea or coffee with milk from allowance.

Mid-afternoon ⅔ oz (20 g) white or brown bread, *or* exchange, with butter from allowance.
or bedtime Salad vegetables from Group A1 if desired.

Evening meal Clear soup, meat or yeast extracts, tomato juice or grapefruit, if desired.
Small helping, 2 oz (60 g) lean meat, ham, poultry, game or offal *or* 3 oz (90 g) white fish (steamed, baked or grilled) *or* 1 egg *or* 1 oz (30 g) cheese.
Salad or vegetables from Group A1 as desired.
1⅓ oz (40 g) bread (white or brown) *or* exchange, with butter from allowance if desired.
1 portion of fruit from list below.
Tea or coffee with milk from allowance.

Before bed Tea or coffee with milk from allowance.

GROUP A: FOODS WHICH MAY BE TAKEN AS DESIRED

1. *Vegetables*
Artichoke, asparagus, aubergine, French beans, runner beans, broccoli, Brussels sprouts, cabbage, carrots, cauliflower, celeriac, celery, chicory, courgette, cucumber, endive, leeks, lettuce, mushrooms, mustard and cress, onions, parsley, pumpkin, raddishes, salsify, seakale, spinach, swede, tomatoes, turnip, turnip tops, vegetable marrow, watercress.

2. *Fruits* (stewed without sugar, or raw)
Gooseberries, grapefruit, lemon, melons (cantaloupe, water or honeydew), rhubarb, blackcurrants, red currants, blackberries, strawberries and raspberries.

3. *Drinks*
Water, soda water, tea or coffee (without milk or sugar), lemon juice, tomato juice, diabetic fruit squash, Marmite, Bovril, Oxo, clear soup (chicken or beef cubes may be used).

4. *Miscellaneous*
Saxine, saccharine or any proprietary sweetening agents except Sucron and sorbitol. Salt, pepper, mustard, vinegar, herbs, spices, gelatine, Worcester Sauce, flavourings and colourings may be used.

GROUP B: FOODS TO BE AVOIDED

Sugar (brown or white), glucose, sorbitol.
Sweets, toffees, chocolates, cornflour, custard powder.
Jam, marmalade, lemon curd, syrup, honey, treacle.
Tinned, frozen or bottled fruits.
Dried fruits, e.g. dates, figs, prunes, apricots, sultanas, currants, raisins, bananas, grapes.
Cakes, buns, pasties, pies, steamed or milk puddings.
Sweet or chocolate biscuits, scones.
Cereals, e.g. rice, sago, macaroni, barley, spaghetti, etc.
Breakfast cereal, porridge.
Cocoa, Ovaltine, Horlicks, etc.
Ice cream, fresh or synthetic cream. Table jelly.
Evaporated or condensed milk.
Peas, parsnips, beetroot, sweetcorn, Haricot beans, butter beans, broad beans, lentils.
Nuts.
Salad cream, salad dressing, mayonnaise.
Tomato and brown sauce or any thickened sauce.
Sweet pickles and chutney.
Thickened soups, gravies, Bisto.
Alcoholic drinks, e.g. beer, wine, sherry, spirits.
Sweetened fruit juices, fruit squash, Coca Cola and other sweet, fizzy, 'soft drinks'.
Lemonades, Lucozade, Ribena.

Starch-reduced products, 'diabetic' foodstuffs.
Sausages.
All Fried Foods.

All foods must be served without thickened gravies and sauces. All foods may be baked, grilled, boiled or steamed—*but not fried.*

DIABETIC DIETS

METHOD OF CONSTRUCTING A DIET RESTRICTED IN CARBOHYDRATE CONTAINING APPROXIMATELY 1,800 KCAL (7,560 kJ) with 210 g CARBOHYDRATE, 80 g PROTEIN AND 70 g FAT

suitable for adults with

DIEBETES MELLITUS

Each *carbohydrate exchange* contains approximately 10 g carbohydrate, 1·5 g protein and 0·3 g fat. Calorie value is about 50 (equivalent to ⅓ oz bread). Use is made of the Atwater calorie conversion factors of 4, 4 and 9 kcal/g for carbohydrate, protein and fat respectively.

Each *protein exchange* contains approximately 7 g protein and 5 g fat. Calorie value is about 70 (equivalent to 1 oz meat).

Each *fat exchange* contains approximately 12 g fat and almost no carbohydrate or protein. Calorie value is about 110 (equivalent to ½ oz butter). One pint of milk contains approximately 30 g carbohydrate, 18 g protein and 24 g fat. Calorie value is about 410.

In practice, for quick construction of a diabetic diet it is usually only necessary to work in terms of grams of carbohydrate and total calories. For this purpose the calorie value of the exchanges can be rounded to the nearest 10, i.e.

1 carbohydrate exchange	= 50 kcal
protein exchange	= 70 kcal
fat exchange	= 110 kcal
one pint of milk	= 410 kcal

Thus, a diet prescription for 210 g carbohydrate, 1,800 kcal would be calculated as follows:

1. The daily intake of carbohydrate (210 g) represents 21 carbohydrate exchanges.
2. The daily allowance of milk is decided, either on the basis of the patient's food habits, or on his special requirements. In this example it is ⅔ pint (400 ml), which contains 2 carbohydrate exchanges, leaving 19 for distribution throughout the day.
3. The daily allowance of protein is then decided. Five protein exchanges will provide 350 kcal.
4. The calories allocated so far amount to 1,580; a further 220 kcal are needed to bring the total up to 1,800 kcal. This must be provided by fat. As one fat exchange provides 110 kcal, two are needed.

Exchanges	Grams of carbohydrate	kcal
⅔ pint milk (400 ml) = 3 carbohydrate exchanges	20	280
19 carbohydrate exchanges	190	950
5 protein exchanges	—	350
Total	210	1,580
2 fat exchanges	—	220
GRAND TOTAL	210	1,800

5. Finally, the exchanges (21 carbohydrate, 5 protein and 2 fat) are distributed throughout the day according to the eating habits and daily routine of the patient. Diet 2 shows a specimen menu and a list of sample exchanges is shown on pp. 942 and 944.

DIETARY EXCHANGES FOR DIABETICS

1. CARBOHYDRATE EXCHANGES

Each item on this list = 1 carbohydrate exchange (10 g CHO).
Calorie value is approximately 50.

	Amount oz	Amount g	Remarks
Bread, Biscuits and Scones—			
Bread (white or brown)	$\frac{2}{3}$	20	$\frac{1}{2}$ slice off a large, cut loaf
Bread (toasted)	$\frac{1}{2}$	15	—
Scones, rolls and oatcakes	$\frac{2}{3}$	20	—
Cream crackers, crispbreads ⎫			
Digestive biscuits ⎬	$\frac{1}{2}$	15	—
Rich Tea biscuits			
Water biscuits ⎭			
Pastry (unsweetened)	$\frac{2}{3}$	20	—
Cereals—			
Porridge	4	120	Cooked
Breakfast cereals			
Arrowroot, barley, cornflour, custard ⎫			
powder, oatmeal, flour, macaroni,	$\frac{1}{2}$	15	All in dry state
rice, sago, semolina, spaghetti,			
tapioca ⎭			
Rice, macaroni, spaghetti	$1\frac{1}{2}$	45	Boiled
Spaghetti in tomato sauce	3	90	Tinned
Miscellaneous—			
Cocoa	1	30	—
Ovaltine, Horlicks, etc.	$\frac{1}{2}$	15	—
Creamed (tinned or packet) soup	4	120	Small teacup
Ice cream (Lyons or Wall's)	2	60	1 Small plain
Packet jelly	2	60	Made up
Milk, fresh	7	210	$\frac{1}{2}$ pint
Milk, evaporated	3	90	—
Milk, condensed (sweetened)	$\frac{2}{3}$	20	—
Ale, lager and draught beer	1 pint	600	—
Stout (Guinness)	$\frac{1}{2}$ pint	300	—
Vegetables—			
Potatoes (raw or boiled)	2	60	—
Potatoes (roast or chipped)	1	30	—
Potato crisps	$\frac{2}{3}$	20	—
Baked beans ⎫			
Butter beans			
Haricot beans ⎬	2	60	—
Sweet corn			
Tinned peas ⎭			
Fresh or frozen peas ⎫	4	120	—
Beetroot ⎭			
Parsnips	3	90	—

CARBOHYDRATE EXCHANGES—*continued*

Each item = 1 Carbohydrate exchange (10 g CHO), approx. 50 kcal.

	Raw		Stewed (without sugar)	
	oz	g	oz	g
Dried Fruits—				
Apricots	⅔	20	2	60
Figs	⅔	20	2	60
Prunes	1	30	2	60
Dates ⎫				
Currants ⎬				
Sultanas ⎬	½	15	—	—
Raisins ⎭				
Fresh Fruits—				
Apples (with skin)	4	120	5	150
Bananas (with skin)	3	90	—	—
Blackcurrants	5	150	7	210
Blackberries (brambles)	6	180	7	210
Cherries	3	90	4	120
Damsons	4	120	6	180
Grapes	2	60	—	—
Oranges and tangerines:				
—with skin	6	180	—	—
—without skin	4	120	—	—
Orange juice	4	120	—	—
Peaches	4	120	—	—
Pears	5	150	5	150
Pineapple (fresh)	3	90	—	—
Plums	4	120	7	210
Raspberries	6	180	7	210
Strawberries	6	180	—	—

2. PROTEIN EXCHANGES

Each item on this list = 1 protein exchange.
Calorie value is approximately 70.

	Amount		Remarks
	oz	g	
Meat, poultry, game and offals	1	30	Cooked weight
Corned beef, corned mutton, tinned meat	1	30	—
Meat paste and pâté	1½	45	—
Egg (1)	2	60	—
Cheese	1	30	—
Fish—white, smoked, cured, oily, shell or tinned and tripe	1½	45	Cooked weight
Sausages (include 1 carbohydrate exchange)	2	60	Cooked weight

Gravies should not contain cornflour or flour. Avoid frying as much as possible.

DIETARY EXCHANGES FOR DIABETICS—*continued*

3. FAT EXCHANGES

Each exchange approximately 12 g fat and almost no
carbohydrate or protein.

Calorie value is approximately 110.

	Amount		Remarks
	oz	g	
Butter, margarine, lard, dripping, cooking fat, olive oil, vegetable oil	½	15	—
Cream (single)	2	60	—
Cream (double)	1	30	—
Salad cream or mayonnaise	1	30	—

INSTRUCTIONS FOR DIABETICS—*continued*

GROUP A: FOODS WHICH MAY BE TAKEN IN ANY QUANTITY

Tea, coffee (milk from allowance, no sugar), Oxo, Bovril, Marmite, etc.
Tomato juice, lemon juice.
Diabetic fruit squashes.
Saccharine preparations.
Clear soup.
Herbs, seasonings and spices.
Brussels sprouts, cabbage, carrots, cauliflower, celery, cucumber, French beans, leeks, lettuce, mushrooms, mustard or cress, onions, spring onions, runner beans, swedes, spinach, tomatoes, turnips, watercress.
Cranberries, grapefruit, gooseberries, lemon, melon, loganberries, redcurrants, rhubarb.

GROUP B: TO BE TAKEN IN STRICT MODERATION IN CONSULTATION WITH THE DOCTOR

Spirits, dry wines, dry sherries.

GROUP C: FOODS NOT ALLOWED

Sugar, glucose, sweets, chocolate, honey, syrup, treacle, jam, marmalade, cakes, biscuits (except those specified), pies, fruit tinned in syrup, fruit squash, lemonade, or similar aerated drinks.

Note.—Most 'Diabetic' foodstuffs on sale at chemists and health food stores *do* contain some carbohydrate and must therefore *not* be taken without consulting your doctor or dietitian.

AN EXAMPLE OF THE DISTRIBUTION OF EXCHANGES FOR A DIET RESTRICTED IN CARBOHYDRATE

suitable for adults with

DIABETES MELLITUS

Approximately: Protein 80 g, Carbohydrate 210 g, Fat 70 g, Energy 1,800 kcal (7,560 kJ).

Breakfast   1 protein exchange.*
                4 carbohydrate exchanges.*
                Butter and milk from allowance.†
                Tea or coffee (no sugar).

Mid-morning   2 carbohydrate exchanges.
                Butter and milk from allowance.
                Tea or coffee (no sugar).

Mid-day meal	Clear soup if desired.
	2 protein exchanges.
	4 carbohydrate exchanges.
	Vegetables if desired (group A, p. 944).
	Butter and milk from allowance.

Mid-afternoon	2 carbohydrate exchanges.
	Butter and milk from allowance.
	Tea (no sugar).

Evening meal	2 protein exchanges.
	5 carbohydrate exchanges.
	Vegetables if desired (group A, p. 944).
	Tea or coffee (no sugar).

Before bed	2 carbohydrate exchanges.
	Remainder of butter and milk from allowance.

* A list of suitable exchanges is given on pages 941 to 944.
† Allowance for day: ⅔ pint (400 ml) whole milk.
        1 oz (30 g) butter or margarine.

DIET 2

AN EXAMPLE OF A MENU RESTRICTED IN CARBOHYDRATES, BASED ON DISTRIBUTION OF EXCHANGES
suitable for adults with
DIABETES MELLITUS

Approximately: Protein 80 g, Carbohydrate 210 g, Fat 70 g, Energy 1,800 kcal (7,560 kJ).

Breakfast	4 oz (120 g) porridge with milk from allowance.
	1 egg.
	2 oz (60 g) bread with butter from allowance.*
	Tea or coffee with milk from allowance.

Mid-morning	1 oz (30 g) Rich tea biscuits.
	Tea or coffee with milk from allowance.

Mid-day meal	Clear soup with shredded vegetables.
	2 oz (60 g) lean meat.
	4 oz (120 g) boiled potatoes.
	2 oz (60 g) tinned peas.
	Salad or other unrestricted vegetables from group A if desired.
	4 oz (120 g) orange (peeled weight).
	Milk from allowance with coffee.

Mid-afternoon	1 oz (30 g) Digestive biscuits.
	Tea or coffee with milk from allowance.

Evening meal	3 oz (90 g) fish.
	Tomato or other unrestricted vegetables from group A if desired.
	2 oz (60 g) bread with butter from allowance.
	3 oz (90 g) banana (weight with skin).
	2 oz (60 g) ice cream.
	Tea or coffee with milk from allowance.

Before bed	Remainder of milk from allowance and ½ oz Ovaltine.
	⅓ (20 g) bread, toasted with butter from allowance.

* Allowance for day: ⅔ pint milk (400 ml).
           1 oz (30 g) butter or margarine.

DIET 3

UNMEASURED DIET suitable for adults with DIABETES MELLITUS

Patients who are unable to weigh their diet or for whom this is unnecessary, are given a list of foods which are grouped into three categories.

I. *Foods to be avoided altogether.*

1. Sugar, glucose, jam, marmalade, honey, syrup, treacle, tinned fruits, sweets, chocolate, lemonade, glucose drinks, proprietary milk preparations and similar foods which are sweetened with sugar.

2. Cakes, sweet biscuits, chocolate biscuits, pies, puddings, thick sauces.

3. Alcoholic drinks unless permission has been given by the doctor.

II. *Foods to be eaten in moderation only.*

1. Breads of all kinds (including so-called 'slimming' and 'starch-reduced' breads, brown or white, plain or toasted).

2. Rolls, scones, biscuits and crispbreads.

3. Potatoes, peas and baked beans.

4. Breakfast cereals and porridge.

5. All fresh or dried fruit.

6. Macaroni, spaghetti, custard and foods with much flour.

7. Thick soups.

8. Diabetic foods.

9. Milk.

III. *Foods to be eaten as desired.*

1. All meats, fish, eggs.

2. Cheese.

3. Clear soups or meat extracts, tomato or lemon juice.

4. Tea or coffee.

5. Cabbage, Brussels sprouts, broccoli, cauliflower, spinach, turnip, runner or French beans, onions, leeks or mushrooms. Lettuce, cucumber, tomatoes, spring onions, radishes, mustard and cress, asparagus, parsley, rhubarb.

6. Herbs, spices, salt, pepper and mustard.

7. Saccharine preparations for sweetening.

For overweight diabetics butter, margarine, fatty and dried foods must be restricted.

DIET 4

Low in saturated fats and cholesterol with increased amounts of polyunsaturated fat, see pages 589 and 937.

Foods to be avoided

Butter and hydrogenated margarines. Use polyunsaturated margarine, e.g. 'Flora'.

Lard, suet, shortenings and cakes, biscuits and pastries made with these.

Fatty meat and visible fat on meat. Meat pies, sausages and luncheon meats.

Whole milk and cream.

Chocolate, ice cream (except water ices). Cheese, except low fat cottage cheese.

Coconut, coconut oil and 'Coffee mate'.

Eggs—no more than 1 to 2 egg yolks per week, including that used in cooking.

Organ meats—liver, kidneys and brain.

Shelfish and fish roes.

Fried foods unless fried in polyunsaturated oil (like sunflower or corn oil).

Potato crips and most nuts.

Gravy unless made with polyunsaturated oil, and tinned soups.

Salad dressing unless made with polyunsaturated oil.

Further reading about dietetics and additional diets:

Davidson, Sir Stanley, Passmore, R., Brock, J. F. & Truswell, A. S. (1975) *Human Nutrition and Dietetics.* 6th edition. Edinburgh: Churchill Livingstone.—For additional diet sheets.

TABLE 18.1

WEIGHTS FOR AGE—BIRTH TO 5 YEARS, SEXES COMBINED[1]

Age (months)	Standard[2]	80% Std	60% Std	Age (months)	Standard[2]	80% Std	60% Std
0	3·4	2·7	2·0				
1	4·3	3·4	2·5	31	13·7	11·0	8·2
2	5·0	4·0	2·9	32	13·8	11·1	8·3
3	5·7	4·5	3·4	33	14·0	11·2	8·4
4	6·3	5·0	3·8	34	14·2	11·3	8·5
5	6·9	5·5	4·2	35	14·4	11·5	8·6
6	7·4	5·9	4·5	36	14·5	11·6	8·7
7	8·0	6·3	4·9	37	14·7	11·8	8·8
8	8·4	6·7	5·1	38	14·85	11·9	8·9
9	8·9	7·1	5·3	39	15·0	12·05	9·0
10	9·3	7·4	5·5	40	15·2	12·2	9·1
11	9·6	7·7	5·8	41	15·35	12·3	9·2
12	9·9	7·9	6·0	42	15·5	12·4	9·3
13	10·2	8·1	6·2	43	15·7	12·6	9·4
14	10·4	8·3	6·3	44	15·85	12·7	9·5
15	10·6	8·5	6·4	45	16·0	12·9	9·6
16	10·8	8·7	6·6	46	16·2	12·95	9·7
17	11·0	8·9	6·7	47	16·35	13·1	9·8
18	11·3	9·0	6·8	48	16·5	13·2	9·9
19	11·5	9·2	7·0	49	16·65	13·35	10·0
20	11·7	9·4	7·1	50	16·8	13·5	10·1
21	11·9	9·6	7·2	51	16·95	13·65	10·2
22	12·05	9·7	7·3	52	17·1	13·8	10·3
23	12·2	9·8	7·4	53	17·25	13·9	10·4
24	12·4	9·9	7·5	54	17·4	14·0	10·5
25	12·6	10·1	7·6	55	17·6	14·2	10·6
26	12·7	10·3	7·7	56	17·7	14·3	10·7
27	12·9	10·5	7·8	57	17·9	14·4	10·75
28	13·1	10·6	7·9	58	18·05	14·5	10·8
29	13·3	10·7	8·0	59	18·25	14·6	10·9
30	13·5	10·8	8·1	60	18·4	14·7	11·0

[1] Based on table by Jelliffe (1966).
[2] Boston standards (Stuart & Stevenson, 1959), taking mean of boys and girls. Boys are 0·05 to 0·15 kg heavier and girls 0·05 to 0·15 kg lighter.

TABLE 18.2

DESIRABLE WEIGHTS OF ADULTS
According to height and frame

Height without shoes (approximate equivalents)			Desirable weight in kilograms and pounds (in indoor clothing), ages 25 and over					
			Small frame		Medium frame		Large frame	
metres	ft	in	kg	lb	kg	lb	kg	lb
Men								
1·550	5	1	50·8–54·4	112–120	53·5–58·5	118–129	57·2–64	126–141
1·575	5	2	52·2–55·8	115–123	54·9–60·3	121–133	58·5–65·3	129–144
1·600	5	3	53·5–57·2	118–126	56·2–61·7	124–136	59·9–67·1	132–148
1·625	5	4	54·9–58·5	121–129	57·6–63	127–139	61·2–68·9	135–152
1·650	5	5	56·2–60·3	124–133	59 –64·9	130–143	62·6–70·8	138–156
1·675	5	6	58·1–62·1	128–137	60·8–66·7	134–147	64·4–73	142–161
1·700	5	7	59·9–64	132–141	62·6–68·9	138–152	66·7–75·3	147–166
1·725	5	8	61·7–65·8	136–145	64·4–70·8	142–156	68·5–77·1	151–170
1·750	5	9	63·5–68	140–150	66·2–72·6	146–160	70·3–78·9	155–174
1·775	5	10	65·3–69·9	144–154	68 –74·8	150–165	72·1–81·2	159–179
1·800	5	11	67·1–71·7	148–158	69·9–77·1	154–170	74·4–83·5	164–184
1·825	6	0	68·9–73·5	152–162	71·7–79·4	158–175	76·2–85·7	169–189
1·850	6	1	70·8–75·7	156–167	73·5–81·6	162–180	78·5–88	173–194
1·875	6	2	72·6–77·6	160–171	75·7–83·9	167–185	80·7–90·3	178–199
1·900	6	3	74·4–79·4	164–175	78·0–86·2	172–190	82·6–92·5	182–204
Women								
1·425	4	8	41·7–44·5	92–98	43·5–48·5	96–107	47·2–54	104–119
1·450	4	9	42·6–45·8	94–101	44·5–49·9	98–110	48·1–55·3	106–122
1·475	4	10	43·5–47·2	96–104	45·8–51·3	101–113	49·4–56·7	109–125
1·500	4	11	44·9–48·5	99–107	47·2–52·6	104–116	50·8–58·1	112–128
1·525	5	0	46·3–49·9	102–110	48·5–54	107–119	52·2–59·4	115–131
1·550	5	1	47·6–51·3	105–113	49·9–55·3	110–122	53·5–60·8	118–134
1·575	5	2	49 –52·6	108–116	51·3–57·2	113–126	54·9–62·6	121–138
1·600	5	3	50·3–54	111–119	52·6–59	116–130	56·7–64·4	125–142
1·625	5	4	51·7–55·8	114–123	54·4–61·2	120–135	58·5–66·2	129–146
1·650	5	5	53·5–57·6	118–127	56·2–63	124–139	60·3–68	133–150
1·675	5	6	55·3–59·4	122–131	58·1–64·9	128–143	62·1–69·9	137–154
1·700	5	7	57·2–61·2	126–135	59·9–66·7	132–147	64 –71·7	141–158
1·725	5	8	59 –63·5	130–140	61·7–68·5	136–151	65·8–73·9	145–163
1·750	5	9	60·8–65·3	134–144	63·5–70·3	140–155	67·6–76·2	149–168
1·775	5	10	62·6–67·1	138–148	65·3–72·1	144–159	69·4–78·5	153–173

Based on weights of insured persons in the United States associated with lowest mortality (*Statist, Bull. Metrop. Life Insur. Co.*, 40, Nov.–Dec. 1959).

Notes on International System of Units (SI Units)

Examples of Basic SI Units

Length	metre (m)
Mass	kilogram (kg)
Amount of substance	mole (mol)
Energy	joule (J)
Pressure	pascal (Pa)

Examples of Decimal Multiples and Submultiples of SI Units

Factor	Name	Symbol
10^6	mega-	M
10^3	kilo-	k
10^{-1}	deci-	d
10^{-2}	centi-	c
10^{-3}	milli-	m
10^{-6}	micro-	μ
10^{-9}	nano-	n
10^{-12}	pico-	p

Units of Volume and Concentration.

Volume. The basic SI unit of volume is the cubic metre (1,000 litre). Because of its convenience the litre is used as the unit of volume in laboratory work.

Amount of Substance ('*Molar*') *Concentration* (e.g., mol/l, μmol/l) is used for substances of defined chemical composition. It replaces equivalent concentration (mEq/l) which is not part of the SI system—for reporting measurements of sodium, potassium, chloride and bicarbonate (the numerical value of these four measurements is unchanged because the ions are univalent).

Mass Concentration (e.g., g/l, μg/l) is used for all protein measurements, for substances which do not have a sufficiently well defined composition and for plasma vitamin B_{12} and folate measurements. The numerical value in SI units will change by a factor of 10 in those instances previously expressed in terms of 100 ml.

Haemoglobin is an exception. It is agreed internationally that meantime haemoglobin should continue to be expressed in terms of g/dl (g/100 ml).

Non-SI units are employed for enzymes and immunoglobulins.

BIOCHEMICAL AND HAEMATOLOGICAL VALUES
(Examples of conversion to SI Units)

B = Blood F = Faeces P = Plasma S = Serum U = Urine	Reference Values *Approximate normal ranges (adults)*		Multiplication factors for converting from other units to SI units
	SI Units	Other Units	
B Ammonium	23–47 μmol/l	40–80 μg/100 ml	0·587
B Ascorbate	45–80 μmol/l	0·8–1·4 mg/100 ml	56·8
U Ascorbate	114–284 μmol/24 h	20–50 mg/24 h	5·68
B Base Excess	$\pm$ 2 mmol/l	$\pm$ 2 mEq/l	No change
P Bicarbonate	24–32 mmol/l	24–32 mEq/l	No change
P Bilirubin (total)	5–17 μmol/l	0·3–1·0 mg/100 ml	17·1
S Caeruloplasmin	300–600 mg/l	30–60 mg/100 ml	10
P Calcium (total)	2·12–2·62 mmol/l	8·5–10·5 mg/100 ml	0·250
B Carbon dioxide (Pco_2)	4·5–6·1 kPa	34–46 mm Hg	0·133
P β-Carotene	0·9–5·6 μmol/l	50–300 μg/100 ml	0·0186
U Catecholamines (as adrenalin)	0·05–0·55 μmol/24 h	10–100 μg/24 h	0·00546

(Continued)

BIOCHEMICAL AND HAEMATOLOGICAL VALUES—*continued*

B = Blood F = Faeces P = Plasma S = Serum U = Urine	Reference Values *Approximate normal ranges (adults)*		Multiplication factor for converting from other units to SI units
	SI Units	Other Units	
P Chloride	95–105 mmol/*l*	95–105 mEq/*l*	No change
P Cholesterol	3·6–7·8 mmol/*l*	140–300 mg/100 ml	0·0259
P Copper	13–24 µmol/*l*	80–150 µg/100 ml	0·157
U Coproporphyrins	0·15–0·31 µmol/24 h	100–200 µg/24 h	0·00153
P Cortisol	276–690 nmol/*l*	10–25 µg/100 ml	27·6
U Creatine	0–400 µmol/24 h	0–50 mg/24 h	7·69
P Creatinine	62–124 µmol/*l*	0·7–1·4 mg/100 ml	88·4
F Fat (as stearic acid)	11–18 mmol/24 h	3–5 g/24 h	3·52
P Fibrinogen	1·5–4·0 g/*l*	150–400 mg/100 ml	0·01
S Folate	3–20 µg/*l*	3–20 ng/ml or µmg/ml	No change
B Glucose	2·5–4·7 mmol/*l*	45–85 mg/100 ml	0·0555
B Haemoglobin	14·4 g/dl	14·4 g/100 ml or g%	No change
S Haptoglobins (Hb binding)	0·3–2·0 g/*l*	30–200 mg/100 ml	0·01
S Iron	14–29 µmol/*l*	80–160 µg/100 ml	0·179
S Total iron binding capacity (as iron)	45–72 µmol/*l*	250–400 µg/100 ml	0·179
B Lactate	0·4–1·4 mmol/*l*	3·6–13·0 mg/100 ml	0·111
B Lead	0·5–1·9 µmol/*l*	10–40 µg/100 ml	0·0483
B Leucocytes (total) (WBC)	4·0–11·0 × 10⁹/*l*	4,000–11,000/µl or 4·0–11·0 × 10³/mm³	10⁶
P Lipids (total)	4·0–10·0 g/*l*	400–1,000 mg/100 ml	0·01
P Magnesium	0·7–1·0 mmol/*l*	1·8–2·4 mg/100 ml	0·411
B Mean Corpuscular Haemoglobin (MCH)	27–32 pg	27–32 pg or µµg	No change
B Mean Corpuscular Haemoglobin Concentration (MCHC)	30–35 g/dl	30–35%	No change
B Mean Corpuscular Volume (MCV)	75–95 fl	75–95 µ³ or µm³	No change
F Nitrogen	71–143 mmol/24 h	1–2 g/24 h	71·4
P Non-protein nitrogen	14–21 mmol/*l*	20–30 mg/100 ml	0·714
U Oestriol	7–173 µmol/24 h	2–50 mg/24 h	3·47
B Oxygen (Po₂)	12–15 kPa	90–110 mm Hg	0·133
U 17 Oxogenic steroids	35–69 µmol/24 h	10–20 mg/24 h	3·47
B Packed Cell Volume (PCV)	0·41	41%	0·01
B Platelets	150–400 × 10⁹/*l*	150,000–400,000/µl or/mm³	10⁶
P Phosphate (as inorganic P)	0·8–1·4 mmol/*l*	2·5–4·5 mg/100 ml	0·323
U Porphobilinogen	0·9–8·8 µmol/24 h	0·2–2 mg/24 h	4·42
P Potassium	3·8–5·0 mmol/*l*	3·8–5·0 mEq/*l*	No change
U Pregnanediol	0–3·1 µmol/24 h	0–1 mg/24 h	3·12

(*Continued*)

B = Blood F = Faeces P = Plasma S = Serum U = Urine	Reference Values *Approximate normal ranges (adults)*		Multiplication factor for converting from other units to SI units
	SI Units	Other Units	
U Pregnanetriol	0·3–8·9 µmol/24 h	0·1–3 mg/24 h	2·97
S Proteins—total	62–82 g/l	6·2–8·2 g/100 ml	10·0
S —albumin	36–52 g/l	3·6–5·2 g/100 ml	10·0
S —globulins	24–37 g/l	2·4–3·7 g/100 ml	10·0
CSF Proteins	0·1–0·4 g/l	10–40 mg/100 ml	0·01
S Protein bound iodine	315–590 nmol/l	4·0–7·5 µg/100 ml	78·8
B Pyruvate	45–80 µmol/l	0·4–0·7 mg/100 ml	113
B Red Cell Count	$4·5 \times 10^{12}/l$	$4·5 \times 10^6/µl$	10^6
(RBC)		or/mm^3	
B Red Cell Diameter	6·7–7·7 µm	6·7–7·7 µ	No change
		or µm	
B Reticulocytes	0·2–2·0%	0·2–2·0%	No change
	or	or	10^6
	$10–100 \times 10^9/l$	$10–100 \times 10^3/µl$	
P Sodium	136–148 mmol/l	136–148 mEq/l	No change
S Thyroxine-iodine	244–465 nmol/l	3·1–5·9 µg/100 ml	78·8
S Transferrin	1·2–2·0 g/l	120–200 mg/100 ml	0·01
P Triglyceride	0·28–1·69 mmol/l	25–150 mg/100 ml	0·0113
(as triolein)			
P Urate	0·12–0·42 mmol/l	2–7 mg/100 ml	0·0595
B Urea	2·5–6·6 mmol/l	15–40 mg/100 ml	0·166
F Urobilinogen	50–504 µmol/24 h	30–300 mg/24 h	1·68
P Vitamin A	0·7–1·7 µmol/l	20–50 µg/100 ml	0·0349
S Vitamin B$_{12}$	160–925 ng/l	160–925 pg/ml	No change
(as cyanocobalamin)		or µµg/ml	
B White Cell Count	$4·0–10·0 \times 10^9/l$	1,000–10,000/mm^3	10^6
B Xylose	0·33–3·33 mmol/l	5–50 mg/100 ml	0·0667
U Xylose	1·3–2·6 mmol	0·2–4·0 g	6·66

Notes on Drug Nomenclature and Prescription

Australia, Britain, Canada, Denmark, Finland, France, Iceland, Italy, Japan, Norway, Pakistan, Korea, Sweden, and the United States all list their own national non-proprietary names for drugs. Some insist on the use of these names or of the international non-proprietary names of the World Health Organisation. The latter are often the same as the national names. In Britain the names of proprietary alternatives for the more commonly used drugs can be obtained by consulting the British National Formulary (1967–78). In this textbook proprietary names have been used only in exceptional circumstances.

Abbreviations used in relationship to the administration of drugs are i.m. (intramuscular injection), i.v. (intravenous injection), s.c. (subcutaneous injection), b.d. (twice daily by mouth) and t.i.d. (thrice daily by mouth). Throughout the book polypharmacy has been avoided in view particularly of the risk of interaction between drugs and because patient 'compliance', i.e. the taking of medicines as prescribed, is improved if instructions are simple and specific.

Further reading about drugs:

Girdwood, R. H. (Ed.) (1976) *Clinical Pharmacology*. 23rd edition. London: Baillière Tindall.

Index